Davy C. H. Cheng
Tirone David

Editors

Evidence-Based Practice in Perioperative Cardiac Anesthesia and Surgery

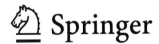 Springer

Editors
Davy C. H. Cheng
Distinguished University Professor
Department of Anesthesia
and Perioperative Medicine
and Department of Medicine
Division of Critical Care Medicine
London Health Sciences Center
and St Joseph's Healthcare London
Centre for Medical Evidence, Decision
Integrity and Clinical Impact (MEDICI)
Western University
London, ON
Canada

Janet Martin
Associate Professor
Department of Anesthesia and
Perioperative Medicine and
Department of Epidemiology
and Biostatistics, Schulich School of
Medicine and Dentistry
Centre for Medical Evidence, Decision
Integrity and Clinical Impact (MEDICI)
Western University
London, ON
Canada

Tirone David
Professor of Surgery
University of Toronto
Melanie Munk Chair of Cardiovascular
Surgery
University Health Network
Toronto, ON
Canada

ISBN 978-3-030-47886-5   ISBN 978-3-030-47887-2   (eBook)
https://doi.org/10.1007/978-3-030-47887-2

This Springer imprint is published by the registered company Springer Nature Switzerland AG
The registered company address is: Gewerbestrasse 11, 6330 Cham, Switzerland

Preface

Cardiac physiology began with the seminal discovery of circulation by William Harvey (1578–1657). The vital connection between circulation and ventilation was also noted by Harvey "There is nothing living which does not breathe nor anything which breathing which does not live." (*Prelectiones Anatomiae Universalis, 1616*). Surgery on the heart in the nineteenth century began with congenital correction of septal defect and mitral and pulmonic stenosis by deep hypothermic beating heart surgery with volatile inhalational anesthetics. This illustrated the early vital actions of surgery and anesthesia together.

Since the successful use of cardiopulmonary bypass circuit in 1953, advances in anesthesia, membrane oxygenators, temperature regulation, and myocardial protection have challenged surgeons to invent new procedures for all kinds of cardiac congenital anomalies. These include heart transplantation, minimally invasive and robotic assisted cardiac surgery, and interventional procedures. Coupled with the advancement of cardiac surgery, cardiac anesthesia has progressed from high-dose narcotic to balanced narcotic-inhalational anesthesia with safer and effective anesthetic agents, regional anesthesia, and standard practice of fast-track recovery or enhanced cardiac surgery recovery. There are continuing advancements in perioperative monitoring of myocardial (transesophageal echocardiography, intraoperative epiaortic scan), cerebral (electroencephalogram, oxygen saturation), coagulation, transfusion practice, organ protection, and cardiac support systems (IABP, left/right ventricular assist devices). I would like to express my personal gratitude to Dr. Tirone David, a legendary cardiac surgeon, a dear friend and colleague, who has been instrumental in coediting earlier books on perioperative care in cardiac anesthesia and surgery with me.

The modern era of cardiac anesthesia and surgery team care is characterized by value-based and evidence-based practice in drugs, techniques, procedures, and perioperative process of care supported by digital data. I appreciate greatly Dr. Janet Martin, a prominent leader in clinical epidemiology, evidence synthesis, health technology assessment, and knowledge translation, joining as coeditor in this new textbook. Renowned experts in anesthesiology, cardiac surgery, cardiology, and critical care medicine around the world pen this evidence-based and state-of-the art management in perioperative cardiac anesthesia and surgery. This textbook aims to provide a succinct, practical management on cardiac anesthesia and surgery from preoperative risks assessment to postoperative critical care until surgical ward and home discharge. All the latest cardiac surgical procedures are concisely written by leading cardiac surgeons, so that the cardiac anesthesiologists and critical care consultants have full comprehension of the perioperative surgical considerations in the management of these patients. The appendices section summarizes the medical orders, protocols, clinical guidelines, and algorithms from leading cardiac programs and professional societies. This will be an invaluable reference resource for any cardiac surgical programs or centers.

The editors gratefully acknowledge the impactful contributions by our eminent authors of these chapters to improve the care and outcomes of our patients, for the consultants and trainees in cardiac anesthesia and surgery, cardiologists, nurses, and other allied cardiac healthcare team.

London, ON, Canada   Davy C. H. Cheng

Acknowledgements

The editors wish to thank those who contributed to the completion of this textbook. The editors gratefully acknowledge Cheryl Kee, NP CSRU, for providing the Cardiac Surgery Recovery Unit postoperative protocols, order sets, and standard operating procedures documents that form the Appendix, as well as LHSC staff responsible for developing and updating these clinical care documents. The editors express their utmost thanks to Jessica Moodie, MLIS, for her role in technical editing, language editing, proofreading, and administrative support, and to Amy Sterkenburg, MLIS, for her role in technical editing, language editing, and proofreading.

Contents

Part I

Introduction

Overview of a Modern Cardiac Surgical Centre

Tirone David

Main Messages

1. All variables that affect patient clinical outcomes must be considered when providing care
2. Modern cardiac units consist of patient care teams that are complex, interdisciplinary and rely on the expertise of every medical specialty
3. Integrating the expertise of surgeons, cardiologists, anesthesiologists, intensivists, radiologists, neurologists, nephrologists, technicians, nurses, and consultants from all medical subspecialties, surgical complications can be promptly identified and managed, reducing morbidity and mortality

Improving Patient Care

The management of cardiovascular diseases continues to evolve and cardiac surgery as a therapeutic option continues to change. However, a new treatment must be better than the natural history of the disease, and better than the alternative treatments available. Clinical improvement is not always simple and many clinical investigators continue to search for the correct answer. During my surgical residency, my mentors impressed upon me the importance of recognizing the potential impact my clinical decisions would have for my patients; not only perioperatively, but during their lifetime.

I had learned a basic computer language during my training and when I started independent practice I developed an elementary program to enter pertinent clinical, hemodynamic and imaging data on each of my surgical patients, and monitored their evolution by periodically collecting information related to their health status. That database also served for quality assurance improvement, which was aimed at perfection. However, since perfection cannot be attained, we settled for excellence. This process of constant improvement in clinical outcomes continues today in our unit and I believe that it is essential in every cardiac surgical unit. Thus, a comprehensive database containing all variables that affect clinical outcomes and patient satisfaction is indispensable and periodical reviews and analyses are necessary to measure and improve quality.

T. David (✉)
The University Health Network,
Toronto, ON, Canada
e-mail: Tirone.David@uhn.ca

© Springer Nature Switzerland AG 2021
D. C. H. Cheng et al. (eds.), *Evidence-Based Practice in Perioperative Cardiac Anesthesia and Surgery*, https://doi.org/10.1007/978-3-030-47887-2_1

Multi-disciplinary Cardiac Units

Cardiac surgical patient care has become increasingly more complex and dependent on a dedicated team as opposed to one individual. The days of a single discipline approach in surgical treatment has been replaced by a multitude of committed experts in the modern cardiac unit. Surgeons, cardiologists, anesthesiologists, intensivists, dedicated nurses and technicians as well as a cadre of teams of radiologists and intervention radiologists, neurologists, nephrologists, and consultants from every sub-specialty in medicine are now part of this complex medical enterprise.

There is no substitute for an operation perfectly and expeditiously performed but when complications occur, prompt corrective management reduces mortality and morbidity. An electrocardiogram that suggests myocardial ischemia soon after discontinuation of cardiopulmonary bypass must be taken very seriously unless an intraoperative echocardiogram shows no new wall motion abnormality. If there is new wall motion abnormality, the mechanism for segmental ischemia must be readily determined and corrected. The same applies for a postoperative new electrocardiographic abnormality which should prompt at least an echocardiogram and possibly immediate coronary angiogram. This aggressive and effective management has been facilitated by the creation of teams of cardiac interventionalists that treat acute myocardial infarction and are continuously available to manage patients with acute cardiac syndromes. The availability and the appropriate use of intra-aortic balloon pump, ECMO and ventricular assist devices may further reduce mortality, but the root cause of acute cardiac dysfunction should be determined and corrected whenever possible. ECMO is also useful for acute pulmonary failure that cannot be managed by conventional methods of assisted ventilation.

Acute stroke teams now can intervene and reduce the devastating effects of cerebral thromboembolism and arterial thrombosis. Here, time is crucial and "fast-track anesthesia" has improved the timing to assess neurologic outcomes in cardiac surgery. The benefit of neurovascular interventions is reduced when the stroke occurred more than 3 h duration.

The main reason cardiac surgical patients are nursed in an intensive care unit during the first hours or days after surgery is to closely monitor vital signs, electrocardiogram, mediastinum bleeding and have periodical assessment of all organs: heart, lungs, brain, kidneys, liver and gastrointestinal, and musculoskeletal systems. Nurses are often the first ones to detect changes and their experience is invaluable. An intensivist must be physically present in the intensive care unit and start immediate management of any complication.

Aiming for perfection we will attain excellence. This manual was written to assist you in providing care to cardiac surgical patients in the operating room, interventional suite, intensive care unit, and ward in the modern era.

Prognostic Risks and Preoperative Assessment

2

Karim S. Ladha and Duminda N. Wijeysundera

Main Messages

1. An accurate estimate of a patient's expected risk of future adverse events can inform decision-making throughout the perioperative period.
2. Quantification of risk, through methods such as risk scores, is not meant to supersede clinical judgment, but rather to serve as a supplemental tool for decision making.
3. No single metric can determine the quality of risk score; rather, several factors are used in combination, including discrimination, risk reclassification, calibration, and generalizability.
4. The EuroSCORE (European System for Cardiac Operative Risk Evaluation) II and STS (Society of Thoracic Surgeons) risk scores are the most commonly employed risk prediction tools in cardiac surgery, with each score having its own advantages and limitations.
5. Future improvements in risk prediction tools may be facilitated by better integrating data from electronic medical records, incorporating predictive information from intraoperative variables or novel biomarkers, and considering prediction of patient-centered outcomes.

The preoperative assessment and optimization of cardiac surgical patients present unique challenges to the perioperative physician. Despite advances in medical therapies and surgical techniques, these patients' risk for adverse events often remains substantial during and after surgery. Indeed, it is worthwhile remembering that most patients presenting for cardiac surgery have pathology that would typically preclude them from undergoing anesthesia for elective non-cardiac surgical procedures. Thus, the preoperative period is a crucial time to ensure: patients are suitable for surgery; all reasonable opportunities for preoperative optimization are identified; and patients have an informed understanding of the potential risks associated with their upcoming procedures.

While each type of cardiac surgical procedure has specific preoperative considerations that are discussed in detail in subsequent chapters, the importance of risk prognostication is a universal concept that should be considered in every patient being considered for surgery. In this chapter, we

K. S. Ladha · D. N. Wijeysundera (✉)
Department of Anesthesia, St. Michael's Hospital and University of Toronto, Toronto, Ontario, Canada
e-mail: karim.ladha@mail.utoronto.ca;
d.wijeysundera@utoronto.ca

© Springer Nature Switzerland AG 2021
D. C. H. Cheng et al. (eds.), *Evidence-Based Practice in Perioperative Cardiac Anesthesia and Surgery*, https://doi.org/10.1007/978-3-030-47887-2_2

aim to provide the reader with general concepts related to the goals and methods of risk stratification, as well as provide selected examples of some common risk scores used in cardiac surgery. Our aim is to present the reader with the benefits and limitations of risk scores and their utility in routine clinical practice.

Why Estimate Risk?

A patient's expected risk of future adverse events can inform almost every aspect of the perioperative period. Prior to surgery, expected risk may influence the type of procedure chosen—e.g. open versus catheter-based approaches to aortic valve replacement. In some cases, this information may lead to the cancellation of the planned procedure if the perioperative team feels that the risks of major adverse events outweigh any potential benefits. Communication of risk to patients also allows them to retain their autonomy in decision-making, improve the informed consent process, and facilitate shared-decision making. In the preoperative setting, estimates of risk can inform decision-making related to further investigations—e.g., pulmonary function testing—or optimization of severe comorbid conditions.

With respect to the intraoperative period, information on expected risk garnered in the preoperative period can influence planning, such as the placement of invasive lines prior to the induction of anesthesia, or the specific choice of vasoactive medications available in anticipation of hemodynamic instability during surgery. One of the most common justifications for preoperative risk stratification for non-cardiac surgery is planning for postoperative disposition or monitoring. While the typical cardiac surgical patient will be transferred immediately after surgery to a critical care unit, preoperative risk stratification can still help with anticipated resource utilization—e.g., expected length of stay; predicting the need for prolonged mechanical ventilation; or planning availability of specialized organ support therapies—e.g., renal replacement therapy.

Risk stratification also has important roles in quality assurance initiatives and research. For example, this information allows for benchmarking to compare outcomes across institutions and providers by enabling adjustment for differences in surgical case-mix. It is interesting to note that the use of risk scores in cardiac surgery was prompted by the desire to explain an increase in mortality after coronary artery bypass grafting (CABG) [1]. In addition, estimates of expected risk allow for risk adjustment in observational—i.e., non-randomized—studies that examine the effectiveness of particular interventions.

The Art and Science of Risk Estimation

Expected risk can be determined both implicitly and explicitly. An experienced clinician who regularly manages cardiac surgical patients can readily use clinical information and judgment to make implicit risk determinations when delivering clinical care. This is done without a pencil and paper, or an online calculator. As an example, experienced cardiac anesthesiologists will immediately recognize that a patient with severe chronic obstructive pulmonary disease and a left ventricular ejection fraction of 20% who is scheduled to have an urgent double cardiac valve replacement procedure is more likely to suffer a major postoperative complication than an otherwise healthy individual scheduled to have an elective CABG. This subjective assessment of risk is a valuable tool in perioperative decision making, especially in dynamic and time-limited circumstances.

The basis for these subjective assessments comes from both experience and previous research examining individual predictors of poor outcomes. The major challenge with subjective assessment, aside from its reliance on sufficient prior experience and potential for inter-rater variability, is how best to integrate available information on various different risk factors to generate an overall estimate of risk for any given patient. Specifically, prior research has identified a multitude of factors that can contribute to risk, including but not limited to: demographic characteristics—i.e., age, sex; functional capacity; presence and severity of comorbid conditions;

complexity and urgency for the planned procedure; and laboratory values.

Risk Scores

Risk scores are a commonly used tool in perioperative medicine that can encapsulate a patient's overall expected risk for specific outcomes of interest—e.g., death, stroke—into a single number or probability. Patients are allocated points or weights based on the presence of certain risk factors. These overall point scores can be then converted into a probability of a certain event, such as 30-day mortality. It should be noted that risk scores and quantification of risk are not meant to supersede clinical judgment, but rather should be used as supplemental tools in decision making.

The scores are developed or derived in a cohort of patients in whom potential predictors—e.g., age, sex, comorbidity, surgical procedure—are measured and where clinically relevant outcome data—e.g. 30-day mortality—are available. Thus, risk scores are typically derived using research or administrative databases. Statistical methods are applied to determine the choice and relevant weighting of risk factors that will go into a score. While there are many techniques that can used to perform this analysis, such as recursive partitioning and machine learning, the most commonly employed approach is multivariable logistic regression modeling. A complete description of these statistical techniques, including their advantages, disadvantages and underlying assumptions, is beyond the scope of this chapter. Thus, we refer readers interested in this more detailed information to other comprehensive reviews dedicated to this topic [2].

Before delving into specific scores, it is important to briefly describe what constitutes a good risk score. The first criterion is that it needs to work, or in other words, be accurate. While this may seem like a straight-forward concept, in reality, there is no single metric that summarizes prognostic accuracy. Rather, there are several factors that are used in combination to assess the quality of a risk score: discrimination, risk reclassification, calibration, and generalizability.

Discrimination refers to the extent to which risk scores correctly assign different distributions of predicted risk estimates to individuals who eventually develop the outcome of interest as compared to those who do not. A "good" risk score is one that generally assigns higher predicted probabilities to individuals who develop the outcome versus those who did not. It should be noted that discrimination does not evaluate whether the actual predicted probability is correct—rather that the distribution of predicted probabilities is higher in people who develop the outcomes—thus, this is essentially an evaluation of correct rank ordering. A commonly used measure of discrimination is the area under the curve (AUC) of the receiver operating characteristic (ROC) curve, which is also identical to the c-statistic of a logistic regression model. The AUC is a function of the sensitivity and specificity of a given test, with possible values ranging from 0 to 1. One way to think about the AUC is as a probability that an individual with an outcome event had a higher predicted risk than an individual without an event. Therefore, if a score is no better than flipping a coin—i.e. 50/50—the AUC would be 0.5. Values higher than 0.5 indicate that the score fares better than chance and many people cite a minimum value of at least 0.7 to have reasonable predictive ability. However, there is no straightforward clinical interpretation of what the AUC means, and there is no single universally accepted value that denotes "good" discrimination.

Calibration is a measure of how well observed outcome rates matched the rates predicted by the risk score. While this may seem similar to discrimination, it is a different concept. For example, if a group of individuals within a cohort had a calculated risk of 20% based on their risk score, did 20% of them actually experience the outcome? Calibration can be assessed by statistical tests such as the Hosmer-Lemeshow statistic, but it can also be graphically depicted. This involves plotting a comparison of the expected versus observed rates that allows for a more nuanced understanding of a score's performance when compared to a single statistic. For example, a score may simply over predict an outcome at higher scores, but otherwise performs well. This could only be determined from plotting the data, rather than interpreting a statistical term. Furthermore, part of calibration pertains to what prediction means in clinical practice—that is that it applies to the prediction of event rates in groups, not individuals. Any specific individual either has either 0% or a 100% probability of developing a specific outcome of interest. Even with genetic data, predictive ability is still limited at the level of an individual. For example, the concordance rate for schizophrenia in monozygotic twins, who would share essentially identical genetic information and very similar socio-economic characteristics, is only about 40–65% [3]. The different concepts encapsulated by discrimination versus calibration are further described in Figs. 2.1 and 2.2.

It should be noted that comparing calibration between risk scores is difficult. However, a similar concept is the idea of risk reclassification. Risk reclassification is often used to determine the value of adding another predictor or biomarker to a particular risk score to see if it improves risk estimation; in addition, risk reclassification can be used to compare two different scores [4]. The basic premise is that the population is divided into strata based on clinically relevant expected outcome event rates, such as <5, 5–15 and >15% event rates. An improvement in risk classification for a risk score would mean that patients who had the outcome were more likely to be reclassified into strata with a higher predicted probability, while those who did not have the outcome were more likely to be reclassified into lower risk strata. An indexed score can be calculated to summarize the overall net improvement in risk classification, which is known as the net reclassification improvement (NRI). A continuous variant of the NRI can also be calculated, which is not reliant on the specific definitions of risk

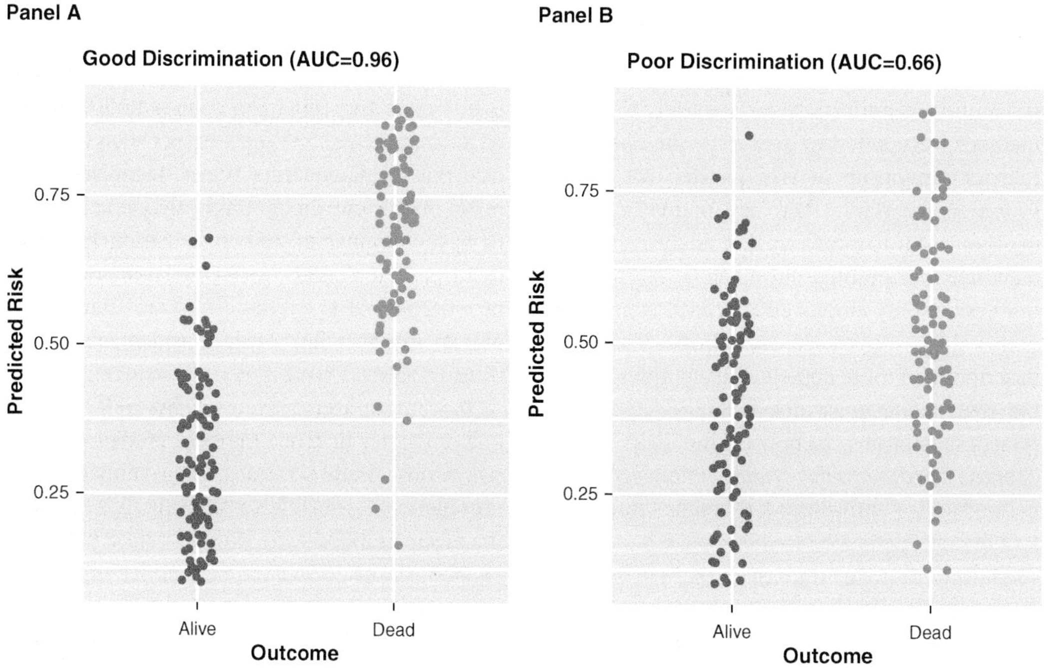

Fig. 2.1 Graphical depiction of the discrimination of two hypothetical risk scores used to predict postoperative 30-day mortality. To help readers to better understand the concept of discrimination, we have graphically depicted this concept using theoretical data. This figure presents two hypothetical risk scores for predicting postoperative mortality, one of which has excellent discrimination (Panel A) while the other has poor-to-fair discrimination (Panel B). The risk score with excellent discrimination (AUC 0.96) has relatively little overlap in the distributions of predicted probabilities between individuals who were alive versus dead at 30-day postoperative follow-up. By comparison, the risk score with poor discrimination (AUC 0.66) shows significant overlap between the two groups (dead and alive) in terms of their predicted probabilities. The R (Version 3.4.1) statistical language (Vienna, Austria) was used to randomly generate these data, and produce the figures (*ggplots2* package)

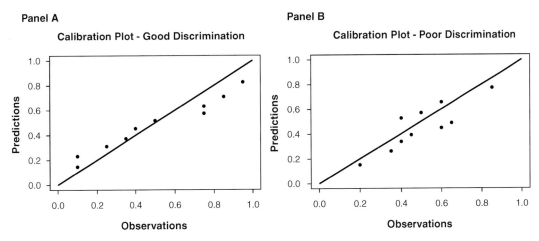

Fig. 2.2 Graphical depiction of calibration using the same theoretical risk scores and randomly generated data depicted in Fig. 2.1. These calibration plots are based on the same theoretical risk scores and randomly generated data depicted in Fig. 2.1. These same data were divided into ten equally sized groups, each of which is represented by a dot that was plotted separately in two plots pertaining to the risk score with good discrimination (Panel A) or poor discrimination (Panel B). The straight line in each plot represents perfect calibration, with points further away from the line indicating worse calibration. It is noteworthy that despite the very different discrimination of the two risk scores (AUC values of 0.96 vs. 0.66), their calibration does not appear to significantly differ. The R (Version 3.4.1) statistical language (Vienna, Austria) was used to randomly generate these data, and produce the figures (*PredictABEL* package)

strata—that themselves can influence the statistical significance of the categorical NRI [5]. While the use of the NRI is increasing in the literature, it is not always applied appropriately and caution should be taken with its interpretation [6].

The generalizability of a risk score must be assessed to determine whether it can be readily applied in samples aside from the one in which it was originally derived. In general, the best estimates of accuracy are obtained from the sample or cohort in which the score was created. Assessment over generalizability involves what is termed '*validation*'. Some components of validation—i.e. 'internal validation'—can take place within the same cohort used to derive the risk score. Internal validation typically involves techniques such as data splitting or bootstrap resampling. However, all risk scores should ideally undergo external validation in a separate cohort to ensure that calibration and discrimination hold and are not degraded when applied in a separate group of patients. In general, discrimination is better preserved than calibration in external validation.

Beyond these measures, a good risk score needs to be easy to implement in clinical practice. If a score is too complicated or time consuming to calculate for a busy clinician with 20 patients waiting to be seen in the preoperative assessment clinic, it will have limited utility regardless of its prognostic accuracy. Additionally, the score must have good inter-rater reliability, meaning that the same patient should be assigned generally similar risk scores by several different raters. The easiest example for considering the importance of inter-rater reliability is the American Society of Anesthesiologists Physical Status classification system [7]. Even in a score with only six categories, there can be discrepancies between providers as to how to categorize a patient. Similarly, if a risk score does not clearly define a predictor or outcome, then its utility in practice is limited [8]. For example, acute kidney injury can be defined multiple ways, including by an increase in creatinine concentration of a specific magnitude, a creatinine concentration exceeding a specific threshold, the need for dialysis, clinical judgment, or a set of criteria. If acute kidney injury is defined differently in clinical practice compared to the method used when a risk score was derived, then the score's predictive ability is unclear.

Risk Scores Used in Cardiac Surgery

There is no shortage of risk scores to choose from when evaluating the cardiac surgical patient. While initial models were built to exclusively predict postoperative mortality in CABG surgery, subsequently developed scores now cover a variety of both procedures and outcomes. For example, a previous study compared 19 different risk scores, each of which was derived from a different cohort of patients [9]. Notably, even this list of assessed scores was not exhaustive. Thus, a complete description of every possible risk score for cardiac surgical patients is beyond the scope of what can be feasibly included in this chapter. Rather, we will focus on and describe three popular risk scores for cardiac surgical patients, namely the Parsonnet score, the Society of Thoracic Surgeons (STS) risk score, and the European System for Cardiac Operative Risk Evaluation (EuroSCORE).

Parsonnet Score

The Parsonnet score is regarded as the first validated, additive scoring system for predicting mortality in patients undergoing cardiac surgery. The impetus for its development came in the 1980s when the operative mortality risks of patients undergoing CABG rose from less than 2% to almost 6% [10]. Surgeons were left struggling to explain the underlying basis for this increase in mortality, and it became apparent that understanding the underlying risk of surgical patients through statistical modeling was the key [1]. Thus, Parsonnet et al. proposed a preoperative score for adult cardiac surgery in 1989 based on 14 risk factors that classified patients into five categories of risk [11]. While the score was simple and performed well according to the metrics discussed above, its major critique was that two factors (catastrophic states and other rare circumstances) had fairly arbitrary definitions. Given the significant weighting of these factors, the reliability of the score was severely limited. In addition, given the age of the score, its relevance to modern practice has also been questioned since it tends to overestimate mortality—i.e., suboptimal calibration [12].

Since its original development, the score has been modified to improve its reliability and predictive ability. In 1997, a modified Parsonnet score was derived that included 44 variables, thereby increasing its accuracy but also its complexity [13]. We include a description of the Parsonnet score in this chapter principally for historic purposes since it was the first score to be derived in cardiac surgical patients. In addition to being the first score, it has often been used as a benchmark against which other newer scores are compared. In our experience, its use in routine clinical practice is fairly limited, especially in comparison to the two other scores described below.

Society of Thoracic Surgeons

For over two decades, the Society of Thoracic Surgeons (STS) National Adult Cardiac Database has been widely regarded as the benchmark for systematic data collection on cardiac surgical patients and their outcomes. The STS began examining predictors of mortality in 1994 in approximately 80,000 patients who had CABG [14]. Since their initial development, these risk models have undergone periodic adjustments to maintain the relevance and accuracy, in addition to adaptation for six types of procedures. Furthermore, the scope of these risk models has expanded to include risk estimates for multiple outcomes beyond mortality, including length of stay, need for re-operation, and other complications—e.g., acute stroke, acute kidney injury. While the actual weights assigned to individual risk factors are considered proprietary and therefore not made public, the methods used to develop the score have been published in the literature [15]. Additionally, the scores can be calculated through an easy-to-use—although potentially time consuming—and publicly-available online tool (http://riskcalc.sts.org).

EuroSCORE

The EuroSCORE was first published in 1999 based on a study that assessed the risk of postoperative mortality among approximately 13,000 patients having a variety of surgical procedures [16]. This original model was known as the '*additive*' model since it assigned points to each risk factor, which were then used to calculate a summative overall risk score. The score was later revised in 2003 using a logistic regression model, to address concerns that the original model underestimated risk in high-risk populations. In this revised risk score, the beta-coefficients from the regression model are added and then converted to a probability, which increased the complexity of the score [17]. Despite this modification, there were still concerns that the score overestimates mortality, a problem that has worsened over time as overall operative survival improved. These persistent concerns led to the creation of the EuroSCORE II in 2011, which was developed using data from a cohort of patients undergoing surgery across 43 countries, including seven centers in North America. This new score contains 18 factors, and is based on a logistic regression model [18]. The updated model is also shorter than the current STS calculator and available online in an easy-to-use format (http://euroscore.org/calc.html). However, it is important to note that even the newest version only calculates risk estimates for mortality.

Comparison of Scores

A comparison of the factors used to calculate all three risk scores can be found in Table 2.1. It should be noted that even when the risk scores incorporate a variable such as renal impairment as a predictor of adverse events, the exact definition typically varies between the scores. Similarly, some categories, such as critical illness prior to surgery, are considered as a single factor in one score but broken down into multiple factors in another—i.e., the use of inotropes and resuscitation prior to surgery. Therefore, Table 2.1 is provided as a summary guide for comparison purposes only. For details regarding each score, we refer the reader to the original manuscripts [11, 15, 18].

Table 2.1 Comparison of three cardiac surgical risk scores for patients undergoing coronary artery bypass grafting surgery

	Euro-SCORE II	Society of Thoracic Surgeons	Original Parsonnet
Demographic Variables[a]			
Age	X	X	X
Sex	X	X	X
Ethnicity		X	
Body composition		X	X
Comorbid conditions[a]			
Diabetes mellitus	X	X	X
Chronic lung disease	X	X	
Cerebrovascular disease		X	
Renal impairment	X	X	X
Peripheral arterial disease	X	X	
Immunocompromised		X	
Cardiac History[a]			
Hypertension		X	X
Cardiac arrhythmia		X	
Heart failure	X	X	
Pulmonary hypertension	X		
Previous cardiac surgery	X	X	X
Left ventricular function	X	X	X
Nature of coronary anatomy or disease		X	
Valvular disease		X	
Previous percutaneous coronary intervention		X	X
Left ventricular aneurysm			X
Prior myocardial infarction	X	X	
Endocarditis	X	X	
Clinical Status[a]			
Preoperative intra-aortic balloon pump		X	X
Critically ill preoperatively	X	X	
Angina	X	X	
Urgency of procedure	X	X	X
Other[a]			
Catastrophic states			X
Other rare circumstances			X
Poor mobility	X		

[a]The definition of each factor varies by the risk score used. For a complete description of definitions for each risk factor, the reader is refered to the original articles

From the Database to the Bedside

Based on the discussion above, it is clear that no single score is consistently superior to others in its ability to accurately estimate risk in all patients.

Both the EuroSCORE II and the STS risk score have shown good discrimination, calibration and generalizability across multiple cohorts. While numerous studies have compared the various scores, the ongoing updates to the scores over time make it difficult to keep track of all the possible comparisons. Furthermore, small differences in AUC values are hard to translate in terms of clinical impact. For example, a 2016 study of almost 12,000 patients undergoing cardiac surgery showed that EuroSCORE II and the STS risk score had similar discriminatory abilities with an AUC of 0.84 and 0.85 respectively in a cohort of patients [19].

Therefore, the question remains as to which score to use, and when? Both the EuroSCORE II and STS have the benefits of having been updated since their original derivation, having been developed using large databases from multiple institutions, and being easy to use with free online calculators. They both have excellent documentation that clearly defines the risk factors and outcomes of interest—which should help make scores more reliable across users. Nonetheless, there are some differences between the EuroSCORE II and STS that are worth highlighting. First, STS computes probabilities for several outcomes beyond mortality. This is an important advantage since a permanent stroke may be just as unacceptable to many patients as death. Second, the EuroSCORE II can be applied to a variety of complex cardiac surgical procedures since it incorporates more detailed information on procedure complexity. For example, one could calculate predicted mortality risk after a double valve replacement plus CABG using the EuroSCORE II, but not STS score. Thus, the EuroSCORE II may be a more flexible score in patients undergoing surgical procedures that are considered beyond "typical".

Risk Scores for Specific Populations

Some subgroups of patients may not be well suited to risk estimation by either of these two risk scores. A key example is the adult with repaired congenital heart disease presenting for surgery. Development of a risk score for this population is extremely challenging given the variety of lesions and pathology, as well as the relative rarity of each particular procedure. Additionally, two patients with similar pathologies—e.g., Tetralogy of Fallot—can have drastically different presentations in terms of age, associated comorbidities and sequelae from their heart disease. Thus, attempts to use existing risk scores from pediatric populations or scores developed for adults with more common acquired heart disease—e.g., coronary artery disease—have not resulted in consistently accurate estimates of risk. A new score that combines previous scores has shown good predictive performance [20], but has yet to undergo wider multicenter validation.

Another example of a population that merits special consideration for risk scores are patients having transcatheter aortic valve replacement (TAVR). Many patients considered for TAVR are considered otherwise very high-risk for a typical open aortic valve replacement, yet the TAVR procedure itself likely involves considerably less physiological stress than the standard open procedure. Thus, unsurprisingly, studies that have applied usual cardiac surgical risk scores to TAVR patients have found poor predictive performance [21]. As the overall rate of transcatheter procedures continues to increase, there is an unmet need to develop better methods to estimate risk in these patients. To address this need, several TAVR-specific scores have been developed, such as OBSERVANT [22] and TAVI2-SCORe [23]. While these scores show promise, their performance in external validation has been inconsistent, and further research is still needed [24].

There Are Important Outcomes Beyond Death Alone

While most preoperative risk scores for cardiac surgery patients have focused on predicting mortality, there is now increasing interest in other outcomes relevant to patients, providers, administrators, and payers. Reflecting this trend, the STS risk calculator now estimates risks of other outcomes, such as prolonged length-of-stay or acute stroke.

Nonetheless, simply using an established risk score to predict a new outcome is often problematic. As described above, adaptation of previously developed risk scores to new specific subgroups, such as TAVR patients and patients with repaired congenital heart disease, often results in suboptimal predictive performance. The same problem applies to using a risk score to predict a different set of outcomes. There are numerous studies examining the use of established risk scores with different outcomes such as critical care length-of-stay and hospital charges [25–27]. However, even though these studies may show some promise of risk scores in different scenarios, a single study does not validate the use of a risk score in a new situation and caution must be taken when applying scores in this manner [28].

Given these issues with simple adaptation of existing risk scores to predict different outcomes, there has been increasing efforts to develop specialized risk scores for specific outcomes. For example, several studies have developed risk scores for predicting severe acute kidney injury requiring dialysis after cardiac surgery [29–33]. However, the scores have undergone generally limited validation in other cohorts, making it difficult to recommend their use.

Future of Risk Scores

One of the main limitations of risk scores is that they use predictive information gathered from large cohorts of patients to make infer-

ences regarding an individual patient. Therefore, regardless of how many risk factors are included, they still involve a generalization for an individual. In an effort to create more personalized estimates, there is a push to include biomarkers to supplement prognostic estimates. Biomarkers allow clinicians to detect subclinical disease as well as provide quantitative measurement of clinical phenomenon. The ability of biomarkers such as troponin or B-type natriuretic peptide to augment existing risk scores in cardiac surgery is currently being investigated and not used in routine clinical practice yet [34].

Risk scores are also a static measure of a patient's risk in the preoperative period at a single moment in time. In reality, a patient's expected risk changes through their perioperative period. For example, simply adding cardiopulmonary bypass times typically adds considerably additional prognostic information about a patient's risk of complications. Neither the STS nor the EuroSCORE prediction models incorporate intraoperative variables that can have a profound influence on a patient's postoperative trajectory. With the ubiquity of information technology in health care, one can envision a future where automated tools will adjust initial preoperative risk estimates throughout the perioperative period as additional clinical information—e.g., cardiopulmonary bypass time, hemodynamics—is accumulated.

Finally, the goal of surgery is not only to avoid stroke or death, but also rather to alleviate symptoms and improve quality of life. Outcomes such as disability, functional capacity, ability to independently perform activities of daily living, and disability-free survival are crucial to patients, but missing from risk score predictions. Specifically, a patient may have no interest in pursuing surgery if there is a significant risk of not being able to live at home independently. There is an unmet need for predictive tools that will allow clinicians to have these types of discussions in the perioperative period [35].

Risk scores are useful tools to help providers integrate clinical information and derive quantitative estimates of perioperative risk. While we have discussed the rationale and methods underlying risk assessment tools, the question is whether better estimation of risk matters? It is extremely difficult to prove that risk scores change practice or outcomes, in part related to the paucity of perioperative interventions proven to improve a patient's trajectory. Nonetheless, even in the absence of proven effects on postoperative outcomes, risk tools can still help better convey information about expected perioperative risk to patients. If we are to move towards a model of health care delivery that emphasizes shared-decision making, we must strive to provide more accurate estimates of adverse events to our patients. Risk assessment tools are integral to achieving that objective.

References

1. Kacila M, Tiwari KK, Granov N, Omerbašić E, Straus S. Assessment of the initial and modified Parsonnet score in mortality prediction of the patients operated in the Sarajevo Heart Center. Bosn J Basic Med Sci. 2010;10(2):165–8.
2. Kuhn M, Johnson K. Applied predictive modeling. New York: Springer Science & Business Media; 2013.
3. Cardno AG, Gottesman II. Twin studies of schizophrenia: from bow-and-arrow concordances to star wars Mx and functional genomics. Am J Med Genet. 2000;97(1):12–7.
4. Ladha KS, Zhao K, Quraishi SA, Kurth T, Eikermann M, Kaafarani HMA, et al. The Deyo-Charlson and Elixhauser-van Walraven comorbidity indices as predictors of mortality in critically ill patients. BMJ Open. 2015;5(9):e008990.
5. Pencina MJ, D'Agostino RB, Steyerberg EW. Extensions of net reclassification improvement calculations to measure usefulness of new biomarkers. Stat Med. 2011;30(1):11–21.
6. Leening MJG, Vedder MM, Witteman JCM, Pencina MJ, Steyerberg EW. Net reclassification improvement: computation, interpretation, and controversies: a literature review and clinician's guide. Ann Intern Med. 2014;160(2):122–31.
7. Sankar A, Johnson SR, Beattie WS, Tait G, Wijeysundera DN. Reliability of the American Society of Anesthesiologists physical status scale in clinical practice. Br J Anaesth. 2014;113(3):424–32.
8. Laupacis A, Sekar N, Stiell IG. Clinical prediction rules. A review and suggested modifications of methodological standards. JAMA. 1997;277(6):488–94.
9. Nilsson J, Algotsson L, Höglund P, Lührs C, Brandt J. Comparison of 19 pre-operative risk stratification models in open-heart surgery. Eur Heart J. 2006;27(7):867–74.
10. Geraci JM, Johnson ML, Gordon HS, Petersen NJ, Shroyer AL, Grover FL, et al. Mortality after cardiac bypass surgery: prediction from administrative versus clinical data. Med Care. 2005;43(2):149–58.
11. Parsonnet V, Dean D, Bernstein AD. A method of uniform stratification of risk for evaluating the results of surgery in acquired adult heart disease. Circulation. 1989;79(6 Pt 2):I3–12.
12. Granton J, Cheng D. Risk stratification models for cardiac surgery. Semin Cardiothorac Vasc Anesth. 2008;12(3):167–74.
13. Gabrielle F, Roques F, Michel P, Bernard A, de Vicentis C, Roques X, et al. Is the Parsonnet's score a good predictive score of mortality in adult cardiac surgery: assessment by a French multicentre study. Eur J Cardiothorac Surg. 1997;11(3):406–14.
14. Edwards FH, Clark RE, Schwartz M. Coronary artery bypass grafting: the Society of Thoracic Surgeons National Database experience. Ann Thorac Surg. 1994;57(1):12–9.
15. Shahian DM, O'Brien SM, Filardo G, Ferraris VA, Haan CK, Rich JB, et al. The Society of Thoracic Surgeons 2008 cardiac surgery risk models: part 1— coronary artery bypass grafting surgery. Ann Thorac Surg. 2009;88(1 Suppl):S2–22.
16. Nashef SA, Roques F, Michel P, Gauducheau E, Lemeshow S, Salamon R. European system for cardiac operative risk evaluation (EuroSCORE). Eur J Cardiothorac Surg. 1999;16(1):9–13.
17. Roques F, Michel P, Goldstone AR, Nashef SAM. The logistic EuroSCORE. Eur Heart J. 2003;24(9):881–2.
18. Nashef SAM, Roques F, Sharples LD, Nilsson J, Smith C, Goldstone AR, et al. EuroSCORE II. Eur J Cardiothorac Surg. 2012;41(4):734–44.
19. Ad N, Holmes SD, Patel J, Pritchard G, Shuman DJ, Halpin L. Comparison of EuroSCORE II, original EuroSCORE, and the society of thoracic surgeons risk score in cardiac surgery patients. Ann Thorac Surg. 2016;102(2):573–9.
20. Hörer J, Kasnar-Samprec J, Cleuziou J, Strbad M, Wottke M, Kaemmerer H, et al. Mortality following congenital heart surgery in adults can be predicted accurately by combining expert-based and evidence-based pediatric risk scores. World J Pediatr Congenit Heart Surg. 2016;7(4):425–35.
21. Wang TKM, Wang MTM, Gamble GD, Webster M, Ruygrok PN. Performance of contemporary surgical risk scores for transcatheter aortic valve implantation: a meta-analysis. Int J Cardiol. 2017;236:350–5.
22. Capodanno D, Barbanti M, Tamburino C, D'Errigo P, Ranucci M, Santoro G, et al. A simple risk tool (the OBSERVANT score) for prediction of 30-day mortal-

ity after transcatheter aortic valve replacement. Am J Cardiol. 2014;113(11):1851–8.

23. Debonnaire P, Fusini L, Wolterbeek R, Kamperidis V, van Rosendael P, van der Kley F, et al. Value of the "TAVI2-SCORe" versus surgical risk scores for prediction of one year mortality in 511 patients who underwent transcatheter aortic valve implantation. Am J Cardiol. 2015;115(2):234–42.

24. Collas VM, Van De Heyning CM, Paelinck BP, Rodrigus IE, Vrints CJ, Bosmans JM. Validation of transcatheter aortic valve implantation risk scores in relation to early and mid-term survival: a single-centre study. Interact Cardiovasc Thorac Surg. 2016;22(3):273–9.

25. Lawrence DR, Valencia O, Smith EE, Murday A, Treasure T. Parsonnet score is a good predictor of the duration of intensive care unit stay following cardiac surgery. Heart. 2000;83(4):429–32.

26. Nilsson J, Algotsson L, Höglund P, Lührs C, Brandt J. EuroSCORE predicts intensive care unit stay and costs of open heart surgery. Ann Thorac Surg. 2004;78(5):1528–34.

27. Kurki TS, Häkkinen U, Lauharanta J, Rämö J, Leijala M. Evaluation of the relationship between preoperative risk scores, postoperative and total length of stays and hospital costs in coronary bypass surgery. Eur J Cardiothorac Surg. 2001;20(6):1183–7.

28. Badreldin AM, Doerr F, Kroener A, Wahlers T, Hekmat K. Preoperative risk stratification models fail to predict hospital cost of cardiac surgery patients. J Cardiothorac Surg. 2013;8(1):126.

29. Pannu N, Graham M, Klarenbach S, Meyer S, Kieser T, Hemmelgarn B, et al. A new model to predict acute kidney injury requiring renal replacement therapy after cardiac surgery. CMAJ. 2016;188(15):1076–83.

30. Thakar CV, Arrigain S, Worley S, Yared J-P, Paganini EP. A clinical score to predict acute renal failure after cardiac surgery. J Am Soc Nephrol. 2005;16(1):162–8.

31. Brown JR, Cochran RP, Leavitt BJ, Dacey LJ, Ross CS, MacKenzie TA, et al. Multivariable prediction of renal insufficiency developing after cardiac surgery. Circulation. 2007;116(11 Suppl):I139–43.

32. Mehta RH, Grab JD, O'Brien SM, Bridges CR, Gammie JS, Haan CK, et al. Bedside tool for predicting the risk of postoperative dialysis in patients undergoing cardiac surgery. Circulation. 2006;114(21):2208–16.

33. Wijeysundera DN, Karkouti K, Dupuis J-Y, Rao V, Chan CT, Granton JT, et al. Derivation and validation of a simplified predictive index for renal replacement therapy after cardiac surgery. JAMA. 2007;297(16):1801–9.

34. Shahian DM, Grover FL. Biomarkers and risk models in cardiac surgery. Circulation. 2014;130(12):932–5.

35. Myles PS. Meaningful outcome measures in cardiac surgery. J Extra Corpor Technol. 2014;46(1):23–7.

Part II

Perioperative Anesthesia Techniques and Management

Perioperative Management of Cardiac Surgical Patients Receiving Antithrombotic Agents

3

Pulkit Bhuptani, Alexander T. H. Suen, and C. David Mazer

Main Messages

1. Appropriate perioperative antithrombotic management is essential prior to cardiac surgery to attain the optimal balance between prevention of thrombosis and minimization of surgical bleeding.
2. Whether and for how long antithrombotic therapy is held perioperatively will depend on the duration and magnitude of risks of thrombosis and bleeding, the half-life of the drug and the renal function of the patient.
3. Patients with the highest risk of perioperative thrombosis will requiring bridging anticoagulation with a parenteral anti-coagulant such as a low molecular weight heparin.
4. The management of perioperative bleeding may require a multidisciplinary approach with a combination of prevention strategies, hemostatic agents, blood products and reversal agents as available.
5. Routine laboratory tests such as aPTT and INR may detect the presence of a NOAC, but normal results do not completely exclude a residual anticoagulant effect. Specialized testing may be required.
6. Resumption of antithrombotic therapy postoperatively is guided by the bleeding and thrombosis risks of the patient. In most cases, such therapy can be resumed 1–2 days post hemostasis.

P. Bhuptani
Pharmacy Department, St. Michael's Hospital, Toronto, ON, Canada

A. T. H. Suen
Department of Anesthesia, St. Michael's Hospital, University of Toronto, Toronto, ON, Canada

C. D. Mazer (✉)
Department of Anesthesia, Keenan Research Center, Li Ka Shing Knowledge Institute, St. Michael's Hospital, University of Toronto, Toronto, ON, Canada
e-mail: David.Mazer@unityhealth.to

There are two primary classes of antithrombotic drugs: antiplatelet and anticoagulant agents. The management of patients undergoing cardiac surgery on antithrombotic therapy is challenging because temporary cessation of such agents increases the risk of thrombosis. On the other hand, cardiac surgery, a highly invasive surgical procedure, is associated with bleeding risks that can be amplified by antithrombotic agents. Both of these outcomes are associated with a significant risk of morbidity and mortality. Therefore, it is essential to seek an optimal balance between reducing the risk of thrombosis/embolism and minimizing risk of periprocedural bleeding.

Achieving this clinical balance between thrombosis and bleeding has recently become more challenging, primarily due to the introduction and widespread use of several new direct oral anticoagulants. While these novel agents have more predictable anticoagulation effects and shorter onset/offset effects, they pose a perioperative conundrum as antidotes are not cur-

rently readily available for all agents. Consequently, an increasing number of patients who are on antiplatelet agents, anticoagulants, or a combination of both are presenting for surgery. The perioperative management of antithrombotic therapy for cardiac surgery needs to take into account the specific agent a patient is on (refer to Table 3.1 for an overview of antithrombotic agents); their individualized risk of thrombosis and bleeding; and whether temporary bridging is required.

Table 3.1 Antithrombotic agent overview

Drug	Clinical indication	Dose	Mechanism of action	Renal clearance	Onset of action	Half-life[a]
Direct Oral Anticoagulants (DOACs)						
Apixaban	Atrial fibrillation	2.5 or 5 mg BID	Factor Xa inhibitor	25%	3–4 h	8–17 h
	VTE treatment	10 mg BID × 7 day then 5 mg BID				
	VTE prevention	2.5 mg BID				
Betrixaban	VTE prevention	160 mg × 1 then 80 mg daily or 80 mg × 1 then 40 mg daily	Factor Xa inhibitor	11%	3–4 h	19–27 h
Edoxaban	Atrial fibrillation	30 or 60 mg daily	Factor Xa inhibitor	50%	1–2 h	10–14 h (for CrCL >50 ml/min)
	VTE treatment					
Rivaroxaban	Atrial fibrillation	15 or 20 mg daily	Factor Xa inhibitor	33% (active drug)	1–3 h	7–15 h
	VTE treatment	15 mg BID × 3 weeks then 20 mg daily				
	VTE prevention	10 mg daily				
Dabigatran	Atrial fibrillation	110 or 150 mg BID	Direct thrombin inhibitor	80%	1–3 h	7–35 h
	VTE treatment					
	VTE prevention	110 mg × 1 then 220 mg daily				
Vitamin K antagonists						
Warfarin	Thromboembolic complications (treatment or prevention)	Variable: 2–10 mg daily	Vitamin K epoxide reductase (factors II, VII, IX, X)	Minimal renal clearance of active drug	4 h (3–7 days to get INR within therapeutic range)	20–60 h
Antiplatelet agents						
Aspirin	CAD PVD Stroke prevention Atrial fibrillation Valvular surgery	80–325 mg	Irreversible COX-1 and COX-2 inhibitor	Minimal	1 h	3 h Impaired platelet function for up to 7 days

Table 3.1 (continued)

Drug	Clinical indication	Dose	Mechanism of action	Renal clearance	Onset of action	Half-life[a]
Aspirin-dipyridamole (ASA/DIP)	Stroke prevention	25/200 mg BID	Dipyridamole: inhibits uptake of adenosine into platelets	Minimal	1–2 h	ASA: 3 h DIP: 10–12 h Impaired platelet function for up to 7 days
Clopidogrel	CAD PVD Stroke prevention	Load: 300–600 mg then 75 mg daily	Irreversible platelet inhibition by blockade of P2Y12 component of adenosine receptors	Minimal	2 h with load	6 h. Activity persists for 5 day after stopping
Prasugrel	ACS	Load: 60 mg then 5 or 10 mg daily			<30 min with load	7 h. Activity persists for 5–9 days after stopping
Ticagrelor		Load: 180 mg then 90 mg BID			30 min with load	58% of anti-platelet activity at 24 h and 10% at 110 h
Abciximab	ACS PCI	Load: 0.25 mg/kg then 0.125 mcg/kg/min (max: 10 mcg/min)	Inhibition of platelets through GP IIb/IIIa receptors	Minimal	10 min	30 min–4 h
Eptifibatide		Load: 180 mcg/kg IV bolus (max 22.6 mg) then 1–2 mcg/kg/min based on renal function		Extensive	5 min	4–8 h
Parenteral anticoagulants						
Argatroban	HIT PCI	0.2–2 mcg/kg/min then titrated to aPTT	Reversible thrombin inhibitor	Minimal	Rapid	40–50 min. 180 min with liver dysfunction
Danaparoid	VTE prophylaxis following orthopedic, abdominal or thoracic surgery	750 units SC Q12H	Factor IIa and Xa inhibitor	Extensive	Peak activity at 4–5 h	25 h (up to 35 h with impaired renal function)
	HIT treatment	Load: 1250–3750 units IV then 150–400 units/h or 3000–5250 units/day SC div. Q8-12H				
	VTE prophylaxis in HIT patients	750–1250 units SC Q8-12H				
Fondaparinux	VTE prophylaxis VTE treatment ACS	2.5 mg SC daily 5–10 mg SC daily 2.5 mg SC daily	Factor Xa inhibitor	77% as unchanged drug	Peak activity at 2–3 h	17–21 h (prolonged with renal impairment and in the elderly)

(continued)

Table 3.1 (continued)

Drug	Clinical indication	Dose	Mechanism of action	Renal clearance	Onset of action	Half-life[a]
Low molecular weight heparin Dalteparin (D) Enoxaparin (E) Tinzaparin (T)	VTE prophylaxis	D: 2500–7500 units SC Q24H E: 40 mg SC Q24H or 30 mg SC Q12H T: Orthopedic: 75 anti-Xa units/kg daily, general surgery: 3500 anti-Xa units/kg daily	Factor IIa and Xa inhibitor (higher ratio of Xa activity)	D,E and T: primarily renal elimination	D: 1–2 h E: 3–5 h T: peak in 4–6 h	D: 3–5 h (SC route) E: 4.5–7 h T: 82 min [a]Prolonged in renal impairment
	VTE treatment	D: 100 units/kg SC Q12H **or** 200 units/kg SC Q24H E: 1 mg/kg SC Q12H or 1.5 mg/kg SC Q24H T: 175 units/kg SC daily				
	ACS	D: 120 units/kg (max: 10,000 units) SC Q12H E: 0.75–1 mg/kg SC Q12H				
	Mechanical heart valve bridging	D: 100 units/kg SC Q12H				
Unfractionated heparin	VTE prophylaxis	5000 units SC Q8-12H	Factor thrombin (IIa) inhibitor and to a lesser extent factors IXa, Xa, XIa and XIIa	Minimal renal elimination at therapeutic doses. Renal elimination may play a role at very high doses	IV: immediate SC: 20–30 min	1–2 h
	VTE treatment	IV: bolus then 18 units/kg/h then titrated to target aPTT SC: 333 units/kg then 250 units/kg Q12H				
	Atrial fibrillation	IV infusion to maintain an aPTT equivalent to 0.3–0.7 units/ml anti-Xa activity				
	ACS	Bolus then 12 units/kg/h then titrated to target aPTT				

[a]Half-lives are provided as ranges as it is variable depending on renal function

Abbreviations: *ACS* acute coronary syndrome, *CAD* coronary artery disease, *COX* cyclooxygenase enzyme, *CrCL* creatinine clearance, *GP* glycoprotein, *HIT* heparin induced thrombocytopenia, *PCI* percutaneous coronary intervention, *PVD* peripheral vascular disease, *SC* subcutaneous, *VTE* venous thromboembolism

Perioperative Considerations

The guiding principle in perioperative antithrombotic management is to ensure interruption such that there is minimal drug exposure at the time of surgery and careful reintroduction such that there is negligible risk of bleeding.

There are several different patient and drug characteristics that will dictate the approach to management. Unfortunately, at present time there is a lack of reliable and easily accessible laboratory tests that are able to quantify the exposure of many antithrombotic agents. In addition, antidotes to immediately reverse the effect of all agents in use are not available on the market. In light of this the perioperative administration of these agents in cardiac surgery patients will largely depend on the following:

- Type of agent the patient is on (different pharmacokinetic/pharmacodynamic profiles)
- Renal function of the patient
- Bleeding risk of the surgical procedure
- Patient comorbidities
- Bleeding risk of the patient
- Thromboembolic risk of the patient
- Timing of last thromboembolic event
- Use of neuraxial anesthesia

Preoperative Management: Antiplatelet Agents

Most antiplatelet drugs work by irreversibly binding to platelets so their effects will only completely wear off by the re-generation of new platelets, which can take 7–10 days. Ticagrelor is a reversible platelet inhibitor and a specific reversal agent for it is under development.

The decision to continue or to hold antiplatelet therapy in the perioperative period will be determined both by the severity of the patient's underlying cardiovascular disease, as well as the placement of recent coronary stents.

- Patients undergoing cardiac surgery for coronary artery bypass grafting (CABG) are deemed as having a high risk for developing cardiovascular events in the absence of antiplatelet therapy; therefore, these patients are usually continued on aspirin.
- For patients on dual antiplatelet therapy (DAPT), the usual recommendation is to hold the P2Y12 receptor blocker for 3–7 days leading up to surgery (as outlined in Table 3.2) and to continue aspirin.
- For patients with coronary stents requiring surgery, guidelines recommend deferring surgery by at least 6 weeks in patients with bare

Table 3.2 Interruption of anticoagulants/antithrombotics prior to elective surgery

Drug	Creatinine clearance (mL/min)	Last dose prior to elective surgery:	# of skipped doses prior to surgery (not including day of surgery)
Direct Oral Anticoagulants			
Apixaban (twice daily)	Greater than 50	3 days	4
	30–50	4 days	6
	15–29	5 days	8
	Less than 15	Consider hematology consultation	–
Betrixaban (once daily)	Greater than 30	4 days	3
	Less than 30	Consider hematology consultation	–
Edoxaban (once daily)	Greater than 30	3 days	2
	Less than 30	Consider hematology consultation	–
Rivaroxaban (once daily)	Greater than 30	3 days	2
	Less than 30	4 days	3
Dabigatran (twice daily)	Greater than 50	3 days	4
	30–50	5 days	8
	Less than 30	7 days	12
Vitamin K antagonist			
Warfarin	–	6 days	5
Antiplatelets			
Aspirin (once daily)	–	5–7 days In patients WITHOUT coronary artery, cerebrovascular or peripheral vascular disease	6
		No interruption In patients WITH known coronary artery, cerebrovascular or peripheral vascular disease	0

(continued)

Table 3.2 (continued)

Drug	Creatinine clearance (mL/min)	Last dose prior to elective surgery:	# of skipped doses prior to surgery (not including day of surgery)
Clopidogrel	–	5–6 days[a,b] 2–3 days based on urgency of surgery or other high risk characteristics	5
Prasugrel	–	7–8 days[a,b]	7
Ticagrelor	–	5–6 days[a,b] 2–3 days based on urgency of surgery or other high risk characteristics	10
Abciximab IV	–	24–48 h	–
Eptifibatide	–	Stop infusion 3–4 h prior to surgery	–
Parenteral anticoagulants			
Danaparoid	Greater than or equal to 30	5 days	4
	Less than 30	Consider hematology consultation	
Fondaparinux	Greater than or equal to 30	4–5 days	4
	Less than 30	Consider hematology consultation	
Low molecular weight heparins (LMWH) Dalteparin Enoxaparin Tinzaparin	Greater than or equal to 30	**Prophylactic doses:** Give in the morning of the day prior to the surgery, hold the day of surgery **Treatment doses:** 24 h prior to surgery give HALF of the total daily dose. If patient receiving twice daily dosing give only on morning prior to surgery, hold evening dose	–
	Less than 30	Consultation with hematology service recommended	
Unfractionated heparin			
Unfractionated heparin Prophylactic doses	–	Hold on the morning of surgery	–
Therapeutic dosing		Heparin subcutaneous: 24 h prior to surgery, give HALF the total daily dose—given in the AM and hold evening dose	
IV infusion as per nomogram		Discontinue IV heparin infusion on call to OR	
Argatroban	–	Discontinue 4 h prior to procedure—prolonged in patients with hepatic insufficiency	–

These recommendations are applicable for patients in whom it is safe to wait the suggested time off the listed antithrombotic agents. The goal is to ensure the patient has less than 10% drug exposure at the time of surgery

[a]High risk characteristics can include: severe left main coronary stenosis, high risk 3 vessel disease, recent bare metal stents or drug-eluting stents. Consider consultation with the patient's cardiologist

[b]In general it may be acceptable to undergo urgent cardiac surgery with 72 h off ticagrelor or clopidogrel, or even less (24–48 h) if the urgency warrants. For emergency patients the benefits of operating on antiplatelet agents may outweigh risk of bleeding

Adapted from [1, 2]

metal stents and for 3–6 months in patients with drug-eluting stents. This is to ensure adequate time for stent endothelialization and to reduce the mortality risk from stent thrombosis.

- In patients with bare metal stent placement greater than 6 weeks ago or drug-eluting stents more than 6 months ago, the recommendation is to continue aspirin and to temporarily discontinue the thienopyridine at an appropriate interval prior to surgery (Table 3.2).
- If emergent surgery is required, the usual recommendation is to continue DAPT in the perioperative period due to the high risk of stent thrombosis.

Preoperative Management: Anticoagulants

Estimate Thromboembolic Risk

The guidelines of the American College of Chest Physicians stratify patients into the following thrombotic risk categories:

- High risk (greater than 10% risk of thrombotic events per year).
- Moderate risk (5–10% risk of thrombotic events per year).
- Low risk (<5% risk of thrombotic events per year).

Table 3.3 Recommendations for bridging for elective cardiac surgery patients

Risk stratum	Indications for oral anticoagulation therapy			Bridging recommended?
	Mechanical heart valve	Atrial fibrillation	VTE	
High	• Any mechanical mitral or tricuspid valve prosthesis • Any caged-ball or tilting disc aortic valve prosthesis • Recent (within 6 months) stroke or TIA	• CHADS$_2$ score of 5 or 6 • Recent (within 3 months) stroke or TIA • Rheumatic valvular heart disease	• Recent—within 3 month—VTE • Severe thrombophilia (e.g. deficiency of protein C, protein S or antithrombin, antiphospholipid antibodies, or multiple abnormalities)	Yes
Moderate	• Bileaflet mechanical aortic valve prosthesis and one of the following: atrial fibrillation, prior stroke or TIA, hypertension, diabetes, CHF, age > 75 year	• CHADS2 score of 3 or 4	• VTE within the past 3–12 months • Non severe thrombophilic conditions (e.g. heterozygous factor V Leiden or prothrombin gene mutation) • Recurrent VTE • Active cancer (treated within 6 months or palliative)	Not routinely required, especially with moderate risk atrial fibrillation. Decision made on a patient specific basis weighing the risks versus the benefits
Low	• Bileaflet mechanical aortic valve prosthesis without atrial fibrillation and no other risk factors for stroke	• CHADS2 score of 0–2 (assuming no prior stroke or TIA)	• Single VTE occurred >12 months ago and no other risk factors	No

Adapted from [1]

A higher thromboembolic risk makes it imperative to both shorten the duration off anticoagulation as well as consider bridging anticoagulation where applicable (see Table 3.3). Where possible consider delaying surgery if not medically urgent. Patients with a low thromboembolic risk usually do not require bridging anticoagulation and can be safely managed by temporary cessation of their anticoagulant a few days leading up to surgery.

Atrial Fibrillation

The CHADS2 score is the mostly commonly used tool in clinical practice to estimate thromboembolic risk in patients with atrial fibrillation [3]. The CHADS2-VASc score is better at discriminating risk among patients at the lower risk strata (i.e. patients with a CHADS2 score of 0) as it accounts for additional factors not captured by the former (Table 3.4).

Venous Thromboembolism (VTE)

In individuals with a history of VTE, the risk of developing another thromboembolic event is primarily dependent on how far out from the original episode the patient is. Risk is categorized as follows:

- High risk if event was less than 3 months ago
- Intermediate risk if event was 3–12 months
- Low risk if event was more than 12 months

Table 3.4 CHADS2 score and CHADS2-VASC score

CHADS2 Score	Points	CHADS2-VASC Score	Points
C = Congestive heart failure*	1	**C** = Congestive heart failure*	1
H = Hypertension	1	**H** = Hypertension	1
A = Age	1	**A** = Age 65-74 years = Age ≥ 75 years	1 2
D = Diabetes mellitus	1	**D** = Diabetes mellitus	1
S = Prior Stroke or TIA	2	**S** = Prior stroke or TIA	2
History of heart failure, clinical findings of heart failure or cardiac imaging showing reduction of left ventricular ejection fraction		**VASC** = Vascular Disease History	1
		Female Sex = 1 point	1

* For CHADS2 Score			* For CHADS2 -VASC Score			
Points	Annual Stroke Risk		Points	Annual Stroke Risk	Points	Annual Stroke Risk
1	2.8%		1	1.3%	6	9.8%
2	4.0%		2	2.2%	7	9.6%
3	5.9%		3	3.2%	8	6.7%
4	8.5%		4	4%	9	15.2%
5	12.5%		5	6.7%		
6	18.2%					

Patients with a history of thrombophilia can either be classified as high or intermediate risk category depending on the nature of their particular condition see (Table 3.3).

Prosthetic Heart Valves

Warfarin is the primary long-term oral anticoagulant used to prevent thromboembolic complications in patients with prosthetic valves. The oral direct thrombin inhibitors are contraindicated for use in this patient population due to an increased risk of thromboembolic events and the likelihood of more major bleeding in the early postoperative period.

In patients with mechanical valves, thromboembolic risk is determined by both the position and type of valve as well as if they have experienced a recent event. In general, patients with a mechanical valve in the mitral or tricuspid position are at a higher risk of thrombosis than aortic valves. Certain types of older generation aortic valves, such as caged-ball or tilting disc valves also place patients in the highest risk strata. See Table 3.3 for specific recommendations around bridging anticoagulation.

Estimate Bleeding Risk

Cardiac surgery using cardiopulmonary bypass is categorized as a high bleeding risk procedure—2 day risk of major bleeding is estimated to be 2–4% [4].

Patient risk factors can also contribute to the bleeding risk associated with cardiac surgery. Scoring systems can help to quantify the risk of major bleeding in patients on antithrombotic therapy as well as identify modifiable risk factors that can be intervened upon prior to surgery. A higher bleeding risk score usually mandates a greater need for perioperative anticoagulant cessation.

The HAS-BLED score (Table 3.5) or a similar bleeding scoring system can be used to determine the patient's risk of bleeding. It is important to note that currently no bleeding scoring system has been validated for perioperative use.

Table 3.5 HAS-BLED scoring system

HAS-BLED score	Points
H = Hypertension (SBP > 160 mmHg)	1
A = Abnormal renal (dialysis, transplant or SCr > 200 μmol/L) or liver function (cirrhosis or bili >2 × ULN with AST/ALT/alk phos >3 × ULN (1 point each)	1 or 2
S = Stroke	1
B = Bleeding history (e.g. anemia, bleeding diathesis)	1
L = Labile INRs (frequent or unstable INRs)	1
E = Elderly (>65 years)	1
D = Drugs (concomitant antiplatelet or anticoagulants) or alcohol use (1 point each)	1 or 2
A score of ≥ 3 indicates patient is at a high risk of a bleeding event	Maximum = 9

Agents that can inhibit platelet function are generally held prior to cardiac surgery to minimize risk of bleeding. Examples include: non-steroidal anti-inflammatory drugs (NSAIDs) and supplements/herbal products that have anticoagulant or antiplatelet properties

Determine Timing of Antithrombotic Interruption

Table 3.2 outlines suggested timing for interrupting these agents prior to elective surgery. This is primarily dependent on the elimination half-life of the particular drug and the patient's renal function, especially for those agents that are extensively cleared through the kidney.

Determine Whether Bridging Anticoagulation Is Required

Bridging anticoagulation usually involves using a shorter-acting anticoagulant—in most cases a LMWH—for a short pre-defined period of time immediately preceding surgery while the maintenance anticoagulant is held. The intent of bridging is to shorten the timeframe a patient at a high thromboembolic risk has antithrombotic interruption, thereby reducing the risk of a perioperative thrombotic event [3]. Table 3.3 can be used as a general guide to stratify a patient into one of three risk categories to ultimately establish if bridging therapy is required.

Management of Perioperative Bleeding Due to Antithrombotic Therapy

Despite preoperative cessation of antiplatelets and anticoagulants, patients can still present to the operating room with inadequate optimization, or they may require urgent/emergency surgery. This can lead to challenges intraoperatively for hemostasis management. The mainstay of therapy is the use of blood components or derivatives; however, some anticoagulants may also allow for targeted therapy.

Transfusion of plasma or related products is reasonable in patients bleeding due to coagulation factor deficiencies, and is established in massive transfusion protocols. In those with specific factor deficiencies, it may be safer to administer fractionated products when available rather than expose the patient to the allogenic complications associated with plasma. For urgent warfarin reversal, it is recommended to use prothrombin complex concentrate (PCC) as it contains concentrated factors II, IX, X, and in some formulations, factor VII. In the event that PCC is unavailable and severe bleeding is present, then plasma transfusion may be considered. Prophylactic administration of plasma has not been found to result in reduced blood loss or transfusion requirements.

Many patients are currently on oral direct thrombin and factor Xa inhibitors for stroke prevention in atrial fibrillation and treatment of venous thromboembolisms (VTEs). The latest CHEST guidelines recommend dabigatran, rivaroxaban, apixaban, or edoxaban over vitamin K antagonist therapy in patients with VTEs and no cancer. However, in contrast to warfarin, these non-vitamin K oral anticoagulants (NOACs) remain largely without an effective reversal agent. Currently, only idarucizumab is available for reversal of dabigatran, a direct thrombin inhibitor. This monoclonal antibody fragment binds dabigatran with high affinity and specificity. In patients receiving dabigatran with uncontrolled bleeding or requiring urgent surgery, a multicenter, prospective, single-cohort study demonstrated the effectiveness and safety of idarucizumab 5 g. Recurrence of elevated clotting time was observed in 23% of patients between 12 and 24 h, and was associated with bleeding in two% of patients, suggesting redistribution of extravascular dabigatran and need for additional dosing.

Reversal agents for factor Xa inhibitors are under various stages of development. Andexanet alfa is approved for patients treated with rivaroxaban and apixaban, when reversal of anticoagulation is needed due to life-threatening or uncontrolled bleeding. Andexanet alfa is a recombinant mimic of factor Xa with no intrinsic activity and binds to apixaban, rivaroxaban, and edoxaban, and was found to decrease anti-factor Xa activity. Current data suggest that andexanet alfa may also inhibit the anti-factor Xa activity of betrixaban as well. Ciraparantag is being developed as a universal anticoagulant reversal agent for Xa inhibitors, direct thrombin inhibitors, and unfractionated and low molecular weight heparin. While ciraparantag interferes with prothrombin time and anti-factor Xa assays, it was able to return whole blood clotting time to baseline within 30 min in healthy patients given edoxaban.

Factor XIII is necessary for the cross-linking and stabilization of fibrin. Increased bleeding is observed with activity levels <60% in surgical patients, and is decreased by 30–50% after cardiopulmonary bypass. However, in a recent phase two, large multi-center randomized controlled trial, replenishment of factor XIII levels after cardiopulmonary bypass did not reduce transfusion rates in moderate-risk cardiac surgery.

Recombinant Factor VIIa is used in patients with hemophilia, inhibitory antibodies, and congenital factor VII deficiency. It has been studied in clinical trials with conflicting results on transfusion requirements in bleeding cardiac surgical patients. Simpson et. al reference to Cochrane review found that in surgical patients without hemophilia, factor VIIa reduced transfusions and blood loss, but there was a trend towards increased thromboembolic events [5]. Current guidelines suggest that the use of factor VIIa can be considered if bleeding is refractory to conventional hemostatic therapy [6].

An intraoperative algorithm for the management of bleeding patients with antithrombotic agents is available as Fig. 3.1.

Reliable laboratory tests to quantify the exposure of antithrombotic agents are currently not widely available. Table 3.6 is a rough guide to

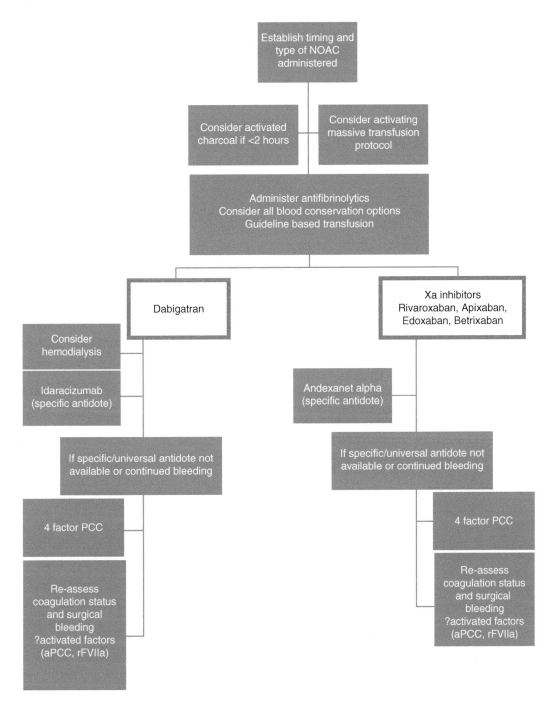

Fig. 3.1 Intraoperative algorithm for management of bleeding patient with antithrombotic agent. Abbreviations: *PCC* prothrombin complex concentrate, *aPCC* activated PCC, *rFVIIa* recombinant factor VIIa

Table 3.6 Interpretation of coagulation tests in patients on oral anticoagulants [2]

Drug	Lab Test					
	Prothrombin time (PT)/International normalized ratio (INR)	Activated partial thromboplastin time (aPTT)	Thrombin clotting time (TCT)	Anti-factor Xa level	Dilute thrombin time	Ecarin clotting time (ECT)
Apixaban	↑ minimal effect	↑ dose dependent effect	No effect	↑↑[a]	No effect	No effect
Dabigatran	↑	↑↑ non-linear increase	↑↑↑	No effect	↑↑[a]	↑↑
Edoxaban	↑ minimal effect	↑ dose dependent effect	No effect	↑↑[a]	No effect	No effect
Rivaroxaban	↑	↑ dose dependent effect	No effect	↑↑[a]	No effect	No effect
Warfarin	↑[a] dose dependent increase	↑ non-linear increase	Not routinely recommended for monitoring effect			

[a]Preferred test
Adapted from [7]

interpretation of what laboratory markers can be used as surrogate.

Postoperative Management

Whether or not to resume antithrombotic therapy is largely determined by the bleeding risk of the patient post-cardiac surgery. Antiplatelet therapy and venous thromboembolism prophylaxis can be resumed within 12–24 hours after surgery provided that adequate hemostasis has been achieved. Since warfarin can take several days to establish its full therapeutic effect, it is usually resumed 12–24 h postoperatively anticipating it to provide a therapeutic effect in 3–5 days.

Factors that may delay antithrombotic initiation include:

- Major bleeding intraoperatively.
- Indication for reoperation.
- High chest tube output.
- Severe thrombocytopenia.
- Imminent requirement of further invasive procedures—e.g. permanent pacemaker insertion, pleural drains, pericardial effusion drainage.
- Anticipated delay in removal of epicardial pacer wires or other devices—e.g. intra-aortic balloon pump.

If the patient is at a high thromboembolic risk and hemostasis has not been achieved, mechanical venous thromboembolism prophylaxis should be considered.

In patients requiring bridging anticoagulation with therapeutic doses of LMWH or intravenous heparin post-cardiac surgery, anticoagulation therapy may not be re-initiated for 24–48 h from the time of surgery, weighing the risk of major bleeding—such as pericardial collections requiring intervention—against the benefits of preventing a thromboembolic event.

In patients who are on DOACs preoperatively for a non-valvular heart valve indication, resumption postoperatively is generally delayed by at least 48 h after cardiac surgery. This is to balance the rapid onset of full anticoagulation effects of such drugs, and the bleeding and thrombosis risks.

Table 3.7 outlines the recommended antithrombotic agents in patients undergoing cardiac surgery for valvular heart disease. Only patients with the highest risk of a thromboembolic complication are bridged in the immediate postoperative phase, primarily patients with mechanical mitral valves. For the remaining vast majority of patients requiring anticoagulation with a vitamin K antagonist, warfarin is started postoperatively with the knowledge that the full anticoagulant effect of the drug will take at least 3–5 days. This window of time allows

Table 3.7 Anticoagulation in postoperative patients following valvular heart surgery

Valve position	Increased thrombotic risk?[a]	Antiplatelet	Anticoagulation[b]	Bridging required?	Warfarin INR target
Tissue/bioprosthetic valves					
Aortic	No	Aspirin 75–100 mg daily for all types of valves, started postoperative Day 1	Usually not recommended. Can be considered for patients with low bleeding risk for 3–6 months	No	2.5 (2.0–3.0)
Aortic	Yes			No	2.5 (2.0–3.0)
Mitral replacement/repair	–		Recommended for patients with low risk of bleeding for 3–6 months	No	2.5 (2.0–3.0)
Mechanical valves					
Aortic	No	Aspirin 75–100 mg daily for all types of valves, started postoperative Day 1	Warfarin started on postoperative Day 1. If in ICU setting and/or potential for invasive procedure anticoagulation with a LMWH or IV heparin may be warranted in lieu of warfarin	No	2.5 (2.0–3.0)
Aortic	Yes			Yes, usually starting postoperative Day 1 or 2 depending on risk versus benefit	3.0 (2.5–3.5)
Mitral	–				
Mitral					

[a]Increased thrombotic risk includes one or more of the following: Atrial fibrillation, previous thromboembolism, left ventricular dysfunction, hypercoagulable states or older generation mechanical AVR (e.g. ball-in-cage) or more than one mechanical valve
[b]Anticoagulant therapy with oral direct thrombin inhibitors (DOACs) should not be used in patients with mechanical valves
Adapted from [8–10]

for closer monitoring for bleeding complications and facilitates the safe implementation of procedures, such as removal of epicardial pacer wires.

References

1. Douketis J, Spyropoulos A, Spencer F, Mayr M, Jaffer A, Eckman M, et al. Perioperative management of antithrombotic therapy. Chest. 2012;141(2):e326S–50S.
2. Spyropoulos A, Douketis J. How I treat anticoagulated patients undergoing an elective procedure or surgery. Blood. 2012;120(15):2954–62.
3. Baron T, Kamath P, McBane R. Management of antithrombotic therapy in patients undergoing invasive procedures. N Engl J Med. 2013;368(22):2113–24.
4. Leitch J, van Vlymen J. Managing the perioperative patient on direct oral anticoagulants. Can J Anaesth. 2017;64(6):656–72.
5. Simpson E, Lin Y, Stanworth S, Birchall J, Doree C, Hyde C. Recombinant factor VIIa for the prevention and treatment of bleeding in patients without haemophilia. Cochrane Database Syst Rev. 2012;14(3):CD005011. https://doi.org/10.1002/14651858.CD005011.pub4.
6. 2011 update to the Society of Thoracic Surgeons and the Society of Cardiovascular Anesthesiologists blood conservation clinical practice guidelines. Ann Thorac Surg. 2011 Mar;91(3):944–82. https://doi.org/10.1016/j.athoracsur.2010.11.078
7. Dale B, Chan N, Eikelboom J. Laboratory measurement of the direct oral anticoagulants. Br J Haematol. 2015;172(3):315–36.
8. Nishimura R, Otto C, Bonow R, Carabello B, Erwin J, Guyton R, et al. 2014 AHA/ACC guideline for the management of patients with valvular heart disease: executive summary. J Am Coll Cardiol. 2014;63(22):2438–88.
9. Nishimura R, Otto C, Bonow R, Carabello B, Erwin J, Fleisher L, et al. 2017 AHA/ACC focused update of the 2014 AHA/ACC guideline for the management of patients with valvular heart disease. J Am Coll Cardiol. 2017;70(2):252–89.
10. Dubois V, Dincq A, Douxfils J, Ickx B, Samama C, Dogné J, et al. Perioperative management of patients on direct oral anticoagulants. Thromb J. 2017;15(1):15.

CHADS2 Score

Gage B. Selecting patients with atrial fibrillation for anticoagulation: stroke risk stratification in patients taking aspirin. Circulation. 2004;110(16):2287–92.

CHEST 2012 Guidelines

Guyatt G, Akl E, Crowther M, Gutterman D, Schuünemann H. Executive summary. Chest. 2012;141(2):7S–47S.

CHADS2-VASC SCORE

Lip G, Nieuwlaat R, Pisters R, Lane D, Crijns H. Refining clinical risk stratification for predicting stroke and thromboembolism in atrial fibrillation using a novel risk factor-based approach. Chest. 2010;137(2):263–72.

Thrombosis Canada

Clinical Guides. Thrombosis Canada [Internet]. Thrombosiscanada.ca. 2017 [cited 12 September 2017]. Available from: http://thrombosiscanada.ca/clinicalguides/#

Fast-Track Cardiac Anesthesia and Early Tracheal Extubation

4

Janet Martin and Davy C. H. Cheng

Main Messages

1. Fast-track management with the goal of early extubation and discharge is now a routine standard of cardiac surgery care. All patients should be considered eligible for fast-track cardiac care and extubation, until proven otherwise.

2. Fast-track care refers to a full program across the continuum of care, involving 'fast-track' anesthesia with balanced anesthesia using reduced doses of opioids (sufentanil, fentanyl) or short-acting opioids (remifentanil) along with short-acting anesthetics and hypnotics (inhaled or intravenous anesthetics, benzodiazepines), usually with the goal of extubation within 1–6 h postoperatively.

3. Fast-track cardiac anesthesia is just one component of care which itself does not guarantee reduced length of stay and reduced complications without other supporting components of care; this starts with appropriate preoperative planning and patient optimization,

This chapter is an updated version of Martin J, Cheng D. "Fast-track cardiac anesthesia and early extubation," in Taggart D and Puskas J (eds.) Coronary Artery Bypass Grafting, Oxford University Press (forthcoming 2020) 3,793w, by permission of Oxford University Press.

J. Martin (✉)
Department of Anesthesia and Perioperative Medicine, Schulich School of Medicine and Dentistry, Western University, London, ON, Canada

Department of Epidemiology and Biostatistics, Schulich School of Medicine and Dentistry, Western University, London, ON, Canada

Centre for Medical Evidence, Decision Integrity and Clinical Impact (MEDICI), Schulich School of Medicine and Dentistry, Western University, London, ON, Canada

WHO Collaborating Centre for Global Surgery, Anesthesia and Perioperative Care, Schulich School of Medicine and Dentistry, Western University, London, ON, Canada
e-mail: jmarti83@uwo.ca

D. C. H. Cheng
Department of Anesthesia and Perioperative Medicine, Schulich School of Medicine and Dentistry, Western University, London, ON, Canada

Centre for Medical Evidence, Decision Integrity and Clinical Impact (MEDICI), Schulich School of Medicine and Dentistry, Western University, London, ON, Canada

WHO Collaborating Centre for Global Surgery, Anesthesia and Perioperative Care, Schulich School of Medicine and Dentistry, Western University, London, ON, Canada

© Springer Nature Switzerland AG 2021
D. C. H. Cheng et al. (eds.), *Evidence-Based Practice in Perioperative Cardiac Anesthesia and Surgery*, https://doi.org/10.1007/978-3-030-47887-2_4

through to fast-track cardiac anesthesia, mildly hypothermic or normothermic surgical technique, and subsequent postoperative protocols for monitoring, extubation, and discharge based on patient milestones.

4. A multimodal approach to managing sedation and analgesia postoperatively is also an integral component of fast-track cardiac care. Devoted postoperative cardiac recovery units allow protocols and patient flow to be maximized in order to achieve efficiencies that are more difficult to coordinate in a generalized intensive care unit.

Rationale for Fast-Track Cardiac Anesthesia

'Fast-track' cardiac anesthesia and recovery is the term given to a multi-component intervention during cardiac surgery and postoperatively, with the ultimate goal of early extubation (within 1–6 h) in order to reduce mechanical ventilation duration, length of stay in the ICU, postoperative recovery and overall resource utilization. Key components of fast-track cardiac care include balanced anesthesia (low-dose opioids together with inhaled or intravenous anesthetics) and a goal-directed extubation protocol in the recovery unit.

While it is often assumed that 'fast-tracking' cardiac surgical patients would be primarily dependent on anesthetic technique, in reality, a focus on anesthesia is not enough. Fast-track cardiac recovery also requires a coordinated, multi-component approach across the full spectrum of intraoperative and postoperative care pathways in order to successfully achieve reduced time to extubation and ICU length of stay without increasing the risk of patient adverse events such as hemodynamic instability, respiratory distress, reintubation, and readmission.

In the 1970s and 1980s, cardiac surgery was conducted under deep hypothermia and high-dose opioids which required prolonged intubation times, often exceeding 24 h. Throughout the 1990s, in response to the economic pressures of increased demand for cardiac surgery that outpaced available ICU capacity, Westaby and colleagues showed that the use of a dedicated cardiac recovery area outside an ICU setting provided improved efficiency of care with faster times to extubation, low rates of reintubation or unplanned ICU admission, and improved overall resource utilization [1, 2].

Evidence for Fast-Track Cardiac Anesthesia

This paradigm shift and fast-track cardiac recovery care was consolidated when randomized trials by Cheng and colleagues showed that a strategy of balanced anesthesia with low-dose opioids and inhaled anesthesia together with an early weaning protocol significantly reduced time to extubation and hospital length of stay, with favorable clinical and resource-related outcomes, when compared to high-dose opioid-based anesthesia [3]. In addition, ICU costs were reduced by 53%, and cost of hospital stay was decreased by 17% [4]. In a subsequent 1–year follow-up of this study, there was no increased risk of readmission in the fast-track group, and total cost of care was lower in the fast-track group compared with conventional high-dose anesthesia [5].

Throughout the late 1990s and 2000s, further randomized trials of fast-track anesthesia were conducted, which eventually paved the evidence base for universal acceptance of the fast-track recovery model as standard of care [6]. A 2006 meta-analysis of 27 RCTs showed that, while low-dose opioids and normothermia were important, the use of an early extubation protocol was the most important predictor of time to extubation and ICU length of stay [7]. Recently updated meta-analyses of 28–30 RCTs, involving approximately 4000 patients, have confirmed that fast-track cardiac recovery models are safe, and reduce time to extubation and ICU length of stay, but with variable net impact on hospital stay and resource utilization [8]. The lack of consistent impact on hospital stay across RCTs, however, re-emphasizes the fact that reductions in opioid dose and extubation time do not alone guarantee improvements in down-stream efficiencies such as ICU and hospital length of stay. This requires changes to discharge policies, and interdisciplinary alignment toward achieving efficiency of patient flow as a routine component of fast-track cardiac recovery.

Safety and Efficiency in Fast Track Cardiac Anesthesia

Tables 4.1 and 4.2 summarize the expected benefits of the fast-track recovery approach to care in cardiac patients, from meta-analyses of randomized trials focused on trials of fast-track anesthesia primarily involving reduced-dose anesthesia (Table 4.1) and time-based weaning protocols

Table 4.1 Meta-analysis of fast-track anesthesia defined as 'reduced-dose opioid anesthesia' (adapted from Wong et al. [8])

Outcome	Number of studies	OR [95% CI] or RR [95% CI]	I^2 (heterogeneity)
Clinical outcomes			
Death, in hospital	7	OR = 0.58 [0.24, 1.39]	0%
Death, at end of study	8	OR = 0.53 [0.25, 1.12]	0%
Myocardial infarction	8	RR = 0.98 [0.48, 1.99]	6%
Stroke	5	RR = 1.17 [0.36, 3.78]	0%
Renal failure, acute	4	RR = 1.19 [0.33, 4.33]	0%
Bleeding, major	4	RR = 0.48 [0.16, 1.44]	27%
Reintubation	5	RR = 1.77 [0.38, 8.27]	0%
Resource-related outcomes		**Mean difference [95% CI]**	
Time to extubation	14	**−7.4 h [−10.5, −4.3 h]**[a]	99%
ICU length of stay	12	**−3.7 h [−7.0, −0.4 h]**[a]	98%
Hospital length of stay	8	−0.3 days [−1.0, +0.4]	85%

[a]p < 0.05

Table 4.2 Meta-analysis of fast-track anesthesia defined as 'time-based weaning protocol' (adapted from Wong et al. [8])

Outcome	Number of studies	OR [95% CI]	I^2 (heterogeneity)
Clinical outcomes			
Death, in hospital	5	OR = 0.23 [0.05, 1.04]	0%
Death, at end of study	10	OR = 0.80 [0.45, 1.45]	37%
Myocardial infarction	8	RR = 0.59 [0.27, 1.31]	39%
Stroke	11	RR = 0.85 [0.33, 2.16]	0%
Renal failure, acute	9	RR = 1.11 [0.42, 2.91]	0%
Bleeding, major	10	RR = 0.92 [0.53, 1.61]	0%
Reintubation	12	RR = 1.34 [0.74, 2.41]	0%
Resource-related outcomes		**Mean difference [95% CI]**	
Time to extubation	16	**−6.3 h [−8.8, −3.7 h]**[a]	99%
ICU length of stay	13	**−7.2 h [−10.5, −3.9 h]**[a]	94%
Hospital length of stay	8	−0.4 days [−1.0, +0.2]	77%

[a]p < 0.05

Since the accumulation of supporting evidence from randomized trials in the 1990s and 2000s, fast-track cardiac anesthesia and surgical management has become the standard of cardiac surgical care

(Table 4.2). As the evidence base has grown and matured, concerns about inducing complications of myocardial ischemia, hemodynamic instability, respiratory distress, reintubation, and intraoperative awareness have been allayed. Contemporary "real-world" evidence from observational studies has confirmed faster times to extubation, reduced ICU length of stay, and improvements in cost-effectiveness [9]. Since the accumulation of supporting evidence from randomized trials in the 1990s and 2000s, fast-track cardiac anesthesia and surgical management has become the standard of care.

Fast Track Cardiac Anesthesia: Drugs and Techniques

In the current paradigm of universal acceptance of fast-track recovery, balanced anesthesia has become the norm, and it is expected that most cardiac surgical patients will be extubated within 1–6 h. It is also expected that fast-track recovery will be attempted on all patients as routine practice, even in very elderly patients, unless there are good reasons to do otherwise. Very rarely, comorbidities or preoperative conditions may preclude a fast-track weaning protocol from the outset.

General Anesthesia

Most anesthetics in current use have been available for several years, and yet the optimal anesthetic regimen for cardiac surgery continues to be a subject of ongoing research. Few trials have specifically addressed optimal doses of each individual component of balanced anesthesia, though general guidelines for practice have been derived from the convergence of balanced regimens used across clinical trials, which have subsequently been refined during evolving practical experience in the contemporary setting of fast-track cardiac care.

Table 4.3 outlines commonly used components of a balanced anesthesia regimen, derived from existing randomized trials. Well-designed randomized controlled trials have generally failed to convincingly demonstrate that selection of different components within each category across those represented in Table 4.3 makes a meaningful difference in terms of clinical outcomes and recovery time. As a result, the choice between these agents has largely been based on local availability, familiarity, and cost.

Short-Acting Versus Long-Acting Opioids

Meta-analysis of head-to-head comparisons of fentanyl, sufentanil and remifentanil as a component of balanced anesthesia in cardiac surgery suggests that the shorter-acting opioid (remifent-

Table 4.3 Fast-track cardiac anesthesia regimens (adapted from Bainbridge and Cheng [10])

Induction (opioid + hypnotic + muscle relaxant)	Opioid • Fentanyl 5–10 mcg/kg • Sufentanil 1–2 mcg/kg • Remifentanil infusion 0.5–1.0 mcg/kg/min Hypnotic • Propofol 0.5–1.5 mg/kg • Midazolam 0.05–0.1 mg/kg Muscle relaxant • Rocuronium 0.5–1 mg/kg • Vecuronium 1–1.5 mg/kg
Maintenance (opioid + hypnotic)	**Opioids** • Fentanyl 1–5 mcg/kg • Sufentanil 1–1.5 mcg/kg • Remifentanil infusion 0.25–0.5 mcg/kg/min **Hypnotic** • Inhaled anesthetic 0.5–1.0 MAC • Propofol infusion 50–100 mcg/kg/min
Transfer to cardiac recovery area (opioid + hypnotic)	Opioid • Morphine 2–10 mg/kg Hypnotic • Propofol infusion 25–50 mcg/kg/min

Derived from the following: Cheng DC, Newman MF, Duke P, et al. The efficacy and resource utilization of remifentanil and fentanyl in fast-track coronary artery bypass graft surgery: a prospective randomized, double-blinded controlled, multi-center trial. Anaesth Analg 2001;92:1094 [11]; Engoren M, Luther G, Fenn-Buderer N. A comparison of fentanyl, sufentanil, and remifentanil for fast-track cardiac anesthesia. Anesth Analg 2001;93:859 [12]; Mollhoff T, Heregods L, Moerman A, et al. Comparative efficacy and safety of remifentanil and fentanyl in 'fast track' coronary artery bypass graft surgery: a randomized, double-blind study. Br J Anaesth 2001;87:718 [13]; Wong WT, Lai VK, Chee YE, Lee A. Fast-track cardiac care for adult cardiac surgical patients. Cochrane Database Syst Rev. 2016 Sep 12;9:CD003587 [8]; Abbreviations: *MAC* minimum alveolar concentration

anil) may reduce time to extubation and hospital length of stay; though caution is warranted regarding this conclusion as there was significant heterogeneity across the trials in morphine delivered postoperatively and adequacy of follow-up with respect to analgesia and need for reintubation [14]. In RCT comparisons of remifentanil and fentanyl, measurable benefit has not been proven for ultra-short acting narcotics [11].

The challenge with ultra-short-acting opioids such as remifentanil is that additional analgesia is required postoperatively to cover for the rapid offset of effect of remifentanil.

Inhaled Versus Intravenous Anesthetics

Meta-analysis of head-to-head comparisons of inhaled versus intravenous anesthesia as a component of balanced anesthesia during cardiac surgery have suggested that use of inhaled anesthesia reduces ICU stay (−16 h, 95% CI −24 to −7 h), and overall risk of mortality in cardiac surgical patients. However, caution is warranted regarding this conclusion, as the number of studies reporting on ICU length of stay was small, even after combination through systematic review and meta-analysis. Head-to-head comparisons of different inhaled agents (isoflurane, desflurane, and sevoflurane) have not definitively shown important differences for cardiac surgery, and the choice should be determined by local availability and costs [15].

Neuromuscular Blockers/Muscle Relaxants

Since the use of long-acting neuromuscular blocking agents may increase the risk of residual muscle weakness and can delay extubation in the recovery period, the choice of muscle relaxant (and reversal agent) remains a key consideration in fast-track recovery patients. Rocuronium (0.5–1 mg/kg, as a single dose) has been shown to reduce time to extubation when compared with pancuronium (0.1 mg/kg, as a single dose) in randomized trials [16, 17]. For this reason shorter acting neuromuscular blockers (rocuronium, vecuronium) have generally replaced pancuronium for fast-track cardiac surgery.

Regional Anesthesia Supplemental to General Anesthesia

Thoracic epidural analgesia has been proposed for improvement of intraoperative and postoperative pain control in cardiac surgical patients. Recent meta-analyses of RCTs suggest that epidural analgesia for cardiac surgery reduces time to extubation (−2.1 h; 95% CI −2.7 to −1.5 h), ICU stay (−2.4 h; 95% CI −4.2 to −0.52 h), and VAS pain scores (0.8–1.1 point on 10-point VAS), as well as risk of supraventricular arrhythmias and pulmonary complications, though without measurable differences on hospital length of stay [18, 19].

Meta-analyses of RCTs of intrathecal analgesia added to general anesthesia versus general anesthesia alone in cardiac surgery suggested that there was increased risk of respiratory depression in intrathecal analgesia, and no important differences in time to extubation, ICU length of stay, or any other clinically relevant outcomes; although VAS scores were reduced [20, 21].

In clinical practice, regional anesthesia is generally not commonly used because of the risk of bleeding and neurological concerns in cardiac surgical patients who are in anti-platelet treatments and undergoing heparization during surgery.

Criteria for Extubation and Predictors of Failure to Extubation

Table 4.4 outlines the initial parameters for stabilization of cardiac surgical patients after entry to the cardiac recovery unit, and suggested criteria

Table 4.4 Extubation criteria for fast-track cardiac recovery

Initial ventilation parameters	A/C Ventilation with pressure support of 10–12 cm H_2O Tidal Volume 8–10 mL/kg PEEP 5 cm H_2O
Maintain ABGs	pH 7.35–7.45 $PaCO_2$ 35–45 PaO_2 > 90 O_2 sats > 95%
Extubation criteria	Awake and alert ABGs as above Hemodynamically stable No significant ECG abnormalities No active bleeding Temperature > 36 °C Muscle strength (>5 s head lift and strong hand grip)

Abbreviations: *A/C* assisted control, *ABG* arterial blood gas, *PEEP* positive end-expiratory pressure

for extubation. Patients should achieve normo-thermia, hemodynamic stability, and normal blood gases before extubation is considered.

There are a number of patient characteristics that predict higher risk of failure to achieve early extubation postoperatively. Predictors have included increased age, female sex, postoperative use of intra-aortic balloon pump, inotropic, bleeding, and atrial arrhythmia, renal failure, hypertension, prolonged CPB time, base deficit after surgery, prolonged clamp time, and advanced age [22].

Fast-Track Versus Ultra-Fast Track Extubation

The increasing trend in OPCAB surgery challenges our techniques, and compels us to streamline our anesthetic and recovery pathways. In terms of routine OR extubation post OPCAB surgery, current evidence suggests that it is feasible. However, we await further randomized controlled studies to confirm relevant benefits for patients (improved outcomes), practitioners (improved quality of care; improved support in decision-making), and providers (improved cost-effectiveness).

A number of studies have evaluated 'ultra-fast track' extubation (within the operating room) in conventional coronary artery bypass surgery to further reduce the extubation time to less than 1 h. While some centres have adopted such an approach as a uniform goal, the practice has not achieved widespread acceptance since ultra-fast track extubation has not been shown to further reduce resource utilization and improve safety beyond that provided by fast-track extubation in the recovery unit (within 1–6 h postoperatively). In fact, ultra-fast track extubation may increase the risk of delaying operating room time, which is the scarcest resource within the chain of resources required for cardiac surgery. Furthermore, ultra-fast track extubation pre-empts the ability to stabilize patient hemodynamics and initial recovery parameters in the 'golden hour' postoperatively.

However, with the advancements in minimally invasive cardiac surgery, and in particular less invasive catheter-based TAVI, the practice of ultra-fast track is gaining popularity with increasing evidence to support its safety and efficiency. More detail regarding anesthetic management of the ultra-fast track approach in minimally invasive and catheter-based TAVI procedures is presented in Chaps. 5, 7, 27 and 35.

References

1. Westaby S, Pillai R, Parry A, O'Regan D, Giannopoulos N, Grebenik K, et al. Does modern cardiac surgery require conventional intensive care? Eur J Cardiothoracic Surg. 1993;7(6):313–8; discussion 8.
2. Chong JL, Pillai R, Fisher A, Grebenik C, Sinclair M, Westaby S. Cardiac surgery: moving away from intensive care. Br Heart J. 1992;68(4):430–3.
3. Cheng DC, Karski J, Peniston C, Asokumar B, Raveendran G, Carroll J, et al. Morbidity outcome in early versus conventional tracheal extubation after coronary artery bypass grafting: a prospective randomized controlled trial. J Thorac Cardiovasc Surg. 1996;112(3):755–64.
4. Cheng DC, Karski J, Peniston C, Raveendran G, Asokumar B, Carroll J, et al. Early tracheal extubation after coronary artery bypass graft surgery reduces costs and improves resource use. A prospective, randomized, controlled trial. Anesthesiology. 1996;85(6):1300–10.
5. Cheng DC, Wall C, Djaiani G, Peragallo RA, Carroll J, Li C, et al. Randomized assessment of resource use in fast-track cardiac surgery 1-year after hospital discharge. Anesthesiology. 2003;98(3):651–7.
6. Myles PS, Daly DJ, Djaiani G, Lee A, Cheng DC. A systematic review of the safety and effectiveness of fast-track cardiac anesthesia. Anesthesiology. 2003;99(4):982–7.
7. van Mastrigt GA, Maessen JG, Heijmans J, Severens JL, Prins MH. Does fast-track treatment lead to a decrease of intensive care unit and hospital length of stay in coronary artery bypass patients? A meta-regression of randomized clinical trials. Crit Care Med. 2006;34(6):1624–34.
8. Wong WT, Lai VK, Chee YE, Lee A. Fast-track cardiac care for adult cardiac surgical patients. Cochrane Database Syst Rev. 2016;9:Cd003587.
9. Svircevic V, Nierich AP, Moons KG, Bruinsma GJBB, Kalkman CJ, van Dijk D. Fast-track anesthesia and cardiac surgery: a retrospective cohort study of 7989 patients. Anesth Analg. 2009;108(3):727–33.
10. Bainbridge D, Cheng DC. Postoperative cardiac recovery and outcomes. In: Kaplan JA, Reich DL,

Savino JS, editors. Kaplan's cardiac anesthesia: the echo era. St. Louis: Saunders; 2011. p. 1010–24.

11. Cheng DC, Newman MF, Duke P, Wong DT, Finegan B, Howie M, et al. The efficacy and resource utilization of remifentanil and fentanyl in fast-track coronary artery bypass graft surgery: a prospective randomized, double-blinded controlled, multi-center trial. Anesth Analg. 2001;92(5):1094–102.

12. Engoren M, Luther G, Fenn-Buderer N. A comparison of fentanyl, sufentanil, and remifentanil for fast-track cardiac anesthesia. Anesth Analg. 2001;93(4):859–64.

13. Mollhoff T, Herregods L, Moerman A, Blake D, MacAdams C, Demeyere R, et al. Comparative efficacy and safety of remifentanil and fentanyl in 'fast track' coronary artery bypass graft surgery: a randomized, double-blind study. Br J Anaesth. 2001;87(5):718–26.

14. Greco M, Landoni G, Biondi-Zoccai G, Cabrini L, Ruggeri L, Pasculli N, et al. Remifentanil in cardiac surgery: a meta-analysis of randomized controlled trials. J Cardiothorac Vasc Anesth. 2012;26(1):110–6.

15. Zangrillo A, Musu M, Greco T, Di Prima AL, Matteazzi A, Testa V, et al. Additive effect on survival of anaesthetic cardiac protection and remote ischemic preconditioning in cardiac surgery: a Bayesian network meta-analysis of randomized trials. PLoS One. 2015;10(7):e0134264.

16. Murphy GS, Szokol JW, Marymont JH, Avram MJ, Vender JS, Rosengart TK. Impact of shorter-acting neuromuscular blocking agents on fast-track recov-

ery of the cardiac surgical patient. Anesthesiology. 2002;96(3):600–6.

17. Murphy GS, Szokol JW, Marymont JH, Vender JS, Avram MJ, Rosengart TK, et al. Recovery of neuromuscular function after cardiac surgery: pancuronium versus rocuronium. Anesth Analg. 2003;96(5):1301–7, table of contents.

18. Svircevic V, Passier MM, Nierich AP, van Dijk D, Kalkman CJ, van der Heijden GJ. Epidural analgesia for cardiac surgery. Cochrane Database Syst Rev. 2013;6:Cd006715.

19. Landoni G, Isella F, Greco M, Zangrillo A, Royse CF. Benefits and risks of epidural analgesia in cardiac surgery. Br J Anaesth. 2015;115(1):25–32.

20. Liu SS, Block BM, Wu CL. Effects of perioperative central neuraxial analgesia on outcome after coronary artery bypass surgery: a meta-analysis. Anesthesiology. 2004;101(1):153–61.

21. Meylan N, Elia N, Lysakowski C, Tramer MR. Benefit and risk of intrathecal morphine without local anaesthetic in patients undergoing major surgery: meta-analysis of randomized trials. Br J Anaesth. 2009;102(2):156–67.

22. Wong DT, Cheng DC, Kustra R, Tibshirani R, Karski J, Carroll-Munro J, et al. Risk factors of delayed extubation, prolonged length of stay in the intensive care unit, and mortality in patients undergoing coronary artery bypass graft with fast-track cardiac anesthesia: a new cardiac risk score. Anesthesiology. 1999;91(4):936–44.

Anesthetic Management in Robotic Hybrid Coronary Artery Bypass Surgery

Keita Sato and Daniel Bainbridge

Main Messages

1. In addition to standard monitors in cardiac surgery, a method to confirm one lung ventilation (OLV) and defibrillator pads should be applied in robotic hybrid coronary artery bypass surgery (CABG).
2. CO_2 insufflation during robotic-assisted CABG can result in significant hemodynamic depression.
3. Concomitant percutaneous coronary intervention (PCI) requires a loading dose of a $P2Y_{12}$ receptor antagonist before PCI, which may increase the risk of bleeding.
4. A direct thrombin inhibitor, bivalirudin, may be used in hybrid revascularization.
5. Ultra-fast track management is considered in selected patients—maintenance of body temperature is extremely important.
6. Pain control should be well-planned since left mini-thoracotomy for robotic-assisted CABG potentially results in more pain than sternotomy.
7. Urgent conversion to sternotomy or initiation of CPB may be needed and should always be anticipated.

Robotic-assisted hybrid coronary artery bypass surgery (CABG) is a form of minimally invasive coronary revascularization combining robotic-assisted coronary artery bypass grafting without full sternotomy—left internal thoracic artery (LITA)—to left anterior descending artery (LAD) with percutaneous coronary intervention (PCI) to non-LAD lesions. The impetus for adopting this approach include: (1) unsatisfied patency of saphenous vein grafts to non-LAD targets in conventional CABG with as many as 50–60% after 10 years of CABG, indicating the best revascularization is LITA to LAD anastomosis (10 years patency >90%) and potential alternatives to non-LAD lesions by PCI [1]; (2) the need to hasten early recovery after surgery avoiding full sternotomy and the associated complications; (3) patient satisfaction with enhanced cosmetic; and (4) the emergence of new-generation drug eluting stents

K. Sato
Department of Anesthesia and Perioperative Medicine, Schulich School of Medicine and Dentistry, Western University, London, ON, Canada

D. Bainbridge (✉)
Department of Anesthesia and Perioperative Medicine, Schulich School of Medicine and Dentistry, Western University, London, ON, Canada

London Health Sciences Centre, University Hospital, London, ON, Canada
e-mail: Daniel.Bainbridge@lhsc.on.ca

© Springer Nature Switzerland AG 2021
D. C. H. Cheng et al. (eds.), *Evidence-Based Practice in Perioperative Cardiac Anesthesia and Surgery*, https://doi.org/10.1007/978-3-030-47887-2_5

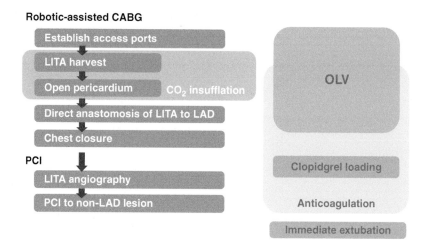

Fig. 5.1 Flow of robotic hybrid CABG

to reduce intra-stent restenosis and to avoid late stent thrombosis.

Hybrid coronary revascularization may offer similar outcomes as conventional CABG, but have reductions in the proportion of patients who require blood transfusion and shorter hospital stays [2]. Although the integrated procedure of robotic-assisted CABG and PCI can be performed as a staged procedure, integrated coronary revascularization in a single operative sequence is feasible and safe in selected patients [3]. The typical flow of robotic hybrid CABG is shown in Fig. 5.1.

Here, anesthetic considerations for robotic-assisted CABG followed by PCI immediate after surgery in a hybrid suite in a single operative setting will be discussed. These include the preoperative and intraoperative managements of robotic-assisted CABG and subsequent PCI, and postoperative ultra-fast track pathway (see also Chap. 36 *Robotic Coronary Artery Revascularization Surgery*).

What Is 'Robotic-Assisted CABG'?

Robotic-assisted CABG is coronary revascularization targeting LAD/diagonal lesion with LITA graft, and performed with the following sequences [3]; first, the LITA is dissected from the anterior thoracic wall and harvested using the da Vinci surgical system (Intuitive Surgical; Sunnyvale, CA) with three ports at the left intercostal spaces—the endoscope port, fifth intercostal space; the other two ports, third and seventh

intercostal space—CO_2 insufflation is required to have good surgical exposure of the internal mammary artery (IMA) during harvesting. Second, the pericardium is opened and the LAD identified, and the site of thoracotomy for surgical anastomosis located. Finally, the endoscope port is extended to create a small left anterior thoracotomy to provide direct vision of the anastomosis site of LAD, and LITA which is manually anastomosed to the LAD with the support of a stabilization device on the beating heart. Total endoscopic anastomosis may be performed but frequently require the use of special anastomotic devices, with mini-thoracotomy and direct anastomosis being the more frequent approach.

The Addition of PCI to Robotic-Assisted CABG as a Single Operative Setting: Does It Change Anything? The addition of PCI with concomitant angiography provides patients with complete revascularization at one time and enables the evaluation of the LITA to LAD anastomosis quality and patency, but the procedure time is prolonged by 1–2 h depending on the complexity of the PCI procedure. Also, special considerations should be taken for anticoagulation strategy during both robotic CABG and PCI, and antiplatelet therapy before PCI, in order to prevent acute stent thrombosis, balancing the risk of surgical bleeding. Alternatively, the PCI may be completed in the catheterization suite after the surgical procedure either with the patient awake or still under GA—a two staged procedure—although this requires the transport of an anesthetized patient and therefore is not routinely done. The disadvantage of this approach is it exposes the patient to potential complications of incomplete revascularization prior to PCI, and does not confirm the quality and patency of the LITA-LAD graft within the operating room.

Preoperative Assessment of Robotic Hybrid CABG

Preoperative Assessment and Plan

The evaluation of patients undergoing robotic hybrid CABG should include the assessment of cardiac function and comorbidities. Robotic-assisted CABG requires one lung ventilation (OLV), therefore respiratory problems such as smoking, asthma, COPD and intestinal lung diseases must be evaluated. In addition, OLV requires a double-lumen tube (DLT), large single lumen tube—usually at least a size 8 tube—or a uninvent tube—which has a large outside diameter—therefore careful attention must also be paid to the airway and ease of intubation.

Robotic hybrid CABG is typically performed in a hybrid operating room (OR), where an operation theatre is combined with fluoroscopy equipment. The robotic system is also placed in the same OR, so the position and traffic line of these systems and anesthetic equipment including ventilator and transesophageal echocardiography (TEE) machine need to be well-planned. An example of the OR arrangement is shown in Fig. 5.2.

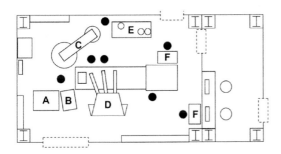

Fig. 5.2 Example of operating room setup . **A** Anesthetic Machine. **B** Echocardiography machine. **C** Fluroscopy Machine. **D** Surgical Robot. **E** Cardiopulmonary Bypass Machine. **F** Imaging viewers

Eligibility for Ultra-Fast Track Management

Robotic hybrid CABG is a procedure without cardiopulmonary bypass (CPB) and is aimed to minimize patient hospitalization and to enhance early recovery. Thus, an ultra-fast track pathway with immediate extubation in the operation room (OR) followed by direct or early transition to the general ward is feasible [4]. The eligibility for immediate extubation must be evaluated precisely before surgery. The benefit of immediate extubation with ultra-fast track pathway in cardiac surgery has not been completely established, but the main advantage appears to be the decreased cost related with shorter ICU stay. Contraindications for ultra-fast track pathway are:

- Difficult intubation
- Severe lung disease
- Severely reduced left ventricular systolic function
- Significant inotropic support
- IABP
- End-stage renal dysfunction
- Morbid obesity
- Emergent surgery/redo surgery

Ultra-fast track management includes preoperative assessment for eligibility, intraoperative anesthetic management focusing on extubation in the OR, and postoperative management including postoperative pain control.

Intraoperative Management

Monitors and Equipment

Intraoperative monitoring for robotic hybrid surgery includes standard monitoring for general anesthesia—ECG, SpO2, non-invasive blood pressure, nasal/esophageal temperature—radial arterial pressure line, central venous line and transeophageal echocardiography. Right radial artery pressure line is preferred to the left side, the right semi-lateral position (30°) with lowered left arm and left shoulder retraction during

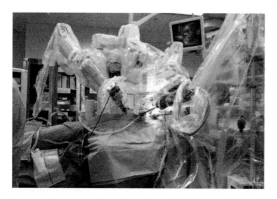

Fig. 5.3 Monitors and equipment

robotic-assisted CABG may compromise the waveform of a left radial pressure line (Fig. 5.3).

A pulmonary artery catheter is rarely needed, but may be useful in a patient with low cardiac function, or with known pulmonary hypertension, in which exacerbations of pulmonary hypertension may warrant abandoning a minimally invasive approach. Defibrillator pads should be placed before the patient is positioned and draped since access to the heart is limited in robotic-assisted CABG. In all cases, nearly the whole the body is prepped and draped, so patients are prone to lose body heat. Maintenance of body temperature is extremely important, especially in elderly patients; otherwise immediate extubation is not feasible. Air warming blankets—whole body and/or upper body—and fluid warmers are beneficial for keeping the patient normothermic.

One Lung Ventilation

OLV is required to achieve surgical visualization during LITA harvest by the robotic system and direct anastomosis of LITA to LAD. Either a double lumen tube or a single lumen tube with a bronchial blocker placed in the left main stem can be applied. Univent tubes may also be considered but it is more difficult to place the blocker as there is no fiber optic scope to guide the blocker, and so the process is predominantly trial and error. Considering the influence of gravity on the distribution of pulmonary perfusion between dependent and non-dependent lungs, semi-lateral

position during robotic-assisted CABG may not be as ideal as the lateral decubitus position for OLV. However, oxygenation of the semi-lateral position has been reported to be similar as lateral position [5], and rarely is robotic CABG complicated by significant hypoxemia during OLV in robotic-assisted CABG unless severe lung disease is present. More common is a failure to appropriately separate the two lungs. Inappropriate lung separation may lead to difficulty in dissecting the LITA, which can result in the surgeons using higher CO_2 insufflation pressures—typically pressures should not exceed 10 mmHg—in the left thoracic cavity followed by hemodynamic compromise. Thus, confirmation of the right placement of double lumen tube or bronchial blocker by bronchoscopy is essential. Other potential methods to confirm lung separation include using the TEE to examine pulmonary vein flow involving both the right and left lung, or the use of surface ultrasound to look for lung sliding.

Anesthetics for Induction and Maintenance for Robotic Hybrid CABG

Balanced anesthesia with either volatile agents or propofol, and low to moderate dose opioid is preferred in ultra-fast track or fast track anesthesia. High dose narcotics or paralyzing agents are not used because of the risk of failed extubation after surgery.

Unlike conventional CABG, the prevention of postoperative nausea and vomiting (PONV) is taken into consideration during cardiac anesthesia in ultra-fast track management. When the estimated risk for PONV is intermediate or high, the following antiemetic doses for the prevention of PONV should be considered either as a single dose or in combination: at induction, dexamethasone 4–5 mg IV, dimenhydrinate 1 mg/kg IV; end of surgery, ondansetron 4 mg IV [6]. 5-HT_3 receptor antagonists have the risk of QTc prolongation, thus they are contraindicated if the patient has a history of torsade de pointes or preexisting QTc prolongation.

Hemodynamic Depression in Robotic-Assisted CABG and Its Management

Hemodynamic fluctuation can often occur during LITA harvest since right OLV with intrathoracic CO_2 insufflation is applied in this phase. CO_2 insufflation pressure is typically below 10 mmHg, but likely contributes more to hemodynamic instability than OLV [7]. Central venous pressure and pulmonary artery pressure are significantly increased, and mediastinal shift, reduced venous return and direct compression of the right heart can be the result of intrathoracic CO_2 insufflation [8]. Regional wall motion abnormalities (RWMA) in both of left and right ventricle are frequently observed by TEE, but the clinical importance of this observation is unclear since these typically resolve after revascularization [8] and may be the result of the physical effects of CO_2 insufflation on the heart. Hemodynamic compromise due to high intrathoracic pressure can be attenuated by volume administration, and vasopressors such as phenylephrine or norepinephrine which can be titrated to maintain blood pressure and coronary perfusion pressure during LITA harvest.

After the completion of LITA harvest using a robotic system, CO_2 insufflation is discontinued and the anastomosis of the LITA to LAD is performed with a stabilizer device through a left mini-thoracotomy. Transient LAD occlusion followed by shunt insertion at the anastomosis site may cause small ST change in the ECG, but usually do not lead to significant depression nor need intervention. Hemodynamic instability in the anastomosis phase is minimal [9], thus less frequently requires vasopressor support.

Conversion to Sternotomy

Since robotic-assisted CABG is minimally invasive it has limited access to the heart, therefore conversion to median sternotomy during the procedure may be required either urgently or non-urgently. The conversion rate is reported to be 3–6%, with the most common reasons for conversion including: technically difficult anastomosis; LITA graft problem; ventricular fibrillation and cardiac arrest; right ventricular injury; and equipment failure [3, 10]. Of these, urgent conversion may be relatively rare, but ventricular fibrillation has been constantly described in the literatures; therefore, defibrillator pads have to be placed. Even when the decision to perform a sternotomy is made, there may be difficulties in establishing CPB with sternotomy in patients prepared for robotic-assisted CABG. First, the robotic system needs to be moved away. Second, the patient is in 30-degree right semi-lateral position with a roll placed beneath the left back of the patient—which is not an ideal situation for surgeons to perform sternotomy—and the roll may need to be removed. In addition, there is not enough time to carefully dissect the cannulation site for CPB in the case of urgent conversion. These can predispose the patient to further complications. Anticipating the above mentioned difficulties, the strategy for urgent conversion and communication among the team is crucial. The marking for sternotomy at the sternum is recommended and CPB should be primed and on standby in the OR.

Communication Among the Team

Because hybrid revascularization is a unique procedure combining minimally invasive surgical CABG with PCI, the communication among the team including surgeons, cardiologists, anesthesiologists, nurses, perfusionists, and intensivists is important. During the LITA harvest of robotic-assisted CABG, the main operator sits in the console of the robotic system separated from the actual surgical site. Therefore, sharing of information regarding the hemodynamic changes and the CO_2 insufflation pressure is critical. Although this procedure is performed without CPB, the availability of perfusionists and the primed pump must be confirmed before surgery in preparation for emergency sternotomy.

Anticoagulation and Antiplatelet Therapy

Anticoagulation in patients undergoing off pump CABG is an area of controversy. Some surgeons prefer a low target activated clotting time (ACT) of 250–300 s with 100–200 U/kg heparin while others choose ACT's above 480 s with a dose of roughly 300 U/kg heparin. Meanwhile, an ACT of 300–350 s is recommended in patients undergoing PCI without intravenous glycoprotein inhibitor to prevent thrombus formation at the site of arterial injury, on the coronary guide wire, and in the catheters used for PCI. This target is based on tradition and experience rather than clear evidence [11]. Since hybrid revascularization is a procedure that combines off pump CABG with PCI, an ACT higher than 300 is a reasonable target throughout the procedure. It should be repeated every 30–45 min. Clear communication between cardiac surgeon, perfusionist and anesthesiologist needs to be maintained as the ability to successfully initiate CPB is strongly dependent on the ACT. A plan about the target ACT and plan to increase the ACT to a CPB target needs to be discussed prior to starting the procedure. Protamine may be used to reverse heparin after the completion of PCI.

In patients undergoing PCI, loading doses of oral $P2Y_{12}$ receptor antagonist before the procedure is recommended in order to reduce the rate of major adverse cardiac events after PCI including acute stent thrombosis or myocardial infarction [11], as in hybrid revascularization. In robotic hybrid CABG, loading dose of clopidogrel 600 mg may be provided through a gastric tube after the completion of the robotic-assisted CABG, but before PCI. The loading dose of clopidogrel is ideally given after fluoroscopic confirmation of a patent LITA anastomosis to the LAD. Clopidogrel needs to be crushed before administration via a gastric tube. An orogastric tube may be preferable to a nasogastric tube in order to avoid epistaxis.

Not surprisingly, heparinization followed by loading dose of clopidogrel poses a potentially increased risk for surgical bleeding. In addition, PCI trials have suggested that heparin use alone is inferior to the use of heparin plus IIb/IIIa antagonists. Therefore, the use of other anticoagulants has been explored. Bivalirudin was shown to be non-inferior to heparin plus a IIb/IIIa inhibitor when both were used in combination with clopidogrel. Bivalirudin is a direct thrombin inhibitor, and the binding of bivalirudin to thrombin is reversible and slowly cleaved by thrombin itself, which may contribute to reduced bleeding risk [12]. Bivalirudin has an immediate onset of action, a half-life of 25 min, and is mainly cleared by proteolytic cleavage and hepatic metabolism. Severe renal insufficiency is considered a contraindication to bivalirudin. The use of bivalirudin has been associated with reduced bleeding compared with unfractionated heparin plus a GP IIb/IIIa inhibitor in PCI [11]. Anticoagulation of bivalirudin during hybrid revascularization followed by loading dose of clopidogrel before PCI is reported to be feasible and safe [3]. The proposed dose of bivalirudin in hybrid revascularization is the same as PCI, which is 0.75 kg/mg bolus IV followed by continuous infusion of 1.75 mg/kg/h [3, 11]. The effect of bivalirudin can be monitored by the ACT and maintained for more than 300 s, but kaolin-ACT should be applied rather than Actalyke-ACT which results in consistently lower ACT measures [13]. Bivalirudin is usually started before the clips are placed at the distal end of the LITA, and is discontinued once the PCI is completed. As no reversal agent exists for bivalirudin, its reversal is dependent on its short elimination half-life.

Postoperative Pain Control

While postoperative pain control is surgery postoperative consideration, the strategy to mitigate postoperative pain should be planned before the procedure starts. Robotic-assisted CABG provides shorter hospital stay and earlier recovery from surgery than conventional CABG with sternotomy. However, this unfortunately does not mean less pain after surgery. Rather, anterolateral thoracotomy can result in much more pain than sternotomy. Superior pain control is the key to enhance early mobilization and avoid pulmonary complication, which maximize the merits of minimally invasive hybrid revascularization. The management of postoperative pain for cardiac surgery can include opioids, nonsteroidal anti-inflammatory drugs (NSAIDs), acetaminophen, and regional analgesia such as intrathecal morphine, epidural analgesia, thoracic paravertebral block, intercostal nerve block, intrapleural analgesia, and intra local infiltration (see also Chap. 29 in Part III, *Regional anesthesia techniques and management in cardiothoracic surgery*). In patients undergoing robotic hybrid CABG where anticoagulation and loading dose of $P2Y_{12}$ receptor antagonist are needed, neuraxial techniques—intrathecal morphine and epidural analgesia—should be avoided [14]. Likewise, the current American Society of Regional Anesthesia (ASRA) guidelines recommend that deep plexus/peripheral techniques such as paravertebral block should be treated in the same way as neuraxial block, thus paravertebral block may be contraindicated in this cohort. Patient controlled analgesia with intravenous opioids with multimodal methods may provide the best analgesic options.

Immediate Extubation in the OR

At the end of the operation, the safety and feasibility of extubation should be judged by standard extubation criteria. Body temperature, hemodynamic stability, pain control and absence of bleeding are especially important.

Postoperative Management

Postoperative care for patients undergoing robotic hybrid CABG is similar to conventional CABG or off pump CABG, which include the management of airway/ventilation, hemoglobin level, bleeding, electrolyte, glucose, and pain control. In the case of re-exploration for bleeding, full sternotomy may be needed. To prevent acute stent thrombosis, aspirin 81 mg should be given after the operation (e.g. 6 h after surgery) followed by dual antiplatelet therapy of aspirin

81 mg and clopidogrel 75 mg once daily as recommended by the current guidelines [11].

Evidence-Based Best Practice Management

Double Lumen Tube Versus Bronchial Blocker for OLV in Robotic-Assisted CABG

Lehmann et al. reported that either double lumen tube or bronchial blocker provided satisfactory lung separation for harvesting LITA in robotic-assisted CABG in a prospective randomized study [15]. In thoracic surgery, most studies has reported that double lumen tube had similar lung collapse quality, shorter time to achieve OLV, and less need for repositioning [16–19] although more laryngoscope attempts to intubate and additional time for tube exchange at the end of surgery may be needed if immediate extubation is not chosen [20]. Another study found that bronchial blockers gave better lung collapse with shorter time to lung collapse [21]. Overall, the choice of double lumen tube for OLV appears to be equivocal if there is no concern for difficult intubation and immediate extubation is planned.

Choice of Anesthetics for Immediate Extubation in the OR in Cardiac Surgery

There is no study in which the comparison of any anesthetics was performed for immediate extubation in robotic-assisted CABG. Any combinations of sevoflurane/isoflurane/desflurane/propofol and fentanyl/sufentanil/remifentanil with or without epidural analgesia have been reported to be feasible for ultra-fast track anesthesia [22–26]. Remifentanil may provide more stable hemodynamics in cardiac surgery than fentanyl and sufentanil [27, 28] although the concerns of postoperative hyperalgesia followed by chronic pain exist when higher doses of remifentanil (>0.1 mcg/kg/min) are used [29, 30]. Hemmerling et al. described that sevoflurane had shorter extubation time than isoflurane (10 ± 5 min vs. 18 ± 4 min) in patients undergoing off-pump CABG with ultra-fast track anesthesia in a prospective randomized trial [31]. Thus, the feasibility of immediate extubation after cardiac surgery does not depend on the types of anesthesia.

Heparin Versus Bivalirudin for Anticoagulation in Robotic Hybrid CABG

There is no study which compares bivalirudin with heparin in hybrid revascularization. In PCI, bivalirudin has been compared with heparin as an anticoagulation therapy. However, the interpretation of these studies are complicated because many studies were conducted: (1) before the routine use of radial-artery access; (2) before the introduction of potent $P2Y_{12}$ inhibitors; or (3) using heparin with glycoprotein IIb/IIIa inhibitor as the control instead of the monotherapy of heparin compared with bivalirudin [32]. In patients undergoing PCI, some studies have shown the risk of bleeding associated with bivalirudin therapy is lower than that associated with heparin therapy [33, 34], whereas others have demonstrated no significant differences [32, 35]. The use of bivalirudin for robotic hybrid CABG should be judged by each institution's policy with expert cardiologists.

References

1. Hillis LD, Smith PK, Anderson JL, Bittl JA, Bridges CR, Byrne JG, et al. 2011 ACCF/AHA guideline for coronary artery bypass graft surgery. A report of the American College of Cardiology Foundation/ American Heart Association task force on practice guidelines. Developed in collaboration with the American Association for Thoracic Surgery, Society of Cardiovascular Anesthesiologists, and Society of Thoracic Surgeons. J Am Coll Cardiol. 2011;58(24):e123–210.
2. Sardar P, Kundu A, Bischoff M, Chatterjee S, Owan T, Nairooz R, et al. Hybrid coronary revascularization versus coronary artery bypass grafting in patients with multivessel coronary artery disease: a meta-analysis. Catheter Cardiovasc Interv. 2017;10:S20–1.
3. Kiaii B, McClure RS, Stewart P, Rayman R, Swinamer SA, Suematsu Y, et al. Simultaneous integrated coronary artery revascularization with long-term angiographic follow-up. J Thorac Cardiovasc Surg. 2008;136(3):702–8.
4. Tarola CL, Al-Amodi HA, Balasubramanian S, Fox SA, Harle CC, Iglesias I, et al. Ultrafast track robotic-assisted minimally invasive coronary artery surgical revascularization. Innovations (Philadelphia, Pa). 2017;12(5):346–50.
5. Watanabe S, Noguchi E, Yamada S, Hamada N, Kano T. Sequential changes of arterial oxygen tension in the supine position during one-lung ventilation. Anesth Analg. 2000;90(1):28–34.
6. Gan TJ, Diemunsch P, Habib AS, Kovac A, Kranke P, Meyer TA, et al. Consensus guidelines for the management of postoperative nausea and vomiting. Anesth Analg. 2014;118(1):85–113.
7. Brock H, Rieger R, Gabriel C, Polz W, Moosbauer W, Necek S. Haemodynamic changes during thoracoscopic surgery the effects of one-lung ventilation compared with carbon dioxide insufflation. Anaesthesia. 2000;55(1):10–6.
8. Mierdl S, Byhahn C, Lischke V, Aybek T, Wimmer-Greinecker G, Dogan S, et al. Segmental myocardial wall motion during minimally invasive coronary artery bypass grafting using open and endoscopic surgical techniques. Anesth Analg. 2005;100(2):306–14.
9. Nierich AP, Diephuis J, Jansen EW, Borst C, Knape JT. Heart displacement during off-pump CABG: how well is it tolerated? Ann Thorac Surg. 2000;70(2):466–72.
10. Daniel WT, Puskas JD, Baio KT, Liberman HA, Devireddy C, Finn A, et al. Lessons learned from robotic-assisted coronary artery bypass surgery: risk factors for conversion to median sternotomy. Innovations (Philadelphia, Pa). 2012;7(5):323–7.
11. Levine GN, Bates ER, Blankenship JC, Bailey SR, Bittl JA, Cerceck B, et al. 2011 ACCF/AHA/SCAI guideline for percutaneous coronary intervention. A report of the American College of Cardiology Foundation/American Heart Association task force on practice guidelines and the Society for Cardiovascular Angiography and Interventions. J Am Coll Cardiol. 2011;58(24):e44–122.
12. Lee CJ, Ansell JE. Direct thrombin inhibitors. Br J Clin Pharmacol. 2011;72(4):581–92.
13. Jones PM, Bainbridge D, Dobkowski W, Harle CC, Murkin JM, Fernandes PS, et al. Comparison of MAX-ACT and K-ACT values when using bivalirudin anticoagulation during minimally invasive hybrid off-pump coronary artery bypass graft surgery. J Cardiothorac Vasc Anesth. 2011;25(3):415–8.
14. Horlocker TT, Wedel DJ, Rowlingson JC, Enneking FK, Kopp SL, Benzon HT, et al. Regional anesthesia in the patient receiving antithrombotic or thrombolytic therapy: American Society of Regional Anesthesia and Pain Medicine evidence-based guidelines (third edition). Reg Anesth Pain Med. 2010;35(1):64–101.

15. Lehmann A, Zeitler C, Lang J, Isgro F, Kiessling AH, Boldt J. A comparison of the Arndt endobronchial blocker with a double lumen tube in robotic cardiac surgery. Anasthesiol Intensivmed Notfallmed Schmerzther. 2004;39(6):353–9.

16. Campos JH, Reasoner DK, Moyers JR. Comparison of a modified double-lumen endotracheal tube with a single-lumen tube with enclosed bronchial blocker. Anesth Analg. 1996;83(6):1268–72.

17. Bauer C, Winter C, Hentz JG, Ducrocq X, Steib A, Dupeyron JP. Bronchial blocker compared to double-lumen tube for one-lung ventilation during thoracoscopy. Acta Anaesthesiol Scand. 2001;45(2):250–4.

18. Campos JH, Kernstine KH. A comparison of a left-sided Broncho-Cath with the torque control blocker univent and the wire-guided blocker. Anesth Analg. 2003;96(1):283–9, table of contents.

19. Narayanaswamy M, McRae K, Slinger P, Dugas G, Kanellakos GW, Roscoe A, et al. Choosing a lung isolation device for thoracic surgery: a randomized trial of three bronchial blockers versus double-lumen tubes. Anesth Analg. 2009;108(4):1097–101.

20. Grocott HP, Darrow TR, Whiteheart DL, Glower DD, Smith MS. Lung isolation during port-access cardiac surgery: double-lumen endotracheal tube versus single-lumen endotracheal tube with a bronchial blocker. J Cardiothorac Vasc Anesth. 2003;17(6):725–7.

21. Bussieres JS, Somma J, Del Castillo JL, Lemieux J, Conti M, Ugalde PA, et al. Bronchial blocker versus left double-lumen endotracheal tube in video-assisted thoracoscopic surgery: a randomized-controlled trial examining time and quality of lung deflation. Can J Anaesth. 2016;63(7):818–27.

22. Djaiani GN, Ali M, Heinrich L, Bruce J, Carroll J, Karski J, et al. Ultra-fast-track anesthetic technique facilitates operating room extubation in patients undergoing off-pump coronary revascularization surgery. J Cardiothorac Vasc Anesth. 2001;15(2):152–7.

23. Straka Z, Brucek P, Vanek T, Votava J, Widimsky P. Routine immediate extubation for off-pump coronary artery bypass grafting without thoracic epidural analgesia. Ann Thorac Surg. 2002;74(5):1544–7.

24. Hemmerling TM, Le N, Olivier JF, Choiniere JL, Basile F, Prieto I. Immediate extubation after aortic valve surgery using high thoracic epidural analgesia or opioid-based analgesia. J Cardiothorac Vasc Anesth. 2005;19(2):176–81.

25. Horswell JL, Herbert MA, Prince SL, Mack MJ. Routine immediate extubation after off-pump coronary artery bypass surgery: 514 consecutive patients. J Cardiothorac Vasc Anesth. 2005;19(3):282–7.

26. Dorsa AG, Rossi AI, Thierer J, Lupianez B, Vrancic JM, Vaccarino GN, et al. Immediate extubation after off-pump coronary artery bypass graft surgery in 1,196 consecutive patients: feasibility, safety and predictors of when not to attempt it. J Cardiothorac Vasc Anesth. 2011;25(3):431–6.

27. Howie MB, Cheng D, Newman MF, Pierce ET, Hogue C, Hillel Z, et al. A randomized double-blinded multicenter comparison of remifentanil versus fentanyl when combined with isoflurane/propofol for early extubation in coronary artery bypass graft surgery. Anesth Analg. 2001;92(5):1084–93.

28. Mollhoff T, Herregods L, Moerman A, Blake D, MacAdams C, Demeyere R, et al. Comparative efficacy and safety of remifentanil and fentanyl in 'fast track' coronary artery bypass graft surgery: a randomized, double-blind study. Br J Anaesth. 2001;87(5):718–26.

29. van Gulik L, Ahlers SJ, van de Garde EM, Bruins P, van Boven WJ, Tibboel D, et al. Remifentanil during cardiac surgery is associated with chronic thoracic pain 1 yr after sternotomy. Br J Anaesth. 2012;109(4):616–22.

30. Fletcher D, Martinez V. Opioid-induced hyperalgesia in patients after surgery: a systematic review and a meta-analysis. Br J Anaesth. 2014;112(6):991–1004.

31. Hemmerling T, Olivier JF, Le N, Prieto I, Bracco D. Myocardial protection by isoflurane vs. sevoflurane in ultra-fast-track anaesthesia for off-pump aortocoronary bypass grafting. Eur J Anaesthesiol. 2008;25(3):230–6.

32. Erlinge D, Omerovic E, Frobert O, Linder R, Danielewicz M, Hamid M, et al. Bivalirudin versus heparin monotherapy in myocardial infarction. N Engl J Med. 2017;377(12):1132–42.

33. Han Y, Guo J, Zheng Y, Zang H, Su X, Wang Y, et al. Bivalirudin vs heparin with or without tirofiban during primary percutaneous coronary intervention in acute myocardial infarction: the BRIGHT randomized clinical trial. JAMA. 2015;313(13):1336–46.

34. Valgimigli M, Frigoli E, Leonardi S, Rothenbuhler M, Gagnor A, Calabro P, et al. Bivalirudin or unfractionated heparin in acute coronary syndromes. N Engl J Med. 2015;373(11):997–1009.

35. Stone GW, McLaurin BT, Cox DA, Bertrand ME, Lincoff AM, Moses JW, et al. Bivalirudin for patients with acute coronary syndromes. N Engl J Med. 2006;355(21):2203–16.

Anesthetic Management in On-Pump Valvular Heart Surgery

6

Steven Konstadt, Walter Bethune, and Jason Fu

Main Messages
1. Regardless of the specific cardiac valvular lesion, a slow and careful anesthetic induction is important. A strategy which takes into account individualized hemodynamic management goals based on the unique pathophysiology of each patient is key to a successful anesthetic and perioperative course
2. Severe aortic stenosis deserves particularly careful attention as it is the valvular lesion to have been most clearly associated with sudden death, and increased perioperative morbidity and mortality
3. Appropriate vigilance must extend beyond the OR into the postoperative period where issues such as hypoxia, dysrhythmias, decreased cardiac output, and fluid shifts often require careful consideration and aggressive management.
4. PA catheter data must be carefully interpreted in the perioperative setting in order to avoid overtreatment and interventions such as fluid or inotrope administration, which may be unnecessary or even harmful
5. Fast track cardiac anesthesia, facilitating early extubation and shorter length of stay in the ICU postoperatively, has many benefits and appears to be safe

On-pump cardiac valvular surgery, performed since the development of Gibbon's pump oxygenator and cardiopulmonary bypass in 1953, presents several unique challenges. Understanding the etiologies and pathophysiology of stenotic and regurgitant lesions is essential to proper perioperative management of patients undergoing cardiac valve repair or replacement. Pathophysiologic pressure and volume loads imposed on the heart by diseased valves lead initially to structural and functional compensation. Pressure overload—secondary to stenotic valvular disease—typically results in concentric ventricular hypertrophy, in which increased ventricular wall thickness enables the heart to preserve forward flow through a stenotic valve orifice. Volume overload—secondary to regurgitant valvular disease—typically results in eccentric hypertrophy, in which chamber dilation occurs without a proportional increase in wall thickness.

S. Konstadt · W. Bethune (✉) · J. Fu
Department of Anesthesiology, Maimonides Medical Center, Brooklyn, NY, USA

© Springer Nature Switzerland AG 2021
D. C. H. Cheng et al. (eds.), *Evidence-Based Practice in Perioperative Cardiac Anesthesia and Surgery*, https://doi.org/10.1007/978-3-030-47887-2_6

Over time, as compensatory mechanisms are overwhelmed, complications occur. Arrhythmias result from atrial stretch and distortion of conduction tissue. Myocardial ischemia along with subsequent systolic and/or diastolic heart failure results from the increased energy requirements of an enlarged heart. The goals of valvular surgery include not only relief of symptoms but also the reversal or prevention of heart failure.

Perioperative Considerations

A careful history and physical exam as well as a thorough review of the patient's chart, including assessment of any preoperative studies—e.g. ECG, CXR, TTE, TEE, cardiac catheterization, etc.—are important both to confirm the operative diagnosis(es) as well as to formulate an anesthetic plan. Mechanism and severity of valvular dysfunction should be ascertained as well as the degree of physiologic compensation and any pathophysiologic sequelae that have occurred—e.g. systolic and/or diastolic dysfunction, eccentric versus concentric hypertrophy, dysrhythmias, ectopic atrial activity, etc. Patients with valvular disease may report symptoms including fatigue, poor exercise tolerance, orthopnea, chest pain, dizziness or syncope. Patients with endocarditis may present with sepsis and its sequelae, including vasodilatory shock. Signs of heart failure may also be present, including jugular venous distension, peripheral edema and pulmonary rales. Important information to ascertain for common lesions is as follows.

Aortic Stenosis

Aortic stenosis (AS) is the most common cardiac valve lesion. Two % of people aged more than 65 years and 4% of those aged more than 85 have severe AS [1]. The normal aortic valve area is 3–5 cm^2. Valvular AS can be caused by calcification, fibrosis and degeneration of either a normal trileaflet AV or a congenitally bicuspid AV. Rheumatic disease is a less common etiology since the advent of antibiotics. Subvalvular AS

(due to a subaortic membrane, hypertrophic cardiomyopathy) and supravalvular AS caused by a congenital syndrome are less prevalent than true valvular AS. Rate of progression is an average valve-area reduction rate of 0.1 cm^2/year with an associated yearly gradient increase of 10–15 mmHg. Progression may be more rapid in patients with heavily calcified or bicuspid valves, in those greater than 50 years of age, and in patients with ischemic heart disease or renal failure [2]. Symptoms including angina, syncope and congestive heart failure typically develop when AV area is reduced to approximately 1 cm^2 and indicate a life expectancy of less than 3 years [3]. It appears safe however to delay surgery until symptoms develop [4]. Advanced AS results in diastolic dysfunction and, ultimately, ischemic contractile dysfunction. Surgical aortic valve replacement (SAVR) remains the gold standard intervention for improving life expectancy and quality. However, for patients whose operative risk is prohibitive, or where technical limitations to SAVR exist, newer minimally invasive interventions such as transcatheter aortic valve replacement (TAVR) are now considered.

Severe aortic stenosis deserves particular attention because it is the only valvular lesion that has been clearly associated with an increased risk of perioperative myocardial ischemia, myocardial infarction and mortality [5]. Hence, careful anesthetic management is imperative. Perioperative hypotension should be avoided whenever possible and must be treated immediately and aggressively as it may critically compromise coronary perfusion in a concentrically hypertrophied left ventricle, resulting in myocardial ischemia. An infusion of an alpha receptor agonist, such as phenylephrine or norepinephrine, may be started prior to induction of general anesthesia in order to decrease the risk of developing significant hypotension. Should hypotension develop anyway, it should be treated aggressively with bolus doses of vasoconstrictors such as phenylephrine, calcium chloride, ephedrine, or vasopressin. Maintenance of normal sinus rhythm with coordinated atrial contraction is critical to ensuring adequate ventricular filling and stroke volume. Maintenance of adequate preload is important in the setting of the diastolic dysfunction that typically accompanies long-standing concentric hypertrophy due to AS. Finally, tachycardia should be avoided as this both increases myocardial oxygen demand and decreases diastolic filling time, hence increasing the risk of myocardial ischemia.

Low-flow, low-gradient AS exists when the mean aortic valve gradient is less than 30 mmHg, most commonly due to a low ejection fraction, while other echocardiographic indices suggest severe AS. The measured gradient depends on both flow and valve area. In this setting, the response to a dobutamine stress test can help to differentiate pseudo-AS—increased valve area without an increased gradient—from true AS—fixed valve area with increased stroke volume and gradient.

Aortic Regurgitation

Aortic regurgitation (AR) results from inadequate coaptation of the AV leaflets during diastole. The most common etiologies are aortic root dilatation and cusp prolapse secondary to hypertension, ascending aortic dissection, cystic medial necrosis, Marfan syndrome, syphilitic aortitis, ankylosing spondylitis or osteogenesis imperfect [6]. Other causes include deformity and thickening of the leaflets due to rheumatic disease, infective endocarditis or a bicuspid AV. Chronic AR develops slowly over many years, allowing for LV compensation to take place as patients remain asymptomatic. The LV dilates and increases its compliance in response to volume and pressure overload. Eventually decompensation occurs with rising left ventricular end diastolic pressure (LVEDP), decreased systolic function, congestive heart failure, dysrhythmias, subendocardial ischemia and a risk of sudden death. Acute AR is usually very poorly tolerated as the LV is unable to dilate acutely, resulting in volume overload and pulmonary edema.

Key goals of anesthetic management include maintenance of a normal to slightly elevated heart rate to minimize regurgitation, maintenance of adequate preload and augmentation of forward flow with vasodilators. Pacing may be helpful in the setting of conduction abnormalities, which often occur secondary to myocardial stretch in a dilated, eccentrically hypertrophied heart. Finally, intra-aortic counter pulsation is generally contraindicated in the setting of hemodynamically significant AR, as it would worsen it.

Mitral Stenosis

The most common etiology of mitral stenosis (MS) by far is rheumatic disease, characterized by thickening, calcification and fusion of valve leaflets and commissures [6]. The normal mitral valve area is 3.5–5.5 cm^2 with surgery indicated when mitral valve area is <1 cm^2 [7]. MS creates a pressure gradient between the left atrium and left ventricle, preventing normal LV filling and leading to atrial stretch, atrial arrhythmias and pulmonary hypertension with eventual RV dysfunction. This in turn may lead to tricuspid regurgitation, RV failure and decreased cardiac output.

In terms of anesthetic management, avoidance of tachycardia is important as this may compromise diastolic filling time when LV filling is already compromised due to flow restriction through the stenotic mitral valve. It is also important to avoid worsening pulmonary hypertension due to hypoxia, hypercarbia, acidosis, atelectasis or increased sympathetic tone. Acute pulmonary hypertension may result in RV failure, in turn leading to hypotension. Inotropic support for the RV may be useful—e.g. epinephrine, dobutamine, milrinone—as well as agents that lower the pulmonary vascular resistance—e.g. milrinone, prostaglandin E$_1$, inhaled nitric oxide.

Mitral Regurgitation

Mitral regurgitation (MR) etiologies include primary valve disorders such as myxomatous degeneration of the mitral valve leaflets and leaflet perforation due to endocarditis. MR can also occur despite structurally normal MV leaflets;

ischemic—functional—MR is a consequence of papillary muscle dysfunction, annular dilatation or left ventricular dysfunction. Progressive volume loading results in LV and LA dilatation, atrial arrhythmias and, eventually, LV decompensation and systolic dysfunction.

Anesthetic considerations include maintenance of adequate preload and relative reduction of afterload in order to promote forward flow. Sudden increases in systemic blood pressure—due to increased sympathetic tone caused by direct laryngoscopy, endotracheal intubation or a surgical incision, for example—can increase the degree of MR and cause acute pulmonary edema and heart failure. A normal to slightly elevated heart rate is desirable as this decreases ventricular filling time and volume, thus decreasing the amount of regurgitation—where the ventricle is already enlarged and eccentrically hypertrophied due to chronic volume overload in the setting of chronic MR.

Of note, the left ventricular ejection fraction (LVEF), which is calculated by dividing the difference between the LV end-diastolic and end-systolic volumes by the LV end-diastolic volume, can significantly overestimate actual LV systolic function. This is due to the fact that LVEF is a simplified estimate that doesn't take into account the relative percentage of LV ejection that represents effective forward flow across the aortic valve versus regurgitant flow backwards across the mitral valve. Hence, in the preoperative assessment of the patient with MR and the formulation of an anesthetic plan, LVEF should be considered in context with other measures including systemic BP, cardiac output and pulmonary pressures in order to properly assess the degree of LV decompensation that has occurred due to chronic MR [8].

Tricuspid Regurgitation

The most common etiology of tricuspid regurgitation (TR) is functional TR—long-standing left-sided valvular disease resulting in pulmonary vascular congestion followed by pressure/volume overload of the right ventricle and subsequent RV dilatation. TR may also be a primary valvular disease caused by rheumatic disease, infective endocarditis, carcinoid syndrome, Ebstein's anomaly or trauma. Normal tricuspid valve area is 7–9 cm^2.

Other Lesions

Tricuspid stenosis and diseases of the pulmonic valve are less prevalent. These are discussed in the chapter on congenital cardiac disease.

Intraoperative Considerations

Regardless of the specific valvular lesion, slow, careful anesthetic induction with particular attention to hemodynamic goals is important. For stenotic lesions, maintenance of forward flow is generally enhanced by sinus rhythm and relatively lower heart rates. For regurgitant lesions, relatively higher heart rates and lower afterload will minimize backward flow and promote cardiac ejection. These goals remain important throughout the maintenance phase of the anesthetic during the pre-bypass period. In general however, the choice of anesthetic agent is less important than having clear hemodynamic management goals and carefully titrating drug doses with attention to these goals. "Keep them where they live."

Management of patients with mixed/multiple lesions is dictated by the relative severity of each lesion. In general the most severe lesion(s) should determine the optimal management.

For valvular operations involving a traditional sternotomy and cardiopulmonary bypass (CPB), typical intraoperative monitoring includes standard ASA monitors in addition to TEE, an arterial line, central venous access and a pulmonary artery catheter (PAC). On-pump valvular surgery performed through minimally invasive incisions—e.g. anterior thoracotomy, parasternal incision or 'mini-sternotomy'—typically involves increased reliance on TEE to facilitate proper positioning of surgical cannulae and may also require lung isolation to facilitate surgical exposure. For procedures such as TAVR and mitraclip that do not require the use of CPB, many institutions have transitioned to a less invasive approach, foregoing endotracheal intubation, internal jugular venous cannulation and TEE in favor of monitored anesthesia care, femoral venous access and TTE [9].

Initiation of CPB for valvular surgery traditionally involves cannulation of the ascending aorta and right atrium. The aortic cannula is typically placed first so that it can be used to provide fluid resuscitation in the event of hemodynamic instability that may ensue during venous cannulation or other surgical manipulation at this stage of the procedure. To prevent the patient's blood from clotting in the CPB circuit, heparin must be administered—the typical dose is 300 units per kg—prior to commencement of CPB with a goal ACT in most institutions of >400 s. The arterial blood pressure is lowered to approximately 100 mmHg prior to cannulation in order to minimize the risk of an iatrogenic aortic dissection.

Separation from CPB is a particularly important part of the intraoperative surgical course. A number of issues must be attended to in order to facilitate a smooth transition. At many institutions a pre-weaning checklist has been implemented to ensure that all pertinent issues are addressed. Appropriate personnel must be present in the OR, including the attending surgeon and anesthesiologist as well as perfusion and nursing staff. Patients are typically cooled to at least 32 °C during CPB for valvular surgery and must be adequately rewarmed, typically to 36 °C, prior to separation from CPB. Hypothermia predisposes to cardiac dysrhythmias, coagulopathy and issues with wound healing and infection. Anesthetic drugs—including amnestic agents, analgesics, muscle relaxants, etc.—should be re-dosed in order to ensure adequate amnesia, analgesia and immobility during the post-CPB period. The patient's metabolic milieu must be optimized, including correction of abnormalities involving acid/base status, oxygen carrying capacity—e.g. serum Hgb/Hct and PaO2—and serum electrolytes—particularly serum potassium, as both hyper- and hypokalemia predispose to significant dysrhythmias. Optimal functioning of monitors and alarms, which may have been disabled during CPB, must be ensured.

Proper ETT position and normal pulmonary compliance should be verified by bag ventilation prior to initiating mechanical ventilation. The appropriate dose of protamine should be prepared—typically 1 mg of protamine per 100 units of heparin administered—in order to be able to quickly reverse heparin and restore normal coagulation function after cessation of CPB. If the need for blood products is anticipated—e.g. packed red blood cells, platelets, FFP, etc.—these should also be ordered and made available in advance.

Perhaps most importantly, attention must be paid to overall cardiovascular function—including cardiac rate and rhythm, contractility, preload and afterload. If normal sinus rhythm at an appropriate heart rate does not spontaneously occur then establishment of a stable rhythm requires pacing via epicardial leads. Atrial pacing is closest to normal physiology and should be employed whenever possible. In the setting of a conduction block, atrioventricular pacing is an acceptable alternative. Ventricular pacing is a last resort, used only when atrial pacing is not possible, e.g. due to refractory atrial fibrillation. With attention to the CVP, PA diastolic pressure, degree of cardiac filling noted on TEE and direct observation in the surgical field, preload is continuously assessed and optimized. Crystalloids, colloids and/or blood products may be administered as needed in addition to incremental boluses of blood which can be given by the perfusionist via the aortic cannula until it is removed. A regimen of vasoactive infusions including vasopressors—e.g. phenylephrine, norepinephrine or vasopressin—and/or inotropes—e.g. epinephrine, milrinone or dobutamine—is started empirically prior to separation from CPB and then titrated aggressively in the immediate post-CPB period in order to optimize cardiac performance and maintain acceptable hemodynamic parameters. Finally, thorough de-airing of the cardiac chambers is necessary to prevent systemic air embolization after all open cardiac surgical procedures; this process is facilitated by careful TEE examination immediately prior to separation from CPB.

Upon separation from CPB and thereafter, attention must also be paid to the functioning of the valve prosthesis or repaired native valve. Surgical decision-making as to whether to repair a diseased native valve versus replace it with a mechanical or biological prosthesis is individualized depending on many factors including patient age and comorbid illnesses as well as both patient and surgeon preference. Biological prostheses have a relatively more limited lifespan but do not require long-term anticoagulation whereas mechanical valves can last indefinitely but require anticoagulation, with its attendant risks and considerations. TEE evaluation of mechanical valvular prostheses may reveal small closing or "washing" jets at the hinge or coaptation points, which is a normal finding, and must be distinguished from abnormal paravalvular regurgitation at or outside the sewing ring. A high pressure gradient through the prosthesis must also be addressed [10].

Postoperative Considerations

Patients who have had open-heart valve surgery are transported to the intensive care unit (ICU) for close monitoring. The goal of postoperative care for these patients is to maintain perfusion and oxygen delivery to vital organs until the patient is recovered and stable enough to be discharged from the ICU. Some common postoperative issues are bleeding, tamponade, poor heart function, and vasodilation, all of which result in hypotension.

In order to understand how these relate to each other, it is important to first understand Ohm's law $V = IR$, where V is voltage, I is current, and R is resistance. The variables in Ohm's law can be rearranged as $R = V/I$. This is analogous to the equation for systemic vascular resistance,

$$SVR = [(MAP - CVP)/CO] \times 80$$

where SVR is systemic vascular resistance, MAP is mean arterial pressure, CVP is central venous pressure, and CO is cardiac output. If 80, which is a conversion unit, is eliminated, and CVP is

eliminated as well—since CVP is normally much less than MAP—the equation can be restated as

$$MAP = CO \times SVR.$$

CO is stroke volume (SV) times heart rate (HR), and stroke volume is equal to ejection fraction (EF) multiplied by left ventricular end diastolic volume (LVEDV). Knowing this, the equation can be further broken down:

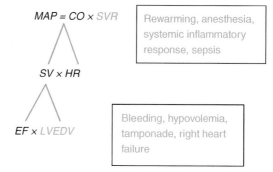

A low MAP on the left side of the equation necessitates one or more low variables on the right side of the equation. Some of the more common causes of postoperative hypotension are listed next to the corresponding variable, and will be discussed in more detail below.

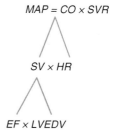

Postoperative bleeding can be divided into surgical or non-surgical bleeding. Surgical bleeding is secondary to surgical trauma, and can occur at vascular anastomoses, prosthetic valve suture lines, cannulation sites, or small blood vessels injured during the procedure. If it does not resolve on its own, it requires mediastinal re-exploration to locate and address the problem. Non-surgical bleeding encompasses all other causes, which include pre-existing coagulopathy due to patient comorbidities or anticoagulants, hypothermia, insufficient heparin reversal with protamine, platelet and clotting factor destruction and fibrinolysis from CPB. Bleeding from hypothermia or insufficient heparin reversal can be treated by warming the patient or giving additional protamine, respectively. Otherwise, the patient may benefit from a transfusion of platelets, fresh frozen plasma, cryoprecipitate, or other procoagulants. Reducing the blood pressure if the patient is hypertensive may also help control the bleeding. Patients with mechanical valves, atrial fibrillation, or history of thromboembolic events are all at increased risk of thromboembolic events, and therefore must be anticoagulated. This must be balanced with the increased risk of bleeding.

Postoperative bleeding is usually evidenced by increased output via chest tubes. However, if there is clot in the tubes or the tubes are not properly positioned, the blood can accumulate in the chest. Continued bleeding can lead to increased intrathoracic pressure and eventually cause cardiac tamponade. Tamponade is classically signified by Beck's triad, which consists of hypotension, distended neck veins and muffled heart sounds. Dyspnea and orthopnea may not be seen in the ventilated patient. Cardiac tamponade results in low SV and CO, which is evidenced by narrow pulse pressure, hypotension and signs of poor perfusion. Other methods of diagnosis include transthoracic or transesophageal echocardiography, which would reveal compressed heart chambers, right atrial or ventricular diastolic collapse, and even LV diastolic collapse. Increased pressure on the heart can cause an equalization of diastolic pressures across the CVP and PA pressures, as well as pulsus paradoxus, which is an exaggerated (>10 mmHg) decrease in systolic blood pressure with inspiration. Under normal physiological conditions a small decrease in blood pressure is observed during inspiration. This is due to the negative intrathoracic pressure during inspiration causing an increase in venous return, which causes the interventricular septum to bow slightly to the left, decreasing LV filling and CO. The negative intrathoracic pressure also causes blood to pool in the lungs, which also decreases LV filling. During cardiac tamponade, because of the equalization

of pressures across the cardiac chambers, this septal bowing is more pronounced, causing an exaggerated drop in cardiac output and blood pressure. In the mechanically ventilated patient, because of increased—instead of decreased—intrathoracic pressure during inspiration, a reverse pulsus paradoxus takes place—the increased intrathoracic pressure squeezes blood out of the pulmonary circulation and improves LV filling, thereby increasing blood pressure. The higher intrathoracic pressure also increases RV afterload and decreases RV preload, which, because of an approximately 2 s pulmonary transit time of blood, translates to less LV filling and lower blood pressure during the following expiration [11].

Another possible cause of decreased CO in patients who have had valve surgery is systolic anterior motion (SAM) of the mitral valve. SAM occurs when the anterior leaflet of the mitral valve obstructs the left ventricular outflow tract (LVOT) during systole, causing severe MR and also decreasing systemic blood flow. This is thought to occur due to the Venturi effect; a reduction in the LVOT cross sectional area increases the flow velocity through it, thereby dragging the anterior leaflet towards the LVOT. Therefore, any factors that reduce LVOT area or bring the mitral valve closer to the LVOT can increase risk of SAM and LVOT obstruction. SAM tends to occur in patients who have had mitral valve annuloplasties for mitral regurgitation; the mitral ring reduces the annular circumference and can decrease the distance between the anterior leaflet and the LVOT. SAM is also seen in patients with concentric LVH who have undergone aortic valve replacements; with the AS fixed, the LV can now contract much more easily and often becomes hyperdynamic, bringing the hypertrophied interventricular septum closer to the mitral annulus and making LVOT obstruction more likely. Medical treatment of SAM involves increasing the size of the LV to make LVOT obstruction less likely; increasing the preload and afterload, and decreasing inotropy all serve this purpose. If medical treatment does not work, surgical intervention may be necessary.

Table 6.1 Risk factors associated with ventricular dysfunction after CPB [12]

Valvular hessart disease requiring repair or replacement
Pre-existing ventricular dysfunction
Long aortic cross clamp or CPB time
Inadequate revascularization after CABG
Residual effects of cardioplegia
Poor myocardial preservation during CPB
Ischemia reperfusion injury

Decreased cardiac function often occurs after open-heart surgery. This is especially true after on-pump valvular surgery, because patients often have pre-existing ventricular dysfunction due to chronic volume or pressure overload from longstanding regurgitant or stenotic lesions, respectively. In addition, aortic cross clamp and CPB have adverse effects on the heart (Table 6.1). Ventricular dysfunction can be diagnosed by echocardiography. It is treated with inotropes, such as epinephrine, milrinone or dobutamine. Non-pharmacological treatment modalities include intra-aortic balloon pump counterpulsation, extracorporeal membrane oxygenation, or a temporary ventricular assist device.

Vasodilation is common after open-heart surgery. It can occur as a result of rewarming, anesthesia, or the systemic inflammatory response associated with CPB, the surgery itself, or sepsis. Aside from using antimicrobials for an infection, vasodilation is treated with vasopressors such as phenylephrine, norepinephrine or vasopressin to cause vasoconstriction and maintain perfusion pressure.

Evidence-Based Best Practice Medicine

Cardiac surgery and cardiac anesthesiology are both constantly evolving specialties. As new technology and techniques are developed, new trials and evidence are produced either supporting or refuting them, in turn changing the way we practice medicine.

Pulmonary Artery Catheters

Pulmonary catheterization has existed since the 1920s, but it was not popularized until Jeremy Swan came up with the idea of flow-directed catheters, after going to the beach with his children and observing a sailboat with a spinnaker move with the wind. With the help of his colleague William Ganz, he constructed a prototype of a long thin flexible catheter with an inflatable balloon at the end, which allowed it to move with blood flow. They conducted successful clinical trials, eventually publishing a case series in 1970, which demonstrated their prototype could be successfully advanced without fluoroscopy, thus heralding the advent of the modern Swan-Ganz catheter, or pulmonary artery catheter (PAC) [13].

Since then, the PAC has evolved into an omnipresent monitor in both the ICU and operating room, especially in patients receiving open-heart surgeries. It provides a multitude of useful information such as CO, mixed venous oxygen saturation, pulmonary artery pressure, and pulmonary capillary wedge pressure, which in turn yields important information about volume status, ventricular function, and tissue perfusion and oxygenation in critically ill patients.

However, despite the PAC's widespread adoption, there has been much controversy surrounding its use as well. Multiple studies have shown no decrease, and even an increase, in morbidity and mortality in patients with PACs [14, 15]. There are several potential reasons. First is the risk of inserting PACs; potential complications range from pulmonary artery thrombosis and rupture to catheter related bloodstream infections and arrhythmias. Secondly, the information gained from a PAC may be inaccurate, and even if it is accurate, can be misinterpreted. Thirdly, if the PAC data is accurate and interpreted correctly, it can lead to overtreatment and interventions such as fluid or inotrope administration, which may be unnecessary and even harmful [16]

In recent years, more advanced modalities such as echocardiography and pulse oximeter waveform analysis have supplemented and in some cases replaced the PAC. However, even amidst controversy, the PAC is still routinely used in the operating room and ICU for open-heart patients, especially those with elevated pulmonary artery pressure due to severe aortic or mitral insufficiency, or intrinsic pulmonary hypertension.

TAVR Versus SAVR

Aortic stenosis is the most common valve disease in North America, and it presents primarily as calcific aortic stenosis in the elderly population [17]. As our population ages, the frequency of calcific aortic stenosis will continue to increase. However, the risk of morbidity and mortality with open SAVR increases with patient age and comorbidities, and often times SAVR is withheld from patients who are considered too high risk. In the last decade and a half however, a new technique called transcatheter aortic valve replacement (TAVR) has emerged, first described by Cribier, in a patient who was refused for SAVR because he was deemed too sick [18]. In this case, femoral venous access and a trans-septal approach was performed, with a bovine pericardial valve mounted on a balloon-expandable stent. Since then, multiple iterations involving different types of vascular access and bioprosthetic aortic valves have evolved. Studies have shown that TAVR significantly reduces the rate of death compared to standard therapy—which includes balloon valvuloplasty—for patients who are not surgical candidates, and that TAVR has similar survival rates as SAVR for patients who are high or intermediate risk surgical candidates [19–21]. TAVR will be discussed in more detail in a later chapter.

Fast Track Cardiac Anesthesia

Since its inception, cardiac anesthesia has evolved from a high-dose opiate and benzodiaz-

epine anesthetic to a relatively lower dose, shorter acting one. Like the anesthetics performed for non-cardiac surgeries, the goal of anesthesia for cardiac surgery has shifted to expediting recovery and decreasing length of stay, without jeopardizing patient safety. There are many benefits of fast track cardiac anesthesia. Earlier extubation results in enhanced patient comfort, improved respiratory mechanics and clearing of secretions, and decreased incidence of ventilator associated pneumonia. A shorter length of stay in the ICU translates to lower health care costs. However, these benefits must be weighed against potential risks of fast tracking; earlier extubation can result in respiratory failure and reintubation, and more aggressive discharge from the ICU before patients are ready can result in readmission. Overall, studies have shown that fast track cardiac anesthesia is not associated with a worsened morbidity or mortality rate [22].

References

1. Carabello BA, Paulus WJ. Aortic stenosis. Lancet. 2009;373:956–66.
2. Lester SJ, Heilbronn B, Gin K, Dodek A, Jue J. The natural history and rate of progression of aortic stenosis. Chest. 1998;113:1109–14.
3. O'Keefe JH Jr, et al. Natural history of candidates for balloon valvuloplasty. Mayo Clin Proc. 1987;62:986.
4. Bono RO, et al. ACC/AHA guidelines for the management of patients with valvular heart disease: executive summary. J Heart Valve Dis. 1998;7:672.
5. Keratin MD, Bountioukos M, Boersma E, et al. Aortic stenosis: an underestimated risk factor for perioperative complications in patients undergoing non cardiac surgery. Am J Med. 2004;116:8–13.
6. Schoen FJ. Cardiac valves and valvular pathology: update on function, disease, repair, and replacement. Cardiovasc Pathol. 2005;14:189–94.
7. Carabello BA. Modern management of mitral stenosis. Circulation. 2005;112:432–7.
8. Rosen SF, Borer JS, Hochteiter C, et al. Natural history of the asymptomatic patient with severe mitral regurgitation secondary to mitral valve prolapse and normal right and left ventricular performance. Am J Cardiol. 1994;74:374.
9. Kasel AM, Shivaraju A, Schneider S, et al. Standardized methodology for transferal transcatheter aortic valve replacement with the Edwards Sapien XT

valve under fluoroscopy guidance. J Invasive Cardiol. 2014;26:451–61.

10. Wernly JA, Crawford MH. Choosing a prosthetic heart valve. Cardio Clin. 1998;16:491.

11. Michard F. Changes in arterial pressure during mechanical ventilation. Anesthesiology. 2005;103:419–28.

12. Kaplan J, Reich D, Savino J. Kaplan's cardiac anesthesia: the echo era. 6th ed. St. Louis: Saunders; 2011. p. 1028.

13. Swan HJ, Ganz W, Forrester J, Marcus H, Diamond G, Chonette D. Catheterization of the heart in man with use of a flow-directed balloon-tipped catheter. N Engl J Med. 1970;283:447–5.

14. Connors AF Jr, Speroff T, Dawson NV, Thomas C, Harrell FE Jr, Wagner D, Desbiens N, Goldman L, Wu AW, Califf RM, Fulkerson WJ Jr, Vidaillet H, Broste S, Bellamy P, Lynn J, Knaus WA. The effectiveness of right heart catheterization in the initial care of critically ill patients. SUPPORT Investigators. JAMA. 1996;276(11):889–97.

15. Sandham JD, Hull RD, Brant RF, Knox L, Pineo GF, Doig CJ, Laporta DP, Viner S, Passerini L, Devitt H, Kirby A, Jacka M, Canadian Critical Care Clinical Trials Group. A randomized, controlled trial of the use of pulmonary-artery catheters in high-risk surgical patients. N Engl J Med. 2003;348(1):5–14.

16. Marik PE. Obituary: pulmonary artery catheter 1970 to 2013. Ann Intensive Care. 2013;3(1):38.

17. Lung B, Baron G, Butchart EG, Delahaye F, GohLke-Barwolf C, Levang OW, et al. A prospective survey of patients with valvular heart disease in Europe: the Euro heart survey on valvular heart disease. Eur Heart J. 2003;24:1231–43.

18. Cribier A, Eltchaninoff H, Bash A, Borenstein N, Tron C, Bauer F, et al. Percutaneous transcatheter implantation of an aortic valve prosthesis for calcific aortic stenosis: first human case description. Circulation. 2002;106(24):3006–8.

19. Leon MB, Smith CR, Mack M, Miller DC, Moses JW, Svensson LG, et al. Transcatheter aortic-valve implantation for aortic stenosis in patients who cannot undergo surgery. N Engl J Med. 2010;363:1597–607.

20. Leon MB, Smith CR, Mack M, et al. Transcatheter versus surgical aortic-valve replacement in high-risk patients. N Engl J Med. 2011;364(23):2187–98.

21. Leon MB, Smith CR, Mack M, et al. Transcatheter or surgical aortic-valve replacement in intermediate-risk patients. N Engl J Med. 2016;374(17):1609–20.

22. Cheng DCH, Karski J, Peniston C, Asokumar B, Raveendran G, Carroll J, Nierenberg H, Roger S, Mickle D, Tong J, Zelovitsky J, David T, Sandler A. Morbidity outcome in early versus conventional tracheal extubation following coronary artery bypass graft (CABG) surgery: a prospective randomized controlled trial. J Thorac Cardiovasc Surg. 1996;112:755–64.

Anesthetic Management for Transcatheter Aortic Valve Implantation (TAVI)

Lachlan F. Miles and Andrew A. Klein

Main Messages

1. Recently published results of multi-centre RCTs suggest widening indications for TAVI beyond aortic valve stenosis in high-risk surgical candidates
2. Best practice guidelines support multidisciplinary decision making regarding referral for TAVI; where anesthesiology support is required, it is preferable that a cardiac anesthesiologist be present
3. Conduct of anesthesia for TAVI varies between centers, with most institutions using a general anesthesia approach until proceduralist comfort is gained, followed by a local anesthetic approach with or without sedation
4. Non-randomized trials suggest that local anesthetic approaches are superior, both with respect to hemodynamic stability and patient centred outcomes such as length of hospital stay; a large,

multicentre RCT is required to confirm these results

5. The development of newer technologies including retrievable valve prostheses promises to decrease procedural trauma, complications and recovery times

On April 16th 2002, Alain Cribier and his collaborators Helene Eltchaninoff and Christophe Tron performed the first, in-human, percutaneous aortic valve replacement at the hôpital Charles-Nicolle in Rouen, France [1]. It was the most momentous leap forward in structural cardiology since percutaneous coronary intervention. Today, transcatheter aortic valve implantation (TAVI) continues to undergo rapid innovation. The results of the PARTNER-II trial suggest transfemoral TAVI is superior to traditional, surgical aortic valve replacement (SAVR) with respect to the primary study end-point of death or disabling stroke (hazard ratio 0.79; 95% CI 0.62–1.0; $p = 0.05$) in intermediate risk patients [2], and upcoming studies aim to assess the role of this technology in low-risk surgical candidates.

For the anesthesiologist, TAVI represents both challenge and opportunity. The challenge arises from providing adequate anesthesia or sedation to a potentially critically unwell patient in an environment remote from the operating room, as

L. F. Miles
Department of Anesthesia, Austin Health, Melbourne, Australia

A. A. Klein (✉)
Department of Anesthesia and Intensive Care, Papworth Hospital, Cambridge, UK
e-mail: andrew.klein@nhs.net

© Springer Nature Switzerland AG 2021
D. C. H. Cheng et al. (eds.), *Evidence-Based Practice in Perioperative Cardiac Anesthesia and Surgery*, https://doi.org/10.1007/978-3-030-47887-2_7

well as a host of peri-procedural considerations unique to TAVI. However, the multidisciplinary approach employed in a number of centres, and which is advocated as best practice [3, 4], provides the opportunity for the anesthesiologist to become an integral member of the group involved in the assessment and selection of patients [5].

This chapter aims to provide an overview of candidate evaluation, the procedure itself and the attendant complications, and the conduct of safe anesthesia and sedation for TAVI.

Multidisciplinary Decision Making

The Heart Valve Team

Expert consensus guidelines have advocated that successful management of patients with aortic valve disease is best achieved through the use of a collaborative, decision making body. This "heart valve team" ideally consists of a structural or interventional cardiologist with direct experience in TAVI, a cardiac surgeon, cardiac anesthesiologist, cardiovascular imaging expert, gerontologist and intensivist [3, 4]. The objective of this multidisciplinary group is to maximise the prognostic benefit of the procedure, and to address patient-centred outcomes such as symptomatology and quality of life. Ultimately, the team must decide which treatment pathway offers the patient the longest life with the fewest symptoms: traditional SAVR, TAVI (with or without prior balloon valvuloplasty to determine responsiveness), or medical management/palliative therapy [3, 4].

Patient Selection and Evaluation

The initial assessment of the patient is focussed on obtaining a thorough understanding of the patient's medical condition, the severity of their valve abnormality, and the extent to which it influences their physical fitness (Table 7.1). This process determines the relative risk of SAVR and

Table 7.1 Preoperative imaging measurements for TAVI

Technique	Area of interest	Specific measurement
Echocardiography	Ventricle	LVEF and dimensions
		Estimated pulmonary artery pressure
		Regional wall motion abnormalities
	Valve	Mean pressure gradient
		Estimated valve area
		Dimensionless pressure/volume index
		Abnormalities of other valves (e.g. mitral)
Computed tomography (CT)	Annulus	Major/minor dimensions
		Area/circumference
	Aortic root	Coronary ostia height
		Aortic calcification
		Aortic root and ascending aortic anatomy
	Coronary arteries	Coronary anatomy
		Concomitant coronary artery disease
	Peripheral vasculature	Femoral vessel calibre, course and atheromatous disease
		Thoracoabdominal aorta calibre, course and atheromatous disease

Computed tomography may be supplemented with conventional angiography where appropriate, and in the case of renal impairment, cardiac MRI

TAVI, and informs the patient and treating team of the best option for ongoing care.

Aortic Stenosis Severity and Symptoms

A thorough history and physical examination is mandatory. Exercise tolerance and the speed of any temporal changes as valve area decreases are particularly relevant, specifically the classical features of aortic stenosis: exertional dyspnoea, chest pain or discomfort and syncope. Echocardiographic measurements such as continuity equation derived valve area and mean pressure gradient should be considered with and against the reported symptomatology, bearing in mind that poor left ventricular function may cause the valve area to be underestimated. In this scenario, metrics which take into account left ventricular outflow tract velocities and can correct for a low cardiac output state—such as dimensionless pressure/velocity indices—assume greater significance.

Major Cardiovascular Comorbidities

Major cardiovascular comorbidities such as previous cardiac surgery or the presence of substantial coronary artery disease are important for procedural selection and stratification of procedural risk. Computer tomographic or fluoroscopic coronary angiography is required, in part due to the high burden of concomitant coronary artery disease seen in this cohort (40–75%) [3]. There is limited evidence at present to suggest what the influence of simultaneous revascularisation at the time of TAVI is on morbidity and mortality.

Previous cardiac surgery or other percutaneous intervention is particularly relevant. Redo sternotomy carries its own, not insubstantial risks, with scarring and fibrosis of the chest cavity resulting in vital structures such as the aorta or right ventricle becoming adherent to the sternum. Similarly, the presence of extensive ascending aorta and arch atheroma or "porcelain aorta" markedly increases the risk of embolic phenomena from aortic cross-clamping. Some "low-risk" surgical candidates may have anatomical factors that increase the risk of sternotomy, such as pectus excavatum or carinatum, or a history of mediastinal irradiation. TAVI may be recommended as lower risk approach in these circumstances.

Major Non-cardiovascular Comorbidities

Other medical comorbidities are used as part of the determination of the prognostic benefit an intervention may offer, as well as the influence any such condition may have on recovery. These include:

- Respiratory—Chronic obstructive airways disease, pulmonary fibrosis or other chronic pathology. Domiciliary oxygen therapy, $FEV_1 < 50\%$ predicted and TLCO <50% predicted are particularly concerning. $FEV_1 < 30\%$ is associated with very poor long-term survival, regardless of which form of intervention is chosen.
- Gastrointestinal—Hepatic cirrhosis with Child-Pugh B or C severity, oesophageal varices, or active intestinal or gastric bleeding with inability to take anti-platelet agents.
- Neurological—Presence of pre-existing cognitive impairment due to dementia or other pathology, movement disorders such as Parkinson's disease.
- Renal—Chronic renal impairment with eGFR <30 ml min^{-1}, or dialysis dependence.
- Musculoskeletal—Joint degeneration or inflammatory arthropathy with specific positional requirements.
- Other—Any active malignancy—particularly metastatic disease—with limited life expectancy.

Risk Assessment

Estimation of risk requires integration of various factors, specifically the results of the cardiac risk estimate score used, frailty testing, major organ system dysfunction and technical considerations that may preclude a particular approach. The cardiac risk estimate score used is region specific; North American guidelines recommend the use of the Society of Thoracic Surgeons scoring system [3], and European guidelines recommend EuroSCORE-2 [4]. It should be noted that neither of these scoring systems performs well in the estimation of TAVI risk, but serve as a starting point by describing hazards of traditional surgical approaches [6]. The current AHA/ACC Guidelines for Management of Patients with Valvular Heart Disease use these factors to stratify candidates for aortic valve intervention into four categories [3]:

1. Low risk—STS predicted mortality <4%, no frailty, no comorbidity and no procedure-specific impediment.
2. Intermediate risk—STS predicted mortality 4–8% with no more than mild frailty or single major organ system compromise not to be improved postoperatively, and minimal procedure specific impediments.
3. High risk—STS predicted mortality >8%, or moderate-severe frailty, no more than two major organ systems compromised that will not be improved postoperatively, or a possible procedure specific impediment.
4. Prohibitive risk—Preoperative risk of mortality/major morbidity >50% at 1 year, or three or more major organ systems compromised that will not be improved postoperatively, or severe frailty, or severe procedure specific impediments.

Imaging Assessment for TAVI

In order to determine the feasibility of TAVI, comprehensive vascular imaging is required. The complex anatomy of the aortic root and valve is best assessed using ECG-gated, multidetector computed tomography to create a three-dimensional data set to delineate the relationships of the aortic root and coronary arteries, the course and tortuosity of the aorta, iliac and femoral arteries, as well as assessing the atherosclerotic burden affecting these vessels. This permits accurate balloon and prosthesis sizing, and minimises vascular complications.

Where the use of iodinated contrast is contraindicated, integration of magnetic resonance imaging and transesophageal echocardiography can be used to provide similar information.

Procedural Considerations for TAVI

Location and Personnel

Considerable inter-institutional variation exists regarding the location and conduct of TAVI. This is reflective of regional preference, and no specific approach is demonstrated to have greater safety relative to other operating environments. Described techniques range from interventional cardiologists alone [7], with no support from other specialities, to a full operating theatre with a cardiac anesthesiologist providing sedation, and cardiac surgeon and clinical perfusionist in the room in the case of major procedural complication [8].

The limiting factor on location has tended to be the availability of permanent fluoroscopy to generate static or dynamic imaging of the femoral vasculature, the aortic root and the thoracoabdominal aorta proper. Practically, this restricts the conduct of the procedure to a dedicated cardiac catheterization laboratory, an angiography suite, or a hybrid operating theatre. The environment chosen frequently reflects the speciality of the primary operator—interventional cardiologist or cardiac surgeon. Additional considerations that determine environment include:

- Adequate space for the housing of equipment and staff. This includes the anesthetic machine and apparatus, and the cardiopulmonary bypass pump if the institution in question operates a "perfusion on standby" model.
- Proximity to operating theatre or intensive care unit in the event of major complication.

Valve Choice

At present, there are two major valve delivery platforms that are FDA approved for TAVI. These are the Medtronic CoreValve® (Medtronic, Fridley, MN) and Edwards SAPIEN® (Edwards

LifeSciences, Irvine, CA) families of valves. The Boston Scientific LOTUS® platform (Boston Scientific, Marlborough, MA) is gaining increasing prominence, but at the time of writing is yet to receive regulatory approval in Europe or North America.

Several factors require consideration when choosing the most appropriate valve platform. These include:

- Institutional preference and training.
- Route of device delivery.
- Aortic annular dimensions and calcification.
- Position of the coronary arteries relative to the valve.
- Degree of annular calcification.

The proceduralist must also consider whether to use a balloon-expandable or self-expandable device. Balloon expandable platforms can be used in a larger number of clinical situations—including transapical approach, high aorto-ventricular angle and dilated ascending aorta—but carry an increased risk of annular rupture in the setting of heavy calcification, and cannot be retrieved once deployed. The newer generation of self-expanding valves can be recaptured and repositioned prior to full deployment, giving additional versatility in the setting of difficult annular anatomy or malposition.

Approach Choice

Comprehensive imaging of the peripheral vasculature prior to the procedure should determine the feasibility of pursuing a transfemoral route.

Transfemoral Approach

The first TAVI procedure was undertaken with venous access and a trans-septal puncture [1], but 80–90% of modern procedures use a retrograde approach via the femoral artery. Over time, there has been a decrease in the size of sheath required for device deployment, from 24Fr down to 14Fr for some of the newer systems, and a reduction in vascular complications. Depending on the device involved, these prostheses can be delivered through a femoral artery as small as 5–6 mm in diameter. Once this sheath is placed, the patient is anticoagulated to an ACT of 250–300 s with unfractionated heparin.

In addition to the sheath through which the device is deployed, an additional 7–8Fr sheath is inserted into the radial or contralateral femoral artery. A venous sheath is placed in the contralateral femoral vein by the proceduralist, or the internal jugular vein by the anesthesiologist to allow passage of a pacing wire. These additional sheaths may be available to the anesthesiologist for central infusion of vasoactive drugs, or invasive pressure monitoring.

Transapical Approach

If there is substantial femoral or aortic occlusive disease, a transapical approach may be used, although advances in transfemoral approaches means that this technique is increasingly rare. It requires a left mini-thoracotomy, and surgical exposure of the apex of the left ventricle. The apex of the ventricle is then punctured, and a guide wire is fed through the left ventricular outflow tract and across the aortic valve. This allows the placement of a deployment sheath and other apparatus into the left ventricle. Following deployment of the valve, the sheath and guide wires are removed, and the apex is closed by the surgeon with a purse-string suture, the placement and tightening of which can be made easier with rapid ventricular pacing. Intercostal, paravertebral or serratus plane blocks may be used to provide intra and postoperative analgesia.

Conduct of Anesthesia for TAVI

The use of general anesthesia, as well as a wide variety of different local anesthesia with variable sedation techniques have been described, each of which carries its own risks and benefits (Table 7.2).

Data reported in 2014 suggested that more than 95% of TAVI in the United Kingdom and the United States was performed under general anesthesia, whilst centres in Germany and Israel performed virtually all transfemoral TAVI under

Table 7.2 Relative benefits and drawbacks for the most commonly used anesthetic techniques for transfemoral TAVI

General anesthesia	Local anaesthetic ± sedation
Benefits	**Benefits**
Definitive airway control	Minimisation of invasive procedures
Enables transesophageal echocardiography	Less hemodynamic instability and lower inotrope requirement
Optimal positioning for valve deployment (i.e. breath holding, etc.)	Shorter length of recovery and hospital stay
Drawbacks	**Drawbacks**
Additive risk of further invasive procedures	Unprotected and remote airway with attendant risk of obstruction
Increased risk of hemodynamic instability and higher inotrope requirement	Unable to use transesophageal echocardiography
Higher risk of malignant arrhythmia on valve deployment	Increased patient distress and discomfort
Prolonged recovery and hospital stay	Higher incidence of pacemaker insertion and paravalvular leak

These should be viewed in the light of a limited evidence base and marked heterogeneity in institutional practice, particularly in the local anesthetic techniques employed

local anesthesia [9, 10]. These demographics have almost certainly changed and, to a large extent, reflect increased maturation of institution-specific TAVI programs: many institutions will begin with a general anesthetic technique to allow the use of transesophageal echocardiography for valve assessment, and allow for additional experience with the technology to be gained. As experience in trans-thoracic echocardiographic and fluoroscopic techniques for post-deployment assessment are gained, practice evolves to a local anesthetic-based approach [8].

It has been observed in multiple non-randomized trials that general anesthesia is associated with a higher rate of certain complications relative to local anesthetic techniques. These include longer total procedural time, increased length of hospital and ICU stay, and an increased incidence of cardiopulmonary complications [11, 12]. Whilst these findings were not replicated in

all studies, it is a consistent finding in the literature that general anesthetic techniques for TAVI are associated with a higher degree of hemodynamic instability [11–15], and in one small, retrospective study, a higher incidence of malignant arrhythmia on valve deployment [8]. This is reflected in narrative and systematic reviews, which note that high-volume centres are able to achieve very satisfactory results with both techniques [9, 12, 16]. However, most non-randomized studies in this area are afflicted by a degree of chronological bias. The only randomised trial in this area showed no difference between general anesthesia or local anesthesia/sedation groups with respect to cerebral desaturation, and found a higher composite incidence of "adverse events" in the sedation group (p < 0.001, fragility index = 19). These were largely defined by airway and respiratory compromise, and included requirement for intra-procedural airway support, desaturation and hypopnea [17]. This trial compared general anesthesia with deep sedation with propofol, and an adequately powered randomized controlled trial using lighter sedation and a responsive patient may yield a different result.

Monitoring

While the precise choice of monitoring modalities is, to a large extent, institute- and technique-dependent, there is a basic standard that should be met for all TAVI cases, regardless of whether or not a general or local anesthetic technique is used. These include:

- 5 electrode electrocardiogram.
- Invasive arterial pressure monitoring—This may utilise a radial or brachial arterial line controlled by the anesthesiologist, or the side arm of an arterial sheath deployed by the proceduralist. The major advantage of the former technique is a dedicated line for monitoring and sampling is made available, although this may be considered an additional procedure with attendant risk of infection and trauma to surrounding structures.

- Invasive central venous pressure monitoring—Again, this may utilise a dedicated internal jugular or subclavian line controlled by the anesthesiologist, or a femoral venous sheath in the surgical field. Some form of central access for the use of potent inotropic or vasoactive agents is considered desirable for any TAVI procedure, particularly in those patients considered high-risk.

Additional monitoring that may be used at the discretion of the treating team include:

- Cerebral and somatic oximetry—useful for determining adequacy of perfusion in the setting of hemodynamic instability.
- Bispectral index or other depth of anesthesia monitor—useful for the titration of anesthetic in the high-risk or hemodynamically unstable patient.

Invasive pulmonary artery pressure monitoring is considered unnecessary in uncomplicated patients. This is because echocardiographic assessment of cardiac output and pulmonary artery systolic pressure through interrogation of the tricuspid regurgitant signal is available at short notice during the procedure. Patients presenting for TAVI frequently have poor left ventricular systolic function and bundle branch block, and the floatation of a pulmonary artery catheter may precipitate complete heart block and hemodynamic collapse.

Venous Access

Despite the evolution of the technology, TAVI remains a highly invasive procedure. Catastrophic bleeding, either from femoral arterial instrumentation, or from perforation of the ventricular wall and resultant tamponade is well recognized. Large bore venous access (at least 16G) is considered mandatory. This may be achieved through a dedicated peripheral cannula, or via a sheath placed in the groin by the proceduralist.

Transvenous Pacing

To facilitate valve deployment, transvenous pacing is deployed to induce a high ventricular rate and minimise cardiac ejection, thus ensuring optimal positioning. This is achieved through a balloon-tipped pacing wire positioned in the right ventricle under fluoroscopic control. This may be introduced through a right internal jugular sheath by the anesthesiologist, or through the femoral vein by the proceduralist. Such a pacing wire can be inserted through a sheath as small as 7Fr, although some centres employ a larger sheath to enable floatation of a pulmonary artery catheter in an emergency.

General Anesthesia

Early TAVI procedures required general anesthesia. This was a reflection of the large calibre sheaths required for device deployment, and the need for transesophageal echocardiography for assessment of valve positioning after deployment. Current practice recommendations from the AHA and EHA suggest that if an anesthesiologist is to be present, they should have specific sub-specialty training in cardiac anesthesia. A general anaesthetic technique is mandatory if a transapical approach is used.

Initially, general anaesthesia techniques utilized neuromuscular blockade with tracheal intubation to provide maximal support for the remote airway in case of procedural complication. Certain proceduralists may require cessation of diaphragmatic movement during valve positioning, which cannot be accomplished with the patient spontaneously ventilating. Some institutions are beginning to perform the procedure using a supraglottic airway device and no neuromuscular blockade.

The standard approach to the patient with severe aortic stenosis applies, with preservation of myocardial perfusion through the use of vasopressors, and use of positive inotropic agents to maintain cardiac output (bearing in mind the limitations of a fixed left ventricular outflow tract obstruction). Sinus rhythm should be maintained, as loss of atrial contraction in the setting of ventricular hypertrophy and uncontrolled ventricular rate can be catastrophic. Many inotropic agents have been associated with atrial dysrhythmia, and balancing defence of cardiac output with preservation of sinus rhythm can be challenging.

Judicious, titrated induction of anesthesia is required, and in the severely impaired left ventricle, ketamine or etomidate may prove useful. Protracted mechanical ventilation is not required if the procedure is successful, and high doses of long-acting opioids, benzodiazepines, or neuromuscular blockade as part of a more traditional cardiac anesthetic are not appropriate, and may impair postoperative recovery. Reasonable analgesia can be achieved through infiltration of local anesthetic into the groin.

Local Anesthesia With or Without Sedation

Evidence based assessment of local anesthetic-based techniques is challenging because of substantial heterogeneity in the literature. A multitude of different approaches have been described, including:

- Deep propofol sedation with oropharyngeal or nasopharyngeal airway support if necessary [17].
- Regional anesthesia with or without low dose remifentanil [8].
- Piritramide, metoclopramide and dimenhydrinate and no anesthesiologist present [7].

Despite this variation, a consistent finding in the limited literature published to date has been the lower incidence of cardiorespiratory complications, increased catheter laboratory efficiency, and shorter hospital stay associated with a local anesthetic technique. However, these approaches have been associated with a higher incidence of permanent pacemaker implantation and prosthetic paravalvular leak [12]. This may reflect malposition on implantation due to patient movement or discomfort during rapid ventricular pac-

ing or breathing artefact. The development of retrievable TAVI platforms will likely reduce the incidence of these complications, as the permanence of balloon-expandable valves prevents re-deployment after initial positioning. A large randomised, controlled trial is required to determine superiority of one anesthetic technique over the other.

Whilst a similar monitoring and vascular access setup may be used in both methods, local anesthetic techniques tend to take a more minimalist approach than general anesthesia (Table 7.3).

The anesthesiologist may only have dedicated access to a single peripheral intravenous cannula for the control of sedation, and utilise the

Table 7.3 Comparison of institution-specific (Royal Papworth Hospital, Cambridge, UK) monitoring and vascular access setups for transfemoral TAVI under general anesthetic or local anesthetic ± sedation

General anesthesia	Local anesthetic ± sedation
Volatile anesthesia with sevoflurane at 1 MAC	Remifentanil infusion at 0–0.1 µg kg^{-1} min^{-1}
5 electrode ECG	5 electrode ECG
Radial arterial cannula for invasive arterial pressure monitoring	Invasive arterial pressure monitoring from femoral sheath ± non-invasive blood pressure monitoring
Internal jugular CVC for sedation administration, inotrope administration and central venous pressure monitoring	Central venous pressure monitoring and inotrope administration from femoral sheath
Dedicated large bore, peripheral, intravenous access for volume administration	Volume administration via femoral sheath
Cerebral ± somatic oximetry monitoring	Dedicated small bore, peripheral intravenous access for sedation administration
Bispectral index	Cerebral ± somatic oximetry monitoring
Transvenous pacing via internal jugular or femoral sheath	Transvenous pacing via internal jugular or femoral sheath
Infiltration of local anaesthetic	Ilioinguinal and fascia iliaca block ± infiltration of local anaesthetic

Tremendous variability in practice exists between institutions, and there is no definitive evidence favouring one technique over another with respect to outcome

side-arm of the sheaths in the procedural field for arterial pressure monitoring, administration of inotropic or vasoactive drugs, and volume resuscitation if required. This requires sterile giving sets to be primed and connected by the proceduralist, but minimises the number of interventions that a patient requires.

Similar to the general anaesthetic approach, post-procedural analgesia is provided through the infiltration of local anesthetic into the groin. Some centres have made use of regional anesthesia as part of this process with a combined fascia iliac and ilioinguinal nerve block, which has previously been described for the commencement of awake cardiopulmonary bypass or ECMO [8].

Conversion to General Anesthesia

Given the frailty of many TAVI candidates, sedation may not provide adequate procedural conditions, and conversion to general anesthesia may be required during the case. A plan should be agreed upon by the proceduralist and the anesthesiologist about how this will be undertaken expeditiously if necessary. The incidence of this varies between series. In the absence of an anesthesiologist, Greif et al. reported a conversion rate of 0.4%, but also noted that deepening of sedation was required in 1.5%, and emergent transfer to the operating theatre for management of complication—and general anesthesia—was required in 4.6% [7]. In those series where an anesthesiologist was present, the rate of conversion to general anesthesia ranges between 0 and 17%, with data sets averaging 6.2% (95% CI 5.3–7.3%) [12]. Common reasons for conversion to general anesthesia include:

- Patient distress or agitation.
- Respiratory failure.
- Management of pericardial tamponade.
- Management of vascular access complications.
- Cardiac arrest.

Valve Deployment

Assuming an absence of other procedural complications (Table 7.4), valve deployment represents the time of greatest physiological trespass during transfemoral TAVI. After positioning of the guide wire across the aortic valve, balloon dilatation of the native valve, with subsequent prosthetic valve deployment is undertaken as a two-stage process.

The prosthesis should be available and preloaded onto to the deployment platform prior to balloon dilatation of the annulus, as this part of the procedure may cause acute, severe aortic regurgitation and hemodynamic compromise. Correct device positioning is essential to mini-

Table 7.4 Reported complications of transfemoral TAVI [18] and ACC/AHA recommendations for immediate management [3]

Category	Complication	Management options
Peripheral vascular	Access site-related complications	Urgent surgical consultation ± repair
Guide wire and balloon related	Ventricular perforation	Administer protamine sulphate in consultation with proceduralist
		Percutaneous pericardial drainage
		Surgical repair (may require emergency sternotomy in catheter laboratory)
	Annular rupture	Administer protamine sulphate in consultation with proceduralist
		Pericardial drainage and cell salvage for autotransfusion
		Surgical repair (may require emergency sternotomy in catheter laboratory)
Prosthetic embolization	Aorta	Recapture or deploy in descending aorta (self-expanding)
		Endovascular retrieval (balloon-expandable)
	Left ventricle	Surgical extraction of prosthesis and AVR

(continued)

Table 7.4 (continued)

Category	Complication	Management options
Prosthetic malposition	Central aortic regurgitation	Reposition prosthetic leaflets with soft guide wire
		Valve-in-valve rescue if severe and intractable
	Paravalvular aortic regurgitation	Recapture and repositioning of prosthesis (self-expanding)
		Valve-in-valve rescue (balloon expandable)
		Percutaneous vascular closure device
		Post-deployment balloon dilatation
		Surgical extraction of prosthesis and AVR
	Coronary occlusion	Recapture and reposition prosthesis (self-expanding)
		Percutaneous coronary intervention
		Coronary artery bypass grafting
Other circulatory compromise	Complete heart block	Transvenous pacing in first instance
		PPM insertion if persistent (at 24–48 h)
	Haemorrhage	Identify site (peripheral vascular vs. central) and obtain surgical control if able
		Administer protamine sulphate in consultation with proceduralist
		Allogeneic blood transfusion or cell salvage
	Haemodynamic collapse	Assess and treat underlying cause
		Inotropic support
		Intra-aortic balloon counterpulsation
		ECMO or cardiopulmonary bypass
Stroke	Embolic	Mechanical clot retrieval (thrombolysis contraindicated)
	Haemorrhagic	Conservative management

mise complications such as prosthetic paravalvular leak, complete heart block and coronary occlusion. This requires temporary cessation of cardiac output through rapid ventricular pacing for approximately 20 s at a time. For the patient under general anesthesia, a rate of 180 beats/min is usually adequate. However, for patients with preserved left ventricular function, particularly those under local anesthesia, a rate of 210 beats/min may be required [8]. Conditions are considered adequate for device deployment when systolic blood pressure is less than 70 mmHg, and pulse pressure is less than 20 mmHg [3].

The sudden cessation of cardiac output manifests in varying ways. In the patient receiving local anesthetic and sedation, reported features range from transient dizziness to loss of consciousness. From a monitoring perspective, blood pressure immediately and precipitously falls, with associated changes in cerebral and somatic oxygenation and bispectral index [17]. The leading predictors for prolonged hemodynamic instability following valve deployment in general anesthesia patients include low mixed venous oxygen saturation and high left ventricular end-diastolic diameter [19]. Recovery is usually fairly rapid, although the anesthesiologist must be prepared to provide immediate support if this is not the case. Malignant dysrhythmia is well described in high-risk patients during valve deployment [8], and provision for immediate defibrillation must also be made as part of preparation for this phase of the procedure.

Following deployment, the prosthesis positioning and performance is assessed using echocardiography—transthoracic or transesophageal depending on the technique used—hemodynamics and fluoroscopy. Key features to evaluate include:

- Valve positioning and opening.
- Transprosthesis gradient and the presence of paravalvular or transvalvular regurgitation.
- Mitral valve function.
- Left ventricular size and function including new regional wall motion abnormality.
- Pericardial effusion.

The guide wire used to facilitate final positioning and deployment of the valve can generate severe aortic regurgitation due to leaflet restriction. Prosthetic assessment can only take place once this is removed.

Balloon-expandable platforms are permanent, and cannot be retrieved unless they are incompletely deployed, with a substantial risk of embolic stroke. Prosthetic failure can be salvaged with a valve-in-valve deployment, the placement of a second balloon expandable valve within the first. The newer, self-expanding stents will be able to be retrieved following deployment, allowing repositioning of prosthesis.

Immediate Post-procedural Care for TAVI

The arterial sheaths are usually removed at the conclusion of the procedure, either with percutaneous closure or direct surgical repair depending on the patient or approach used. Anticoagulation is reversed using protamine sulphate. Rapid emergence from anesthesia is preferred to allow assessment for embolic stroke. Whilst the patient will need to remain supine for a variable period of time to prevent bleeding or pseudo-aneurysm formation at the arterial puncture site, early mobilisation is encouraged.

Assuming a straightforward, uncomplicated device deployment, the immediate postprocedural management of the transfemoral TAVI patient can be undertaken in the recovery room (Post-Anaesthesia Care Unit), and subsequently in an environment that allows continuous electrocardiographic monitoring and transvenous pacing, such as the coronary care unit. Complete heart block may be noted on device deployment, but may also be a late complication, particularly with the Medtronic CoreValve. The majority of cases emerge within the first 3–7 days, emphasising the importance of close postoperative monitoring. Major risk factors for AV block are patient age more than 75 years, valve oversizing greater than 4 mm and preoperative/immediate postoperative bradycardia (less than 55 beats/min) [20].

If the patient retains a normal heart rhythm, with an adequate rate, without transvenous pacing or chronotropic support, continuous ECG monitoring can be ceased within 24 h. Hospital length of stay is usually between 4 and 6 days [12]. As the size of vascular access sheaths decreases, and the incidence of AV block diminishes, shorter lengths of stay are becoming possible, with 24-h hospital stays for transfemoral and 2–3 day hospital stays for transapical approaches in some centres. Lifelong aspirin is recommended, as is 3–6 months dual antiplatelet therapy.

References

1. Cribier A. Development of transcatheter aortic valve implantation (TAVI): a 20-year odyssey. Arch Cardiovasc Dis. 2012;105(3):146–52. https://doi.org/10.1016/j.acvd.2012.01.005.
2. Leon MB, Smith CR, Mack MJ, Makkar RR, Svensson LG, Kodali SK. Surgical or transcatheter aortic-valve replacement in intermediate-risk patients. N Engl J Med [Internet]. 2016;374(17):1609–20. https://doi.org/10.1056/NEJMoa1700456.
3. Otto CM, Kumbhani DJ, Alexander KP, Calhoon JH, Desai MY, Kaul S, et al. 2017 ACC expert consensus decision pathway for transcatheter aortic valve replacement in the management of adults with aortic stenosis. J Am Coll Cardiol. 2017;69(10):1313–46. https://doi.org/10.1016/j.jacc.2016.12.006.
4. Vahanian A, Alfieri O, Andreotti F, Antunes MJ, Barón-Esquivias G, Baumgartner H, et al. Guidelines on the management of valvular heart disease. Eur Heart J. 2012;33(19):2451–96.
5. Klein AA, Webb ST, Tsui S, Sudarshan C, Shapiro L, Densem C. Transcatheter aortic valve insertion: anaesthetic implications of emerging new technology. Br J Anaesth. 2009;103(6):792–9.
6. Cockburn J, Dooley M, de Belder A, Trivedi U, Hildick-Smith D. A comparison between surgical risk scores for predicting outcome in patients undergoing transcatheter aortic valve implantation. J Cardiovasc Surg (Torino). 2017;58(3):467–72.
7. Greif M, Lange P, Näbauer M, Schwarz F, Becker C, Schmitz C, et al. Transcutaneous aortic valve replacement with the Edwards SAPIEN XT and Medtronic CoreValve prosthesis under fluoroscopic guidance and local anaesthesia only. Heart. 2014;100(9):691–5.
8. Miles LF, Joshi KR, Ogilvie EH, Densem CG, Klein AA, O'Sullivan M, et al. General anaesthesia vs. conscious sedation for transfemoral aortic valve implantation: a single UK centre before-and-after study. Anaesthesia. 2016;71(8):892–900.

9. Dall'Ara G, Eltchaninoff H, Moat N, Laroche C, Goicolea J, Ussia GP, et al. Local and general anaesthesia do not influence outcome of transfemoral aortic valve implantation. Int J Cardiol. 2014;177(2):448–54.

10. Bufton KA, Augoustides JG, Cobey FC. Anesthesia for transfemoral aortic valve replacement in North America and Europe. J Cardiothorac Vasc Anesth [Internet]. 2013;27(1):46–9. https://doi.org/10.1053/j.jvca.2012.08.008.

11. Bergmann L, Kahlert P, Eggebrecht H, Frey U, Peters J, Kottenberg E. Transfemoral aortic valve implantation under sedation and monitored anaesthetic care—a feasibility study. Anaesthesia. 2011;66(11):977–82.

12. Ehret C, Rossaint R, Foldenauer AC, Stoppe C, Stevanovic A, Dohms K, et al. Is local anesthesia a favorable approach for transcatheter aortic valve implantation? A systematic review and meta-analysis comparing local and general anesthesia. BMJ Open. 2017;7(9):e016321.

13. Motloch LJ, Rottlaender D, Reda S, Larbig R, Bruns M, Müller-Ehmsen J, et al. Local versus general anesthesia for transfemoral aortic valve implantation. Clin Res Cardiol. 2012;101(1):45–53.

14. Goren O, Finkelstein A, Gluch A, Sheinberg N, Dery E, Matot I, et al. Sedation or general anesthesia for patients undergoing transcatheter aortic valve implantation—does it affect outcome? An observational single-center study. J Clin Anesth. 2015;27(5):385–90.

15. Yamamoto M, Meguro K, Mouillet G, Bergoend E, Monin J-L, Lim P, et al. Effect of local anesthetic management with conscious sedation in patients undergoing transcatheter aortic valve implantation. Am J Cardiol. 2013;111(1):94–9.

16. Mayr NP, Michel J, Bleiziffer S, Tassani P, Martin K. Sedation or general anesthesia for transcatheter aortic valve implantation (TAVI). J Thorac Dis. 2015;7(9):1518–26.

17. Mayr NP, Hapfelmeier A, Martin K, Kurz A, Van Der Starre P, Babik B, et al. Comparison of sedation and general anaesthesia for transcatheter aortic valve implantation on cerebral oxygen saturation and neurocognitive outcome. Br J Anaesth. 2016;116(1):90–9.

18. Klein AA, Skubas NJ, Ender J. Controversies and complications in the perioperative management of transcatheter aortic valve replacement. Anesth Analg. 2014;119(4):784–98.

19. Iritakenishi T, Kamibayashi T, Torikai K, Maeda K, Kuratani T, Sawa Y, et al. Predictors of prolonged hemodynamic compromise after valve deployment during transcatheter aortic valve implantation. J Cardiothorac Vasc Anesth. 2015;29(4):868–74.

20. Neragi-Miandoab S, Michler RE. A review of most relevant complications of transcatheter aortic valve implantation. ISRN Cardiol. 2013;2013:956252.

Anesthetic Considerations for Non-Robotic-and Robotic Minimally Invasive Mitral Valve Surgery

8

M. Ackermann, W. Zakhary, and J. Ender

Main Messages
1. Placement of an intrajugular venous drainage cannula is indicated when the right atrium will be opened during the procedure and in patients with a body surface area > 2 m^2
2. Intraoperative transesophageal echocardiography is essential to ensure correct placement of cannulas and the endoaortic balloon occlusion catheter to detect possible complications
3. Endoaortic balloon occlusion catheter warrants left and right sided arterial pressure monitoring
4. Lung isolation techniques are mandatory for Robotic-Assisted Minimally Invasive Mitral Valve Surgery
5. Hemodynamics may be affected by capnothorax during Robotic-Assisted Minimally Invasive Mitral Valve Surgery mandates

Minimally invasive mitral valve surgery (MIMVS) presents patients with a less invasive alternative compared to the traditional sternotomy for procedures to the mitral valve [1] and has become the preferred approach in many centers [2]. Compared to sternotomy, the minimally invasive approach is comparable with regards to mortality [3, 4], repair rate and the durability of the repair [1]. MIMVS does not refer to a single approach, but rather to a collection of techniques and operation-specific technologies [5].

Surgery can be done through a lower hemisternotomy, with the operative strategy, setup and anesthetic technique similar to that of mitral valve surgery through a full sternotomy. The more commonly used technique is that of a right mini-thoracotomy in the fourth or fifth intercostal space. After access to the heart is gained with this technique, surgery can then be performed either by direct vision or endoscopically with the Port access system.

The total endoscopic robotic technique for mitral valve surgery—robotic-assisted minimally invasive mitral valve surgery (RAMIMVS)—has numerous advantages when compared to the conventional approach. This includes a reduction in postoperative pain, wound infections, shorter hospital stay and faster return to activities of daily living with a higher patient satisfaction [6]. On the other hand, RAMIMVS consumes more anesthetic resources compared to conventional surgery in the form of increased anesthesia

M. Ackermann · W. Zakhary · J. Ender (✉)
Department of Anesthesiology and Intensive Care Medicine, Herzzentrum Leipzig GmbH, Leipzig, Germany
e-mail: Joerg.Ender@medizin.uni-leipzig.de

© Springer Nature Switzerland AG 2021
D. C. H. Cheng et al. (eds.), *Evidence-Based Practice in Perioperative Cardiac Anesthesia and Surgery*, https://doi.org/10.1007/978-3-030-47887-2_8

induction time, total anesthesia time and anesthetic staffing costs [7].

This chapter focuses on specific perioperative anesthesia related aspects unique to MIMVS and RAMIMVS, in which the anesthesiologist plays a central role. When comparing the anesthetic management of robotic-assisted MIMVS to *non*-robotic MIMVS, many aspects are exactly the same. The discussion to follow is therefore applicable to both techniques. Where important differences do exist, this will be highlighted appropriately.

Preoperative Management

Preoperative Evaluation

Patient Selection: General

One should be cognizant of significant patient comorbidities such as morbid obesity, significant lung disease, peripheral vascular disease, advanced renal dysfunction, advanced liver disease, significant pulmonary hypertension, severe left ventricular dysfunction as well as more than mild aortic regurgitation, when selecting patients for MIMVS [2]. For planned RAMIMVS the procedure, when performed in smaller patients with insufficient intercostal thoracic spaces (<3 cm), with a high body mass index, prior thoracic surgery or radiation, is expected to be more difficult [8].

Previous Right Sided Chest Interventions

Previous interventions to the right hemithorax or adhesions might complicate and add time or morbidity to the operation [9]. This includes a history of pneumothorax, chest trauma, and/or insertion of chest tubes or surgery to the right hemithorax. There is no reliable way to predict the presence or absence of significant adhesions in the right pleural space [10]. Direct visualization through the working port, or a right-sided thoracoscopy through a 5 mm port could be used to deter-

mine if a right-sided approach is safe [2, 10]. Abnormal anatomy that may possibly complicate or preclude the use of a minimally invasive technique, such as deformities to the chest wall, ribs and diaphragm can also be evaluated by means of preoperative computed tomography.

Planning the Vascular Access

In addition, preoperative CT-Angiography can provide valuable information with regards to the aorta, great vessels, mitral calcification and iliofemoral vessels, and has become routine in the preoperative evaluation in patients presenting for a minimally invasive approach [2].

Perfusion strategies and clamping techniques should be carefully selected following preoperative screening of the aorto-iliac-femoral axis.

Intraoperative Management

Appropriate Theatre and Patient Preparation: Room Layout

For MIMVS there are no special considerations to be addressed, whereas in RAMIMVS the anesthetic workspace is greatly affected by the huge robotic equipment. The anesthetic and transesophageal echocardiography (TEE) machines should be moved as cephalad as possible to facilitate robotic arms movement (Fig. 8.1). The endotracheal tube must be well secured, as access to the patient will be limited. In addition, the robotic arms often obstruct the patient monitors. In case of a surgical emergency, all of the staff should be trained to gain access to the patient, quickly detach and remove the robot from the patient and re-position him for a sternotomy [8].

Positioning

For MIMVS through a right mini-thoracotomy and RAMIMVS, the need of exposure to the right hemithorax necessitates placing the patient

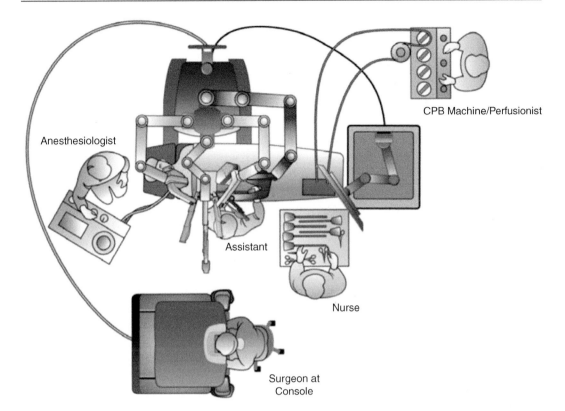

© 2013 Intuitive Surgical Inc,

Fig. 8.1 Operating room setup for RAMIMVS

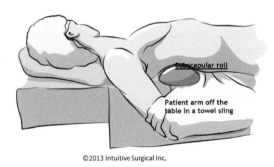

©2013 Intuitive Surgical Inc,

Fig. 8.2 Positioning of the patient

in a partial left lateral position of about 30°. The patient should be placed on the right side of the operating table with a roll underneath the right scapula, with the right arm slightly flexed (Fig. 8.2). This should improve access to the anterior axillary line. One should remember that this position might place considerable stress on the neck and brachial plexus [9].

Monitoring General

Monitoring should be placed according to institutional practice for mitral valve surgery through a median sternotomy. This usually consists of:

- Multi-lumen central venous line in the right internal jugular vein.
- Peripheral venous access.
- Urinary catheter.
- Two temperature probes—nasopharyngeal and bladder.
- Transesophageal echocardiography (TEE).
- Convective warming device.

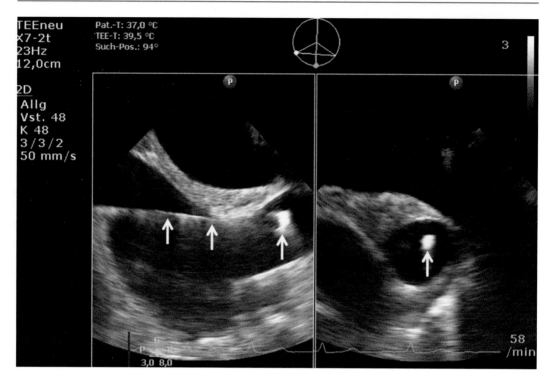

Fig. 8.3 Visualization of the guide wire in the superior vena cava by TEE—the right arrow in the bicaval view indicates the J tip of the wire

Specific additional patient preparations:

- External defibrillator paddles should be placed prior to the draping of the patient.
- Bilateral radial or brachial arterial pressure monitoring is obligatory when endoclamp is used for aortic occlusion (for details see below).
- One-lung ventilation using either a double-lumen tube or a bronchial blocker is mandatory for RAMIMVS and often used for MIMVS.

Pre-Bypass TEE

A standard pre-bypass TEE exam should be performed for conventional mitral valve sur-

gery. It is important to exclude significant annular calcification, as this may not only increase the risk for atrioventricular disruption, but also make suture placement with single shaft instruments more difficult. More than mild aortic regurgitation may limit myocardial protection and should be approached with caution [2].

In addition to providing information with regards to the specific valvular pathology present and the grading thereof, transesophageal echocardiography is essential during MIMVS to confirm correct placement of the:

- Guide wire and the venous cannula (Figs. 8.3 and 8.4)
- Guide wire of the arterial cannula (Fig. 8.5)
- Endoballoon if used (Fig. 8.6)

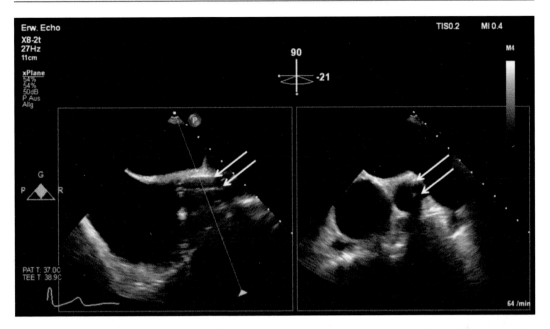

Fig. 8.4 Visualization of the multi-lumen venous cannula by TEE, white arrows indicating the double contour of the cannula in long (left side) and in short axis (right side)

Fig. 8.5 Guide wire of the femoral aortic cannula in descending aorta (white arrow)

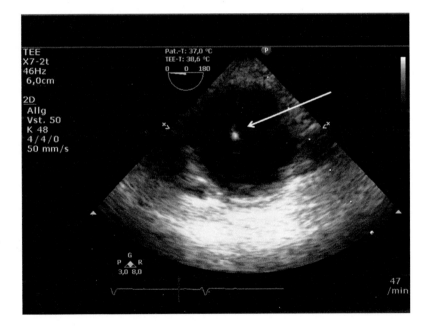

The guide wire from the venous multi-lumen cannula placed from the groin can migrate through an existing patent foramen ovale (Fig. 8.7) or can be seen in the right atrial appendage (Fig. 8.8) with potential perforation when advancing the cannula in that position.

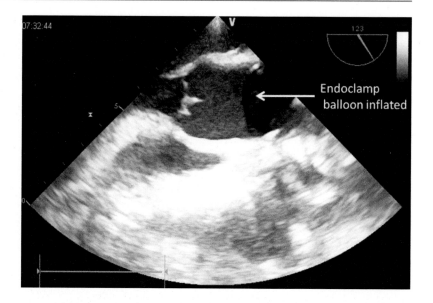

Fig. 8.6 Endoclamp balloon inflated. With courtesy of Dr. Alexander Mladenow

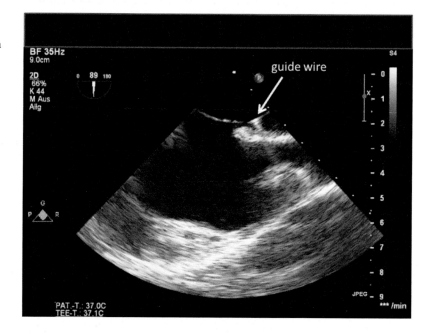

Fig. 8.7 ME bicaval view showing guide wire migrating through a patent foramen ovale

Anesthetic Technique

Choice of Agents

Specific drugs used are not dictated by MIMVS, but is dependent by specific practitioner and institutional preferences [9]. Adequate muscle paralysis is of special importance during RAMIMVS to avoid injuries to the myocardium, great ves-

sels and other structures when the robotic arms are engaged [11]. Should a fast track protocol be used or patients are extubated in theatre, drugs should be selected with these goals in mind.

There may be concerns that inhalational anesthetics may impair hypoxic pulmonary vasoconstriction and thereby increase shunt. There is very little evidence suggesting that there is a difference with regards to patient outcomes when

Fig. 8.8 ME bicaval view showing guide wire in the right atrial appendage (see white arrows)

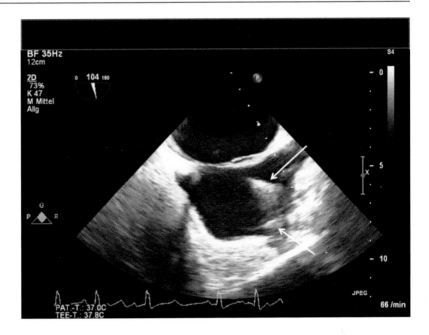

maintenance of general anesthesia is done by inhalational anesthetics compared to intravenous anesthetics, during one-lung ventilation [12].

Analgesia

RAMIMVS is not pain-free. Similar postoperative pain scores have been noted regardless of whether a minimally invasive approach or standard sternotomy was used. Systemic opioids may be used in either approach, but this may hinder prompt extubation and decrease patient satisfaction due to postoperative nausea and vomiting.

Several regional techniques can be utilized as part of a balanced anesthetic technique including intercostal nerve blocks, paravertebral blocks [13] and local wound infiltration with long acting liposomal bupivacaine [6]. Intrathecal morphine at a dose of $1–5~\mu g.kg^{-1}$ [14] *or a standard dose of 300 μg* [6] can reduce additional opioid requirements in the immediate postoperative period without delaying extubation, but does not reduce the incidence of postoperative nausea and vomiting when compared to systemic opioids alone [14]. Since a large volume of local anesthetic is not used—as is the case with a paravertebral block—the surgeon can then inject a larger volume of local anesthetic at the end of the procedure in combination with this technique [6].

The PECS II block, that reliably blocks the T2–4 dermatomes with variable coverage to T6 as well as the serratus plane block, that reliably covers the T2–7 dermatomes with variable coverage to the level of T9 are used for RAMIMVS [6].

Endotracheal Tube and Ventilation Strategy

While not mandatory, one-lung ventilation is central to anesthetic management during the minimally invasive approach. Common techniques include a left-sided double-lumen endotracheal tube or a right-sided bronchus blocker. Exposure can also be achieved by either holding ventilation or intermittently ventilating both lungs with a normal single lumen endotracheal tube at commencement and end of cardiopulmonary bypass [9]. One-lung ventilation is usually mandatory during the robotic procedure [1].

Compared to values during the induction of general anesthesia with two-lung ventilation, the $P_aO_2: F_iO_2$ ratio is significantly decreased during separation from cardiopulmonary bypass with one-lung ventilation after MIMVS. It is also significantly reduced compared to two-lung ventilation after cardiopulmonary bypass following conventional sternotomy [7]. One should keep the deleterious effect of hypoxia and hypercarbia on the pulmonary vascular resistance in mind and also that of the increased sympathetic tone on the occurrence of arrhythmias [9].

Cannulation

Since peripheral cannulation rather than central cannulation forms part of most MIMVS-procedures, familiarity with the principles thereof and adequate planning is essential [15].

Venous Drainage During Cardiopulmonary Bypass

There are several techniques to establish venous return to the cardiopulmonary bypass circuit. The anesthesiologist is always essential for either the placement of the cannula or performing the monitoring confirming correct placement.

Long Multiport Femoral Venous Cannula

A common method utilized is the placement of a long venous cannula through the femoral vein. A long guide wire is advanced to the right atrium and superior vena cava after access to the femoral vein is established. Confirming advancement of the wire by means of (TEE) is essential.

The guide wire J-tip should be visible within the superior vena cava by all team members (Fig. 8.3). The guide wire should be visible during the entire period of catheter-advancement. This minimizes the possibility of the guide wire kinking and therefore the possible perforation of the femoral vein. TEE is used to confirm placement of the catheter tip 2–3 cm within the superior vena cava with the typical railroad track appearance confirming optimal placement. The development of an acute pericardial effusion should alert the team of a possible perforation of an intrapericardial structure [9].

With the tip of femoral cannula in the SVC and the multiple orifices located within the right atrium, adequate venous drainage of the entire body can usually be established. Kinetic or vacuum assisted venous drainage can increase flow dynamics by 20–40%.

Endopulmonary Vent Catheter

An Endopulmonary Vent Catheter (Edward Lifesciences, Irvine, CA) can also be used in conjunction with a femoral cannula. The appearance is similar to that of pulmonary artery catheter. The placement 1–2 cm within the main pulmonary artery can be guided and confirmed either by TEE or fluoroscopy. Since vacuum assisted venting of the pulmonary artery at a rate of only 50 ml/min can usually be established, this technique is currently seldom used [8, 9].

Superior Vena Cava Venous Drainage Cannula

Indications for its use: Cannulation strategies have evolved over time with dual stage femoral cannulation being preferred over percutaneous neck and femoral cannulation [16]. The use of a single femoral venous catheter is usually sufficient for MIMVS through a left atriotomy. When the right atrium is opened to close an atrial septal defect or a concomitant tricuspid valve repair is performed, bicaval cannulation with occlusion is usually performed [9]. This can also be indicated when single cannula venous drainage might be insufficient due to a large body surface area. A body surface area of greater than 2.0 m^2 is considered as an indication for the placement of a percutaneous superior vena cava cannula during robotic mitral valve surgery [17].

Some centers routinely place a percutaneous superior vena cava cannula [2]. However, there is risk of vascular injury associated with the placement of these cannulas [9]. Incomplete cardiac emptying may result in suboptimal surgical visualization. The primary benefit of a percutaneous superior vena cava cannula is better surgical visualization of the mitral valve. One study has demonstrated no effect on brain near-infrared spectroscopy (NIRS) with the use of a percutaneous superior vena cava cannula. The lower central venous pressure associated with the use of this cannula likely reflected better venous drainage. It should be noted that the difference in cerebral perfusion pressure in this study was only 5 mmHg [18] and therefore higher central venous pressures might impair cerebral perfusion pressure resulting in decreased NIRS values. Left atrial retraction may also partially impede superior vena cava drainage [2], which might reduce brain perfusion during long operations.

Technique for placement: A large bore (15 or 18 French) percutaneous venous drainage catheter can be placed in the right internal jugular vein due to its direct course to the superior vena cava. After guide wire placement, the completion of the procedure is determined by the preference of the specific center. It may be placed entirely by the anesthesiologist [2]. Alternatively, a 5Fr single-lumen cannula is inserted in the right internal jugular vein close to the clavicle by the anesthesiologist. It is then flushed, capped and prepared as part of the surgical field. The surgeon then later uses this cannula to introduce guide wires, followed by dilators and finally the cannula [6].

The following important steps minimize the possibility of vascular perforation during placement:

- A strict Seldinger technique should be used. An assistant should be available to establish the midesophageal bicaval view in TEE. In this view the guide wire should be visible during the entire process.
- Sequential dilators of increasing size should be used to facilitate placement of the cannula.
- Correct placement is usually confirmed by the presence of air-bubbles in the mid-esophageal bicaval view, after commencement of an infusion directly after placement of the cannula. Continuing the infusion through the cannula helps to prevent the formation of clots.

If a long time-interval exists between cannula placement and systemic heparinization, a small dose of heparin (i.e. 5000 IE) should be administered just before its placement [9].

Femoral Arterial Cannulation

The descending aorta should be visualized during cannulation of the femoral artery with TEE. Not only should the presence of the guide wire (Fig. 8.5) within the aorta be confirmed, but also the rare occurrence of a false lumen upon the initiation of cardiopulmonary bypass should be excluded by TEE [2].

Endoaortic Balloon Occlusion

Monitoring during placement and utilization: Arterial pressure monitoring catheters should be placed in both the left and right upper extremities prior to the use of the Endoclamp Aortic Catheter (Edwards Life Sciences). If catheter placement in the left arm is not possible, pressure monitoring in the lower extremities can be used as an alternative [9].

Significant TEE guidance is required with the use of the Endoclamp. The first step is to confirm appropriate size of the ascending aorta—a diameter greater than 35 mm may limit endo-occlusion and too small a size may increase the probability of balloon migration or aortic injury [9]. Additionally, inflating the balloon with 1 ml saline per 1 mm aortic diameter will usually result in sufficient occlusion in most cases. This volume should be administered incrementally, anticipating an occlusion pressure of 350–450 mmHg [15].

The anesthesiologist is central to confirm correct initial placement and monitoring for migration during usage of the Endoclamp [9]. After advancement over the guide wire, the tip of the catheter should be confirmed to be just above the sinotubular junction (Fig. 8.6). Emptying the venous circulation and thereby diminishing left ventricular stroke volume will mitigate migration during balloon inflation. Additionally, Adenosine (20–30 mg) may be administered during deployment [15].

Once the left atrium is opened, visualization of the ascending aorta is limited by air interposition. This can partially be limited by filling the left atrium with blood or another fluid if required

[9]. With the use of the Endoclamp, proximal or distal balloon migration may occur during the procedure.

Flow from the aortic cannula, increased arterial perfusion pressure and active aortic root venting will all promote proximal migration—migration towards the aortic valve. This should be diagnosed by TEE and active traction on the catheter should maintain the balloon at the rim of the sinotubular junction. Migration towards the valve might result in circumferential leak or iatrogenic injury to the aortic valve or root [15].

Residual cardiac contraction, administration of antegrade cardioplegia and decreased arterial perfusion all promote distal migration—the migration away from the aortic valve. A sudden isolated drop in the arterial pressure monitor from the right upper extremity usually indicate distal balloon migration with subsequent occlusion of the innominate artery [9, 15].

Alternatives to the Endoclamp

Many centers avoid the use of an Endoclamp not necessarily due to an increased rate of complications, but because of increased cost, infrastructural demands and longer cross-clamp and operative times associated with its use. In this scenario an angled Chitwood Transthoracic Aortic Cross Clamp (Scanlan International Inc.) is usually utilized and a separate root vent catheter is then placed [9]. A long Chitwood clamp can also be used during RAMIMVS [6]. This is placed through a stab wound in the second intercostal space, 8–10 cm posterior to the left robotic arm to avoid internal and external conflict with the robotic arms [10].

Cardiopulmonary Bypass

Cardioplegia Administration

There are many methods to deliver cardioplegia to the heart during MIMVS. The easiest and most common way is the direct antegrade route. The surgeon uses a transthoracic aortic cross clamp and then the cardioplegia is administered by a cannula placed in ascending aorta via a small incision. Cardioplegia can otherwise be delivered either antegradely if an endoaortic balloon occlusion is used, or via the retrograde route through a coronary sinus catheter placed percutaneously.

Retrograde cardioplegia is used if aortic regurgitation is present. A percutaneous coronary sinus catheter is inserted from the right internal jugular vein and advanced in RA guided by TEE modified bicaval view with or without fluoroscopy and contrast administration. If the catheter moves toward the tricuspid valve or the right atrial appendage, it is rotated anticlockwise, and if the catheter is directed toward IVC, it is rotated clockwise and then advanced. Once the catheter is in position, inflating the coronary sinus catheter balloon will change the pressure waveform from the right atrial to a right ventricular trace form. Heparin 100 mg/kg must be administrated to prevent coronary sinus thrombosis [6, 8]. If cardioplegia administration is impossible, non-cardioplegic myocardial protection may be provided.

Capnothorax During RAMIMVS

In addition to one-lung ventilation, insufflation of the right hemithorax with CO_2 is performed to facilitate surgical exposure and prevent smoke formation during cautery usage. The usual safe insufflation pressure is between 5 and 10 mmHg and insufflation rate below 2–3 L/min. Hemodynamic parameters may be affected with higher pressures (10–15 mmHg) [6]. Cardiac index, mean blood pressure and mixed venous oxygen values will be decreased, which will be more obvious in patients with reduced ventricular function. $PaCO_2$ can significantly increase with subsequent coronary vasoconstriction. Monitoring of intrathoracic pressure is mandatory and can be done by 18G venous cannula in the pleural space, which can also act as a vent for the excess CO_2, in order to avoid a tension pneu-

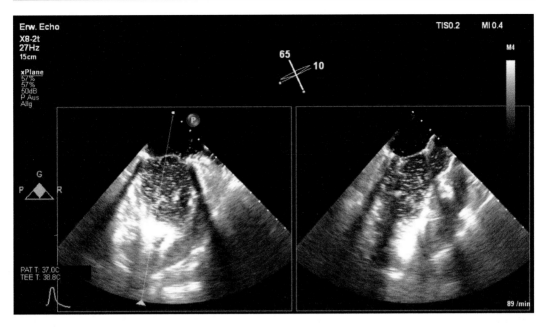

Fig. 8.9 Demonstrating importance of correct de-airing with a huge amount of air in left ventricle after release of the aortic cross clamp

mothorax/capnothorax. Communication between the anesthesiologist and the surgeon is essential in this phase. To wash out arterial CO_2 during one-lung ventilation is difficult, and a return to ventilating both lungs may be warranted. The hemodynamic effects can be treated with fluids, transfusion, inotropic agents, vasopressors and decreasing the insufflation pressure [8]. As CO_2 acts as an electrical insulator, defibrillation using external pads is sometimes ineffective and mandates resuming two-lung ventilation before another attempt at defibrillation [6].

De-Airing

Routine use of CO_2 insufflation during MIMVS will minimize residual intracardiac air. Before separating from cardiopulmonary bypass, sufficient de-airing of the left ventricle should be confirmed [19]. TEE should be used in this context (Fig. 8.9). The primary means for de-airing are vents in the ascending aorta and left ventricle that are either placed through the thoracotomy or working port, or that reside inside the endoballoon [10].

Post-Bypass TEE

The post-bypass TEE exam should exclude residual mitral regurgitation, paravalvular leaks and mitral stenosis. Complications such as systolic anterior motion of the mitral valve in the case of hemodynamic instability—especially in patients identified to be at risk in the preoperative TEE exam—and iatrogenic injury to circumflex artery should be excluded [20].

Postoperative Management

Preparing for Transfer to the Intensive Care Unit

Unless immediate extubation is planned, the double-lumen endotracheal tube should be exchanged to a single lumen tube to facilitate respiratory weaning. This is best done with an airway exchange catheter—especially if upper airway edema is present. If a second arterial catheter or a venous drainage catheter in the internal jugular vein was used, this should be removed prior to the transfer to the intensive care unit [9].

Suitability for a Fast-Track Protocol

The following strategies have been used as part of a balanced anesthetic technique in order to facilitate a fast tract protocol. Although paravertebral blocks decrease the intraoperative use of opioids and facilitate early extubation in theatre, the hospital length of stay remains unchanged [21, 22]. They may shorten ICU- and hospital stay after a robotic procedure [13].

The evidence suggests that compared to conventional sternotomy, MIMVS might reduce the duration of mechanical ventilation. However, other institutional factors may play a greater role in the time to extubation [1].

Complications and MIMVS

Neurological: There are concerns regarding the increased risk for neurological complications during MIMVS when compared to conventional sternotomy. Possible explanations for the increased risk of stroke include restricted access to the surgical site, difficulties with de-airing, increased crossclamp and cardiopulmonary bypass times, the use of different perfusion strategies—antegrade and retrograde—and the use of an endoclamp. Introduction of a guide wire with the resultant mobilization of emboli or iatrogenic aortic dissection and catheter migration are the proposed method by which an endoclamp can result in stroke.

Although an earlier meta-analysis showed an increased stroke rate in patients undergoing MIMVS compared to conventional sternotomy, a more recent meta-analysis failed to show this difference [23]. With regards to stroke, not only is the specific route for surgical access of importance, but also the technique utilized for aortic cross-clamping. There is a trend towards a higher risk of stroke in studies exclusively using an endoclamp for aortic occlusion and hence many institutions favor the use of the transthoracic clamp [1]. In a recent meta-analysis however, there was no significant difference between the use of an endoclamp and transthoracic aortic clamp with regards to the occurrence of cerebrovascular accidents, all-cause mortality and acute kidney injury at 30 days [5].

The use of retrograde perfusion is an independent risk factor for stroke and postoperative delirium. This can be avoided by the use of central aortic cannulation when feasible or when mandated by contraindications to femoral cannulation [24].

Vascular: Endoartic balloon occlusion is associated with a 5-fold increase in the relative risk of aortic dissection (4-fold for Type A dissection) and a numerical higher risk of leg ischaemia, necessitating active monitoring therefore in the intra- and postoperative periods [5].

Bleeding, transfusions and reoperation for bleeding: Compared to conventional surgery, MIMVS shows a clear benefit with regards to blood loss and transfusion requirements. Possible explanations include the lack of sternal marrow bleeding, minimal dissection and smaller incisions. However, this benefit is only evident once the learning curve has been completed [1, 4].

Unilateral pulmonary edema: The incidence of unilateral pulmonary edema (UPE) varies according to the definition used. When defined by radiological features, the incidence reported is 12.9–25% [25, 26]. When clinical features are incorporated in the definition, the incidence is between 1.2–4% [17, 26]. This complication is of importance as it carries a mortality rate of up to 33% [17]. The exact mechanism of UPE is unknown, but an ischemic-reperfusion injury is postulated. UPE is associated with chronic obstructive pulmonary disease, pre-existing pulmonary hypertension, moderate to severe right ventricular dysfunction and longer cardiopulmonary bypass times. There is no association between the occurrence of UPE and the method used for lung-isolation, the intraoperative administration of blood products and left ventricular function [25].

Phrenic nerve palsy: Phrenic nerve palsy is more common in patients undergoing the minimally invasive approach compared to a sternotomy [4].

References

1. Nagendran J, Catrip J, Losenno KL, Adams C, Kiaii B, Chu MW. Minimally invasive mitral repair surgery: why does controversy still persist? Expert Rev Cardiovasc Ther. 2017;15(1):15–24.
2. Ailawadi G, Agnihotri AK, Mehall JR, Wolfe JA, Hummel BW, Fayers TM, et al. Minimally invasive mitral valve surgery I: patient selection, evaluation, and planning. Innovations (Phila). 2016;11(4):243–50.
3. Falk V, Cheng DC, Martin J, Diegeler A, Folliguet TA, Nifong LW, et al. Minimally invasive versus open mitral valve surgery: a consensus statement of the international society of minimally invasive coronary surgery (ISMICS) 2010. Innovations (Phila). 2011;6(2):66–76.
4. Cheng DC, Martin J, Lal A, Diegeler A, Folliguet TA, Nifong LW, et al. Minimally invasive versus conventional open mitral valve surgery: a meta-analysis and systematic review. Innovations (Phila). 2011;6(2):84–103.
5. Kowalewski M, Malvindi PG, Suwalski P, Raffa GM, Pawliszak W, Perlinski D, et al. Clinical safety and effectiveness of Endoaortic as compared to transthoracic clamp for small thoracotomy mitral valve surgery: meta-analysis of observational studies. Ann Thorac Surg. 2017;103(2):676–86.
6. Rehfeldt KH, Andre JV, Ritter MJ. Anesthetic considerations in robotic mitral valve surgery. Ann Cardiothorac Surg. 2017;6(1):47–53.
7. Kottenberg-Assenmacher E, Kamler M, Peters J. Minimally invasive endoscopic port-access intracardiac surgery with one lung ventilation: impact on gas exchange and anaesthesia resources. Anaesthesia. 2007;62(3):231–8.
8. Bernstein WK, Walker A. Anesthetic issues for robotic cardiac surgery. Ann Card Anaesth. 2015;18(1):58–68.
9. Vernick W, Atluri P. Robotic and minimally invasive cardiac surgery. Anesthesiol Clin. 2013;31(2):299–320.
10. Lehr EJ, Guy TS, Smith RL, Grossi EA, Shemin RJ, Rodriguez E, et al. Minimally invasive mitral valve surgery III: training and robotic-assisted approaches. Innovations (Phila). 2016;11(4):260–7.
11. Chauhan S, Sukesan S. Anesthesia for robotic cardiac surgery: an amalgam of technology and skill. Ann Card Anaesth. 2010;13(2):169–75.
12. Modolo NS, Modolo MP, Marton MA, Volpato E, Monteiro Arantes V, do Nascimento Junior P, et al. Intravenous versus inhalation anaesthesia for one-lung ventilation. Cochrane Database Syst Rev. 2013;7:CD006313.
13. Neuburger PJ, Ngai JY, Chacon MM, Luria B, Manrique-Espinel AM, Kline RP, et al. A prospective randomized study of paravertebral blockade in patients undergoing robotic mitral valve repair. J Cardiothorac Vasc Anesth. 2015;29(4):930–6.
14. Mukherjee C, Koch E, Banusch J, Scholz M, Kaisers UX, Ender J. Intrathecal morphine is superior to intravenous PCA in patients undergoing minimally invasive cardiac surgery. Ann Card Anaesth. 2012;15(2):122–7.
15. Wolfe JA, Malaisrie SC, Farivar RS, Khan JH, Hargrove WC, Moront MG, et al. Minimally invasive mitral valve surgery II: surgical technique and postoperative management. Innovations (Phila). 2016;11(4):251–9.
16. Chan EY, Lumbao DM, Iribarne A, Easterwood R, Yang JY, Cheema FH, et al. Evolution of cannulation techniques for minimally invasive cardiac surgery: a 10-year journey. Innovations (Phila). 2012;7(1):9–14.
17. Moss E, Halkos ME, Binongo JN, Murphy DA. Prevention of unilateral pulmonary edema complicating robotic mitral valve operations. Ann Thorac Surg. 2017;103(1):98–104.
18. Bainbridge DT, Chu MW, Kiaii B, Cleland A, Murkin J. Percutaneous superior vena cava drainage during minimally invasive mitral valve surgery: a randomized, crossover study. J Cardiothorac Vasc Anesth. 2015;29(1):101–6.
19. Ender J, Sgouropoulou S. Value of transesophageal echocardiography (TEE) guidance in minimally invasive mitral valve surgery. Ann Cardiothorac Surg. 2013;2(6):796–802.
20. Ender J, Selbach M, Borger MA, Krohmer E, Falk V, Kaisers UX, et al. Echocardiographic identification of iatrogenic injury of the circumflex artery during minimally invasive mitral valve repair. Ann Thorac Surg. 2010;89(6):1866–72.
21. Neuburger PJ, Chacon MM, Luria BJ, Manrique-Espinel AM, Ngai JY, Grossi EA, et al. Does paravertebral blockade facilitate immediate extubation after totally endoscopic robotic mitral valve repair surgery? Innovations (Phila). 2015;10(2):96–100.
22. Rodrigues ES, Lynch JJ, Suri RM, Burkhart HM, Li Z, Mauermann WJ, et al. Robotic mitral valve repair: a review of anesthetic management of the first 200 patients. J Cardiothorac Vasc Anesth. 2014;28(1):64–8.
23. Cao C, Gupta S, Chandrakumar D, Nienaber TA, Indraratna P, Ang SC, et al. A meta-analysis of minimally invasive versus conventional mitral valve repair for patients with degenerative mitral disease. Ann Cardiothorac Surg. 2013;2(6):693–703.
24. Murzi M, Cerillo AG, Gasbarri T, Margaryan R, Kallushi E, Farneti P, et al. Antegrade and retrograde perfusion in minimally invasive mitral valve surgery with transthoracic aortic clamping: a single-institution experience with 1632 patients over 12 years. Interact Cardiovasc Thorac Surg. 2017;24(3):363–8.
25. Tutschka MP, Bainbridge D, Chu MW, Kiaii B, Jones PM. Unilateral postoperative pulmonary edema after minimally invasive cardiac surgical procedures: a case-control study. Ann Thorac Surg. 2015;99(1):115–22.
26. Keyl C, Staier K, Pingpoh C, Pache G, Thoma M, Gunkel L, et al. Unilateral pulmonary oedema after minimally invasive cardiac surgery via right antero-lateral minithoracotomy. Eur J Cardiothorac Surg. 2015;47(6):1097–102.

Anesthetic Management in Aortic Arch Surgery and Neuroprotection

Alexander J. Gregory and Albert T. Cheung

Main Messages

1. Major thoracic aortic operations require temporary interruption of blood flow to the brain and body producing physiologic alterations that affect every organ system.
2. Contributions toward improved outcomes include the use of extracorporeal circulation to deliver therapeutic hypothermia to protect organs from ischemic injury, development and refinement of surgical techniques to provide selective antegrade cerebral perfusion, and advanced physiologic monitoring and intraoperative imaging to optimize the conditions necessary to perform the operation and detect complications.

A. J. Gregory
Department of Anesthesiology, Perioperative and Pain Medicine, Cumming School of Medicine, University of Calgary, Calgary, AB, Canada

A. T. Cheung (✉)
Department of Anesthesiology, Perioperative and Pain Medicine, Stanford University School of Medicine, Stanford, CA, USA
e-mail: ATCheung@stanford.edu

Aortic arch surgery presents a unique challenge due to the obligatory alteration or cessation of blood flow to the brain and the rest of the body to accomplish the repair. The cells of the central nervous system (CNS) have a high metabolic activity and are exquisitely sensitive to even brief periods of ischemia that can lead to neuronal injury and apoptosis. The successful outcome of operations involving the aortic arch depends in large part on effective strategies for neuroprotection.

Traditionally, the principal method of neuroprotection was deep hypothermic circulatory arrest (DHCA) that relied on the metabolic suppression by deliberate hypothermia. Although deliberate hypothermia remains a reliable neuroprotective strategy, surgical neurocirculatory techniques to partially or fully maintain cerebral perfusion during aortic arch operations has permitted operations to be performed under moderate hypothermic conditions. There has also been a concurrent evolution of surgical techniques including multiple variations on total arch repairs, hybrid arch repairs with endovascular grafts, and even total endovascular aortic arch repairs to decrease the duration and risk of cerebral ischemia during operation. The combination of neuroprotective strategies that include deliberate hypothermia, neurocirculatory management, and surgical techniques are often used together and have expanded variations in clinical practice because no single approach has been proven to be superior.

© Springer Nature Switzerland AG 2021
D. C. H. Cheng et al. (eds.), *Evidence-Based Practice in Perioperative Cardiac Anesthesia and Surgery*, https://doi.org/10.1007/978-3-030-47887-2_9

Preoperative Evaluation

Aortic Pathology

Aortic arch pathology requiring surgical intervention can generally be divided into two categories; those that require emergency surgery and those that can be completed in a semi-urgent or elective timeframe. See the following list of major thoracic aortic operations that may require deep hypothermic circulatory arrest or selective antegrade cerebral perfusion:

Operation
- Composite Aortic Root Replacement—*when combined with ascending aorta or proximal aortic arch graft.*
- Aortic Valve Replacement and Ascending Aortic Graft.
- Valve-Sparing Aortic Root Replacement— *when combined with ascending aorta or proximal aortic arch graft.*
- Bicuspid Aortic Valve and Ascending Aortic Repair.
- Acute Stanford Type A Aortic Dissection— *when combined with ascending aorta or proximal aortic arch graft.*
- Stanford Type B Aortic Dissection—*when combined with graft repair of the distal aortic arch.*
- Total Aortic Arch Replacement.
- Descending Thoracic Aortic Aneurysm Repair—*when combined with graft repair of the distal aortic arch.*
- Crawford Extent I Thoracoabdominal Aortic Aneurysm Repair—*when combined with graft repair of the distal aortic arch.*
- Crawford Extent II Thoracoabdominal Aortic Aneurysm Repair—*when combined with graft repair of the distal aortic arch.*

Conditions that require emergency surgery are often referred to as "acute aortic syndromes" that include acute type-A aortic dissection (ATAAD), penetrating aortic ulcer, intramural hematoma, contained rupture, or pseudo-aneurysm (Fig. 9.1).

The common aspect that binds these acute conditions together is the potential for unpredict-able and rapid progression with a high risk of sudden death. Aortic aneurysms make up the largest proportion of elective procedures. Aneurysms may be hereditary or acquired and can be characterized based on the location and extent of abnormality relative to the aortic arch. Examples of other aortic arch diseases that may require operation include chronic type-A dissection, aneurysmal growth of diseased aortic segments after prior ATAAD repair, reoperations for progression of disease after a primary surgical repair, and failed surgical or medical management of an acute aortic syndrome.

Aortic aneurysms may be associated with aortic regurgitation if it involves the aortic root or cause compression of mediastinal structures. Patients with degenerative aneurysms may have a high burden of atherosclerotic and peripheral vascular disease. Preoperative evaluation should include cardiac catheterization to detect significant coronary artery disease, echocardiography to evaluate cardiac and valve function, computed tomography (CT) imaging of the chest to evaluate the thoracic aorta, carotid Duplex imaging to detect cerebral vascular disease, and laboratory testing to detect pre-existing chronic kidney disease. Patients should be examined for signs of peripheral arterial disease that may increase the difficulty of peripheral vascular access as well as the risk of limb ischemia or thromboembolism.

Hereditary or familial aortic syndromes may be associated with bicuspid aortic valves and other congenital defects. Genetic mutations such as Loeys-Deitz syndrome may have associated cervical spine instability, Ehlers-Danlos syndrome may have co-existing platelet dysfunction, and Marfan's patients will be more susceptible to spontaneous pneumothorax with positive pressure ventilation or joint dislocations during positioning.

In patients with acute Stanford type A or DeBakey type I or II aortic dissection the mortality and morbidity associated with surgical repair is largely determined by the preoperative condition of the patient. Two principal drivers of outcome are the presence of proximal complications resulting in circulatory shock—aortic regurgitation, myocardial ischemia, and

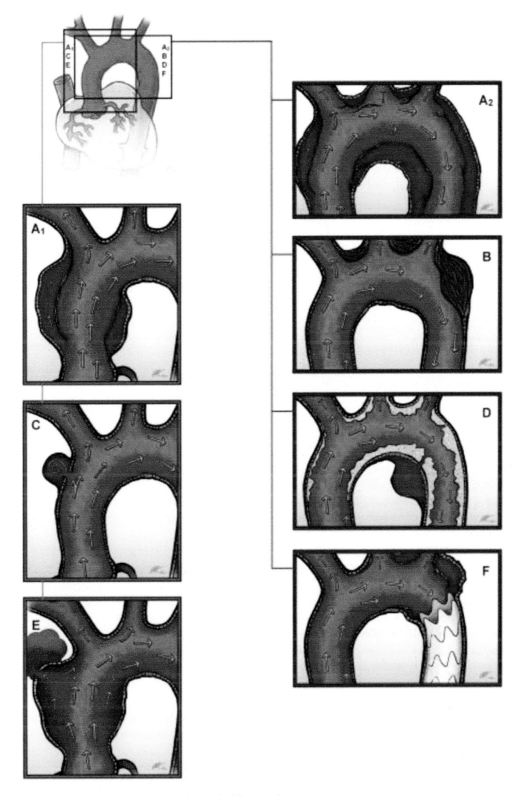

Fig. 9.1 Aortic syndromes that may require surgical intervention

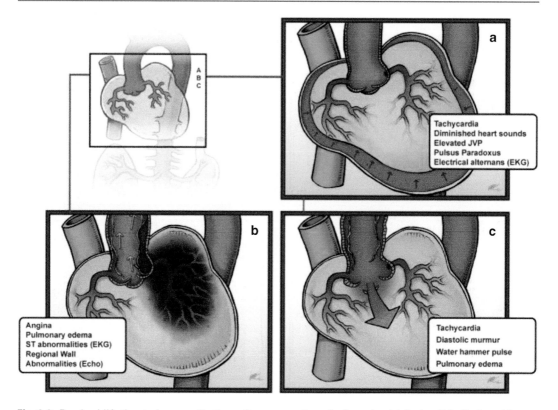

Fig. 9.2 Proximal life-threatening complications of acute type-A aortic dissection (**a**) Pericardial effusion with tamponade, (**b**) Coronary dissection or occlusion with myocardial ischemia, (**c**) Acute aortic regurgitation

pericardial tamponade—and malperfusion syndromes (Figs. 9.2 and 9.3).

The Penn Classification highlights the importance of these presenting features and their relation to operative mortality. In patients with neither circulatory shock nor organ malperfusion (Penn Class A) the operative mortality was 3.1%. The mortality increased to 25.6% once malperfusion was present (Penn Class B), to 17.6% in patients with circulatory shock (Penn Class C), and to 40% when both conditions were present (Penn Class BC) [1]. Additional published data support the notion that the presence of both cerebral and systemic malperfusion increases the mortality of patients presenting with ATAAD [2–6]. The presence of proximal circulatory compromise and distal malperfusion are also important risk factors that dictate specific intraoperative management decisions. Patients with severe aortic regurgitation, pericardial tamponade, or myocardial ischemia may decompensate in response to beta-blocker or antihypertensive therapy and

may manifest hemodynamic instability upon induction of general anesthesia. Patients with malperfusion require decisions to be made regarding: selecting the appropriate arterial pressure monitoring site, strategies to cannulate for CPB, ensuring cerebral perfusion during CPB, the need for an extended aortic arch repair, or use of endovascular adjuncts.

History, Physical Exam, and Investigations in ATAAD

The history and physical exam should be focused to detect signs and symptoms of proximal circulatory complications and malperfusion (Figs. 9.2 and 9.3). Angina, dyspnea, abdominal pain, or limb pain may indicate underlying malperfusion. A brief neurologic exam should be performed to assess for altered consciousness, evidence of stroke, loss of limb sensation, or any focal neurologic abnormalities including paraplegia that

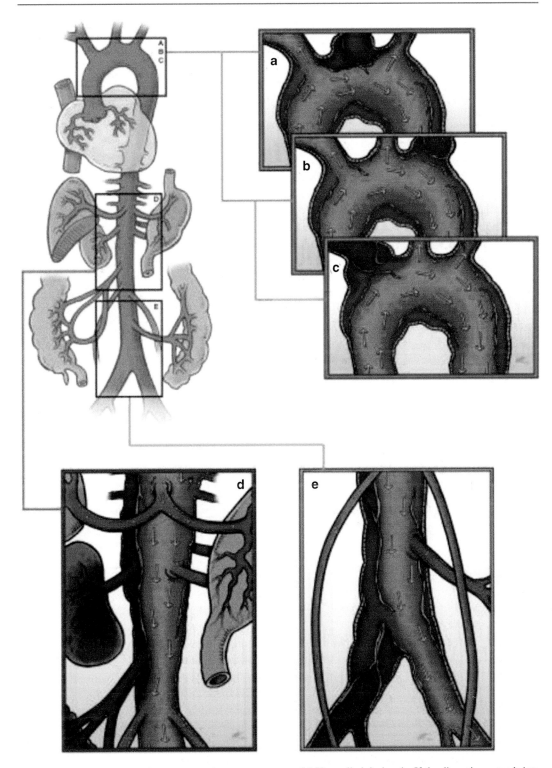

Fig. 9.3 Malperfusion syndromes secondary to acute type-A aortic dissection. Dissection involvement of the arch vessels may result in (**a**) cerebral, (**b**) Spinal chord, or (**c**) Upper limb ischemia. If the dissection extends into the abdomen and beyond there may also be (**d**) Visceral; or (**e**) Lower limb ischemia

may indicate cerebral or spinal cord malperfusion. Tachycardia, distended jugular veins, exaggerated pulsus paradoxus, diastolic murmur, rales, or diminished heart sounds are findings that may indicate pericardial tamponade or congestive heart failure from acute aortic regurgitation or myocardial ischemia. Abdominal tenderness or oliguria may indicate visceral ischemia with renal malperfusion although chronic renal dysfunction and contrast-induced nephropathy are commonly associated with ATAAD. Pulse deficits or pale, cool, and painful limbs indicate limb malperfusion. The CT angiogram, ECG, chest radiograph, laboratory tests (such as elevated troponin, creatinine or lactate), bedside transthoracic echocardiography, and point-of-care ultrasound assessment of carotid and peripheral arteries can all assist in identifying the presence and severity of dissection-related complications (Table 9.1).

Table 9.1 Preoperative testing for major thoracic aortic operations

Test	Clinically relevant findings
Computed tomographic angiography (CTA)	Aneurysm location
	Aneurysm size
	Aortic dissection
	Location of intimal tears
	Extent of disease
	Location and patency of aortic branch vessels
	Pericardial effusion or hemopericardium
	Pleural effusion or hemothorax
	Compression of mediastinal structures
Echocardiography including transesophageal echocardiography (TEE)	Aortic dissection
	Location of intimal tears
	Aneurysm size
	Aortic regurgitation
	Ventricular function
	Cardiac tamponade
	Valvular heart disease
Chest roentgenogram (CXR)	Pleural effusion
	Pulmonary edema
	Lung disease
	Widened mediastinum
Cardiac catheterization	Coronary artery disease
Carotid Duplex	Carotid artery disease
	Dissection involving the carotid arteries

Imaging Considerations for Aortic Surgery

Surgical diseases of the thoracic aorta are primarily structural problems so preoperative imaging studies are important for diagnosis, determining the anatomic location and extent of disease, surgical planning, and assessing the potential for complications (Table 9.1).

Computed tomography angiography (CTA), magnetic resonance angiography (MRA), or echocardiography can all be used to diagnose thoracic aortic diseases, with CTA being the most available and frequently used initial diagnostic technique, particularly in the emergency setting [7]. The widespread availability of cardiac-gated CTA has improved the diagnostic accuracy of CTA imaging for the detection of aortic dissection. CTA and MRA will provide precise information on aneurysm size, location, and its proximity to the aortic arch. CTA will also demonstrate anatomic variants such as bovine aortic arch or an aberrant origin of the left vertebral artery off the aortic arch that is important for planning a perfusion strategy. If a dedicated CTA or MRA of the head is performed, it can provide information on pre-existing cerebrovascular disease, stroke, the presence of dissection or thrombus in the aortic arch branch vessels, and patency of the Circle of Willis. In the assessment of aneurysmal disease one should examine imaging for any features of mediastinal mass effect causing compression of the right ventricular outflow track, trachea, right pulmonary artery, or left mainstem bronchus (Fig. 9.4) [7–11].

In the setting of ATAAD, imaging will provide vital information regarding the extent of the dissection, presence of distal re-entry tears, identification of which organs are perfused from the true- or false-lumens together with radiographic evidence of malperfusion. Additional information provided by imaging studies include coronary calcification that may indicate significant coronary artery disease, left ventricular hypertrophy indicating pre-existing hypertension, pericardial effusion that may cause cardiac tamponade, and pulmonary congestion indicating heart failure.

Fig. 9.4 Giant ASC AO
Aneurysm.
*Intraoperative
transesophageal
echocardiographic
(TEE) image of the
ascending aorta (Ao) in
short-axis in a patient
with a 9.0 cm diameter
ascending aortic
aneurysm causing a
mediastinal mass effect
and compression of the
right pulmonary artery
(RPA)*

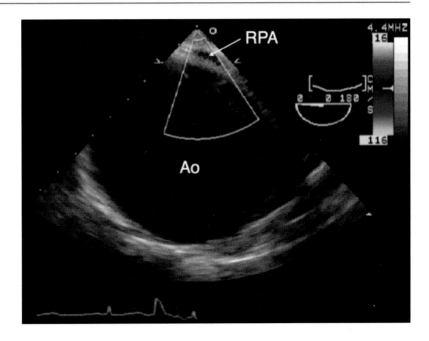

Considerations for Neuroprotection

Pathophysiology of Brain Injury and Rationale for Hypothermia

The human brain is exquisitely sensitive to ischemia, receives approximately 20% of total cardiac output and uses 50% of the body's glucose requirements [12]. By measuring cerebral metabolism in canines using electroencephalography (EEG), it was determined that 60% of the brain's energy needs are for generating and transmitting electrical impulses. The remaining 40% is for processes that maintain cellular integrity [13]. When blood supply is compromised, the brain becomes ischemic and neuronal electrical activity decreases. Under normothermic conditions, the brain manifests EEG evidence of ischemic dysfunction with 60 seconds after the interruption of blood flow. Irreversible ischemic injury occurs at 4–5 min after the interruption of blood flow upon activation of a complex cascade of pathways resulting in neuronal damage, necrosis and apoptosis. This cascade can be summarized by three main steps: (1) the consequences of oxygen and glucose deprivation, (2) inability to remove toxic cellular waste products and (3) reperfusion injury once blood flow resumes (Table 9.2) [14–16]. Intracellular acidosis, inflammation,

Table 9.2 Metabolic, cellular, and biochemical events leading to neuronal injury in response to ischemia

STEP 1: $CBF < CMR_{GLC} + CMRO_2$
ATP deficit
Failure of Na^+/K^+-ATPase pump
Accumulation of intracellular Na^+ and Ca^{2+}
Excessive cell depolarization
STEP 2: Continued lack of CBF
Additional release of Ca^{2+}
Elevated intracellular levels of glutamate
Intracellular acidosis
Protein degradation
Free fatty acid and free radical formation
Inflammatory pathways activated
Immune system activated
Disruption of blood: Brain barrier
Alteration of genetic transcription and translation
STEP 3: Reperfusion
Increased free radicals
Escalation of inflammatory pathways
Excessive nitric oxide
Tissue edema
Hyperthermic injury

Summary of the mechanisms of neuronal injury from ischemia
ATP adenosine triphosphate, *Ca2+* calcium, *CBF* cerebral blood flow, CMR_{GLC} cerebral metabolic rate of glucose utilization, $CMRO_2$ cerebral metabolic rate of oxygen utilization, *K+* potassium, *Na+* sodium, *Na+/K+-ATPase* sodium-potassium adenosine triphosphatase

immune activation, calcium, glutamate, enzyme activation and free radicals all play important roles [17, 18]

In 1950, Bigelow hypothesized that deliberate hypothermia could be used to extend the scope of operations by decreasing the oxygen requirements of tissues and allowing organs to be temporarily excluded from the circulation [19]. The primary neuroprotective action of deliberate hypothermia was believed to be due to the reduction in cellular metabolic activity and a proportional increase in ischemic tolerance. In response to hypothermia, energy demands are suppressed leading to a relative energy surplus [20]. Temperature dependent metabolic rate reduction can be quantified by the temperature coefficient Q_{10}, defined as the ratio between two measured rates of metabolism at a temperature difference of 10 °C [21]. Humans have a Q_{10} ratio of 2.3 based on measurements of cerebral metabolic oxygen consumption that can be used to estimate a "safe" duration of ischemia in relation to temperature in response to deliberate hypothermia [22]. Clinical experience has demonstrated the effectiveness of deliberate hypothermia for cerebral protection. The relationship between body temperature and the corresponding projected ischemic tolerance has been endorsed by an international group of cardiothoracic surgeons specializing in aortic surgery (Fig. 9.5) [23].

It should be emphasized that the ischemic tolerance of the brain represents an estimate, does not necessarily guarantee protection against ischemic neuronal injury, and that individual variability may exist. Furthermore, it should be recognized that brain temperature cannot be measured directly. In addition to metabolic suppression, hypothermia likely provides additional protection by mitigating many of the injurious processes that occur once ischemia is triggered [24–27]. Brain energetics, oxygen consumption and normalization of tissue pH occurs faster following an ischemic period in the presence of hypothermia [28–30]. Finally, hypothermia may also attenuate reperfusion injury by attenuating post-ischemic hyperperfusion, blood-brain barrier disruption, and edema [31].

Pharmacologic Neuroprotection

A wide array of adjunct pharmacologic neuroprotective adjuncts has been studied and are routinely used to supplement the protective effects of hypothermia [32]. In general, the putative pharmacologic actions parallel the neuroprotective mechanisms of hypothermia: to reduce cerebral cellular metabolic rate or to attenuate the injuri-

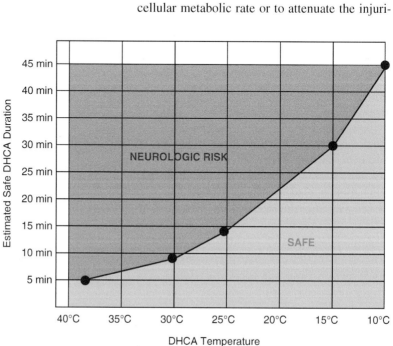

Fig. 9.5 Summary of temperature-based reduction of cerebral metabolism and estimated "safe-times" for circulatory arrest

ous pathways that are initiated following ischemic injury. Agents that have been used include barbiturates, volatile anesthetic agents, propofol, benzodiazepines, N-methyl-D-aspartate (NMDA) antagonists, corticosteroids, calcium channel and sodium channel blockers [14, 33]. In general, although many of these agents have beneficial effects in experimental studies, no high level evidence supports their efficacy in humans [14]. Furthermore, it is important to recognize that pharmacologic-induced neuro suppression should not be considered the equivalent of hypothermia-induced neuroprotection even though they may have similar effects on the electrical activity of the brain.

Hypothermic Circulatory Arrest Techniques for Open Aortic Arch Surgery

Hypothermia has been the mainstay of neurologic and organ protection in aortic arch surgery for decades. The first successful aortic arch replacement employed deep hypothermic circulatory arrest (DHCA) delivered with extracorporeal circulation [34]. Surface cooling by packing the body and head in ice has been successfully employed for DHCA, but the use of CPB is more efficient, reliable, and provides a greater margin of safety [35]. Packing the head in ice for DHCA continues to be performed in many centers, but its effectiveness for cooling or maintaining brain hypothermia varies depending on the quality of ice and technique that is used because of the thermo-insulating properties of the skull and soft tissues [36, 37]. A major limitation of DHCA is that the safe duration of DHCA appears to be less than 45 min even though clinical series have reported successful outcomes after DHCA times of greater than 45 min. At DHCA durations beyond 45 min, the incidence of complications such as postoperative seizures, transient neurologic deficits, and stroke increase [38–41]. The 45-min safe duration of DHCA also corresponds to experimental evidence of neuronal injury after 30–60 min of DHCA [42]. Retrograde cerebral perfusion (RCP) was developed to increase the

safe duration of DHCA. Though it has been shown that RCP does not provide adequate blood flow to prevent cerebral ischemia, it may still be beneficial for increasing the safe duration of DHCA, maintaining cerebral hypothermia and decreasing the risk of thromboembolism upon the restoration of antegrade perfusion. RCP is performed by snaring the superior vena cava cannula between the right atrium and the azygous vein then perfusing the superior vena cava cannula with cold oxygenated blood at a rate of 150–250 ml/min (Fig. 9.6).

During RCP, the superior vena cava pressure is monitored and kept less than 25–30 mm Hg to prevent cerebral edema. The patient is maintained in a 10° Trendelenburg position to decrease the risk of cerebral air embolism into the open aortic arch. During RCP, blood perfused into the superior vena cava can be observed to flow out of the open ends of the aortic arch branch vessels. The clinical advantage of DHCA with or without RCP is it is a simple technique that does not require cannulation or instrumentation of aortic arch vessels and may decrease the risk of thromboembolic stroke. The clinical efficacy of DHCA used alone or in combination with RCP is well established for aortic arch operations [43–46].

The optimal temperature for DHCA remains to be established and temperatures that have been reported for the conduct of DHCA in clinical series have ranged from 12 to 25 °C. Because brain temperature cannot be measured directly, and individual variability may exist on the rate and uniformity of brain cooling, several studies have used EEG criteria as a physiologic surrogate for cerebral metabolic suppression as an endpoint for the initiation of DHCA. The application of clinical protocols to ensure the achievement of temperatures that produce electrocortical silence in an effort to provide uniform conditions for DHCA have been shown to generate consistent clinical outcomes [47–49]. Although lower temperatures may be advantageous for providing a greater and more uniform degree of cerebral metabolic suppression, the incremental advantages of achieving a temperature associated with electrocortical silence for DHCA is not known. The use of lower temperatures for DHCA shifts the

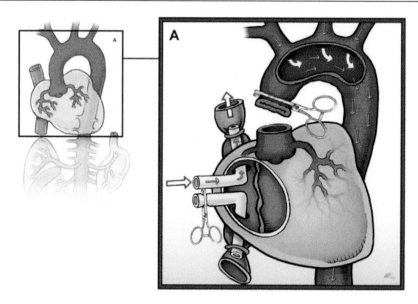

Fig. 9.6 CPB circuit for RCP. Retrograde cerebral perfusion can be provided by modifying the cardiopulmonary bypass circuit. After the initiation of deep hypothermic circulatory arrest a bridge is made between the arterial and superior vena cava venous cannulae and a snare is placed around the superior vena cava cannula (**a**). The inferior vena cava cannula is then clamped, and the arterial-venous bridge is opened to infuse cold oxygenated blood via the superior vena cava. Retrograde blood flow from the aortic arch branch vessels may be observed

oxygen-hemoglobin dissociation curve to the left and increases the risks associated with cardiopulmonary bypass by increasing the duration of cardiopulmonary bypass necessary to cool and rewarm the patient. Finally, few centers have the resources to provide routine intraoperative EEG monitoring for thoracic aortic operations.

Selective antegrade perfusion (SACP) refers to intraoperative neurocirculatory techniques to provide full or partial antegrade cerebral arterial blood flow during open aortic or arch operations. SACP was initially developed for procedures where the anticipated circulatory arrest time exceeded the safe duration of DHCA. In contemporary practice, the general trend has been towards the increased use of SACP for ascending aorta and arch operations [50]. This change in practice reflects new surgical techniques to safely deliver SACP, increased experience with the use of SACP for aortic arch reconstruction, and the added margin of safety SACP provides for operations that take longer than 30 min to complete [51]. There are a wide variety of approaches described to perform SACP, but in general they can be grouped into two categories: (1) unilateral SACP or (2) bilateral SACP (Fig. 9.7).

Unilateral SACP is the most common neurocirculatory strategy used for aortic arch procedures [50]. Unilateral SACP is performed by perfusion via the right axillary artery while the base of the innominate artery is clamped or by direct cannulation of the innominate artery itself. Oxygenated blood is then directed into the right carotid and vertebral arteries, typically at a flow rate of 5–7 ml/kg/min and a pressure of 60–70 mm Hg measured in the ipsilateral radial artery. Blood flow to the contralateral side of the brain is provided by collateral circulation via the circle of Willis. The base of the left carotid artery and the left subclavian artery can also be clamped during unilateral SACP to prevent vascular steal. Because up to 15% of patients may not have a patent circle of Willis, bilateral SACP may be necessary to ensure global perfusion of the brain. Bilateral SACP is achieved during unilateral SACP by placing an additional perfusion cannula into the left carotid artery. Bilateral SACP can also be performed by direct cannulation of innominate, left carotid, and subclavian arteries in the open aortic arch. The advantages of SACP include the ability to precisely control blood flow, perfusion pressure, and perfusate temperature to

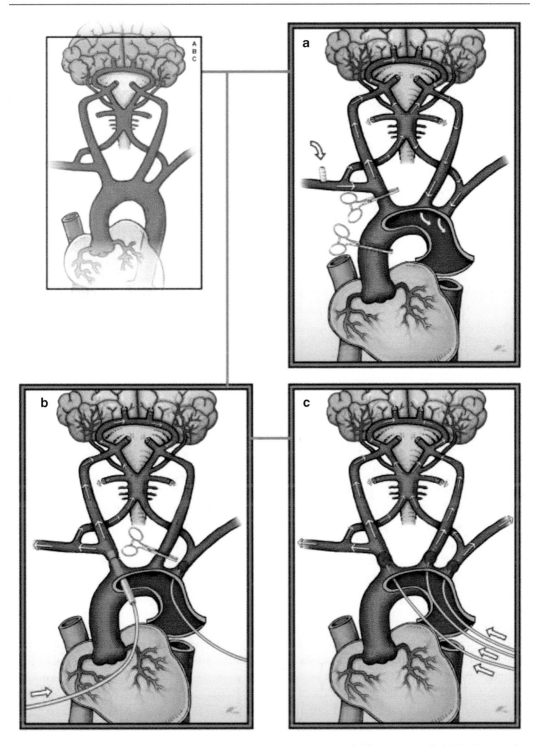

Fig. 9.7 Examples of techniques for selective antegrade perfusion (SACP). (**a**) Unilateral ACP (uACP) via a graft sewn onto the right axillary artery. The innominate artery is clamped. Blood flow is delivered through the right common and right vertebral arteries. Retrograde blood is seen exiting the left common carotid and left subclavian arteries. (**b**) Direct cannulation of the innominate artery provides uACP with the same blood flow pattern as in (**a**). In this example a clamp has been placed on the left carotid and an occlusive balloon placed in the left subclavian artery, both options which may be used to minimize retrograde steal. (**c**) Bilateral ACP (bACP) with balloon-tipped cannulae placed in the innominate, left common carotid, and left subclavian arteries. Fully physiologic blood flow is delivered to the brain

the brain. SACP can provide full metabolic substrate delivery to the brain to prevent ischemia. The operative time thus becomes limited by the "lower body circulatory arrest-time" that can tolerate a longer duration of ischemia.

SACP can be performed in a variety of ways and controversies pertaining to its conduct include defining the maximum safe systemic temperature for operations, the optimal temperature of the cerebral perfusate, the need for bilateral SACP, and the safe duration of SACP. In one systematic review, the core temperature of patients undergoing SACP ranged from 16 to 25.6 °C, although many centers have moved towards even warmer temperatures [43]. A recent large clinical series suggested that moderate hypothermia in the range of 24–28 °C had a similar degree of safety compared to patients managed at lower temperatures in the range of 20–23.9 °C when SACP was used [52]. Another clinical series also suggested that moderate hypothermia afforded adequate ischemic protection for visceral organs during SACP in the absence of distal aortic perfusion [53]. In contrast, a recent meta-analysis examining unilateral versus bilateral SACP for aortic surgery in 5100 patients found no differences in outcome among patients who received unilateral vs. bilateral SACP, but found a significant correlation between postoperative mortality with the temperature or duration of circulatory arrest [54]. Although the analysis did not factor in the temperature of the cerebral perfusate in the individual studies, the findings suggest that deliberate hypothermia remains an important adjunct for cerebral and lower body organ protection when SACP is used, particularly when the duration of circulatory arrest is prolonged. Although existing studies have not demonstrated differences in outcome between the use of unilateral and bilateral SACP, the decision to use bilateral SACP may be made based on the anticipated duration of the operation, the complexity of the operation, or the presence of asymmetry in the cerebral oximetry rSO_2 values during unilateral SACP indicating reduced cerebral perfusion to the contralateral cerebral hemisphere. Although it is generally believed that SACP affords a greater degree of safety for operations

that require a greater duration of circulatory arrest, there is limited data available to support this rationale. The risks associated with SACP include the need to access the axillary artery or the aortic arch branch vessels, the need to instrument or cross-clamp the aortic arch branch vessels, and the potential for arterial embolization.

Published retrospective studies comparing outcomes with SACP to DHCA in combination with RCP have generally demonstrated shorter CPB and operating room times with SACP. Select publications have also found that SACP may decrease mortality, the risk of bleeding, and the incidence of neurologic complications [40, 55–59]. However, when all available studies were systematically incorporated into a meta-analysis, there was a failure to reproduce any of the neurologic or mortality benefits of SACP [43, 60]. Further prospective research will be required to determine conclusively if there is an advantage of any specific technique, particularly since there is considerable variation in current practice amongst institutions. The American College of Cardiology Foundation and American Heart Association Guidelines on the management of patients with thoracic aortic diseases published in 2010 recommended that a brain protection strategy should be a key element of the surgical, anesthetic, and perfusion techniques for ascending aorta and arch repairs, but the recommendation was qualified with the statement that institutional experience and preferences were important factors in selecting a specific technique for clinical use [61].

Re-warming

In contrast to the debate over neurocirculatory techniques and optimum circulatory arrest temperatures, one area of general agreement is on the importance of preventing cerebral hyperthermia during the re-warming phase [62]. Once circulation is restored, the brain will go through a transient period of hyperperfusion [63]. In addition to the risk of thromboembolism and cerebral edema, the re-warming period coincides with reperfusion which may trigger injury pathways. Even mild hyperthermia may cause or worsen brain injury during reperfusion [64, 65]. During the re-warming phase, extracranial temperature monitoring sites may underestimate brain temperature by several degrees [66]. It is for these reasons that a 2015 set of guidelines, endorsed by multiple societies, has emphasized the importance of strictly controlling the rate of rewarming and avoiding excessive patient temperatures or temperature gradients between the patient and blood in the CPB circuit [67]. Near infra-red spectroscopy (NIRS), jugular venous bulb oxygen saturation (SJVO$_2$), or EEG monitoring for desaturation or hyperactivity, may be of additional help in determining need for increasing oxygen delivery, slowing the rate of re-warming, or increasing the depth of anesthesia. There may also be a protective benefit to a period of hypothermic reperfusion of the brain prior to initiating rewarming [68].

Systemic Organ Protection

Systemic or distal aortic blood flow is temporarily interrupted during the period of DHCA or SACP. Under this condition, deliberate hypothermia serves also to protect other vital organs such as the kidneys and spinal cord during the period of ischemia. The optimal temperature for systemic organ protection and the safe duration of circulatory arrest for organs besides the brain has not been extensively studied. In general, moderate hypothermia in the range of 25–30 °C appears to be sufficient for providing organ protection during the period of DHCA or SACP [69]. Preoperative hydration or intravenous mannitol are reasonable interventions to preserve renal function in response to hypothermic circulatory arrest, but the administration of furosemide, mannitol, or dopamine for the sole purpose of renal protection has not been justified. Lactic acidosis is common during reperfusion and should be expected after DHCA or SACP with lactate peaking approximately 4–5 h after DHCA and pH normalizing 8–10 h after DHCA [70]. The severity of metabolic acidosis after uncomplicated elective operations performed using DHCA did not correlate with hospital or ICU length of stay, but the administration of sodium bicarbonate to treat metabolic acidosis was associated with postoperative hypernatremia [71].

Intraoperative Monitoring

Invasive Pressure Monitoring

Invasive arterial pressure monitoring is a particularly important consideration in the perioperative management of patients undergoing both emergent and elective aortic arch procedures. The surgical plan regarding cannulation for CPB, use of SACP, and extension or presence of disease involving aortic branch vessels need to be considered when choosing the best site for arterial pressure monitoring. If unilateral SACP via the right axillary or innominate artery is planned, a right radial catheter can be used to measure cerebral perfusion pressure during SACP. However, pressures in the right radial artery may not accurately reflect cerebral or systemic perfusion pressures if the right axillary artery is directly cannulated. In contrast, a right radial artery pressure may overestimate systemic perfusion pressure during CPB if the right axillary artery is perfused through a side-branch graft. Additionally, the right axillary artery is often temporarily occluded to construct a side-branch graft onto the axillary artery. Placement of an additional left radial or femoral artery catheter may be necessary to provide continuous arterial pressure monitoring. In the case of aortic dissection, any clinical or radiographic features of limb malperfusion may impact the choice of site for arterial pressure measurement. An effort should be made to choose a location that will most likely reflect the true central aortic pressure and it is not uncommon in this scenario to require arterial pressure monitoring from multiple sites.

Temperature Monitoring

Continuous temperature monitoring is important during the delivery of deliberate hypothermia on cardiopulmonary bypass, rewarming on cardiopulmonary bypass, and recovery to normothermia after separation from cardiopulmonary bypass. Common monitoring sites include the nasopharynx, esophagus, tympanic membrane, bladder, rectum, pulmonary artery catheter, as well as the

CPB circuit venous return and arterial inflow cannulae. When compared to a thermocouple sensor embedded in the cerebral cortex, all sites of temperature monitoring showed some discrepancy during cooling and re-warming from deep hypothermia. The nasopharynx, pulmonary artery and esophagus provided the most accurate estimation of brain temperature, differing by approximately 1–2 °C during periods of stable temperature and by 2–3 °C during active cooling or warming. The tympanic membrane, bladder, rectum, axilla and skin had a much greater discrepancy with actual brain temperature, differing by up to 9 °C from the brain [72]. The nasopharyngeal temperature is the most commonly used site in reports on studies involving DHCA [66, 73, 74]. Furthermore, clinical experience in patients undergoing DHCA has demonstrated a correlation between nasopharyngeal temperature and hypothermia-induced neurophysiologic events [47, 48]. Other monitoring sites provide different information. The bladder, rectal, and CPB venous return temperatures at the conclusion of re-warming can be used to estimate the final systemic body temperature at thermal equilibrium following separation from CPB.

Neurophysiologic Monitoring

Intraoperative neurophysiologic monitoring has some unique applications in the setting of aortic arch surgery. Although neurophysiologic monitors can be employed as part of a brain protection strategy, its clinical application is contingent on the institutional experience and the availability of equipment and personnel where the operation is being performed. In general, neurophysiologic monitors are particularly useful in aortic arch surgery for one of two main purposes: (1) to track and monitor the expected changes in neurophysiologic activity in response to cooling and rewarming and (2) detection of cerebral malperfusion during SACP (Fig. 9.8). The two most familiar monitoring modalities are electroencephalography (EEG) and near-infrared spectroscopy (NIRS). Somatosensory Evoked Potentials (SSEP), trans-cranial Doppler (TCD), and jugu-

lar venous bulb oxygen saturation are additional modalities that may be used for the same purposes as EEG and NIRS, but there is less available literature on their use.

Intraoperative EEG can detect cerebral hypoperfusion, seizure, or be used to establish an endpoint for DHCA. Cerebral hypoperfusion will appear as a decrease in the amplitude and frequency of the EEG. Deliberate hypothermia causes incremental changes in the EEG that correlate with the reduction of cerebral metabolic rate associated with hypothermia (Figure 9.9) [47]. Assessing temperature-induced changes in the EEG and using electrocortical silence on the EEG as an endpoint for deliberate hypothermia may provide a more consistent and accurate physiologic surrogate of cerebral metabolic suppression for brain protection prior to the initiation of deep hypothermic circulatory arrest. Clinical studies have demonstrated that pre-determined standard nasopharyngeal temperature for all patients will not reliably predict the onset of electrocortical silence or maximum suppression of cerebral metabolic activity (Figure 9.9) [47, 48]. At a nasopharyngeal temperature of 18 °C, a commonly used cooling endpoint, only 50% of patients had electrocortical silence. A temperature of 12.5 °C was necessary to ensure that all individual patients had achieved EEG silence.

Anesthetic agents can affect the EEG independent of cerebral perfusion, temperature, or cerebral metabolic rate. Inhaled anesthetic agents cause a dose-dependent decrease in EEG amplitude and frequency. Intravenous anesthetic agents such as propofol or barbiturates will temporarily suppress EEG activity while narcotic analgesics have minimal effects on the EEG. When intraoperative EEG monitoring is performed to detect cerebral hypoperfusion or to assess suppression of cerebral metabolism during deliberate hypothermia, maintaining the dose of the inhaled anesthetic at a fixed end-tidal concentration and avoiding intravenous bolus administration of propofol or other central nervous system depressant drugs will increase the sensitivity and specificity of EEG for detecting physiologic events or complications corresponding to the conduct of the operation. Anesthetic agents can be safely

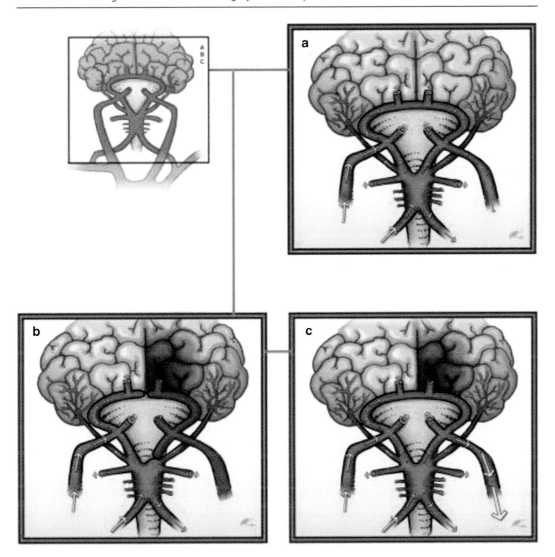

Fig. 9.8 Examples of the clinical utility of neurophysiologic monitoring in aortic arch surgery with uACP. (**a**) In uACP blood is being delivered to the right side of the brain via the right common and right vertebral arteries. After crossing the circle of Willis blood perfuses the left hemisphere. The NIRS and EEG monitors display symmetric regional tissue saturation and electrical activity respectively. (**b**) Due to an abnormal circle of Willis or because of insufficient uACP pressure/flow there is no perfusion to the contralateral hemisphere. This ischemia is detected by the NIRS and EEG monitors. (**c**) Despite a normal circle of Willis and appropriate uACP pressure/flow there is contralateral ischemia due to left carotid steal. The resulting left hemisphere ischemia is again detected by the NIRS and EEG monitors

discontinued at the onset of EEG slowing or burst suppression during deliberate hypothermia to avoid interfering with detecting the onset of electrocortical silence prior to initiating deep hypothermic circulatory arrest.

Commercially available instruments to monitor depth of anesthesia based on processed EEG using proprietary or published algorithms are available for clinical use to guide dosing of anesthetic drugs to decrease the risk of intraoperative awareness or anesthetic overdose [75]. These depth of anesthesia monitors record a limited EEG montage from the prefrontal cortex and may provide a display of the raw EEG, processed EEG, or a numerical value associated with anesthetic-induced EEG suppression. The moni-

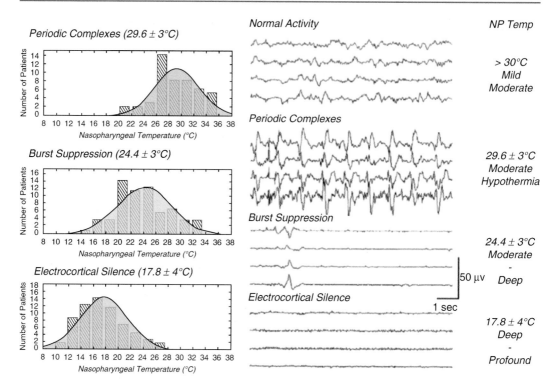

Fig. 9.9 EEG and temperature. Brain temperature cannot be measured directly during deliberate hypothermia on cardiopulmonary bypass. Temperature measured within the nasopharynx (NP) or ear canal near the tympanic membrane are often used as surrogate indicator of brain temperature. Hypothermia produces characteristic changes in the electroencephalogram (EEG) that can also be used as a physiologic surrogate of the suppression of cerebral metabolism in response to deliberate hypothermia. Based on intraoperative EEG monitoring, electrocortical silence occurs at an average NP temperature of 18 °C in adults, but a NP temperature in the range of 12.5 °C is necessary to ensure electrocortical silence in more than 95% of patients. (Adapted from Stecker MM, et al. Ann Thorac Surg 2001;71:14)

tors also incorporate algorithms to exclude artifacts from electrocautery and muscle activity. Because anesthetic-induced EEG changes mimic and follow a similar pattern to hypothermia-induced EEG changes, these monitors are sometimes applied in the setting of thoracic aortic operations to guide cerebral metabolic suppression or detect electrocortical silence during deliberate hypothermia. No direct comparisons have been performed between full montage unprocessed EEG monitoring and depth of anesthesia monitors to detect hypothermia-induced burst suppression or electrocortical silence. One study suggests the two monitoring techniques correlate, where a bispectral index value (BIS) of less than 15 correlated with barbiturate-induced burst suppression on the EEG [76]. However, it is important to recognize that discrepancies among

individual patients may occur because the depth of anesthesia monitors are designed to detect changes produced by anesthetic agents and EEG signals from only a limited region of the cerebral cortex are monitored.

Near infrared spectroscopic cerebral oximetry (NIRS) is a non-invasive technique that permits the continuous monitoring of oxygen saturation in the cerebral cortex in the presence of both pulsatile or non-pulsatile flow. The regional cerebral oxygen saturation value generated (rSO_2) by the instrument is a function of the venous oxygen saturation, arterial oxygen saturation, hemoglobin concentration, and cerebral blood flow from a sample of the first several centimeters of the frontal cortex immediately below the forehead probes. The positioning of dual oximetry probes on either side of the forehead also provides the ability to detect right and left asymmetry that may indicate differences in cerebral blood flow to each side of the brain. The typical pattern of cerebral oxygen saturation during the conduct of deep hypothermic circulatory arrest is an increase in rSO_2 during deliberate hypothermia, a gradual decrease rSO_2 during periods of circulatory arrest, an increase in response to SACP, and recovery during reperfusion. Cerebral oxygen saturation typically increases or remains at baseline during SACP. Decreases in cerebral oxygen saturation may indicate cerebral hypoperfusion, venous hypertension, hypoxemia, hypocarbia, or anemia. Baseline rSO_2 values may vary among individual patients, but a 10–20% decrease in rSO_2 is usually considered to be clinically significant. The clinical application of NIRS does not require specialized institutional expertise and is not affected by anesthetic agents. The specific clinical application of NIRS for aortic arch operations is based on its reported ability to detect cerebral hypoperfusion as a consequence of dissection extending into an aortic arch branch vessel, arterial cannula malposition during SACP, carotid artery graft thrombosis, and Circle of Willis insufficiency during unilateral SACP via the right subclavian artery [77–79].

Intraoperative Transesophageal Echocardiography (TEE) and Ultrasound Imaging

Intraoperative transesophageal echocardiography (TEE) and the application of intraoperative ultrasound imaging has had a major impact on the clinical care of patients undergoing thoracic aortic operations. TEE provides a means to diagnose acute aortic syndromes in emergency situations, to confirm and characterize surgical pathology, to assess myocardial function, to quantify the severity of underlying cardiac disease, to guide cannula placement for cardiopulmonary bypass, and to detect complications associated with aortic dissection. In patients with Stanford type A aortic dissection, TEE can be used to diagnose and quantify the severity of aortic regurgitation, detect the presence of cardiac tamponade, assess ventricular function for suspected coronary artery involvement, characterize the extent of the dissection flap, and characterize the presence and location of intimal tears (Fig. 9.10).

During the initiation of cardiopulmonary bypass, intraoperative TEE can also be used to detect left ventricular distension due to aortic regurgitation. Prior to the separation from cardio-

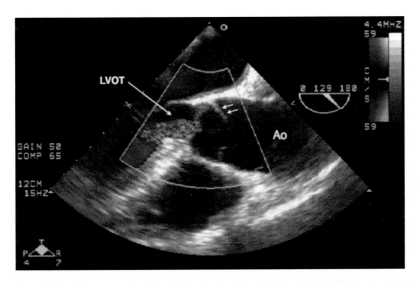

Fig. 9.10 Type A aortic dissection and aortic regurgitation. Intraoperative TEE image of the aortic valve, aortic root, and proximal ascending aorta (Ao) in long-axis with color Doppler flow imaging in diastole demonstrating severe aortic regurgitation in a patient with an acute Stanford type A aortic dissection. The presence of an inti- mal flap in the aortic root (arrows) was diagnostic for a Stanford type A aortic dissection. Severe aortic regurgitation is present as a mosaic regurgitant jet in the left ventricular outflow tract (LVOT) that was caused by acute enlargement of the aortic root by the dissection

pulmonary bypass, intraoperative TEE can be used to detect the presence of trapped air within the cardiac chambers and to detect the presence of aortic regurgitation after aortic valve-sparing operations. Intraoperative ultrasound imaging can also be performed using the same imaging platform to examine the carotid arteries in the neck to detect extension of the dissection into the carotid arteries and to confirm that blood flow in the carotid arteries is not compromised with the initiation of cardiopulmonary bypass or upon application of a cross clamp on the ascending aorta.

In patients with aortic dissection who require direct cannulation of the thoracic aorta or cannulation of the femoral artery for cardiopulmonary bypass, TEE can be used to guide cannula insertion, ensure that the true lumen of the aorta is cannulated, and verify blood flow within the true lumen of the aorta during cardiopulmonary bypass. When using the Seldinger technique for arterial cannulation, TEE is used to confirm that the guide wire is within the true lumen of the dissection before advancing the cannula into the vessel (Figure 9.11).

Definitive criteria do not exist to positively identify the true lumen of the dissected aorta in all patients and some typical features may be misleading. Despite these limitations TEE is often helpful for correctly identifying the true- and false-lumens. The true lumen is typically smaller than the false lumen, is in continuity with the aortic valve, expands during systole, has rounded borders due to the continuity of the intimal layer, and the direction of blood flow through intimal fenestrations is from the true lumen into the false lumen. The false lumen is typically larger than the true lumen, shaped like a crescent with a sharp edge where the intimal flap joins the adventitia, and may contain spontaneous echocardiographic contrast or thrombus. If a CTA is available, referencing the echocardiographic images to the CTA images is also useful to assist in identifying the true and false lumens of the aortic dissection.

In the presence of aortic regurgitation, left ventricular distention can occur following the onset of asystole but before aortic cross clamping during deliberate hypothermia on cardiopulmonary bypass. TEE imaging of the left ventricle during hypothermia together with monitoring the pulmonary artery pressure can be used to detect left ventricular distension. Similarly, TEE can also be used to detect left ventricular distension prior to ventricular contraction after the removal of the aortic cross clamp during rewarming on cardiopulmonary bypass. Finally, TEE can be used to detect and guide the removal of intracavitary air within the cardiac chambers and the aorta during reperfusion, as well as detect endo-leaks if a concurrent endovascular technique has been employed [80, 81].

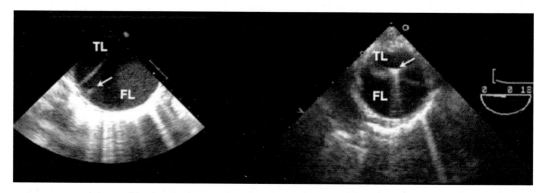

Fig. 9.11 Intraoperative TEE can be used to guide aortic cannulation for cardiopulmonary bypass in patients with aortic dissection to ensure that the true lumen of the aorta is cannulated. TEE short-axis image of the aortic arch (left panel) showed that the arterial guide wire (arrow) was inadvertently inserted into the false lumen of the aortic dissection (FL). TEE short-axis image of the descending thoracic aorta in another patient with an acute aortic dissection (right panel) showed proper position of the arterial guide wire in the true lumen (TL) of the aortic dissection

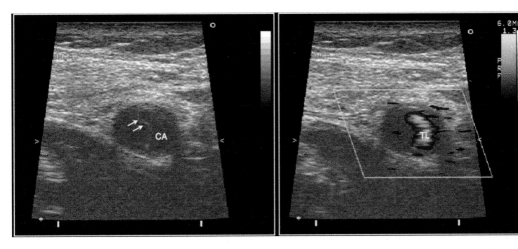

Fig. 9.12 Carotid dissection. Intraoperative Duplex ultrasound imaging of the right common carotid artery in short-axis in a patient with an acute Stanford type A aortic dissection demonstrating dissection extending into the right common carotid artery as evidenced by the presence of an intimal flap within the vessel (arrow, left panel). Doppler flow imaging during cardiopulmonary bypass was used to confirm blood flow within the true lumen (TL) of the carotid artery dissection

The carotid artery can be imaged by ultrasound with a surface ultrasound transducer placed on the neck and color Doppler flow imaging can be used to assess blood flow in the vessel. Dissection extending into the carotid arteries can usually be diagnosed by imaging a thin intimal flap within the carotid artery and observing reduced or absent blood flow in the false lumen (Figure 9.12).

Intraoperative imaging of the carotid arteries during thoracic aortic operations is useful for detecting cerebral malperfusion caused by dissection involving or extending into the branch vessels of the aortic arch, inadvertent placement of the arterial cannula in the false lumen of the dissection, occlusion of the aortic arch branch vessels by the intimal flap, or arterial cannula malposition. The risk of cerebral malperfusion is greatest during the initiation of cardiopulmonary bypass, application of the aortic cross clamp, and during selective antegrade cerebral perfusion by direct cannulation of the aortic arch branch vessels.

Postoperative Complications

Neurologic

Postoperative neurologic complications include stroke, encephalopathy, delirium, neurocognitive dysfunction, spinal cord ischemia, and peripheral nerve injuries. The incidence of stroke ranges between 3 and 10% depending on pre-existing risk factors and on the whether the operation is elective or emergent [52, 60, 62]. Postoperative stroke manifests as a focal neurologic deficit that is most commonly the consequence of thrombo-embolism. Pre-existing cerebrovascular disease or perioperative hypoperfusion may contribute to the severity of the ischemic infarct. Postoperative brain imaging should be performed when stroke is suspected to confirm the diagnosis, characterize the location of injury, and to detect intracranial hemorrhage or cerebral edema. Augmenting the arterial pressure immediately after stroke in the absence of hemorrhagic transformation or cerebral edema may be effective for limiting the size of the infarct.

Global brain ischemia from hypoperfusion or circulatory arrest may manifest as encephalopathy, delirium, neurocognitive dysfunction, or a transient neurologic deficit. Anoxic encephalopathy is a likely contributor to postoperative encephalopathy, but its etiology may be multifactorial. The incidence of transient neurologic deficits ranges from 2.5 to 10% [52, 60]. Severe anoxic encephalopathy may manifest as postoperative seizures, coma, or myoclonus. There is no specific therapy for postoperative encephalopathy or delirium except for supportive care with the anticipation that full or partial recovery will occur over time. Delirium often improves over time, but may require treatment with antipsychotic drugs such as haloperidol or quetiapine to facilitate patient care and to treat symptoms. If seizures or myoclonus is present, EEG should be performed for diagnosis and anticonvulsants prescribed according to recommendations from a neurologist.

Spinal cord ischemia is rare after isolated thoracic aortic and aortic arch operations, but is a notable complication of thoracoabdominal aortic operations. Paraplegia from spinal cord ischemia may also complicate extended arch or frozen elephant trunk procedures for the repair of type A aortic dissection [82–84]. The treatment of spinal cord ischemia is directed at increasing the arterial pressure together with reducing the central venous and lumbar cerebrospinal fluid pressure to improve spinal cord perfusion pressure [85]. The treatment of spinal cord ischemia is most effective when treatment is initiated immediately upon the first signs of lower extremity weakness.

Peripheral nerve injuries may occur as a consequence of surgical traction at vascular access sites and typically improves over time with conservative management. Operations involving the distal aortic arch are associated with a risk of injury to the recurrent laryngeal nerve that may cause hoarseness or vocal cord paralysis. Injuries to the phrenic nerve may contribute to postoperative respiratory failure caused by diaphragmatic paralysis.

Bleeding

One of the earliest and most challenging issues is postoperative hemorrhage and the establishment of hemostasis. Surgical bleeding at major vascular anastomoses and vascular access sites for cardiopulmonary bypass is potentiated by coagulopathy caused by endothelial injury, from the disease process itself, surgical instrumentation of vessels, the inflammatory responses to CPB, blood loss, hemodilution, the metabolic consequences of circulatory arrest, renal dysfunction, or hypothermia. Antifibrinolytic ther-

apy with aminocaproic acid or tranexamic acid has been proven to be safe and effective in cardiac operations and is routinely administered as prophylactic agents [86, 87]. The initial treatment of coagulopathy is to replace red blood cells and factor deficiencies with fresh frozen plasma, cryoprecipitate, and platelets. If microvascular bleeding persists despite blood product administration and the correction of factor deficiencies, procoagulant agents such as recombinant activated Factor VIIa, anti-inhibitor coagulation complex (FEIBA), or prothrombin complex concentrates are often necessary to achieve hemostasis [88]. Fibrinogen concentrate should also be considered to maintain levels >2.0 g/L. [89, 90] Point of care testing of coagulation function may also be helpful to guide blood product and factor replacement in response to refractory hemorrhage [91, 92]. The treatment of perioperative hypertension and the control of arterial pressure with vasopressor and vasodilator therapy are critical to maintain satisfactory organ perfusion without increasing the risk of hemorrhage. Re-exploration for bleeding complications after thoracic aortic operations may be necessary in 3% of elective operations and up to 10% for emergency operations [93]. Complications related to postoperative bleeding include cardiac tamponade, hemothorax, hypovolemia, anemia, thrombocytopenia, dilutional coagulopathy, and transfusion-related acute lung injury (TRALI).

Malperfusion

Postoperative malperfusion, limb ischemia, or mesenteric ischemia may be a consequence of aortic dissection and remain problematic after operative repair. Thromboembolism, technical problems with a vascular anastomosis, or vascular access site complications may also contribute to postoperative complications. Limb ischemia can be assessed by peripheral arterial pulses and the presence of cold and mottled extremities with delayed capillary refill. Mesenteric ischemia can be assessed by tenderness on the abdominal exam and progressive worsening metabolic acidosis beyond 6–8 h after operation accompanied by an increasing lactate concentration. If the diagnosis of limb ischemia is delayed or if the patient had preoperative malperfusion on presentation, reperfusion after operative repair can cause hyperkalemia, rhabdomyolysis, or compartment syndrome in the affected extremity.

Renal Injury

Acute kidney injury or postoperative renal failure may be a consequence of renal malperfusion, pre-existing renal disease, thromboembolism, or radiographic contrast nephropathy. Circulatory arrest and hypotension during the course of operation may contribute to postoperative renal dysfunction as a consequence of visceral ischemia. Risk factors for postoperative renal injury include advanced age, peripheral vascular disease, chronic renal disease, and recent exposure to radiographic contrast agents. Postoperative renal dysfunction combined with reperfusion may cause hyperkalemia. Insulin therapy to treat hyperglycemia may contribute to hypokalemia. Sodium bicarbonate administration to treat metabolic acidosis may contribute to hypernatremia [71].

References

1. Augoustides JG, Geirsson A, Szeto WY, Walsh EK, Cornelius B, Pochettino A, Bavaria JE. Observational study of mortality risk stratification by ischemic presentation in patients with acute type a aortic dissection: the Penn classification. Nat Clin Pract Cardiovasc Med. 2009;6:140–6.
2. Geirsson A, Szeto WY, Pochettino A, McGarvey ML, Keane MG, Woo YJ, Augoustides JG, Bavaria JE. Significance of malperfusion syndromes prior to contemporary surgical repair for acute type a dissection: outcomes and need for additional revascularizations. Eur J Cardiothorac Surg. 2007;32:255–62.
3. Mehta RH, Suzuki T, Hagan PG, Bossone E, Gilon D, Llovet A, Maroto LC, Cooper JV, Smith DE, Armstrong WF, Nienaber CA, Eagle KA, International Registry of Acute Aortic Dissection (IRAD) Investigators. Predicting death in patients with acute type a aortic dissection. Circulation. 2002;105:200–6.
4. Immer FF, Grobety V, Lauten A, Carrel TP. Does malperfusion syndrome affect early and mid-term outcome in patients suffering from acute type a aorticdissection? Interact Cardiovasc Thorac Surg. 2006;5:187–90.
5. Czerny M, Schoenhoff F, Etz C, et al. The impact of pre-operative Malperfusion on outcome in acute type a aortic dissection: results from the GERAADA registry. J Am Coll Cardiol. 2015;65:2628–35.
6. Goldberg JB, Lansman SL, Kai M, et al. Malperfusion in type a dissection: consider reperfusion first. Semin Thorac Cardiovasc Surg. 2017;29:181–5.
7. Pape LA, Awais M, Elise M, Woznicki EM, et al. Presentation, diagnosis, and outcomes of acute aortic dissection 17-year trends from the international registry of acute aortic dissection. J Am Coll Cardiol. 2015;66:350–8.
8. Kimitoshi N, et al. Severe tracheal compression caused by false aneurysm arising from the ascending aorta: successful airway management using induced hypotension and bronchoscopy. Anesthesiology. 1990;73:1073.
9. MacGillivray RG. Tracheal compression caused by aneurysms of the arotic arch. Anaesthesia. 1985;40:270.
10. Kutchner WL, et al. Occlusion of the right pulmonary artery by and acute dissecting aneurysm. Crit Care Med. 1988;16:564–5.
11. Downey RJ, et al. Right ventricular obstruction in aortic dissection: a mechanism of hemodynamic collapse. Ann Thorac Surg. 1996;61:988–90.
12. Lord LD, Expert P, Huckins JF, et al. Cerebral energy metabolism and the brain's functional network architecture: an integrative review. J Cereb Blood Flow Metab. 2013;33:1347–54.
13. Michenfelder JD. The interdependency of cerebral functional and metabolic effects following massive doses of thiopental in the dog. Anesthesiology. 1974;41:231–6.
14. Conlon N, Grocott HP, Mackensen G. Neuroprotection during cardiac surgery. Expert Rev Cardiovasc Ther. 2008;6:503–20.
15. Erecinska M, Silver IA. Tissue oxygen tension and brain sensitivity to hypoxia. Respir Physiol. 2001;128:263–76.
16. Sims NR, Muyderman H. Mitochondria, oxidative metabolism and cell death in stroke. Biochim Biophys Acta. 2010;1802:80–91.
17. Hou ST, MacManus JP. Molecular mechanisms of cerebral ischemia-induced neuronal death. Int Rev Cytol. 2002;221:93–148.
18. Nakka VP, Gusain A, Mehta SL, et al. Molecular mechanisms of apoptosis in cerebral ischemia: multiple neuroprotective opportunities. Mol Neurobiol. 2008;37:7–38.
19. Bigelow WG, Lindsay WK, Greenwood WF. Hypothermia. Its possible role in cardiac surgery: an investigation of factors governing survival in dogs at low body temperatures. Ann Surg. 1950;132:849–66.
20. Erecinska M, Thoresen M, Silver IA. Effects of hypothermia on energy metabolism in mammalian

central nervous system. J Cereb Blood Flow Metab. 2003;23:513–30.

21. Michenfelder JD, Milder JH. The relationship among canine brain temperature, metabolism, and function during hypothermia. Anesthesiology. 1991;75:130–6.

22. McCullough JN, Zhang N, Reich DL, Juvonen TS, Klein JJ, Spielvogel D, Ergin MA, Griepp RB. Cerebral metabolic suppression during hypothermic circulatory arrest in humans. Ann Thorac Surg. 1999;67:1895–9.

23. Yan TD, Bannon PG, Bavaria J, et al. Consensus on hypothermia in aortic arch surgery. Ann Cardiothorac Surg. 2013;2:163–8.

24. Bickler PE, Buck LT, Hansen BM. Effects of isoflurane and hypothermia on glutamate receptor-mediated calcium influx in brain slices. Anesthesiology. 1994;81:1461–9.

25. Busto R, Globus M, Dietrich W, et al. Effect of mild hypothermia on ischemia-induced release of neurotransmitters and free fatty acids in rat brain. Stroke. 1989;20:904–10.

26. Globus M, Busto R, Lin B, et al. Detection of free radical activity during transient global ischemia and recirculation: effects of intraischemic brain temperature modulation. J Neurochem. 1995;65:1250–6.

27. Popovic R, Liniger R, Bickler PE. Anesthetics and mild hypothermia similarly prevent hippocampal neuron death in an in vitro model of cerebral ischemia. Anesthesiology. 2000;92:1343–9.

28. Aoki M, Nomura F, Stromski ME, et al. Effects of pH on brain energetic after hypothermic circulatory arrest. Ann Thorac Surg. 1993;55:1093–103.

29. Chopp M, Knight R, Tidwell CD, et al. The metabolic effects of mild hypothermia on global cerebral ischemia and recirculation in the cat: comparison to normothermia and hyperthermia. J Cereb Blood Flow Metab. 1989;9:141–8.

30. Conroy BP, Lin CY, Jenkins LW, et al. Hypothermic modulation of cerebral ischemic injury during cardiopulmonary bypass in pigs. Anesthesiology. 1998;88:390–402.

31. Karibe H, Zarow GJ, Graham SH, et al. Mild intraischemic hypothermia reduces postischemic hyperperfusion, delayed postischemic hypoperfusion, blood brain barrier disruption, brain edema and neuronal damage volume after temporary focal cerebral ischemia in rats. J Cereb Blood Flow Metab. 1994;14:620–7.

32. Dewhurst AT, Moore SJ, Liban J. Pharmacological agents as cerebral protectants during deep hypothermic circulatory arrest in adult thoracic aortic surgery. A survey of current practice. Anaesthesia. 2002;57:1016–21.

33. Svyatets M, Tolani K, Zhang M, et al. Perioperative Management of Deep Hypothermic Circulatory Arrest. J Cardiothorac Vasc Anesth. 2010;24:644–55.

34. Griepp RB, et al. Prosthetic replacement of the aortic arch. J Thorac Cardiovasc Surg. 1975;70:1051–63.

35. Guvakov DV, Cheung AT, Weiss SJ, Kalinin NB, Fedorenko NO, Shunkin AV, Lomivorotov VM, Karaskov AM. Effectiveness of forced air warming after pediatric cardiac surgery employing hypothermic circulatory arrest without cardiopulmonary bypass. J Clin Anesthesia. 2000;12:519–24.

36. Grocott HP, Andreiw A. Con: topical head cooling should not be used during deep hypothermic circulatory arrest. J Cardiothorac Vasc Anesth. 2012;26:337–9.

37. Xu X, Tikuisis P, Giesbrecht G. A mathematical model for human brain cooling during cold-water near-drowning. J Appl Physiol (Bethesda, Md: 1985). 1999;86:265–72.

38. Chau KH, Ziganshin BA, Elefteriades JA. Deep hypothermic circulatory arrest: real life suspended animation. Prog Cardiovasc Dis. 2013;56:81–9.

39. Gaynor JW, Nicolson SC, Jarvik GP, Wernovsky G, Montenegro LM, Burnham NB, Hartman DM, Louie A, Spray TL, Clancy RR. Increasing duration of deep hypothermic circulatory arrest is associated with an increased incidence of postoperative electroencephalographic seizures. J Thoracic Cardiovasc Surg. 2005;130:1278–86.

40. Okita Y, Minatoya K, Tagusari O, Ando M, Nagatsuka K, Kitamura S. Prospective comparative study of brain protection in total aortic arch replacement: deep hypothermic circulatory arrest with retrograde cerebral perfusion or selective antegrade cerebral perfusion. Ann Thorac Surg. 2001;72(1):72–9.

41. Fleck TM, Czerny M, Hutschala D, Koinig H, Wolner E, Grabenwoger M. The incidence of transient neurologic dysfunction after ascending aortic replacement with circulatory arrest. Ann Thorac Surg. 2003;76:1198–202.

42. Cheung AT, Bavaria JE, Pochettino A, Weiss SJ, Barclay DK, Stecker MM. Oxygen delivery during retrograde cerebral perfusion in humans. Anesth Analg. 1999;88:8–15.

43. Hu Z, Wang Z, Ren Z, et al. Similar cerebral protective effectiveness of antegrade and retrograde cerebral perfusion combined with deep hypothermia circulatory arrest in arch surgery: a meta-analysis and systematic review of 5060 patients. J Thorac Cardiovasc Surg. 2014;148:544–60.

44. Gega A, Rizzo JA, Johnson MH, et al. Straight deep hypothermic arrest: experience in 394 patients supports its effectiveness as a sole means of brain preservation. Ann Thorac Surg. 2007;84:759–67.

45. Percy A, Widman S, Rizzo JA, et al. Deep hypothermic circulatory arrest in patients with high cognitive needs: full preservation of cognitive abilities. Ann Thorac Surg. 2009;87:117–23.

46. Svensson LG, Crawford ES, Hess KR, et al. Deep hypothermia with circulatory arrest. Determinants of stroke and early mortality in 656 patients. J Thorac Cardiovasc Surg. 1993;106:19–31.

47. Stecker MM, Cheung AT, Pochettino A, Kent G, Patterson T, Weiss SJ, Bavaria JE. Deep hypothermic circulatory arrest: I. Effects of cooling on EEG and evoked potentials. Ann Thorac Surg. 2001;71:14–21.

48. James ML, Andersen ND, Swaminathan M, et al. Predictors of electrocerebral inactivity with deep hypothermia. J Thorac Cardiovasc Surg. 2014;147:1002–7.

49. Appoo JJ, Augoustides JG, Pochettino A, et al. Perioperative outcome in adults undergoing elective deep hypothermic circulatory arrest with retrograde cerebral perfusion in proximal aortic arch repair: evaluation of protocol-based care. J Cardiothorac Vasc Anesth. 2006;20:3–7.

50. De Paulis R, Czerny M, Weltert L, et al. Current trends in cannulation and neuroprotection during surgery of the aortic arch in Europedaggerdouble dagger. Eur J Cardiothorac Surg. 2015;47:917–23.

51. Bachet J. What is the best method for brain protection in surgery of the aortic arch? Selective antegrade cerebral perfusion. Cardiol Clin. 2010;28:389–401.

52. Preventza O, Coselli JS, Garcia A, et al. Moderate hypothermia at warmer temperatures is safe in elective proximal and total arch surgery: results in 665 patients. J Thorac Cardiovasc Surg. 2017;153:1011–8.

53. Pacini D, Pantaleo A, Di Marco L, et al. Visceral organ protection in aortic arch suergery: safety of moderate hypothermia. Eur J Cardiothorac Surg. 2014;46:438–43.

54. Angeloni E, Benedetto U, Takkenberg JJM, et al. Unilateral versus bilateral antegrade cerebral protection during circulatory arrest in aortic surgery: a meta-analysis of 5100 patients. J Thorac Cardiovasc Surg. 2014;147:60–7.

55. Hagl C, Ergin MA, Galla JD, et al. Neurologic outcome after ascending aorta-aortic arch operations: effect of brain protection technique in high-risk patients. J Thorac Cardiovasc Surg. 2001;121:1107–21.

56. Halkos ME, Kerendi F, Myung R, et al. Selective antegrade cerebral perfusion via right axillary artery cannulation reduces morbidity and mortality after proximal aortic surgery. J Thorac Cardiovasc Surg. 2009;2009:1081–9.

57. Misfeld M, Leontyev S, Borger MA, et al. What is the best strategy for brain protection in patients undergoing aortic arch surgery? A single center experience of 636 patients. Ann Thorac Surg. 2012;93:1502–9.

58. Shihata M, Mittal R, Senthilselvan A, et al. Selective antegrade cerebral perfusion during aortic arch surgery confers survival and neuroprotective advantages. J Thorac Cardiovasc Surg. 2011;141:948–52.

59. Vallabhajosyula P, Jassar AS, Menon RS, et al. Moderate versus deep hypothermic circulatory arrest for elective aortic transverse hemiarch reconstruction. Ann Thorac Surg. 2015;99:1511–7.

60. Tian DH, Wan B, Bannon PG, et al. A meta-analysis of deep hypothermic circulatory arrest versus moderate hypothermic circulatory arrest with selective antegrade cerebral perfusion. Ann Cardiothorac Surg. 2013;2:148–58.

61. Hiratzka LF, Bakris GL, Beckman JA, et al. ACCF/AHA/AATS/ACR/ASA/SCA/SCAI/SIR/STS/SVM guidelines for the diagnosis and management of patients with thoracic aortic disease: executive summary. A report of the American College of Cardiology Foundation/American Heart Association Task Force on Practice Guidelines, American Association for Thoracic Surgery, American College of Radiology, American Stroke Association, Society of Cardiovascular Anesthesiologists, Society for Cardiovascular Angiography and Interventions, Society of Interventional Radiology, Society of Thoracic Surgeons, and Society for Vascular Medicine. Circulation. 2010;121(13):e266–369.

62. Grigore AM, Grocott HP, Mathew JP, et al. The rewarming rate and increased peak temperature alter neurocognitive outcome after cardiac surgery. Anesth Analg. 2002;94:4–10.

63. Kawata H, Fackler J, Aoki M, et al. Recovery of cerebral blood flow and energy state in piglets after hypothermic circulatory arrest versus recovery after low-flow bypass. J Thorac Cardiovasc Surg. 1993;106:671–85.

64. Busto R, Dietrich WD, Globus MYT, et al. Small differences in Intraischemic brain temperature critically determine the extent of ischemic neuronal injury. J Cereb Blood Flow Metabol. 1987;7:729–38.

65. Campos F, Blanco M, Barral D, et al. Influence of temperature on ischemic brain: basic and clinical principles. Neurochem Int. 2012;60:495–505.

66. Kaukuntla H, Harrington D, Bilkoo I, et al. Temperature monitoring during cardiopulmonary bypass-do we undercool or overheat the brain? Eur J Cardiothorac Surg. 2004;26:580–5.

67. Engelman R, Baker RA, Likosky DS, et al. The Society of Thoracic Surgeons, the Society of Cardiovascular Anesthesiologists, and the American society of ExtraCorporeal technology: clinical practice guidelines for cardiopulmonary bypass--temperature management during cardiopulmonary bypass. Ann Thorac Surg. 2015;100:748–57.

68. Ehrlich MP, McCullough J, Wolfe D, et al. Cerebral effects of cold reperfusion after hypothermic circulatory arrest. J Thorac Cardiovasc Surg. 2001;121:923–31.

69. Pacini D, Pantaleo A, Di Marco L, et al. Visceral organ protection in aortic arch suergery: safety of moderate hypothermia. Eur J Cardiothorac Surg. 2014;46:438–43.

70. Ghadimi K, Gutsche JT, Setegne SL, et al. Severity and duration of metabolic acidosis after deep hypothermic circulatory arrest for thoracic aortic surgery. J Cardiovasc Thorac Anesthes. 2015;29:1432–40.

71. Ghadimi K, Gutsche JT, Ramakrishna H, et al. Sodium bicarbonate use and the risk of hypernatremia in thoracic aortic surgical patients with metabolic acidosis following deep hypothermic circulatory arrest. Ann Card Anaesth. 2016;19:454–62.

72. Stone GS, Young WL, Smith CR, et al. Do standard monitoring sites reflect true brain temperature when profound hypothermia is rapidly induced and reversed? Anesthesiology. 1995;82:344–51.

73. Akata T, Setoguchi H, Shirozu K, et al. Reliability of temperatures measured at standard monitoring sites as an index of brain temperature during deep hypo-

thermic cardiopulmonary bypass conducted for thoracic aortic reconstruction. J Thorac Cardiovasc Surg. 2007;133:1559–65.
74. Cambonia D, Philippa A, Schebeschb KM, et al. Accuracy of core temperature measurement in deep hypothermic circulatory arrest. Interact Cardiovasc Thorac Surg. 2008;7:922–92.
75. Avidan 2009.
76. Cottonceau V, Petit L, Masson F, et al. The use of bispectral index to monitor barbiturate coma in severely brain-injured patients with refractory intracranial hypertension. Anesth Analg. 2008;107:1676–82.
77. Janelle GM, Mnookin S, Gravenstein N, Martin TD, Urdaneta F. Unilateral cerebral oxygen desaturation during emergent repair of a DeBakey type 1 aortic dissection: potential aversion of a major catastrophe. Anesthesiology. 2002;96:1263–5.
78. Rubio A, Hakami L, Munch F, Tandler R, Harig F, Weyand M. Noninvasive control of adequate cerebral oxygenation during low-flow antegrade selective cerebral perfusion on adults and infants in the aortic arch surgery. J Card Surg. 2008;23:474–9.
79. Santo KC, Barrios A, Dandekar U, Riley P, Guest P, Bonser RS. Near-infrared spectroscopy: an important monitoring tool during hybrid aortic arch replacement. Anesth Analg. 2008;107(3):793–6.
80. Fattori R, Caldarera I, Rapezzi C, et al. Primary endoleakage in endovascular treatment of the thoracic aorta: importance of intraoperative transesophageal echocardiography. J Thorac Cardiovasc Surg. 2000;120:490–5.
81. Rocchi G, Lofiego C, Biagini E, et al. Transesophageal echocardiography-guided algorithm for stent-graft implantation in aortic dissection. J Vasc Surg. 2004;40:880–5.
82. Lin HH, Liao SF, Wu CF, et al. Outcome of frozen elephant trunk technique for acute type a aortic dissection. A systematic review and Meta-analysis. Medicine. 2015;94:e694.
83. Takagi T, Umemoto T, ALICE Group. A meta-analysis of total arch replacement with frozen elephant trunk in type a aortic dissection. Vasc Endovasc Surg. 2016;50:33–46.

84. Katayama K, Uchida N, Katayama A, et al. Multiple factors predict the risk of spinal cord injury after the frozen elephant trunk technique for extended thoracic aortic disease. Eur J Cardiothorac Surg. 2015;47:616–20.
85. Cheung AT, Weiss SJ, McGarvey ML, et al. Interventions for reversing delayed-onset postoperative paraplegia after thoracic aortic reconstruction. Ann Thorac Surg. 2002;74:413–21.
86. Myles PS, Smith JA, Andrew Forbes A, et al. Tranexamic acid in patients undergoing coronary-artery surgery. N Engl J Med. 2017;376:136–48.
87. Brown JR, Birkmeyer NJO, O'Connor GT. Meta-analysis comparing the effectiveness and adverse outcomes of antifibrinolytic agents in cardiac surgery. Circulation. 2007;115:2801–13.
88. Ghadimi K, Levy JH, Welsby IJ. Prothrombin complex concentrates for bleeding in the perioperative setting. Anesth Analg. 2016;122:1287–300.
89. Rahe-Meyer N, Solomon C, Hanke A, et al. Effects of fibrinogen concentrate as first-line therapy during major aortic replacement surgery: a randomized, placebo-controlled trial. Anesthesiology. 2013;118:40–50.
90. Solomon C, Rahe-Meyer N. Fibrinogen concentrate as first-line therapy in aortic surgery reduces transfusion requirements in patients with platelet counts over or under 100×10(9)/L. Blood Transfus = Trasfusione del sangue. 2015;13:248–54.
91. Karkouti K, Callum J, Wijeysundera DN, et al. Point-of-care hemostatic testing in cardiac surgery: a stepped-wedge clustered randomized controlled trial. Circulation. 2016;134:1152–62.
92. Karkouti K, McCluskey SA, Callum J, et al. Evaluation of a novel transfusion algorithm employing point-of-care coagulation assays in cardiac surgery: a retrospective cohort study with interrupted time-series analysis. Anesthesiology. 2015;122:560–70.
93. Achneck HE, Risso JA, Tranquilli M, et al. Safety of thoracic aortic surgery in the present era. Ann Thorac Surg. 2007;84:1180–5.

Anesthetic Management in Open Descending Thoracic Aorta Surgery

10

Sreekanth Cheruku and Amanda Fox

Main Messages

1. Open repair of the descending aorta is performed to repair a spectrum of aortic diseases including aneurysms, penetrating atherosclerotic ulcers, intramural hematomas and aortic dissections

2. Techniques used for descending aorta repair include 'clamp-and-sew,' left heart bypass, partial or complete cardiopulmonary bypass and deep hypothermic circulatory arrest

3. Anesthetic management during open descending aortic repair includes improving surgical exposure, optimizing end-organ perfusion, maintaining hemodynamic stability, monitoring extra-corporeal circulation and correcting coagulopathy

4. Trans-esophageal echocardiography is helpful in confirming the pre-operative diagnosis, evaluating for progression of the known aortic disease and optimizing cardiac preload, afterload and contractility

5. Descending aorta repair is associated with range of complications including stroke, paraplegia, myocardial ischemia, lung injury and renal failure. The incidence of each complication is dependent on the location and extent of the aortic pathology as well as the surgical technique utilized

6. Perioperative strategies to decrease the incidence of paraplegia include the use of lumbar spinal drains to optimize spinal cord perfusion pressure by increasing mean arterial pressure and draining cerebrospinal fluid

S. Cheruku (✉)
Department of Anesthesiology and Pain Management, UT Southwestern Medical Center, Dallas, TX, United States
e-mail: Sreekanth.Cheruku@UTSouthwestern.edu

A. Fox
Department of Anesthesiology and Pain Management, McDermott Center for Human Growth and Development, UT Southwestern Medical Center, Dallas, TX, United States
e-mail: Amanda.Fox@UTSouthwestern.edu

Aneurysmal disease of the thoracic aorta has an incidence of approximately six per 100,000 person-years and contributes disproportionately to morbidity, mortality and cost of healthcare in the United States [1, 2]. About 40% of thoracic aortic aneurysms affect the descending thoracic aorta [1]. The complexity of the descending thoracic aortic pathologies that warrant open surgical repairs in combination with major presenting comorbidities that patients who have thoracic aortic disease frequently have means that this surgical population is at particularly high risk for developing significant postoperative neurologic, pulmonary and cardiovascular complications. These surgeries therefore present unique challenges for the anesthesiologist and the rest of the perioperative care team with regards to mitigating risks and preventing complications.

The descending thoracic aorta is anatomically defined as beginning immediately distal to the origin of the left subclavian artery. These aneurysms can further be localized within the descending thoracic and abdominal aorta and are often characterized using the Crawford classification scheme (Fig. 10.1).

The etiology of aneurysmal disease is thought to begin with the degeneration of connective tissue in the aortic tunica media due to aging, hypertension, or connective tissue disorders or a combination of these. The relationship between atherosclerosis and development of thoracic aortic aneurysms (TAAs) has not been conclusively determined, but the two are frequently known to coexist and share several risk factors [2].

Aortic dissection involves an intimal tear that results in blood flow through the medial layer of the aorta, resulting in separation of the medial layer to create a true and a false lumen within the aorta. A comprehensive natural history study conducted at Yale University revealed that descending TAAs grow more than twice as fast as ascending aortic aneurysms and are significantly more likely to dissect or rupture once they reach a critical dimension [3]. Based on this and other population studies, recent guidelines recommend repairing descending TAAs electively when they measure 5.5–6.0 cm in diameter and to repair at even smaller diameters in patients who have known genetic connective tissue disorders [4, 5]. Intramural hematomas (IMH) and penetrating atherosclerotic ulcers (PAU) are distinct from aneurysmal disease but can also progress to aortic dissection or aortic rupture. IMH results from bleeding from the vasa vasorum into the tunica media without intimal disruption. PAU results from an atherosclerotic plaque that erodes through the layers of the aorta, leading to hematoma formation and rupture.

Open surgical repair of descending TAAs began in the 1950s when Drs. Gross, Swan, Lam

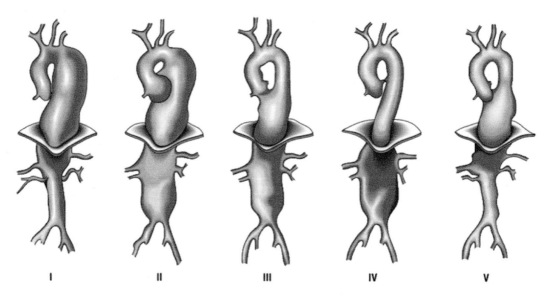

| I | II | III | IV | V |

Fig. 10.1 Crawford classification of thoracoabdominal aneurysms, modified by Safi. Black S.A., Brooks M.J., Wolfe J.H.N. (2007) Thoracoabdominal Aneurysms. In: Liapis C.D., Balzer K., Benedetti-Valentini F., Fernandes e Fernandes J. (eds) Vascular Surgery. European Manual of Medicine. Springer, Berlin, Heidelberg. With Permission of Springer

and Debakey pioneered the techniques of resecting diseased portions of the descending aorta and replacing them with synthetic grafts [6]. Over the next four decades, a variety of techniques were developed to improve upon this general procedure in order to reduce associated complications. These enhancements included utilizing left atrial cannulation with perfusion to the distal aorta, partial cardiopulmonary bypass (CPB) through bifemoral cannulation, and complete cardiopulmonary bypass (CPB) combined with hypothermic circulatory arrest (HCA). The development of endovascular stent-grafts in the 1990s has further decreased the complications associated with descending TAA repair and the 2014 European Society of Cardiology guidelines recommend this as the primary approach in suitable candidates [5]. In patients with familial connective tissue disorders and those with anatomy precluding endovascular repair, open surgical repair can provide a durable therapeutic option.

Perioperative Management

The Preoperative Evaluation

A detailed assessment of preoperative physical condition and associated anesthetic risk is an essential part of perioperative planning for patients presenting for open descending TAA repair. Appropriate surgical candidates require a versatile anesthetic plan that addresses their presenting aortic disease process, coexisting medical conditions and the implications of surgical approach. A thorough history and physical examination should take place before surgery with a focus on cardiovascular, neurologic, pulmonary and renal conditions.

Cardiovascular

Given many overlapping risk factors for coronary artery disease and for development of TAAs, it is not surprising that most patients representing for repair of descending TAAs have a history of hypertension [7] and one-third have concurrent coronary artery disease [7, 8]. A comprehensive evaluation of cardiac function and risk for postoperative adverse cardiovascular events is therefore necessary. An electrocardiogram can provide information about the patient's baseline heart rhythm, new EKG changes, and any pre-existing arrhythmias. Transthoracic echocardiography is useful to evaluate for cardiac ventricular dysfunction and valvular pathology, both of which may influence the perioperative selection of pre-induction monitors and induction agents. Patients who are at increased risk for coronary artery disease may have poor functional capacity and may require pharmacologic stress testing and coronary angiography to evaluate and treat flow limiting coronary artery lesions prior to elective surgery [9].

Pulmonary

A history and physical exam can offer significant insight into the pulmonary status of most patients. For example, wheezing or a persistent cough may signify tracheal compression by the aneurysm, while hemoptysis can indicate communication between the aneurysm and the lungs. Patients with suspected pulmonary disease should undergo pulmonary function testing (PFTs) for risk stratification and to guide post-operative rehabilitation. Poor PFT results can indicate intolerance of one lung ventilation (OLV) and may necessitate cardiopulmonary bypass. Smokers should be counseled to stop at least 4 weeks before the date of surgery and should be referred to smoking cessation resources [10]. Computerized tomography (CT) or magnetic resonance imaging (MRI) is always performed for diagnosis and surgical planning, and the astute anesthesiologist should also evaluate these studies for potential impingement of the aneurysm on airway, esophagus and vascular structures. Impingement on the esophagus may be a relative contraindication to intraoperative monitoring with transesophageal echocardiography (TEE), and in this situation TEE monitoring should be a risk benefit balance weighed by the anesthesiologist—i.e. consider risk for aortic rupture secondary to TEE probe placement and manipulation.

Neurologic

Paraplegia and stroke are recognized as significant complications of descending TAA repair. The possibility of postoperative neurologic injury in the context of patient-specific risk factors should be discussed with the patient and family members. The preoperative exam should focus on establishing a neurologic baseline so that subtle postoperative changes indicative of spinal cord ischemia can be recognized readily. Recurrent laryngeal nerve (RLN) palsy is another complication of either the existence of a large descending TAA or as a consequence of injury during descending TAA repair [11]. Hoarseness or stridor should alert the perioperative physician to consider the possibility of this neurologic complication.

Renal

Preoperative renal insufficiency is an independent predictor of postoperative major morbid events and operative mortality after open surgical descending TAA repair [12]. Preoperative optimization of renal function includes intravenous hydration, minimizing the use of nephrotoxic contrast agents and correction of electrolyte abnormalities. All patients scheduled for open surgical descending TAA repair should undergo a serum chemistry evaluation. In patients with significantly impaired kidney function (e.g. GFR < 30 ml/min), renally cleared medications should be dosed appropriately and nephrotoxic medications should be substituted for alternative agents. The intraoperative mean arterial pressure (MAP) should be maintained above 65 mm Hg and perhaps higher in hypertensive patients to ensure kidney perfusion [13].

Intraoperative Monitors

Selection of hemodynamic monitors placed for intraoperative and postoperative management is influenced by individualized patient and procedural concerns, but hemodynamic monitoring should generally aim to track cardiac function, end organ perfusion and central neurologic function.

Blood Pressure Monitoring

Hemodynamic monitoring is an essential component of goal-directed intraoperative management. Both the aneurysm itself and the introduction of the aortic cross clamp can create zones of differential perfusion pressure along the aorta. Invasive arterial catheters ideally should be placed to measure the blood pressure in each zone (i.e. proximal and distal to the aneurysm and then proximal and distal to the aortic cross-clamp) to best optimize tissue perfusion. The right radial artery is ideally suited to measure blood pressure proximal to the more proximal aortic cross-clamp. Alternatively, a right radial arterial line can also be used to monitor anterograde cerebral blood flow administered via the right axillary artery if this technique is employed in conjunction with deep hypothermic circulatory arrest (DHCA). A second arterial line can be placed in the left radial artery if right axillary cannulation is employed so as to get accurate blood pressure monitoring on cardiopulmonary bypass. A femoral arterial line can be used to measure blood pressure distal to the aortic cross-clamp. It is particularly helpful to employ arterial blood pressure monitoring in both a radial and femoral artery if left heart bypass is utilized, as this will guide degree of bypass in balancing cerebral perfusion with perfusion distal to the aneurysm. The left radial artery is susceptible to inaccurate or redundant blood pressure readings if the aneurysm involves the left subclavian artery.

Cardiac Output Monitoring

A central venous line is necessary both to provide large-bore, central access and to monitor central venous pressure (CVP). CVP assessment can be used as a continuous monitor of right ventricular preload. Both a pulmonary artery catheter (PAC) and trans-esophageal echocardiography (TEE) may be used to monitor cardiac function. In contrast to the PAC which may not provide accurate measurements of pulmonary artery (PA) pressures during OLV and lateral positioning, TEE often can provide adequate direct visualization of right and left heart function. Doppler interrogation of a tricuspid regurgitation jet can be used to assess PA pressures. TEE can be used to confirm preoperative cardiac and aortic pathologies, but can also be used to evaluate for any intraoperative progression of aortic pathology or changes in right and left ventricular function, volume status, or changes in estimated pulmonary arterial systolic pressures. It can also be used as a continuous monitor to evaluate for left ventricular volume changes as well as for new regional wall motion abnormalities. The PAC is arguably more useful for postoperative monitoring than intraoperative monitoring if intraoperative TEE is concurrently used, but postoperatively a PAC may be useful for guiding fluid management, particularly in patients with reduced ejection fraction and/or marginal renal function.

Neurologic Monitoring

Intraoperative somatosensory evoked potentials (SSEP) and motor evoked potentials (MEP) are often used to monitor function in the sensory and motor spinal columns, respectively. MEP monitoring directly measures motor column function and potential poor perfusion but requires use of a balanced low dose volatile-intravenous anesthetic technique with sparing use of neuromuscular blockers. Both SSEP and MEP signal attenuation that remains abnormal after removal of the aortic clamp strongly correlates with postoperative paraplegia [14].

Stroke detected after descending TAA repair typically results from embolic phenomena during CPB or aortic cross-clamping and/or cerebral hemorrhage secondary to higher cerebral perfusion pressures occurring proximal to the aortic cross clamp. Cerebral oximetry, which uses infrared spectroscopy to determine the oxygen saturation of cerebral blood is often used during aortic surgery. Because measurements are limited to a small sampling region on the forehead, the cerebral oximeter is an unreliable monitor for focal ischemia but may be a relatively sensitive indicator of global hemispheric perfusion.

pressures during intubation and for overall hemodynamic monitoring in patients with reduced ejection fraction. Induction is generally performed using a combination of sedative hypnotics and opioids to accomplish two competing goals: the avoidance of myocardial depression and hypotension—which can result in tissue ischemia—and the prevention of tachycardia and hypertension—which can contribute to aortic wall stress and precipitate aneurysm rupture or propagate dissection. Esmolol, a short acting beta blocker, can also be administered immediately prior to periods of anticipated adrenergic stimulation, such as those that may occur with direct laryngoscopy.

Airway considerations in patients with large, proximal descending TAAs differs from those for patients with other aortic aneurysms due to the need for lung isolation for surgical exposure and because they may involve and distort the trachea, left main bronchus and pulmonary parenchyma. For this reason, radiologic studies delineating the anatomy of the aneurysm should be reviewed prior to surgery. Both compression and distortion of the left bronchial tree and rightward deviation of tracheobronchial structures by large aneurysms can occur. A left sided double lumen tube (DLT) is most commonly used for lung isolation to facilitate OLV, but a right sided DLT can be used when the aneurysm impinges upon the left main stem bronchus. A single lumen tube with a bronchial blocker or Univent (Teleflex Medical, Morrisville, NC) tube may be preferable when airway deviation complicates DLT placement [1]. However, bronchial blockers may be easily displaced throughout the case when the surgeons manipulate the left lung and the anesthesiologist may have to frequently reposition the bronchial blocker. Fiber-optic bronchoscopy should be performed after endotracheal intubation to confirm correct placement of the double lumen tube or bronchial blocker and to evaluate for airway deviation and aortobronchial fistulae.

Induction of Anesthesia

At least one intra-arterial catheter should be placed prior to induction of general anesthesia for hemodynamic monitoring to avoid excessively high

Intraoperative Management

The anesthetic management during descending TAA repair focuses on allowing optimal surgical exposure, monitoring and optimizing end-organ perfusion, maintaining hemodynamic stability, replacing blood loss, correcting coagulopathy and generally mitigating risk for developing adverse postoperative outcomes. Common to all currently utilized surgical techniques for open repair of descending TAAs is a left posterolateral thoracotomy incision that requires right lateral decubitus positioning. An axillary roll should be used to protect the right brachial plexus, and pressure points must be covered with soft padding. The main surgical approaches to open descending thoracic aortic repair are outlined below with emphasis on their implications for anesthetic management.

"Clamp-and-sew"

Clamping the aorta proximal and distal to the aneurysm and repairing it without establishing distal perfusion is the earliest developed surgical approach to repairing descending TAAs (Fig. 10.2a). Because of the large hemodynamic swings typically associated with clamping and unclamping the aorta as well as distal ischemia, this technique is mostly reserved for expedient repairs of small, focal aneurysms [15]. The anesthesiologist should anticipate that the application of the aortic cross clamp can result in proximal hypertension, an increase in cardiac afterload and

distal hypotension [16]. The placement of a Gott shunt, a small heparinized piece of tubing which allows passive aorto-aortic flow across the cross-clamp can be used to provide distal perfusion. Using blood pressure measurements from both a radial and femoral arterial line—i.e. proximal and distal to the aneurysm—and assessing TEE-measured indices of cardiac filling and contractility will allow vasoactive infusions to be titrated to optimize perfusion pressure on both sides of the aortic cross clamp.

With the clamp-and-sew approach, aortic cross clamp times are planned to be short—i.e. less than 30 min—to mitigate effects of distal ischemia. Thus, the anesthesiologist should be ready for quick release of the clamp and the consequent hypotension that can occur from redistribution of blood flow, possible bleeding and vasodilation that can occur from metabolites from ischemia-reperfusion. Goal-directed replacement of fluid loss with crystalloids, colloids and blood products should be undertaken so that the patient is euvolemic prior to release of the clamp. After the clamp is released, the patient's blood pressure should be supported with short acting vasopressors and inotropes as needed. A brief period of hyperventilation and infusion of sodium bicarbonate may be necessary to counteract the acidemia generated from anaerobic metabolism.

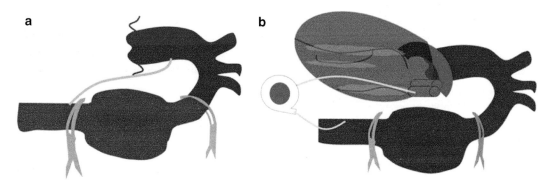

Fig. 10.2 Illustration of 'clamp-and-sew' and left heart bypass surgical techniques. (**a**) (left): The clamp-and-sew technique involves the application of proximal and distal clamps. A Gott shunt, which is a small length heparinized polyvinylchloride tube, can be used to provide passive flow distal to the clamp. (**b**) (right): Left heart bypass involves active direction of oxygenated blood from the left atrium or one of its pulmonary veins into the distal aorto-iliac system by means of a centrifugal pump

Left Heart Bypass

Complications associated with distal ischemia occurring with the clamp-and-sew technique led to the development of left heart bypass, during which blood from one of the pulmonary veins is directed to the distal aortoiliac system by an extracorporeal centrifugal pump (Fig. 10.2b). A moderate dose of heparin (typically 100 U/kg) targeting an activated clotting time (ACT) of 180–200 is necessary to facilitate left heart bypass. Because the distal organs and lower extremities receive oxygenated blood, they do not transition to anaerobic metabolism and the metabolic acidemia frequently seen with the clamp-and-sew technique is largely avoided. The perfusionists should work together with the anesthesiologist to adjust left heart bypass flows to prioritize proximal perfusion to the brain while also ensuring as much distal perfusion as possible. Proximal perfusion of the brain is favored preferentially to distal perfusion, and in the setting of hypovolemia the flow rates of left heart bypass may need to be slowed while the patient is volume resuscitated. The volume status of the heart should be monitored on TEE and pump flows can be adjusted depending on cardiac preload, and left heart bypass flows may be increased in the setting of cardiac volume overload or proximal hypertension. The left heart bypass approach is most beneficial in patients with Extent I and II aneurysms, those with impaired cardiac function and those at a higher risk of renal failure or paraplegia [17].

Partial CPB

In patients with impaired cardiac function or in extensive, complex or reoperative descending aneurysm repairs, partial CPB can be used to reduce cardiac stress and end organ ischemia even further. To facilitate partial bypass, the venous cannula is generally placed in either the right atrium or a femoral vein and the arterial cannula is placed in the distal aorta or femoral artery. After the proximal aorta is clamped, CPB is initiated and pump flow is titrated to produce adequate perfusion as measured in both an upper extremity and femoral arterial lines. Partial CPB requires full systemic heparinization (typically ~300 U/kg) and is associated with more bleeding and coagulopathy when compared to left heart bypass. Because the heart continues to eject blood into the pulmonary circulation with partial flow CPB, ventilation of the right lung must continue. Partial CPB can be increased to full CPB as needed during aortic repair.

Full CPB with DHCA

In cases where there is not an adequate location for placement of a proximal aortic clamp—e.g. aortic pathology involves the left subclavian take-off or there is significant complex aortic disease that does not allow aortic clamp placement distal to the left subclavian—CPB with DHCA allows aneurysm repair in a bloodless field with cerebral and other end-organ protection. By reducing oxygen demand in the brain, spinal cord, kidneys and gut, DHCA has an organ protective effect and has been shown to reduce the incidence of postoperative paraplegia and renal failure [18]. However, DHCA is associated with significant coagulopathy due to platelet dysfunction and consumption of clotting factors. When aneurysm repair under DHCA is expected to take longer than 30 min, anterograde cerebral perfusion (ACP) should be considered [19]. If ACP is utilized, cerebral oximetry monitoring can be used to help assess if both sides of the brain are being perfused or if additional efforts need to be introduced to perfuse the left brain—this likely occurs in patients without an intact Circle of Willis [20].

Transesophageal Echocardiography

Most patients presenting for open descending TAA repair have extensive preoperative imaging by CT or MRI. Contrast-enhanced MRI provides excellent delineation of aneurysm and other aortic pathologic anatomy while MR angiography (MRA) can be used to map branch vessels arising from the aorta. Because the esophagus runs parallel to the aorta, trans-esophageal echocardiography can usually be used to image the entire length of the descending thoracic aorta. Transthoracic echocardiography imaging is frequently done in the preoperative setting to define cardiac function. While TEE is generally not needed for preoperative assessment, if there are no contraindications to placing a TEE probe, the intraoperative use of TEE can be very useful during open descending TAA surgery. Before placing the TEE probe in patients with large descending TAAs, preoperative imaging studies should be reviewed to determine esophageal proximity to avoid potential aortic rupture.

Intraoperative TEE Imaging

After induction of general anesthesia and endotracheal intubation, TEE should be used to confirm the preoperative diagnosis and to evaluate for any progression of the aneurysm, significant atheroma within the aneurysm, or propagation of an aortic dissection flap. From the mid-esophageal four chamber view, the TEE probe should be rotated leftward until the descending aorta appears in short axis. The probe should then be withdrawn until the takeoff of the left subclavian artery appears on the screen (Fig. 10.3a). The imaging depth should be reduced to exclude the area beneath the aorta and the probe should be gradually advanced, while carefully evaluating the imaged cross section of the aorta for pathology. Simultaneous bi-plane can be used to display the orthogonal view of each cross section (Fig. 10.3b). Color Doppler should also be used to evaluate for abnormalities of flow. The presence of an intimal flap in the aorta can signify aortic dissection and should be confirmed using bi-plane and color Doppler in multiple views in order to distinguish it from artifact (Fig. 10.3c). TEE should also be used to assess for a left pleural effusion, which will appear as an anechoic space below the aorta and curve to the left, as this may signify aneurysmal rupture (Fig. 10.3d).

The TEE probe can also be withdrawn up the esophagus to visualize some of the distal aortic arch proximal to the takeoff of the left subclavian. The bulk of the aortic arch cannot be well visualized on TEE examination because of interposition of the tracheal and left main bronchus between the esophagus and the heart. The ascending aorta should also be viewed, as concurrent involvement of the ascending aorta can sometimes occur. After performing a comprehensive examination of the aorta, the TEE exam should continue to evaluate cardiac structures and valve and ventricular function. Ventricular and valvular function can dictate choice of vasopressors and inotropes used during critical portions of the case and may influence choice of surgical technique.

It is generally helpful to use TEE throughout surgery for continuous monitoring of cardiac function—i.e. when not on full CPB or DHCA. When the clamp-and-sew technique or left heart bypass is utilized for descending TAA repair, TEE can be a useful monitor of left and right ventricular filling and function. Left ventricular end-diastolic volume is best assessed in the transgastric mid-papillary short axis view. Volume overload can result from translocation of venous capacitance from the lower extremities and may necessitate the use of venodilators to reduce cardiac preload. When left heart bypass or partial CPB is used to offload the volume proximal to the aortic cross-clamp and to provide perfusion distal to the aortic cross-clamp, TEE is helpful in guiding bypass pump flow rate. Left ventricular distension on TEE should prompt increasing bypass flow rates, while decreased ventricular volume should prompt decreasing pump output or administering intravascular volume. When complete CPB is used, TEE is helpful for assessing ventricular function while separating from CPB. Prior to separation from CPB, the long axis views of the aortic valve and left ventricle are valuable for assessing for intracardiac air. Along with available hemodynamic monitors, TEE should be used to ensure that cardiac preload, afterload and contractility are optimal.

Postoperative Outcomes

Improving postoperative outcomes after open descending TAA surgery requires the perioperative team—i.e. the surgeon, anesthesiologist and

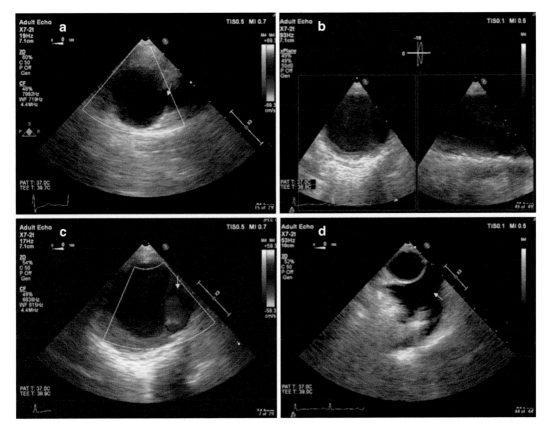

Fig. 10.3 Transesophageal echocardiography for evaluation of the thoracic aorta. (**a**) Color flow Doppler demonstrating flow to the left subclavian artery from the aortic arch. (**b**) 2D Biplane used to evaluate orthogonal aspects of descending thoracic aorta. (**c**) Color Doppler used to evaluate flow within the true lumen of an aortic dissection. (**d**) Left-sided pleural effusion from ruptured aortic aneurysm

intensivist—to recognize patients who are at risk for complications and to initiate appropriate perioperative measures to prevent or mitigate them.

Paraplegia

Paraplegia can be a devastating complication after descending TAA repair, with a reported incidence of 3–10% [21, 22]. The mechanism of spinal cord injury is thought to result from a combination of hypoperfusion distal to the aortic clamp, elevated cerebrospinal fluid (CSF) pressure and individual variability in collateral arterial flow. The spinal cord receives its blood supply from a single anterior spinal artery and paired posterior spinal arteries. The artery of Adamkiewicz, which originates from an intercostal artery between T9-T12 in most individuals, makes an important contribution to the blood supply of the thoracolumbar spinal cord. Injury to this vessel can result in ischemia of the anterior spinal cord and consequent motor deficits. Additionally, in patients with atherosclerotic disease, the smaller segmental arteries may not be patent, resulting to ischemia during aortic clamping [23].

Surgical strategies to decrease the incidence of paraplegia include the use of passive or active aorto-femoral bypass, re-implantation of arterial spinal segmental vessels and the induction of hypothermia during the clamping period. The anesthesiologist can contribute to this strategy by optimizing spinal cord perfusion pressure (SCPP).

$$SCPP = Mean\ Arterial\ Pressure\ (MAP)$$
$$- Cerebrospinal\ Fluid\ (CSF)\ Pressure$$

Increasing SCPP can be done using two mechanisms: raising MAP with use of vasopressor drugs and volume resuscitation and reducing CSF pressure by draining CSF via a lumbar spinal drain. Placement of a lumbar spinal drain allows the measurement of SCPP as well as the drainage of CSF. In patients without contraindications, a large bore Touhy needle is inserted into a lumbar interspace below the termination of the spinal cord (i.e. L1/L2) and is used to access the intrathecal space. A catheter is then threaded through the Touhy needle into the intrathecal space. This intrathecal catheter can now be connected to a manometer to allow transduction of CSF pressure. While the utilization of lumbar spinal drains in open descending TAA surgery has resulted in better outcomes in some studies, they are also associated with a host of complications including neuraxial and subdural hematomas, persistent CSF leak, infection and retained catheter. Patients at greatest risk for postoperative paraplegia include those with ruptured aneurysms, those with extensive aneurysms, previous aneurysm repair and those with numerous medical comorbidities [24]. In lower risk patients, an alternative strategy may be postoperative drain placement in patients who develop concerning intraoperative motor evoked potential (MEP) signals, those who emerge from anesthesia with paraplegia or those who develop delayed postoperative paraplegia.

Renal Failure

Acute kidney injury (AKI) after descending TAA repair occurs as frequently as 29% and is associated with increased incidence of need for long-term dialysis as well as higher mortality [25]. Multiple studies have found that a history of chronic kidney disease and prolonged aortic clamping are the strongest predictors of postoperative AKI [12, 25]. The etiology of postoperative AKI after TAA repair likely involves renal hypoperfusion due to aortic clamping, systemic hypotension and embolization of cellular debris. Prospective data suggests surgical techniques that may prevent AKI include extracorporeal circulation that allows perfusion of the kidneys below the aortic cross-clamp; local or systemic hypothermia; and selective renal perfusion with cold crystalloid solution [26, 27]. Additional anesthetic management strategies to reduce AKI require goal-directed intravenous hydration, limiting intra-operative hypotension and avoidance of nephrotoxic medications. There is some suggestion from the cardiac surgical literature that goal-oriented management of CPB and other parameters can help to mitigate AKI, but this has not been studied to date for descending aortic surgery [28].

Coagulopathy

Coagulopathy after descending TAA repair is related to blood loss and transfusion of packed red blood cells and cell saver, inflammatory responses to surgery, and extent and duration of extracorporeal circulation of DHCA. The clamp-and-sew technique, which does not rely on active bypass flow, is associated with decreased clotting factor activity and an increase in fibrinolysis [29]. The use of left heart bypass requires a smaller dose of heparin than is required for full CPB and may avoid some of the associated coagulopathy. CPB with DHCA is often associated with the most coagulopathy resulting from platelet dysfunction, thrombocytopenia, consumption of clotting factors and hypofibrinogenemia. Antifibrinolytics such as the lysine analog, ε-aminocaproic acid can be used prophylactically in all patients in whom bypass flow is established. Thrombo-elastography assessment can be used throughout the intraoperative period to evaluate for etiologies of bleeding. The transfusion of blood products should be guided not only by laboratory results, but also by vigilantly observing the surgical field and communicating with the surgical team regarding concerns related to potential ongoing surgical bleeding. A massive transfusion involves the replacement of one or more of a patient's blood volume and is associated with a unique set of complications. These include lung injury, hypocalcemia, hyperkalemia, hypothermia and dilutional coagulopathy. To mitigate these complications, we recommend a goal directed transfusion strategy guided by thrombo-elastography, platelet count, INR measurement and frequent measurement of electrolytes.

Postoperative Care

After open surgical repair of descending thoracic aortic disease patients should be transferred to the postoperative intensive care unit (ICU) for continued hemodynamic and neurologic monitoring, and for respiratory monitoring. In the absence of significant head and neck edema—which could cause concern regarding successful endotracheal tube exchange—the DLT should be exchanged for a single lumen endotracheal tube at the end of surgery. Both the use of an airway exchange catheter and a videolaryngoscope may be helpful in enhancing the safety of exchanging the endotracheal tube. Frequently there is enough hemodynamic instability or pulmonary edema that patients are left intubated after surgery and weaned from the ventilator and extubated after a few hours in the postoperative intensive care unit.

Aggressive postoperative pulmonary and physical rehabilitation is very useful for avoiding common postoperative complications such as atelectasis, pneumonia, deep venous thromboses and pulmonary thromboemboli. Common enhanced rehabilitation approaches in the ICU include early extubation, mobilization from the ICU bed and frequent ambulation as tolerated by the patient. As renal failure occurs in approximately one-third of these patients, acid-base and electrolyte laboratory tests should be monitored frequently. Renal replacement therapy may be necessary to correct severe metabolic abnormalities.

Patients undergoing open descending TAA repair have an increased risk of perioperative stroke, owing to patient and procedural factors. Thus, these patients should be extubated as soon as possible in the ICU to allow for optimal neurologic monitoring and early detection of perioperative stroke. If they cannot be extubated early, then periodically reducing sedation to perform neurologic checks can be helpful. Hourly examination by the ICU nursing staff for detection of spinal cord ischemia is necessary to detect neurologic changes early and institute acute interventions. Because paraplegia can occur hours or days after surgery, the spinal drain should be left in and CSF pressure should be monitored postoperatively. In the setting of paraplegia MAP should be increased using vasoactive drugs and CSF should be drained from the spinal drain. If the patient does not have a lumbar spinal drain and develops postoperative paraplegia, strong consideration should be given to placing a lumbar spinal drain and draining CSF to enhance arterial spinal cord perfusion. The CSF drainage strategy employed in the majority of published studies includes the drainage for a CSF pressure between 10–15 mm Hg [24]. To avoid the excessive drainage of CSF, we advocate the drainage of no more than 10–15 mL of CSF hourly for an institutionally designated maximum CSF pressure. CSF drainage should be performed in accordance with strict institutional guidelines by nursing staff who are familiar with the drain and potential complications associated with its management. In patients without paraplegia, the drain should be removed within 72 h of placement to avoid infectious complications.

References

1. Puchakayala MR, Lau WC. Descending thoracic aortic aneurysms. Continuing Education in Anaesthesia, Crit Care Pain. 2006;6(2):54–9.
2. Coady MA, Ikonomidis JS, Cheung AT, Matsumoto AH, Dake MD, Chaikof EL, et al. Surgical management of descending thoracic aortic disease: open and endovascular approaches. Circulation. 2010;121(25):2780–804.
3. Elefteriades JA. Natural history of thoracic aortic aneurysms: indications for surgery, and surgical versus nonsurgical risks. Ann Thorac Surg. 2002;74(5):S1877–S80.

4. Coady MA, Rizzo JA, Hammond GL, Mandapati D, Darr U, Kopf GS, et al. What is the appropriate size criterion for resection of thoracic aortic aneurysms? J Thorac Cardiovasc Surg. 1997;113(3):476–91.

5. Erbel R, Aboyans V, Boileau C, Bossone E, Bartolomeo R, Eggebrecht H, et al. ESC Committee for practice guidelines. 2014 ESC guidelines on the diagnosis and treatment of aortic diseases: document covering acute and chronic aortic diseases of the thoracic and abdominal aorta of the adult. The task force for the diagnosis and treatment of aortic diseases of the European Society of Cardiology (ESC). Eur Heart J. 2014;35(41):2873–926.

6. Kouchoukos NT, Dougenis D. Surgery of the thoracic aorta. N Engl J Med. 1997;336(26):1876–89.

7. Svensson LG, Crawford ES, Hess KR, Coselli JS, Safi HJ. Variables predictive of outcome in 832 patients undergoing repairs of the descending thoracic aorta. Chest. 1993;104(4):1248–54.

8. Greenberg RK, Lu Q, Roselli EE, Svensson LG, Moon MC, Hernandez AV, et al. Contemporary analysis of descending thoracic and thoracoabdominal aneurysm repair. Circulation. 2008;118(8):808–17.

9. Fleisher LA, Fleischmann KE, Auerbach AD, Barnason SA, Beckman JA, Bozkurt B, et al. ACC/AHA guideline on perioperative cardiovascular evaluation and management of patients undergoing noncardiac surgery. Circulation. 2014;130(24):2215–45. https://doi.org/10.1161/CIR.0000000000000105.

10. Vaughn SB, LeMaire SA, Collard CD. Case scenario anesthetic considerations for Thoracoabdominal aortic aneurysm repair. J Am Soc Anesthesiol. 2011;115(5):1093–102.

11. Teixido MT, Leonetti JP. Recurrent laryngeal nerve paralysis associated with thoracic aortic aneurysm. Otolaryngol Head Neck Surg. 1990;102(2):140–4.

12. Girardi LN, Ohmes LB, Lau C, Di Franco A, Gambardella I, Elsayed M, et al. Open repair of descending thoracic and thoracoabdominal aortic aneurysms in patients with preoperative renal failure. Eur J Cardiothorac Surg. 2017;51(5):971–7.

13. Webb ST, Allen JSD. Perioperative renal protection. Continuing Education in Anaesthesia, Crit Care Pain. 2008;8(5):176–80.

14. Bicknell C, Riga C, Wolfe J. Prevention of paraplegia during thoracoabdominal aortic aneurysm repair. Eur J Vasc Endovasc Surg. 2009;37(6):654–60.

15. Mauney MC, Tribble CG, Cope JT, Tribble RW, Luctong A, Spotnitz WD, et al. Is clamp and sew still viable for thoracic aortic resection? Ann Surg. 1996;223(5):534–43.

16. Kahn RA, Stone ME, Moskowitz DM, editors. Anesthetic consideration for descending thoracic aortic aneurysm repair. Seminars in cardiothoracic and vascular anesthesia. Los Angeles, CA: Sage; 2007.

17. Coselli JS. The use of left heart bypass in the repair of thoracoabdominal aortic aneurysms: current techniques and results. Seminars in thoracic and cardiovascular surgery. New York: Elsevier; 2003.

18. Fehrenbacher JW, Siderys H, Terry C, Kuhn J, Corvera JS. Early and late results of descending thoracic and thoracoabdominal aortic aneurysm open repair with deep hypothermia and circulatory arrest. J Thorac Cardiovasc Surg. 2010;140(6):S154–S60.

19. Di Mauro M, Iacò AL, Di Lorenzo C, Gagliardi M, Varone E, Al Amri H, et al. Cold reperfusion before rewarming reduces neurological events after deep hypothermic circulatory arrest. Eur J Cardiothorac Surg. 2012;43(1):168–73.

20. Fischer GW, Lin H-M, Krol M, Galati MF, Di Luozzo G, Griepp RB, et al. Noninvasive cerebral oxygenation may predict outcome in patients undergoing aortic arch surgery. J Thorac Cardiovasc Surg. 2011;141(3):815–21.

21. Livesay JJ, Cooley DA, Ventemiglia RA, Montero CG, Warrian RK, Brown DM, et al. Surgical experience in descending thoracic aneurysmectomy with and without adjuncts to avoid ischemia. Ann Thorac Surg. 1985;39(1):37–46.

22. Estrera AL, Miller CC, Chen EP, Meada R, Torres RH, Porat EE, et al. Descending thoracic aortic aneurysm repair: 12-year experience using distal aortic perfusion and cerebrospinal fluid drainage. Ann Thorac Surg. 2005;80(4):1290–6.

23. Jacobs MJ, Elenbaas TW, Schurink GW, Mess WH, Mochtar B. Assessment of spinal cord integrity during thoracoabdominal aortic aneurysm repair. Ann Thorac Surg. 2002;74(5):S1864–S6.

24. Fedorow CA, Moon MC, Mutch WA, Grocott HP. Lumbar cerebrospinal fluid drainage for thoracoabdominal aortic surgery: rationale and practical considerations for management. Anesth Analg. 2010;111(1):46–58.

25. Safi HJ, Harlin SA, Miller CC, Iliopoulos DC, Joshi A, Mohasci TG, et al. Predictive factors for acute renal failure in thoracic and thoracoabdominal aortic aneurysm surgery. J Vasc Surg. 1996;24(3):338–45.

26. MacArthur RG, Carter SA, Coselli JS, LeMaire SA, editors. Organ protection during thoracoabdominal aortic surgery: rationale for a multimodality approach. Seminars in cardiothoracic and vascular anesthesia. New York: Westminster Publications; 2005.

27. LeMaire SA, Jones MM, Conklin LD, Carter SA, Criddell MD, Wang XL, et al. Randomized comparison of cold blood and cold crystalloid renal perfusion for renal protection during thoracoabdominal aortic aneurysm repair. J Vasc Surg. 2009;49(1):11–9.

28. Magruder JT, Crawford TC, Harness HL, Grimm JC, Suarez-Pierre A, Wierschke C, et al. A pilot goal-directed perfusion initiative is associated with less acute kidney injury after cardiac surgery. J Thorac Cardiovasc Surg. 2017;153(1):118–25. e1

29. Gertler JP, Cambria RP, Brewster DC, Davison JK, Purcell P, Zannetti S, et al. Coagulation changes during thoracoabdominal aneurysm repair. J Vasc Surg. 1996;24(6):936–45.

Anesthetic Management of Thoracic Endovascular Aortic Repair

Mariya Geube and Christopher Troianos

Main Messages

1. TEVAR has evolved as a less invasive alternative treatment than the open aortic repair in a wide range of aortic diseases, including thoracic descending and abdominal aortic aneurysms, aortic dissections, penetrating aortic ulcers, acute pathologies of the ascending aorta and aortic arch, and traumatic aortic injury

2. TEVAR is associated with lower rate of blood transfusions, spinal cord ischemia, kidney insufficiency and short term mortality compared with open surgical repair of descending thoracic aortic aneurysms; however, TEVAR is associated with a higher re-intervention rate than open aortic repair, mostly due to occurrence of endoleak

3. TEVAR is safely performed under general, regional or local anesthesia, with similar rates of technical success, conversion to open repair, operative mortality and acute kidney insufficiency; the most common anesthetic technique used for TEVAR is general anesthesia, which has certain advantages—ability to control ventilation during the apnea periods, limited patient movement, improved patient tolerance, creation of iliac conduits, and the use of transesophageal echocardiography

4. TEE is a sensitive tool for assessing aortic pathology, such as aortic dissection, size of the aortic aneurysm, presence of intramural thrombus; it has a great value intraoperatively for detecting early myocardial ischemia in high risk patients or for assessment of intravascular volume status, and can also help guiding wire placement in the true lumen of the aorta and detection of small endoleaks.

5. Spinal cord protection in TEVAR is indicated when there is an extensive aortic coverage of the stent graft, left subclavian occlusion affecting the flow in the cervical spinal network, prior abdominal aortic aneurysm repair; inte-

M. Geube (✉)
Department of Cardiothoracic Anesthesiology,
Cleveland Clinic Foundation, Cleveland, OH, USA
e-mail: Geubem@ccf.org

C. Troianos
Anesthesiology Institute, Cleveland Clinic
Foundation, Cleveland, OH, USA
e-mail: troianc@ccf.org

© Springer Nature Switzerland AG 2021
D. C. H. Cheng et al. (eds.), *Evidence-Based Practice in Perioperative Cardiac Anesthesia and Surgery*, https://doi.org/10.1007/978-3-030-47887-2_11

grated approach to spinal cord protection includes placement of subarachnoid drain, blood pressure augmentation, treatment of blood loss anemia, frequent neurologic status monitoring in the postoperative period

6. Endoleaks present a complication unique to endovascular aneurysm repair; they are identified as the most common cause of aneurysm rupture after TEVAR, and the most common indication for reintervention

7. Type I and III endoleak warrant surgical intervention, while type II and IV may be treated expectantly and require long term follow up

Descending thoracic aortic aneurysms have a high prevalence in the modern society and are frequently discovered incidentally as a consequence of cardiovascular workup for another medical problem. They are classified by location, extent of the disease, size and shape, which determines the complexity of the surgical procedure, and the clinical outcome [1]. Isolated descending thoracic aneurysm is confined to the aorta between the left subclavian artery and the diaphragm, while the thoracoabdominal aneurysm is an extensive disease of the aorta between the left subclavian artery and the aortic bifurcation. Indications for repair of descending thoracic aortic aneurysms are rupture or impending rupture, malperfusion syndrome, refractory pain, rapid growth of aneurysm (> 1 cm per year) or an absolute aneurysm dimension of >6.5 cm or 6.0 cm in connective tissue disorders [2, 3].

Conventional open surgical repair has been the gold standard for treatment of symptomatic descending thoracic aortic disease for many years. It is associated with substantial morbidity and mortality in an aged population with multiple coexisting conditions. TEVAR was initially reserved for patients considered very high risk for open surgery or in difficult-to-reach aortic segments. Currently, this has evolved as a less invasive alternative treatment modality with an excellent perioperative morbidity profile in a

wide range of aortic diseases. Technological evolution in medical imaging and devices has enabled TEVAR to be used in more proximal—aortic arch and ascending aorta—or more distal—thoracoabdominal aortic disease.

Indications for TEVAR

The indications for TEVAR are listed in Table 11.1.

Despite the favorable safety profile and multiple applications of TEVAR, the endovascular approach should be considered with caution in patients with connective tissue disorders. Progression of the aortic disease is expected and associated with high re-intervention rate in these patients.

Outcome Comparison of TEVAR Versus Open Repair

Comparative studies of TEVAR versus open surgical repair [13–15] favor TEVAR for reduced 30-day mortality, shorter intensive care unit stay, and shorter hospital length of stay. The incidence of spinal cord ischemia, blood transfusions and acute kidney insufficiency is lower in TEVAR, however, the long-term need for re-intervention is higher, mainly due to the occurrence of endoleaks. The incidence of stroke and myocardial infarction is similar between the two techniques. Despite the low intraoperative morbidity and mortality, the late complications from TEVAR outnumber those in open surgical repair. These include endoleaks, aneurysm progression-related death, and stent graft migration. TEVAR is associated with significantly higher health care costs, determined by the price of the device, the number of stent grafts placed, and the extensive lifelong follow-up [3]. Treating ruptured thoracic aortic aneurysms with TEVAR present another expanding field for the endovascular approach. Several large studies examining the outcomes after endovascular versus open surgery for ruptured aneurysms have confirmed a slightly reduced mortality [16] and improved composite outcomes—death, stroke, paraplegia—with TEVAR [17, 18].

Table 11.1 Common indications and outcomes for TEVAR [4]

Indication for TEVAR	Outcomes and evidence
Descending thoracic aortic aneurysm	Lower rate of blood transfusions, spinal cord ischemia, and short term mortality compared with open surgical repair. Equal rate of all-cause mortality at 5 years
Thoraco-abdominal aneurysm	Fenestrated graft stenting is feasible in patients with significant comorbidity who are considered high risk for open surgical repair [5]
Acute type B* aortic dissection with complications (20%)— Rupture, malperfusion, refractory pain	Indicated for urgent repair. High procedural success rate and low intraoperative mortality, and emergency conversion. Proximal entry coverage reduces the flow to the false lumen and improves perfusion to spinal cord, kidneys and lower extremities
Acute type B aortic dissection without complications (80%)	Similar survival at 2 years compared with patients on optimal medical therapy, but enhanced true lumen remodeling and delayed aneurysm dilatation with TEVAR [6, 7]. Elective procedure or conservative management with follow-up are both reasonable options
Chronic type B aortic dissection	Stent graft treatment does not reduce the risk of rupture nor has a survival benefit. Lower success rate of excluding completely the false lumen than in acute dissection [8]
Acute type A* aortic dissection	Evidence is limited to case series as a salvage procedure in patients at very high risk for open repair [9]
Penetrating aortic ulcer and intramural hematoma	No consensus on first line therapy. Progression of intramural hematoma to dissection is observed in 16–36%. TEVAR should be considered in symptomatic patients with refractory chest pain, increasing size, formation of pseudoaneurysm or contained rupture
Traumatic aortic transection	Associated with dismal prognosis due to multiorgan injuries. TEVAR has shown superior to open repair due to the localized aortic pathology, with significantly lower early mortality and paraplegia rate [10]
Ruptured thoracic descending aortic aneurysm	60% pre-hospital mortality and 30–50% 30-day mortality after TEVAR [11]. Coverage of left subclavian artery may be required to achieve good proximal seal. Management of spinal cord ischemia is expectant and spinal drain may be placed after hemodynamic stability has been achieved [12]

According to the Stanford classification, type A aortic dissection refers to a dissection with origin in the ascending aorta or aortic arch. Type B aortic dissection refers to a tear originating in the descending aorta distal to the left subclavian artery

Preoperative Assessment and Optimization of the Patient

Patients presenting for TEVAR undergo extensive preoperative work-up, because they have a high prevalence of cardiovascular disease, chronic pulmonary disease, and chronic renal insufficiency.

Cardiovascular Assessment

Based on the perioperative risk of major adverse cardiac events greater than 5%, TEVAR is considered a high risk surgery. The most common cardiovascular complications after TEVAR are myocardial infarction, arrhythmias, and conges-

tive heart failure. There is a high (30–70%) prevalence of coronary artery disease among patients with aortic aneurysms [19]. Testing and medical optimization are thus warranted prior to the procedure in symptomatic patients and should be tailored to their existing comorbidities and the risk of aortic rupture [20]. Preoperative electrocardiography and transthoracic echocardiography are important studies used to assess the perioperative risk for cardiovascular complications. Stress testing is reserved for patients with poor functional capacity—less than four metabolic equivalents (METS) on exercise testing [21, 22]. Routine revascularization in patients with stable coronary artery disease before elective vascular surgery does not improve mortality or reduce postoperative adverse cardiac events, and is currently not recommended [23]. Cardiac optimization includes life style modifications and medical optimization such as smoking cessation, blood pressure and serum glucose control, and continuation of statin, beta blocker, and aspirin therapy. In case of emergent TEVAR with unknown cardiac status, intraoperative transesophageal echocardiography can be used to facilitate intraoperative cardiovascular assessment and management.

Renal Injury Risk Assessment

Baseline renal function should be determined preoperatively, because renal insufficiency is a known risk factor for postoperative cardiovascular complications. The strongest predictors for acute kidney insufficiency (AKI) after TEVAR are preexisting renal dysfunction, increased age, involvement of the renal arteries in the acute aortic pathology with evidence of malperfusion, preoperative exposure to radiocontrast agents, high complexity and prolonged procedures, emergency surgery, and perioperative hypotension [24]. These factors reflect the larger dose of intraoperative contrast, renal microembolism, and inflammatory response. Adequate hydration before radiocontrast imaging studies and planning the surgery several days after the contrast load, are strategies to minimize the risk of contrast induced renal injury. The use of intravascular ultrasound during TEVAR can significantly reduce the total dose of intravenous contrast administered during the procedure [25].

Surgical Considerations for TEVAR

Preoperative Imaging and Evaluation

Contrast enhanced computed tomography of the aorta extending from supra-aortic vessels to the femoral arteries with three-dimensional volumetric reconstruction of the image is routinely performed preoperatively. This provides important information on the location and shape of the aneurysm, tortuosity of the thoracic descending

aorta, and the origin of the aortic branches. Computed tomographic angiography (CTA) guides the surgeon to determine whether the patient's anatomy is suitable for endograft placement, the size of the stent graft, and the need for custom designed stent grafts. This imaging has the advantage of rapid acquisition, high spacial resolution, and provides the ability to image heavy calcifications and to detect the location of contrast extravasation in aortic rupture or endovascular leak. If coverage of the left subclavian artery is planned, head and neck CTA is obtained to determine the presence of a complete circle of Willis and patent vertebral arteries.

Devices for Thoracic Endovascular Aortic Repair

Stent grafts are composed of a metal skeleton attached to an impermeable fabric deployed proximally into a healthy aortic segment and distally beyond the degenerated segment, thus excluding the diseased aortic wall from the circulation. A landing zone map divides the aortic arch and descending aorta into five segments, which are used as landmarks for endograft seal zone [26] (Fig. 11.1).

At least 2 cm of normal aortic wall are required on the proximal and distal end of the aortic pathology for successful stent graft deployment. There are several devices approved by Federal Drug Administration for use in thoracic endovascular aortic aneurysm repair [3]. TEVAR has been performed with success in thoracic aortic pathologies other than aortic aneurysms. Examples include acute and chronic aortic dissection, ascending aortic or arch pathologies, penetrating aortic ulcers, traumatic aortic injury, thoracoabdominal aneurysms and ruptured aortic aneurysms [27]. In the presence of aortic dissection, the goal of the endovascular repair is to cover the proximal intimal tear, to exclude the aneurysmal segment of the aorta, and to ensure distal perfusion of the major aortic side branches [3]. TEVAR can be performed in high risk patients with complex aortic aneurysms involving the origin of major aortic branches (landing

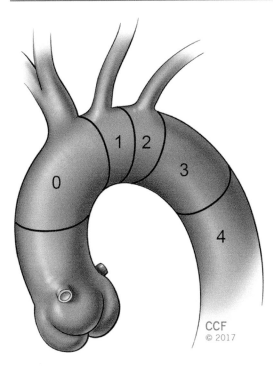

Fig. 11.1 Landing zone map of the thoracic aorta. The classic TEVAR seal zones extend from the left carotid artery to the celiac artery (landing zone 2 and 4). Reprinted with permission, Cleveland Clinic Center for Medical Art and Photography © 2017. All Rights Reserved

zones 0 and 1, or below zone 4, Fig. 11.1). These are best managed with fenestrated or branched endografts. Fenestrated endografts are custom made grafts that accommodate the specific anatomy of the patient and have openings in the endograft fabric that are positioned over the origin of the visceral arteries. Branched endografts have small side arm grafts constructed into the main endograft, which are then extended into the artery to maintain its patency [28]. Follow-up CTA after TEVAR is required before discharge, at 3 months, and annually thereafter to assess repair stability, device integrity, presence of endoleaks, and size of the aortic aneurysm.

Choice of Anesthetic Techniques

Various anesthetic techniques can be used for TEVAR. The EUROpean collaborators on Stent-graft Techniques for abdominal aortic Aneurysm

Repair registry [29] reported that 69% of cases were performed with general anesthesia (GA), 25% with regional anesthesia (RA) and 6% with local anesthesia (LA). Early reports failed to show any difference in the technical success of the endovascular repair, the rate of conversion to open surgical repair, mortality rate, or the incidence of acute kidney injury among different anesthetic techniques [30]. A more recent registry study reported decreased pulmonary complications and length of hospital stay with local/regional technique compared to GA [31]. TEVAR is most commonly performed with GA. The advantages include the ability to control ventilation during the required periods of apnea, limited patient movement, improved patient tolerance in prolonged procedures, creation of iliac conduits, and use of transesophageal echocardiography (TEE).

TEVAR can be performed with spinal or epidural anesthesia, which allows the patient to remain awake and avoid tracheal intubation, which is especially important in patients with severe chronic lung disease. The patient's breathing can be assisted with non-invasive ventilation, if the supine position increases their breathing difficulty. Regional anesthetic techniques can also provide optimal pain control in the early postoperative period. The disadvantages of regional anesthesia are patient discomfort and movement, poor compliance with breath holds during the procedure, sympathectomy with hypotension, and inability to obtain a timely neurological exam after the procedure. Regional anesthesia is performed with success in the authors' institution among patients with advanced lung disease who are considered high risk for postoperative pulmonary complications and prolonged intubation. After subarachnoid catheter placement, a local anesthetic is injected into the catheter and capped until stent deployment. After deployment, the SA catheter is opened and cerebrospinal fluid (CSF) is drained. The concentration of the local anesthetic in the CSF decreases quickly after opening the SA drain, necessitating supplementation of the regional anesthetic with light sedation at a time when the procedure is near completion.

The use of local anesthetic alone for TEVAR is possible when a percutaneous approach is planned [32]. There are certain advantages of local anesthesia, such as avoidance of inhalational agents, muscle paralysis, airway manipulation, and mechanical ventilation, while allowing for early detection of neurological impairment due to stroke or spinal cord ischemia.

Intraoperative Monitoring and Management

Invasive Hemodynamic Monitoring

The need for invasive monitoring during TEVAR is determined by the potential for catastrophic bleeding and cardiovascular collapse during the procedure. Although TEVAR is theoretically less invasive than an open surgical repair, the anesthetic planning should include intraoperative monitoring and vascular access adequate to manage the patient in case of emergent conversion to open repair (about 2%). Arterial, central venous and large bore peripheral venous catheters are routinely placed. The preferred site for placement of the arterial catheter is the right radial artery, in case of left subclavian artery involvement. Surgeons frequently access the left brachial artery for placing ancillary devices, leaving the right side available for blood pressure monitoring. In aortic dissection, accessing the true lumen may be difficult. In this circumstance, the wire can be placed through the arterial access of the right arm, which needs to be free of intravascular devices and monitors, and prepped in the surgical field. Central venous access is indicated for administration of vasoactive medications and for central venous pressure monitoring.

Role of TEE

TEE is a sensitive tool for diagnosing aortic pathology. It can be used to evaluate and confirm significant atheroma burden, aortic dissection, size of the aortic aneurysm, and presence of intraluminal thrombus. Patients who present for elective aortic surgery have already undergone various imaging modalities to determine the type and extent of the aortic pathology, and provide information about the individual's aortic anatomy. One important shortcoming of TEE is the difficulty in visualizing the distal ascending aorta and proximal aortic arch, because of the interposition of the left mainstem bronchus between the esophagus and this portion of the thoracic aorta. Important applications of TEE in TEVAR are for patients with high risk for serious cardiovascular adverse events, for early detection of myocardial ischemia, and for volume assessment. The intraoperative use of TEE is especially helpful in emergent TEVAR, because usually the patients have insufficient preoperative cardiac work-up. TEE is an invaluable imaging tool to distinguish between true and false lumens and to guide placement of wires in the aorta and to detect distal dissection flap fenestrations. Although the standard for intraoperative endoleak diagnosis is angiography, small leaks may be missed. TEE in color flow Doppler mode is more sensitive for detecting type I endoleak after stent deployment than angiography [33].

Hemodynamic Goals During Induction and Maintenance of Anesthesia

The ultimate intraoperative anesthetic goals are to provide adequate oxygen delivery, maintain normovolemia, optimize perfusion to vital organs, and maintain normal body temperature. The main concern during induction of general anesthesia is to maintain tight blood pressure control and avoid a sympathetic surge during laryngoscopy and intubation. Placement of pre-induction arterial catheter, use of anxiolytics and pain medications are useful to help achieve these goals.

Hemodynamic Management During Aortic Endograft Deployment

Endograft deployment is difficult in the proximal descending thoracic aorta or aortic arch in normal hemodynamic conditions because of the high velocity blood flow in this part of the aorta. There are certain techniques that can be used to decrease the cardiac output to facilitate stent deployment. Frequently used pharmacologic agents are adenosine (which causes a brief asystolic pause), esmolol (which decreases the heart rate and has transient effect on the blood pressure), propofol and nitroglycerin. Other non-pharmacologic techniques include rapid transvenous pacing of the right ventricle at a rate 130–180 beats per minute. This causes loss of atrioventricular synchrony, severe decrease of ventricular filling and ejection, and dramatic decrease in the stroke volume and blood pressure. Cessation of flow can also be achieved by temporary balloon occlusion of the aorta proximally to the landing zone. Balloon expansion is accompanied by significant proximal hypertension, which is transient and should not prompt correction. Any pharmacological manipulation during this time can lead to prolonged hypotension after the stent deployment, which is detrimental for the brain and spinal cord perfusion.

Body Temperature Control

Body temperature control and prevention of hypothermia during TEVAR is of paramount importance. The chest, abdomen and legs are exposed to the ambient temperature and predisposed to rapid heat loss. Although mild hypothermia may benefit spinal cord protection, more severe hypothermia must be avoided because of the risk for adverse intraoperative and postoperative cardiac events, coagulopathy, and residual muscle paralysis, which preclude timely extubation and the ability to perform an early neurological exam. The use of devices for active rewarming, such as fluid warmer, a heated airway circuit and forced air warming devices on the upper body, along with higher room temperature are recommended. Lower body warming devices or underbody warm mattresses should be avoided due to local hyperthermia in the area of the spinal cord and lower extremities, which can exacerbate ischemia of the spinal cord and the legs.

Spinal Cord Ischemia

TEVAR, as opposed to open surgical repair, avoids many of the critical intraoperative insults that contribute to the development of spinal cord ischemia (SCI), such as aortic cross clamping, severe hemodynamic perturbations, cardiopulmonary bypass, reperfusion injury, and deep hypothermic circulatory arrest, when used. Nevertheless, placement of a stent graft leads to abrupt exclusion of the segmental blood supply to the spinal cord and is associated with 1–10% incidence of ischemic spinal cord injury [34].

Spinal cord perfusion is dependent on a single anterior and two posterior spinal arteries, and on a complex arterial network at the proximal—cervical vascular network—and distal portion of the spinal cord—pelvic vascular network [35]. The cervical vascular network originates from the subclavian arteries, which give rise to the vertebral arteries, then to the anterior spinal artery. The anterior spinal artery receives blood supply from the thoracic intercostal arteries, which arise directly from the thoracic descending aorta. Perfusion of the distal portion of the spinal cord arises from the lumbar and sacral arteries, which form a collateral network with branches of the inferior mesenteric and hypogastric arteries, which in turn are branches of the internal iliac arteries. The most vulnerable segment of the spinal cord is between T4 and L2, where sacrificing the intercostal arteries may significantly disrupt the perfusion to the spinal cord and lead to watershed infarction. The pathogenesis of SCI after TEVAR is multifactorial with the following contributing factors:

1. Extensive aortic coverage of the stent graft with complete exclusion of the intercostal arteries. Stent graft length more than 20 cm is associated with significant increase in the incidence of SCI [36]
2. Extension of the stent graft into normal aorta because of proximal and distal landing zones, thus increasing the length of the aorta excluded from direct spinal cord perfusion
3. Destabilization and embolization of atheromatous debris from the aortic wall due to guide wire manipulation and stent deployment

4. Left subclavian artery occlusion affecting blood flow in the proximal cervical network;
5. Back flow from the interrupted segmental arteries into the aneurysmal sac, which causes "steal" from the spinal cord collateral network
6. Prior abdominal aortic aneurysm repair
7. Intraoperative hypotension
8. Hypogastric artery occlusion
9. Emergent surgery [37, 38]

Integrated Strategy for Spinal Cord Protection

Paraplegia and paraparesis due to SCI remain the most feared complications of endovascular repair of descending thoracic or thoracoabdominal aortic aneurysms. A variety of strategies have been described to reduce the ischemic insult to the spinal cord with varying degrees of efficacy [39].

Subarachnoid (SA) Drain

Strategies to reduce the incidence of SCI are directed towards optimizing spinal cord perfusion pressure, which is the difference between the mean arterial pressure and either the CSF pressure or central venous pressure—whichever is higher. Spinal cord perfusion is improved by draining CSF, augmentation of arterial pressure, reducing central venous pressure, or a combination. Common indications for placement and the clinical management of SA drain are explained in Table 11.2.

There are two different approaches to intraoperative management of the subarachnoid drain. One is to measure the SCF pressure continuously and to drain intermittently to maintain a CSF pressure of 10 mmHg [41, 42]. The other approach is to drain continuously with a system that allows drainage with CSF pressure over 10 mmHg and to measure pressure intermittently. Risks from SA drain placement are spinal headache, subarachnoid hemorrhage, subdural and epidural hematoma, infection, and catheter fracture [43].

Table 11.2 Placement and clinical management of subarachnoid drain during TEVAR

Indication for SA drain
• Type I or type II aneurysm (Crawford classification)
• Stent graft length > 20–25 cm
• Hybrid procedures including the aortic arch or visceral branches
• Previous surgery of the abdominal aorta
Placement technique
• Seated or latero-decubital position
• Preferably awake patient
• Insertion at L3–4 or L4–5 level
• Intrathecal length > 5 cm
Management of SA drain [40]
• Connection to a non-pressurized transducer
• Zero-point at ear lobe
• Continuous drainage to maintain CSF pressure at 10 mmHg
• Limit drainage to 25 ml per hour
• Intermittent monitoring of CSF pressure with transducer
• Avoid elevated central venous pressure
• Clamp the SA drain during patient transport
Additional measures
• Maintain mean arterial pressure 85–100 mmHg
• Maintain spinal cord perfusion pressure > 70 mmHg
• Maintain hemoglobin >10 g/dL
• Maintain normal cardiac output/index
• Avoid underbody or lower body forced air warming devices

Blood Pressure Augmentation

Augmentation of the mean arterial pressure can be achieved with fluid administration and/or use of vasopressor agents. A targeted mean arterial pressure of 85–100 mmHg is typically well tolerated. The ultimate goal is to ensure a spinal cord perfusion pressure above 70 mmHg [44], which is achieved when the CSF pressure 15 or less with a mean arterial pressure of 85 mmHg. Vasopressor support is sometimes required to achieve a higher mean arterial pressure. Another important intervention is to maintain low central venous pressure, which reduces venous congestion. If the central venous pressure is higher than the CSF pressure, the spinal cord perfusion gradient becomes dependent on the difference between the mean arterial and central venous pressures.

Surgical Interventions

New endovascular techniques have evolved to decrease the insult on spinal cord perfusion. These include coil embolization of large lumbar arteries to prevent reverse flow from the collateral network into the aneurysmal sac, and use of branched stent grafts to preserve perfusion into larger intercostal arteries. Another approach includes a staged procedure consisting of coil embolization of feeding arteries, followed by stenting of the aorta. This aims to improve the ischemic tolerance and allow remodeling of the collateral network of the spinal cord before the stent placement [45]. Temporary aortic sac perfusion is another approach, in which a fenestrated stent graft is placed, allowing flow into the aneurysmal sac to supply the segmental arteries during the most vulnerable period. Coil embolization is performed at a later date. Lastly, staged operations of long segments of the descending aorta with or without hybrid techniques have become popular. Stenting smaller segments at each stage allows for excluding vital feeding vessels over a longer period of time, which promotes the development of the spinal cord collateral network [46].

Neurophysiologic Monitoring

Intraoperative monitoring of spinal cord integrity with motor- and somatosensory evoked potentials is used in some institutions. Although these methods are very sensitive to detect early spinal cord ischemia, they are complex, require trained specialists to interpret the findings and can be influenced by anesthetic agents. In addition, they cannot be used in the postoperative period. The anesthetic management must be tailored to minimize interference of this monitoring technique by limiting the alveolar concentration of inhaled agent to 0.5 MAC, supplemented by intravenous anesthetics, and withholding paralytic agents, if motor evoked potentials are monitored. Recent experience with the use of near infrared spectroscopy has been described as a noninvasive trend monitor of paraspinal vasculature perfusion, which is part of the spinal cord collateral network [47].

Postoperative Considerations

Although TEVAR is less invasive than open surgical repair, the advanced age and multiple comorbidities that typically comprise these patients' clinical profile, make them susceptible to a variety of postoperative complications. The intensive care management of patients with TEVAR aims to optimize end organ function and to identify and manage complications early in their course.

Spinal Cord Ischemia Detection and Rescue Treatment

The choice of anesthetic agents should provide a fast emergence that allows for immediate neurological assessment after TEVAR. A rapid wean of respiratory support and extubation of the patient's trachea in the operating room is the goal. SCI is suspected in the presence of a motor or sensory deficit not attributable to intracranial pathology. The clinical presentation of SCI is a spectrum of motor and sensory impairment, which vary in severity and onset. It is important to examine the quadriceps flexion controlled by the lumbar plexus, as opposed to toe flexion and extension, controlled by the sacral plexus. There is sometimes a presentation of SCI with sacral sparing. This presents with proximal muscle weakness, but preserved toe movement. It is important to differentiate SCI from acute leg ischemia due to vascular occlusion, which can also present with sensory and motor deficit, but the management is much different. Vascular occlusion is usually unilateral, associated with severe pain and profound loss of sensory and motor function of the ipsilateral limb, and lack of peripheral pulses. This mandates emergent intervention for revascularization. There are several helpful interventions in the event of spinal cord ischemia with new motor deficit (see Fig. 11.2).

Blood pressure augmentation (to a target of mean arterial pressure 85–100 mmHg) is accomplished with fluid volume expansion and vasopressor agents—phenylephrine, norepinephrine, and/or vasopressin. Spinal cord infarction that

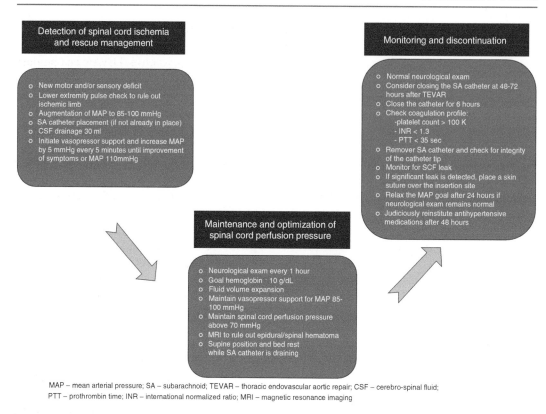

Detection of spinal cord ischemia and rescue management

- o New motor and/or sensory deficit
- o Lower extremity pulse check to rule out ischemic limb
- o Augmentation of MAP to 85-100 mmHg
- o SA catheter placement (if not already in place)
- o CSF drainage 30 ml
- o Initiate vasopressor support and increase MAP by 5 mmHg every 5 minutes until improvement of symptoms or MAP 110mmHg

Monitoring and discontinuation

- o Normal neurological exam
- o Consider closing the SA catheter at 48-72 hours after TEVAR
- o Close the catheter for 6 hours
- o Check coagulation profile:
  -platelet count > 100 K
  - INR < 1.3
  - PTT < 35 sec
- o Remover SA catheter and check for integrity of the catheter tip
- o Monitor for SCF leak
- o If significant leak is detected, place a skin suture over the insertion site
- o Relax the MAP goal after 24 hours if neurological exam remains normal
- o Judiciously reinstitute antihypertensive medications after 48 hours

Maintenance and optimization of spinal cord perfusion pressure

- o Neurological exam every 1 hour
- o Goal hemoglobin ˙ 10 g/dL
- o Fluid volume expansion
- o Maintain vasopressor support for MAP 85-100 mmHg
- o Maintain spinal cord perfusion pressure above 70 mmHg
- o MRI to rule out epidural/spinal hematoma
- o Supine position and bed rest while SA catheter is draining

MAP – mean arterial pressure; SA – subarachnoid; TEVAR – thoracic endovascular aortic repair; CSF – cerebro-spinal fluid; PTT – prothrombin time; INR – international normalized ratio; MRI – magnetic resonance imaging

Fig. 11.2 Algorithm for rescue management of spinal cord ischemia in the postoperative period

occurs as a consequence of intraoperative embolization is often irreversible, and may not improve with blood pressure augmentation. If not already present, a subarachnoid catheter should be placed and 25–40 ml of CSF fluid should be drained immediately. Hemoglobin should be maintained to a level of 10 g/dL in the event of SCI to ensure adequate oxygen delivery. Magnetic resonance imaging is used to detect spinal cord infarction and spinal/epidural hematoma. The duration of CSF drainage is empirical and based on the patient's clinical signs, however, experimental studies have shown that the zenith of the spinal cord blood supply is in the first 48 h after the aortic stenting. After that period, the blood supply slowly recovers, suggesting augmentation of the existing collateral network [48].

Postoperative Stroke

The incidence of stroke after TEVAR is about 4% [49]. The stroke risk is increased with severe atheromatous aortic disease, guide wire instru-

mentation of the aortic arch, history of stroke, landing zone for the stent graft in the aortic arch, and left subclavian artery occlusion [50]. More often the embolic shower involves the posterior cerebral circulation (60%) rather than the anterior circulation (40%) [51]. The immediate management of the postoperative stroke is focused on the prevention of secondary ischemic insult, thus avoidance of hypercarbia, hypoxemia, hyperglycemia, hyperthermia, hyponatremia, anemia and hypotension are of paramount importance.

Contrast Induced Nephropathy and Postoperative AKI

Acute kidney injury (AKI) after TEVAR is associated with increased morbidity and mortality [52]. The treatment is largely supportive and consists of hemodynamic optimization, restoration of euvolemia, correction of anemia, and avoidance of nephrotoxic agents. Long term, there is a risk of worsening kidney function several months after TEVAR, which is often due to the repetitive administration of radiocontrast during surveillance studies and to the progression of the atherosclerotic disease. Contrast induced nephropathy has a known insulting factor and highly predictable timing and thus, it is a modifiable cause of post-procedural AKI. The strongest predictor for contrast induced nephropathy is preexisting renal insufficiency. The principal intervention that reduces the incidence of contrast induced nephropathy is fluid volume expansion. Cumulative data from randomized studies have established the attenuating effect of isotonic fluid administration, several hours before and after the injection of radiocontrast agent [53]. The concomitant use of loop diuretics, mannitol or dopamine receptor agonists is not supported by the current evidence. Recently, the theory of contrast associated kidney injury in other fluoroscopic procedures, such as transfemoral aortic valve replacements, has been challenged in the absence of an association between the dose of radiocontrast agent and development of AKI [54].

Hybrid Procedures

A hybrid surgery involves TEVAR and an open surgical approach in a concurrent or staged procedure of extra-anatomic vascular transposition to expand the safe length of the stent graft without causing occlusion of important aortic branches.

Aortic Arch Debranching and Bypass Procedures

Hybrid procedures are performed when aortic pathology involves the aortic arch, and allow stent graft coverage of the supra-aortic branch vessels. These techniques are attractive alternative to the open arch replacement under deep hypothermic circulatory arrest. The most common example of a hybrid aortic arch procedure is the left carotid-subclavian artery bypass followed by TEVAR (Fig. 11.3a). It is considered when the proximal landing zone is expected to cover the origin of left subclavian artery (in 40% of the patients presenting for TEVAR). The technique

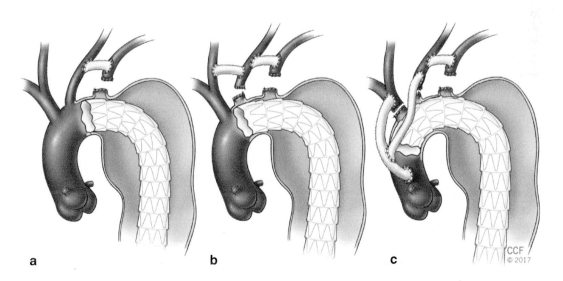

a   b   c

Fig. 11.3 Common aortic arch debranching procedures are used to ensure an adequate landing zone for endovascular stent grafting in proximal arch pathology. (**a**) Endograft with proximal seal in landing zone 2, requiring left carotid-subclavian artery bypass. (**b**) Endograft with proximal seal in landing zone 1, which requires carotid- to-carotid and left carotid-subclavian artery bypass graft. (**c**) Endograft with proximal seal in landing zone 0, and full arch debranching with extra-anatomical bypass graft attached to the ascending aorta. Reprinted with permission, Cleveland Clinic Center for Medical Art and Photography © 2017. All Rights Reserved

includes a carotid-subclavian artery bypass graft placement with ligation of the left subclavian artery proximally, to prevent back flow into the aneurysm sac. Left carotid-subclavian artery bypass is indicated prior to TEVAR when the proximal end of the stent graft causes left subclavian occlusion and in the presence of any of the following high risk conditions: a left dominant vertebral artery, an occluded right vertebral artery, a patent left internal mammary coronary artery bypass graft, use of long segment (>20 cm) stent graft, previous abdominal aortic repair, and/ or hypogastric artery occlusion [55]. If the stent landing zone is even more proximal into the aortic arch, a right-to-left carotid-carotid and left carotid-subclavian artery bypass grafting is plausible to allow aortic stent placement between the innominate and the left carotid artery (Fig. 11.3b). A full arch debranching with grafting of all three supra-aortic vessels into the ascending aorta allows the aortic stent coverage of the entire aortic arch (Fig. 11.3c) [56]

Hybrid Elephant Trunk Procedure

The classic approach for pathology involving the transverse arch with inadequate proximal landing zone is to perform a stage I elephant trunk procedure—total arch replacement—to create a proximal landing zone. A second stage procedure addresses the descending thoracic aortic aneurysm with endovascular stent grafting.

Frozen Elephant Trunk Procedure

Frozen elephant trunk (FET) is a newer technique, which extends the repair of the aorta beyond the arch into the proximal descending aorta within a single stage operation [57]. It includes ascending aortic replacement with a surgical graft, along with total arch and proximal descending repair with direct attachment of a thoracic stent graft sutured to the proximal surgical graft. The stent device is delivered in antegrade fashion through the open aorta. The length of the stent graft is 10–15 cm and the distal end is positioned in the proximal descending aorta [58].

This procedure is followed by TEVAR, and the frozen stent graft serves as a proximal landing zone. The site for intraoperative arterial line monitoring during a FET procedure presents a challenge for the anesthesiologist. The most common surgical arterial cannulation site is the right axillary artery, making right upper extremity arterial pressure monitoring inaccurate during cardiopulmonary bypass. The arterial catheter can be placed in the left arm, assuming that the surgical plan includes left subclavian artery revascularization. It is common practice to have a lower extremity arterial catheter in addition to the upper extremity arterial catheter, to detect elephant trunk graft kinking. In this case, the femoral catheter will have lower blood pressure than the upper extremity arterial catheter. Spinal cord ischemia is reported in 6% of the patients undergoing a FET technique [58]. The risk of spinal cord ischemia precludes the placement of longer stent grafts in these hybrid procedures. In high risk patients, a preoperative subarachnoid drain is placed to decrease the risk of ischemic spinal cord injury.

Aortic Visceral Debranching Procedures

Similar to the aortic arch debranching techniques, hybrid procedures can also be used to treat distally extending aortic disease involving the visceral aortic segment. Aortic visceral debranching with extra-anatomic bypasses allows for retrograde perfusion of the visceral and renal arteries from the lower aorta or iliac arteries, during endovascular stent grafting of thoracoabdominal aorta. This technique has the advantage of avoiding a thoracoabdominal incision, visceral and renal ischemic time, and the use of left heart bypass. It can be performed as a single or two-stage procedure. The advantage of the single stage surgery is to avoid a possible aneurysm rupture between the interventions. The two stage procedure allows for a shorter interventional procedure, a lower incidence of acute kidney injury by avoiding administration of a contrast load immediately after an ischemic episode, and avoiding ischemia reperfusion injury with hypotension [59]. Reno-visceral debranching combined with TEVAR is preserved for patients at very high risk for open surgical repair.

Complications Unique to Endovascular Aneurysm Repair

Complications unique to TEVAR include the development of endoleaks, stent graft migration, occlusion of aortic branches with acute ischemic complications, access site complications, post-implantation syndrome, and cumulative radiation exposure.

Classifications of Endoleaks and the Need for Repeat Interventions

Endoleaks occur with incomplete exclusion of the aortic aneurysm by the stent graft, due to the continued flow into the aneurysmal sac. They are the most common cause of aneurysm rupture after endovascular aortic repair, and the most common indication for reintervention (7%) [60]. Endoleaks may occur immediately or late after surgery, therefore, long term follow-up with aortic imaging is required for patients after TEVAR. There are five types of endoleaks, which differ in their mechanism, prognosis and clinical management (Table 11.3) [61, 62].

Stent Graft Migration

Stent graft migration occurs when the stent changes its position over time due to inappropriate seal at the proximal landing zone. The most common causes for migration are suboptimal graft sizing—graft is under-sized—and landing on diseased aorta.

Access Site Complications

Arterial access for endovascular aortic repair can be performed via percutaneous or cut-down techniques. Percutaneous access has a lower rate of

Table 11.3 Types of endoleaks associated with TEVAR, mechanism and clinical management

Type of endoleak	Mechanism	Clinical management
Type I, Ia, Ib	At the landing zone of the endograft Proximal seal zone Distal seal zone	Repair is warranted in order to prevent pressurization of the aneurysmal sac with angioplasty or stent graft extension
Type II	Retrograde filling into the aneurysmal sac from aortic branch vessels	Observation with serial imaging, majority resolve spontaneously. If persistent, treatment is recommended due to aneurysm sac expansion. Most common technique is arterial coil embolization
Type III	Component separation in the endograft, more common in the thoracic region, because of greater hemodynamic stress	Repair is indicated due to "endograft fatigue" and high risk of aneurysm rupture. Most common intervention is additional stent placement across the fabric disruption
Type IV	Graft porosity	Rare type, does not increase the risk of rupture and intervention is not recommended
Type V	Expansion of the sac with no detectable endoleak	Poorly understood mechanism, may represent unidentified type I or type III. If sac expansion is detected, treatment options include additional stent placement or open surgical repair

complications, and is associated with faster recovery and patient ambulation, and lower pain scores. The presence of arterial calcifications, prior groin exploration, and small vessel caliber may preclude the use of a percutaneous approach. Arterial thrombosis with acute leg ischemia, pseudoaneurysm formation, bleeding, infection, and arterial dissection are among the most common vascular site complications. These may require additional interventions such as thrombectomy, endarterectomy, and angioplasty to ensure arterial patency and hemostasis [28]. Iliac surgical conduit is commonly used for entry point and passage of the endovascular device into heavily diseased iliac arteries. Arterial rupture most commonly occurs during insertion or removal of the delivery system [63].

Post-implantation Syndrome

Post-implantation syndrome is a self-limited inflammatory phenomenon, which occurs several days to several weeks after endovascular stent grafting of the aorta. It presents with fever, malaise, increased white blood cell count and C-reactive protein, and may be difficult to distinguish from infection. Factors contributing to the development of post-implantation syndrome are the stent graft material, and ongoing thrombosis of the excluded aneurysmal sac. Careful inspection of the wound sites, negative blood cultures and low procalcitonin level can help to distinguish from blood stream infection.

References

1. Gutsche J, Szeto W, Cheung A. Endovascular stenting of thoracic aortic aneurysm. Anesth Clin. 2008;26:481–99.
2. Elefteriades J, Botta D. Indications for the treatment of thoracic aortic aneurysms. Surg Clin North Am. 2009;89:845–67.
3. Bavaria J, Coselli J, Curi M, Eggebrecht H, Elefteriades J, Erbel R, Gleason T, Lytle B, Mitchell S, Nienaber C, Roselli E, Safi H, Shemin R, Sicard G, Sundt T, Szeto W, Wheatley G. Expert consensus document on the treatment of descending thoracic aortic disease using endovascular stent-grafts. Ann Thorac Surg. 2008;85:S1–41.
4. Cao C, Bannon P, Shee R, Yan T. Thoracic endovascular repair – indications and evidence. Ann Thorac Cardiovasc Surg. 2011;17:1–6.
5. Roselli E, Greenberg R, Pfaff K, Francis C, Svensson L, Lytle B. Endovascular treatment of thoracoabdominal aortic aneurysm. J Thorac Cardiovasc Surg. 2007;133:1474–82.
6. Brunkwall J, Kasprzak P, Verhoeven E, Heijmen R, Taylor P, The ADSORB Trialists. Endovascular repair of acute uncomplicated aortic type B dissection promotes aortic remodeling: 1 year results of the ADSORB trial. Eur J Vasc Endovasc Surg. 2014;48:285–91.
7. Nienaber C, Rousseau H, Eggebrecht H, et al. Randomized comparison of strategies for type B aortic dissection: the investigation of STEnt grafts in aortic dissection (INSTEAD) trial. Circulation. 2009;120:2519–28.
8. Nienaber C, Kische S, Rousseau H, Eggebrecht H, Rehders T, Kundt G, et al. Endovascular repair of type B aortic dissection: long term results of the randomized investigation of stent grafts in aortic dissection trial. Circ Cardiovasc Interv. 2013;6:407–16.
9. Roselli E, Idrees J, Greenberg R, Johnston D, Lytle B. Endovascular stent grafting for ascending aorta repair in high risk patients. J Thorac Cardiovasc Surg. 2015;149:144–51.
10. Jonker F, Giacovelli J, Muhs B, et al. Trends and outcomes of endovascular and open treatment for traumatic thoracic aortic injury. J Vasc Surg. 2010;51:565–71.
11. Powell J. IMPROVE trial investigators. Endovascular or open repair strategy for ruptured abdominal aortic aneurysm: 30 day outcomes from IMPROVE randomized trial. BMJ. 2014;348:f7661.
12. Hogendoorn W, Schlosser F, Muhs B, Popescu W. Surgical and anesthetic considerations for the endovascular treatment of ruptured descending thoracic aortic aneurysms. Curr Opin Anesthesiol. 2014;27:12–20.
13. Cheng D, Martin J, Shennib H, Dunning J, Muneretto C, Schueler S, Segesser L, Sergeant P, Turina M. Endovascular aortic repair versus open surgical repair for descending thoracic aortic disease. J Am Coll Cardiol. 2010;55:986–1001.
14. Goodney P, Travis L, Lucas F, et al. Survival after open versus endovascular thoracic aortic aneurysm repair in an observational study of the Medicare population. Circulation. 2011;124:2661–9.
15. Gopaldas R, Huh J, Dao T, et al. Superior nationwide outcomes of endovascular versus open repair for isolated descending thoracic aortic aneurysm in 11 669 patients. J Thorac Cardiovasc Surg. 2010;140:1001–10.
16. Gopaldas R, Dao T, LeMaire S, et al. Endovascular versus open repair of ruptured descending thoracic aortic aneurysms: a nationwide risk-adjusted study of 923 patients. J Thorac Cardiovasc Surg. 2011;142:1010–8.
17. Jonker F, Verhagen H, Lin P, et al. Open surgery versus endovascular repair of ruptured thoracic aortic aneurysms. J Vasc Surg. 2011;53:1210–6.
18. Jonker F, Verhagen H, Heijmen R, et al. Endovascular repair of ruptured thoracic aortic aneurysms: predictors of procedure-related stroke. Ann Vasc Surg. 2011;25:3–8.
19. Berg K, Janelle G. Descending thoracic aortic surgery: update on mortality, morbidity, risk assessment and management. Curr Opin Crit Care. 2012;18:393–8.
20. Bub G, Greenberg R, Mastracci T, et al. Perioperative cardiac events in endovascular repair of complex aortic aneurysms and association with preoperative studies. J Vasc Surg. 2011;53:21–7.

21. Fleisher L, Fleischmann K, Auerbach A, et al. American College of Cardiology; American Heart Association. 2014 ACC/AHA guideline on perioperative cardiovascular evaluation and management of patients undergoing noncardiac surgery: a report of the American College of Cardiology/American Heart Association task force on practice guidelines. J Am Coll Cardiol. 2014;64(22):e77–e137.

22. Singh S, Maldonado Y, Taylor M. Optimal perioperative medical management of the vascular surgery patient. Anesthesiol Clin. 2014;32:615–37.

23. Zhan H, Purcell S, Bush R. Preoperative optimization of the vascular surgery patient. Vasc Health Risk Manage. 2015;11:379–85.

24. Ikeda S, Hagihara M, Kitagawa A, Izumi Y, Suzuki K, Ota T, Ishiguchi T, Ishibashi H. Renal dysfunction after abdominal and thoracic endovascular aortic aneurysm repair: incidence and risk factors. Jpn J Radiol. 2017;35:562–7.

25. Pisimisis G, Khoynezhad A, Bashir K, Kruse M, Donayre C, White R. Incidence and risk factors of renal dysfunction after thoracic endovascular aortic repair. J Thorac Cardiovasc Surg. 2010;140:S160–7.

26. Ishimaru S. Endografting of the aortic arch. J Endovasc Ther. 2004;11(suppl 2):II62–71.

27. Nicolaou G, Ismail M, Cheng D. Thoracic endovascular aortic repair: update on indications and guidelines. Anesthesiol Clin. 2013;31:451–78.

28. Chung C, Fremed D, Han D, Faries P, Marin M. Update on the use of abdominal and thoracic endografts for treating aortic aneurysms. Expert Rev Med Devices. 2016;13(3):287–95.

29. Ruppert V, Leurs L, Steckmeier B, Buth J, Umscheid T. Influence of anesthesia type on outcome after endovascular aortic aneurysm repair: an analysis based on EUROSTAR data. J Vasc Surg. 2006;44:16–21.

30. Kim M, Brady J, Li G. Anesthetic technique and acute kidney injury in endovascular abdominal aortic aneurysm repair. J Cardiothorac Vasc Anesth. 2014;28(3):572–8.

31. Edwards M, Andrews J, Edwards A, Ghanami R, Corriere M, Goodney P, Godshall C, Hansen K. Results of endovascular aortic aneurysm repair with general, regional, and local/monitored anesthesia care in the American College of Surgeons National Surgical Quality Improvement Program database. J Vasc Surg. 2011;54(5):1273–82.

32. van Drop M, Gilbers M, Lauwers P, von Schil PE, Hendriks J. Local anesthesia for percutaneous thoracic aortic repair. AORTA. 2016;4(3):78–82.

33. Hughes C, Sulzer C, McCann R, Swaminathan M. Endovascular approaches to complex thoracic aortic disease. Semin Cardiothorac Vasc Anesth. 2008;12(4):298–312.

34. Scott D, Denton M. Spinal cord protection in aortic endovascular surgery. BJA. 2016;117(S2):26–31.

35. Ullery B, Wang G, Low D, Cheung A. Neurological complications of thoracic endovascular aortic repair. Semin Cardiothorac Vasc Anesth. 2011;15(4):123–40.

36. Feezor R, Martin T, Hess P, Daniels M, Beaver T, Klodell C, et al. Extend of aortic coverage and incidence of spinal cord ischemia after thoracic endovascular aneurysm repair. Ann Thorac Surg. 2008;86:1809–14.

37. Ullery B, Cheung A, Fairman R, et al. Risk factors, outcomes and clinical manifestations of spinal cord ischemia following thoracic endovascular aortic repair. J Vasc Surg. 2011;54:677–84.

38. Drinkwater S, Goebells A, Haydar A, et al. The incidence of spinal cord ischaemia following thoracic and thoracoabdominal aortic endovascular intervention. Eur J Vasc Endovasc Surg. 2010;40:729–35.

39. Matsuda H, Ogino H, Fukuda T, Iritani O, Sato S, Iba Y, Tanaka H, Sasaki H, Minatoya K, Kobayashi J, Yagihara T. Multidisciplinary approach to prevent spinal cord ischemia after thoracic endovascular aneurysm repair for distal descending aorta. Ann Thorac Surg. 2010;90:561–5.

40. Rizvi A, Sullivan T. Incidence, prevention and management in spinal cord protection during TEVAR. J Vasc Surg. 2010;52:86S–90S.

41. Arnaoutakis D, Arnaoutakis G, Beaulieu R, Abularrage C, Lum Y, Black J. Results of adjunctive spinal drainage and/or left Subclavian artery bypass in thoracic endovascular aortic repair. Ann Vasc Surg. 2014;28:65–73.

42. Hnath J, Mehta M, Taggert J, Sternbach Y, Roddy S, Kreinberg P, Ozsvath K, Chang B, Shah D, Darling C. Strategies to improve spinal cord ischemia in endovascular thoracic aortic repair: outcomes of a prospective cerebrospinal fluid drainage protocol. J Vascul Surg. 2008;48:836–40.

43. Cheung A, Pochettino A, Guvakov D, et al. Safety of lumbar drains in thoracic aortic operations performed with extracorporeal circulation. Ann Thorac Surg. 2003;76(4):1190–6.

44. Bobadilla J, Wynn M, Tefera G, Acher C. Low incidence of paraplegia after thoracic endovascular aneurysm repair with proactive spinal cord protective protocols. J Vasc Surg. 2013;57:1537–42.

45. Foley L, Reece B. Advances in spinal cord protection for complex aortic repairs. J Thorac Cardiovasc Surg. 2016;151:614–5.

46. Etz C, Weigang E, Hartert M, Lonn L, Mestres C, Bartolomeo R, Bachet J, Carrel T, Grabenwoger M, Schepens M, Czerny M. Contemporary spinal cord protection during thoracic and thoracoabdominal aortic surgery and endovascular repair: a position paper of the vascular domain of the European Association for Cardio-Thoracic Surgery. European J Cardiothorac Surg. 2015;47:943–57.

47. Aspern K, Luehr M, Mohr F, Etz C. Spinal cord protection in open- and endovascular Thoracoabdominal aortic aneurysm repair: critical review of current concepts and future perspectives. J Cardiovasc Surg. 2015;56:745–9.

48. Etz C, Kari F, Mueller C, Brenner R, Lin H, Griepp R. The collateral network concept: remodeling of the arterial collateral network after experimental seg-

mental artery sacrifice. J Thorac Cardiovasc Surg. 2011;141:1029–36.

49. Feezor R, Martin T, Hess P, Klodell C, Beaver T, Huber T, Seeger J, Lee A. Risk factors for perioperative stroke during thoracic endovascular aortic repairs (TEVAR). J Endovasc Ther. 2007;14:568–73.

50. Cole S. Intensive care management of thoracic aortic surgical patients, including thoracic and infradiaghragmatic endovascular repair (EVAR/TEVAR). Semin Cardiothorac Vasc Anesth. 2015;19(4):331–41.

51. Ullery B, McGarvey M, Cheung A, Fairman R, Jackson B, Woo E, Desai N, Wane G. Vascular distribution f stroke and its relationship to perioperative mortality and neurologic outcome after thoracic endovascular aortic repair. J Vasc Surg. 2012;56:1510–7.

52. Chang C, Chuter T, Niemann C, Shlipak M, Cohen M, Reilly L, Hiramoto J. Systemic inflammation, coagulopathy and acute renal insufficiency following endovascular thoracoabdominal aortic aneurysm repair. J Vasc Surg. 2009;49(5):1140–6.

53. Weisbord S, Palevsky P. Prevention of contrast-induced nephropathy with volume expansion. Clin J Am Soc Nephrol. 2008;3:273–80.

54. Elhmidi Y, Bleiziffer S, Piazza N, Hutter A, Opitz A, Hettich I, Kornek M, Ruge H, Brockman G, Mazzitelli D, Lange R. Acute kidney injury after transcatheter aortic valve replacement: incidence, predictors and impact on mortality. Thorac Cardiovasc Surg. 2011;161(4):735–9.

55. Matsumura J, Lee A, Mitchell S, Farber M, Murad M, Lumsden A, Greenberg AR, Safi H, Fairman R. The Society for Vascular Surgery Practice Guidelines: management of the left subclavian artery with thoracic endovascular aortic repair. J Vasc Surg. 2009;50:1155–8.

56. Bicknell C, Powell J. Aortic disease: thoracic endovascular aortic repair. Heart. 2015;101:586–91.

57. Roselli E, Tong M, Bakaeen F. Frozen elephant trunk in DeBakey type 1 dissection: the Cleveland Clinic technique. Ann Cardiothorac Surg. 2016;5(3):251–5.

58. Roselli E, Rafael A, Soltesz E, Canale L, Lytle B. Simplified frozen elephant trunk repair for acute DeBakey type I dissection. J Thorac Cardiovasc Surg. 2013;145:S197–201.

59. Perez M, Coto J, Madrazo J, Prendes C, Al-Sibbai A. Debranching aortic surgery. J Thorac Dis. 2017;9:S465–77.

60. Ranney D, Cox M, Yerokun B, Benrashid E, McCann R, Hughes G. Long-term results of endovascular repair for descending thoracic aortic aneurysms. J Vasc Surg. 2017, Aug 25;67(2):363–368 (Epub ahead of print).

61. Green N, Sidloff D, Stather P, et al. Endoleak after endovascular aneurysm repair: current status. Rev Vasc Med. 2014;2:43–4.

62. Schlosser F, Muhs B. Endoleaks after endovascular abdominal aortic aneurys repair: what one needs to know. Curr Opin Cardiol. 2012;27:598–603.

63. Cheshire N, Bicknell C. Thoracic Endovasculr aortic repair: the basics. J Thorac Cardiovasc Surg. 2013;145:S149–53.

Non-Operating Room Anesthesia for Electrophysiology Procedures

12

Janet Martin and Davy C. H. Cheng

Main Messages
1. Provision of anesthesia services outside the setting of the operating room, also known as non-operating room anesthesia (NORA), is growing due to increased demand for less invasive interventions that occur in suites specifically devoted to non-operative interventional procedures.

2. This chapter focuses on NORA for electrophysiologic procedures for cardioversion and cardiac ablation.
3. NORA anesthetic interventions for non-operative cardiac interventions may include monitored care, sedation, regional anaesthesia or general anaesthesia.

Provision of anesthesia services outside the setting of the operating room, also known as non-operating room anesthesia (NORA), is growing due to increased demand for less invasive cardiac interventions. Recent advances in technology allows for increasingly complex cases, which may not otherwise be eligible for conventional surgery. Together with concomitant increases in co-morbidity burden and an aging population, the challenge of providing safe NORA is also rising. NORA anesthetic interventions for non-operative cardiac interventions may include monitored care, sedation, regional anaesthesia or general anaesthesia. Since anaesthesia for transcatheter procedures and percutaneous coronary intervention (PCI) have been covered elsewhere in this book, this chapter focuses on NORA for electrophysiologic procedures for cardioversion and cardiac ablation.

J. Martin (✉)
Centre for Medical Evidence, Decision Integrity and Clinical Impact (MEDICI), Department of Anesthesia and Perioperative Medicine, Schulich School of Medicine and Dentistry, Western University, London, ON, Canada

Department of Epidemiology and Biostatistics, Schulich School of Medicine and Dentistry, Western University, London, ON, Canada
e-mail: jmarti83@uwo.ca

D. C. H. Cheng
Centre for Medical Evidence, Decision Integrity and Clinical Impact (MEDICI), Department of Anesthesia and Perioperative Medicine, Schulich School of Medicine and Dentistry, Western University, London, ON, Canada

© Springer Nature Switzerland AG 2021
D. C. H. Cheng et al. (eds.), *Evidence-Based Practice in Perioperative Cardiac Anesthesia and Surgery*, https://doi.org/10.1007/978-3-030-47887-2_12

Anesthesia in Electrophysiologic Procedure Rooms

Anesthesia practice has expanded to support interventions beyond the operating room. Cardiac anesthesiologists may be particularly suited to providing anesthesia care during electrophysiologic (EP) procedures such as atrial ablation or cardioversion procedures given their familiarity with ventricular assist devices (VAD), intra-aortic balloon pumps (IABP), and other drugs, technologies and procedures for hemodynamic management, anticoagulation, and cardiac resuscitation. In addition, there is an increasing role for transesophageal echocardiography (TEE) to detect and navigate potential intracardiac thrombus, septal puncture, and other complications such as cardiac tamponade [1]. However, there are many aspects of anesthesia care provision in the EP suite that may be unfamiliar to the cardiac anesthesiologist, including management of the airway without intubation, deep sedation monitoring, high-frequency jet ventilation, and managing decompensating patients without the safety net of the well-equipped operating room.

General Issues of Safety and Competency in NORA Settings

Anesthesiologists are responsible for developing and implementing a framework that supports a culture of safety for non-operating room anesthesia (NORA). In addition, proactive monitoring and reporting NORA outcomes is essential for quality assurance and continued improvement [2]. Patients undergoing NORA procedures are at risk of serious injury and death if support structures and standards for NORA are inadequately implemented [3–5].

Closed claims analysis of NORA patients suggests that 25% of claims occurred in cardiac catheterization or EP laboratories. The most commonly reported claims involved death, permanent brain damage, or airway damage due to inadequate oxygenation and/or ventilation after substandard anesthesia care that could have been prevented by appropriate respiratory monitoring techniques [4, 6, 7].

NORA for EP procedures is often performed in suboptimal conditions, with crowded rooms,

Table 12.1 Challenges to providing safe care in NORA settings

NORA-specific challenges
Remote location far from pharmacy and supplies
Noisy environments
Limited workspace, small procedure room
Inadequate lighting
Minimal temperature regulation
Electrical/magnetic interference
Older, possibly unfamiliar equipment
Lack of skilled anesthesia support staff
Limited patient access during procedures
Inadequate power supply
Radiation safety
Challenges relevant to NORA and OR anesthesia
Supply of equipment
Appropriate monitoring devices
Inadequate support staff
Patient-related illness
More cases after normal working hours
Increased percentage of "emergency" procedures

Reproduced with permission from [8]

overhead equipment and C-arms, limited patient access, and with equipment that may be less familiar or suboptimal for the intended purpose (Table 12.1). While newer anesthesia equipment has been developed to support procedure-specific NORA settings, some settings rely on older or non-ideal equipment, which may have been modified or retrofitted for anesthesia in the EP laboratory setting.

In addition, many EP procedure rooms have not been proactively designed to support anesthesia equipment and added anesthesia personnel. As a result, power supply for anesthesia equipment may be inadequate, and lighting and patient access may be geared toward the EP procedure needs rather than that required for optimal patient monitoring by the anesthesiologist. Furthermore, EP labs may be remotely located, and comprehensive back-up equipment and protocols for all emergency contingencies must be proactively planned for.

Guidelines for NORA

Anesthesia provision for EP procedures must meet the same standards of safety as the OR setting. Anesthesia providers of NORA should be certified and competent resuscitation providers.

Deep sedation should be considered with the same regard for monitoring standards as for anesthesia [2]. Recommendations for NORA have been published by the ASA (Table 12.2). Readers are also referred to the extensive Royal College of Anaesthetists (RCoA) guidelines for non-operating room anesthesia which are routinely updated online [2].

Table 12.2 ASA Statement for Non-Operating Room Anesthesia (NORA) [9]

Background

These guidelines apply to all anesthesia care involving anesthesiology personnel for procedures intended to be performed in locations outside an operating room. These are minimal guidelines which may be exceeded at any time based on the judgment of the involved anesthesia personnel. These guidelines encourage quality patient care but observing them cannot guarantee any specific patient outcome. These guidelines are subject to revision from time to time, as warranted by the evolution of technology and practice. ASA standards, guidelines and policies should be adhered to in all nonoperating room settings except where they are not applicable to the individual patient or care setting.

Oxygen

1. There should be in each location a reliable source of oxygen adequate for the length of the procedure. There should also be a backup supply. Prior to administering any anesthetic, the anesthesiologist should consider the capabilities, limitations and accessibility of both the primary and backup oxygen sources. Oxygen piped from a central source, meeting applicable codes, is strongly encouraged. The backup system should include the equivalent of at least a full E cylinder.

Suction

2. There should be in each location an adequate and reliable source of suction. Suction apparatus that meets operating room standards is strongly encouraged.

Scavengers for inhaled anesthetics

3. In any location in which inhalation anesthetics are administered, there should be an adequate and reliable system for scavenging waste anesthetic gases.

Ventilation and Back-up

4. There should be in each location: (a) a self-inflating hand resuscitator bag capable of administering at least 90% oxygen as a means to deliver positive pressure ventilation; (b) adequate anesthesia drugs, supplies and equipment for the intended anesthesia care; and (c) adequate monitoring equipment to allow adherence to the "standards for basic anesthetic monitoring." in any location in which inhalation anesthesia is to be administered, there should be an anesthesia machine equivalent in function to that employed in operating rooms and maintained to current operating room standards.

Electrical outlets and suitable power supply

5. There should be in each location, sufficient electrical outlets to satisfy anesthesia machine and monitoring equipment requirements, including clearly labeled outlets connected to an emergency power supply. In any anesthetizing location determined by the health care facility to be a "wet location" (e.g., for cystoscopy or arthroscopy or a birthing room in labor and delivery), either isolated electric power or electric circuits with ground fault circuit interrupters should be provided[a]

Lighting and Back-up

6. There should be in each location, provision for adequate illumination of the patient, anesthesia machine (when present) and monitoring equipment. In addition, a form of battery-powered illumination other than a laryngoscope should be immediately available.

Space

7. There should be in each location, sufficient space to accommodate necessary equipment and personnel and to allow expeditious access to the patient, anesthesia machine (when present) and monitoring equipment.

Emergency resuscitation cart

8. There should be immediately available in each location, an emergency cart with a defibrillator, emergency drugs and other equipment adequate to provide cardiopulmonary resuscitation.

Emergency support

9. There should be in each location adequate staff trained to support the anesthesiologist. There should be immediately available in each location, a reliable means of two-way communication to request assistance.

Building and safety codes

10. For each location, all applicable building and safety codes and facility standards, where they exist, should be observed.

Post-anesthesia care

11. Appropriate post-anesthesia management should be provided (see standards for post-anesthesia care). In addition to the anesthesiologist, adequate numbers of trained staff and appropriate equipment should be available to safely transport the patient to a post-anesthesia care unit.

[a]See National Fire Protection Association. Health Care Facilities Code 99; Quincy, MA: NFPA, 2012

Anesthetic Considerations for EP Procedures

EP procedures, such as cardioversion and AF ablation, may be performed as elective procedures for patients with chronic arrhythmia. However, as population demographics change, and as indications for EP services expand, there has been an increasing demand for anesthesia support for emergent and urgent EP procedures.

To ensure adequate training and standards of care are implemented and adhered to, all NORA programs should appoint a lead clinical anesthesiologist to oversee program standards, training, and quality assurance [2]. Simulation training for crisis management should be provided.

Communication between the anesthesiologist, proceduralist, nursing and other support staff is essential, at all stages including before the procedure begins (anesthetic choice and safety concerns), during the procedure, and throughout recovery. An adaptation of the safe surgery checklist should be routinely used for all NORA procedures [2].

Preprocedural Anesthesia Considerations

Before anesthesia is provided in the EP suite, preparation should include review of equipment, space, and team roles. Preplanning for catastrophic cardiac emergences including cardiac arrest or rapid decompensation due to tamponade or unstable arrhythmias is essential [1, 2, 9, 10]. Communication and planning between the EP physician and anesthesiologist is critical.

Equipment Considerations

Before starting the procedure, check whether full facilities for resuscitation are available including functioning defibrillator, external pacing equipment, rapid infuser, pressors prepared, blood products in the room, large bore intravenous access oxygen supply (with back-up cylinders), airway devices, suction, and ventilation equipment. Ensure that pulse oximetry is available for conscious sedation. For general anesthesia and deep sedation, ensure continuous waveform capnography is available.

If surgical rescue might be provided within the EP lab setting, ensure the surgical instruments and anesthesia support measures for sternotomy have been prepared. If surgical rescue would be provided in the OR setting, ensure the protocol for rapid transport is discussed by the team before the procedure begins [1, 2, 9].

Emergency drugs including dantrolene for malignant hyperthermia, intralipid for local anaesthetic toxicity, and other reversal agents (naloxone, sugammadex, flumazenil) should also be available [2].

Before anesthesia is started, all anesthetic equipment should be checked. NORA equipment and medications should be part of a routine maintenance and quality assurance program [2].

Patient Considerations

On average, patients undergoing NORA for EP procedures are at higher risk than patients traditionally encountered in the operating room, due to advanced age, medical complexity (ASA III-IV), and may be undergoing NORA specifically because their complexity deems them ineligible for conventional surgical approaches.

To ensure safety and feasibility of NORA, patients should undergo pre-procedural work-up by the anesthesiologist in order to plan the best anesthetic approach based on the patient's medical history (type of arrhythmia, history of MI, stroke, heart failure, valvular disease, previous cardiac revascularization, previous ablation attempts, OSA, COPD, esophageal stricture, difficult intubation), physical examination (including presence of devices such as IABP, VAD, other implantable cardiac devices; surgical scars; signs of decompensated heart failure; vital signs, electrolytes, renal function; fasting status; TEE or TTE to rule out cardiac thrombus and assess ventricular function and valvular disease), ECG, current medications (anticoagulants, antithrombotics, antihypertensive agents, rate control agents, antiarrhythmic agents, diuretics; any drug associated with VT prolongation).

Perioperative Medication Considerations

For elective EP procedures, careful preoperative assessment of patient medications is essential. Medications with relevant cardiovascular effects including beta-blockers, calcium channel blockers, Class I and III antiarrhythmics, and digoxin are generally discontinued before the ablation or cardioversion procedure (Table 12.3). Discontinuation is recommended in order to allow for unimpeded diagnosis and monitoring of natural heart rhythm in order to guide the ablation or cardioversion procedure.

For emergent EP procedures, planned discontinuation of influential medications is not possible, and their impact will need to be considered in planning the anesthetic regimen and interpretation of rhythms throughout the procedure.

Pre-procedural assessment of the patient's current medication list for other agents which may affect cardiac arrhythmogenesis should be considered. Assessment should include whether the patient is taking any QTc-prolonging medications, which could predispose to added risk of torsades de pointes peri-procedurally (Table 12.4).

Intra-Procedural Anesthesia Considerations

Patients should be monitored by telemetry, with non-invasive blood pressure monitoring (NIBP), pulse oximetry, and capnography. Supplemental

Table 12.3 Antiarrhythmic drugs, half-lives, and when to discontinue before ablation procedures

Drug	Half-life (hour)	Time to discontinue before ablation (day)
Procainamide	3–4	1
Flecainide	12–27	3–5
Bisoprolol	9–12	2–3
Atenolol	6–7	2
Sotalol	10–20	3–5
Amiodarone	15–142 days	30–90
Diltiazem	4–9	1–2
Verapamil	3–7	1–2

Reprinted from the Journal of Cardiothoracic and Vascular Anesthesia, 2018, Vol 33, Pages 1892–1910, with permission from Elsevier [1]

Table 12.4 Drugs which may prolong QT interval

Drug Class	Examples[a, b, c, d]	
Class I antiarrhythmic agents	Procainamide Disopyramide	Quinidine
Class III antiarrhythmic agents	Amiodarone Ibutilide	Dofetilide Sotalol
Adrenergics	Epinephrine	
Antipsychotics	Haloperidol Droperidol Thioridazine Chlorpromazine Pimozide	Iloperidone Risperidone Paliperidone Quetiapine Ziprasidone
Antidepressants	Amitriptyline Nortriptyline Desipramine Imipramine Trimipramine Clomipramine Maprotiline Mirtazapine	Doxepin Fluoxetine Fluvoxamine Citalopram Escitalopram Sertraline Venlafaxine Trazodone
Antihistamines	Diphenhydramine Terfenadine	Astemizole Loratadine
Antifungals	Ketoconazole Fluconazole	Itraconazole
Antibiotics	Erythromycin Clarithromycin Levofloxacin Ciprofloxacin Pentamidine	Gatifloxacin Moxifloxacin Grepafloxacin Sparfloxacin
Antimalarials	Halofantrine	
Diuretics	Indapamide	
GI stimulant	Cisapride	
Antiemetics	Dolasetron	
Other	Tacrolimus	Tamoxifen

[a]This list is not comprehensive
[b]In general, first generation antipsychotics, antidepressants, and antihistamines have a higher risk of QT prolongation that newer-generation agents
[c]Risk of QT prolongation may be dose-dependent
[d]Digoxin may also predispose to torsades de pointes, though it does not itself lead to QT prolongation

oxygen should be administered via non-rebreather mask [1]. Transesophageal echocardiography (TEE) may be useful to guide hemodynamics and titration of drug infusions, fluid resuscitation, monitor for valvular or ventricular dysfunction, and detect pericardial fluid accumulation, or LA thrombus formation [1, 10].

Anticoagulation

Despite continuation of patient's usual anticoagulants warfarin or novel oral anticoagulants (NOACs), additional anticoagulation is essential for left heart procedures in order to prevent stroke, TIA, and LA thrombus. Current guidelines suggest administering unfractionated heparin to provide anticoagulation throughout EP procedures as shown in Table 12.5 [1, 11–15]. Anticoagulation loading dose should be administered at the time of intra-arterial sheath insertion and transseptal puncture, followed by continuous infusion [10].

Choice of Anesthetic

Since there remains a lack of definitive evidence from adequately designed and powered clinical

trials comparing different anesthesia and sedation regimens in the context of EP procedures, decisions related to which drug and dose rely on extrapolation of evidence from underpowered clinical trials together with theoretical knowledge from pharmacologic mechanisms of action, in vitro studies, clinical experience, and procedural-technical information. (Table 12.6).

1. **Cardioversion Procedures**

   For cardioversion procedures, the procedure is painful, but lasts only a short period of time (usually a few seconds). The goal for

Table 12.5 Heparin dosing for atrial ablation

Procedure	Heparin bolus	Heparin infusion	Target ACT
Atrial fibrillation	130 U/kg for patients receiving NOAC	2000–2500 U/h	300–400 s
	100 U/kg for patients receiving warfarin	10 U/kg/h	300–400 s
Ventricular tachycardia	50–100 U/kg	1000–1500 U/h	>250 s

Reprinted from the Journal of Cardiothoracic and Vascular Anesthesia, 2018, Vol 32, Pages 1892–1910, with permission from Elsevier [1]

Table 12.6 Anesthetic agents and their electrophysiologic effects

Anesthetic agent	EP effects	Special considerations
Sevoflurane	↑ QTc Enhances ectopic atrial rhythms No effect on SA and AV nodes No effect on accessory pathway	Safe to use
Desflurane	↑ QTc Inhibitory effect on AV node Tachycardia	Sympathomimetic ?Arrhythmogenic
Propofol	Inhibitory or no effects on SA and AV nodes No effect on accessory pathway Bradycardia	May not be suitable for ectopic atrial tachycardia ablation; suppresses electrical storm
Midazolam	? Vagolysis ? Tachycardia	
Rocuronium	Minimum effects on automaticity	Avoid during phrenic nerve pacing
Vecuronium	Minimum effects on automaticity Bradycardia	Avoid during phrenic nerve pacing
Succinylcholine	Inhibitory effects on AV node Bradycardia or tachycardia	
Remifentanil	Inhibitory effects on SA and AV nodes Bradycardia	May not be optimal for AVRT and AVNRT ablation in pediatric patients.
Fentanyl	↑ vagal tone	Safe to use in EP procedures when combined with midazolam
Sufentanil	May ↑ QTc No effect on accessory pathway	
Dexmedetomidine	Enhances vagal activity Bradycardia ↓ norepinephrine release ↓ sympathetic tone	May not be suitable for EP procedures. Antiarrhythmic in pediatric patients
Ketamine	Minimal effect on SA and AV nodes ↑atrial conduction time	↑ heart rate ± blood pressure

AV Atrioventricular, *AVNRT* Atrioventricular nodal re-entrant tachycardia, *AVRT* Atrioventricular re-entrant tachycardia, *SA* Sinoatrial

Reprinted from the Journal of Cardiothoracic and Vascular Anesthesia, 2018, Vol 33, Pages 1892–1910, with permission from Elsevier [1]

direct current (DC) cardioversion will be to provide short-term general anesthesia (GA), such as with a propofol bolus (30-50 mg), or short term deep sedation using benzodiazepines and opioids. Propofol has been proposed as the preferred agent in order to ensure rapid onset and offset, blunt laryngeal reflexes, and prevent patient recall, though clinical trials have been sparse. Etomidate can be used if hemodynamic instability precludes the use of propofol; however, etomidate may induce myoclonus. Episodes of hypotension may be managed with fluids and phenylephrine. Regardless of which anesthetic approach is used, the patient should be continuously monitored for airway obstruction and adverse respiratory events. If chin-lift, jaw thrust, or nasal airway are unhelpful to relieve obstruction, emergency airway should be immediately available [1, 16].

2. **Ablation Procedures**

Cardiac ablation is achieved using catheter-based radiofrequency, cryoablation, ultrasound, or other forms of energy. Since the procedure is typically prolonged and uncomfortable, and requires mandatory periods of patient immobility, anesthesia requires appropriate levels of monitored anesthesia care (MAC) or GA. Preliminary evidence that GA may improve outcomes for AF ablation, requires assessment in larger randomized trials [17].

Depending on which anesthetic agents are used, GA may adversely affect hemodynamic stability and decrease the inducibility of VT. While MAC may provide some advantage in this regard, titration is challenging, and appropriate monitoring to ensure adequate sedation, while balancing risks of over-sedation and respiratory depression, must be guaranteed with appropriate equipment and monitoring staff devoted solely to the purpose of monitoring respiration. Furthermore, patient mobility and respiration may interfere with the quality and precision of the ablation field.

Since arrhythmias may be sensitive to sedation, over-sedation should be avoided. When intra-procedural testing for arrhythmia inducibility is required (i.e., ablation for focal PVCs), it is essential to use an approach to sedation or anesthesia that minimally interferes with inducibility.

GA may be preferred when complex ablation procedures with unstable rhythms, lack of cardiorespiratory reserve, or difficult airway is anticipated [1]. GA may also be preferred when control of ventilation is essential, such as during septal puncture or sheath exchange (to reduce risk of air embolism). Whether GA is provided with volatile or intravenous anesthetics remains an area of controversy, which will not be resolved until adequately powered trials of clinically-relevant outcomes have been completed.

GA with propofol is commonly used to balance patient comfort with level of sedation, but requires adequate monitoring for respiratory events, hypoxia, and if longer infusions are required: propofol infusion syndrome or metabolic acidosis. Use of ketamine (anesthetic, analgesic, and sympathomimetic properties) and dexmedetomidine have been described for ablation procedures; however, dexmedetomidine may induce hypotension and bradycardia through depressed nodal function (and unknown clinical relevance on arrhythmia inducibility), albeit with lesser risk of respiratory depression.

GA with inhaled anesthetics remains somewhat controversial. While in vitro studies suggest that sevoflurane and isoflurane might interfere with arrhythmia inducibility by prolonging action-potential duration and delaying atrial and ventricular repolarization, the clinical implications of this for EP procedures remain uncertain, and many centres continue to use volatile anesthetics in this setting [1]. Less information is available for the role of nitrous oxide in the EP setting. Scavenging systems and appropriate protections to reduce exposure of staff and the environment to inhaled anesthetic agents should be in place.

Monitored anesthesia care (MAC) may be preferred for procedures where GA suppression of arrhythmia inducibility must be avoided. For EP procedures under MAC, midazolam combined with short-acting opioids have typically been used, with selection and administration based on their respective dose-dependent EP effects [1].

Overall, the balance of existing evidence suggests that the nuances between theoretical differences anesthetic or sedation regimens are less important than the clinical acumen and safety structures in place to support the approach to anesthesia and sedation through adequate monitoring and management of adverse events as they arise [16]. Overall, similar to anesthesia in the operating room, monitoring of depth of anesthesia and use of muscle relaxants (and associated monitoring) should be directed on a case-by-case basis, depending on the concomitant patient characteristics, the complexity of procedure, and approach to ventilation.

Ventilation

High-frequency jet ventilation (HFJV) may be useful to improve conditions for ablation as it provides an apnea-quality stability for cardiac ablation, while minimizing the risk of hypoxia, hypercarbia, and atelectasis that is associated with apneic manoeuvres [1]. Serial blood gas measurements, and punctuated ETCO2 measurements can be used to guide ventilatory settings throughout the procedure. While HFJV may improve stability of tissue targets and LA or PV dimensions with less risk of catheter displacements, caution is warranted since it may increase risk of inadequate ventilation, barotrauma, pneumothorax, and pneumo-mediastinum [1]. Conversion to conventional ventilation may be required.

Since other forms of ventilation, including spontaneous ventilation and conventional mechanical ventilation, allows for cardiac excursion and changing LA and PV dimensions, which provides additional challenges for accuracy of ablation procedures, the ventilation strategy will need to be modified throughout the critical stages of the procedure. For mechanical ventilation with endotracheal intubation, using intermittent positive pressure to reduce atelectasis, and using appropriate settings for inspiratory-to-expiratory ratios, lung-volume, and PEEP will be essential to mitigate pulmonary excursion during critical ablation periods [1]. If an apneic period is required for the ablation procedure, hypoxia can be minimized by increasing the fraction of inspired oxygen before apnea onset, followed by performing recruitment maneuvers after the apneic period [1].

Radiation Exposure

Risk of radiation exposure during fluoroscopy-guided ablation procedures is relevant for patients and all team members present during the procedure. Female patients should be screened for pregnancy prior to EP procedures. Healthcare team members should be apprised of appropriate radiation protection strategies for EP procedures, as outlined in recent guidelines [18].

Post-Procedure Considerations

The usual standards of post-anesthesia monitoring are required post-EP procedures, typically occurring within the post-anesthesia recovery unit, cardiac intensive care unit, or equivalent. Most hemodynamically stable patients are extubated in the EP lab, particularly if there is low concern for catecholamine surge during emergence. Patients should be monitored for hypoxia, apnea, new arrhythmias, cardiac tamponade, fluid overload (crystalloid overload), heart failure, and groin or retroperitoneal bleeding.

Complications and Surgical Back-Up

Potential complications should be anticipated and planned for (Table 12.7).

Risk of death or conversion to surgery has been reported to be >4%. Together with the EP team, the anesthesiologist is responsible for setting up the EP lab to accommodate sudden cata-

Table 12.7 Potential complications of EP ablation

1. **Vascular complications**
   - (a) Hematoma
   - (b) Retroperitoneal bleeding
   - (c) Arteriovenous fistula
   - (d) Pseudoaneurysm
   - (e) Hemothorax
   - (f) Extrapericardial pulmonary venous perforation
2. **Transseptal puncture**
   - (a) Failure to puncture
   - (b) Puncture of adjacent structures
     (Aortic root, right atrium, coronary sinus, or circumflex artery)
   - (c) Cardiac perforation with tamponade
3. **Complications during catheter navigation and ablation**
   - (a) Transient ischemic attack or stroke due to thromboembolism
   - (b) Cardiac perforation
   - (c) PV stenosis
   - (d) Circumflex artery occlusion
   - (e) Esophageal perforation and atrioesophageal fistula
   - (f) Postablation atrial remodeling
4. **Pulmonary complications**
   - (a) Phrenic nerve palsy (more common with cryoablation)
   - (b) Pulmonary hypertension secondary to PV stenosis
   - (c) Pneumothorax
5. **Radiation hazards**
6. **Miscellaneous**
   - (a) High-grade AV block and inappropriate sinus tachycardia
   - (b) Pericarditis
   - (c) Valve trauma
   - (d) Coronary artery spasm and thrombosis
   - (e) Acute pyloric spasm and gastric hypomotility
   - (f) Infection

Abbreviations: *EP* electrophysiologic, *PV* pulmonary vein
Reprinted from the Journal of Cardiothoracic and Vascular Anesthesia, 2018, Vol 33, Pages 1892–1910, with permission from Elsevier [1]

strophic cardiac complications that may arise intra-procedurally (ie, tamponade, destabilizing arrythmias). Simulation training for catastrophic cardiac complications is encouraged. If conversion to surgery is required and must occur in the OR, the transportation plan must be preplanned and communicated, including the plan for adequate patient support and monitoring during transport (ECG, oxygen saturation, BP monitoring), along with dedicated OR capacity, OR personnel, and guaranteed elevator and hallway access. If surgical rescue for complications is possible within the EP lab, adequate supplies (surgical instruments, sternotomy tray on standby) and protocols should be part of the preprocedure checklist, to ensure preparation. In some cases, overly complex EP procedures may be performed in the OR instead of the EP lab or in hybrid OR settings, to offset the need for emergency conversion or transfer, which are often associated with poor outcomes [1, 10, 16].

Complications may occur during the procedure, during the recovery period, and others may arise after discharge. Patients should be constantly monitored for potential loss of airway, respiratory drive, or airway obstruction throughout the procedure and during recovery [1]. During recovery, the patient is at risk for new arrhythmias, tamponade, and fluid overload, heart failure, and bleeding from the sheath. If catecholamine surge is a risk, continued intubation and sedation may be required [10].

Summary

Demand for NORA for elective and emergent EP procedures is growing, and patient complexity is increasing due to patient factors including inherent cardiac and thrombotic risk, often alongside a complicated medical history and advanced age. Provision of NORA requires significant attention to patient safety, including proactive management of equipment, medications, and a clear executable plan for the decompensating patient. Additional preparation measures should include the routine maintenance of all anesthesia related equipment, an adequate supply of rescue medications, development of appropriate safety protocols, and routine use of a safety checklist and continuous real-time communication As in the operating room, routine use of safe surgery checklists and protocols ensuring availability of personnel and equipment and contingency plans are essential produce reliable and consistently safe results.

Evidence suggests that many NORA-related complications could have been prevented through appropriate, vigilant monitoring and maintaining the same standard of care as used in the operating room. The majority of adverse outcomes in closed claims related to NORA are related to respiratory depression and inadequate monitoring, which are preventable with adequate vigilance and preparation. Monitoring standards such as those outlined by ASA or RCoA should be instituted in all NORA environments, specifically emphasizing the assurance of continuous monitoring of adequate ventilation through clinical evaluation, pulse oximetry, and monitoring expired carbon dioxide.

References

1. Fujii S, Zhou JR, Dhir A. Anesthesia for cardiac ablation. J Cardiothorac Vasc Anesth. 2018;32(4):1892–910.
2. Royal College of Anaesthetists. Chapter 7 guidelines for the provision of anaesthesia services (GPAS) guidelines for the provision of anaesthesia services in the Non-theatre Environment 2019. Available at: https://www.rcoa.ac.uk/system/files/GPAS-2019-07-ANTE.pdf
3. Melloni C. Anesthesia and sedation outside the operating room: how to prevent risk and maintain good quality. Curr Opin Anaesthesiol. 2007;20:513–9.
4. Metzner J, Posner KL, Domino KB. The risk and safety of anesthesia at remote locations: the US closed claims analysis. Curr Opin Anaesthesiol. 2009;22:502–8.
5. Metzner J, Domino KB. Risks of anesthesia or sedation outside the operating room: the role of the anesthesia care provider. Curr Opin Anaesthesiol. 2010;23:523–31.
6. Chang B, Kaye AD, Diaz JH, et al. Interventional procedures outside of the operating room: results from the National Anesthesia Clinical Outcomes Registry. J Patient Saf. 2018;14:9–16.
7. Woodward ZG, Urman RD, Domino KB. Safety of non-operating room anesthesia: a closed claims update. Anesthesiol Clin. 2017;35:569–81.
8. Walls JD, Weiss MS. Safety in non-operating room anesthesia (NORA). APSF Newsletter. 2019;34(1):3–4.
9. American Society of Anesthesiologists Committee on Standards and Practice Parameters (CSPP). Statement on nonoperating room anesthetizing locations. October 17, 2018. Available at: https://www.asahq.org/standards-and-guidelines/statement-on-nonoperating-room-anesthetizing-locations. Accessed 23 Dec 2018.
10. Deng Y, Naeini PS, Razavi M, Collard CD, Topin DA, Anton MJ. Anesthetic management in radiofrequency catheter ablation of ventricular tachycardia. Tex Heart Inst J. 2016;43(6):496–502.
11. Calkins H, Kuck KH, Cappato R, et al. 2012 HRS/EHRA/ECAS expert consensus statement on catheter and surgical ablation of atrial fibrillation: recommendations for patient selection, procedural techniques, patient management and follow-up, definitions, endpoints, and research trial design. J Interv Card Electrophysiol. 2012;33:171–257.
12. Ren JF, Marchlinski FE, Callans DJ, et al. Increased intensity of anticoagulation may reduce risk of thrombus during atrial fibrillation ablation procedures in patients with spontaneous echo contrast. J Cardiovasc Electrophysiol. 2005;16:474–7.
13. Yamaj H, Murakami T, Hina K, et al. Adequate initial heparin dosage for atrial fibrillation ablation in patients receiving non-vitamin K antagonist oral anticoagulants. Clin Drug Investig. 2016;36:837–48.
14. Enriquez AD, Churchill T, Gautam S, et al. Determinants of heparin dosing and complications in patients undergoing left atrial ablation on uninterrupted rivaroxaban. Pacing Clin Electrophysiol. 2017;40:183–90.
15. Calkins H, Brugada J, Packer DL, et al. HRS/HERA, ECAS expert consensus statement on catheter and surgical ablation of atrial fibrillation: recommendations for personnel, policy, procedures and follow-up. A report of the Heart Rhythm Society (HRS0 task force on catheter and surgical ablation). Europace. 2007;9:335–79.
16. Gerstein NS, Young A, Schulman PM, Stecker EC, Jessel PM. Sedation in the electrophysiology laboratory: a multidisciplinary review. J Am Heart Assoc. 2016;5:e003629.
17. Di Biase L, Conti S, Mohanty P, et al. General anaesthesia reduces the prevalence of pulmonary vein reconnection during repeat ablation when compared with conscious sedation: results from a randomised study. Heart Rhythm. 2011;8:368–72.
18. Miller DL, Vano E, Bartal G, et al. Occupational radiation protection in interventional radiology: a joint guideline of the cardiovascular an interventional radiology Society of Europe and the Society of Interventional Radiology. J Vasc Interv Radiol. 2010;21:607–15.

Anesthesia for Combined Cardiac and Thoracic Procedures

13

Nathan Ludwig, Marcin Wasowicz, and Peter Slinger

Main Messages

1. Single stage combined cardiac and thoracic surgical procedures are high risk interventions, especially with regard to post-operative pulmonary complications and bleeding.
2. Anesthesiologists involved in these cases require expertise in lung isolation, one-lung ventilation, coagulopathy, right ventricular support and extracorporeal life support
3. In patients with intrathoracic malignancy there are specific considerations that need to be considered.
4. Lung transplantation patients with significant cardiac disease are a particularly challenging patient population
5. In some cases, two staged procedures involving non-invasive cardiac interventions may be ideal.

N. Ludwig (✉)
Department of Anesthesia & Perioperative Medicine, Western University, London, ON, Canada
e-mail: nathan.ludwig@lhsc.on.ca

M. Wasowicz · P. Slinger
Department of Anesthesia, University of Toronto, Toronto, ON, Canada
e-mail: marcin.wasowicz@uhn.ca;
peter.slinger@uhn.ca

Combined cardiac and thoracic procedures are rare, however due to progress of surgical techniques and recent advances in use of extracorporeal life support (ECLS) techniques the number of these procedures is increasing [1].

Anesthesia and optimal perioperative management for these complex, high-risk surgical interventions requires an expertise in both cardiac and pulmonary physiology, lung isolation techniques, the multi-organ impact of cardiopulmonary bypass (CPB) and additional monitoring techniques—e.g. transesophageal echocardiography (TEE). Combined procedures may include excision of invasive tumors, pulmonary endarterectomy, cardiac revascularization combined with lung resection, and cardiac procedures combined with lung transplantation (e.g. PFO closure).

There is no agreement amongst experts whether a one-stage or a two-stage procedure is ideal patients who are found to have both cardiac and thoracic lesions. The literature is mainly limited to case reports [2, 3]. A single stage procedure will have the advantages of avoiding of a second anesthetic, incision and hospital stay. One the other hand, a single stage procedure may be associated with excessive surgical trauma, blood loss, and ICU morbidity [4]. Combined pulmonary resection with cardiopulmonary bypass may be associated with post-operative pulmonary morbidity. In addition, possible immunological consequences regarding completing cancer surgery with cardio-pulmonary bypass have to be

© Springer Nature Switzerland AG 2021
D. C. H. Cheng et al. (eds.), *Evidence-Based Practice in Perioperative Cardiac Anesthesia and Surgery*, https://doi.org/10.1007/978-3-030-47887-2_13

considered. This text contains much discussion of various cardiac pathologies and their treatments in other chapters; therefore, this chapter will focus on the assessment of respiratory function in the preoperative setting. This will be followed by the specific anesthetic considerations of pulmonary malignancies. The relationship between cardiac surgery, CPB, and post-operative pulmonary dysfunction will then be explored. Finally, the anesthetic management for various combined thoracic and cardiac procedures will be discussed.

Patient Presentation

There are several clinical scenarios to consider:

1. An asymptomatic lung lesion is found during evaluation for cardiac surgery
2. A patient being investigated for lung pathology is found to have significant cardiac disease
3. A patient with an intrathoracic malignancy that is invading cardiac or major vascular structures
4. A previously undetected lung lesion is found intraoperatively after sternotomy for cardiac surgery

In scenarios one through three, there will likely be time for patient evaluation and multidisciplinary decision making to guide anesthetic and perioperative management. In scenario number four, anesthetic management will be more ad hoc. However, many of these "surprise" lesions are benign—i.e. granulomas or bullae—and require only simple wedge resection without intraoperative lung isolation or significant loss of postoperative pulmonary function.

Preoperative Evaluation

In order to decide if a patient is a candidate for a combined cardiac and thoracic procedure it is important to first consider some concepts that apply to all thoracic surgery patients. This section will focus primarily on the pre-anesthetic assessment for pulmonary resection in cancer patients [5].

A patient with a "resectable" lung cancer has a disease that is still local or local-regional in scope and can be encompassed in a plausible surgical procedure. An "operable" patient is someone who can tolerate the proposed resection with acceptable risk. The anesthesiologist is often seeing the patient at the end of the referral chain which may include family physicians, chest physicians, medical oncologists, radiation oncologists, critical care specialists and surgeons. There are situations when an anesthesiologist is asked to give his/her opinion on specific high-risk patients. However, the primary role of the anesthesiologist in the preoperative setting is to risk stratify patients and focus resources on the high-risk patients to improve their outcome.

Respiratory Function

One of the major causes of perioperative morbidity and mortality in the thoracic surgical population is respiratory complications—atelectasis, pneumonia, and respiratory failure. An assessment of respiratory function in three domains can help risk stratify patients: lung mechanical function, pulmonary parenchymal function, and cardio-pulmonary interaction.

Lung Mechanical Function

Many tests of respiratory mechanics and volumes show correlation with post-thoracotomy outcome: forced expiratory volume in 1 s (FEV1), forced vital capacity (FVC), maximal voluntary ventilation (MVV), and residual volume/total lung capacity ratio (RV/TLC). For preoperative assessment, these values should always be expressed as a percent of predicted volumes corrected for age, sex and height (e.g.: FEV1%). Of these the most valid single test for post-thoracotomy respiratory complications is the predicted postoperative FEV1 (ppoFEV1%) which is calculated as:

$$\text{ppoFEV1\%} = \text{preoperative FEV1\%} \times$$
$$(1 - \%\text{functional lung tissue removed} / 100)$$

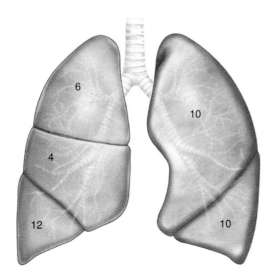

Fig. 13.1 Lung sub-segments. Copied with permission from Peter Slinger (Ed) 2011 "Principles and Practice of Anesthesia for Thoracic Surgery." Springer-Verlag New York

One method of estimating the percent of functional lung tissue is based on a calculation of the number of functioning sub-segments of the lung removed (Fig. 13.1). Patients with a ppoFEV1% > 40% can generally be considered low risk of post resection respiratory complications [6]. More recent improvements in surgical technique and postoperative analgesia can allow for patients to be operated on with a ppoFEV1% as low as 30 with an acceptable risk. 20% has been proposed as an absolute lower limit of acceptability for ppoFEV1% [7].

Pulmonary Parenchymal Function
As important to the process of respiration as the mechanical delivery of air to the distal airways is the subsequent ability of the lung to exchange oxygen and carbon dioxide between the pulmonary vascular bed and the alveoli. Traditionally arterial blood gas data such as $PaO_2 < 60$ mmHg or $PaCO_2 > 45$ mmHg have been used as cut-off values for pulmonary resection. Cancer resections have now been successfully done or even combined with volume reduction in patients who do not meet these criteria, although they remain useful as warning indicators of increased risk. The most useful test of the gas exchange capacity of the lung is the diffusing capacity for carbon monoxide (DLCO). The DLCO is a reflection of the total functioning surface area of alveolar-capillary interface. The corrected DLCO can be used to calculate a post-resection (ppo) value using the same calculation as for the FEV1 (Fig. 13.1). A ppoDLCO <40% predicted correlates with both increased respiratory and cardiac complications and is, to a large degree, independent of the FEV1. The National Emphysema Treatment Trial has shown that patients with a preoperative FEV_1 or DLCO <20% had an unacceptably high perioperative mortality rate [8].

Cardio-Pulmonary Interaction
The final and perhaps most important assessment of respiratory function is an assessment of the cardio-pulmonary interaction. Formal laboratory exercise testing is currently the "Gold Standard" for assessment of cardio-pulmonary function [9] and the maximal oxygen consumption (VO2 max) is the most useful predictor of post-thoracotomy outcome. The risk of morbidity and mortality is unacceptably high if the preoperative VO_2 max is <15 ml/kg/min [10]. Few patients with a VO_2 max >20 ml/kg/min have respiratory complications. Exercise testing is particularly useful to differentiate between patients who have poor exercise tolerance due to respiratory vs. cardiac etiologies.

Combination of Tests
No single test of respiratory function has shown adequate validity as a sole preoperative assessment. Prior to surgery, an estimate of respiratory function in all three areas: lung mechanics, parenchymal function and cardio-pulmonary interaction should be made for each patient. These three aspects of pulmonary function form the "3-legged Stool" and together they form the foundation of pre-thoracotomy respiratory testing (Fig. 13.2). The 3-legged stool can also be used to guide intra and postoperative management and also to alter these plans when intraoperative surgical factors necessitate that a resection becomes more extensive than foreseen.

Fig. 13.2 3-Legged
stool of pre-thoracotomy
respiratory assessment

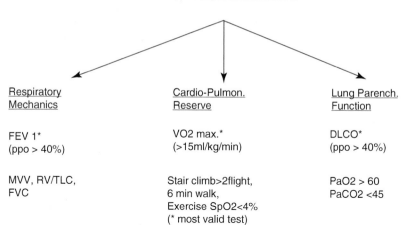

Fig. 13.2 3-Legged stool of pre-thoracotomy respiratory assessment

Preoperative Considerations in Thoracic Malignancies

At the time of initial assessment, cancer patients should be assessed for the "4-M's" associated with malignancy (mass effects, metabolic abnormalities, metastases, and medications). Mass effect relates to clinical syndromes such as obstructive pneumonitis, superior vena cava syndrome and Pancoast syndrome. Metabolic effect relates to clinical syndromes such as Eaton-Lambert syndrome, syndrome of inappropriate antidiuretic hormone (SIADH), and hypercalcemia. Pulmonary malignancies may metastasize to the brain, bone, liver, and adrenal glands and have effects on other organ systems. Medication effect relates to preoperative chemotherapy agents to consider in the perioperative period including bleomycin and cisplatin. Bleomycin is not used to treat primary lung cancers but patients presenting for excision of lung metastases from germ-cell tumors will often have received prior bleomycin therapy. Although the association between previous bleomycin therapy and pulmonary toxicity from high inspired oxygen concentrations is well documented, none of the details of the association are understood—i.e. safe doses of oxygen or safe period after bleomycin exposure. The safest anesthetic management is to use the lowest FiO2 consistent with patient safety and to closely monitor oximetry in any patient who has received bleomycin. We have seen lung cancer patients who received preoperative chemotherapy with cisplatin, which is mildly nephrotoxic, and then developed an elevation of serum creatinine when they received non-steroidal anti-inflammatory analgesics (NSAIDs) postoperatively. For this reason, we do not routinely administer NSAIDs to patients who have been treated recently with cisplatin.

Tobacco smoke—both primary and second-hand—is responsible for approximately 90% of all lung cancers. Other environmental causes include asbestos and radon gas—a decay product of naturally occurring uranium—which act as co-carcinogens with tobacco smoke. Lung cancer is broadly divided into small cell lung cancer (SCLC) and non-small cell lung cancer (NSCLC), with about 75–80% of these tumors being NSCLC. Other less common and less aggressive tumors of the lung include the carcinoid tumors—typical and atypical—and adenoid cystic carcinoma. In comparison to lung cancer, primary pleural tumors are rare. They include the solitary fibrous tumors of pleura (previously referred to as benign mesotheliomas) and malignant pleural mesothelioma (MPM). Asbestos exposure is implicated as a causative effect in up to 80% of MPM.

Although it is not always possible to be certain of the pathology of a given lung tumor preoperatively, many patients will have a known tissue diagnosis at the time of pre-anesthetic assessment on the basis of prior cytology, bronchos-

Table 13.1 Anesthetic considerations for different types of lung cancer

Type of Lung Cancer	Considerations
Squamous cell	Central lesions (predominantly)
	Mass effects: obstruction, cavitation
	Hypercalcemia
	Hypertrophic pulmonary osteoarthropathy
Adenocarcinoma	Peripheral lesions
	Metastases (distant)
	Growth hormone, corticotropin
Small cell	Central lesions (predominantly)
	Few surgically treatable
	Para-neoplastic syndromes
	Lambert-Eaton syndrome
	Fast growth rate
	Early metastases
Carcinoid	Proximal, intra-bronchial
	Benign (predominantly)
	No association with smoking
	5 year survival >90%
	Carcinoid syndrome (rarely)
Mesothelioma	Intra-operative hemorrhage
	Direct extension to diaphragm, pericardium, etc.

Copied with permission from Peter Slinger (Ed) 2011 "Principles and Practice of Anesthesia for Thoracic Surgery." Springer-Verlag New York.

copy, endobronchial ultrasound (EBUS) and sometimes mediastinoscopy or trans-thoracic needle aspiration. This is useful information for the anesthesiologist to obtain preoperatively. Specific anesthetic implications of the different types of lung cancer are listed in Table 13.1.

Non-small cell lung cancer is a pathologically heterogeneous group of tumors including squamous cell, adenocarcinoma and large-cell carcinoma with several sub-types and combined tumors. This represents the largest grouping of lung cancers and the vast majority of those that present for surgery. They are grouped together because the surgical therapy, and by inference the anesthetic implications, is similar and depends on the stage of the cancer at diagnosis. Survival can approach 80% for stage I lesions. Unfortunately, 70–80% patients present with advanced disease at stage III or IV.

Small cell lung cancer is neuroendocrine in origin and is considered metastatic on presentation

and is usually regarded as a medical, not a surgical disease. SCLC is known to cause a variety of paraneoplastic syndromes due to the production of peptide hormones and antibodies. The commonest of these is hyponatremia usually caused by an inappropriate production of anti-diuretic hormone (SIADH). Cushing's syndrome and hypercortisolism through ectopic production of adrenocorticotropic hormone (ACTH) are also commonly seen.

A well-known but rare neurologic paraneoplastic syndrome associated with small cell lung tumors is the Eaton-Lambert syndrome due to impaired release of acetylcholine from nerve terminals. This typically presents as proximal lower limb weakness and fatigability that may temporarily improve with exercise. Similar to true Myasthenia Gravis patients, myasthenic syndrome patients are extremely sensitive to non-depolarizing muscle relaxants. However, unlike true myasthenics, they respond poorly to anticholinesterase reversal agents [11].

Carcinoid tumors are low grade neuroendocrine malignancies and may be typical or atypical. These tumors can precipitate an intraoperative hemodynamic crisis or coronary artery spasm even during bronchoscopic resection [12]. The anesthesiologist should be prepared to manage severe hypotension that may not respond to the usual vasoconstrictors and will require the use of the specific antagonists Octreotide or Somatostatin [13].

Solitary fibrous tumors of pleura are usually large, space occupying masses that are usually attached to visceral pleura. They can be either benign or malignant, but most are easily resected with good results. Malignant pleural mesotheliomas are strongly associated with exposure to asbestos fibers. Their incidence in Canada has almost doubled in the past 15 years. With the phasing out of asbestos-containing products and the long latent period between exposure and diagnosis, the peak incidence is not predicted for another 10 to 20 years. The tumor initially proliferates within the visceral and parietal pleura, typically forming a bloody effusion.

Malignant pleural mesotheliomas respond poorly to therapy and the median survival is less than 1 year. In patients with very early disease, extra-pleural pneumonectomy may be considered. Alternatively, pleurectomy/decortication has been increasingly used.

Lung Injury Associated with Cardiac Surgery and CPB

Respiratory complications occurring after cardiac surgery with use of CPB are relatively common but the vast majority are mild and self-limiting [14, 15]. It is important to emphasize that the cause of lung failure after operations involving CPB is multifactorial [16, 17]; patient factors combine with the direct detrimental effects of CPB to compromise pulmonary function in the early postoperative period. A second insult to the respiratory system, such as loss of part of the pulmonary parenchyma, can be detrimental and lead to acute lung injury and unfavourable outcomes. If a cardiac procedure is performed with the use of CPB and is combined with thoracic surgery, which involves resection of lung parenchyma—lobectomy or pneumonectomy—respiratory complications may reach an incidence as high as 49% [18, 19].

Most patients who undergo cardiac surgery with the use of CPB present some degree of histological lung injury. Microscopic observations reveal a range of injuries detected within the structures of the air-blood barriers [20]. CPB causes a systemic inflammatory response syndrome (SIRS) [21]. This leads to the activation of neutrophils, macrophages and multiple cytokines including complement, and is commonly associated with free radical formation [22].

Prolonged mechanical ventilation after cardiac surgery occurs in about 6–7% of patients and the strongest predictors of this complication are: previous cardiac surgery, lower left ventricular ejection fraction, shock, surgery involving repair of congenital heart disease, and cardiopul-

monary bypass time [15]. The most severe form of injury to respiratory system-Acute Respiratory Distress Syndrome (ARDS)—occurs in 1–2% of cardiac cases with a very high mortality rate (40%) [23].

It should be noted that not all respiratory dysfunction after cardiac surgery is related to CPB. Other common factors include:

- Changes in lung mechanics related to sternotomy, internal mammary artery harvesting and other surgical manipulations. This presents as an increased elastance of the pulmonary tissue (decreased compliance).
- Atelectasis is a common postoperative complication after any major, prolonged surgery performed under general anesthesia. Atelectasis occurs in up to 70% of patients undergoing cardiac surgery with or without the use of CPB [17]. Atelectasis is also thought to be one of the main factors leading to further inflammatory injury leading to further deterioration in pulmonary function during the recovery phase after cardiac surgery.
- Phrenic nerve injury leading to poor diaphragmatic function. The most common cause of phrenic nerve injury is the use of cold saline flush or ice slush as a method of additional cardiac preservation. Fortunately, most of centers have abandoned this method of cardio-protection.
- Postoperative infections including pneumonia. All the aforementioned factors impairing pulmonary mechanics and ciliary clearance increase the risk of postoperative infections. Moreover, if a patient remains intubated for a prolonged period of time after any cardiac procedure the risk of ventilator associated pneumonia (VAP) increases to 44% (after 7 days of intubation) [24]. Other significant risk factors for postoperative pulmonary infectious complications include cigarette smoking (a very common habit in patients undergoing combined cardiac and thoracic surgery) and the use of H_2 blockers [25].
- Massive transfusions of red blood cells and other blood products also contribute to respiratory dysfunction postoperatively [26].

Overview of Anesthetic Management

The anesthesiologist providing care during combined cardiac-thoracic procedures faces multiple challenges. Quite often she/he must simultaneously manage hemodynamic instability, hypoxemia, problems with ventilation and excessive bleeding. The author will discuss only the most important problems occurring during combined thoracic and cardiac procedures.

Airway Management

If pulmonary resection is performed before or after CPB, the patient will require lung isolation. Options for lung isolation include the use of double lumen endotracheal tubes, single lumen endobronchial tubes, as well as bronchial blockers such as the Arndt blocker, Cohen blocker, Fuji uniblocker, or the EZ blocker. Regardless of device chosen, appropriate placement should be confirmed by the use of bronchoscopy. The most commonly used device for lung isolation is the left sided double lumen endotracheal tube. This versatile device is relatively easy to place, is more stable intraoperatively, allows access to both mainstem bronchi for suction, bronchoscopy, and application of continuous positive airway pressure (CPAP). In addition, double lumen endotracheal tubes allow for differential lung ventilation if required.

Management of one Lung Ventilation

The goals of one lung ventilation include the maintenance of adequate oxygenation and ventilation while also preventing the development perioperative lung injury. A full discussion of one lung ventilation is beyond the scope of this chapter but will be briefly described.

Hypoxemia with one lung ventilation may be difficult to manage. Risk factors for hypoxemia under one lung ventilation include high percentage of perfusion to the operative lung on preoperative V/Q scan, poor PaO2 during two lung ventilation, right sided procedure, normal or restrictive spirometry pre-op, and supine position during one lung ventilation [5].

The key maneuvers to be considered to improve oxygenation under one lung ventilation include: correct positioning of the lung isolation device; increasing FiO2; treatment of pulmonary edema; bronchospasm; blood and mucous plugging; CPAP to the operative lung; positive end expiratory pressure (PEEP) titration to the ventilated lung; recruitment maneuvers to the ventilated lung; selective lobar ventilation of the operative lung; decreasing volatile anesthetic concentration (or other vasodilators); increasing hemoglobin; optimizing cardiac output; temporary clamping the operative side main pulmonary artery (decreasing shunt); combination inhaled pulmonary vasodilator and systemic vasoconstrictor therapy (decreasing shunt); and return to two lung ventilation. If oxygenation is proving difficult with the maneuvers, it is likely that extracorporeal support will be necessary.

The ventilation strategy chosen for one lung ventilation must take into account the prevention of perioperative acute lung injury. The known factors associated with acute lung injury following pulmonary resection include: large pulmonary resection; large tidal volumes during one lung ventilation; excessive fluid administration; decreased lung function preoperatively; long duration of one-lung ventilation; preoperative chemotherapy; restrictive lung disease; administration of blood products; advanced age; and preoperative alcohol abuse [27]. One lung ventilation should include tidal volumes 4–6 ml/kg ideal body weight, PEEP and recruitment maneuvers titrated to optimal compliance, peak airway pressures less than 35 cm H20, plateau airway pressures less than 25 cm H20, minimizing FiO2 to the extent safely possible, as well as permissive mild hypercapneia.

Transesophageal Echocardiography

The use of TEE is one of the key components of intraoperative anesthetic management of patients undergoing combined cardiac and thoracic procedures. The important information obtained from intraoperative TEE during combined cardiac and thoracic procedures includes: assessment of left and right ventricular function (especially important after pneumonectomy); diagnosis of new wall-motion abnormalities (coronary artery bypass surgery); evaluation of effects of valve repair / replacement; and extension of the disease—for example lung tumor invading left atrium or pulmonary vein.

The Use of a Pulmonary Artery Catheter (PAC) in the Assessment of RV Function

The PAC is an excellent tool for combined cardiac and thoracic procedures as it will allow for continuous monitoring of hemodynamic status, particularly RV function and afterload for RV. It is particularly useful in the postoperative period when continuous TEE monitoring may not always be available. Warning signs of RV dysfunction include: high CVP, low PAD pressures or presence of square root sign when an RV channel is available [28]. During surgery, the anesthesiologist must remember to ask the surgeon to palpate the PA and its major branches catheter before clamping any part of the pulmonary arterial system. If necessary the PA line must be pulled back prior resection. RV failure may also be identified by a direct visual assessment of right ventricular distension. It is commonly caused by a rapid increase in the afterload (pressure) for the right side of the heart, especially after major resection of the pulmonary parenchyma—e.g. pneumonectomy.

Treatment includes:

- Reduction of RV preload—e.g. promotion of diuresis with diuretics—or early introduction of renal replacement therapy if there is no response to diuretics.

- Maneuvers to decrease the pressure in the pulmonary circulation—hyperventilation, hyperoxia, and pharmacological support. First line intravenous agents which decrease RV afterload and improve its contractility are dobutamine and milrinone. Inhalational pulmonary vasodilators—nitric oxide or prostacycline—are used when a lack of response to intravenous agents occurs.
- Preservation of good perfusion pressure to the right ventricle and ventricular interdependence— norepinephrine or vasopressin, and/or the use of an intra-aortic balloon pump.
- Since stroke volume is usually fixed in RV dysfunction, pacing (e.g. A-V pacing) can be used to increase heart rate and cardiac output.

Veno-Arterial ECMO

Due to advancement in development of extracorporeal techniques and better availability of ECLS perfusion, in some cases venoarterial ECMO might be used instead of full CPB. It allows for using relatively small doses of heparin (typically ACT is between 160–200 s) and subsequently it leads to less significant disturbances in coagulation. On the other hand, ECLS can still cause systemic inflammatory reaction and subsequent vasoplegia. When veno-arterial ECMO is used we must remember that it is entirely closed system, which does not allow the perfusionist to add any volume. When used in venoarterial configuration it allows to offload the heart; however, it does not allow full circulatory arrest.

Treatment of Coagulopathy

Combined cardio-thoracic procedures performed with the use of CPB are frequently complicated by excessive bleeding, which can have two possible causes: surgical (extensive surgery) and coagulopathy related to prolonged CPB. Treatment of CPB related coagulopathy is covered in more detail elsewhere in this book. In the context of high likelihood of massive bleeding and coagulopathy in our institution, for most of the combined cardiac-thoracic cases we secure at least two, large bore venous catheters to be able to transfuse large volumes of blood products in relatively short period of time.

Postoperative Pain Management

Postoperative pain control in the form of thoracic epidural analgesia remains the ideal technique for post thoracotomy pain. However, with many combined cardiac and thoracic procedures there is a distinct possibility of ECLS with resultant coagulopathy. Therefore, it is usually not advisable to place a thoracic epidural preoperatively. Instead thoracic epidural analgesia can be initiated in the postoperative period once bleeding has been stabilized and there is an absence of coagulopathy.

Anesthetic Management of Various Clinical Scenarios

Patients with Intrathoracic Malignancy Requiring Cardiac Surgery

Due to the above-mentioned concerns of postoperative pulmonary dysfunction many surgeons are reluctant to perform one stage cardiac-thoracic operations in the case of intrathoracic malignancy. Moreover, surgical access to the lung structures might be difficult if surgical incision and subsequent CPB cannulation are performed via median sternotomy. Additionally, there is anxiety regarding heparin use and the possibility of excessive bleeding. Apart from the injury to respiratory system, the possibility of dissemination of pulmonary malignancy through the use of CPB is a concern [29–31]. On the other hand, a one-stage combined procedure avoids the need for a second major thoracic surgery. Because of the risk of contamination of the operative field from an open bronchus, it is recommended to complete the cardiac procedure, wean from CPB, and close the pericardium before the pulmonary resection. Lung isolation and one lung ventilation will therefore be required in these cases. A dou-

ble lumen endobronchial tube placed at induction is an optimal way to manage these patients.

In the case of coexisting pulmonary malignancy and coronary artery disease the answer seems to be straightforward [30, 32]. Preoperative revascularizations performed by interventional cardiologists (PCI- primary coronary intervention) may cause significant time delays for subsequent cancer surgery and/or lead to in-stent thrombosis [33]. Thus, combined surgical coronary revascularization and resection of the lung cancer may be the optimal management.

Whenever possible, off pump coronary artery grafting (OPCABG) is the preferred surgical management of coronary artery disease in patients who require pulmonary resection at the same time as coronary revascularization. Revascularization is usually performed as the first part of the procedure followed by the resection of the pulmonary pathology. The most important principles of anesthetic management for OPCABG are covered in more detail in other chapters of this text. Significant considerations include aggressive maintenance of normothermia to prevent bleeding and/or acidosis, and preservation of hemodynamic stability during surgical manipulation of the heart. The results of these combined thoracic-cardiac surgeries are encouraging, however published results usually involve a small number of patients [19, 34].

In the case of open heart valve repair/replacement, CPB cannot be avoided. Thus, the decision to proceed with single versus two-staged procedures is more difficult. Consideration should be given to a two-staged procedure involving transcatheter valve repair/replacement such as TAVR and TMVR.

Lung Transplantation Combined with Cardiac Surgery

In the course of the extensive work up conducted in patients being considered for lung transplantation it is not uncommon to discover significant cardiac comorbidities. The usual options of single and dual stage procedures exist in the case of coronary artery disease. If the patient's respiratory status allows for some time before transplant listing, it is often possible to proceed with PCI prior to lung transplantation. This will allow for the patient to come off of duel anti-platelets therapy as per AHA/ACC guidelines [35] and then be listed for lung transplantation.

If the patient is in more urgent need of lung transplantation, single stage coronary artery bypass grafting and lung transplantation can be carried out. Options in increasing order of invasiveness include:

- Off pump coronary artery bypass grafting followed by lung transplantation. The transplant can be completed on or off centrally cannulated venoarterial extracorporeal membrane oxygenation (VA ECMO)
- Coronary artery bypass grafting completed on VA ECMO followed by lung transplantation (on or off VA ECMO)
- CPB facilitated coronary artery bypass grafting followed by lung transplantation (on or off VA ECMO)
- A prolonged CPB run with combined coronary artery bypass grafting and lung transplantation

The decision of which option to utilize will vary based on the specifics of the coronary lesions and experience of available surgeons. The use of CPB will significantly increase coagulopathy and bleeding during lung transplantation. This will similarly be true if lung transplantation is combined with other cardiac procedures including PFO closure or valve repair/replacement.

Intrathoracic Lesion with Invasion of Cardiac or Major Vascular Structures

When considering proper management of thoracic malignancies invading heart structures, surgical resection remains the only curative option for most intrathoracic malignancies. Sometimes conventional thoracic surgical techniques do not allow complete resection of a pulmonary tumor which is invading the heart or large vessels,

therefore radical surgical removal may necessitate the use of CPB [31].The most common examples are tumors involving left atrium, pulmonary artery or infiltrating the descending portion of the aorta [29, 36].

Most of the procedures involving resection or opening of the heart structures are performed via median sternotomy. Surgical exposure to some of the hilar structures is more difficult when compared to a lateral thoracotomy approach. Left lower lobectomy and mediastinal lymph nodes dissection are especially technically challenging when performed via median sternotomy. In many cases, EBUS or mediastinoscopy is indicated initially to rule out mediastinal spread of the disease and/or provide a tissue diagnosis. All these concerns raise the question as to whether aggressive treatment including surgical resection of lung parenchyma and cardiac or major vascular structures should be routine management. Clearly aggressive surgical treatment should be only performed in departments that are prepared for the complexity of those cases, can offer expertise in both cardiac and thoracic surgery, and provide anesthesia and postoperative ICU care for these patients. Moreover, the functional status of the patient prepared for this type of surgery should be excellent to allow them to survive a potential prolonged stay within an intensive care setting.

References

1. Wasowicz M. Anesthesia for combined cardiac and thoracic procedures. In: Slinger P, editor. Principles and practice of anesthesia for thoracic surgery. New York: Springer; 2011. p. 453–64.
2. Marseu K, Minkovich L, Zubrinic M, Keshavjee S. Anesthetic considerations for Pneumonectomy with left atrial resection on cardiopulmonary bypass in a patient with lung cancer: a case report. A & A case reports. 2017;8(3):61–3.
3. Rao V, Todd TR, Weisel RD, Komeda M, Cohen G, Ikonomidis JS, et al. Results of combined pulmonary resection and cardiac operation. Ann Thorac Surg. 1996;62(2):342–6. Discussion 6–7.
4. Ciriaco P, Carretta A, Calori G, Mazzone P, Zannini P. Lung resection for cancer in patients with coronary arterial disease: analysis of short-term results. Eur J Cardiothorac Surg. 2002;22(1): 35–40.

5. Slinger P, Darling G. Preanesthetic assessment for thoracic surgery. In: Slinger P, editor. Principles and practice of anesthesia for thoracic surgery. New York: Springer; 2011. p. 11–34.
6. Nakahara K, Ohno K, Hashimoto J, Miyoshi S, Maeda H, Matsumura A, et al. Prediction of postoperative respiratory failure in patients undergoing lung resection for lung cancer. Ann Thorac Surg. 1988;46(5):549–52.
7. Linden PA, Bueno R, Colson YL, Jaklitsch MT, Lukanich J, Mentzer S, et al. Lung resection in patients with preoperative FEV1 < 35% predicted. Chest. 2005;127(6):1984–90.
8. Fishman A, Martinez F, Naunheim K, Piantadosi S, Wise R, Ries A, et al. A randomized trial comparing lung-volume-reduction surgery with medical therapy for severe emphysema. N Engl J Med. 2003;348(21):2059–73.
9. Weisman IM. Cardiopulmonary exercise testing in the preoperative assessment for lung resection surgery. Semin Thorac Cardiovasc Surg. 2001;13(2):116–25.
10. Walsh GL, Morice RC, Putnam JB Jr, Nesbitt JC, McMurtrey MJ, Ryan MB, et al. Resection of lung cancer is justified in high-risk patients selected by exercise oxygen consumption. Ann Thorac Surg. 1994;58(3):704–10. Discussion 11.
11. Levin KH. Paraneoplastic neuromuscular syndromes. Neurol Clin. 1997;15(3):597–614.
12. Mehta AC, Rafanan AL, Bulkley R, Walsh M, DeBoer GE. Coronary spasm and cardiac arrest from carcinoid crisis during laser bronchoscopy. Chest. 1999;115(2):598–600.
13. Vaughan DJ, Brunner MD. Anesthesia for patients with carcinoid syndrome. Int Anesthesiol Clin. 1997;35(4):129–42.
14. Clark SC. Lung injury after cardiopulmonary bypass. Perfusion. 2006;21(4):225–8.
15. Sharma V, Rao V, Manlhiot C, Boruvka A, Fremes S, Wasowicz M. A derived and validated score to predict prolonged mechanical ventilation in patients undergoing cardiac surgery. J Thorac Cardiovasc Surg. 2017;153(1):108–15.
16. Picone AL, Lutz CJ, Finck C, Carney D, Gatto LA, Paskanik A, et al. Multiple sequential insults cause post-pump syndrome. Ann Thorac Surg. 1999;67(4):978–85.
17. Weissman C. Pulmonary complications after cardiac surgery. Semin Cardiothorac Vasc Anesth. 2004;8(3):185–211.
18. Danton MH, Anikin VA, McManus KG, McGuigan JA, Campalani G. Simultaneous cardiac surgery with pulmonary resection: presentation of series and review of literature. Eur J Cardiothorac Surg. 1998;13(6):667–72.
19. Wiebe K, Baraki H, Macchiarini P, Haverich A. Extended pulmonary resections of advanced thoracic malignancies with support of cardiopulmonary bypass. Eur J Cardiothorac Surg. 2006;29(4):571–7. Discussion 7–8.
20. Wasowicz M, Sobczynski P, Drwila R, Marszalek A, Biczysko W, Andres J. Air-blood barrier injury during cardiac operations with the use of cardiopulmonary bypass (CPB). An old story? A morphological study. Scand Cardiovasc J. 2003;37(4):216–21.
21. Tonz M, Mihaljevic T, von Segesser LK, Fehr J, Schmid ER, Turina MI. Acute lung injury during cardiopulmonary bypass. Are the neutrophils responsible? Chest. 1995;108(6):1551–6.
22. Kawamura T, Wakusawa R, Okada K, Inada S. Elevation of cytokines during open heart surgery with cardiopulmonary bypass: participation of interleukin 8 and 6 in reperfusion injury. Canadian journal of anaesthesia. Can J Anaesth. 1993;40(11):1016–21.
23. Ng CS, Wan S, Yim AP, Arifi AA. Pulmonary dysfunction after cardiac surgery. Chest. 2002;121(4):1269–77.
24. Rady MY, Ryan T, Starr NJ. Early onset of acute pulmonary dysfunction after cardiovascular surgery: risk factors and clinical outcome. Crit Care Med. 1997;25(11):1831–9.
25. Gaynes R, Bizek B, Mowry-Hanley J, Kirsh M. Risk factors for nosocomial pneumonia after coronary artery bypass graft operations. Ann Thorac Surg. 1991;51(2):215–8.
26. Karkouti K, Wijeysundera DN, Yau TM, Beattie WS, Abdelnaem E, McCluskey SA, et al. The independent association of massive blood loss with mortality in cardiac surgery. Transfusion. 2004;44(10):1453–62.
27. Slinger P. Perioperative lung injury. In: Slinger P, editor. Principles and practice of anesthesia for thoracic surgery. New York: Springer; 2011. p. 143–51.
28. Denault AY, Haddad F, Jacobsohn E, Deschamps A. Perioperative right ventricular dysfunction. Curr Opin Anaesthesiol. 2013;26(1):71–81.
29. de Perrot M, Fadel E, Mussot S, de Palma A, Chapelier A, Dartevelle P. Resection of locally advanced (T4) non-small cell lung cancer with cardiopulmonary bypass. Ann Thorac Surg. 2005;79(5):1691–6. Discussion 7.
30. Dyszkiewicz W, Jemielity MM, Piwkowski CT, Perek B, Kasprzyk M. Simultaneous lung resection for cancer and myocardial revascularization without cardiopulmonary bypass (off-pump coronary artery bypass grafting). Ann Thorac Surg. 2004;77(3):1023–7.
31. Klepetko W. Surgical intervention for T4 lung cancer with infiltration of the thoracic aorta: are we back to the archetype of surgical thinking? J Thorac Cardiovasc Surg. 2005;129(4):727–9.
32. Mariani MA, van Boven WJ, Duurkens VA, Ernst SM, van Swieten HA. Combined off-pump coronary surgery and right lung resections through midline sternotomy. Ann Thorac Surg. 2001;71(4):1343–4.
33. Marcucci C, Chassot PG, Gardaz JP, Magnusson L, Ris HB, Delabays A, et al. Fatal myocardial infarction after lung resection in a patient with prophylactic preoperative coronary stenting. Br J Anaesth. 2004;92(5):743–7.
34. Dyszkiewicz W, Jemielity M, Piwkowski C, Kasprzyk M, Perek B, Gasiorowski L, et al. The early and late results of combined off-pump coro-

nary artery bypass grafting and pulmonary resection in patients with concomitant lung cancer and unstable coronary heart disease. Eur J Cardiothorac Surg. 2008;34(3):531–5.

35. Levine GN, Bates ER, Bittl JA, Brindis RG, Fihn SD, Fleisher LA, et al. ACC/AHA guideline focused update on duration of dual antiplatelet therapy in patients with coronary artery disease: a report of the American College of Cardiology/American Heart Association task force on clinical practice guidelines: an update of the 2011 ACCF/AHA/SCAI guideline for percutaneous coronary intervention, 2011 ACCF/AHA guideline for coronary artery bypass graft surgery, 2012 ACC/AHA/ACP/AATS/PCNA/SCAI/STS guideline for the diagnosis and Management of Patients with Stable Ischemic Heart Disease, 2013 ACCF/AHA guideline for the management of ST-elevation myocardial infarction, 2014 AHA/ACC guideline for the Management of Patients with non-ST-elevation acute coronary syndromes, and 2014 ACC/AHA guideline on perioperative cardiovascular evaluation and Management of Patients Undergoing Noncardiac Surgery. Circulation. 2016;134(10):e123–55.

36. Nakajima J, Morota T, Matsumoto J, Takazawa Y, Murakawa T, Fukami T, et al. Pulmonary intimal sarcoma treated by a left pneumonectomy with pulmonary arterioplasty under cardiopulmonary bypass: report of a case. Surg Today. 2007;37(6):496–9.

Anesthetic Management of Heart Transplantation

14

A. Stéphane Lambert and Mark Hynes

Main Messages

1. Successful heart transplantation is a multidisciplinary collaboration
2. The considerations of patients with a "virgin chest" differ from those of patients on an LVAD
3. Perioperative events should be coordinated around the need to minimize the ischemic time to the transplanted heart
4. The transplanted heart is extremely sensitive to preload conditions and does not tolerate overloading very well
5. Pharmacologic support of the right ventricle is important
6. Echocardiography is critical to the success of heart transplantation, both intraoperatively and in the postoperative period
7. The new heart remains vulnerable to acute dysfunction for days to weeks following transplant and should be managed carefully

Much has changed since Professor Christiaan Barnard performed the first successful orthotopic human heart transplant in December 1967 at the University of Cape Town in South Africa [1]. Nevertheless, while it has become relatively common across the world, heart transplantation has never quite become a routine procedure and its success depends on a coordinated multidisciplinary approach involving careful patient selection and preparation, meticulous surgical technique, expert perioperative management and well-orchestrated long-term medical follow up and immunosuppressive therapy.

Heart transplantation can occur in isolation, or in combination with lung transplantation. Since combined procedures only account for about 10% of all heart transplantations, this chapter will focus on the management of isolated adult heart transplantation.

Successful organ transplantation begins with the careful management of the brain-dead donor, including careful consideration for oxygenation and organ perfusion during organ harvesting at the donor site. The detailed management of these patients is beyond the scope of this chapter, but good reviews have been written on the subject [2].

Epidemiology

Recent data from the International Society for Heart and Lung Transplantation shows that as of June 2015, about 55,795 isolated heart and 3879

A. S. Lambert (✉) · M. Hynes
Division of Cardiac Anesthesiology,
University of Ottawa Heart Institute,
Ottawa, ON, Canada
e-mail: slambert@ottawaheart.ca

© Springer Nature Switzerland AG 2021
D. C. H. Cheng et al. (eds.), *Evidence-Based Practice in Perioperative Cardiac Anesthesia and Surgery*, https://doi.org/10.1007/978-3-030-47887-2_14

heart-lung transplantations have been reported to their Registry, from 457 centers across the world [3]. In the United States, the number of isolated heart transplantations has steadily increased from about 2100 in the year 2000 to just a little under 3200 in 2016, according to the United Network for Organ Sharing [4]. As of August 2017, the number of people awaiting heart transplantation was just over 3900.

In Canada, 125 isolated heart transplantations were performed in 2015, according to the Canadian Institute for Health Information, a number that has remained relatively constant for the past 10 years. As of December 312,015, the wait list had steadily grown to 137 patients [5].

With constant improvement in the matching process, better surgical techniques and more effective immunosuppressive agents, the survival of heart transplant patients is well over 90% at 1 year and 80-85% at 5 years [4, 5].

The major indication for heart transplantation remains end-stage heart failure from chronic, acquired cardiomyopathy, which accounted for roughly 80% of all heart transplant recipients according to 2015 CIHI data (ischemic 36.8%, dilated 20.7%, idiopathic 11.8% and unspecified 11.8%). Other less common indications include refractory malignant ventricular arrhythmias—specifically VT storm—acute viral myocarditis, and post-partum cardiomyopathy.

Available donor organs are one of the most valuable resources in health care due to their paucity, and careful patient selection for transplantation is therefore critical. Specific selection criteria are beyond the scope of this chapter, but patients tend to be relatively young—although many centers will not hesitate to transplant patients well into their 60's—and free of major co-morbidities [6].

Preoperative Evaluation

Advanced Evaluation

While the availability of a donor heart and the timing of the surgical procedure itself are unpredictable, the planning of most heart transplanta-

tions is done in an elective fashion and there is time for a detailed work-up of the patient by the various teams involved: cardiology/heart failure, cardiac surgery and cardiac anesthesiology.

The etiology of the heart failure and the patient's comorbidities are carefully evaluated, along with the patient's psychosocial situation, since he/she will be subjected to a close postoperative follow-up and will have to be compliant with various immunosuppressive regimens.

Preoperative investigations usually cover all major organ systems: patients undergo detailed transthoracic and/or transesophageal echocardiography as well as left and right-heart catheterization; head, chest and abdominal computerized tomography (CT) scans are usually performed to assess various organ systems and rule out occult malignancy. Patients also undergo pulmonary function tests, complete hematology and biochemistry profiles, renal, hepatic and thyroid function tests, as well as blood type and HLA typing. Of particular importance is the assessment of the pulmonary vascular resistance (PVR), which may be elevated in response to chronic heart failure. Elevated PVR, greater than 5 Woods units, is generally considered a contraindication to heart transplantation, because the thin-walled right ventricle of a healthy transplanted heart would quickly fail in that environment [6].

Patients with pulmonary hypertension in response to chronic heart failure may still be candidates for heart transplantation eventually, but only if their PVR can be lowered to near normal levels. If reversibility in PVR can be demonstrated at the time of right heart catheterization—by administering vasodilators of the pulmonary circulation—a left ventricular assist device (LVAD) may be inserted, in the hope that improved effective left ventricular function will lead to regression of the pulmonary vascular remodeling over weeks to months, at which time the patient can be listed for transplantation. This is commonly referred to as a "bridge to transplant candidacy". Patients whose pulmonary hypertension is believed to be irreversible should be considered for combined heart-lung transplantation.

The details of specific organ matching and selection are outside the scope of this chapter, but it is important to mention that, besides human leukocyte antigen (HLA) typing and blood grouping, the matching process also takes into consideration the patient's heart size [7]. A heart must obviously fit well in the recipient's chest, but some believe that a slightly larger heart may be better able to better withstand elevated PA pressures, if present. An important consideration when deciding whether to bridge a patient with an LVAD is the expected availability of organs for this particular patient. For example, a very large man with group O blood may face a relatively limited pool of donors, and he may fare better with an LVAD. Finally, some reports suggest that matching the gender of donor and recipient also plays a role in outcomes [8].

A consultation by a cardiac anesthesiologist familiar with the procedure should be sought in all patients being considered for transplantation. This not only ensures that all aspects of care are adequately planned for, but it also greatly facilitates the work of the anesthesiology team when the patient eventually presents for surgery. As for all anesthetics, the goal of the preoperative evaluation is to identify patient conditions and surgical factors that may impact the overall success of the procedure. It should include a detailed history—past anesthetics, family history, allergies, medications, review of systems—and a careful physical examination, including airway, cardiorespiratory system and careful consideration of all sites of potential intravenous and intra-arterial access. Some patients have never had surgery ("virgin" chest), but many others have had one or more prior sternotomy, even if they do not have an LVAD. It is common for transplant patients to have undergone coronary artery bypass surgery or valve repair/replacement. Many heart transplant candidates also have an automatic implanted cardioverter defibrillator (AICD), and note should be made of its make/model if possible. As for all cardiac surgeries, a history of dysphagia or other contraindications to transesophageal echocardiography (TEE) should be elicited. Finally, all laboratory results and preoperative investigations should be carefully reviewed and noted.

The Day of Surgery

When a heart becomes available and a potential match has been identified, a complex sequence of events must quickly be set in motion: the recipient is called to the hospital and the operative team is quickly assembled.

Before surgery, the anesthesiologist should review all preoperative documentation—most cardiac transplant centers have well organized record keeping systems that contain all relevant information, including the elective anesthesia consult—and ask the patient about any recent change in his or her condition/symptoms. Recent worsening of heart failure/pulmonary edema may dictate the need for special precautions at the time of induction or in the pre-bypass period. Depending on the timing of the last investigations—some patients can be on the wait list for months to years—repeat blood samples should be obtained for complete blood count, extended electrolytes, renal and hepatic function, coagulation parameters, as well as cross matching of blood products.

Patients on warfarin, which targets vitamin-K dependent coagulation factors, should be given intravenous vitamin K before surgery—because it takes hours for the vitamin K to take effect, and because of the urgent nature of transplant surgery, most of these patients will still require intraoperative blood products to reverse their anticoagulation.

Arrangements should be made to turn off the anti-tachycardia functions of the patient's AICD, to prevent its inadvertent activation by electrocautery.

Finally, the anti-rejection drug regimen is initiated before surgery with the first dose of corticosteroids—commonly methylprednisolone—administered on call to the operating room (OR). Since most transplant patients are nervous before the procedure, they often appreciate an anxiolytic premedication—benzodiazepines work well if the anesthesiologist feels that it is safe to use them—along with supplemental oxygen, to be administered after all consent forms and other instructions have been completed.

The Importance of Timing

Heart transplantation is a race against time. The total ischemic time experienced by the donor heart (= from the aortic cross-clamping time in the donor to the moment of reperfusion in the recipient's chest) is one of the most critical determinants of the immediate and long-term success of a heart transplantation. Consequently, every decision regarding the timing of surgery must be centered on the need to minimize the ischemic time of the donor heart.

Much experimental work is being done in the field of ex-vivo perfusion of human donor hearts and beating heart transportation systems for donated organs [9], but at the time of this writing, most transplant centers still base their practices on the "*clamp and run*" principle.

Since donor hearts usually come from another hospital—and often from another city/state/province—frequent communications and careful coordination between the harvesting team and the transplant team should take place: the start time of transplant surgery should be adjusted so that the recipient is ready to go on cardiopulmonary bypass (CPB) when the donor heart arrives at the transplant center. *As a general rule, it is better for the transplant team to be ready too early and have to wait for the donor heart to arrive, than to prolong the ischemic time because the recipient is not ready.* This is an extremely important consideration that *both* the surgeon and the anesthesiologist should bear in mind before surgery, especially in cases of redo-sternotomy, when the time needed to open the chest and go on CPB may be uncertain, or when additional time may be needed for the anesthesia preparation and induction—for example, if one anticipates difficult IV/arterial access, or a difficult airway requiring awake fiberoptic intubation. Once again, good communication is critical.

Intraoperative Management

Monitoring

The preparation of heart transplantation patients does not differ significantly from other cardiac surgeries. Standard anesthesia monitors, with or

without a cerebral saturation monitor depending on institutional practices; an intra-arterial cannula—radial, brachial or femoral depending on the anesthesiologist's preference and the specifics of the patient; and a jugular central venous catheter are standard practice in most centers. Since the surgery involves major vascular anastomoses and brisk bleeding is always a possibility, at least two large-bore peripheral and/or central intravenous cannulas are recommended. Of note, most LVADs currently on the market deliver continuous flow, which means that these patients may not have any palpable pulses. Ultrasound guidance for line insertion is indispensable in such instances. Tonometric based noninvasive blood pressure measurement systems will not function properly in such patients and cannot be relied upon.

Once standard practice in most cardiac surgery cases, pulmonary artery (PA) catheters have fallen out of fashion in some cardiac surgical centers in recent years, because of the risk of complications and the lack of conclusive evidence that their use positively affects outcomes. PA catheters are used in all heart transplantation cases at our institution: we believe that PA catheters provide the most benefit in cases where right ventricular function is compromised and heart transplantation is the paramount example. Special PA catheters that display continuous cardiac output, continuous mixed venous oxygen saturation and/or right ventricular ejection fraction, may be particularly helpful in these cases but are not necessary.

Induction

As for every cardiac surgery, the goal of induction is to render the patient unconscious and secure the airway while maintaining oxygenation and hemodynamic stability. From a hemodynamic point of view, much of the approach will depend on whether one is dealing with a native heart or an LVAD. Induction of general anesthesia in a patient with a failing native heart often means trying not to upset the precarious balance of a compensated cardiovascular system, using a carefully titrated administration of anesthetics, often in conjunction with boluses/infusions of inotropic agents. By contrast, the patient with an

LVAD has a normal *effective* left ventricular function and usually tolerates induction well.

Specific anesthetic agents reflect institutional practices and personal preference of the anesthesiologist but, as a general rule, combinations of benzodiazepines—e.g. midazolam—and opioids—e.g. fentanyl, sufentanil—are the mainstay of induction, because these agents have a relatively small impact on hemodynamic stability. Judicious doses of other induction agents like propofol, ketamine, etomidate or vapor anesthetics can also be used, depending on preference and availability. The decision to begin infusions of inotropes or vasopressors before induction should be made based on the patient's hemodynamics and the potential for acute cardiovascular decompensation.

The need for rapid sequence induction depends on the circumstances: in many cases, the organ matching process and the patient preparation take several hours, allowing patients to meet the *NPO* requirements for regular induction of general anesthesia. If a patient has a full stomach, however, precautions should be taken to minimize the risk of aspiration—pro-motility agents, antacids, and cricoid pressure. The rate of administration of induction drugs should obviously try to balance the risk of aspiration and the risks associated with poor cardiac function/precarious hemodynamics.

Pre-Bypass Period

The goals of anesthetic care in the pre-bypass period are to maintain hemodynamic stability and to help get the patient on cardiopulmonary bypass (CPB) in a safe and timely manner. The importance of the baseline TEE examination at this stage is not so much to establish/confirm the preoperative diagnosis—the heart will be removed—but rather to identify factors that may influence the bypass and post-bypass periods (see later section on TEE).

On CPB

The management of these patients on bypass is not significantly different from other types of cardiac surgery. In our institution, we routinely use hemofiltration on CPB during heart transplantation, as it is a highly effective way to deal with the large volumes of blood contained in these often severely dilated hearts. It also permits highly efficient fluid removal should it be necessary to transfuse large volumes of plasma during reperfusion to correct coagulopathy while maintaining euvolemia and preventing hemodilution in those cases at a high risk of bleeding—redosternotomy, LVAD, and patients on warfarin [10]. It is also important for the anesthesiologist/echocardiographer to understand how the anastomosis of the new heart is made, in order to interpret the post-bypass TEE images.

Reperfusion

Reperfusion time is important to the recovery of an ischemic organ, but it is also a time of significant disturbances at the cellular level, during which the organ is vulnerable to additional injury. Several factors can mitigate, or worsen the potential for reperfusion injury.

The duration of reperfusion is probably the most important factor, and it should be adjusted to the ischemic time. There are no hard and fast rules, but the longer the organ was ischemic, the longer it needs to be re-perfused to allow it to recover. The decision is usually made in collaboration with the surgical team. Temperature and perfusion pressure, oxygenation and acid/base balance are all very important at this stage, as is the avoidance of hyperglycemia. While hypocalcemia is detrimental to cardiovascular function and coagulation in the post-CPB period, the decision to administer boluses of calcium during reperfusion should be carefully considered, because of the risk that a high extracellular calcium environment may potentiate reperfusion injury of the cardiac myocytes [11].

Reperfusion is also the time when, depending on institutional anti-rejection protocols, additional doses of corticosteroids are given—e.g. methylprednisolone—and infusions of other immunosuppressant agents are started—e.g. antithymocyte globulin—ATG—a detailed discussion of which is outside the scope of this chapter.

Separation from CPB

Separating from bypass after any cardiac surgery is a traumatic time for the heart. Weaning techniques are described in other parts of this book and many others, and the basic principles do not differ from any other cardiac procedure. In fact, it may be much more difficult to wean a bad native heart from CPB than a good transplanted one. The aim of this section is to point out to discuss some of the concerns and factors pertaining to the freshly transplanted heart, and to offer some practical insight into how to manage them.

Hyper-acute graft rejection will make it essentially impossible to separate from CPB, but fortunately this is an extremely rare event. Much more common is myocardial dysfunction due to severe stunning, which usually resolves over time: sometimes this improvement takes place over minutes to hours, and sometimes it may take days to weeks. This recovery will determine in large part how quickly the patient will get out of the OR and out of the intensive care unit.

Several factors are well known to be associated with graft dysfunction and difficulty separating from CPB: technical problems with the anastomosis of the heart; insufficient reperfusion time; and prolonged total ischemic time—especially if greater than 5 hrs. While the first two are usually preventable or correctable, the latter is beyond the control of the anesthesiologist and should prompt him/her to prepare for a difficult wean. Note that, even in the absence of any of these factors, some hearts may unexpectedly suffer severe stunning and be difficult to manage.

Preparing for weaning should follow the same checklist as any other cardiac procedures: careful de-airing of the graft is important to prevent air embolism to the coronaries and/or other organs (see section on TEE); adequate ventilation with 100% oxygen; correction of acid-base disturbances and excessive anemia; and treatment of hyperkalemia and hyperglycemia—severe hypocalcemia should also be treated, in spite of the concerns expressed above.

Freshly denervated hearts have no parasympathetic input (vagus nerve) and tend to beat at a resting rate of 90–110 beats per minute. This helps to reduce chamber distension. If for some reason the heart rate is slow or even normal, it is often helpful to pace the heart at a faster rate. Atrio-ventricular pacing—sequential A-V or DDD—is the preferred mode, to take advantage of the atrial contraction and maximize the filling of the stiff ventricles recovering from ischemia. Denervated hearts also tend to be very preload dependent and the Starling curve can be grossly distorted in these patients.

"It's about the RV!" Experienced cardiac anesthesiologists know that right ventricular (RV) performance often determines the success and/or ease of weaning from CPB: the universal challenge in this context is to adequately fill the left ventricle (LV) without overloading the struggling RV. Because the RV is so sensitive to ischemia, and because PVR is often not normal in chronic heart failure patients, heart transplantation is probably one of the situations where this struggle is most evident. Therapeutic priorities for the RV include the following:

1. *Avoidance of anything that can increase PVR*: Avoiding hypoxia, hypercarbia, acidosis, extremes of positive end expiratory pressure (PEEP) and hemoglobin may seem obvious, but such details can sometimes be overlooked in a busy environment and can make a huge difference to RV function. Thankfully, they are usually relatively easy to correct when abnormal.
2. *Judicious fluid management*: Immediately post-transplant, RV volume status is extremely important. The RV often rests on a knife-edge, teetering between under-filling and volume overload. Attempting to optimize LV preload may be difficult, and this is one situation where one may have to accept an under-filled, hyper-dynamic LV in order to prevent RV over-stretching. If the RV becomes over-distended, reverse Trendelenburg, venodilating agents like nitroglycerin, or even phlebotomy—draining blood back into the CPB reservoir—may be required to correct the situation. It is important to remember that even a "good looking" RV can quickly fail if challenged with too much preload.

3. *Pharmacologic support*: While the LV may sometimes require inotropic support, especially in cases of excessively long ischemic time, the RV almost always needs some pharmacologic assistance, even if it appears to be doing well. Beta agonists like dobutamine or epinephrine, and phosphodiesterase-III inhibitors like milrinone, are often used for this purpose. Because they work synergistically through different mechanisms—by increasing production of intracellular cyclic-AMP in the case of beta agonists, or decreasing its breakdown in the case of phosphodiesterase-III inhibitors—their combination can be extremely effective.

The balance between inotropic/vasopressor support is dictated by the clinical situation, but it is useful to keep in mind that vasopressors (like norepinephrine and vasopressin) increase systemic and pulmonary afterload, which can increase ventricular workload, but they also increase coronary perfusion to both ventricles, which may be extremely important in patients with RV dysfunction and pulmonary hypertension where maintenance of an RV perfusion pressure is critical.

Nitric oxide (NO) is a vasodilator that works through the production of cyclic GMP [12]. If given by inhalation it can be "functionally" a selective pulmonary vasodilator as it is usually broken down before it reaches the systemic circulation. NO is useful to reduce PVR in situations of severe RV failure. Other selective pulmonary vasodilators like iloprost, a synthetic analogue of prostaglandin PGI_2, or inhaled milrinone can also be used to reduce PVR in such situations.

4. *Mechanical support*: In cases of severe myocardial dysfunction, mechanical support may have to be considered as a last resort. The type of support will be dictated by the clinical situation, depending on which ventricle requires support. Intra-aortic balloon counter-pulsation (IABP) causes a decrease in LV afterload, an increase in coronary perfusion pressure to both ventricles and an overall improvement in the myocardial oxygen supply/demand of the failing heart. Temporary ventricular assist devices—like percutaneous temporary intravascular pumps—may be needed for the left, right or both ventricles. Rarely, arteriovenous extra-corporeal membrane oxygenation (ECMO) may be necessary to support the patient until the failing heart improves, or another definitive solution—like re-transplant—is found.

Severe anemia is undesirable in this context, because it imposes an additional workload on the recovering heart. Much work has been published on optimal transfusion thresholds in critically ill patients. In the post-transplantation context, one must balance the potential risk of exposing a patient to immunogenic blood products with the need to maintain adequate oxygen carrying capacity. In patients subject to systemic inflammatory response, with potentially leaky capillary beds, blood cells are also reliable volume expanders when preload is important. Finally, it is important to remember that red blood cells also play a role in hemostasis—by supplying the ADP necessary in platelet activation and occupying the center of blood vessels, which displaces platelets toward their site of action at the vessel walls. As a result, actively bleeding patients may need higher hematocrit levels than non-bleeding patients.

Massive bleeding and coagulopathy can occur after heart transplantation for many reasons: preoperative warfarin therapy; redo-sternotomy requiring a long and complex dissection; long bypass runs resulting in platelet dysfunction and dilution of coagulation factors. Regardless of the cause, it is always easier to anticipate than to catch up. Hence prophylactic transfusion of clotting factors may be necessary in patients with a very high risk of bleeding—patients on warfarin. The widespread use of devices that evaluate various coagulation parameters at the point of care—e.g. activated clotting time, point of care hematology, international normalized ratio or functional assays of coagulation like thromboelastography/rotation thromboelastometry—has greatly facilitated the management of coagulopathy in cardiac surgery. In the context of cardiac transplantation, it is critical to remember the delicate balance between the need to treat a coagulopathy with blood products and the ability of the fragile RV to cope with large volumes of factors. Careful consideration should be given to using concentrated preparation—like prothrombin complex concentrates and fibrinogen concentrates—rather than larger volumes of fresh frozen plasma or cryoprecipitate. For more details, the reader is referred to other sections of this book and specialized texts on the subject.

Transesophageal Echocardiography

Even though it will soon be removed from the patient, it is important to perform a comprehensive examination of the original heart, as recommended in the ASE/SCA published guidelines [13]. The goals of the pre-bypass TEE assessment are to assist in the anesthetic management of the patient—chamber size, myocardial contractility, valvular function, pericardial effusions—and to diagnose issues that may affect the surgery in the pre-bypass period. For example, the presence of a left ventricular thrombus may prompt the surgeon to limit cardiac manipulations until the aortic cross-clamp is on—or even the management surgery itself. The authors once found an unexpected persistent left superior vena cava in a transplant recipient, which completely changed the surgical plan for anastomosis of the new heart.

Before separation from CPB, careful de-airing of the new heart must be achieved and TEE plays a crucial role in making sure no air is left in any of the cardiac chambers. Air rises to the top of any blood filled cavity: In "normal" cardiac surgical patients in the supine position, this is usually: (1) the roof of the left atrium in an area adjacent to the aorta and the superior vena cava—best visualized in the long axis at 110 to 135 degrees of transducer rotation, by gently rotating the probe between the two structures; (2) the LV apex and anteroseptal wall—best visualized in the mid-esophageal long axis view. In heart transplantation, it is important to remember that the heart was manipulated *outside* of the body and

rotated in many different ways, so air may accumulate in many unusual recesses/areas of the transplanted heart. This requires a complete careful assessment.

Post-bypass, a careful and comprehensive examination of the new heart must again be performed. Each part of the new heart must be evaluated for its structure and function. Every suture line must be surveyed, ensuring that the vessels are patent and that flow is unobstructed. The presence of aliasing on color flow Doppler or high gradients on spectral Doppler should prompt a more detailed assessment, and a warning to the surgeon about the possible need to revise an anastomosis. It is important to note that the size of the new heart does not always perfectly match that of the recipient's great vessels and that the new atria—comprised of parts of native and donor tissue—are typically enlarged. Some mild kinks that do not restrict flow, as well as changes in vessel caliber at the various anastomotic sites are to be expected.

Left and right ventricular filling and function should be repeatedly evaluated throughout the post-bypass period, as the patient's condition evolves in the operating room. Systolic function typically improves over time and in response to inotropic support. Diastolic dysfunction should be expected in a heart recovering from an ischemic insult, and it is difficult to interpret in this context.

Immediate Postoperative Management

The immediate postoperative management of heart transplant patients generally resembles that of other cardiac surgical patients, with a few important distinctions:

Inotropic support may be required for longer than usual periods of time, and one should be careful not to upset a steady state with excessively aggressive weaning regimens.

Volume management should take into account the fact that the denervated heart is very dependent on proper preload, but at the same time, the RV can be quite sensitive to excessive volume challenges. The authors' institution routinely uses PA catheters to help monitor central venous pressure, pulmonary artery pressures and, if necessary, right ventricular pressure, as well as measurement of mixed venous saturation. Pulmonary arterial occlusion pressure (PAOP) is notoriously unreliable and should be interpreted with great caution.

The immediate post-transplant period is very dynamic and unpredictable. Acute deterioration should prompt an immediate transthoracic or transesophageal echocardiographic evaluation (TTE or TEE), looking for signs of tamponade and/or ventricular—especially RV—dysfunction.

The changes in intrathoracic pressure associated with weaning and extubation result in increased right-ventricular preload and an increased left-sided afterload. The magnitude of such acute changes in loading conditions is variable, but they can in turn lead to acute changes in cardiac function. In the post-transplant setting, a right ventricle that had apparently been well-functioning until then may suddenly deteriorate following extubation, sometimes associated with the development of significant tricuspid regurgitation. This vulnerability of the RV remains apparent throughout the postoperative period, where the mobilization of accumulated edema and/or other fluid shifts can lead to acute changes in RV loading conditions. The aggressiveness with which inotropic support is titrated/withdrawn over the hours/days following surgery should take all these factors into consideration, and some patients may need inotropic support for days to weeks following transplant.

Immunosuppressive agents are very important in the immediate post-transplant period. A detailed discussion of these agents is beyond the scope of this discussion, but it is important for the anesthesiologist to remember that immunosuppressive agents can interact with many drugs used in the perioperative period. Also the choice and dosage of various agents is dictated by the patient's renal and hepatic function, as well as various hematologic parameters.

Serial echocardiography examinations and myocardial biopsies are important in the long-term management of heart transplant patients, and this is usually started in hospital.

References

1. Barnard MS. Heart transplantation: an experimental review and preliminary research. S Afr Med J. 1967 Dec 30;41(48):1260–2.
2. Anderson TA, Bekker P, Vagefi PA. Anesthetic considerations in organ procurement surgery: a narrative review. Can J Anaesth. 2015 May;62(5):529–39.
3. Yusen R, et al. Journal of Heart and Lung Transplantation Available from: doi:https://doi.org/10.1016/j.healun.2016.09.001. Accessed 2nd September 2017.
4. Available from https://www.unos.org/data/transplanttrends/#transplants_by_organ_type+year+2016. Accessed 20th August 2017.
5. Available from: https://www.cihi.ca/en/corr-annual-statistics-2017. Accessed 20th August 2017.
6. Mehra MR, Kobashigawa J, Starling R, Russell S, Uber PA, Parameshwar J, et al. Listing criteria for heart transplantation: International Society for Heart and Lung Transplantation guidelines for the Care of Cardiac Transplant Candidates—2006. J Heart Lung Transplant. 2006;25:1024–42.
7. Hunt SA, Haddad F. The changing face of heart transplantation. J Am Coll Cardiol. 2008;52:587–98.
8. Reed RM, Netzer G, Hunsicker L, Mitchell BD, Rajagopal K, Scharf S, et al. Cardiac size and sex-matching in heart transplantation: size matters in matters of sex and the heart. JACC: Heart Failure. February 2014;2(1):73–83.
9. Ardehali A, Esmailian F, Deng M, Soltesz E, Hsich E, Naka Y, et al. Ex-vivo perfusion of donor hearts for human heart transplantation (PROCEED II): a prospective, open-label, multicentre, randomised non-inferiority trial. Lancet. 2015 Jun 27;385(9987):2577–84.
10. Babaev A, Saczkowski R, Hynes M, Boodhwani M, Hudson CC. Use of plasma "reconstitution" during cardio pulmonary bypass for a heart transplant after previous left ventricular assist device implant surgery. Perfusion. 2014 Jan;29(1):29–31.
11. Chen RH. The scientific basis for hypocalcemic cardioplegia and reperfusion in cardiac surgery. Ann Thorac Surg. 1996 Sep;62(3):910–4.
12. Green JB, Hart B, Cornett EM, Kaye AD, Salehi A, Fox CJ. Pulmonary vasodilators and anesthesia considerations. Anesthesiol Clin. 2017 Jun;35(2):221–32.
13. Hahn RT, Abraham T, Adams MS, Bruce CJ, Glas KE, Lang RM, et al. Guidelines for performing a comprehensive transesophageal echocardiographic examination: recommendations from the American Society of Echocardiography and the Society of Cardiovascular Anesthesiologists. J Am Soc Echocardiogr. 2013;26:921–64.

The LVAD-Supported Patient Presenting for Non-Cardiac Surgery

15

Marc E. Stone and Tanaya Sparkle

Main Messages

1. Mechanical circulatory support (MCS) with an left ventricular assist device has become the standard management for patients with chronic refractory Heart Failure (HF). Survival following implantation with a modern, durable device is now approximately 80% at 1 year, 70% at 2 years, 60% at 3 years and 50% at 4 years.

2. Regardless of the operative/procedural venue or level of complexity or invasiveness of the planned procedure, the removal of sympathetic tone by sedation or induction of general anesthesia exerts the same initial effect on the physiology of the LVAD-supported patient. Therefore, the perioperative considerations and the anesthetic approach to the LVAD supported patient remain similar for all cases.

3. An INR of approximately 2–3x normal is required for the HeartMate (HM) II, the HM 3 and the HVAD to prevent thrombus formation and potential thromboembolism. Thus, a multidisciplinary decision must be made in advance regarding management of anticoagulation for the perioperative period, in conjunction with the surgeon, the cardiologist managing the VAD, and the anesthesiologist.

4. The anesthetic management of a VAD-supported patient for a sedation case or a general anesthetic is not different than that for a non-supported patient. One must simply ensure continued optimization of the usual determinants of biventricular hemodynamics, namely preload, afterload, heart rate and contractility.

5. Standard ACLS protocols should be initiated if a VAD-supported patient experiences cardiac arrest but the issue of performing chest compressions has been a matter of debate for decades. Recently, however, the American Heart Association released a scientific statement in which chest compressions are now advocated in the case of mechanical VAD failure, especially if the ETCO2 is <20. Per their recommendations, if the ETCO2 is >20, the mean arterial pressure is >50 mmHg and the VAD appears to be functioning, then compressions should be withheld

M. E. Stone (✉) · T. Sparkle
Program Director, Fellowship in Cardiothoracic Anesthesiology Icahn School of Medicine, New York, NY, USA
e-mail: marc.stone@mountsinai.org

© Springer Nature Switzerland AG 2021
D. C. H. Cheng et al. (eds.), *Evidence-Based Practice in Perioperative Cardiac Anesthesia and Surgery*, https://doi.org/10.1007/978-3-030-47887-2_15

Introduction

The prevalence of heart failure (HF) worldwide is estimated to be about 26 million people, with 5.7 million adults in the US [1]. Since 2001, when the REMATCH trial demonstrated superiority of left ventricular assist devices (LVADs) over medical therapy in advanced heart failure patients not eligible for transplantation [2, 3], mechanical circulatory support (MCS) with an LVAD has become the standard management for patients with chronic refractory HF. The progressive advent of miniaturized "next generation devices" has now resulted in further improved MCS survival rates approaching 80% at 1 year and 50% at 4 years. According to the latest data, there are currently 2000–3000 LVAD implantations annually at approximately 160 centers in the United States alone and this number continues to rise [3]. Thus, the number of patients supported by an LVAD that require interventional and diagnostic non-cardiac surgical procedures (NCS) is also increasing.

Several anecdotal experiences and small studies evaluating perioperative outcomes of NCS in LVAD patients have suggested that for routine procedures (e.g., endoscopies, cystoscopies, etc) and straightforward routine NCS, there is no significant difference in outcomes between the anesthetic care provided by a cardiac trained, and a non-cardiac trained anesthesiologist who has been educated regarding the anesthetic considerations for the LVAD-supported patient [4, 5]. As there is no objective "evidence" or hard data on which to base the anesthetic management of a given patient, a didactic educational program targeting general anesthesiologists could be useful to train and prepare general anesthesiologists for the projected sheer increase in the number of NCS that will be required by the ever increasing number of LVAD patients [6]. That said, most authors agree that it is prudent for a cardiac and transesophageal echocardiography (TEE) trained anesthesiologist to be involved in those major cases with potential for significant hemodynamic compromise or large fluid shifts, as well as for patients who are not stable at baseline.

Types of Mechanical Circulatory Support Devices

MCS devices can be divided into short- and long-term devices. Short-term MCS devices used to rescue patients from acute cardiac failure are often paracorporeal, with an external pump connected to cannulas in the heart and great vessels, though catheter-based short-term MCS devices also exist that are positioned within the heart during support. Such short-term devices (including extracorporeal membrane oxygenation, ECMO) are beyond the scope of this chapter, and the concepts discussed herein pertain to long-term support with durable, implantable LVADs.

An LVAD receives blood returning to the left side of the heart through an inflow cannula in the apex of the left ventricle and ejects it through an outflow cannula to the aorta, thereby considerably reducing the LV workload. The goals of LVAD support are twofold:

1. to relieve the pressure and volume overload of the failing left ventricle, thereby reducing LV myocardial oxygen demand (which may promote recovery in a small percentage of patients by reverse remodeling [7, 8].)
2. to maintain adequate systemic perfusion to avert cardiogenic shock and potentially improve multisystem organ function over time.

Indications for Long-Term MCS

Table 15.1 outlines recent data for durable LVADs in the US. Until 2009, Bridge-to-Transplantation (BTT) was the most common indication for implantation of a durable LVAD, but the approval of the HeartMate II for Destination Therapy (DT) in 2010 heralded a new era of MCS because of its durability and seemingly lower rate of adverse events compared to first-generation devices. Continuous flow (CF) devices (e.g., the HeartMate II) have been used to provide support for 100% of patients implanted for DT since 2010, as well as for more than 95% of all other LVAD indications.

Table 15.1 Indications for long-term mechanical circulatory support, current frequencies of use and current rates of success

Indication	Explanation	Current US frequency	Current US success
Bridge-to-transplantation	The LVAD is implanted to "bridge" the patient with chronic, progressive heart failure to transplantation.	26%	86% alive at 1 yr. 31% transplanted 55% still supported
Bridge-to-candidacy	The LVAD is implanted to maintain systemic perfusion at an adequate level which, over time, will improve multisystem organ failure such that the patient might become an acceptable transplant candidate.	37%	84% alive at 1 yr. 20% transplanted 64% still supported
Destination therapy	The LVAD is implanted as a final, permanent management strategy for end-stage, refractory heart failure in a transplant ineligible patient.	46%	>75% alive at 1 yr. > 50% alive at 3 yrs

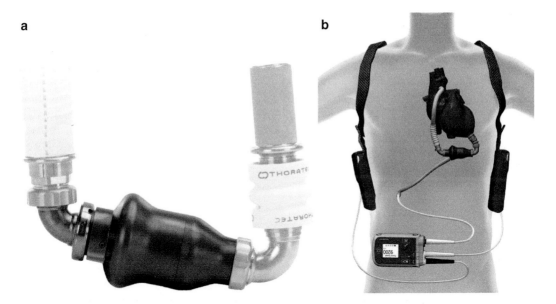

a   b

Fig. 15.1 HEARTMATE® II (Abbott). (**a**) The HeartMate II. (**b**) The HeartMate II implanted. Note the driveline that emerges from the device and is tunneled through the skin of the abdomen to connect to the system controller and power supply. Images provided courtesy of Abbott

First generation implantable LVADs were large, mechanically complex devices that captured an entire potential stoke volume from the LV and produced a pulsatile output. Second generation devices are smaller, less noisy and produce a continuous flow output. Third generation devices also produce continuous flow but design advancements utilize magnetic and hydrodynamic technology to potentially reduce shear stress and thrombus formation. The two most commonly implanted FDA-approved durable devices in the US at the time of this writing are the Heartmate II (Abbot, Chicago, IL; Fig. 15.1a and b) and the Heartware HVAD (Medtronic, Framingham, MA; Fig. 15.2). The HeartMate 3 (Abbot, Fig. 15.3a and b) is a more recently FDA-approved implantable, durable device that is rapidly gaining in popularity.

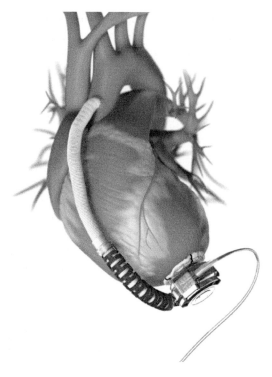

Heart Mate II:

- The HM II is a miniaturized continuous axial flow pump and currently the most commonly implanted durable LVAD around the world.
- The HM II was FDA approved in the US as a BTT in 2008 and as destination therapy in 2010. The longest duration of support exceeds 8 years. The currently reported rate of successful BTT with the HM II is approximately 86%.
- The post-implantation anticoagulation protocol is with warfarin to produce an INR of 2.5–3.5x normal plus aspirin.

HeartWare HVAD:

- The HVAD is a miniaturized continuous flow centrifugal pump with a magnetically driven, magnetically suspended impeller. This device is implanted within the pericardium without any significant intervening "inflow cannula"; it directly abuts the LV apex. This design provides potential for use in patients with smaller body surface areas and ostensibly results in shorter surgical implantation times.
- The HVAD was FDA approved in the US as a BTT in 2012 and as DT in 2017, with the lon-

Fig. 15.2 The HeartWare® HVAD™ (HeartWare, Framingham, MA, USA). The HeartWare HVAD implanted. Note that the device is implanted within the pericardium, directly abutting the apex of the left ventricle, and the driveline that emerges from the device and is tunneled through the skin of the abdomen to connect to the system controller and power supply. Image provided courtesy of HeartWare

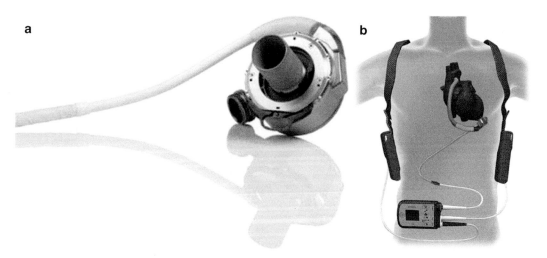

Fig. 15.3 HEARTMATE® 3 (Abbott). (**a**) The HM 3. (**b**) The HM 3 implanted. Note that the device is implanted within the pericardium, directly abutting the apex of the left ventricle, and the driveline that emerges from the device and is tunneled through the skin of the abdomen to connect to the system controller and power supply. Images provided courtesy of Abbott

gest duration of support over 7 years. The currently reported rate of successful BTT with the HVAD is 88–90%.

- Post-implantation anticoagulation protocol is with warfarin to an INR of 2.0–3.0x normal plus aspirin. The manufacturer also recommends testing for aspirin resistance and if detected, the adjunctive use of clopidogrel and/or dipyridamole.
- The HVAD is also being used as an implantable right ventricular assist device (RVAD).

HeartMate 3:

- The HM 3 is a miniaturized continuous flow centrifugal pump implanted within the pericardium with a magnetically driven, magnetically suspended impeller with design features intended to improve hemocompatibility and reduce the risk of thrombus formation.
- This third-generation device was approved for "short term indications" in August 2017, and for "long term indications" (including DT) in October 2018.
- The HM 3 was demonstrated to be non-inferior to the HM II in the MOMENTUM 3 trial [9] regarding survival free from either disabling stroke or reoperation for device malfunction at 6 months after implantation, and has now been declared "superior" to the HM II based on the observed lower incidence of need for pump replacement.

INTERMACS

The Interagency Registry for Mechanically Assisted Circulation (INTERMACS) is a North American registry database sponsored by the National Heart, Lung and Blood Institute, the FDA, and the centers for Medicare and Medicaid Services. It was established in 2005 to collect clinical data about patients receiving long-term MCS therapy with implantable, durable devices. Such data includes both major outcomes (such as death, transplant, explant, re-hospitalization and adverse events) and more "complex" endpoints

such as the patient's level of function and quality of life. With improved survival and new devices, outcomes beyond simple survival are becoming important. A similar European-based database called EuroMACS exists in Europe, a database of pediatric MCS called PEDIMACS and a new international database maintained by the International Society for Heart and Lung Transplantation (ISHLT) called IMACS now exists. Reports from international experience with MCS will be available soon.

The INTERMACS profile/level describes the clinical condition of the patient on a scale from 1–7 (Table 15.2), with a numerically lower profile indicating more severe illness. An INTERMACS 7 patient is simply in advanced stages of heart failure (e.g., NYHA class III), an INTERMACS 4 has symptoms at rest, an INTERMACS 3 is essentially hemodynamically stable but inotrope dependent, an INTERMACS 2 is deteriorating despite inotropes and an INTERMACS 1 is in cardiogenic shock despite maximal therapy.

The experience has been that if one electively implants a durable LVAD too early, at numerically higher INTERMACS levels, the risks of adverse events outweigh the benefits. Conversely, if one waits to implant the VAD until the patient is already likely developing multisystem organ failure (e.g., INTERMACS 1), benefits are low and survival is poor. Survival data suggests that implantation of durable LVADs when the patient is an INTERMACS 3 or 4 would be ideal to balance the risks and benefits.

Table 15.2 INTERMACS Profiles

INTERMACS 1:	Critical cardiogenic shock
INTERMACS 2:	Deteriorating on inotropes
INTERMACS 3:	Stable, but inotrope dependent
INTERMACS 4:	Symptomatic at rest
INTERMACS 5:	Exertion intolerant
INTERMACS 6:	Limited with exertion
INTERMACS 7:	Advanced NYHA class III

Perioperative Management of the LVAD-Supported Patient

While LVAD patients still tend to receive their care in tertiary/academic VAD centers, there has been expansion into the private practice setting and even some of the larger endoscopy suites.

Regardless of the venue or level of complexity or invasiveness of the planned procedure, the removal of sympathetic tone by sedation or induction of general anesthesia exerts the same initial effect on the physiology of the LVAD-supported patient. Therefore, the perioperative considerations and the anesthetic approach to the LVAD supported patient remain similar for all cases.

Preoperative Considerations

A thorough assessment of the VAD-supported patient is mandatory, even for minor procedures because:

1. even an ambulatory and seemingly uncompromised VAD-supported patient may have some level of underlying renal, hepatic, pulmonary, and/or central nervous system insufficiency,
2. the physiology of the VAD-supported state can be adversely affected by inadequate optimization during the anesthetic, and
3. deterioration in the perioperative period may preclude full recovery, or may disqualify a patient from later heart transplantation.

   It is recommended that these patients undergo an earnest preoperative consultation by an anesthesiologist, the surgeon, a cardiothoracic surgeon, and a heart failure cardiologist and/or a VAD specialist prior to surgery to ensure that they are optimized for any planned procedure [10].

Preoperative History

The importance of a thorough preanesthetic history and physical exam cannot be stressed

enough. The name of the device, baseline stable LVAD parameters (including pulsatility index, pump output, power, and pump speed), baseline functional status, history of other affected organ systems, medications, anticoagulation status, prior surgeries, complications after prior surgeries, data regarding coexisting organ failure, cardiac implanted electronic devices (a.k.a. pacemakers and ICDs; with history of interrogation), prior vascular lines and indication for LVAD (BTT vs DT) should be documented in an organized fashion along with a complete physical exam [10].

It is also imperative to have recent laboratory testing, including a complete blood count, a current electrolyte profile, and a cross match for blood transfusion (due to the use of anticoagulants and a higher rate of transfusion in these patients [11]) prior to any intervention or procedure. A preoperative ECG should be sufficient to determine the preoperative rhythm. The importance of prior discussion about the planned perioperative management with dedicated VAD personnel, the physician managing the VAD, the surgeon, and the cardiothoracic anesthesiologists cannot be over emphasized. Perioperative changes to VAD settings are rarely needed in an optimized stable VAD-supported patient.

Appropriate Perioperative Anticoagulation

A multidisciplinary decision must be made regarding management of anticoagulation for the perioperative period, in conjunction with the surgeon, the cardiologist managing the VAD, and the anesthesiologist. The risk of bleeding must be weighed against the risk of thrombosis. Anticoagulation goals for the procedure must be agreed upon preoperatively and can be ensured with lab values (potentially including PTT, INR, TEG/ROTEM, platelet function analysis, etc).

An INR of approximately 2–3x normal is required for the HM II, the HM 3 and the HVAD to prevent thrombus formation and potential thromboembolism. Maintenance is usually with warfarin and aspirin (and antiplatelet agents in some patients). In elective cases where bleeding risk is substantial, warfarin can be discontinued and the patient bridged to surgery with heparin. Automatic discontinuation of heparin "on call to OR", and the "knee-jerk reflex" stopping of warfarin without preoperative discussion with the physician managing the VAD is imprudent. The risk of bleeding must be weighed against the risk of thrombus formation and thromboembolism. In general, one can usually safely reduce the amount of anticoagulation for the immediate perioperative period to the lower limits of manufacturers' recommendations (which may allow for brief periods without any), but most semi-invasive procedures (e.g., endoscopies) and many general surgical procedures can be safely performed with some degree of anticoagulation. Where needed, infusions of FFP, cryoprecipitate and/or platelets may be guided by POC tests. In a series of 33 axial LVAD-supported patients, anticoagulation was reversed in 32 of 49 procedures with no perioperative thrombotic complications [5]. The administration of vitamin K and/or factor concentrates to reverse anticoagulation is not recommended.

Intra-Operative Management

The safe intraoperative management of the LVAD-supported patient entails both an understanding of the physiology at work and a number of "workflow" related considerations.

Physiology of the LVAD-Supported State

The essential points of physiology of the VAD supported state that must be considered to maintain optimal hemodynamics perioperatively are:

- Ventricular interdependence
- Series circulatory effects
- Ventriculoarterial coupling
- The Frank-Starling mechanism
- The Anrep effect
- The Bowditch effect

Ventricular Interdependence

The muscle fibers of the free wall of the right ventricle (RV), the left ventricle (LV) and the common interventricular septum (IVS) are continuous in nature resulting in mechanical interactions between the ventricles and an anatomic coupling of their contractile function. Changes in the geometry of one ventricle due to volume or pressure overload can affect the effectiveness of contractility of the other ventricle. It has also been demonstrated that with unimpaired septal function, the RV free wall has little contribution to RV pressure development and volume output. Excessive decompression of the LV by LVAD action and/or overfilling of the RV can cause a leftward shift of septum which leads to an induced dysfunction of the IVS, and thereby a deleterious effect on RV contractility and output.

Series Circulatory Effects

It is the output of the RV that eventually fills the LVAD, and the LVAD output subsequently becomes the preload of the RV. Thus, optimal LVAD function requires optimal RV preload and an adequate amount of blood in the LV. This conceptually requires adequate intravascular volume status, adequate RV function and a low enough pulmonary vascular resistance so blood can get across from the right side to the left.

Ventriculoarterial Coupling

Afterload reduction is a key principle in the modern management of both left and right-sided ventricular failure due to improvement in the ability of a ventricle to function as a pump by decreasing the afterload against which it must pump. This has application during both acute and chronic situations. Acute RV dysfunction, for example, responds particularly well to selective pulmonary vasodilators, and chronic LV dysfunction is routinely managed with inodilators, although hypotension may limit the ability to use systemic vasodilators.

The Frank-Starling Mechanism

The Frank-Starling law states that increased stretch on the myocytes, to a certain degree, increases the force of their contraction. Stretching of the left ventricle muscle fibers due to LV filling increases the affinity of troponin C for calcium, causing a greater number of actin-myosin cross-bridges to form within the muscle fibers and thereby increasing the force of the muscle contraction. The force that any single cardiac muscle fiber generates is proportional to the stretch on the individual fibers and their initial length before contraction which is represented by end-diastolic volume of the left and right ventricles. In the human heart, maximal force is generated with an initial sarcomere length of 2.2 microns which is rarely exceeded in the normal heart. Initial lengths larger or smaller than this optimal value will decrease the force the muscle can achieve. At larger sarcomere lengths, there is less overlap of the thin and thick filaments whereas at smaller sarcomere lengths, there is a decreased sensitivity for calcium by the myofilaments.

The Anrep Effect

The Anrep effect is an intrinsic autoregulatory myocardial reflex, maintained even in the denervated heart, in which myocardial contractility increases in a linear proportional fashion with increasing afterload. Initially, increased aortic resistance to ejection results in a decreased stroke volume and an increased end systolic volume which increases the force of contraction through the Frank-Starling mechanism. However, contractility continues to increase starting around 10–15 min after the initial sudden stretch through the Anrep effect, compensating for an increased end-systolic volume present. Without the Anrep effect, an increase in aortic pressure would result in a sustained decrease in stroke volume which might compromise cardiac output. This effect was originally described in 1912 by the Russian physiologist Gleb von Anrep, and investigations into this mechanism are continuing. Modern investigations have revealed the Anrep effect to be a very complex mechanism, involving: angiotensin II, endothelin, the mineralocorticoid receptor, the epidermal growth factor receptor, mitochondrial reactive oxygen species, redox-sensitive kinases upstream myocardial Na+/H+ exchanger (NHE1), NHE1 activation, increase in intracellular Na + concentration, and increase in Ca^{2+} transient amplitude through the Na+ /Ca^{2+} exchanger [12].

The Bowditch Effect

The Bowditch effect is an autoregulatory mechanism by which an increase in heart rate results in an increase in contractility. The mechanism underlying the Bowditch effect is similar to that of digoxin. Increased adrenergic stimulation increases activity of Na+/Ca++ Exchanger which leads to increased Na ions inside the cell. The Na^+/K^+ ATP-ase which pushes this sodium back out is unable to keep up and thereby, leading to decreased efflux of Na and a calcium build up which is inotropic in myocardial tissue. The Bowditch effect also reportedly exerts a lusitropic effect where increase in heart rate improves diastolic function by increased relaxation.

Workflow Considerations

Transport

The baseline parameters of LVAD function should be noted and documented prior to and after transfer. Battery power is used for transportation to and from the operating room. A pair of modern LVAD batteries can last up to 8 h, depending on the charge status, the number of previous charging cycles and the hemodynamic condition of the patient, but the LVAD should ideally be plugged in to mains AC power whenever possible as this will allow the use of the full control console for monitoring of VAD parameters. Care must be taken during transfer of the patient to the OR table due to the potential for circuitry disruption. A VAD knowledgeable person must always be present to assist with and troubleshoot any equipment-related issues in a certified VAD-center, though equipment-related issues will be rare.

Appropriate Antibiotic Coverage

Broad spectrum antibiotics are used in most cases taking local flora into consideration. For intra-abdominal procedures, additional coverage for gram negative and anaerobic bacteria might be needed. Antifungal agents should be considered for high risk patients with longstanding indwelling intravascular access lines, catheters and drains, and for those who have been on antibiotics recently. Though most VAD-associate infections occur within the percutaneous driveline exit tract, it must be considered that LVADs are large foreign bodies that could not be adequately sterilized if infected. Povidone iodine- containing solutions can cause breakdown of the plastic VAD driveline and thus must not be used directly on the driveline. When necessary for surgical procedures, drivelines can be draped out of the field with a sterile incise drape.

Presence of a Cardiac Implantable Electronic Device (CIED)

It is not uncommon for the VAD-supported patient to have a pacemaker or an implantable cardioverter defibrillator (ICD). Preoperatively, for the highest level of patient safety, one must ascertain the type of device present, how it is programmed, that it is functioning as intended, and the level of dependency on the device. Often, one can ascertain the information one needs from the medical record (e.g., from a recent "device check"), but in the absence of a recent interrogation, a review of the CXR can help determine if a device is a pacemaker or an ICD (an ICD has thick "shock coils" on the RV lead and possibly the SVC) and an ECG can help to establish pacemaker dependency (pacemaker spikes before every P wave and/or before every QRS complex suggests dependency on the pacemaker).

One also needs to assess the risk of electromagnetic interference (EMI) with device function during the procedure. The closer the source of EMI to the device (e.g., from the surgical electrocautery unit), the higher the risk of interference. EMI will most likely inhibit/interfere with the intended function of a pacemaker and/or trigger the delivery of antitachycardia therapies from an ICD. Though there is some controversy surrounding when the source of the EMI from the device and/or it's leads is sufficiently far away that no EMI would be manifest (e.g., > 15 cm), current recommendations still hold that ICD therapies should be disabled and pacing settings reprogrammed to an asynchronous mode for pacemaker dependent patients if the source of

EMI is <15 cm from the device and/it's leads. There is NO evidence in favor of empirically reprogramming pacing NON-DEPENDENT patients to an asynchronous mode, as this could be harmful if the asynchronous pacing competes with a spontaneous rhythm (e.g., "R-on-T" phenomenon resulting in ventricular fibrillation).

Temporary reprogramming of a CIED for the perioperative period can be accomplished with a manufacturer-specific programmer or a magnet. Magnet application to most pacemakers should cause a pacemaker to pace asynchronously for as long as the magnet remains in place (there will be no sensing of intrinsic rhythm to direct device activity). This protects the patient from interference with pacing due to EMI. Magnet application to an ICD should disable the antitachycardia therapies, but will have no effect on any pacing settings, which becomes critical if the patient is pacer dependent. *Thus, a patient with an ICD who is pacemaker-dependent will require formal reprogramming of the pacing settings preoperatively.* It is more convenient to use a magnet to control the behavior of an ICD intraoperatively because magnet removal will enable rapid defibrillation if needed perioperatively, and discharge from the monitored recovery setting without the need for formal interrogation and reprogramming. Removal of a magnet from a CIED will restore the baseline settings (e.g., the antitachycardia capability of an ICD, and/or the baseline "sensing" mode of a pacemaker).

Anesthetic Agents and Techniques

No specific anesthetic agents are contraindicated because of the presence of a VAD, but one must consider the potentially dysfunctional unsupported right ventricle, as well as any other existing comorbidities. Most VAD-supported patients will receive a general anesthetic due to the requisite anticoagulation required for LVAD-support, but in selected cases, superficial regional blocks under ultrasound guidance, or a regional intravenous technique (e.g., a Bier block) may be appropriate. Neuraxial anesthesia is generally contraindicated due to the anticoagulated state. *Intubation and extubation criteria are the same as for any other patient.* An LVAD by itself does not warrant intubation for cases where intubation would not normally be required, and it does not preclude a patient from being promptly extubated. Prolonged intubation predisposes to pulmonary infection.

Monitoring

Standard ASA monitoring applies, but the non-pulsatile nature of the outflow of currently used CF devices may pose a challenge to hemodynamic monitoring if pulsatility is low at baseline or is lost following anesthetic induction. Pulsatility of the circulation in a CF VAD-supported patient is due to the contractility of the LV either through the LVAD, out the aortic valve, or both. It is not unusual for the baseline pulsatility to decrease after induction (and possibly during surgery) due to the vasodilation and relative hypovolemia that accompanies anesthetic induction and mainte-

nance, and/or fluid shifts and blood loss during surgery. A standard oscillometric NIBP cuff and pulse oximeter will work if one maintains sufficient pulsatility of the circulation through optimization of the volume status presented to the LV. An arterial line (often requiring ultrasound for placement when baseline pulsatility is low) is needed for more complicated cases. Another noninvasive (but cumbersome) option is manual assessments of blood pressure using Doppler modalities. Cerebral oximetry is increasingly being used as an alternative to pulse oximetry in LVAD patients to monitor oxygenation perioperatively. TTE and/or TEE are not generally necessary, but may provide valuable information if questions regarding clinical management arise. In addition to standard monitors, the clinical control screens of the HM II, the HVAD and the HM 3 (Figs. 15.4, 15.5, 15.6, 15.7 and 15.8, respectively) show several parameters of LVAD function that can be very helpful to guide management, as discussed in the figure legends.

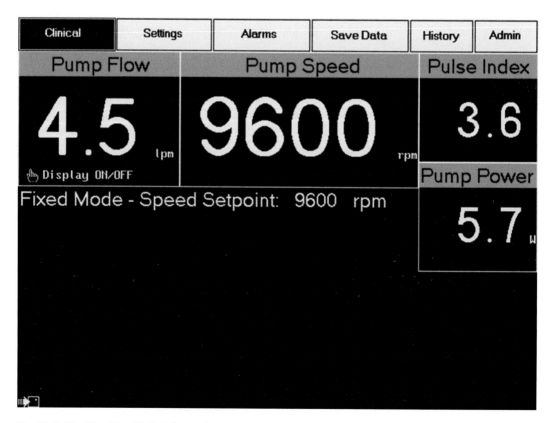

Fig. 15.4 The HeartMate II clinical control screen

Parameter	Description
Pump flow	A continuous estimate of the output from the device (derived from the speed of the impeller and the power it takes to achieve that speed). Flows encountered clinically usually range from 4–6 L/min. If the estimated outflow is less than the lower limit set as the alarm condition, three minus signs will be displayed in this box instead of a number. This does not mean there is no outflow. It only means there is less flow than the lower limit set for the alarm.
Pump speed	Pump speed is the number of revolutions per minute at which the impeller is rotating. In most situations, this is a set and fixed value. Speeds encountered clinically are usually in the range of 9000–10,000 RPM, though some centers use speeds in the 8000 s. increases in speed will facilitate ventricular unloading by increasing flow through the pump. If the amount of flow exceeds the available volume in the ventricle, a "suckdown" will occur. Where volume infusion (and/or support of RV function and minimizing of pulmonary vascular resistance as applicable) fail to correct the situation, temporarily decreasing the pump speed will increase the volume in the left ventricle, thereby breaking the suckdown. However, this is not usually necessary, and should be used as a last resort.
Pulse index	A unitless index of how much pulsatility the device senses as a result of ventricular contractions. As the excessive LV wall tension is decreased as a result of VAD action, the LV begins to recover, and as long as preload is optimized, the ventricle will again begin to contract, forcing little pulses through the VAD, as well as through the aortic valve. PI values around 2–3 are typical when there is little pulsatility and the VAD is doing most or all of the work. *PI values around 4–6 are typical when the partially decompressed ventricle recovers and volume status is optimized.* The PI will decrease with hypovolemia and will increase with myocardial recovery. Thus, a low (or falling) PI likely indicates the need to increase the volume status, or possibly to increase contractility. One should also always bear in mind that RV dysfunction can lead to a decreased filling of the LV.
Pump power	The power required to spin the impeller at the set speed. Increases in speed or flow or resistance to flow will require increased power. Power is generally in the range of 5–7 W. A sudden increase in the power requirement may suggest significantly increased afterload (perhaps your patient is very light?), but it can also suggest thrombus or other obstruction to rotor rotation. These will be exceedingly rare events. One should always investigate abrupt increases in power not explainable by an intentional increase in pump speed. A gradual increase in power to high levels over time suggests developing thrombus in the pump.

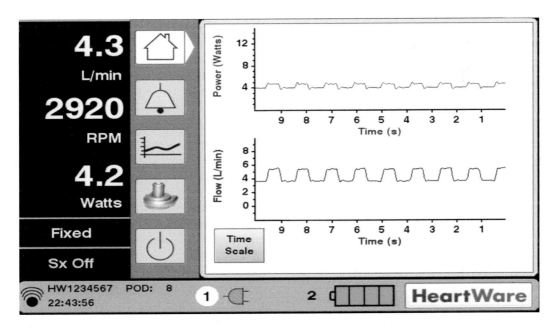

Fig. 15.5 The HeartWare HVAD clinical screen

Parameter	Description
Pump flow	According to the manufacturer, the flow estimation should be used as a trending tool only. The readout of device flow is derived from the speed of the impeller, the power it takes to achieve that speed, and the blood viscosity. The viscosity is calculated from the patient's hematocrit. To obtain the most accurate estimate of flows with this device, one must input the patient hematocrit into the monitor, and one must update the hematocrit whenever it changes by 5% or more in either direction. Flows encountered clinically usually range from 4–6 L/min, but the device is capable of flowing up to 10 LPM. The amount of flow a centrifugal pump can generate is dependent on a number of factors to do with the diameter and geometry of the impeller, the capacity of the motor, and the pressure differential across the pump between the volume available to the pump (the "preload" and the "afterload").
Pump speed	The number of revolutions per minute at which the impeller is rotating. In most situations, this is a set and fixed value. Speeds encountered clinically are usually in the range of 2400–3200 RPM, but the device range is from 1800–4000 RPM. Increases in speed will facilitate ventricular unloading by increasing flow through the pump. If the amount of flow exceeds the available volume in the ventricle, a "suckdown" will occur. Infusing volume (and supporting RV function and decreasing PVR, as applicable) and/or decreasing the speed will increase the volume in the left ventricle. As with the HM II, a change to previously stable pump settings will rarely be the appropriate first action to take to correct hemodynamic aberrations induced by the anesthetic.
Pump power	The power required to spin the impeller at the set speed. Increases in speed or flow or resistance to flow will require increased power. A sudden increase in the power requirement may suggest significantly increased afterload (and the centrifugal pumps are at least temporarily relatively more sensitive to significant increases in afterload than axial devices). One should always investigate abrupt increases in power not explainable by an intentional increase in pump speed. A gradual increase in power to high levels over time suggests developing thrombus in the pump.

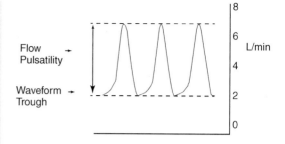

Fig. 15.6 HVAD flow waveform

Flow waveforms	The peaks are the flow during systole and the troughs during diastole, so the difference, in effect, reflects the "pulse pressure" or "pulsatility" of the patient during support. The difference in velocity is coming from LV contraction, forcing blood through the pump at a higher velocity during systole. This waveform can help greatly with fluid management in real time because just as in a patient without a VAD, one can increase the pulse pressure by administering fluid to optimize volume status. In general, one wants to maintain the diastolic flows >2 LPM and there should be at least 2 LPM difference between systolic and diastolic flows. Maintenance of a pulse pressure is also important to prevent retrograde flow through the pump, as well as to prevent suction events.

Central Venous Access

Since the VAD console tells about cardiac output and LV volume status, the actual utility of a central venous access and/or pulmonary artery catheter should be carefully assessed for a given patient, particularly for non-major procedures. The risks of line sepsis, dysrhythmias/arrhythmias, pneumothorax, etc., from central line placement must be weighed against the potential utility of following the trends of cardiac output and derived hemodynamic indices to help guide fluid management and inotropic support, the ability to measure SVO_2, the ability to assess the efficacy of interventions to lower PA pressures, the ability to provide pacing, etc. Echocardiography, especially TEE, is likely to be the most helpful monitor if a management dilemma arises.

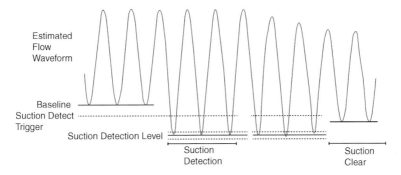

Fig. 15.7 HVAD suction detection

Suction detection	The HVAD controller establishes a diastolic flow baseline. If the diastolic flow falls to <40% of the established baseline for >10 s, the suckdown detection alarm will be annunciated. Observed decreases in the diastolic flow should prompt volume infusion to proactively prevent suckdown events from occurring. If RV dysfunction results in underfilling of the LV, then one would support RV function with inotropes and/or decrease the PVR.

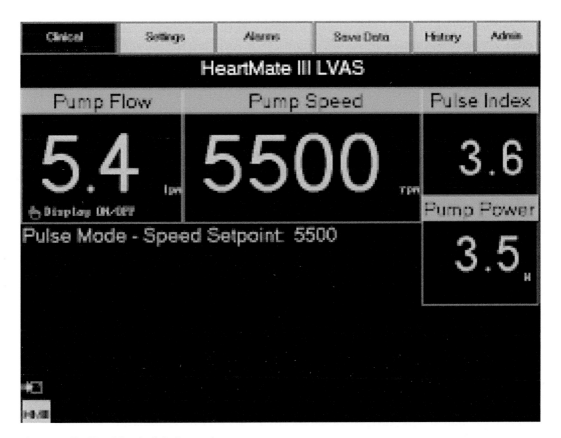

Fig. 15.8 The HeartMate 3 clinical control screen

Parameter	Description
Pump flow	A continuous estimate of the output from the device (derived from the speed of the impeller and the power it takes to achieve that speed). Flows encountered clinically usually range from 4–6 L/min. If the estimated outflow is less than the lower limit set as the alarm condition, three minus signs will be displayed in this box instead of a number. This does not mean there is no outflow. It only means there is less flow than the lower limit set for the alarm.
Pump speed	Pump speed is the number of revolutions per minute at which the impeller is rotating. In most situations, this is a set and fixed value. Speeds encountered clinically are usually in the range of 5000–5500 RPM. Increases in speed will facilitate ventricular unloading by increasing flow through the pump. If the amount of flow exceeds the available volume in the ventricle, a "suckdown" will occur. Where volume infusion (and/or support of RV function and minimizing of pulmonary vascular resistance as applicable) fail to correct the situation, temporarily decreasing the pump speed will increase the volume in the left ventricle, thereby breaking the suckdown. However, this is not usually necessary, and should be used as a last resort. The pump speed of the HM 3 will automatically decrease somewhat 30 times per minute to impart an artificial pulsatility.
Pulse index	A unitless index of how much pulsatility the device senses as a result of ventricular contractions. As the excessive LV wall tension is decreased as a result of VAD action, the LV begins to recover, and as long as preload is optimized, the ventricle will again begin to contract, forcing little pulses through the VAD, as well as through the aortic valve. PI values around 2–3 are typical when there is little pulsatility and the VAD is doing most or all of the work. *PI values around 4–6 are typical when the partially decompressed ventricle recovers and volume status is optimized.* The PI will decrease with hypovolemia and will increase with myocardial recovery. Thus, a low (or falling) PI likely indicates the need to increase the volume status, or possibly to increase contractility. One should also always bear in mind that RV dysfunction can lead to a decreased filling of the LV.
Pump power	The power required to spin the impeller at the set speed. Increases in speed or flow or resistance to flow will require increased power. Power is generally in the range of 3–7 W. A sudden increase in the power requirement may suggest significantly increased afterload (perhaps your patient is very light?), but it can also suggest thrombus or other obstruction to rotor rotation. These will be exceedingly rare events. One should always investigate abrupt increases in power not explainable by an intentional increase in pump speed.

Optimization

Experience has shown that the anesthetic management of a VAD-supported patient for a sedation case or a general anesthetic is not different than that for a non-supported patient. One must ensure continued optimization of the usual determinants of hemodynamics namely preload, afterload, heart rate and pump function. In general, maintaining an adequate volume status is the priority if one is to maintain hemodynamic stability and pulsatility by optimizing Starling's forces.

The goal for perioperative fluid management is to maintain a euvolemic, if not slightly hypervolemic state, provided the right ventricle is able to handle the fluid load. Small (usual) boluses of vasoconstrictors at the time of induction are usually enough to compensate the relative vasodilatation that accompanies sedation/induction if volume status is kept optimized.

Positioning can have an effect on the LV preload and afterload, thereby causing hemodynamic changes in an LVAD patient. Reverse-Trendelenberg's position and abdominal insufflation can cause transient decreases in preload, which could trigger a suction event (discussed in detail below). Lateral positioning may cause decreased LVAD outflow due to decreased preload and/or increased pulmonary pressures associated with hypercarbia and hypoxemia. Optimizing preload with fluid administration, slow abdominal insufflation and avoiding sudden changes in positioning are some helpful measures to mitigate the adverse effect of positioning on the hemodynamic parameters of the patient.

Suction Events

A suction event can happen when a significant decrease in the volume in the left ventricle results in total LV decompression by the LVAD. Though suction events will be rare if the patient is kept optimized, the most common cause of this rare event will be hypovolemia (e.g., resulting from sudden blood loss), or relative hypovolemia due to sudden vasodilatation (e.g., at the time of induction) in a non-optimized patient. The legends accompanying Figs. 15.4 and 15.5 describe how parameters on the VAD clinical screens can be used to anticipate and avert suction events. Management of suction events depends on the cause of the decreased volume in the LV. Infusion of volume is usually going to be the first line action. As well, tidal volumes can be adjusted and PEEP set to low levels to allow for good venous return. Blood losses must be replaced in an aggressive fashion. If RV failure is suspected, inotropic support with milrinone or epinephrine might be used in conjunction with pulmonary vascular dilators to support the right heart. In some cases, the pump speed might have to be decreased to prevent excessive unloading of the LV until the volume status can be optimized. TEE/TTE can help to determine the etiology where needed.

ACLS and the VAD-Supported Patient

Standard ACLS protocols should be used if a VAD-supported patient experiences cardiac arrest but the issue of performing chest compressions has been a matter of debate for decades. The consensus with the prior generation of devices (which tended to have longer and more rigid apical inflow cannulas) was that compressions risked cardiac perforation and/or dislodgement of VAD components. Even in the era of the current devices, many experts have tended to caution against chest compressions due to the risk of LVAD cannula and equipment dislodgement [11]. Recently, however, the American Heart Association released a scientific statement in which chest compressions are now advocated in the case of mechanical VAD failure, especially if the ETCO$_2$ is <20 [13]. Per their recommendations, if the ETCO$_2$ is >20, the mean arterial pressure is >50 mmHg and the VAD appears to be functioning, then compressions should be withheld.

Post-Operative Management

Appropriate Recovery Setting

The location of patient recovery must be decided prior to surgery. (e.g., PACU vs ICU vs VAD floor, if available) It is important to ensure that the receiving staff on duty are trained and able to take care of an LVAD patient.

Plug it in!

The patient will be transported on battery power from the OR to the recovery location. When available, it is prudent to reconnect the VAD to mains A/C power and the system base unit on arrival. Backup batteries should be maintained in their chargers.

Optimization

Optimization of all parameters of hemodynamics must continue into the postoperative period. Volume status must be maintained and all factors avoided that could contribute to elevated PVR such as hypercarbia, hypothermia and acidemia should be mitigated.

Pain Management

Effective pain management is essential not only for patient comfort, but to avoid increases in the pulmonary vascular resistance that might put a strain on the potentially dysfunctional, unsupported right ventricle.

CIEDs

Baseline pacemaker or ICD settings should be restored prior to discharge from a monitored setting. A formal interrogation of a CIED is generally not necessary postoperatively (especially if a magnet had been used to temporarily control the

CIED behavior intraoperatively), but there are some clinical situations in which a formal device interrogation is recommended postoperatively, including:

1. patients who had formal reprogramming of their device preoperatively to restore baseline settings
2. patients who underwent long and complex procedures, involving large fluid shifts and/or transfusions that may have resulted in altered lead impedances
3. patients who experienced a cardiac arrest intraoperatively requiring resuscitation, defibrillation, etc.
4. patients who underwent cardiac or thoracic surgery, where the possibility exists that leads may have been dislodged or injured, or the device affected by high levels of EMI close to the device.

Coordination with Knowledgeable VAD Personnel

The transportation of the VAD-supported patient from one location to another should be coordinated with and assisted by knowledgeable personnel who can ensure the batteries are correctly hooked up and that the system is functioning as intended prior to and after transport.

References

1. Ambrosy AP, Fonarow GC, Butler J, et al. The global health and economic burden of hospitalizations for heart failure: lessons learned from hospitalized heart failure registries. J Am Coll Cardiol. 2014;63(12):1123–33. https://doi.org/10.1016/j.jacc.2013.11.053.
2. Slaughter MS, Rogers JG, Milano CA, et al. Advanced heart failure treated with continuous-flow left ventricular assist device. N Engl J Med. 2009;361(23):2241–51. https://doi.org/10.1056/NEJMoa0909938.
3. Kirklin JK, Naftel DC, Pagani FD, et al. Seventh INTERMACS annual report: 15,000 patients and counting. J Hear Lung Transplant. 2015;34(12):1495–504. https://doi.org/10.1016/j.healun.2015.10.003.
4. Goudra BG, Singh PM. Anesthesia for gastrointestinal endoscopy in patients with left ventricular assist devices: initial experience with 68 procedures. Ann Card Anaesth. 2013;16(4):250–6. https://doi.org/10.4103/0971-9784.119167.
5. Barbara DW, Wetzel DR, Pulido JN, et al. The perioperative management of patients with left ventricular assist devices undergoing noncardiac surgery. In: Mayo Clinic Proceedings.Vol 88.; 2013:674–682. doi:https://doi.org/10.1016/j.mayocp.2013.03.019.
6. Stone M, Hinchey J, Sattler C, Evans A. Trends in the Management of Patients with Left Ventricular Assist Devices Presenting for noncardiac surgery: a 10-year institutional experience. Semin Cardiothorac Vasc Anesth. 2016;20(3):197–204. https://doi.org/10.1177/1089253215619759.
7. Guglin M, Miller L. Myocardial recovery with left ventricular assist devices. Curr Treat Options Cardiovasc Med. 2012;14(4):370–83. https://doi.org/10.1007/s11936-012-0190-9.
8. Wohlschlaeger J, Schmitz KJ, Schmid C, et al. Reverse remodeling following insertion of left ventricular assist devices (LVAD): a review of the morphological and molecular changes. Cardiovasc Res. 2005;68(3):376–86. https://doi.org/10.1016/j.cardiores.2005.06.030.
9. Heatley G, Sood P, Goldstein D, et al. Clinical trial design and rationale of MOMENTUM 3: multi-center study of MagLev Technology in Patients Undergoing MCS therapy with HeartMate 3™ IDE clinical study protocol. J Hear Lung Transplant. 2016; https://doi.org/10.1016/j.healun.2016.01.021.
10. Roberts SM, Hovord DG, Kodavatiganti R, Sathishkumar S. Ventricular assist devices and noncardiac surgery. BMC Anesthesiol. 2015;15(1):185. https://doi.org/10.1186/s12871-015-0157-y.
11. Garatti A, Bruschi G, Colombo T, et al. Noncardiac surgical procedures in patient supported with long-term implantable left ventricular assist device. Am J Surg. 2009;197(6):710–4. https://doi.org/10.1016/j.amjsurg.2008.05.009.
12. Cingolani HE, Perez NG, Cingolani OH, Ennis IL. The Anrep effect: 100 years later. AJP Hear Circ Physiol. 2013;304(2):H175–82. https://doi.org/10.1152/ajpheart.00508.2012.
13. Peberdy MA, Gluck JA, Ornato JP, et al. Cardiopulmonary resuscitation in adults and children with mechanical circulatory support. A scientific statement from the American Heart Association. Circulation. 2017;135:e1115–34.

Anesthesia in Pediatric Cardiac Surgery

16

Eric L. Vu and Pablo Motta

Main Messages
1. Pediatric cardiac surgery involves a heterogenous group of lesions with mortality risk influenced by both procedure complexity and age
2. Congenital heart disease can be grouped into five broad categories: lesions with increased pulmonary blood flow, lesions with decreased pulmonary blood flow, lesions with obstructive blood flow, circulations incompatible with life, and lesions silent until adulthood. A close understanding of the pathophysiology guides hemodynamic management
3. Early extubation in the operating room or intensive care unit is possible after routine pediatric cardiopulmonary bypass cases
4. With increasing survival in patients with congenital heart disease, the cardiac anesthesiologist will likely encounter and should be familiar with both congenital heart lesions and congenital heart disease for non-cardiac procedures

Congenital heart surgery (CHS) involves a heterogeneous group of patients requiring procedures of variable complexity. The Society of Thoracic Surgeons-European Association for Cardiothoracic Surgery (STAT) ranks procedures in complexity and mortality risk [1]. On one end of the spectrum, simple procedures are classified as STAT 1—e.g. Atrial septal defect closure—with almost no expected mortality. Extremely complicated procedures are classified as STAT 5—e.g. Norwood Procedure for single ventricle palliation—with mortality risk greater than 20% (Tables 16.1 and 16.2).

In addition to procedure type, age has important prognostic implication in pediatric cardiac surgery. The neonatal period is the one with highest mortality (9%), followed by infancy (2.8%), and decreasing in childhood (1.1%) according to data from the Society of Thoracic Surgeons in 2015 [2].

Preoperative Evaluation

CHD can be grouped into five broad categories [3]: lesions with increased pulmonary blood flow; decreased pulmonary blood flow; obstructive blood flow; circulations incompatible with life; and lesions silent until adulthood (Table 16.3).

E. L. Vu · P. Motta (✉)
Baylor College of Medicine–Texas Children's Hospital, Pediatric Cardiovascular Anesthesiology, Houston, TX, USA
e-mail: pxmotta@texaschildrens.org

© Springer Nature Switzerland AG 2021
D. C. H. Cheng et al. (eds.), *Evidence-Based Practice in Perioperative Cardiac Anesthesia and Surgery*, https://doi.org/10.1007/978-3-030-47887-2_16

Group 1

*CHD with increased pulmonary blood flow involves **left-to-right shunts** caused by septal defects—atrial, ventricular, or atrioventricular level shunting; or, shunting at the great vessels—aorto-pulmonary window or patent ductus arteriosus* (Fig. 16.1).

The clinical presentation is characterized by increased pulmonary blood flow and heart failure. In infants, heart failure presents as difficulty feeding and failure to thrive. The severity of symptoms is dependent upon the shunt size and pressure gradient between the cardiac chambers. The ventricular septal defect (VSD) can be classified as pressure restrictive or non-restrictive. Non-restrictive VSDs are large and present early in life requiring repair in infancy. Restrictive VSDs and atrial septal defects (ASDs) are usually better tolerated in infancy and early childhood. The medical management of heart failure due to pulmonary over-circulation is diuretics and afterload reduction with angiotensin-converting enzyme (ACE) inhibitors. In severe cases, the patient may need preoperative mechanical ventilation. The ventilatory strategy is to reduce left to right shunting by maintaining or increasing pulmonary vascular resistance with mild hypoventilation and low fraction of inspired oxygen (FiO2). During the preoperative evaluation, it is important to identify and correct severe electrolyte abnormalities which could be caused by excessive diuresis. In addition, anemia is a common problem, particularly if poor feeding and nutrition worsens the physiologic hemoglobin nadir that occurs at eight to 12 weeks of age.

Table 16.1 Society of Thoracic Surgeons—European Association for Cardio-Thoracic Surgery (STAT) Score by Procedure

Rank	Procedures
STAT 1	• Atrial septal defect repair • Pacemaker generator change • Vascular ring repair • Ventricular septal defect repair
STAT 2	• Anomalous origin of coronary artery repair • Bi-directional Glenn • Coarctation of aorta repair • Fontan • New pacemaker implantation • Tetralogy of Fallot repair • Valve replacement
STAT 3	• Arterial switch operation for transposition of great arteries • Atrial ventricular septal defect / atrial ventricular canal repair • Conduit placement • Rastelli procedure
STAT 4	• Double outlet right ventricle repair • Interrupted arch repair • Shunt procedures, systemic to pulmonary artery—Central or modified Blalock-Taussig • Total anomalous pulmonary venous connection repair • Transplant, heart • Truncus arteriosus repair
STAT 5	• Damus-Kaye-Stansel procedure • Norwood procedure • Transplant, heart and lung

Group 2

*CHD with decreased pulmonary blood flow are cyanotic lesions which involve lesions with **right-to-left shunts**—VSD with pulmonary obstruction or tetralogy of Fallot.* The most common lesion of this group is tetralogy of Fallot (TOF). TOF is characterized by a non-restrictive VSD, right ventricular outflow tract obstruction (RVOT), right ventricular hypertrophy, and an aorta overriding the interventricular septum (Fig. 16.2).

Table 16.2 Texas Children's Mortalities by STAT Classification in 2016

Primary Procedure	Number of Procedures	Number of Discharge Mortalities	% Mortality	STS National Benchmark[a]
STAT 1	214	0	0.00%	0.50%
STAT 2	219	3	1.40%	1.70%
STAT 3	63	0	0.00%	2.10%
STAT 4	207	11	5.30%	6.80%
STAT 5	25	2	8.00%	17.30%
Grand Total	**728**	**16**	**2.20%**	**3.10%**

[a]*Source for STS National Benchmark is* Table 16.1 *of the Society of Thoracic Surgeons Data Harvest Report Jan. 2015 to Dec. 2015. The source for the overall hospital data is STAT Index Surg CHD Volume; Data pulled 4/14/2017*

Table 16.3 Anatomical and pathophysiological classification of congenital heart disease

Pathophysiology	Anatomy	Presentation	Lesions
CHD with increased pulmonary blood flow	Septal defects without pulmonary obstruction and left-to-right shunt	• Acyanotic heart failure • Increased pulmonary blood flow	ASD, VSD, CAVC, PAVC, PDA or TrA
CHD with decreased pulmonary flow	Septal defects with pulmonary obstruction and right-to-left shunt	• Cyanosis • Decreased pulmonary blood flow	TOF, PS/ASD, TA
CHD with obstruction to blood flow	Obstruction to blood progression and no septal defects (no shunt)	• Ventricular pressure overload • Heart failure	PS, AS, CoA '
CHD incompatible with postnatal blood circulation	Ductal dependent lesions	• Cyanosis in ductal dependent blood flow	PA
		• Heart failure in ductal dependent systemic flow	AA/MA or IAA
	Parallel systemic and pulmonary circulations	• Cyanosis or pulmonary overcirculation (PVR/SVR)	D-TGA or D-TGA/VSD
	Anomalous connection/obstruction of the pulmonary veins	• Cyanosis	TAPVR
CHD silent until adulthood	Variable	• Variable	BAV, AAOCA, WPW or L-TGA

Abbreviations: CHD congenital heart disease, *ASD* atrial septal defect, *VSD* ventricular septal defect, *CAVC* complete auriculoventricular canal, *PAVC* auriculoventricular canal, *PDA* patent ductus arteriosus, *TrA* truncus arteriosus, *TOF* tetralogy of Fallot, *PS/ASD* pulmonary stenosis / atrial septal defect, *TA* tricuspid atresia, *PS* pulmonary stenosis, *AS* aortic stenosis, *CoA* coarctation of the aorta, *PA* pulmonary atresia, *AA/MA* aortic atresia, *IAA* interrupted aortic arch, *D-TGA* D-transposition of the great arteries, *D-TGA/VSD* D-transposition of the great arteries with ventricular septal defect, *TAPVR* total anomalous pulmonary venous return, *BAV* bicuspid aortic valve, *AAOCA* abnormal aortic origin on the coronary arteries, *WPW* Wolf Parkinson White, *L-TGA* L-transposition of the great arteries

The RVOT obstruction may have two components: (1) a fixed obstruction at subvalvar, valvar, or supravalvar level; and (2) a dynamic obstruction caused by infundibular spasm. A feared complication in TOF patients is the triggering of a hypercyanotic or "Tet Spell" during induction of anesthesia due to sympathetic stimulation and infundibular spasm. A hypercyanotic crisis is characterized by acute right-to-left shunting due to a sudden increase in right ventricular afterload and / or decrease in systemic vascular resistance (SVR). It presents with hypoxemia, hypercapnia, and acidosis that further increases the pulmonary vascular resistance and promotes further shunt-ing. To reduce the incidence of hypercyanotic spells, TOF patients are treated with beta-blockers to decrease the catecholamine response and infundibular spasm. Not all the TOF are prone to cyanosis: the TOF patients with minor RVOT obstruction—"Pink TOF"—may present with pulmonary over-circulation symptoms due to a large VSD which would cause left-to-right shunting. The long-term effect of cyanosis is polycythemia due to increased erythropoietin levels in response to chronic hypoxemia. Hematocrit levels >65% increase blood viscosity and may impair microvascular perfusion, predisposing the patient to thrombosis and thrombocy-

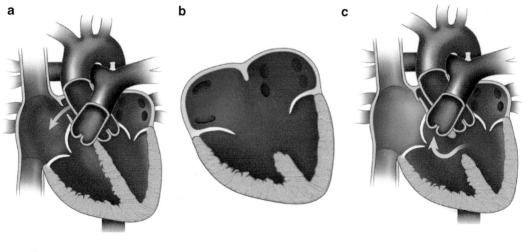

© 2015 Texas Children's Hospital

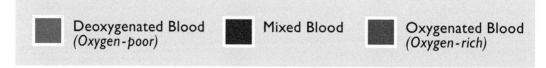

Deoxygenated Blood
(Oxygen-poor)   **Mixed Blood**   **Oxygenated Blood**
                                                  (Oxygen-rich)

Fig. 16.1 Illustration of Acyanotic Lesions. (**a**) ASD with arrow showing the left-to-right flow through the atrial defect. (**b**) CAVC displaying a common atrium, AV valve and incompletely septated ventricular chambers. (**c**) VSD with arrow exhibiting the left-to-right flow across the ventricular communication. Abbreviations: *ASD* atrial septal defect, *CAVC* complete atrioventricular canal, *VSD* ventricular septal defect. [Printed with permissions from Texas Children's Hospital]

topenia. Because bleeding time may be prolonged, these patients are also at risk for coagulation abnormalities and should be evaluated preoperatively with either a coagulation profile or functional coagulation testing—thromboelastography. In the perioperative period it is important to avoid long periods of fasting to minimize risk of hyperviscosity syndrome and/or hypercyanotic spells. Intravenous hydration is recommended once the patient is NPO (nil per os) and beta-blocker administration should be continued on the day of surgery.

Group 3

*The third group of CHD involves **obstructive lesions with no shunting**.* These patients present with an obstruction to systemic or pulmonary blood flow and ventricular pressure overload which leads to heart failure. The obstruction can be in the right or left heart. Pulmonary stenosis (PS) is the most common obstructive lesion of the right heart. PS is considered severe when the peak velocity is >4 m/s (peak gradient >64 mmHg) by echocardiography or cardiac catheterization. The left sided obstructive lesions can present at any level of the left ventricular outflow tract (LVOT): subvalvar, valvular, or supravalvar. Aortic stenosis (AS) is considered severe when the peak velocity is >4 m/s (mean gradient >40 mmHg) and the aortic valve area body surface area index is <0.6 cm^2/m^2. Aortic narrowing is known as coarctation of the aorta (CoA) and can be at any level in relationship to the ductus arteriosus—pre-ductal, ductal, or post-ductal. Presentation is dependent upon the severity and location of the CoA. CoA can be an isolated disease or associated with other CHD such as VSD, bicuspid aortic valve and/or Shone's syndrome—LVOT obstruction, parachute mitral valve, subaortic stenosis, and CoA. William's syndrome

Fig. 16.2 Diagram of
Tetraology of Fallot
exhibiting all hallmarks
of the disease (1) Right
ventricular hypertrophy
(2) RVOT obstruction
(3) Overriding aorta (4)
VSD. Abbreviations:
RVOT, right ventricular
outflow tract; VSD,
ventricular septal defect.
[Printed with
permissions from Texas
Children's Hospital]

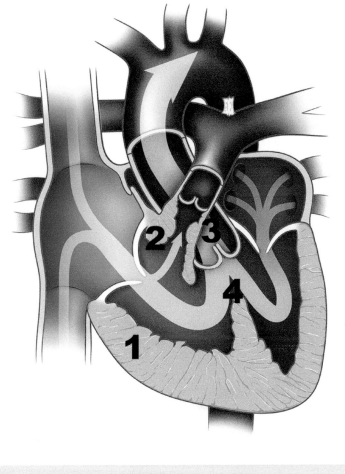

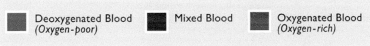

Deoxygenated Blood (Oxygen-poor)	Mixed Blood	Oxygenated Blood (Oxygen-rich)

(deletion of chromosome 7q11.23) presents with supravalvar aortic stenosis, pulmonary branch stenosis, and coronary artery ostial stenosis. This syndrome carries one of the highest risks of sudden death during induction of anesthesia due to the imbalance of oxygen supply and demand to the heart. Most patients with obstructive lesions are managed medically with exercise restriction and beta-blockers; surgical intervention is undertaken with increasing severity of symptoms.

Group 4

The *fourth group of CHD includes patients with lesions incompatible with postnatal circulation*. To better understand this group of CHD, it is important to review the fetal circulation (Fig. 16.3). The fetal circulation involves shunt-ing at four levels: placenta, ductus venosus, fora-men ovale, and ductus arteriosus. In these patients, the patency of the foramen ovale and ductus arteriosus are needed for postnatal survival. To secure patency of these structures shortly after birth, balloon atrial septectomy (BAS) may be performed to assure shunting at the atrial level, and prostaglandin E_1 (PGE_1) may be utilized to maintain a patent ductus arteriosus (PDA).

Group 4a. **Ductal dependent lesions** can be divided in two groups:

- PDA dependent **pulmonary blood flow**—e.g. pulmonary atresia
- PDA dependent **systemic blood flow**—e.g. hypoplastic left heart syndrome (HLHS)

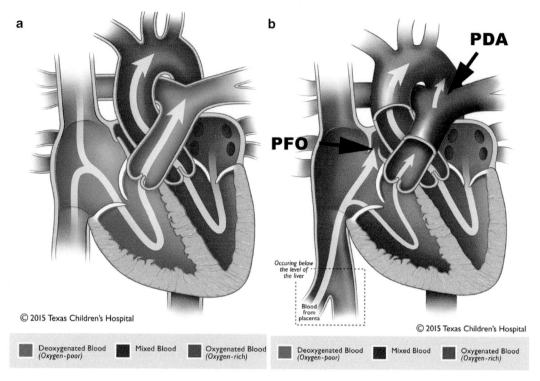

Fig. 16.3 Illustration of Normal and Fetal Circulation displaying (**a**) Normal circulation with deoxygenated blood flowing from the IVC and SVC to the RA, RV and PA (light blue arrows) and oxygenated blood from the PV to the LA, LV and to the aorta (light red arrows). (**b**) Fetal circulation with the oxygenated blood from the placenta to the RA, shunting to the LA through the PFO, LV and to the aorta (light red arrows) and the deoxygenated blood from the RA to the RV and to the PA (purple). Some blood is shunted to the descending aorta by the PDA. Printed with permission from Texas Children's Hospital. Abbreviations: *IVC* inferior vena cava, *SVC* superior vena cava, *RA* right atrium, *RV* right ventricle, *PA* pulmonary artery, *PV* pulmonary vein, *LA* left atrium, *LV* left ventricle, *PFO* patent foramen ovale, *PDA* patent ductus arteriosus. [Printed with permissions from Texas Children's Hospital]

For survival, a mixing lesion must exist—e.g. atrial and ductal level shunting. The amount of pulmonary (Q_p) versus systemic blood flow (Q_s) depends on the ratio of SVR to pulmonary vascular resistance (PVR). Patients with pulmonary atresia are palliated with systemic to pulmonary shunts—e.g. Blalock-Taussig shunt—and HLHS patients are palliated with the Norwood procedure—aortic reconstruction with systemic to pulmonary shunting. Eventually, both groups will continue to stage two of the single ventricle palliation pathway with a bidirectional Glenn shunt—superior cavo-pulmonary anastomosis—at approximately three to 6 months of age. The third and final stage of the palliation pathway—Fontan procedure—is performed at two to 4 years of age in which the systemic venous return (IVC and SVC flow) is directed to the pulmonary arter-

ies. After palliation, antiplatelet agents are used to prevent thrombus formation within the shunts. The antiplatelet agents are typically continued in the preoperative period, which may lead to increased intraoperative bleeding for subsequent procedures.

Group 4b. **When the systemic and pulmonary circulations are in parallel, these are cyanotic lesions incompatible with life.** Transposition of the great arteries (TGA) is the most common of these lesions. In TGA, the aorta arises from the right ventricle (RV) while the pulmonary artery arises from the left ventricle (LV), leading to two parallel circulations. TGA is associated with VSDs in 10–25% of the patients. Even though mixing may occur at any level—atrial, ventricular, or ductal—the most important determinant of oxyhemoglobin saturation is the atrial level shunting. BAS and PGE$_1$ are used in the early management of TGA to not only improve mixing, but also decrease pulmonary venous congestion. The surgical repair for TGA is the arterial switch operation (ASO) performed in the neonatal period. The goal is to time surgical repair before PVR declines or a high degree of LV deconditioning occurs. The ASO consists of a PA anastomosis to the RV, aorta anastomosis to the LV, and coronary artery re-implantation.

Group 4c. **Anomalous connection with obstruction of the pulmonary veins** is a surgical emergency in CHD. The pulmonary veins drain to other structures rather than the left atrium. Drainage can occur at three different levels: supracardiac, cardiac or infracardiac. The infracardiac type is more prone to obstruction. For survival, a mixing lesion must also occur. Typically, these lesions need to be addressed shortly after birth before pulmonary edema and RV dysfunction develops.

Group 5

The last group, **silent CHD until adulthood** is discussed in other chapters of this book.

Intraoperative Management: Monitors

Hemodynamic Monitoring

All pediatric cardiac surgery patients are extensively monitored through the perioperative period. Standard hemodynamic monitoring includes invasive arterial and central venous pressure monitoring. The use of ultrasound for percutaneous vascular access has simplified line placement in infant and children [4]. In infants <5 kg and single ventricle physiology patients, avoiding the internal jugular vein for central access minimizes potential thrombosis of the superior vena cava. Oftentimes, central venous access is obtained through the femoral vein. Percutaneous pulmonary artery catheters, oximetric catheters, and continuous mixed venous oxygen saturation monitoring are typically not utilized in pediatric congenital heart surgery.

When monitoring of left-sided cardiac pressures is required, a left atrial catheter can be placed directly into the left atrium by the surgeon.

Intraoperative Echocardiography

The majority of patients undergoing CHD will have intraoperative evaluation of the surgical repair by transesophageal echocardiography (TEE). Miniaturized TEE probes can be used in patients <3 kg. In patients with contraindication to TEE or patients who do not tolerate probe placement—due to hemodynamic or ventilatory compromise—epicardial echocardiography may be utilized in the surgical field [5]. TEE is often performed before the start of the operation to confirm diagnosis, and may help image structures that are difficult to view with transthoracic echocardiography windows—e.g. pulmonary veins, interatrial septum, etc. A post-repair TEE exam is useful to detect residual defects that may require prompt surgical revision. Common causes to resume CPB include: residual outflow tract gradients, e.g. after TOF repair; persistent shunting, e.g. after VSD closure; and valvar insufficiency / stenosis, e.g. after CAVC repair.

Neurologic Monitoring

Neurologic injury is a significant concern in pediatric heart surgery, particularly in the developing brain. The results of ongoing studies are conflicting. Nonetheless, the Food and Drug Administration issued a "Drug Safety Communication" warning in 2016 that general anesthesia and sedation drugs used in children less than 3 years of age for > 3 h may affect brain development, but that emergency or life-saving surgery should not be delayed for this risk [6, 7]. In procedures that require prolonged periods of circulatory arrest or low flow bypass—e.g. Norwood procedure, aortic arch reconstruction, etc.—close neuromonitoring and neuroprotection become paramount. Cerebral oximetry measured by near infrared spectroscopy (NIRS) can be utilized to detect periods of cerebral hypoperfusion [8–10]. Therapeutic interventions are suggested when baseline values have decreased more than 20%. Methods to improve cerebral oxygenation involve improving oxygen delivery—increasing CPB pump flow, CO_2, hematocrit, blood pressure; or, decreasing oxygen consumption—decreasing temperature, deepening the anesthetic. Transcranial doppler (TCD) can also be utilized in infants to guide CPB flows during regional cerebral perfusion (RCP) and avoid cerebral hypoperfusion / hyperperfusion [11, 12]. One approach is to measure baseline TCD mean velocities and keep velocities within 5–10% during RCP. Surgical approaches to neuroprotection on CPB may include deep hypothermia (18 °C) or RCP and is surgeon / center dependent. At this time, there are no data to suggest which method is superior.

Coagulation Monitoring

The neonatal coagulation system is not mature at birth and the risk of perioperative bleeding is increased. There are decreased levels of factors II, VII, IX, XI, XII, antithrombin III, Proteins C and S, but increased levels of factor VIII and Von Willebrand factor. In comparison to adult patients transitioning on to CPB, the degree of hemodilution is much greater in infants and neonates, which further increases the risk of dilutional coagulopathy. Early, aggressive diagnosis and treatment of coagulopathy after CPB can be achieved with thromboelastography or thromboelastometry testing with associated directed transfusion therapy [13, 14].

Anesthetic Management

Common principles include:

- Avoidance of air in intravenous fluids in patients with shunts to prevent paradoxical emboli
- Prophylactic use of antibiotics
- Invasive monitors
- Postoperative management in the intensive care unit (ICU)

Table 16.4 Hypercyanotic spell management

Objective	Management Strategy
Increase O_2 content	Increase FiO_2
Increase SVR	Phenylephrine 0.5–3 mcg/kg
Decrease infundibular spasm	Volume administration (10 mL/kg); Beta-blockers (Esmolol 0.5–1 mg/kg)
Decrease catecholamine discharge	Increase anesthetic depth (opioid and/or inhalational agent)

The *anesthetic goals* during pediatric cardiac surgery vary depending on the pathophysiology of CHD:

Left-to-right shunt: the aim is to minimize left-to-right shunting by maintaining / increasing PVR—low FiO_2 and mild hypercarbia—and lowering SVR—deep plane of anesthesia.

Right-to-left shunt: the objective is to minimize right-to-left shunting and cyanosis by decreasing RVOT obstruction—volume administration, beta-blockers, narcotics—and maintain SVR at baseline values—alpha-agonist (Table 16.4).

Obstructive lesion with no shunting: the goal is to avoid further increases in ventricular or vascular obstruction during induction and maintenance of anesthesia. It is crucial to keep the heart rate and SVR within 20% of baseline values. A slow and judicious induction to ensure hemodynamic stability with beta-blockers—e.g. esmolol—or alpha-agonists—e.g. phenylephrine—is recommended.

CHD incompatible with postnatal blood circulation: the objective in ductal dependent lesions is to maintain patency of shunts from fetal circulation (PFO and PDA) with PGE_1 and BAS, as necessary

- An adequate Q_p:Q_s ratio close to 1:1 achieves a systemic SpO2 of 80%. Higher SpO_2 values (>90%) indicate luxury pulmonary perfusion at the extent of poor systemic perfusion and the potential development of lactic acidosis
- Lower SaO_2 values (<70%) indicate the opposite: poor pulmonary perfusion with excessive systemic flow
- During induction of anesthesia, higher FiO_2 and hyperventilation will increase pulmonary blood flow, which may be detrimental for

these patients. Close attention to the SVR/PVR ratio is needed during induction and maintenance of anesthesia

Induction should be gradual, especially in patients with decreased ventricular function and/or severe ventricular outflow tract gradients. In patients with no intravenous access, an inhalational induction with sevoflurane is likely well tolerated if the cardiovascular physiology is well compensated. Uncompensated patients need a controlled intravenous induction due to the risk of depressed cardiac function associated with high inhalational anesthetic concentrations. Ketamine (1–2 mg/kg) or etomidate (0.2–0.4 mg/kg) intravenously, with incremental doses of narcotics and non-depolarizing muscle relaxant (NDMR) is often used in these uncompensated patients.

Regional techniques are an evolving field in pediatric cardiac surgery. Single dose caudal morphine (50 mcg/kg) has been used after induction and intubation to decrease intravenous narcotic requirements and facilitate early extubation. Our institution has good experience with ultrasound guided paravertebral blocks in pediatric cardiac thoracotomy cases as an alternative to epidural anesthesia [15].

Maintenance of general anesthesia is implemented with a balanced technique involving inhalational anesthetics, opioids, non-depolarizing muscle relaxants, and vasoactive agents to achieve hemodynamic goals for the cardiac lesion(s).

Cardiopulmonary Bypass Management

The patient size and the starting hematocrit determine the type of prime used in CPB. The goal is to keep the **hematocrit > 25%,** which has been associated with better long-term neurodevelopmental outcomes [16]. General guidelines for CPB include:

- **Less than 20 kg:** packed red blood cells (pRBCs) with albumin and / or fresh frozen plasma (FFP) is used

- **Over 20 kg:** crystalloid prime with Plasma-Lyte and electrolytes—e.g. calcium and glucose—are added to recapitulate physiological levels. Blood conservation techniques, such as intraoperative blood salvage may be considered
- Other prime supplements include:
  - Heparin, buffer solution (e.g. sodium bicarbonate), mannitol, and steroids [17].
  - Antifibrinolytics: ε-aminocaproic acid (EACA) and tranexamic acid (TXA) decrease fibrinolysis by blocking plasminogen binding sites or blocking enzymatic plasminogen activators that convert plasminogen to plasmin [18, 19].
- **Full heparinization** is needed before CPB with a target activated clotting time (ACT) of >380–480 seconds. In infants the dose is higher (400 units/kg) than in adults and older children (300 units/kg) due to the higher body water content and lager volume of distribution
- The suggested calculated **CPB flow** is:

$$Q = Wt \times 150\,mL\,/\,kg\,/\,min\,(\text{for patients} < 10\,kg)$$

$$Q = BSA \times CI\,(\text{for patients} \geq 10\,kg)$$

- Q: flow (mL/min)
- Wt: weight (kg)
- BSA: body surface area (m^2)
- CI: cardiac index (mL/min/m^2)

To achieve higher CPB flows in infants, vasodilators may be used (e.g. phentolamine 0.1–0.2 mg/kg) to target physiological mean arterial pressures. The **degree of hypothermia** on CPB is dependent on the patient's size and type of surgical repair. **CHD incompatible with postnatal blood circulation** is typically performed under deep hypothermia with or without circulatory arrest. The blood gas management utilized in these patients is pH stat where carbon dioxide (CO_2) is introduced to the oxygenator to maintain constant pH and pCO_2 levels while hypothermic. This CPB approach maximizes cerebral blood flow and tissue oxygenation.

Weaning of CPB is attempted once the patient is fully rewarmed, has an adequate hematocrit—

variable with the type of lesion, and is typically higher in cyanotic patients; cardiac chambers have been de-aired, confirmed by TEE; and adequate ventilation has resumed. Optimal ventilation is crucial to avoid increases in PVR. Nitric oxide (NO) should be available for patients prone to develop postoperative pulmonary hypertension—e.g. late repair of **left-to-right shunts** where pulmonary vascular remodeling has occurred after chronic pulmonary over-circulation. TEE is used to examine the repair and assess the ventricular function. If the ventricular function is decreased, inotropes should be initiated—e.g. milrinone 0.375–0.75 mcg/kg/min and/or epinephrine 0.02–0.05 mcg/kg/min. In hypotensive patients with adequate ventricular function, hypotension is likely secondary to decreased SVR and/or vasoplegic syndrome, and vasopressin (0.01–0.06 U/kg/h) can be utilized to increase SVR. Once the ventricular function and blood pressure are stabilized, heparinization is reversed with protamine sulfate (1:1—1:1.3 ratio to heparin). When acute kidney injury is anticipated in neonates, peritoneal dialysis catheters may be placed for fluid removal in the postoperative period.

Postoperative Management

The **emergence of anesthesia** and **extubation in the operating room** is possible in patients after pediatric cardiac surgery if the patient has no severe comorbidities, an uneventful OR course—e.g. no bleeding, no EKG changes, good ventricular function, no residual lesion by TEE—and adequate oxygenation and ventilation [20, 21]. Judicious use of opioids and muscle relaxants is essential to avoid respiratory depression and/or residual muscle relaxation. Because medications administered before CPB tend to be diluted and ultra-filtrated, one strategy may be to administer 15–20 mcg/kg of fentanyl for the case with the majority prior to the pre-CPB period. Another strategy may be to limit fentanyl to 1–3 mcg/kg/hr. during the case. Sufentanil (0.5–2 mcg/kg/min) or remifentanil (0.05–0.2 mcg/kg/min) infusions are valid alternatives to fentanyl. Due to the

extremely short half-life (<5 min) of remifentanil, a longer acting opioid—e.g. morphine or hydromorphone—should be utilized prior to discontinuation of the infusion.

ICU Management and Complications

Patients who do not meet criteria for early extubation in the operating room are kept intubated, ventilated and sedated until the clinical situation improves.

Increased **chest tube output (CTO)** due to mediastinal bleeding is a common cause of re-operation after pediatric cardiac surgery. Normal CTO is less than 1–2 mL/kg/h but could be greater than 3–4 mL/kg/h in the first 2 h. Coagulation point of care testing in the OR and in the ICU allows for prompt diagnosis and decreased use of blood products [13]. Excessive use of blood products has been associated with severe complications including acute renal failure (ARF), transfusion-related immunomodulation (TRIM), transfusion-related acute lung injury (TRALI) and transfusion associated circulatory overload (TACO).

Low cardiac output syndrome (LCOS), a transient decrease in systemic perfusion caused by myocardial dysfunction, is a risk in the immediate postoperative period. Common factors associated with LCOS are long CPB and cross-clamp times; poor myocardial protection—e.g. hypertrophic ventricles and inadequate cardioplegia; hypothermia; and ventriculotomy. Most patients will improve with inotropes and mechanical ventilation if no residual lesion is present. Temporary mechanical support with extracorporeal mechanical oxygenation (ECMO) may be required if no hemodynamic improvement is achieved.

Another feared postoperative complication is **pulmonary hypertension (PHTN),** commonly seen in late repair of **left-to-right shunt lesions**. The management includes sedation; ventilation—a high FiO2 + mild hyperventilation; right ventricular support—e.g. milrinone; and pulmonary vasodilation with nitric oxide. Severe cases of refractory PHTN may require temporary ECMO support.

One of the hallmarks of pediatric cardiac ICU care is the use of **peritoneal dialysis** after neonatal cardiac surgery to help with fluid management due to immature renal function or acute kidney injury (AKI), particularly after prolonged CPB time [22]. Older pediatric patients who develop AKI after cardiac surgery may require continuous venovenous hemodialysis (CVVHD).

References

1. O'Brien SM, Clarke DR, Jacobs JP, Jacobs ML, Lacour-Gayet FG, Pizarro C, et al. An empirically based tool for analyzing mortality associated with congenital heart surgery. J Thorac Cardiovasc Surg. 2009 Nov;138(5):1139–53.
2. Harvest Schedule and Information | STS [Internet]. [cited 2017 Oct 30]. Available from: https://www.sts.org/registries-research-center/sts-national-database/harvest-schedule-and-information
3. Thiene G, Frescura C. Anatomical and pathophysiological classification of congenital heart disease. Cardiovasc Pathol Off J Soc Cardiovasc Pathol. 2010 Oct;19(5):259–74.
4. Lamperti M, Bodenham AR, Pittiruti M, Blaivas M, Augoustides JG, Elbarbary M, et al. International evidence-based recommendations on ultrasound-guided vascular access. Intensive Care Med. 2012 Jul;38(7):1105–17.
5. Practice Guidelines for Perioperative Transesophageal Echocardiography. Anesthesiol J Am Soc Anesthesiol. 2010 May 1;112(5):1084–96.
6. Zhang H, Du L, Du Z, Jiang H, Han D, Li Q. Association between childhood exposure to single general anesthesia and neurodevelopment: a systematic review and meta-analysis of cohort study. J Anesth. 2015 Oct;29(5):749–57.
7. Andropoulos DB, Greene MF. Anesthesia and developing brains—implications of the FDA warning. N Engl J Med. 2017;2017(376):905–7.
8. Steppan J, Hogue CW. Cerebral and tissue oximetry. Best Pract Res Clin Anaesthesiol. 2014 Dec;28(4):429–39.
9. Hogue C, Kraut M, Selnes O. Continuous Cerebral Autoregulation Monitoring to Reduce Brain Injury from Cardiac. Grantome [Internet]. [cited 2016 Nov 3]; Available from: http://grantome.com/grant/NIH/R01-HL092259-02
10. Hoffman GM, Ghanayem NS, Scott JP, Tweddell JS, Mitchell ME, Mussatto KA. Postoperative cerebral and somatic near-infrared spectroscopy saturations and outcome in Hypoplastic left heart syndrome. Ann Thorac Surg. 2017 May;103(5):1527–35.
11. Bathala L, Mehndiratta MM, Sharma VK. Transcranial doppler: technique and common findings (part 1). Ann Indian Acad Neurol. 2013;16(2):174–9.
12. Andropoulos DB, Easley RB, Brady K, McKenzie ED, Heinle JS, Dickerson HA, et al. Neurodevelopmental outcomes after regional cerebral perfusion with Neuromonitoring for neonatal aortic arch reconstruction. Ann Thorac Surg. 2013 Feb;95(2):648–55.
13. Wikkelsø A, Wetterslev J, Møller AM, Afshari A. Thromboelastography (TEG) or thromboelastometry (ROTEM) to monitor haemostatic treatment versus usual care in adults or children with bleeding. Cochrane Database Syst Rev. 2016 Aug 22;8:CD007871.
14. Nakayama Y, Nakajima Y, Tanaka KA, Sessler DI, Maeda S, Iida J, et al. Thromboelastometry-guided intraoperative haemostatic management reduces bleeding and red cell transfusion after paediatric cardiac surgery. BJA Br J Anaesth. 2015 Jan;114(1):91–102.
15. Boretsky K, Visoiu M, Bigeleisen P. Ultrasound-guided approach to the paravertebral space for catheter insertion in infants and children. Paediatr Anaesth. 2013 Dec;23(12):1193–8.
16. Wypij D, Jonas RA, Bellinger DC, Del Nido PJ, Mayer JE, Bacha EA, et al. The effect of hematocrit during hypothermic cardiopulmonary bypass in infant heart surgery: results from the combined Boston hematocrit trials. J Thorac Cardiovasc Surg. 2008 Feb;135(2):355–60.
17. Elhoff JJ, Chowdhury SM, Zyblewski SC, Atz AM, Bradley SM, Graham EM. Intraoperative steroid use and outcomes following the Norwood procedure: an analysis of the pediatric heart Network's public database. Pediatr Crit Care Med. 2016 Jan;17(1):30–5.
18. Eaton MP, Alfieris GM, Sweeney DM, Angona RE, Cholette JM, Venuto C, et al. Pharmacokinetics of ε-aminocaproic acid in neonates undergoing cardiac surgery with cardiopulmonary bypass. Anesthesiol J Am Soc Anesthesiol. 2015;122(5):1002–9.
19. Grassin-Delyle S, Couturier R, Abe E, Alvarez JC, Devillier P, Urien S. A practical tranexamic acid dosing scheme based on population pharmacokinetics in children undergoing cardiac surgery. Anesthesiology. 2013 Apr;118(4):853–62.
20. Mahle WT, Jacobs JP, Jacobs ML, Kim S, Kirshbom PM, Pasquali SK, et al. Early Extubation after repair of tetralogy of Fallot and the Fontan procedure: an analysis of the Society of Thoracic Surgeons congenital heart surgery database. Ann Thorac Surg. 2016 Sep;102(3):850–8.
21. Jacobs ML, Jacobs JP, Hill KD, Hornik C, O'Brien SM, Pasquali SK, et al. The Society of Thoracic Surgeons congenital heart surgery database: 2017 update on research. Ann Thorac Surg. 2017 Sep;104(3):731–41.
22. Santos CR, Branco PQ, Gaspar A, Bruges M, Anjos R, Gonçalves MS, et al. Use of peritoneal dialysis after surgery for congenital heart disease in children. Perit Dial Int J Int Soc Perit Dial. 2012;32(3):273–9.

Congenital Heart Disease and the Adult for Cardiac Surgery and Cardiac Intervention

17

Jane Heggie

Main Messages

1. The increasing prevalence of adult congenital heart disease and the changing demographic of this population will be a challenge for all cardiac programs and health systems management.
2. These patients are living full adult lives with post-secondary education, careers, relationships and children.
3. In planning the management of the ACHD patient electronic resources can be utilized to envision the anatomy and physiology that they were born with and how previous surgery has altered that physiology.
4. If a non-cardiac surgical procedure is planned, the surgical team must review if there a conflict with their adapted physiology and determine how the conflict can be mitigated.
5. Cardiac surgery and cardiac interventions should be planned in a multidisciplinary fashion with perioperative screening and optimization of comorbidities.

6. Patients are frequently lost to follow up for reasons of finances, insurance, distance to the reference center and many due to the fact they believe their CHD is resolved.
7. Patients may return with an arrhythmia, non-cardiac surgical issue or heart failure—these are opportunities to reconnect the patient with the circle of care and improve their quality of life.

The prevalence of patients with congenital heart disease (CHD) surviving past 18 years is increasing. A comprehensive population-based cohort study of patients with CHD in Quebec from 1987 to 2005 demonstrated the median age at death for all CHD increased by 15 years, from 60 years in 1987 to 1993, to 75 years in 1999 to 2005. Patients with severe forms of CHD, the median age at death increased from 2 years in 1987 to 1993, to 23 in 1999 to 2005 [1]. Most patients will have been diagnosed in childhood, however there are simple lesions such as atrial septal defect (ASDs) and complex lesions—cc-TGA and Ebstein's—that present in adulthood. In 2000, 49% of patients living with severe congenital heart disease were adults and in 2010 this increased to 66% of patients [2, 3].

Several regional case series have published 30-day surgical mortality for cardiac surgery in

J. Heggie (✉)
University Health Network - Toronto General Hospital, Toronto, ON, Canada
e-mail: jane.heggie@uhn.ca

© Springer Nature Switzerland AG 2021
D. C. H. Cheng et al. (eds.), *Evidence-Based Practice in Perioperative Cardiac Anesthesia and Surgery*, https://doi.org/10.1007/978-3-030-47887-2_17

ACHD, with results ranging from 3.5% to 7%, with variation in reporting of major adverse events and long-term morbidity [4–6]. Over time there is a shift to higher acuity cases with proportionately less 'simple' cases such as ASDs as many of these are referred to interventionists. These studies detail intraoperative factors that were predictive of outcome but do not account for the organ dysfunction that are a burden of living with congenital heart disease. A recent scientific statement from the American Heart Association (AHA) discusses the diagnosis and management of non-cardiac complications in ACHD [7]. Many of these associated conditions are relevant to surgical and ICU care.

Stratification of perioperative risk will be determined partially by patient factors—anatomical diagnosis, comorbid conditions, acuity of the presenting complaint and cognitive function; and regional or system factors—insurance, prior surgical care in another center, and regional referral patterns. Gaps in care after transition from a pediatric setting are common and reasons to return to care are new symptoms, referral from provider, and desire to prevent problems [8]. Guidelines for ongoing care and referrals to specialized ACHD centers exist, however fewer than one third of patients are actively followed in regional centers in Canada—and less so in the United States—and yet there is a mortality benefit in being followed in a regional center [9, 10].

Perioperative Considerations

The anesthetic considerations for diagnostic procedures, cardioversions, therapeutic interventions and cardiac surgery are all similar for an individual but with escalating risk and at times conflict with the hemodynamic goals of the patient's physiology. Ideally the patient has been presented at multidisciplinary case conference and followed by a cardiologist with an interest in ACHD. Frequently diagnostic procedures, cardioversions and minimal risk surgery may occur at a regional level whereas interventions and complicated surgery will happen at a reference center.

Cardiac red flags for management are as follows:

- Is the lesion dependant on pulmonary vascular resistance (PVR)?
- Septal shunts or fenestrations?
- Preload and afterload dependant?
- Pacemaker dependant?
- Pulmonary function
- Liver disease
- Pulmonary hypertension
- Blood loss anticipated? Massive?
- Cognitive impairment and Syndromes

Detailed management of individual ACHD lesions is beyond the scope of this handbook and the reader is directed to reference texts and reviews, however there are commonalities and hemodynamic considerations unique to ACHD lesions [11].

Ebstein's, repaired Tetralogy of Fallot with a previous transannular patch and free pulmonary regurgitation, and Fontan and Glenn shunts are all dependent on a low pulmonary vascular resistance. They are best managed with spontaneous ventilation for non-cardiac surgery or diagnostic procedures and when mandatory ventilation is needed at volumes close to FRC with little positive end-expiratory pressure (PEEP) and low airway pressures. Maintaining a pH that is not acidotic and well oxygenated as well as a normothermic patient are all important.

Patients with unrestricted intracardiac shunts or large aortopulmonary (AP) collaterals are dependent on a balance between the PVR and systemic vascular resistance (SVR). These patients have found this balance in their ambulatory life and post induction it is wise to target their room air PaO2 and saturations. A pre-existing left to right shunt can be exacerbated by exuberant ventilation and hyperoxygenation. Ironically a pink patient will have a metabolic acidosis. Similarly, cyanotic patients may have temporary increases in saturation but at the expense of systemic oxygen delivery.

Intracardiac shunts—ASD, ventricular septal defect (VSD), fenestrations in ASDs and lateral tunnel Fontans—and great vessel shunts—patent ductus arteriosus (PDA), systemic artery to pulmonary artery (PA) shunts such as Blalock Taussig, Waterston and Potts shunts—will need thoughtful precautions for venous air emboli. Meticulous de-airing of lines in preparation and use of stop cocks is recommended. Filters are problematic in cases using total intravenous anesthesia (TIVA) or blood transfusion as the filters occlude with Propofol and transfusion is problematic. If the lines are tucked and the filters remote from the anesthesiologist, you may be isolated from your patient with loss of venous access.

Examples of preload dependent lesions include Fontan and Glenn circulations, a failing RV in the context of a repaired tetralogy of Fallot with a pulmonary regurgitation due to the transannular patch, lesions with systemic left ventricular outflow tract obstruction—aortic stenosis. Examples of cases where patients are dependent on reduced after load are: the systemic right ventricle (RV) in transposition of the great arteries (d-TGA) post Mustard/Senning repair; congenitally corrected transposition of the great arteries (l-TGA) where the patient is born with a subaortic morphological RV; and the single ventricle patients palliated with a Fontan circulation.

Right sided heart lesions and single ventricle physiology necessitate a high proportion of epicardial pacemakers and many heart failure patients are managed with biventricular pacing. Location of the pulse generator and a plan for back up pacing must be verified prior the case, particularly for non-cardiac surgery.

ACHD patients have decreased static lung function and capacity to augment cardiac output in response to stress, decreased exercise tolerance based on VO2 index, diminished FEV1 and forced vital capacity (FVC) and significant restriction compared to normal [12]. Restriction is strongly associated with the number of previous chest incisions, particularly sternotomies and thoracotomies (>50%). Fontan and Tetralogy of Fallot patients have mean FEV1 and FVC 60% of predicted compared to age matched controls [13, 14]. Moderate to severe impairment of forced vital capacity is a known predictor of mortality in ACHD patients.

The majority of ACHD patients have hepatic congestion from a failing right sided circulation. The MELD score was developed at the Mayo clinic to predict death while waiting for a liver transplant. MELD-xi score, which excludes INR, has been validated to be nearly as accurate as MELD score in predicting short-term survival in cirrhosis [15]. Excluding INR is important because many ACHD patients are on warfarin. MELD-xi score was retrospectively evaluated in a cohort of 96 Fontan patients of which 73 patients were > 18 years old. Creatinine and bilirubin were measured within a seven-day period and the values were compared to control patients with hepatitis C cirrhosis. This study found that Fontan patients exhibited a similar distribution of MELD-xi scores as patients with established Hepatitis C cirrhosis; furthermore, MELD-xi score > 18 was associated with substantially higher risk of sudden cardiac death, death from congestive heart failure and cardiac transplantation [16]. A recent but smaller series from Japan reviewed 32 re-do cardiac surgical ACHD patients of which 38% [12] had documented liver dysfunction, had longer duration of anesthesia, surgery and cardiopulmonary bypass, and higher transfusion requirements [17].

Pulmonary hypertension is an independent risk factor but is managed differently depending on the root cause [18]:

- Eisenmenger's: a consequence of living with a longstanding left to right shunt where the pulmonary arterioles hypertrophy and eventually the pulmonary arterial pressures can match or exceed systemic pressures and the patient is cyanosed; this is a challenge as the anaesthesiologist must deal with both the pulmonary hypertension and the potential to exacerbate the right to left shunt and cyanosis.
- Systemic-to-pulmonary shunt with increased PVR cardiac defect that cannot be closed without high risks; the patients may have a failing right ventricle post closure.
- Primary pulmonary hypertension attributed to CHD and, yet the CHD lesion is quite mild and not the cause—the small patent foramen ovale (PFO) or incidental ASD

- Pulmonary hypertension due to left heart disease such as regurgitant systemic atrioventricular (AV) valve, aortic regurgitation or a failing systemic ventricle.

Blood loss for the procedure and the vulnerability of the ACHD patient to coagulopathy must be anticipated. Risk factors for blood loss include the number of previous chest wall incisions, perioperative anticoagulation, history of a prior massive transfusion, MELDxi score and intraoperative events such as sternal entry injury to the heart or adjoining vessels. The anesthetic and surgical team must assess the anatomy with axial imaging and have contingency plans for sternal entry. There is a risk benefit ratio of accepting that there may be a cardiac injury on entry necessitating femoral cannulation and drop suckers in the wound with the patient head down to reduce air emboli versus pre-emptive femoral bypass and cooling to circulatory arrest prior to sternotomy adding significant morbidity to the operation. Exposing the patient to a major transfusion may sensitize them and limit their options for transplantation in the future.

Patients with cyanosis have their own unique hematological issues. They have an increase in red cells and a relative dilution of platelets and vitamin K dependent clotting factors. They are frequently relatively iron deficient despite their high hemoglobin. Iron deficient red cells are less flexible in the micro circulation exposing the patient to increase risk of stroke. Normal transfusion triggers do not apply to this population and higher postoperative hemoglobin will be necessary [19].

Cognitive impairment and Syndromes such as Downs Syndrome (DS), and 22q11.2 Deletion Syndrome with conotruncal defects add the complexity of managing the environment around the patient in addition to their operative care and ICU recovery. DS comorbidities include deficiencies in cognition, hypothyroidism, tendency towards infection dementia >40 years and prevalence of dementia 50–70% at 60 years, acquired mitral valve disease, atlanto-axial instability, obstructive sleep apnea, and epilepsy [20]. The preoperative visit must include a thorough history and assessment of atlanto-axial instability with recent flexion and extension views of the cervical spine and risk assessment for sleep apnea. Patients with 22q11.2 Deletion Syndrome comorbidities include palatal abnormalities, autism spectrum and or schizophrenia, developmental delay, trachea-esophageal disorders, renal anomalies, seizures, immunodeficiency and hypocalcemia [21]. Whether the patient is living with their family or in a supervised care there will be an investment required by both the perioperative team and the care givers of the patient.

In summary, the preoperative considerations for the ACHD patient are substantial. In addition to complex anatomy and physiology that is often very different form the acquired heart disease patient, their comorbidities and accompanying syndromes add to their complexity and risk. Ideally the patient should be presented to a multidisciplinary case conference and if deemed an operative candidate must then be assessed by a cardiac anesthesiologist with an ICU background and an interest in ACHD a few months prior to the surgical date. Comorbidities can be identified and potentially optimized as well as risks explained to the family and substitute decision maker. A follow up appointment prior to admission is helpful to review risks and optimization. Many of these patients were traumatized by their childhood experiences and are averse to hospitalization. Others perceive themselves as normal with a sternotomy scar and have trouble comprehending the seriousness of the procedure and have never made these decisions for themselves.

ASDs, VSDs and Fenestrations

Atrial Septal Defect

ASD is one of the most common forms of congenital heart disease and is one of the ACHD conditions that commonly presents in adulthood. There are four types, and the majority are: Secundum ASDs followed by Primum ASD—associated with a mitral valve cleft; Sinus Venosus ASD—associated with partial anomalous pulmonary venous drainage; and the rare Unroofed Coronary Sinus defect—associated with a persistent left sided superior vena cava (SVC).

Indications for ASD closure include right atrial or ventricular enlargement, paradoxical embolism or documented orthodeoxia-platypnea—hypoxia and dyspnea while upright. Patients with pulmonary hypertension will be assessed in the cath lab and considered for closure if the pulmonary arterial pressures are less than 2/3 systemic and there is a favourable response to pulmonary vasodilators.

With rare exceptions Secundum ASDs are referred for device closure and rarely need anesthetic care. Surgical closure is needed for large defects and defects that lack an adequate septal rim or for patients who also need an antiarrhythmic intervention (MAZE). The remaining defects are complex and should be referred to a reference center. In pre-cardiopulmonary bypass (CPB) patients, an optimal PVR:SVR ratio needs to be maintained and the usual precautions for paradoxical embolus should be followed. For post-CPB patients, methods to reduce PVR should be utilized, including a normal $PaCO_2$, an alkalotic pH, optimal PaO_2 and ventilating with low tidal volumes and airway pressures. Specific pulmonary vasodilators such as milrinone, inhaled nitric oxide (NO), or inhaled prostacyclin are helpful and agents that promote RV contractility.

Ebstein's

Ebsteins's anomaly is a rare ACHD defect, occurring in less than 1% of all ACHD, that may present in childhood or in adults who are unaware of their diagnosis, with new onset atrial flutter. It is characterized by severe tricuspid regurgitation due to apical displacement of the septal and posterior leaflets of the tricuspid valve (TV) and a small "atrialized" thin walled RV that is dilated and hypokinetic with resulting tricuspid regurgitation and a reduced functional size of the RV. The patient may shunt right to left across a PFO or ASD; these patients require an adequate filling pressure and a technique that minimizes

the PVR and enhances RV function. Operative repair will include repair or re-implantation the tricuspid valve leaflets, plication of the atrialized right ventricle and closure of inter-atrial communications [22]. In addition to the RV dysfunction, RV volume overload and geometrical alteration may impact on the left ventricular function.

Tetralogy of Fallot

Tetralogy of Fallot rarely presents in the adult world uncorrected. The history of the lesion and its repair has changed with each decade [23]. Older adults likely will have had a temporizing systemic artery to pulmonary artery shunt, Blalock Taussig, Potts or Waterston Coley, and a definitive repair as an older child. Younger adults are likely diagnosed in utero and have had a primary correction as a neonate or more recently as an infant three to 6 months. Most patients will have had a transannular patch to widen the right ventricular outflow tract (RVOT) at the time of repair and over time they will develop pulmonary insufficiency, right ventricular dilatation and eventually tricuspid regurgitation due to right ventricular dilatation; however, some centers had a practice of leaving residual outflow tract gradients with less disruption to the annulus. Tetralogy patients are susceptible to ventricular tachycardia, atrial arrhythmias and sudden death and a widened QRS complex >180 ms correlating with an increased risk of sudden death [24]. Pulmonary valve replacement post childhood repair is a common booking in adult reference centers although timing and efficacy remain controversial [25]. Like the Ebstein's patients with repaired tetralogy, these patients require an adequate filling pressure and a technique that minimizes the PVR.

Transposition of the Great Arteries

There are three common presentations of transposition. Dextro-transposition of the great arteries) D-TGA; D-TGA with a VSD and Pulmonary stenosis and Levo-transposition of the great arteries (L-TGA) [26]. Transpositions can also present as a combination with other complex lesions.

D-TGA with a Mustard or Senning Baffle (Fig. 17.1)

D-TGA with an Arterial Switch

Early in the 1980s CHD paediatric centers moved from the above repairs to the Jatene or Arterial

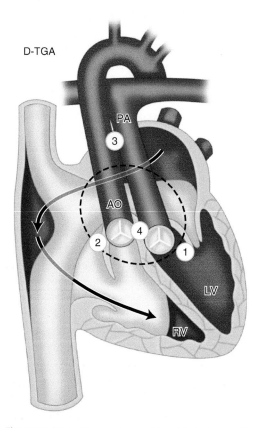

Fig. 17.1 Schematic drawings of the Mustard operation D-TGA have atrial-ventricular concordance and ventricular-great artery discordance and prior to the 1980s had a Mustard or Senning repair. Although rarely performed now there are many adults living with atrial baffles which re-direct atrial blood to the opposite ventricle. The RV remains as the systemic and sub-aortic ventricle. Patients with a Mustard or Senning repair frequently have baffle leaks, sinus atrial arrhythmias, sick sinus syndrome and inevitably systemic ventricular failure. Although their anatomy may be confusing they are managed much like a dilated cardiomyopathy waiting for a heart transplant with an AICD or PPM in-situ. Strategies that optimize function and lower afterload of the systemic ventricle are indicated for operative and ICU management

Switch operation [27]. The aortic and pulmonary arteries are switched with re-implantation of the coronary arteries. Complications include coronary artery perfusion defects and aneurysms of the neo-aortic root. The advantage is that the LV is the systemic ventricle AV and VA synchrony is restored. Urgent non-cardiac surgery can be done safely in the community setting with consultation from cardiac anaesthesia and an ACHD cardiologist.

D-TGA with VSD and Pulmonary Stenosis and a Rastelli Repair

Adults living with D-TGA—AV concordance and VA discordance—having a VSD and Pulmonary stenosis were corrected in childhood with a Rastelli repair which entails a tunnel from the LV through the VSD to the aorta and an extra cardiac conduit that connects the RV to the main PA. A red cell flowing through the heart will travel through all the chambers in an appropriate fashion and the LV is restored as the systemic ventricle. Frequently the RV to PA conduit will become obstructed and require balloon dilatation or replacement. Anesthetic management is likely to occur in the interventional lab for percutaneous PVR within the RV to PA conduit and should account for stenosis of the conduit and occasionally patients will have sub-aortic obstruction. Cases that present to the operating room are likely associated with right endocarditis and there are significant sternal entry risks (Fig. 17.2).

L-TGA is also called congenitally corrected transposition which is a term that confuses many community and non-cardiac anesthesiologists by implying the patients are "born corrected". These patients have both AV discordance and VA discordance. The RA is connected to a morphological LV that is subpulmonic. The LA is connected to a morphological RV which is sub aortic, as the majority of these patients have an Ebstein's like malformation of the tricuspid, systemic AV valve, with moderate to severe systemic AV valve regurgitation. In the absence of associated anomalies these patients present in the second and third

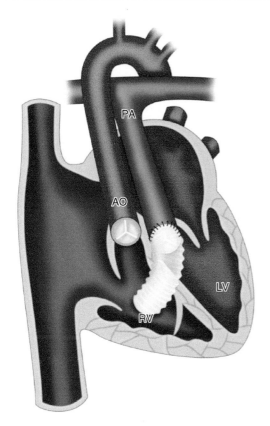

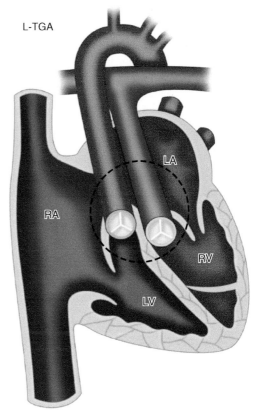

Fig. 17.2 A Rastelli repair [1] VSD Patch with an LV to Aorta tunnel [2] The RV to PA conduit anterior to the heart

Fig. 17.3 L-TGA (Congenitally Corrected)

decade of life with systemic AV valve regurgitation and symptoms of heart failure. They can also present with heart block. As with Mustard patients, they are managed much like that of a dilated cardiomyopathy (Fig. 17.3).

Bicuspid Aortic Valve

Bicuspid aortic valve is very common and may present in childhood or adulthood with stenosis, regurgitation or mixed stenosis/regurgitation with the concomitant concerns about aortopathy. It is associated with coarctation. The valvular issues are straight forward and no different than those of acquired aortic valve disease; however, the aortopathy associated with bicuspid vale disease requires some special consideration particularly in relation to a valve sparing root or Ross

Konno procedures. These topics are dealt with elsewhere in this book.

Coarctation

Coarctation is a narrowing of the aorta, usually near the ductus arteriosus, that requires an intervention for a gradient across the narrowing. It is associated with bicuspid aortic valve. It is usually an interventional procedure of dilation and stenting and occasionally a complicated lesion or an aneurysm associated with a residual coarctation post repair may require surgical intervention. Regardless of the site and type of surgery, monitoring of the blood pressure pre- and post-coarctation is necessary.

Interventional Cath lab management involves stand-by sedation and induction of a brief deeper plane of anesthesia for balloon dilation and stenting. Tear or rupture of the aorta is exceedingly rare; however, attention to back pain post-procedure is very important.

Open repair via a left thoracotomy and with lung isolation is not unique to congenital surgery, but has the advantage of pre-existing pre-ductal collateral flow so that the risk of spinal cord ischemia is reduced. There are similar considerations for a re-do chest incision and femoral cannulation for circulatory arrest. These are not unique to coarctation.

Single Ventricle with Glenn and Fontan Type Connections; Tricuspid Atresia and Pulmonary Atresia; Double Inlet LV; Hypoplastic Left Heart Syndrome.

Adults with single ventricle physiology such as tricuspid atresia, pulmonary atresia, double inlet left ventricle (DILV) and hypoplastic left heart syndrome (HLHS) will likely have had at least a Glenn shunt followed by a form of the Fontan procedure. In the case of HLHS the first stage is a Norwood procedure. This patient population is complex and now living well beyond 18 years and may present to adult centers for cardioversion, diagnostic and interventional procedures as well as non-cardiac surgery. The population of HLHS is now living beyond 18 years and are disadvantage with a morphological RV as their single ventricle. Cardiac surgery, revision of the Fontan circulation or conversion to a cavopulmonary connection, should only be done at reference centers after careful planning and consultation.

A classic Glenn is a superior vena cava (SVC) directly anastomosed to the right pulmonary artery (RPA); a bi-directional Glenn is the SVC anastomosed to the confluence of the LPA and RPA. In each case there is no access to the heart via the SVC as the SVC is disconnected from the RA. Planning for something as simple as a cardioversion must include this important fact as there is no ability to pass a pacing wire and no `pump` for systemic venous return, as well as resuscitation drugs, to get to the left heart. Figure 17.4 Bidirectional Glenn [28].

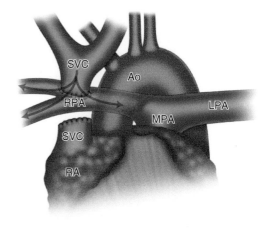

Fig. 17.4 Bidirectional Glenn

For a Glenn shunt patient or a Fontan circulation to be successful the patient must have adequate filling pressures, a low PVR, unobstructed pulmonary veins, compliant LA, AV synchrony, compliant LV without outflow tract obstruction and a low SVR. Hemodynamic considerations of the various versions of the Fontan since its introduction are described in comprehensive reviews [29, 30] (Fig. 17.5).

The Fontan palliation was first described in 1971. Originally the operation was an anastomosis of the RA to main PA and subsequent modifications have included the lateral tunnel Fontan and the total Cavo-pulmonary connection. Arrhythmias and thrombus formation due to the RA dilating over time is what has driven these revisions. Patients may have had a fenestration from the Fontan connection to the systemic or common atrium and precautions for venous emboli to the systemic circulation will be needed. Anesthetic techniques, postoperative recovery and step down planning must consider these goals. Spontaneous respiration is desirable but not always compatible with the surgical plan. Liver dysfunction is common in this population. Non-cardiac surgery should be planned with an ACHD cardiologist involved and preferably at a reference ACHD center or with telephone consultation for urgent non-cardiac surgery.

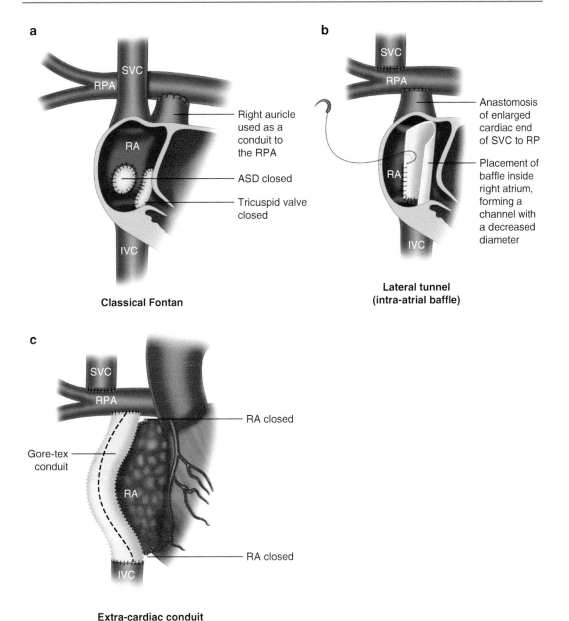

Fig. 17.5 The three most common variations of teh Fontan Circulation. (**a**) The orginal Fontan procedure as described by Dr Fontan in 1971. (**b**) The Lateral Tunnel Modification. (**c**) The Total Cavo-pulomnary Connection or Extra Cardaic Fontan. An illustration of the evolution of the Fontan procedure. d'Udekem, Y et al. The Fontan procedure: contemporary techniques have improved long-term outcomes Circulation 2007

Summary

The Adult congenital heart patient is challenging with unique considerations. Careful consideration of the physiology that existed at birth, its modification with palliative surgery and potential conflicts with future procedures will enable successful management. Working in collaborative teams and with clear referral pathways and follow up are essential.

References

1. Khairy P, et al. Changing mortality in congenital heart disease. JACC. 2010;56(14):1149–57.
2. Marelli A, et al. Congenital heart disease in the general population: changing prevalence and age distribution. Circulation. 2007;115(2):163–72.
3. Marelli A, et al. Lifetime prevalence of congenital heart disease in the general population from 2000 to 2010. Circulation. 2014 Aug 26;130(9): 749–56.
4. Kogon B, et al. Surgery in adults with congenital heart disease: risk factors for morbidity and mortality. AnnThorac Surg. 2013;95(4):1377–82.
5. Padalino MA, et al. Midterm results of surgical intervention for congenital heart disease in adults: an Italian multicenter study. J Thorac Cardiovasc. Surg. 2007;134(1):106–13.
6. Srinathan SK, Bonser RS, Sethia B, Thorne SA, Brawn WJ, Barron DJ. Changing practice of cardiac surgery in adult patients with congenital heart disease. Heart. 2005;91(2):207–12.
7. Liu GK, et al. Diagnosis and Management of Noncardiac Complications in adults with congenital heart disease. Circulation. 2017;136:e348–92.
8. Gurvitz M, et al. Prevalence and predictors of gaps in care among adult congenital heart disease patients (the health, education and access research trial: HEART-ACHD). J Am Coll Cardiol. 2013;61(21): 2180–4.
9. Webb GD, et al. 32nd Bethesda conference: "care of the adult with congenital heart disease". J Am Coll Cardiol. 2001;37(5)
10. Mylotte D, et al. Specialized adult congenital heart disease care-the impact of policy on mortality. Circulation. 2014;129:1804–12.
11. Andropulous DB, et al. Anesthesia for congenital heart disease. 3rd ed. Hoboken: Wiley; 2015.
12. Fredriksen PM, Veldtman G, Hechter S, Therrien J, Chen A, Warsi MA, Freeman M, Liu P, Siu S, Thaulow E, Webb G. Aerobic capacity in adults with various congenital heart diseases. Am J Cardiol. 2001;87(3):310–4.
13. Hawkins SM, Taylor AL, Sillau SH, Mitchell MB, Rausch CM. Restrictive lung function in pediatric patients with structural congenital heart disease. J Thorac Cardiovasc Surg. 2013;
14. Ginde S, Bartz PJ, Hill GD, Danduran MJ, Biller J, Sowinski J, Tweddell JS, Earing MG. Restrictive lung disease is an independent predictor of exercise intolerance in the adult with congenital heart disease. Congenit Heart Dis. 2013;8(3):246–54.
15. Heuman DM, et al. MELD-XI: a rational approach to "sickest first" liver transplantation in cirrhotic patients requiring anticoagulant therapy. Liver Transpl. 2007;13(1):30–7.
16. Assenza GE, et al. MELD-XI score and cardiac mortality or transplantation in patients after Fontan surgery. Heart. 2013;99(7):491–6.
17. Adachi K, et al. The impact of liver disorders on perioperative management of reoperative cardiac surgery: a retrospective study in adult congenital heart disease patients. J Anesth. 2017;31(2):170–7.
18. Gatzoulis MA, et al. Congenital heart disease and pulmonary hypertension: pharmacology and feasibility of late surgery. Eur Respir Rev. 2009;18(113):154–61.
19. Oechslin E. Hematological management of the cyanotic adult with congenital heart disease. Int J Cardiol. 2004;97(Suppl 1):109–15.
20. Malt EA, et al. Health and disease in adults with down syndrome. Tidsskr Nor Laegeforen. 2013 Feb;5:133(3).
21. DM MG, et al. 22q11.2 Deletion Syndrome. Gene. 2013;527(1)
22. Kron IL, et al. Management of Ebstein's anomaly. Ann Cardiothorac Surg. 2017 May;6(3):266–9.
23. Apitz C, et al. Tetralogy of Fallot. Lancet. 2009;374:1462–71.
24. Gatzoulis M. Risk factors for arrhythmia and sudden cardiac death late after repair of tetralogy of Fallot: a multicentre study. Lancet. 2000;356:975–81.
25. Bokma JP, et al. A propensity score-adjusted analysis of clinical outcomes after pulmonary valve replacement in tetralogy of Fallot. Heart. 2017;104(9):738–44.
26. Warnes CA. Transposition of the great arteries. Circulation. 2006;114:2699–709.
27. Jatene AD, et al. Anatomic correction of transposition of the great vessels. J Thorac Cardiovasc Surg. 1976;72:364–70.
28. Neema PK, et al. Annals of cardiac Anaesthesia. 2009;12(1):53–6.
29. d'Udekem Y, et al. The Fontan procedure: contemporary techniques have improved long-term outcomes. Circulation. 2007;116:I-157–64.
30. Ohye RG, et al. Current therapy for Hypoplastic left heart syndrome and related single ventricle lesions. Circulation. 2016 October 25;134(17):1265–79.

Anesthetic Management of Cardiac Surgery Patients with Uncommon Diseases

18

Carlos Galhardo Jr. and Mauricio Daher

Main Messages

1. The appropriate understanding of the underlying pathological disorder and how it affects the anesthetic approach is fundamental for the successful management of cardiac patients with uncommon diseases.
2. Cardiac myxoma is the most common benign cardiac tumor; the majority of primary malignant heart tumors are sarcomas; malignant tumors of the heart are much more likely to be metastatic in origin than primary cardiac tumors.
3. Approximately 75% of cardiac myxomas occur in the left atrium with a stalk frequently attached to the interatrial septum, usually in the fossa ovalis region; typical myxomas are pedunculated, round and gelatinous in consistency.
4. The anesthesiologist must have a comprehensive understanding of the tumor's size, its exact location, and clinical implications to anticipate any complications that may arise during the adminis-

tration of anesthesia and surgical resection of the tumor.

5. Cardiomyopathies exclude heart disorders secondary to known cardiovascular abnormalities and include myocardial diseases that manifest with various structural and functional phenotypes; primary cardiomyopathies describe disorders that are predominantly confined to the heart muscle, while secondary cardiomyopathies are caused by myocardial damage in the context of a systemic disease.
6. Pericardial effusion, constrictive pericarditis and cardiac tamponade can severely compromise cardiac filling and cardiac output, increasing the risk of hemodynamic collapse during induction.
7. Anesthetic concerns for patients with hematological disorders are essential to avoid or reduce perioperative complications related to bleeding or thrombotic events.
8. Cardiac disease is the main cause of non-obstetric mortality related to pregnancy; in most cases, the underlying mechanism is present before the onset of pregnancy but becomes decompensated secondary to gestational hemodynamic changes.

C. Galhardo Jr.
Anesthesiology Division, National Institute of Cardiology, Rua das Laranjeiras 374, Rio de Janeiro, Brazil

M. Daher (✉)
Anesthesiology Division, Faculty of Medicine, Universidade de Brasilia, Brasilia, Brazil

© Springer Nature Switzerland AG 2021
D. C. H. Cheng et al. (eds.), *Evidence-Based Practice in Perioperative Cardiac Anesthesia and Surgery*, https://doi.org/10.1007/978-3-030-47887-2_18

Cardiac Tumors

Primary tumors involving the heart may originate from any cardiac tissue. Although intracardiac tumors represent a rare cardiac pathology, comprehensive knowledge of the implications of specific tumor types is fundamental for the perioperative management. Cardiac masses may produce different symptoms through a variety of mechanisms. The patient may present symptoms of heart failure due to obstruction of blood flow or valve dysfunction; signs of tumor fragmentation and embolization; and constitutional or systemic symptoms. The nature and magnitude of the symptoms are determined by the size of the tumor, invasiveness, friability, and its location in the heart.

Although most cardiac tumors are found incidentally during routine cardiac imaging, recent technological advances in cardiac imaging have resulted in an earlier and more complete assessment of cardiac tumors. The information obtained from echocardiography, cardiac MRI or CT can confirm the presence of a cardiac tumor and provide essential characteristics of a mass such as its anatomic location, mobility, attachment, and potential hemodynamic consequences.

Cardiac tumors can be classified into primary or secondary, depending if they are originating in the heart or have metastasized from different locations to the heart. Primary cardiac tumor can be further categorized into benign tumors or malignant tumors. Roughly 75% of primary cardiac tumors are benign in origin, and 25% are malignant. Approximately 50% of the benign tumors are myxomas, and cardiac sarcomas are the most frequent malignant tumors. Metastatic tumors to the heart are from 20- to 40-fold more common than primary tumors [1].

Benign Tumors

In adults, the majority of benign tumors are myxomas; other common benign neoplasms include papillary fibroelastomas, lipomas, and rhabdomyomas.

Cardiac Myxomas

Cardiac myxomas are the most common primary cardiac tumors in adults. Typically the peak incidence is between the ages of 30 and 60 years, and they are found mainly in women. Approximately 75% occur in the left atrium, with a stalk frequently attached to the interatrial septum, usually in the fossa ovalis region [2]. Macroscopically, typical myxomas are pedunculated, round and gelatinous in consistency, with the surface smooth or slightly lobulated. Mobility depends on the length of the stalk and the extent of attachment to the heart.

As opposed to the rest of cardiac tumors, the majority of patients with myxoma are symptomatic. Clinically, the most common initial symptom is dyspnea on exertion, secondary to mitral valve obstruction. Temporary obstruction of blood flow may cause hypotension, syncopal episodes, arrhythmias, hemolysis as well as other signs and symptoms of heart failure. Further, cardiac myxomas may manifest as recurrent strokes or transient ischemic attacks, peripheral embolization, and constitutional symptoms. Right atrial myxomas can produce clinical features of right ventricular failure, including peripheral edema, hepatomegaly, and ascites.

The Carney complex is a familial syndrome with autosomal dominant inheritance characterized by multiple tumors, including atrial and extracardiac myxomas, schwannomas, and assorted endocrine tumors.

Surgical resection is promptly required once a diagnosis of myxoma is suspected by clinical findings and cardiac imaging because of the risk of embolization, cardiovascular complications, and sudden death. The long-term results of the surgical procedure are good with low operative mortality.

Papillary Fibroelastomas (PFEs)

Papillary fibroelastoma is the second most common benign primary cardiac tumor in adults. PFEs may occur in all age groups but is more prevalent in elderly patients. Morphologically, papillary fibroelastomas are small (<1 cm in diameter), avascular tumors, singular more often than multiple, and derived from the normal components of the endocardium. Their appearance is often compared to sea anemones when viewed under water, with frond-like arms attached to a short pedicle of dense connective tissue [2]. They are most commonly on the valves, usually on the left side, and primarily affecting the aortic surface of the aortic valve followed by the atrial surface of the mitral valve.

Although considered a benign cardiac tumor, PFEs may result in life-threatening conditions due to high risk of embolization to coronary or cerebral circulation. The most common clinical presentation is a stroke or transient ischemic attack, followed by syncope, angina, myocardial infarction, and sudden death.

Surgery is recommended for patients with previous embolic events or complications directly related to tumor mobility—e.g. cerebral infarction or ostial coronary occlusion—and those with highly mobile or large (≥1 cm) tumors.

Lipomas

Lipomas are composed of benign adipose cells. Within the heart, the majority of these tumors occur in the subendocardial region. Tumor size varies and can range from a few to several centimeters. Subendocardial lipomas are often small and sessile. Usually lipomas are asymptomatic, but symptoms when present may manifest as arrhythmias, conduction block or valvular dysfunction. Surgery may be required due to progressive growth of the tumor and clinical symptoms.

Rhabdomyomas

Rhabdomyomas are the most common primary cardiac tumor in children, and the majority is associated with tuberous sclerosis. They are usually located on the ventricular walls or the atrioventricular valves. Diagnosis can be made by the presence of well delineated multiple masses of different sizes on echocardiography. Symptoms may be caused by left-ventricular outflow tract obstruction or arrhythmias. Although most of the cardiac rhabdomyomas tend to regress spontaneously, occasionally, resection is necessary if the cardiac tumor causes symptoms.

Malignant Tumors

Malignant tumors of the heart are rare and much more likely to be metastatic in origin than primary cardiac tumors. Sarcomas are the most common type of primary malignant cardiac neoplasm. Males are more affected than females and typically occur in individuals in their third to fifth decades of life. The clinical presentation is similar to benign lesions. Sarcomas proliferate rapidly, are very aggressive, and they present high incidence of metastasis at the time of diagnosis, most commonly to the lungs. Angiosarcomas are more prevalent in adults, and rhabdomyosarcomas are most common in children.

Cardiac malignant tumors are located predominantly on the right side of the heart, especially in the right atrium. Different from the myxomas and PFEs, they do not have a stalk and tend to involve the pericardium. Clinical manifestations may include right-sided congestive heart failure, superior vena cava obstruction, symptoms consistent with pulmonary emboli, and pericardial effusion or cardiac tamponade. The prognosis of patients with malignant cardiac tumors is critical, and complete surgical resection is the treatment of choice.

Metastatic Heart Tumors

Metastases to the heart are not a rare condition observed late in the course of a primary tumor. Malignant neoplasm may reach the heart through direct invasion from mediastinal tumors, hematogenous dissemination, lymphatic spread, and transvenous extension from the inferior vena cava [3]. Cardiac involvement should be suspected in any patient with a malignant tumor, who develops a pericardial effusion or new cardiovascular symptoms. Echocardiography should be the initial diagnostic test to evaluate the presence of metastatic cardiac disease.

Malignant melanoma has the highest propensity for secondary cardiac involvement. Other solid tumors with metastatic cardiac potential are lung carcinoma, breast cancer, renal cell carcinoma, esophageal carcinoma, malignant lymphoma and thyroid cancer.

Carcinoid syndrome is the most common paraneoplastic syndrome involving the heart secondary to carcinoid tumors. Carcinoid heart disease is a frequent occurrence in patients with hepatic metastases from their primary gastrointestinal carcinoid tumors. Although the pathophysiology of carcinoid heart disease is poorly understood, chronic exposure to excessive circulating vasoactive amines, especially serotonin, may lead to fibrosis and deposition of plaque-like material on the endocardial surfaces of valve leaflets, subvalvular apparatus, and cardiac chambers, mainly on the right side of the heart [4]. Typical echocardiographic findings in carcinoid heart disease demonstrate tricuspid regurgitation and pulmonary valve stenosis.

Perioperative Considerations

Surgical resection of cardiac tumors can pose various anesthetic and surgical challenges. Anesthetic management of patients with heart tumors is mainly guided first by the patient's clinical status and comorbidities, and second by tumor characteristics. The anesthesiologist must have a comprehensive understanding of the tumor's size, its exact location, and clinical implications to anticipate any complications that may arise during the administration of anesthesia and surgical resection of the tumor. Preoperative workup should include the usual investigations before any cardiac surgery. A complete review of the preoperative cardiac imaging will favor an appropriate anesthetic management. Transesophageal echocardiography (TEE) monitoring is crucial during surgical resection of cardiac tumors. It may confirm a total excision of the mass, assesses the valvular repair or replacement, and the absence of shunting or leakage around patch repair, and also guides weaning from cardiopulmonary bypass.

Perioperative concerns and anesthetic considerations associated with surgical resection of the cardiac tumor are described in Table 18.1.

Cardiomyopathies

A contemporary definition for cardiomyopathies refer as a heterogeneous group of myocardial diseases associated with mechanical and/or electri-

Table 18.1 Perioperative concerns and anesthetic considerations associated with surgical resection of cardiac tumors

Perioperative concerns	Anesthetic considerations
Large tumors located in the atrium (left or right) causing atrioventricular valve obstruction and hemodynamic instability	• Management similar to mitral or tricuspid stenosis (adequate preload, avoid tachycardia and hypercontractile states, maintain sinus rhythm and adequate SVR, and avoid any additional increases in PA pressure) • Vasoactive medication ready for use, large-bore intravenous access, surgeon present in the OR during induction, CBP machine primed and ready for use, and careful position of the patient minimizing the risk of impaired venous return • Avoid the use of PA catheter, and cautiously place catheters and cannulas (US-guided) in right atrial tumor surgeries
Tumors with high risk of embolization	• Minimal manipulation of the heart and careful placement of catheters and cannulas (US-guided). • Consider femoral cannulation specially in right side heart tumors
Tumors involving the IVC and RA	• High risk of hypotension during induction (volume and vasoactive drugs ready for use, surgeon in the OR, and CPB machine primed and ready for use) • Major risk of severe obstruction of IVC in case of hypovolemia and PPV • Prepare for excessive bleeding and coagulopathy • Large-bore peripheral intravenous lines should be placed above the diaphragm
Carcinoid heart disease	• Avoiding the administration of drugs or situations that may trigger carcinoid crisis (hypertension, hypercapnia and hypothermia) • Ensure an adequate depth of anesthesia Consider perioperative administration of somatostatin analogues (first-line), interferon alfa or peptide receptor radionuclide therapy

Abbreviations: *SVR* Systemic vascular resistance, *PA* pulmonary artery, *OR* operating room, *CPB* cardiopulmonary bypass, *US* ultrasound, *IVC* inferior vena cava, *RA* right atrium, *PPV* positive pressure ventilation

cal dysfunction that usually exhibit structural myocardial abnormalities and failure of myocardial performance [5]. The current definition of cardiomyopathy excludes heart disease secondary to known cardiovascular abnormalities such as that which occurs with ischemic heart disease, hypertension, congenital heart disease or valvular heart disease. Cardiomyopathies may manifest with various structural and functional phenotypes and frequently has a genetic basis. Primary cardiomyopathies describe disorders that are predominantly confined to the heart muscle, while secondary cardiomyopathies are caused by myocardial damage in the context of a systemic disease [5].

The World Health Organization has defined five subtypes of cardiomyopathies according to anatomical and physiological characteristics: hypertrophic, dilated, restrictive, arrhythmogenic right ventricular dysplasia, and unclassified cardiomyopathies [6]. Posteriorly, the European Society of Cardiology proposed that each category could be subdivided into familiar/genetic or nonfamilial/nongenetic to raise awareness of genetic disease as a cause of dysfunction [7].

Hypertrophic Cardiomyopathy

Hypertrophic cardiomyopathy (HCM) is a genetic cardiac disorder caused by a variety of mutations encoding contractile proteins of the cardiac sarcomere. Familial disease with autosomal dominant inheritance predominates. HCM is one of the most prevalent cardiomyopathy, affecting 1 of every 500 adults in the general population. It is recognized as the most common cause of sudden cardiac death in the young, and a relevant substrate for disability at any age [5]. HCM is characterized by unexplained ventricular hypertrophy, non-dilated ventricle in the absence of pathologic loading conditions—e.g. systemic hypertension or aortic valve disease. The disease is associated with myocardial fiber disarray that predisposes patients to arrhythmias.

Clinical diagnosis is established with transthoracic echocardiogram (TTE) and the patient's clinical presentation or as part of the family screening. Cardiac MRI also has a diagnostic role in determining the location and extent of left ventricular hypertrophy (LVH) and abnormalities of the mitral valve apparatus. Asymmetrical hypertrophy of the basal septum is the most common presentation and predisposes to dynamic left ventricular outflow tract obstruction. Typically, LV systolic function is preserved or even increased, with high ejection fraction.

HCM may affect patients in all age groups with a diverse clinical presentation. However, the majority of patients are asymptomatic throughout life. The pathophysiology of HCM is complex and includes dynamic left ventricular outflow tract (LVOT) obstruction, mitral regurgitation, diastolic dysfunction, myocardial ischemia, and arrhythmias [8]. Symptoms include dyspnea, exercise intolerance, angina, syncope, and/or sudden death. Some patients present signs of myocardial ischemia due to increase in left ventricular mass and myocardial oxygen consumption as well as reduced coronary perfusion. Also, impaired LV diastolic function can occur as a consequence of compromised relaxation and reduced chamber compliance. Loading conditions and ventricular contractility influence the degree of LVOT obstruction. Increased myocardial contractility, decreased ventricular volume, or reduced afterload increases the degree of subaortic obstruction.

Treatment of patients with HCM requires a complete understanding of pathophysiology, clinical status, natural history of disease and experience of the heart team. The initial therapy for symptomatic patients with obstruction is pharmacological therapy with β-blockers as the first-line agent, and calcium channel blockers in patients intolerant to β-blockers. However, there are some patients who are unresponsive to medical therapy who maintain severe symptoms. These patients can be treated with invasive septal reduction therapy, either surgical septal myectomy or alcohol septal ablation [9].

The perioperative hemodynamic management in patients with HCM is similar to those patients with aortic stenosis undergoing cardiac surgery; the main difference is the dynamic obstruction of LVOT presented in HCM patients. No evidence-based data are available to determine the best choice of medications for induction or anesthesia maintenance. Regardless of the drugs chosen, they should be used to avoid or reduce hemodynamic instability. Preoperative echocardiography should be assessed to determine the LV systolic and diastolic function, the severity of LVOT pressure gradient (significant if >30 mmHg peak gradient at rest or >50 mmHg peak gradient provoked), chambers dimension, and abnormality of mitral valve apparatus. Specific perioperative goals for the management of patients with HCM are reported in Table 18.2.

Table 18.2 Perioperative goals for the management of patients with hypertrophic cardiomyopathies

Perioperative period	Goals for management of patients with hypertrophic cardiomyopathies
Preoperative	• Avoid long fasting time • Maintain proper hydration to optimize volume status • Continue β-blockers, calcium channel blockers and/or disopyramide • Anxiolytic premedication is indicated to minimize catecholamine levels • If implantable cardioverter-defibrillator is present, deactivation of anti-tachycardia capabilities is necessary
Intraoperative	• Invasive blood pressure monitoring prior to the induction • CVP and PCWP may not reflect LVEDP (trends are more reliable) • Monitoring for signs of myocardial ischemia (ECG, TEE) • Intraoperative TEE is fundamental (assess volume status, LV contractility, dynamic obstruction, and mitral regurgitation; provides information for septal myectomy and potential complications such as VSD, aortic or mitral valve damage) • Avoid hypovolemia, tachycardia, increased contractility, and hypotension; maintain an adequate systemic vascular resistance (phenylephrine, vasopressin or norepinephrine) and sinus rhythm (direct current cardioversion may be necessary)
Postoperative	• Adequate pain control • Avoid fluid overload, hypovolemia or tachycardia, and maintain sinus rhythm in order to optimize diastolic dysfunction

Dilated Cardiomyopathy

Dilated cardiomyopathy (DCM) is a disease characterized by progressive enlargement of ventricular chamber and systolic dysfunction of one or both ventricles. About 20% to 35% of DCM cases have evidence for familial disease with primarily autosomal dominant inheritance [5]. DMC is a common cause of heart failure, various types of arrhythmias, and thromboembolism. It is also the most frequent cause of heart transplantation. A large number of cases are idiopathic, but the known reasons are related to infectious agents, inflammation, excessive consumption of alcohol, and chemotherapy agents. DCM can also be found in autoimmune disorders, pheochromocytoma, and neuromuscular diseases.

Anesthetic management of patients with DCM is challenging and associated with increased risk of complications. Optimal care of the patient with heart failure should occur before surgery with an adequate clinical evaluation, diagnostic testing, correction of any electrolyte abnormalities, and pharmacological optimization [10]. The essential hemodynamic features of patients with DCM are related to myocardial dysfunction, elevated filling pressures, reduced tolerance of fluid overload and increases in afterload. Therefore, the anesthetic goals include minimizing further myocardial depression, optimizing preload in the presence of elevated left ventricular end-diastolic pressure (LVEDP), ensuring adequate coronary perfusion, and preventing increases in systemic vascular resistance. Maintenance of sinus rhythm and avoidance of tachycardia are essential. Inotrope support and circulatory support with intra-aortic balloon counterpulsation, and short or long-term ventricular assist devices are further options to be considered in patients with severely compromised ventricles and inadequate systemic perfusion.

Restrictive Cardiomyopathy

Primary restrictive cardiomyopathy (RCM) is a rare disease defined by non-dilated ventricles with impaired ventricular filling and reduced diastolic volume of one or both ventricles. The systolic function is usually normal or near normal as well as the wall thickness. RCM may be idiopathic, familial, or is associated with a wide range of different systemic pathologies—e.g. amyloidosis, hemochromatosis, sarcoidosis. Diastolic dysfunction is the principal clinical feature. The condition can affect both ventricles and may cause symptoms and signs of right or left ventricular failure. The initial differential diagnosis should be made with constrictive pericarditis, which results in similar symptomatology to those of RCM. The goal of treatment is to lower the elevated filling pressures caused by impaired ventricular compliance without reducing cardiac output. Perioperative management should focus on maintaining adequate preload and systemic vascular resistance. It is also necessary to preserve sinus rhythm, or at least atrioventricular synchrony to allow for complete ventricular filling and optimized cardiac output.

Arrhythmogenic Right Ventricular Cardiomyopathy

Arrhythmogenic right ventricular cardiomyopathy/dysplasia (ARVC) is an uncommon genetically determined disease. The pathology is associated with sudden death in young people. ARVC is characterized by the presence of progressive replacement of right ventricular myocardium with adipose and fibrous tissue, which leads to regional or global right ventricular dysfunction. Clinical manifestations of the disorder include structural and functional abnormalities of the right ventricle (RV), depolarization/conduction abnormalities, syncope, ventricular tachyarrhythmias, and sudden death. The main perioperative consideration is to avoid trigger factors for arrhythmias such as light anesthesia, hypoxia, hypercarbia, acidosis, and hypovolemia.

Unclassified Cardiomyopathy

Unclassified cardiomyopathies include rare disorders that do not fit into any of the above phenotypic group. Some examples include stress-induced cardiomyopathy (Takotsubo), LV noncompaction, ion channelopathies, and peripartum cardiomyopathy.

Pericardial Heart Disease

The pericardium consists of a 1 to 2 mm thick dual-layered membrane that envelops the heart. The thin visceral pericardium covers the surface of the heart, while the fibrous outer parietal pericardium is attached to the diaphragm, sternum, thoracic vertebrae and great vessels. The lines of reflexion between the two layers form the oblique (a cul-de-sac posterior to the left atrium) and transverse (left-to-right opening posterior to the great vessels) pericardial sinuses [11]. Mesothelial cells of the pericardium produce pericardial fluid which normally amounts to 15 to 50 mL inside the pericardial sac [12].

The pericardium is not essential to life, but it still presents relevant physiological functions. The intrapericardial pressure reflects variations of intrapleural pressure integrating the respiratory and cardiac functions. The negative intrapleural pressure generated by spontaneous breathing is transferred to the pericardium, which facilitates the venous return to the heart. The pericardium is also a key determinant of ventricular interdependency—the coupling of left and right ventricular function [11].

Patients may require anesthetic care for either invasive diagnostic or therapeutic procedures following: acute pericarditis, constrictive pericarditis, pericardial effusion, effusion after cardiac surgery and cardiac tamponade. Other sections of this book address cardiac tamponade pathophysiology following cardiac surgical procedures, and that subject will not be described here.

Acute Pericarditis and Pericardial Effusion

Inflammation of the pericardium is characterized by fibrin deposition and reactive fluid accumulation. Main etiologies can be grouped as infectious, non-infectious and autoimmune. In most cases, however, a definite cause is not determined. Acute pericarditis is associated with fever and pleuritic pain located in the center or left side of the chest. Hemodynamic compromise may ensue if pericardial fluid accumulates faster than the pericardium can stretch or if the effusion becomes large enough. Electrocardiogram shows widespread ST-segment elevation. An echocardiographic examination can indicate if signs of tamponade are present. A combination of NSAIDs and colchicine is usually prescribed for the treatment of uncomplicated cases of acute pericarditis [12, 13].

The intrapericardial compartment has a fixed volume, and fluid accumulation will increase the pressure surrounding the heart producing diastolic impairment. Heart rate and contractility are increased as adaptive sympathetic activation unfolds to maintain cardiac output. Normal respiratory variations of stroke volume are exacerbated as increased intrapericardial pressure decreases the gradient for left atrium filling. If this effect becomes severe enough, it is clinically manifested as pulsus paradoxus (systolic arterial pressure decrease of >10 mmHg during inspiration) and a decrease of mitral inflow E velocity with inspiration. The collapse of the right atrium (in systole) followed by the right ventricle (in diastole) is echocardiographic signs of tamponade denoting severity progression, which can ultimately lead to life-threatening obstructive shock. Urgent decompression of pericardial fluid is performed in cases of hemodynamic instability [11, 14].

Constrictive Pericarditis

Fusion of the pericardium and the epicardial surface of the heart characterize the condition of constrictive pericarditis. It can be the result of a single episode of acute pericarditis or may be the consequence of recurrent or chronic inflammatory disorders of the pericardium. The clinical picture of constrictive pericarditis resembles the congestive states of chronic heart failure or chronic liver disease. Initial symptoms are usually nonspecific and progress slowly over months

to years. Severe diastolic impairment ensues as the heart becomes enclosed in a hard shell [11].

As in pericardial effusion, heart rate and contractility increase as compensatory sympathetic activation develop. Respiratory variations of cardiac filling are also exaggerated, and some patients exhibit pulsus paradoxus. Electrocardiographic findings include nonspecific ST and T wave changes and low QRS voltage. Atrial fibrillation is frequently observed in severe cases. Suggestive echocardiographic changes are 25% inspiratory decrease in mitral inflow E velocity and higher medial mitral annulus e' velocity on tissue Doppler (annulus reversus). Computed tomography and magnetic resonance imaging provide detailed pericardial visualization revealing thickening sites and calcifications. Pericardiectomy is the treatment of choice for patients with severe symptoms of constrictive pericarditis. Depending on severity, the procedure can be performed with or without cardiopulmonary bypass [13].

Perioperative Considerations

The anesthetic approach for patients with pericardial diseases must take into consideration the onset rate of symptoms, hemodynamic status, compensatory responses and surgical planning. Cardiac tamponade signs should be evaluated in all patients with pericardial effusion, preferably by transthoracic echocardiography. An arterial line must be in place before induction of anesthesia, and central venous cannulation should be considered for procedures more complex than minor [14].

Whenever possible, light sedation and local anesthesia should be employed as the institution of positive pressure ventilation may result in considerable reduction of venous return, which may lead to hemodynamic collapse. If mechanical ventilation is necessary, inspiratory pressure should be kept as low as possible. Bradycardia should be avoided as pericardial effusion, or constrictive pericarditis produce a fixed stroke volume and heart rate dramatically impacts cardiac output. Other hemodynamic objectives are the maintenance of myocardial contractility, afterload, and preload. Some cases may respond positively to increases in preload. Drainage procedures for pericardial effusion are usually straightforward. Surgical treatment of constrictive pericarditis, however, is much more challenging. Pericardiectomy can result in arrhythmias, acute hemorrhage and coronary artery lesion, conditions that may require urgent institution of cardiopulmonary bypass [11].

Hematologic Disorders and Cardiac Surgery

The hematological management of patients undergoing cardiac surgery requires a complex balance between the intense amount of anticoagulation and the restoration of normal coagulation after the procedure. Anesthetic concerns for patients with hematological disorders are essential to avoid or reduce perioperative complications related to bleeding or thrombotic events. Hemophilia, von Willebrand disease, heparin-induced thrombocytopenia, antithrombin deficiency and cold agglutinins are a few of the hematological disorders that deserve special consideration in patients undergoing cardiac surgery.

Hemophilia

Hemophilia A and Hemophilia B are X-linked recessive disorders and result in a deficiency of coagulation factor VIII and factor IX, respectively, with consequent failure to generate sufficient thrombin to form a stable hemostatic plug at sites of vascular damage. The natural history of patients without treatment is a progressive loss of mobility from spontaneous joint and muscle bleeding and early death due to uncontrolled bleeding. In patients with hemophilia, standard screening laboratory tests show a prolongation of activate partial thromboplastin time (APTT) with normal prothrombin time (PA). Further, specific factor assays to quantify FVIII and FIX are necessary. Adequate laboratory support is required

for reliable monitoring of clotting factor level and inhibitor testing. Traditionally, clotting factor level VIII or IX <1% of normal is defined as a severe deficiency, 1–5% moderate and 5 to <40% mild deficiency. The perioperative bleeding risk is related to the degree of factor deficiency.

Appropriate treatment of patients with hemophilia A or B primarily depends on replacement of intravenous FVIII and FIX, respectively. There is a low level of evidence in the literature about the best protocol for the management of the hemophilic patient undergoing cardiac surgery. In one case report, Stine and Becton reported a successful management of a patient with hemophilia A who underwent a mitral valve repair and coronary artery bypass. The patient received 50 IU kg^{-1} of FVIII one hour preoperatively and then a continuous infusion of 4 IU/kg per hour for 72 hours to maintain FVIII activity greater than 100% [15]. Desmopressin (DDAVP) has been used successfully to increase FVIII level and decrease transfusion requirements in patients with hemophilia A. Antibodies to FVIII or FIX may occur in patients with hemophilia who have received therapy with factor concentrates. In this situation, the therapy with recombinant factor VIIa is indicated (90 µg/kg as a bolus and repeated at 3-h intervals for a maximum of four times). In general, outcomes across reported cases and series were excellent, considering the high-risk of bleeding diatheses in this group of patients.

von Willebrand Disease

von Willebrand factor (vWF) is a plasma protein that mediates platelet adhesion to injured vascular sites and also binds and stabilizes factor VIII, playing a crucial role in primary hemostasis. von Willebrand disease (vWD) is the most common inherited bleeding abnormality that is caused by deficiency or dysfunction of von Willebrand factor (vWF). The condition may affect up to 1% of the population and is classified into three major categories: partial quantitative deficiency of vWF (type 1), qualitative vWF deficiency (type 2), and total deficiency (type 3). Type 1 vWD is the most common and accounts for more than 70% of all vWD. Qualitative type 2 vWD is divided further into four variants by the clinical phenotype (Subtypes 2A, 2B, 2M, and 2N).

Clinical symptoms usually involve mild to moderate membrane or skin bleeding (epistaxis, skin bruises, hematomas, oral cavity bleeding and excessive menstrual bleeding). Specific tests for vWD include ristocetin cofactor activity (vWF:RCo); collagen-binding activity (vWF:CB); vWF antigen (vWF:Ag); and FVIII level. Acquired von Willebrand syndrome (AvWS) refers to vWF deficiency that is not inherited but secondary to other medical disorders. AvWS is associated with cleavage of the circulating large vWF multimeters by ADAMTS13 (von Willebrand factor cleaving protease) under pathological increases in fluid shear stress. AvWS has been described in patients with chronic aortic stenosis, ventricular septal defect, pulmonary hypertension and ventricular assist devices.

The subtype of vWD, coagulation status, and clinical findings guide the treatment. There are three main therapeutic strategies in patients with vWD. The first is to increase the plasmatic concentration of vWF by releasing endogenous vWF stores with desmopressin (DDAVP). The second is to replace vWF by plasma-derived vWF (FVIII/vWF concentrates, cryoprecipitate). The third is to improve hemostasis with hemostatic agents that do not affect the plasma concentration of vWF (antifibrinolytic agents, topical agents, platelet, recombinant factor VIIa) [16].

Heparin-Induced Thrombocytopenia

Heparin-induced thrombocytopenia (HIT) is a life-threatening immune-mediated adverse effect of heparin therapy. Antibody-mediated platelet activation and consequent thrombin generation can lead to catastrophic prothrombotic complications. HIT is caused by antibodies (IgG) against complexes of heparin-platelet factor 4 (PF4), a primary protein stored in platelet alpha granules. The incidence of HIT is variable and is affected by the clinical scenario (surgical patient > clinical patient, unfractionated heparin > low-

molecular heparin, female > male, and most frequently after 10–14 days of heparin administration). Patients undergoing cardiovascular surgery who received UFH are especially at risk to develop HIT, although the diagnosis is particularly difficult because thrombocytopenia is not uncommon, and may be drug-induced or related to cardiopulmonary bypass. The diagnosis of HIT requires the combination of the clinical score (pretest probability based on the 4Ts score) and a positive test for anti-PF4/heparin antibodies (IgG-specific enzyme-immunoassay). In the case of a patient scheduled for cardiac surgery and presenting HIT, the procedure should be delayed, if possible, until HIT tests negative [17]. The primary objective of the management of HIT is to decrease the thrombotic risk by reducing platelet activation and thrombin generation. It is recommended to discontinue heparin when a patient is strongly suspected or confirmed as having HIT, and alternative anticoagulation therapy should be initiated [18] (Table 18.3).

Antithrombin III Deficiency

Antithrombin III (AT-III), often referred to as antithrombin, is a naturally protease inhibitor that inactivates thrombin and other serine proteases responsible to generate thrombin. AT-III is produced primarily in the liver and is the major coagulation pathway inhibitor. Deficiency of antithrombin can be inherited or acquired, and results in an increased risk of thrombotic complications. Normal AT-III levels are 80% to 120%, with activity less than 50% considered clinically significant. Enhancement of antithrombin III activity is the mechanism by which heparin achieves its anticoagulant effect. Heparin resistance in cardiac surgery is considered when a heparin bolus (300–400 μ/kg) fails to achieve an activated coagulation time beyond 480 s before cardiopulmonary bypass. Inadequate anticoagulation during CPB increases the risk of thrombin generation, platelet activation, clotting factors consumption and fibrinolysis, exposing the patient to an increased risk of thrombotic events and coagulopathy. The

Table 18.3 Alternatives to heparin for the treatment of heparin-induced thrombocytopenia

Agent (Class)	Clearance	Initial dosing	Monitoring
Argatroban (Direct thrombin inhibitors)	Hepatic	Bolus: None Continuous infusion: 1 to 2 mcg/kg/min (normal organ function) or 0.5 to 1.0 mcg/kg/min (liver dysfunction, heart failure, post-cardiac surgery)	Adjust dose to aPTT of 1.5–3.0 times patient baseline Monitor aPTT every 4 h
Bivalirudin (Direct thrombin inhibitors)	Enzymatic (80%) and Renal (20%)	Bolus: None Continuous infusion: 0.15 mg/kg/h (normal organ function) or lower dose (renal or hepatic dysfunction)	Adjust dose to aPTT of 1.5–2.5 times patient baseline Monitor aPTT every 4 h
Lepirudin (Direct thrombin inhibitors)	Renal	Bolus: 0.2 to 0.4 mg/kg IV Continuous infusion: 0.05 to 0.10 mg/kg/h	Adjust dose to aPTT of 1.5–2.0 times patient baseline Monitor aPTT every 4 h
Danaparoid (Indirect FXa inhibitors)	Renal	Bolus: Weight < 60 kg = 1500 U Weight 60–75 kg = 2250 U Weight 75–90 kg = 3000 U Weight > 90 kg = 3750 U Continuous infusion: Cr < 2.5 mg/dL = 200 U/h. Cr $\geq$ 2.5 mg/dL = 150 U/h	Adjust dose to danaparoid-specific anti-Xa level of 0.5–0.8 U/ml (if assay is available)
Fondaparinux (Indirect FXa inhibitors)	Renal	< 50 kg = 5 mg SC daily 50–100 kg = 7.5 mg SC daily > 100 kg = 10 mg SC daily Warning: If Cl_{cr} 30–50 ml use caution, if Cl_{cr} < 30 ml/min is contraindicated	Some experts recommend adjusting dose to a peak anti-Xa activity of 1.5 fondaparinux-specific U/ml. Others do not recommend routine monitoring

Adapted with permission from Linkins et al., Chest 2012;141:e495S
The American College of Chest Physician suggests argatroban or danaparoid over other non-heparin anticoagulants (Grade 2C). Argatroban is preferred in patients with renal insufficiency (Grade 2C)

treatment for patients with AT-III deficiency is the administration of antithrombin III to restore plasma levels to 100%. AT-III is available both in a plasma-derived solution and a recombinant formula. It is also contained in fresh-frozen plasma, but should be avoided due to a higher degree of viral transmission than other replacement options [19].

Cold Agglutinins

Cold agglutinins (CA) are circulating autoantibodies that are activated at the temperature below normal physiologic body temperature. CA are clinically relevant in cardiac surgery cases in which hypothermic cardiopulmonary bypass is required. The CA activation occurs at varying levels of hypothermia and can cause hemolysis, microvascular thrombosis, and end-organ damage. Thermal amplitude is the blood temperature below which the CA will react and cause agglu-tination and hemolysis. When agglutination occurs during on CPB, the perfusionist might notice higher pressure in the cardioplegia circuit and visible blood aggregates, raising the risk for thromboembolic or hemolytic complications. Increasing the temperature will rapidly reverse the activation process. The evaluation of the patient's antibody titer and thermal amplitude are essential in patients with a known diagnosis of the disorder. Patients with antibody titer <1:32 and a thermal amplitude below 20 °C are considered in the low-risk group. In high-risk patients, preoperative plasmapheresis and intravenous IgG are the choices of treatment to reduce or eliminate the antibody titer. The perioperative goal is to avoid body temperature below the thermal threshold. Intraoperative considerations consist of rigorous core temperature monitoring, warming fluids and blood products, prevention of hypothermia in the operating room, and normothermic CPB with warm cardioplegia, if possible [20].

Connective Tissue Disease and Cardiac Surgery

Marfan Syndrome

An autosomal dominant disease with an incidence of 1 in 3000 to 5000 individuals. Most patients with the Marfan syndrome phenotype present mutations involving the gene that encodes fibrillin-1 (FBN1), a protein integral to the structure of elastic fibers. Cardiovascular abnormalities are the main feature of Marfan syndrome and include proximal aortic and main pulmonary artery dilation, thickening and prolapse of atrioventricular valves and mitral annulus calcification. Aortic root aneurysm, aortic regurgitation, and dissection constitute the main cause of morbidity and mortality, and the reason replacement of ascending aorta is frequently performed in these patients. Other relevant manifestations include hyperextensible joints, arched palate, bullous emphysema, pectus excavatum, and kyphoscoliosis. Medical therapy with beta blockers is recommended in most cases to decrease the risk of aortic complications [21].

Perioperative Considerations

Airway abnormalities that may result in difficult intubation should be investigated. Excessive traction of the temporomandibular joint while manipulating the airway *must* be avoided. Thoracic and spine deformities associated with the pulmonary disease can make ventilation challenging (restrictive pattern), and a lung protective strategy may be considered. Moreover, patients with Marfan syndrome have an increased risk of spontaneous pneumothorax. Careful positioning of the patient on the operating table is essential to avoid dislocations and nerve injuries, which may derive from the hyperextensible joints.

Hemodynamic goals must focus on maintaining a low aortic wall tension, thus avoiding catastrophic aortic complications (dissection and rupture). Blood pressure and contractility, therefore, need to be kept stable which can be accomplished with generous doses of opioids.

Aortic cannulation should probably be performed while systolic blood pressure is at lower than usual values during this procedure (80 to 90 mmHg) [22].

Ehlers-Danlos Syndrome

Comprised of a collection of heritable connective tissue disorders, Ehlers-Danlos syndrome presents an average incidence of 1 in 10,000 to 25,000 individuals and originates from mutations in genes that produce or regulate fibrillar collagen proteins. Patients with Ehlers-Danlos syndrome are subdivided into one of six significant subtypes according to presentation (classic, hypermobility, vascular, kyphoscoliotic, arthrochalasis, dermatosparaxis), which can vary from very mild phenotypes to life-threatening conditions. Hyperextensible joints, skin and coagulation anomalies and vascular and internal organ fragility characterize the syndrome. Patients present for cardiovascular surgery typically for mitral regurgitation, aortic aneurysm or aortic dissection [23].

Perioperative Considerations

The preoperative evaluation must assess subtype and known abnormalities. Selection of medical tape must consider the presence of skin fragility, in which case it should be easily removable. Use of ultrasound to guide arterial and central venous catheterization is mandatory, as it will lower the risks of dissection and bleeding. Possible intubation difficulties—temporomandibular dysfunction, premature spondylosis or occipitoatlantoaxial instability—should be anticipated. Lung protective ventilation may be considered as the risk of pneumothorax is increased.

Equivalent hemodynamic measures as described for patients with Marfan syndrome should be employed to decrease the risk of complications for patients with aortic aneurysms. Individuals with Ehlers-Danlos syndrome can present platelet aggregation abnormalities even if regular coagulation tests are normal. Therefore, intraoperative point-of-care coagulation testing and use of cell-saver are recommended. In cases of refractory bleeding, the administration of desmopressin should be considered [23].

Loeys-Dietz Syndrome

Relatively recently described, the Loeys-Dietz syndrome is a connective tissue genetic disorder which shares phenotypic features with Marfan and Ehlers-Danlos syndromes. The presentation, however, is more aggressive with the early development of an aortic aneurysm and dissection. Other presenting features include widely spaced eyes (hypertelorism), cervical spine deformity, bifid uvula, cleft palate, generalized arterial tortuosity and aneurysms of other arteries besides the aorta. Similar anesthetic recommendations as for Marfan and Ehlers-Danlos syndromes can be applied for patients with Loeys-Dietz syndrome and will depend on presenting abnormalities [24].

Cardiac Surgery During Pregnancy

Cardiac disease is the main cause of non-obstetric mortality related to pregnancy. It occurs in one to three percent of gestations and is responsible for 10 to 15% of maternal deaths. In most cases, the underlying mechanism is present before the onset of pregnancy but becomes decompensated secondary to gestational hemodynamic changes. Presently, the two most common etiologies are congenital heart disease and rheumatic heart disease [25].

The increased metabolic demands of pregnancy produce elevations of heart rate, stroke volume, and intravascular volume. Cardiac output, thereby, is increased roughly 50% impacting an increase in myocardial oxygen consumption. In parallel, coronary perfusion pressure decreases as systemic vascular resistance lowers during gestation. Patients with heart problems, mainly valvular stenosis, are heavily burdened by these modifications. Ensuing complications include pulmonary hypertension, pulmonary edema, myocardial infarction, heart failure, arrhythmias, and stroke. Main predictors of maternal compli-

cations are: (1) previous history of transient ischemic attack, stroke or arrhythmia; (2) NYHA heart failure class three or four before the onset of pregnancy; (3) left-heart valvular stenosis; and (4) an ejection fraction lower than 40% [11].

The most common indication for urgent cardiac surgery during pregnancy is worsening heart function related to valvular stenosis. Other less frequent conditions include dissection or rupture of the aorta, pulmonary embolism, closure of patent foramen ovale and cardiac tumors. Maternal outcomes seem comparable to non-pregnant women undergoing cardiac surgery [25]. Nonetheless, surgical treatment during pregnancy should be considered a last resort as cardiac surgery in this context carries prominent fetal risks denoted by mortality rates that range from 16 to 33%. Predictors of worse fetal outcomes are the institution of CPB, duration of surgery and hypothermia [11].

Perioperative Considerations

General management of cardiac surgery during pregnancy mostly depends on the extrauterine viability of the fetus. If maternal conditions allow gestation to be carried until 28 weeks (complete organogenesis), cardiac surgery is probably best performed after a cesarean section in a combined procedure. Delivery should be timed to occur after the steps of heparinization and cannulation are complete. Unfractionated heparin does not cross the placental barrier and can be used safely following the same routine as for non-pregnant individuals. Care should be taken if administration of oxytocin is necessary as it can induce hypotension [25].

In situations of worsening maternal hemodynamics before the fetus becomes viable, cardiac surgery should be carried out following explanation to both parents that the associated risks to the fetus are considerable. Most commonly used drugs appear to be safe but specific information regarding gestational and fetal effects is mainly lacking. High doses of ketamine, however, should probably be avoided. Cardiotocography must be performed continuously, and detection of uterine contractions should prompt the use of tocolytic drugs (ethanol, magnesium sulfate, terbutaline or ritodrine). If necessary, cardiopulmonary bypass should be conducted at higher flow rates (> 2.5 L/min per m^2) and mean arterial pressures (>70 mmHg). Slightly elevated $PaCO_2$ values should be the goal since hypocapnia decreases uterine blood flow. Hypothermia should be avoided whenever possible. The hematocrit should be kept at least at 28%. In case life-threatening conditions arise while cardiac surgery is being performed, obstetric and neonatology teams must be immediately available to perform a cesarean delivery [25].

References

1. Paraskevaidis IA, Michalakeas CA, Papadopoulos CH, Anastasiou-Nana M. Cardiac tumors. ISRN Oncol [Internet]. 2011;2011:1–5. Available from http://www.hindawi.com/journals/isrn/2011/208929/

2. Bruce CJ. Cardiac tumours: diagnosis and management. Heart. 2011;97:151–60.

3. Castillo JG, Silvay G. Characterization and management of cardiac tumors. Semin Cardiothorac Vasc Anesth. 2010;14:6–20.

4. Davar J, Connolly HM, Caplin ME, Pavel M, Zacks J, Bhattacharyya S, et al. Diagnosing and managing carcinoid heart disease in patients with neuroendocrine tumors: an expert statement. J Am Coll Cardiol. 2017;69(10):1288–304.

5. Maron BJ, Towbin JA, Thiene G, Antzelevitch C, Corrado D, Arnett D, et al. Contemporary definitions and classification of the cardiomyopathies: an American Heart Association Scientific Statement from the Council on Clinical Cardiology, Heart Failure and Transplantation Committee; Quality of Care and Outcomes Research and Function. Circulation. 2006;113(14):1807–16.

6. Journal AT, Journals AHA, Issues ALL, Features B. Report of the 1995 World Health Organization/International Society and Federation of Cardiology Task Force on the Definition and Classification of Cardiomyopathies. Circulation [Internet]. 1996;93(5):841–2. Available from http://circ.ahajournals.org/cgi/doi/10.1161/01.CIR.93.5.841

7. Elliott P, Andersson B, Arbustini E, Bilinska Z, Cecchi F, Maisch B, et al. Classification of the cardiomyopathies: a position statement from the European society of cardiology working group on myocardial and pericardial diseases. Eur Heart J. 2008;29:270–6.

8. Gersh BJ, Maron BJ, Bonow RO, Dearani JA, Fifer MA, Link MS, et al. 2011 ACCF/AHA guideline for the diagnosis and treatment of hypertrophic cardiomyopathy. J Am Coll Cardiol [Internet]. 2011;58(25):e212–60. Available from http://linkinghub.elsevier.com/retrieve/pii/S0735109711022753

9. Braunwald EE, Marian AJ, Nishimura RA, Seggewiss H, Schaff HV. Cardiomyopathy compendium hypertrophic obstructive cardiomyopathy surgical myectomy and septal ablation. 2017;121:771–783.

10. Yancy CW, Jessup M, Bozkurt B, Butler J, Casey DE, Colvin MM, et al. 2017 ACC/AHA/HFSA focused update of the 2013 ACCF/AHA guideline for the management of heart failure: a report of the American College of Cardiology/American Heart Association Task Force on Clinical Practice Guidelines and the Heart Failure Society of America. J Am Coll Cardiol. 2017;70(6):776–803.

11. Fox JF, Smith MM, Nuttall GA, Oliver W. Uncommon cardiac diseases. In: Kaplan's cardiac anesthesia: for cardiac and noncardiac surgery. 7th ed. New York: Elsevier; 2017. p. 883–973.

12. Imazio M. Contemporary management of pericardial diseases. Curr Opin Cardiol [Internet]. 2012;27(3):308–17. Available from http://content.wkhealth.com/linkback/openurl?sid=WKPTLP:landingpage&an=00001573-201205000-00017

13. Grocott HP, Gulati H, Srinathan S, Mackensen GB. Anesthesia and the patient with pericardial disease. Can J Anesth. 2011;58(10):952–66.

14. Mittnacht A, Reich DL, Rhee AJ, et al. In: Fleisher L, editor. Anesthesia and uncommon diseases. 6th ed. Philadelphia (PA): Saunders; 2012. p. 28–74.

15. Stine KC, Becton DL. Use of factor VIII replacement during open heart surgery in a patient with haemophilia A. Haemophilia. 2006;12(4):435–6.

16. Nichols WL, Hultin MB, James AH, Manco-Johnson MJ, Montgomery RR, Ortel TL, et al. von Willebrand disease (VWD): evidence-based diagnosis and management guidelines, the National Heart, Lung, and Blood Institute (NHLBI) expert panel report (USA). Haemophilia. 2008;14(2):171–232.

17. Levy JH, Winkler AM. Heparin-induced thrombocytopenia and cardiac surgery. Curr Opin Anaesthesiol [Internet]. 2010;23(1):74–9. Available from http://content.wkhealth.com/linkback/openurl?sid=WKPTLP:landingpage&an=00001503-201002000-00013

18. Linkins L-A, Dans AL, Moores LK, Bona R, Davidson BL, Schulman S, et al. Treatment and prevention of heparin-induced thrombocytopenia. Chest [Internet]. 2012;141(2):e495S–e530S. Available from http://linkinghub.elsevier.com/retrieve/pii/S0012369212601305

19. Rodgers GM. Role of antithrombin concentrate in treatment of hereditary antithrombin deficiency: an update. Thromb Haemost. 2009;101(5):806–12.

20. Patel PA, Ghadimi K, Coetzee E, Myburgh A, Swanevelder J, Gutsche JT, et al. Incidental cold agglutinins in cardiac surgery: intraoperative surprises and team-based problem-solving strategies

during cardiopulmonary bypass. J Cardiothorac Vasc Anesth [Internet]. 2017;31(3):1109–18. https://doi.org/10.1053/j.jvca.2016.06.024.

21. Wright MJ, Connolly H. Management of Marfan syndrome and related disorders. UpToDate [Internet]. Available from http://www.uptodate.com

22. Castellano JM, Silvay G, Castillo JG. Marfan syndrome. Semin Cardiothorac Vasc Anesth [Internet]. 2014;18(3):260–71. Available from http://journals.sagepub.com/doi/10.1177/1089253213513842

23. Wiesmann T, Castori M, Malfait F, Wulf H. Recommendations for anesthesia and periop-erative management in patients with Ehlers-Danlos syndrome(s). Orphanet J Rare Dis [Internet]. 2014;9(1):109. Available from http://ojrd.biomedcen-tral.com/articles/10.1186/s13023-014-0109-5

24. Williams JA, Loeys BL, Nwakanma LU, Dietz HC, Spevak PJ, Patel ND, et al. Early surgical experience with Loeys-Dietz: a new syndrome of aggressive thoracic aortic aneurysm disease. Ann Thorac Surg. 2007;83(2):S757–63.

25. Chandrasekhar S, Cook CR, Collard CD. Cardiac surgery in the parturient. Anesth Analg. 2009;108(3):777–86.

Essence of Cardiopulmonary Bypass Circuit and Intra-Aortic Balloon Pump

19

Jodie Beuth and George Djaiani

Main Messages
1. The CPB circuit is a network of tubing with integrated oxygenators, pumps, filters, heat exchangers and monitoring components, which generates non-pulsatile flow.
2. Systemic heparinization is initiated via central venous line at a dose of 350–400 IU/kg aiming to achieve an Activated Clotting Time (ACT) exceeding 480 s.
3. CPB circuit increases complications in hematological, cardiovascular, renal, neurological, and pulmonary systems.
4. IABP is a mechanical circulatory support device for the management of low cardiac output syndromes, via counterpulsation that results in improvement of the myocardial oxygen supply-demand ratio and coronary perfusion in diastole.

Cardiopulmonary bypass (CPB) has revolutionised cardiac surgery since the successful use of a heart lung machine by Gibbon in 1953. Utilisation of this extracorporeal complete or partial circulatory support has use in cardiac and aortic surgeries, and expanded prolonged circulatory or pulmonary support for cardiogenic shock or respiratory failure. Improvements in technological components as well as advances in surgical instrumentation and techniques have resulted in exponential growth and availability of open-heart surgery internationally with an impressive safety profile. However, utilising mechanical circulation creates a non-physiological perfusion state that alters homeostatic function.

Cardiopulmonary Bypass: Circuit and Components

Pumps

The CPB circuit is essentially a network of tubing with integrated oxygenators, pumps, filters, heat exchangers and monitoring components (Fig. 19.1). Pumps are either roller or centrifugal in mechanism. Roller pumps are a displacement pump, and are the most commonly used type. They consist of polyvinyl chloride (PVC) tubing that resides in a curved 'raceway' which propels blood in a unidirectional manner with rotational compression creating a waveform of approxi-

J. Beuth · G. Djaiani (✉)
Department of Anesthesia and Pain Management, Toronto General Hospital, University Health Network, University of Toronto, Toronto, ON, Canada
e-mail: jodie.beuth@one-mail.on.ca;
George.Djaiani@uhn.ca

© Springer Nature Switzerland AG 2021
D. C. H. Cheng et al. (eds.), *Evidence-Based Practice in Perioperative Cardiac Anesthesia and Surgery*, https://doi.org/10.1007/978-3-030-47887-2_19

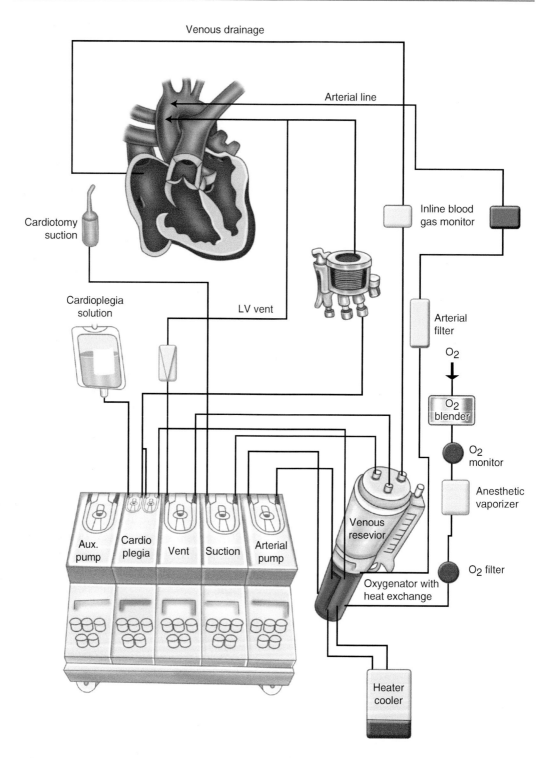

Fig. 19.1 Diagram of a cardiopulmonary bypass circuit. From Allen P. Essence of Cardiopulmonary Bypass Circuit and Intra-aortic Balloon Pump. In Cheng DCH and David TE, Perioperative care in cardiac anesthesia and surgery. Philadelphia, PA: Lippincott Williams & Wilkins; 2006:124, with permission

mately 5 mmHg of non-pulsatile flow [1]. The degree of tubing compression must be optimised to prevent significant backflow of blood, and maintain the integrity of the tubing, minimising potential 'spallation' (formation of particulate emboli) of tubing into the blood stream [1]. The volume displacement mechanism is related to tubing compression and therefore is independent of the afterload of the circuit, such that distal occlusion will result in significant pressure increase and risk component rupture.

Centrifugal pumps are more commonly found in extracorporeal membrane oxygenator (ECMO) circuits or for isolated left heart bypass. These pumps function via an internal impeller, with central blood flow proportionate to internal rotation, which can be maximal at 3000 revolutions per minute. These pumps are affected by the preload and afterload of the circuit, and hence pump flow varies accordingly with predetermined rate of revolutions. Pressure increases distal to the pump—e.g. via clamp or cannula displacement—will result in a reduction in pump flow for a given revolutions rate; therefore, a flow meter is required within the circuitry components.

There has been ongoing debate regarding the ideal pump type for optimal perfusion and minimal trauma to blood [2]. It has been theorised that centrifugal pump systems cause less red blood cell shear stress (and therefore less hemolysis) as there is reduced compression compared to displacement pumps; however, a recent meta-analysis of randomized controlled trials has not shown superiority of either pump type in the management of CPB [3]. When compared to centrifugal pumps, roller pumps are relatively cheaper, more durable, drain under gravity, use smaller priming volumes, and can be used for cardiotomy suction, vent suction, and cardioplegia delivery [1]. However, if negative suction pressure is excessive, the circulation is at risk of cellular trauma, hemolysis and gaseous microemboli formation [1, 4]. A vacuum-assist can be used to supplement venous drainage with roller pump systems and typically it is not associated with increased hemolysis, although, caution should be exercised with negative pressure in excess of 50 mmHg that may cause collapse of

raceway tubing and subsequent pump dysfunction [5].

Cannulas, Vents and Tubing

Configuration of cannulation will vary with surgical procedure and desired technique. Central cannulation is typically performed with an arterial cannula placed in the ascending aorta and a venous drainage cannula placed in the right atrium. The venous cannula is typically a 'two-stage' cannula inserted into the inferior vena cava (IVC) via the right atrium (RA) such that both IVC and RA are drained. Alternatively, bicaval cannulation of the superior and inferior vena cava is performed such that a bloodless surgical field in the RA is created for mitral or tricuspid valve surgery.

Vent cannulas are often placed to prevent distension and improve drainage of the left ventricle (LV). The LV vent is inserted via the right upper pulmonary vein (RUPV), directly via the apex, or alternatively the vent can be placed into the pulmonary artery (PA vent). Vent cannulas are drained via roller pump regulated by the perfusionist.

The CPB conduit is a configuration of sterilised PVC medical grade tubing that is coated with a non-thrombogenic medium, either heparin (bioline) or an alternate biocompatible substrate (polymer, phosphorylcholine, or 2-methoxyethyl acrylate) [6, 7]. These third generation circuits are kink resistant, retard thrombus formation, and reduce systemic inflammatory response caused by blood contact with a foreign surface [8].

Oxygenators and Heat Exchangers

Oxygenators in modern day CPB circuits have evolved significantly from the original bubble oxygenator design allowing for complete separation of blood from gas flow with dramatically improved gas exchange. The modern day oxygenator is a hollow fibre non-porous polymethylpentane membrane oxygenator that has low flow resistance, causing minimal blood trauma and reduced thrombus formation [8]. These oxygenators are used in both CPB and ECMO circuits with excellent durability [9]. Heat exchangers are placed upstream of the oxygenator permitting cooling and heating of the patient whilst on CPB. The temperature gradient between the circuit and the patient must be controlled to prevent the precipitation of gaseous bubbles in the circuit with rewarming, as the solubility of dissolved gases increases with hypothermia. Bubble traps and 40 micron filters are used to avoid systemic exposure to debris and gas emboli [10].

Cardiopulmonary Bypass: Conduct

Preparation for CPB

There is a structured approach for preparation of CPB that requires continuous communication between the surgeon, anesthesiologist, and perfusionist. Prior to initiation of CPB adequate systemic heparinization must be ensured. Heparin is administered by the anesthesiologist typically via central venous access at a dose of 350–400 IU/kg aiming to achieve an Activated Clotting Time (ACT) exceeding 480 s.

Cannulation configuration depends on the type of surgery. Configurations for emergency dissections and re-sternotomies can vary from peripheral femoral veno-arterial cannulation to axillary-femoral cannulation. However, central cannulation technique is the most common and involves cannulation of the ascending aorta followed by the right atrium once the ACT exceeds 300 s. For aortic cannulation the patient's systolic blood pressure should not exceed 100 mmHg to minimize the risk of aortic dissection. Appropriate 'swing' of pulsatile flow is verified at this stage and meticulous examination for potential air entrainment is crucial with removal of any microbubbles which is performed by the surgeon. This is followed by the venous cannulation that is performed via the right atrium either with a two stage venous cannula inserted into the inferior vena cava or bicaval cannulation of the inferior and superior vena cava for procedures requiring bloodless surgical field within the atria (e.g. atrial

septal defect repair, atrioventricular valve surgery, heart transplantation). At this stage, arrhythmias are common and there is a potential for significant blood loss if the placement of venous cannula is technically challenging.

A retrograde cardioplegia cannula may also be inserted into the coronary sinus usually causing a temporary hemodynamic instability with lifting of the heart. A transduced fluid line should demonstrate an appropriate waveform confirming presence of the retrograde cardioplegia cannula in the coronary sinus. An antegrade cardioplegia cannula is placed in the aorta proximal to the arterial cannula.

Commencement of CPB

Upon the surgeon's request, the perfusionist initiates CPB by drainage of the venous line under gravity and into the reservoir. Blood then flows through oxygenator, heat exchanger, bypass filters and pump head with oxygenated blood returning to the patient via the arterial cannula in the ascending aorta. At this stage the anesthesia machine alarms are deactivated, the arterial trace becomes non pulsatile and ventilation is discontinued once 'full flow' is declared by the perfusionist. Generally an initial pump flow of 2.2–2.8 L/min/m^2 is targeted and titrated to surrogate measures of end organ perfusion [11]. Maintenance of anesthesia is continued with intravenous or inhalational agents with addition of titrated opioids and muscle relaxants as required. Depth of anesthesia is usually monitored with entropy or bispectral index (BIS) monitors for the duration of surgery. Antegrade cardioplegia, with or without retrograde cardioplegia is utilized to protect the heart during CPB. A typical initial dose of cardioplegia is 1 to 1.5 L. If retrograde cardioplegia is used, it should be monitored at a delivery pressure not exceeding 40–50 mmHg to prevent rupture of the coronary sinus whilst minimizing edema of myocytes. Cardioplegia is generally readministered every 20–25 min, sooner if the heart electrical activity is detected. Often a 'hot shot' of warm cardioplegia is administered prior to the cross clamp being removed with the aim to flush the coronary circulation of cold cardioplegia solution and reduce ischemia-reperfusion injury.

Maintenance of CPB

Currently, it is a routine practice to use 'non-pulsatile' CPB, with a perfusion pressure that is maintained at 50 to 80 mmHg. Pump flow is based on the estimated cardiac output based on patient's body surface area and is titrated to surrogate markers of appropriate end organ perfusion such as acid-base equation, serial lactate levels, and venous oxygen saturations. Pump flows and perfusion are manipulated by alterations in venous drainage, vascular resistance, and circulating blood volume. Readily titratable vasoactive drugs (Table 19.1) and control of volume status via colloid, crystalloid or red blood cell administration are used to achieve adequate end organ perfusion as determined by frequent assessment of patient metabolic and hemodynamic status.

Weaning from CPB

Weaning from CPB is discussed in detail in Chap. 21. Achieving cardiovascular stability after CPB can be challenging, often requiring pharmacological support, and sometimes mechanical devices. Mechanical circulatory support ranges from the use of an intra-aortic balloon pump (IABP) to extracorporeal membrane oxygenation, and ventricular assist devices. Use of the IABP in cardiac surgery is discussed later in this chapter.

Table 19.1 Determinants of flow on cardiopulmonary bypass

Vasoconstrictors	Vasodilators
– Phenylephrine: bolus 50–100 mcg	– Nitroglycerin: 0.05–3 mcg/kg/min
– Norepinephrine: titration 0.01–0.6 mcg/kg/min	– Volatile anesthetic agent on CPB
– Vasopressin: 2–6 IU/min	– Sodium Nitroprusside: 0.25–1 mcg/kg/min

Pathophysiology and Complications of Cardiopulmonary Bypass

CPB is a pathophysiological state that disrupts cellular activity and alters regional blood flow. When blood contacts non-biological material a cellular inflammatory cascade is triggered which can cause an insult to all organ systems. Altered blood flow that is non-pulsatile, variable, hypothermic, and hemodiluted can also compromise end organ perfusion. The severity of organ dysfunction typically correlates with the extent of surgery and therefore duration of CPB. In addition, patient comorbidities, frailty, critical illness, and older age can also increase perioperative morbidity and mortality.

Hematological System

Patient blood flow through the artificial circuit activates the complement system and stimulates inflammatory mediators. This cascade of events results in endothelial activation leading to capillary leakage and cellular edema [12]. Simultaneously shear stress on platelets and red blood cells causes cellular lysis and release of free hemoglobin into the plasma that may result in hemoglobinuria, and associated renal injury [13]. Furthermore, tissue factor and platelet activation occurs with exposure of blood to the intrapleural and pericardial surfaces. Use of cardiotomy suction exacerbates trauma to red cells and introduces fat globules into the circulation [14]. This can result in significant hyperfibrinolysis and coagulopathy following administration of protamine after separation from CPB. Techniques adopted to minimise these effects include: improved CPB components (e.g. oxygenators, pumps, advanced PVC tubing, leucocyte depletion filters); cell salvage to filter emboli and free haemoglobin; routine administration of antifibrinolytics; and point of care testing [15].

Cardiovascular System

Cardiovascular complications after CPB are relatively common. For the duration of cross clamp, meticulous attention is paid to myocardial protection. The myocardial metabolic demand during this time should be kept to a minimum. Cold cardioplegia that is administered every twenty to thirty minutes is required to maintain electrical silence. Often with coronary disease it is difficult to ensure that cardioplegia penetrates to all regions of the myocardium. Additionally, retrograde cardioplegia often cannot fully protect the right heart, as not all of the coronary circulation drains directly into the coronary sinus. It is the right heart that is more susceptible to dysfunction when weaning from CPB. Often a dose of warm cardioplegia 'hot shot' is administered prior to removal of the cross clamp to minimise the ischemia-reperfusion injury to the myocardium [15]. Following open chamber procedures, air within the heart can be ejected directly into the right coronary artery with resultant arrhythmias and right ventricular dysfunction. Flooding the surgical field with carbon dioxide may minimize the formation of air bubbles during the procedure, and together with thorough de-airing techniques, facilitate successful weaning from CPB. The vascular responses to CPB vary depending on patient's comorbidities, as well as the nature and duration of surgery. Typically with prolonged CPB, systemic vascular resistance reduces due to ongoing systemic inflammatory response necessitating administration of vasopressors, such as norepinephrine and vasopressin [14]. Furthermore, refractory vasoplegia may require administration of methylene blue, a nitric oxide scavenger.

Renal System

Acute kidney injury (AKI) following CPB has a relatively high incidence, ranging from 7–28%, depending on the definition of AKI [16]. The renal medulla is exquisitely sensitive to adequate oxygen delivery. A combination of hemodilution, hypothermia with regional vasoconstriction, relative hypotension, and non-pulsatile perfusion during CPB may threaten renal perfusion and reduce oxygen delivery [17, 18]. Patients with pre-existing renal disease, diabetes, hyperten-

sion, anemia and peripheral vascular disease are at higher risk of renal insult during the perioperative period. In addition, this risk increases proportionately with duration of CPB and complexity of surgery. Renal replacement therapy is required in 1% of patients after coronary surgery compared with 5% of patients following combined coronary and valve surgery [16]. The optimal hematocrit for adequate renal perfusion has been debated; and is a balance between adequate oxygen carrying capacity, prevention of excessive hemodilution and avoidance of transfusion with associated complications. Consensus aims for a hematocrit above 25% to lessen the likelihood of acute renal insult [16, 19]. Techniques to optimise hematocrit and reduce transfusion aim to reduce hemodilution due to non-sanguineous pump prime volume. The methods to reduce the prime include shortening circuit tubing, using smaller bypass circuit components, employing retrograde autologous priming, or considering a blood prime in anemic patients [19]. Recent research has identified that perioperative administration of dexmedetomidine may reduce the incidence and severity of kidney injury after cardiac surgery [20].

Neurological System

The central nervous system injury after cardiac surgery ranges from subtle cognitive impairment, to more evident hyperactive delirium, to devastating frank stroke. Preventive strategies to reduce the incidence of delirium include both non-pharmacological and pharmacological strategies [21, 22]. The incidence of sustained cerebrovascular events after CPB is estimated at 1–2% for coronary revascularisation procedures, and increases to 3–5% for valve surgery [23]. Patients with limited cerebrovascular reserve are more likely to suffer from altered cerebral perfusion during CPB. The risk of neurological sequelae is increased in the elderly, those with a history of previous cerebrovascular event, carotid stenosis, and significant peripheral vascular disease [24]. The majority of perioperative strokes in cardiac surgery are embolic in nature, with the minority being of thrombotic or hemorrhagic origin. Cerebral perfusion can be compromised by: relative hypotension; excessive hemodilution; anemia; and microembolic phenomena from dislodged calcified plaque, often from manipulation of the aorta, as well as fat emboli from suction of scavenged blood via cardiotomy or from air emboli with open chamber procedures [25–27]. The optimal hematocrit for these patients is unknown but there is evidence that a hematocrit below 22% increases the risk of stroke, and that a hemoglobin above 70 g/L should be a target in patients at risk of end organ ischemia [28]. Embolic effects on cerebral circulation can be minimised by use of filters within the CPB circuit, careful de-airing of open chamber procedures, and the use of carbon dioxide to flood the surgical field. In those with severe atheromatous disease of the aorta, an off pump coronary grafting technique can be considered to avoid handling of the aorta in reducing perioperative stroke [23, 29]. Preventative measures to protect the brain include preoperative risk stratification, limiting CPB duration, targeting optimal perfusion pressure, aggressive management of postoperative arrhythmias, and avoidance of rapid rewarming and cerebral hyperthermia which can be associated with adverse neurological outcomes [24, 30, 31]. Management of patients with known high-grade carotid lesions and neurological monitoring during cardiac surgery are discussed in other chapters.

Pulmonary System

During CPB, the transpulmonary circulation is isolated and perfusion via the pulmonary artery ceases. As a result, the perfusion to the pulmonary vasculature is dependent solely on blood supply from the bronchial arteries. The duration of relative lung ischemia can result in a reperfusion injury on resumption of physiological circulation [32]. The incidence of postoperative pulmonary complications is in a range of 5–7%, related to atelectasis and hypoxemia. Recruitment manoeuvres and lung protective ventilation may aid in preventing pulmonary complications [32, 33].

Damage to the microvasculature of the pulmonary circulation due to the systemic inflammatory response related to CPB may contribute to acute lung injury. Severe damage to the lung endothelium manifests as acute respiratory distress syndrome, with an associated mortality rate ranging from 30–70% [34]. Transfusion of blood products, micro-aspiration, pneumonia, barotrauma, pneumothorax, sepsis, prolonged CPB time and sustained hypotension can also exacerbate pulmonic injury [35].

Intra-Aortic Balloon Pump

The IABP is a form of mechanical circulatory support device for the management of low cardiac output syndromes. It is rapid, reliable, relatively cheap and the least invasive of all forms of mechanical circulatory support [36]. Specific indications include preservation of hemodynamic stability for coronary percutaneous interventions, unstable angina, preoperative insertion for high risk patients undergoing cardiac or non-cardiac surgery, refractory cardiogenic dysfunction after CPB or decompensated heart failure as a bridge to intervention [36, 37]. A recent meta-analysis has not demonstrated significant advantages or detriment in long term outcomes related to use of IABP in select patient populations; however, IABP support may negate the need for escalation of inotropic therapy and associated complications [38].

Components of the device include a balloon typically of 35–50 ml attached to a helium gas drive line with an incorporated pressure transducer at the tip of the balloon. The pump unit is a large external component capable of detecting and triggering co-ordinated inflation and deflation of the balloon timed with the cardiac cycle either by electrocardiogram detection or synchronisation with the dichrotic notch on the arterial waveform. Triggering results in a rapid inflation of the balloon which occurs in diastole. Deflation occurs with systole, co-ordinated with the R wave on electrocardiogram. Timing can be synchronised either 1:1, ensuring the balloon inflation/deflation with each beat, 1:2 or 1:3. Often support for alternate beats is used for weaning from the IABP prior to removal. The IABP should never be stopped whilst in situ for longer than a few minutes due to the risk of thrombus formation.

The mechanism of IABP support is via counterpulsation that results in improvement of the myocardial oxygen supply-demand ratio (Fig. 19.2). Coronary perfusion is augmented in

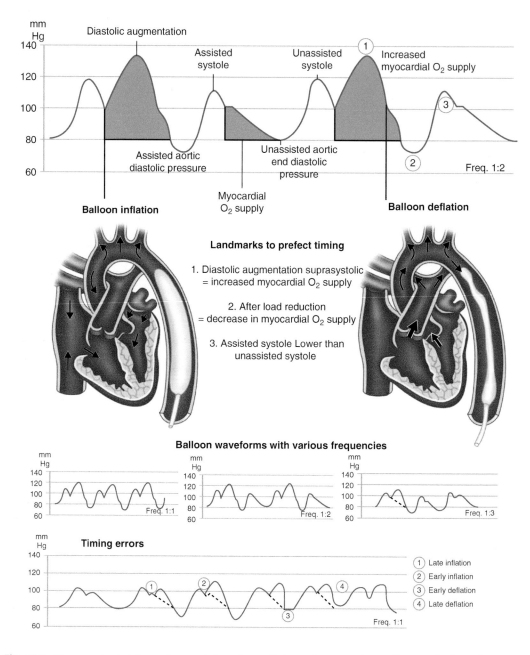

Fig. 19.2 Diagram of arterial waveform variations during intra-aortic balloon pump (IABP) therapy. From Allen P. Essence of Cardiopulmonary Bypass Circuit and Intra-aortic Balloon Pump. In Cheng DCH and David TE, Perioperative care in cardiac anesthesia and surgery. Philadelphia, PA: Lippincott Williams & Wilkins; 2006:133, with permission

diastole and afterload is reduced with subsequent improvement in left ventricular ejection fraction [39, 40].

Insertion of IABP is performed percutaneously via the femoral artery. The tip of the balloon should be positioned in the aortic arch just distal to the left subclavian artery. Appropriate placement is confirmed with radiological imaging or visualised with transesophageal echocardiography.

Contraindications to the Use of IABP	Complications Associated with the Use of IABP

• Significant aortic regurgitation
• Aortic dissection or aneurysm
• Severe peripheral vascular disease
	• Device dysfunction: balloon rupture, gas embolism, pump failure
	• Aortic trauma: dissection
	• Ischemia:
	  – Ipsilateral lower limb
	  – Potential for balloon migration and occlusion of left subclavian or renal arteries causing left arm or renal ischemia
	• Thrombus formation and embolization

References

1. Lafçı G, Budak AB, Yener AÜ, Cicek OF. Use of extracorporeal membrane oxygenation in adults. Heart, Lung Circul. 2014;23(1):10–23.
2. Passaroni AC, Silva MA, Yoshida WB. Cardiopulmonary bypass: development of John Gibbon's heart-lung machine. Rev Bras Cir Cardiovasc. 2015;30(2):235–45.
3. Saczkowski R, Maklin M, Mesana T, Boodhwani M, Ruel M. Centrifugal pump and roller pump in adult cardiac surgery: a meta-analysis of randomized controlled trials. Artif Organs. 2012;36(8):668–76.
4. Toomasian JM, Bartlett RH. Hemolysis and ECMO pumps in the 21st century. Perfusion. 2011;26(1):5.
5. Vercaemst L. Hemolysis in cardiac surgery patients undergoing cardiopulmonary bypass: a review in search of a treatment algorithm. J Extra Corpor Technol. 2008;40(4):257–67.
6. Mahmood S, Bilal H, Zaman M, Tang A. Is a fully heparin-bonded cardiopulmonary bypass circuit superior to a standard cardiopulmonary bypass circuit? Interact Cardiovasc Thorac Surg. 2012;14(4):406–14.
7. McBride WT, Elliott P. Advances in cardiopulmonary bypass circuitry. Curr Opin Anaesthesiol. 2003;16(1):27–31.
8. Rehder K, Turner D, Bonadonna D, Walczak R, Rudder R, Cheifetz I. Technological advances in extracorporeal membrane oxygenation for respiratory failure. Expert Rev Respir Med. 2012;6(4):377–84.
9. Khoshbin JE, Roberts WN, Harvey KC, et al. Polymethyl pentene oxygenators have improved gas exchange capability and reduced transfusion requirements in adult extracorporeal membrane oxygenation. ASAIO J. 2005;51(3):281–7.
10. Mitchell SJ. From trash to leucocytes: what are we filtering and why? J Extra Corpor Technol. 2006;38(1):58–63.
11. De Somer F. What is optimal flow and how to validate this. J Extra Corpor Technol. 2007;39(4):278–80.
12. Yavari M, Becker R. Coagulation and fibrinolytic protein kinetics in cardiopulmonary bypass. J Thromb Thrombolysis. 2009;27(1):95–104.
13. Mao H, Katz N, Ariyanon W, et al. Cardiac surgery-associated acute kidney injury. Cardio Renal Med. 2013;3(3):178–99.
14. De Somer F. Recent advances in the comprehension and the management of perioperative systemic host response during cardiopulmonary bypass. Recent Pat Cardiovasc Drug Discov. 2012;7(3):180–5.
15. Esper SA, Subramaniam K, Tanaka KA. Pathophysiology of cardiopulmonary bypass: current strategies for the prevention and treatment of anemia, coagulopathy, and organ dysfunction. Semin Cardiothorac Vasc Anesth. 2014;18(2):161–76.
16. Di Tomasso N, Monaco F, Landoni G. Hepatic and renal effects of cardiopulmonary bypass. Best Pract Res Clin Anaesthesiol. 2015;29(2):151–61.
17. Karkouti K, Beattie WS, Wijeysundera DN, et al. Hemodilution during cardiopulmonary bypass is an independent risk factor for acute renal failure in adult cardiac surgery. J Thorac Cardiovasc Surg. 2005;129(2):391–400.
18. Ranucci M, Romitti F, Isgrò G, et al. Oxygen delivery during cardiopulmonary bypass and acute renal failure after coronary operations. Ann Thorac Surg. 2005;80(6):2213–20.
19. Long DM, Jenkins E, Griffith K. Perfusionist techniques of reducing acute kidney injury following cardiopulmonary bypass: an evidence-based review. Perfusion. 2015;30(1):25–32.
20. Cho JS, Shim JK, Soh S, Kim MK, Kwak YL. Perioperative dexmedetomidine reduces the incidence and severity of acute kidney injury following valvular heart surgery. Kidney Int. 2016;89(3):693–700.
21. Siddiqi N, Harrison JK, Clegg A, et al. Interventions for preventing delirium in hospitalised non-ICU patients. Cochrane Database Syst Rev. 2016;3:CD005563.
22. Djaiani G, Silverton N, Fedorko L, et al. Dexmedetomidine versus propofol sedation reduces delirium after cardiac surgery: a randomized controlled trial. Anesthesiology. 2016;124(2):362–8.
23. Engelman RM, Engelman DT. Strategies and devices to minimize stroke in adult cardiac surgery. Semin Thorac Cardiovasc Surg. 2015;27(1):24–9.
24. Mao Z, Zhong X, Yin J, Zhao Z, Hu X, Hackett ML. Predictors associated with stroke after coronary

artery bypass grafting: a systematic review. J Neurol Sci. 2015;357(1–2):1–7.

25. Karkouti K, Djaiani G, Borger MA, et al. Low hematocrit during cardiopulmonary bypass is associated with increased risk of perioperative stroke in cardiac surgery. Ann Thorac Surg. 2005;80(4): 1381–7.

26. Djaiani G, Fedorko L, Borger M, et al. Mild to moderate atheromatous disease of the thoracic aorta and new ischemic brain lesions after conventional coronary artery bypass graft surgery. Stroke. 2004;35(9):e356–8.

27. Djaiani G, Fedorko L, Borger MA, et al. Continuous-flow cell saver reduces cognitive decline in elderly patients after coronary bypass surgery. Circulation. 2007;116(17):1888–95.

28. Society of Thoracic Surgeons Blood Conservation Guideline Task F, Ferraris VA, Brown JR, et al. 2011 update to the Society of Thoracic Surgeons and the Society of Cardiovascular Anesthesiologists blood conservation clinical practice guidelines. Ann Thorac Surg 2011;91(3):944–982.

29. Wijeysundera DN, Beattie WS, Djaiani G, et al. Off-pump coronary artery surgery for reducing mortality and morbidity: meta-analysis of randomized and observational studies. J Am Coll Cardiol. 2005;46(5):872–82.

30. McDonagh DL, Berger M, Mathew JP, Graffagnino C, Milano CA, Newman MF. Neurological complications of cardiac surgery. Lancet Neurol. 2014;13(5):490–502.

31. Grigore AM, Murray CF, Ramakrishna H, Djaiani G. A core review of temperature regimens and neuroprotection during cardiopulmonary bypass: does rewarming rate matter? Anesth Analg. 2009;109(6):1741–51.

32. Garcia-Delgado M, Navarrete-Sanchez I, Colmenero M. Preventing and managing perioperative pulmonary complications following cardiac surgery. Curr Opin Anaesthesiol. 2014;27(2):146–52.

33. Minkovich L, Djaiani G, Katznelson R, et al. Effects of alveolar recruitment on arterial oxygenation in patients after cardiac surgery: a prospective, randomized, controlled clinical trial. J Cardiothorac Vasc Anesth. 2007;21(3):375–8.

34. Milot J, Perron J, Lacasse Y, Létourneau L, Cartier PC, Maltais F. Incidence and predictors of ARDS after cardiac surgery. Chest. 2001;119(3):884–8.

35. Huffmyer JL, Groves DS. Pulmonary complications of cardiopulmonary bypass. Best Pract Res Clin Anaesthesiol. 2015;29(2):163–75.

36. Poirier Y, Voisine P, Plourde G, et al. Efficacy and safety of preoperative intra-aortic balloon pump use in patients undergoing cardiac surgery: a systematic review and meta-analysis. Int J Cardiol. 2016;207:67–79.

37. Minha S, et al. Overview of the 2012 Food and Drug Administration circulatory system devices panel meeting on the reclassification of external counterpulsation, intra-aortic balloon pump, and non-roller-type cardiopulmonary bypass blood pump devices. Am Heart J. 2013;166(3):414–20.

38. Grieshaber P, Niemann B, Roth P, Boning A. Prophylactic intra-aortic balloon counterpulsation in cardiac surgery: it is time for clear evidence. Crit Care. 2014;18(6):662.

39. Gravlee GP. Cardiopulmonary bypass: principles and practice. 3rd ed. Philadelphia: Wolters Kluwer Health/Lippincott Williams & Wilkins; 2008.

40. Bia D, Cabrera-Fischer EI, Zocalo Y, Armentano RL. Intra-aortic balloon pumping reduces the increased arterial load caused by acute cardiac depression, modifying central and peripheral load determinants in a time- and flow-related way. Heart Vessel. 2012;27(5):517–27.

Essence of Pacemakers and Its Application After CPB

20

Nathan Waldron and Joseph Mathew

Main Messages

1. The SA and AV nodes are both densely innervated with adrenergic and cholinergic nerve fibers, which co-localize to co-regulate these opposing branches of the autonomic nervous system.
2. Postoperative atrial fibrillation (POAF) is one of the most common perioperative complications of cardiac surgery, occurring in 27–40% of patients, with associated risk of cerebrovascular accidents, myocardial infarction, prolonged length of stay, and mortality.
3. Transient atrioventricular blockade after surgeries utilizing cardiopulmonary bypass is extremely common; however, the need for both temporary epicardial pacing and placement of permanent pacemaker differs based upon surgical procedure.
4. Patients with persistent need for epicardial pacing should have daily checks for lead thresholds to inform the timeframe

for potential permanent pacemaker placement.
5. Troubleshooting Common Problems with Epicardial Pacing: failure to capture, cross talk inhibition, and Pacemaker-mediated tachycardia.

Fundamentals of Pacemakers

Anatomy of the Cardiac Conduction System

The cardiac conduction system consists of highly specialized myocardial tissue that functions to generate and conduct organized electrical impulses. Normal cardiac electrical activity begins with spontaneous diastolic depolarization of cells in the sinoatrial (SA) node, a spindle-shaped structure located at the junction of the superior vena cava and right atrial appendage. Electrical wavefronts then propagate across the atrium toward the atrioventricular (AV) node, located in the Triangle of Koch [1], as well as toward the left atrium via Bachmann's bundle. Purkinje fibers from the AV node then converge to form the His bundle, which runs in the membranous interventricular septum (IVS) before dividing into left and right bundle branches at the superior aspect of the muscular IVS. The left bundle branch then divides again into three fasci-

N. Waldron (✉) · J. Mathew
Department of Anesthesiology, Duke University
Medical Center, Durham, NC, USA
e-mail: nathan.waldron@duke.edu;
joseph.mathew@duke.edu

© Springer Nature Switzerland AG 2021
D. C. H. Cheng et al. (eds.), *Evidence-Based Practice in Perioperative Cardiac Anesthesia and Surgery*, https://doi.org/10.1007/978-3-030-47887-2_20

cles (anterior, medial, posterior), whereas the right bundle branch remains undivided until it reaches the apex of the right ventricle. After dividing, the bundle branch system forms a complex, highly variable network of Purkinje fibers that promote near-synchronous electrical activation of the left and right ventricular myocardium [2].

The SA and AV nodes are both densely innervated with adrenergic and cholinergic nerve fibers, which co-localize—potentially pointing to co-regulation of these opposing branches of the autonomic nervous system. Classically, the SA node is preferentially innervated by branches of the right Vagus nerve and stellate ganglion, while the AV node is preferentially innervated by the left Vagus and stellate ganglion. Past the AV node, autonomic fiber density decreases, though myocardial autonomic innervation may play an important role in both atrial [3] and ventricular [4] dysrhythmias. Overall, the preponderance of acetylcholine and acetylcholinesterase activity in the SA and AV node points toward a baseline vagal predominance to autonomic tone.

Conduction Derangements Associated with Cardiac Surgery

Cardiac surgery is associated with a number of rhythm disturbances, which may potentially necessitate the use of a pacemaker. Atrial dysrhythmias, primarily postoperative atrial fibrillation (POAF), are one of the most common perioperative complications of cardiac surgery, occurring in 27–40% of patients [5, 6]. Unfortunately, POAF is associated with increased risk of cerebrovascular accidents, myocardial infarction, prolonged length of stay, and increased mortality [5, 7–9]. Risk factors for POAF include increased age, history of AF, valvular surgery, left ventricular dysfunction, and medication withdrawal [5]. While highly efficacious preventative strategies for POAF remain elusive, temporary epicardial pacing may play a role in both the prevention and treatment of POAF.

After coronary surgery, there is a high incidence of isolated, transient ventricular dysrhythmias, including premature ventricular beats

(100% incidence) and short runs (<10 s) of ventricular tachycardia (49% incidence) that do not translate into sustained episodes of ventricular arrhythmias [10]. As such, the incidence of sustained ventricular arrhythmias after CABG is considerably lower (1.6%), though linked to a high perioperative mortality [11]. Risk factors for malignant ventricular arrhythmias include female sex, age <65, congestive heart failure, preoperative IABP or inotropes, lower ejective fraction, increased comorbidity burden, and more severe anginal or heart failure symptoms [11]. Additionally, inappropriate ventricular pacing strategies may increase risk of ventricular dysrhythmias after cardiac surgery, and in-depth understanding of epicardial pacemaker modes may reduce this risk.

Transient atrioventricular blockade after surgeries utilizing cardiopulmonary bypass is extremely common. Cold cardioplegia is commonly associated with temporary sinus and/or AV nodal dysfunction, which can compromise hemodynamics during separation from bypass. Additionally, tissue injury causing temporary or permanent sinus node dysfunction is possible during right atrial and/or SVC cannulation. Direct injury to AV nodal or bundle branch structures is also possible during cardiac surgery, particularly surgeries involving the aortic, mitral, or tricuspid annulus.

The need for both temporary epicardial pacing and placement of permanent pacemaker differs based upon surgical procedure. In a retrospective single-center study, 8.6% of patients undergoing coronary artery bypass grafting (CABG) required short-term pacing in the immediate postoperative period. Predictors of the requirement for pacing were preoperative arrhythmias (bundle branch block, atrioventricular block, atrial fibrillation), diabetes, and need for chronotropic pacing to separate from cardiopulmonary bypass. Among patients without these risk factors, only 2.6% required postoperative pacing [12]. Retrospective reviews have placed the incidence of complete heart block after CABG at 2.4%, which translates to a Number Needed to Treat (NNT) of 42 for epicardial wires to prevent significant bradycardia [13].

While very few patients require implantation of a permanent pacemaker (PPM) after CABG, patients undergoing valvular surgery have significantly increased risk of requiring PPM implantation. In a retrospective study of 4694 patients undergoing valvular surgery, 256 (5.5%) patients required PPM implantation. Multivariate modeling revealed age ≥70, prior valve surgery, PR interval >200 ms, multivalve surgery, right bundle branch block (RBBB), and left bundle branch block (LBBB) as independent predictors of need for PPM, with multivalve surgery including the tricuspid valve and RBBB as the strongest predictors [14]. Among patients who experienced high-grade AV block and receive a PPM after valvular surgery, >50% of patients regained AV nodal function and were not pacemaker dependent over a three year follow-up period. The propensity for remaining pacemaker dependence appeared related to the persistence of AV block in the perioperative period, with *transient* postoperative AV block associated with improved recovery of AV nodal function [15].

Transcatheter aortic valve implantation (TAVI) has emerged as a very valuable strategy to treat aortic stenosis in patients deemed unfavorable surgical candidates, but is associated with a notable incidence (6–17%) of AV block requiring permanent pacemaker placement. A recent meta-analysis found that male sex, use of the Medtronic CoreValve® system (versus Edwards Sapien®), pre-existing AV block and intraoperative AV block predicted increased need for postoperative permanent pacemaker implantation [16]. Additionally, new-onset LBBB increased the risk of permanent pacemaker implant and mortality after TAVR [17].

The Role of Epicardial Pacing in Perioperative Care: An Overview

Temporary epicardial pacing may play a role in hemodynamic optimization, as well as the prevention, treatment, and diagnosis of dysrhythmias after cardiac surgery. Cold cardioplegic arrest is associated with a temporary, mixed systolic/diastolic dysfunction, which may compromise separation from cardiopulmonary bypass [18]. Given this temporary decrease in myocardial function, temporary epicardial pacing to maintain a high rate (e.g. 90 BPM) typically improves cardiac output. Prophylactic atrial pacing has been posited as a preventative strategy for POAF by way of reducing atrial conduction delay, dispersion of refractoriness, and premature atrial beats. While isolated right or left atrial pacing do not meaningfully reduce POAF, biatrial overdrive pacing may hold promise as a prevention strategy [19]. Additionally, temporary overdrive pacing may be used as a treatment for reentrant supraventricular tachycardias or Type I atrial flutter [20]. In some patients, pharmacologic treatment (or rarely prophylaxis) for POAF may induce a bradyarrhythmia or atrioventricular block, which can benefit from temporary epicardial pacing. Finally, epicardial pacing wires may play a valuable role in the diagnosis and differentiation of postoperative dysrhythmias. If atrial pacing is not actively being employed, atrial leads may be used to record atrial electrograms (AEGs), which can be invaluable in differentiating between atrial and junctional tachycardias, and in verifying atrioventricular block (Fig. 20.1). AEG recordings may be completed with a standard ECG machine, and are recorded as a bipolar or unipolar recording, based on the lead configuration. A bipolar recording will record primarily atrial depolarization, whereas a unipolar AEG will reflect both atrial and ventricular electrograms.

Basics of Epicardial Pacemaker Leads

There are two types of epicardial leads in common use—bipolar and unipolar. Placing unipolar leads involves carefully suturing a single wire—the negative anode—to the epicardial surface of the heart, while the positive wire is attached to subcutaneous tissues. Bipolar wires, on the other hand, involves placement of a single wire with two conductors (typically the anode is distal and the cathode proximal) separated by an insulator. In both types of leads, pacing results from the generation of a potential difference between the cathode and anode. Given the reduced distance

Atrial Electrograms

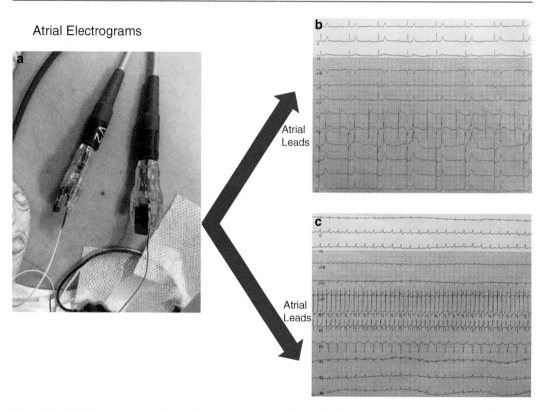

Fig. 20.1 Atrial electrograms—clinical utility and examples. (**a**) Recording an atrial electrogram ("atrial lead study"). Standard ECG patch placement is used except for V1 and V2, which are connected to the atrial wires. A rhythm strip is then obtained for all leads to look for the relationship between atrial depolarizations (visualized as a large biphasic spike in V1 or V2) and the ventricular response, or to determine the mechanism of atrial tachycardia (i.e. atrial fibrillation vs. flutter vs. sinus tachycar- dia). (**b**) Atrial electrogram demonstrating complete heart block in a patient after mitral valve replacement. The atrial leads (V1, V2) clearly demonstrate regular atrial depolarizations with no relationship between atrial and ventricular electrical activity. (**c**) Atrial electrogram demonstrating atrial flutter with 2:1 conduction in a patient with a regular atrial tachycardia after CABG. Atrial leads (V1, V2) demonstrate regular, uniform flutter waves with 2:1 block

between terminals in bipolar systems, less energy is required to generate potential. This results in a smaller pacemaker "spike" on the surface ECG, as well as a lower potential for interference during dual-chamber pacing.

Placement of Epicardial Pacemaker Leads

Placement of epicardial pacemaker leads is variable between individual surgeons and certainly across institutions. Despite the overall low incidence of clinically significant bradyarrhythmias or AV block necessitating rapid epicardial pacing, the placement of at least one ventricular wire is likely advisable as a back-up strategy.

Frequently, two wires are placed in case one fails or becomes dislodged. Atrial wires may be placed on the right atrial appendage or right atrial free wall. Ventricular wires are generally placed on the right ventricular free wall, though the optimal locations for these wires remains a subject of study [21]. In patients with low left ventricular ejective fraction or diastolic dysfunction, placement of atrial leads for dual-chamber pacing is advisable to optimize cardiac function [22].

Epicardial pacing fails to mimic the true efficiency of native cardiac depolarization [20]. In an effort to improve electromechanical synchrony, investigators have examined different lead locations. Placement of the atrial lead along Bachmann's bundle may improve inter-atrial conduction and potentially prevent POAF [23].

Cardiac resynchronization therapy with dual-chamber, biventricular pacing is well-known to improve outcomes in patients with reduced left ventricular ejection fraction (LVEF) and prolonged QRS [24]. Applying these results to cardiac surgery, it would stand to reason that patients with poor myocardial function would benefit from biventricular pacing. Though dual chamber, synchronous biventricular pacing increased cardiac output in a small cohort of patients undergoing valvular surgery [25], it does not appear to meaningfully impact hemodynamics or recovery in patients with reduced LVEF undergoing CABG [26]. This may be due to differences in LV lead placement relative to cardiac resynchronization therapy (CRT), as response to CRT depends on optimal placement of left ventricular leads to restore mechanical synchrony [27]. As such, placement of biventricular wires and synchronized epicardial biventricular pacing is not widely recommended.

Another limitation of epicardial wire placement is the steady deterioration in lead function in the immediate perioperative period, primarily due to ongoing fibrosis and inflammation. Prior studies have found that atrial and ventricular lead impedances begin decreasing on postoperative day one, and that by postoperative day four, wire thresholds have significantly increased [28]. As such, patients with persistent need for epicardial pacing should have daily checks for lead thresholds to inform the timeframe for potential PPM placement. When no longer required for the patient, epicardial leads should be discontinued. To remove leads, gentle traction is applied to wires while allowing intrinsic cardiac motion to dislodge the wires. Rarely, epicardial pacemaker wire placement and/or removal are associated with complications such as myocardial perforation and cardiac tamponade.

Transitioning to a Permanent Pacemaker

The timing of PPM implantation in a patient with a persistent postoperative pacemaker requirement has not been systematically determined, and likely remains a highly individual-

ized decision. Given that many patients with unanticipated temporary AV block will recover function, it is reasonable to wait four to seven days prior to device implantation. This also allows for removal of chest tubes, which may represent a source of infection in the setting of permanent device placement. However, in high-risk patients (i.e. age >70, multi-valve surgery including the tricuspid, those with pre-existing AV or bundle branch block, and prior valve surgery), early PPM placement may be beneficial in reducing length of stay and promoting recovery. Finally, practitioners should consider the steady decrement in epicardial wire function over the postoperative recovery period and the planned duration of pacing when making these decisions.

Common Functions of Intraoperative Pacemakers

The full spectrum of monitoring and treatment options available with modern implantable pacemakers is beyond the scope of this chapter, but is covered in an excellent review series [1, 29]. Below, the common functions of epicardial pacemaker generators will be reviewed. For reference, a common pacemaker interface is displayed (Fig. 20.2). Additionally, we have included the standard generic pacemaker code (the NBG code) endorsed by the North American Society of Pacing and Electrophysiology (NASPE), now Heart Rhythm Society (HRS) as well as the British Pacing and Electrophysiology Group (BPEG; Table 20.1). Additionally, Table 20.2 includes a list of common pacemaker modes utilized after cardiac surgery, and advantages/disadvantages of each.

Commonly Adjusted Pacemaker Generator Parameters

Mode

For temporary epicardial pacing, typically only the first three components of the NBG code are manipulated—chamber paced, chamber sensed,

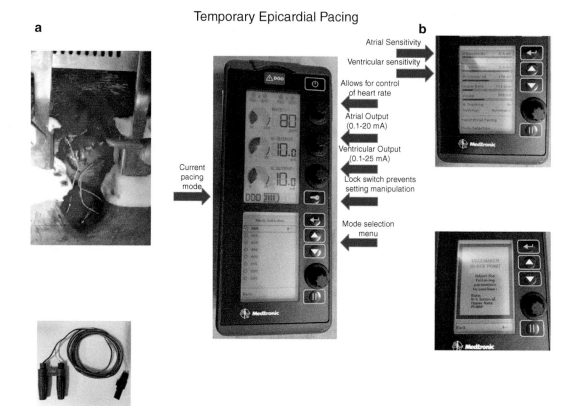

Fig. 20.2 Basic components to temporary epicardial pacemakers. (**a**) Temporary epicardial pacing wires are sutured to the right atrial free wall (image left) and the right ventricular free wall (image right), and then exit the skin. The wires are then connected to a pacemaker adapter (picture below) and plugged into the pacemaker generator. (**a**) Medtronic™5392 Temporary External Pacemaker. This sophisticated dual-chamber pacing system allows for multiple modes of synchronous or asynchronous pacing, as well as rate and output manipulation. (**b**) Common and less-commonly manipulated pacemaker settings, including lead sensitivities, AV interval, and PVARP duration. These settings are adjusted using the dial at the bottom of the generator. (**b**) Pre-programmed safe-guards prevent inappropriate pacemaker settings. In this case, the AV interval was progressively prolonged before the generator recognized the error

Table 20.1 The NASPE/BPEG Generic pacemaker modes

NASPE(HRS)/BPEG Generic Code for Pacemaker Modes				
Position	1	2	3	4	5
Category	Chamber(s) paced	Chamber(s) sensed	Response to sensing	Rate modulation	Multisite Pacing
	A = Atrium	A = Atrium	I=Inhibited	R = Rate modulation	A = Atrium
	V=Ventricle	V=Ventricle	T = Triggered	O=None	V=Ventricle
	D = Dual (A + V)	D = Dual (A + V)	D = Dual (T + I)		D = Dual (A + V)
	O=None	O=None	O=None		O=None

Generic code for Pacemaker Modes. In general, only the first three positions (chambers paced, sensed and response to sensing) apply to temporary epicardial pacemakers

and response to sensing. Specific advantages/disadvantages to each mode are listed in Table 20.2. In general, it is preferable to preserve atrial contraction with the use of a dual- or atrial-pacing mode to optimize cardiac output. Certain cases, however, will necessitate the use of a ventricular pacing strategy. For patients with atrial dysrhythmias or inconsistent atrioventricular conduction, a ventricular pacing strategy is often preferable.

Table 20.2 Commonly used perioperative pacemaker modes

1	2	3	Description	Benefits	Downsides	Notes
D	D	D	AV sequential pacing—both chambers sensed and paced	Allows for intrinsic AV coupling	Potential for rapid ventricular pacing in the setting of atrial arrhythmia	Most common mode of pacing in patients with both atrial and ventricular wires
D	V	I	AV Sequential pacing—ventricular demand pacing	Preserves AV coupling	Can precipitate atrial fibrillation/flutter	(1) Relies on intact atrioventricular conduction (2) Contraindicated in AF/atrial flutter (3) Risk of pacemaker "cross-talk" if ventricular sensitivity too high (4) Immediate treatment of pacemaker-mediated tachycardia (PMT)
D	O	O	AV Sequential pacing—asynchronous/emergency mode	(1) Consistent (programmed) AV coupling interval (2) Not vulnerable to electrocautery interference	Can precipitate ventricular fibrillation via R on T phenomenon	Abnormal dispersion of paced ventricular depolarization reduces mechanical efficiency
V	V	I	Ventricular demand pacing	Consistent ventricular pacing with minimal risk of induced ventricular fibrillation	Negates the atrial contribution to cardiac output	(1) May be used to overdrive suppress ventricular ectopic beats (2) Risk of pacemaker "Cross-talk"
A	A	I	Atrial demand pacing	Preserves AV coupling	Potential risk for precipitating ventricular fibrillation via R on T phenomonon	(1) Relies on intact atrioventricular conduction (2) Contraindicated in AF/Atrial flutter
A	O	O	Asynchronous atrial pacing	(1) Preserves AV coupling (2) Not vulnerable to electrocautery interference	Contraindicated with atrial dysrhythmias	(1) Relies on intact atrioventricular conduction (2) Requires a pacemaker rate that is reliably higher than the intrinsic atrial rate
V	O	O	Asynchronous ventricular pacing	Not vulnerable to electrocautery interference	Can precipitate ventricular fibrillation via R on T phenomenon	May be the "emergency" mode on temporary pacemaker generators

Rate

One of the most basic and frequently manipulated parameters on an epicardial pulse generator is heart rate. Because cardiac output is the product of stroke volume and heart rate, increasing the pacemaker rate (typically to a maximum of 100–110 BPM) is a simple way to increase postoperative cardiac output. Given the combined systolic and diastolic dysfunction that accompanies cardioplegic arrest, a heart rate of 80–90 is likely beneficial while separating from cardiopulmonary bypass. As the patient progresses through the postoperative period, practitioners may desire a period of "back-up" pacing, where the pacemaker is placed into a sensing mode and the programmed rate dropped below the intrinsic rate (e.g. 40 BPM). This allows (A) confirmation that the patient is not experiencing frequent or prolonged bradyarrhythmias and (B) continuous monitoring of the wire sensitivities.

Output/Threshold

The delivered pacemaker stimulus is characterized by amplitude (volts) and pulse duration (ms), both of which impact current utilization and battery life. Stimulation threshold is the minimum amount of energy required to depolarize the myocardium [1]. The pacemaker output, typically measured in milliAmperes (mA), is the amount of current the pacemaker generator directs through the wires. This can be changed independently for the atrial and/or ventricular wires. Output is governed by Ohm's law, whereby I (output) = Voltage across the wires / Resistance across the wires and myocardium. As such, increased resistance, as is seen with aging epicardial wires, will necessitate increases in the output to maintain capture. Unfortunately, increasing the output results in increased fibrosis and hastens decay of lead function.

Pacemaker thresholds are checked by setting the programmed heart rate above the intrinsic rate until consistent pacing is observed. Thereafter, the pacemaker output is progressively reduced until either a P-wave or QRS complex no longer follows each pacer spike for atrial and ventricular wires, respectively. The pacemaker output is then typically set at two times the threshold, or 20 mA, whichever is lower. It is generally inadvisable to check thresholds in patients with an unclear, absent, or non-perfusing underlying rhythm, as loss of capture could result in an inability to regain capture. Practitioners should remember that electrical capture may not reflect mechanical capture, so careful observation of the arterial waveform, pulse oximetry waveform, and/or live echocardiographic images are warranted during threshold checks. Ventricular thresholds >5 mA and/or atrial thresholds >2 mA should promote further investigation [30].

There are multiple clinical conditions and variables that will affect the stimulation threshold of epicardial pacing wires. Myocardial fibrosis, such as in the setting of prior infarction, endo- or epicardial ablations, or longstanding atrial enlargement, will increase stimulation threshold. Metabolic conditions such as hyperkalemia, hyperglycemia, hypoxia, hypercarbia, and metabolic acidosis/alkalosis will all increase stimulation threshold and may cause pacemakers to lose capture. Medications may also affect pacemaker thresholds, with Vaughan Williams Class I agents (e.g. flecainide, propafenone) often increasing thresholds, while catecholamines may decrease stimulation threshold. Additionally, myocardial ischemia alters resting membrane potential and may increase stimulation threshold. In the absence of an obvious cause of increased stimulation thresholds, providers may reverse the polarity of bipolar leads at the level of the pacemaker adapter. This takes advantage of the fact that lead fibrosis is more pronounced at the tip of the electrode, and so changing stimulation polarity may reduce thresholds.

Sensitivity

The pacemaker sensitivity reflects the minimum current that a pacemaker lead will detect, with lower numbers representing better ("higher") sensitivity. In order to test sensitivity, the pacemaker generator has to first be set to a sensing mode, indicated by an A, V, or D in the second column of the pacemaker code—typically AAI, VVI, or DDD. Thereafter, the pacemaker generator's rate is dropped below the intrinsic rate, and the generator examined for the sensing indicator to flash with each intrinsic beat. After this is established, the sensitivity number is increased until (A) the sensing indicator stops and (B) asynchronous pacing begins. The sensitivity number is then reduced until the sensing indicator begins to flash again and asynchronous pacing ceases—an indicator of the sensitivity threshold. The period of asynchronous pacing should be minimized to prevent dysrhythmias resulting from R on T phenomena.

In practice, the sensitivity of each lead is often maintained at half the sensitivity threshold, acknowledging that lead fibrosis will reduce sensed amplitudes. By convention, sensitivities are often empirically set at 2 mV for patients without an intrinsic rhythm, though this low sensitivity can potentially result in inappropriate sensing of T waves. An inappropriately low sensitivity (high sensitivity number) may result in failure to perceive endogenous depolarizations and inappropriate impulse delivery. Conversely, excessively high sensitivity (low sensitivity number) can cause inappropriate pacemaker inhibition due to over-sensing [1].

Less Frequently Adjusted Parameters

AV Interval

Similar to the intrinsic AV interval, the pacemaker generator AV interval represents the longest potential interval between an atrial and ventricular depolarization. Given that the AV interval of a paced beat is generally longer than that of an intrinsic beat, it may be advantageous to make this setting slightly longer than the intrinsic AV interval (denoted on the surface ECG as the PR interval) to achieve similar electromechanical coupling. In practice, AV interval is highly individualized and may be titrated to achieve optimal cardiac output by comparing continuous indices of cardiac performance, such as catheter- or echocardiographically-derived cardiac output [31].

Post-Ventricular Atrial Refractory Period (PVARP) and Upper Tracking Rate

A safeguard against pacemaker-mediated tachycardia, the PVARP is only relevant in atrial-sensed modes of pacing (DDD, VDD), and represents the refractory period of the atria after a ventricular spike. When the PVARP is very low, potential retrograde conduction (or far-field sensing) from ventricular beats may be sensed as an atrial depolarization and trigger a ventricular depolarization. Increasing the PVARP guards against this complication, but may reduce the maximum atrial tracking rate through increasing the total atrial refractory period (TARP, a combination of the programmed AV interval + PVARP). The PVARP may need to be adjusted to account for inter-individual variability in retrograde AV conduction times, though we recommend this be done in concert with Electrophysiology consultants. As a safety measure, the upper tracking rate represents the fastest ventricular rate the generator will deliver in response to atrial depolarizations. At atrial rates above the maximum tracking rate, the pacemaker generator will begin to pro-

gressively lengthen the AV interval (and thus the TARP), introducing a 4:3 "Pseudo-Wenckebach" block. This gradual AV interval lengthening and introduction of AV block prevents a dramatic decrease in cardiac output. As atrial rates increase, the interval between each P wave may shorten below the TARP. In this case, every other P wave falls within the PVARP of the preceding beat, and a 2:1 AV blockade is introduced, resulting in a rate that is equivalent to 60,000/TARP. Appearance of a new AV block in a patient with an epicardial pacemaker should prompt further investigation. Most pacemaker generators will automatically determine maximum tracking rate based upon the PVARP and AVI. However, given the potential detrimental effects of rapid tachycardias in the postoperative cardiac surgical patient, we recommend an upper tracking rate less than 130BPM, and certainly less than the 2:1 block rate (60,000/TARP).

Pulse Duration

In order to propagate an electrical wavefront, an impulse must be delivered not only at the appropriate strength, but for the appropriate duration of time. There is a somewhat complex exponential relationship (Strength-Duration Curve) between delivered electrical impulse strength and pulse duration whereby much higher voltage is required at short pulse durations. Though uncommonly manipulated, clinicians may occasionally increase pulse duration and decrease pulse amplitude in order to minimize far-field sensing or off-target pacing (i.e. phrenic pacing). In the case of implantable pacemakers, pulse duration and amplitude may be manipulated to optimize battery life.

Troubleshooting Common Problems with Epicardial Pacing

Failure to Capture

One of the most common problems with epicardial pacemakers, failure to capture, is the defined

Table 20.3 Troubleshooting common epicardial pacemaker problems

Problem	Differential Diagnosis	Signs	Causes	Troubleshooting
Unexpected bradycardia HR lower than set rate	Output failure ("failure to pace")	Inappropriate lack of pacemaker output *Absence of pacing spikes on surface ECG*	Lead/cable malfunction Depleted generator battery Oversensing Cross-talk	(1) Prepare for an appropriate backup mode of pacing (2) Check generator power, battery life, connections (3) Increase output to maximum (4) Switch to asynchronous mode with appropriate rate (5) EP consultation after stability established
	Failure to capture	Appropriate pacemaker output without measurable cardiac contraction *Pacing spikes visualized on surface ECG*	Fibrosis around pacemaker lead Metabolic abnormalities (hyperkalemia) Acid-base abnormalities (acidosis/alkalosis) Medications (anti-arrhythmics) Myocardial ischemia	(1) Prepare for an appropriate backup mode of pacing (2) Check generator power, battery life, connections (3) Increase output to maximum (4) Stop offending medications, correct metabolic abnormalities (5) Reverse pacemaker lead polarity (6) Create unipolar circuit (7) Consider EP consultation for durable pacing strategy
Unexpected tachycardia HR higher than set rate	Intrinsic change in rate	Gradual increase in rate Sudden increase in rate	Sinus tachycardia Atrial or ventricular dysrhythmia	(1) Ensure hemodynamic stability (2) Investigate underlying causes (1) Ensure hemodynamic stability (2) Treat with appropriate anti-arrhythmics
	Sensing errors	Continued atrial pacing despite intrinsic > set rate Ventricular-paced tachycardia in dual-chamber pacemaker mode (DDD, VDD)	Undersensing Pacemaker-mediated tachycardia	(1) Ensure hemodynamic stability (2) If undersensing suspected, reduce sensitivity of atrial leads (3) If PMT suspected, switch to VVI/DVI mode

as the absence of measurable cardiac contraction in response to a successfully delivered epicardial pulse (Table 20.3). From a practical standpoint, this may be noted as a lack of arterial waveform or photoplethysmographic waveform despite visualization of a pacing spike on the surface ECG. Failure to capture may be caused by a number of processes, including lead fibrosis, electrolyte abnormalities that make the heart refractory to pacing (acidosis, alkalosis, hyperkalemia), myocardial ischemia, and anti-arrhythmic drugs. The first step in troubleshooting failure to capture is to ensure hemodynamic stability and the availability of alternative modes of pacing, should the patient require temporary pacing. After correction of any reversible causes, failure to capture may be mitigated by reversing the polarity of the epicardial leads. In the case of bipolar leads, the distal lead (anode) often experiences more fibrosis than the proximal lead, which can be used as the a negative unipolar electrode, provided a return electrode is placed in the subcutaneous tissues. After acute treatment of failure to capture, providers must predict the anticipated duration of pacing and generate an alternative strategy, such as placing a temporary or permanent transvenous pacer.

Failure to capture must be differentiated from failure to pace, where no electrical impulse is delivered to the tip of the pacing wire and a pacing spike is not seen on the surface ECG. Mechanical causes of failure to pace include depleted generator batteries or lead malfunction, while over-sensing and pacemaker cross-talk (covered below) are other potential cause of failure to pace. In the setting of failure to pace, switching to an asynchronous mode will differentiate mechanical causes (continued failure to pace) from other causes (appropriate pacing delivered).

Cross-Talk Inhibition

Pacemaker cross-talk is a phenomenon of dual-chamber systems that results from inappropriate sensing of a delivered stimulus from one wire as intrinsic electrical activity in the other wire. This is distinguished from over-sensing in which small electrical currents, such as those generated by skeletal muscle contraction, electromagnetic interference, or intermittent contact between pacing wires, are interpreted as intrinsic depolarizations, thus inhibiting appropriate pacing. The most common example of cross-talk occurs in the setting of dual-chamber pacing and ventricular sensing (DDD, DDI, DVI), where the atrial pacemaker spike is detected by the ventricular wire as a ventricular

depolarization, and thus ventricular pacing inhibited. In the setting of complete heart block, this effectively halts cardiac output and is very poorly tolerated. A more benign version occurs in the setting of atrial-sensed dual-chamber modes, where a delivered ventricular pulse is interpreted as an atrial depolarization, and thus atrial pacing inhibited. Basic approaches to reducing cross-talk are to (A) reduce the output of the offending lead or (B) reduce the sensitivity of the inhibited lead. Given the potential disastrous nature of cross-talk, most epicardial pacemaker generators employ a ventricular blanking period immediately following atrial depolarization in which ventricular depolarizations (or inappropriately detected atrial depolarizations) are ignored.

Pacemaker-Mediated Tachycardia (PMT)

Pacemaker-mediated tachycardia becomes a problem with dual-chamber pacemakers in a ventricular pacing mode (DDD or VDD) when a delivered ventricular impulse is sensed by the atrial wires as an intrinsic atrial depolarization, leading to an additional delivered ventricular impulse. Functionally, this may result from either far-field atrial sensing of a ventricular spike or retrograde conduction (through the AV node or an accessory pathway) of a ventricular depolarization. In order to prevent this complication, pacemakers employ a PVARP, which should be programmed to account for the speed of retrograde conduction through an accessory pathway and/or the AV node. Given the inter-individual variability of retrograde conduction speed, the PVARP may need to be adjusted for each individual patient. In general, a longer PVARP guards more effectively against PMT, but also limits the upper atrial tracking rate. In the acute post-surgical period, this does not meaningfully impact recovery, but may impact rate-responsiveness of indwelling pacemakers.

Recommendations for Epicardial Pacing After Cardiac Surgery

Temporary epicardial pacing adds a safety margin to cardiac surgery, allowing providers to manipulate heart rate and guard against temporary disturbances in atrioventricular conduction. However, the epicardial delivery of electrical impulses, though minute, should be viewed as an impactful therapy—similar to prescribing vasoactive medications, and treated with the same weight. Inappropriate epicardial pacemaker settings may decrease the effectiveness of cardiac contractions or even predispose patients to deleterious and potentially fatal cardiac dysrhythmias.

In general, native electrical conduction is more effective than epicardial pacing, so in patients with effective native conduction, pacemakers should be placed in a "backup" sensing mode of pacing at the lowest heart rate deemed acceptable by the care team. This can be accomplished with either atrial or ventricular pacing modes set below the intrinsic rate, though it should be noted that in patients at risk of complete heart block, an atrial backup mode will not guarantee a cardiac output in the setting of bradycardia coupled with AV block. Many providers find that VVI pacing set to a rate of 40 or 50 BPM adequately protects patients from profound bradycardia, provided that wire sensitivities and output settings are appropriate.

No matter the selected location of epicardial pacing (atrial, ventricular, or dual-chamber) a sincere effort should be made to avoid asynchronous modes of pacing. In some circumstances, such as directly after bypass separation and while electrocautery is being used for hemostasis prior to chest closure, an asynchronous mode may avoid missed beats should cautery be sensed as intrinsic depolarizations with the pacemaker in a synchronous mode. However, the hemodynamic consequences of an occasional missed beat are less than that of a provoked arrhythmia, particularly a ventricular arrhythmia. In our practice, pacemakers are switched to a synchronous mode at the time of chest closure, with this setting confirmed by the OR nurses at the time of OR departure.

Care of the cardiac surgical patient with implantable cardiac devices, including pacemakers and/or ICDs, bears special mention. Though guidelines exist for the care of the perioperative patient with a cardiovascular implantable electronic device (CIED) [32], cardiac surgery represents a period in which device parameters are routinely manipulated. At the time of cardiac surgery, it is generally safe to place external defibrillating pads and disable any potential tachytherapies on a patient's device. Similarly, it is reasonable to manipulate the lower rate limit on a patient's indwelling device in order to optimize cardiac output and prepare for bypass separation. However, these changes should be clearly documented in the operative record, reversed as soon as appropriate, and accompanied by a formal device interrogation prior to the patient leaving the intensive care unit. Optimal treatment of these patients is dependent upon the close collaborative relationship between electrophysiologists, cardiothoracic anesthesiologists, cardiac surgeons, and intensivists.

References

1. Mulpuru SK, Madhavan M, McLeod CJ, Cha YM, Friedman PA. Cardiac pacemakers: Function, troubleshooting, and management: Part 1 of a 2-part series. J Am Coll Cardiol. 2017;69:189–210.
2. Ellenbogen KaK, K. Cardiac pacing and icds. 2014.
3. Shen MJ, Zipes DP. Role of the autonomic nervous system in modulating cardiac arrhythmias. Circ Res. 2014;114:1004–21.
4. Fudim M, Boortz-Marx R, Ganesh A, Waldron NH, Qadri YJ, Patel CB, Milano CA, Sun AY, Mathew JP, Piccini JP. Stellate ganglion blockade for the treatment of refractory ventricular arrhythmias: a systematic review and meta-analysis. J Cardiovasc Electrophysiol. 2017;28(12):1460–7.
5. Mathew JP, Fontes ML, Tudor IC, Ramsay J, Duke P, Mazer CD, Barash PG, Hsu PH, Mangano DT, Investigators of the Ischemia R, Education F, Multicenter Study of Perioperative Ischemia Research G. A multicenter risk index for atrial fibrillation after cardiac surgery, Jama. 2004;291:1720–9.

6. Mitchell LB, Exner DV, Wyse DG, Connolly CJ, Prystai GD, Bayes AJ, Kidd WT, Kieser T, Burgess JJ, Ferland A, MacAdams CL, Maitland A. Prophylactic oral amiodarone for the prevention of arrhythmias that begin early after revascularization, valve replacement, or repair: Papabear: a randomized controlled trial. JAMA. 2005;294:3093–100.

7. Kertai MD, Li YW, Li YJ, Shah SH, Kraus WE, Fontes ML, Stafford-Smith M, Newman MF, Podgoreanu MV, Mathew JP, Duke Perioperative G, Safety Outcomes Investigative T. G protein-coupled receptor kinase 5 gene polymorphisms are associated with postoperative atrial fibrillation after coronary artery bypass grafting in patients receiving beta-blockers. Circ Cardiovasc Genet. 2014;7:625–33.

8. Arsenault KA, Yusuf AM, Crystal E, Healey JS, Morillo CA, Nair GM, Whitlock RP. Interventions for preventing post-operative atrial fibrillation in patients undergoing heart surgery. Cochrane Database Syst Rev. 2013:CD003611.

9. LaPar DJ, Speir AM, Crosby IK, Fonner E Jr, Brown M, Rich JB, Quader M, Kern JA, Kron IL, Ailawadi G, Investigators for the Virginia Cardiac Surgery Quality I. Postoperative atrial fibrillation significantly increases mortality, hospital readmission, and hospital costs. Ann Thorac Surg. 2014;98:527–33. discussion 533

10. Mouws E, Yaksh A, Knops P, Kik C, Boersma E, Bogers A, de Groot NMS. Early ventricular tachyarrhythmias after coronary artery bypass grafting surgery: is it a real burden? J Cardiol. 2017;70:263–70.

11. Ascione R, Reeves BC, Santo K, Khan N, Angelini GD. Predictors of new malignant ventricular arrhythmias after coronary surgery: a case-control study. J Am Coll Cardiol. 2004;43:1630–8.

12. Bethea BT, Salazar JD, Grega MA, Doty JR, Fitton TP, Alejo DE, Borowicz LM Jr, Gott VL, Sussman MS, Baumgartner WA. Determining the utility of temporary pacing wires after coronary artery bypass surgery. Ann Thorac Surg. 2005;79:104–7.

13. Khorsandi M, Muhammad I, Shaikhrezai K, Pessotto R. Is it worth placing ventricular pacing wires in all patients post-coronary artery bypass grafting? Interact Cardiovasc Thorac Surg. 2012;15:489–93.

14. Koplan BA, Stevenson WG, Epstein LM, Aranki SF, Maisel WH. Development and validation of a simple risk score to predict the need for permanent pacing after cardiac valve surgery. J Am Coll Cardiol. 2003;41:795–801.

15. Rene AG, Sastry A, Horowitz JM, Cheung J, Liu CF, Thomas G, Ip JE, Lerman BB, Markowitz SM. Recovery of atrioventricular conduction after pacemaker placement following cardiac valvular surgery. J Cardiovasc Electrophysiol. 2013;24:1383–7.

16. Siontis GC, Juni P, Pilgrim T, Stortecky S, Bullesfeld L, Meier B, Wenaweser P, Windecker S. Predictors of permanent pacemaker implantation in patients with severe aortic stenosis undergoing tavr: a meta-analysis. J Am Coll Cardiol. 2014;64:129–40.

17. Regueiro A, Abdul-Jawad Altisent O, Del Trigo M, Campelo-Parada F, Puri R, Urena M, Philippon F, Rodes-Cabau J. Impact of new-onset left bundle branch block and periprocedural permanent pacemaker implantation on clinical outcomes in patients undergoing transcatheter aortic valve replacement: a systematic review and meta-analysis. Circ Cardiovasc Interv. 2016;9:e003635.

18. Wallace A, Lam HW, Nose PS, Bellows W, Mangano DT. Changes in systolic and diastolic ventricular function with cold cardioplegic arrest in man. The multicenter study of perioperative ischemia (mcspi) research group. J Card Surg. 1994;9:497–502.

19. Maisel WH, Epstein AE, American College of Chest P. The role of cardiac pacing: American college of chest physicians guidelines for the prevention and management of postoperative atrial fibrillation after cardiac surgery. Chest. 2005;128:36S–8S.

20. Reade MC. Temporary epicardial pacing after cardiac surgery: a practical review: Part 1: General considerations in the management of epicardial pacing. Anaesthesia. 2007;62:264–71.

21. Hurle A, Gomez-Plana J, Sanchez J, Martinez JG, Meseguer J, Llamas P. Optimal location for temporary epicardial pacing leads following open heart surgery. PACE. 2002;25:1049–52.

22. Curtis J, Walls J, Boley T, Reid J, Flaker G, Madigan N, Alpert M. Influence of atrioventricular synchrony on hemodynamics in patients with normal and low ejection fractions following open heart surgery. Am Surg. 1986;52:93–6.

23. Goette A, Mittag J, Friedl A, Busk H, Jepsen MS, Hartung WM, Huth C, Klein HU. Pacing of Bachmann's bundle after coronary artery bypass grafting. PACE. 2002;25:1072–8.

24. Prinzen FW, Vernooy K, Auricchio A. Cardiac resynchronization therapy: state-of-the-art of current applications, guidelines, ongoing trials, and areas of controversy. Circulation. 2013;128:2407–18.

25. Berberian G, Quinn TA, Kanter JP, Curtis LJ, Cabreriza SE, Weinberg AD, Spotnitz HM. Optimized biventricular pacing in atrioventricular block after cardiac surgery. Ann Thorac Surg. 2005;80:870–5.

26. Eberhardt F, Heringlake M, Massalme MS, Dyllus A, Misfeld M, Sievers HH, Wiegand UK, Hanke T. The effect of biventricular pacing after coronary artery bypass grafting: a prospective randomized trial of different pacing modes in patients with reduced left ventricular function. J Thorac Cardiovasc Surg. 2009;137:1461–7.

27. Seo Y, Ishizu T, Sakamaki F, Yamamoto M, Machino T, Yamasaki H, Kawamura R, Yoshida K, Sekiguchi Y, Kawano S, Tada H, Watanabe S, Aonuma K. Mechanical dyssynchrony assessed by speckle tracking imaging as a reliable predictor of acute and chronic response to cardiac resynchronization therapy. J Am Soc Echocardiogr. 2009;22:839–46.

28. Elmi F, Tullo NG, Khalighi K. Natural history and predictors of temporary epicardial pacemaker wire func-

tion in patients after open heart surgery. Cardiology. 2002;98:175–80.

29. Madhavan M, Mulpuru SK, McLeod CJ, Cha YM, Friedman PA. Advances and future directions in cardiac pacemakers: Part 2 of a 2-part series. J Am Coll Cardiol. 2017;69:211–35.

30. Sullivan BL, Bartels K, Hamilton N. Insertion and management of temporary pacemakers. Semin Cardiothorac Vasc Anesth. 2016;20:52–62.

31. Durbin CG Jr, Kopel RF. Optimal atrioventricular (av) pacing interval during temporary av sequential pacing after cardiac surgery. J Cardiothorac Vasc Anesth. 1993;7:316–20.

32. Crossley GH, Poole JE, Rozner MA, Asirvatham SJ, Cheng A, Chung MK, Ferguson TB Jr, Gallagher JD, Gold MR, Hoyt RH, Irefin S, Kusumoto FM, Moorman LP, Thompson A. The heart rhythm society (hrs)/american society of anesthesiologists (asa) expert consensus statement on the perioperative management of patients with implantable defibrillators, pacemakers and arrhythmia monitors: Facilities and patient management this document was developed as a joint project with the american society of anesthesiologists (asa), and in collaboration with the american heart association (aha), and the society of thoracic surgeons (sts). Heart Rhythm. 2011;8:1114–54.

Weaning from CPB

21

Annette Vegas

Main Messages
1. Successful weaning from CPB requires adequate preparation and a thorough understanding of cardiac physiology, pharmacology and MCS.
2. Low CO, low MAP, high preload and poor myocardial oxygen delivery accompanies the critical period of myocardial dysfunction during CPB weaning.
3. Anticipating the difficult wean and the introduction of timely interventions may alter patient outcomes.
4. Newer therapies to manage acute decompensated heart failure have yet to be studied in the role of weaning.

Weaning from cardiopulmonary bypass (CPB) is the transition during cardiac surgery from temporary total mechanical support back to the patient's native circulation. As there are no universally accepted guidelines, successful weaning is based on institutional practice, teamwork and the experience of the intraoperative team [1].

A. Vegas (✉)
University Health Network, Toronto General Hospital, Toronto, ON, Canada
e-mail: annette.vegas@uhn.ca

Preparation for Weaning from CPB

The goal of CPB is to provide extracorporeal cardiopulmonary support by diverting blood into a heart-lung machine which performs the functions of (A) respiration (ventilation, oxygenation); (B) circulation and (C) temperature regulation. Circulation in the patient depends on the pump flow rate which is adjusted to any level, and in normothermic adults ranges from 2.2–2.5 L/min/$m^2 \times$ BSA (m^2). Maintenance of cardiovascular stability during CPB involves the interplay of machine function and patient factors such as afterload and venous compliance.

In preparation for weaning from CPB attention is paid to the details outlined in Table 21.1 to ensure a safe effective process. Fortunately, many patients require little or no support to successfully wean. Collaboration, communication and a standardized approach are vital to avoiding errors which may expose the patient to serious complications.

Although **temperature** management during CPB varies between institutions, in 90% of patients the temperature drifts to maintain mild hypothermia at 32–34 °C [2]. When indicated, active cooling to 20 °C facilitates deep hypothermic circulatory arrest. Currently there is no recommended temperature to wean; the choice must balance the deleterious effects of cerebral hyperthermia and post-CPB systemic hypother-

© Springer Nature Switzerland AG 2021
D. C. H. Cheng et al. (eds.), *Evidence-Based Practice in Perioperative Cardiac Anesthesia and Surgery*, https://doi.org/10.1007/978-3-030-47887-2_21

Table 21.1 Checklist prior to weaning from CPB

Goal	Action
• Surgery complete	Heart de-aired
• Core temperature	36°–36.5 °C
• Reperfusion time	> 8 min
• Metabolic milieu	HCT > 20%, K^+ < 6.0 meq/L, HCO_3 > 20 mmol
• Stable HR/rhythm	Sinus rhythm 80–100 bpm
• Ventilator on	100% FiO_2, PCO_2 < 40 mmHg
• Monitors re-zeroed	Arterial line discrepancy
• Additional volume	Blood products, colloid, crystalloids
• Additional support	Drugs and mechanical

mia. The absolute temperature for weaning is less important than avoidance of rapid rewarming to prevent inadvertent cerebral hyperthermia. Excessive rewarming (>37 °C) increases morbidities of neurocognitive decline, delirium, mediastinitis, and acute kidney injury. Core temperature values vary with the monitoring site, with nasopharyngeal and bladder temperature sites underestimating cerebral temperature. The blood temperature at the pump arterial outlet better indicates cerebral temperature and is maintained <37 °C to avoid cerebral hyperthermia.

Cardiac **reperfusion time** is the time from aortic clamp removal to weaning. A minimum of eight minutes reperfusion time replenishes myocardial ATP stores and washes out metabolites from the coronary circulation. Different reperfusion strategies have been proposed to minimize myocardial reperfusion injury, although none have proven to be superior [3].

An adequate **metabolic milieu** is essential for myocardial performance and is assessed from the warm arterial blood gas (ABG) drawn by the perfusionist during reperfusion. The optimal hematocrit (Hct) during CPB is ill-defined. Most patients will tolerate a low Hct (20%), but those with compromised ventricular and/or end-organ function may benefit from a higher Hct (>24%). The serum potassium (K^+) should be <6.0 mEq/L at weaning to avoid conduction abnormalities and myocardial dysfunction. Administration of intravenous calcium, insulin (and glucose) or furosemide can reduce hyper-

kalemia. Metabolic and respiratory acidosis is treated to avert myocardial depression, reduced catecholamine activity and increased pulmonary vascular resistance (PVR). Normalizing the blood bicarbonate (HCO_3^-) level to around 20 mmol/L is an important consideration, particularly if a difficult wean is anticipated. Tight control of endogenous hyperglycemia may have some beneficial effects but does not reduce the need for inotropic or anti-arrhythmic therapy post-CPB [4].

During weaning the patient requires a faster **heart rate** (HR) of 80–100 bpm to maintain an adequate cardiac output (CO) as compensation for a lower stroke volume due to myocardial dysfunction. Sinus rhythm is preferred to exploit optimal ventricular filling by the atria. In particular, small hypertrophied or large dilated ventricles with a limited stroke volume benefit from the faster HR and optimal atrial filling. For many patients a stable HR and rhythm is the decisive factor to successful weaning. A slow HR responds to pacing (atrial, sequential atrio-ventricular or ventricular) using temporary epicardial pacer wires placed on the surface of the right atrium and right ventricle (RV). Rarely, alternative pacing options such as LV pacing, multisite RV pacing or atrio-biventricular pacing can facilitate a difficult wean. An intrinsic fast HR often decreases with cardiac filling. Reducing or eliminating exogenous catecholamines, administering beta-blockers or electrical cardioversion of a supraventricular tachycardia may reduce the HR. Persistent ventricular irritability (tachycardia or fibrillation) after aortic unclamping may imply inadequate myocardial protection, hypoperfusion or persisting ischemia. Management options include epicardial defibrillation (5–100 J); raising systemic mean arterial pressure (MAP); correcting the metabolic milieu; and/or administering intravenous antiarrhythmics such as magnesium sulphate (1–2 g), lidocaine (1–1.5 mg/kg) or amiodarone (150 mg). Surgical management of refractory ventricular arrhythmias may involve insertion of a LV vent to decompress the heart or re-arresting the heart with cardioplegia.

The lungs are re-expanded with 2–3 sustained breaths to a peak pressure of 30–40 cmH$_2$O with visual confirmation of bilateral lung expansion. In addition to recruiting atelectatic areas, this maneuver helps remove trapped air in the pulmonary veins. Inspired FiO$_2$ is 90–100% and the minute **ventilation** is adjusted to maintain a PaCO$_2$ of 40 mmHg. Ventilation may resume during pulsatile flow (partial CPB) or just prior to weaning. A recent meta-analysis of RCTs for ventilation during CPB showed immediate improvement in post-CPB oxygenation but no effect on postoperative lung morbidity or long-term prognosis [5].

The choice of monitors during cardiac surgery is often patient specific and based on institutional practice. Invasive **arterial** systolic blood pressure (SBP) or MAP serves as a surrogate for the adequacy of tissue perfusion. There may be an initial discrepancy between a lower peripheral arterial SBP and higher central aortic root pressure, which gradually resolves over the post-CPB period [6]. During this time more accurate BP monitoring may be obtained from (A) non-invasive BP cuff; (B) transducing the aortic root line; or (C) inserting a femoral arterial line. Ventricular filling is invasively monitored using central venous pressure (CVP) or pulmonary artery (PA) diastolic pressure. TEE assesses the adequacy of de-airing during open-heart procedures prior to weaning.

The perfusionist determines whether there is sufficient **volume** in the pump to wean. Pump volume is affected by patient intravascular volume, venous drainage, hemoconcentration or diuresis and the cardioplegia volume. Administration of volume in the form of crystalloids, colloids or blood products may be required to optimize patient preload.

Low CO, low MAP, high preload and poor myocardial oxygen delivery accompanies the critical period of myocardial dysfunction during weaning. Depending on institutional practice, routinely administered **drugs** as well as additional inotropes, vasopressors, vasodilators and mechanical support should be readily available to assist the patient as needed.

Weaning from CPB

For a brief period the perfusionist leaves blood in the patient by partially clamping the venous line. The right heart fills and ejects as the CVP and PA traces become pulsatile. Pump flow in the aortic cannula is reduced as the patient's native circulation gradually begins to function. Patients with preserved heart function will tolerate a rapid wean with abrupt clamping of the venous line, while those with poor heart function benefit from a stepwise reduction in pump flows. In the presence of an adequate BP (SBP > 80 mmHg, MAP >60 mmHg) and reasonable preload CPB is discontinued. The venous line is completely clamped and the aortic pump head is turned off. The patient is now off CPB. An algorithm for weaning from CPB is provided as Fig. 21.1.

Integration of hemodynamic parameters with TEE assessment provides information about the cardiac status of the patient. During weaning cardiac filling is monitored by visual inspection of the RV, TEE examination of the LV and measurement of CVP or PA pressures, which should approximate pre-CPB values. Patients with a stiff or a dilated ventricle require additional volume, transfused in100cc increments through the aortic root line, to increase filling pressures and optimize preload immediately after weaning. Titration of volume is important to limit cardiac overdistension which further compromises ventricular contractility. Most patients tolerate a low SBP (60–80 mmHg) for 5 min before the hemodynamics improve, often without any support. In the setting of low SBP and adequate filling pressures the measured CO and calculated systemic vascular resistance (SVR) provide further data on whether to manipulate contractility or afterload.

Failure to Wean from CPB

If the patient is doing poorly the most expedient solution is to go back on CPB for reperfusion. Investigations by TEE, ECG, ABG, and Doppler of coronary graft patency may identify the etiology of a failed wean as: (A) incomplete surgery;

Fig. 21.1 Algorithm weaning from CPB. *CI* cardiac index, *ECMO* extracorporeal membrane oxygenation, *IABP* intra-aortic balloon pump, *HR* heart rate, *MAP* mean arteral pressure, *NO* nitric oxide, *NTG* nitroglycerin, *PDI* phosphodiesterase inhibitor, *PVR* pulmonary vascular resisitance, *SNP* sodium nitroprusside, *SvO₂* venous oxygen saturation, *SVR* systemic vascular resistance, *VAD* ventricular assist device

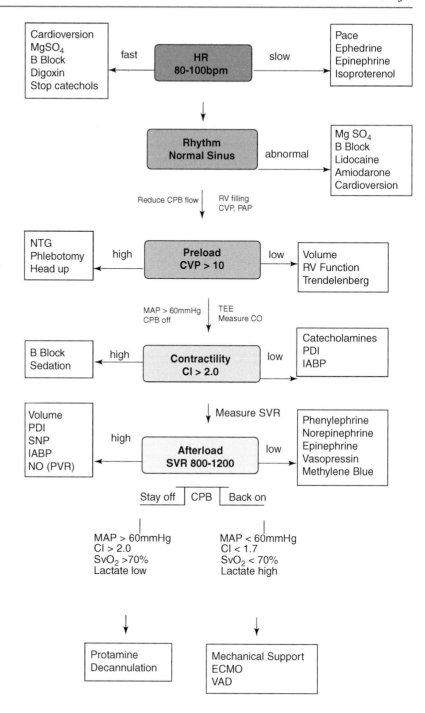

(B) ventricular dysfunction; (C) inadequate or excessive preload; (D) inadequate HR and rhythm; or (E) abnormal SVR. There is no simple recipe of drugs or magic formula to memorize; instead, the management options for these patients are individualized (Table 21.2). In the absence of a clear etiology the patient may simply benefit from additional reperfusion time prior to another attempt to wean. Specific surgical interventions may entail revision or additional bypass graft, valve replacement, paravalvular leak repair or management of surgical bleeding.

Table 21.2 Management options for difficult wean from CPB

Left ventricular failure	Right ventricular failure	Vasoplegia	Dynamic outflow
Catecholamine	Catecholamine	Catecholamine	Additional surgery
Dobutamine	Norepinephrine ± NTG	Norepinephrine	MV Repair/Replace
Epinephrine	Epinephrine	Epinephrine	Septal myectomy
Norepinephrine	Isoproterenol	Phenylephrine	Increase preload
Dopamine	Non-catecholamine	Non-catecholamine	Slow HR
Non-catecholamine	Milrinone	Vasopressin	Stop inotropes
Milrinone	Nitric oxide	Methylene blue	Phenylephrine
Levosimendan	PGE_1		Beta blockers
Mechanical	Avoid N_2O, acidosis, low PO_2		
IABP	Mechanical		
VAD	± IABP		
ECMO	VAD		
	ECMO		

Table 21.3 Risk Factors for LCOS and Vasoplegia

Low Cardiac Output (LCOS)		Vasoplegia	
Patient	Procedure	Patient	Procedure
Low EF	Emergency	High EuroScore	Protamine
Recent MI	Redo surgery	Myocardial dysfunction	Long CPB time
Female	± Valve surgery	Diabetes	Transfusion
Older	X-clamp time	Thyroid disease	IABP
Diabetes		BMI > 30	Surgical Procedure
Left Main, 3 Vessel		Heparin IV	VAD
Disease		ACEI, ARB	Heart transplant
		B Blockers	Endocarditis
		CCB	

Difficult to Wean Patient

There is no agreed upon definition for the difficult to wean patient, though hemodynamic instability obliges the use of more than one pharmacologic agent or mechanical circulatory support (MCS) to achieve adequate tissue perfusion. Identifying patients at risk for a difficult wean may prevent a failed wean leading to prolonged CPB duration with the probability for more myocardial damage, coagulopathy and shock. A precise definition of post-cardiotomy cardiogenic shock (PCCS) is lacking but involves failure to wean from CPB and the need for major pharmacologic and MCS. PCCS is a difficult to manage often lethal form of acute heart failure that occurs in 0.2–6% of cardiac surgery patients.

Recognized risk factors associated with the perioperative use of inotropes to manage low cardiac output syndrome (LCOS) [7] and vasopressors for vasoplegia [8] have been identified (Table 21.3). The recognition and institution of any pharmacotherapy to manage LCOS or vaso-plegia increases morbidity and mortality in this surgical population. Contributing factors to a difficult wean include existing and developing problems with (A) systolic myocardial function; (B) vasoplegia; (C) diastolic dysfunction; and (D) pulmonary hypertension.

Myocardial dysfunction after cardiac surgery is a common problem, with initial preserved function, deterioration over 4–6 h, then gradual to complete recovery within 24 h. Preoperative myocardial dysfunction prolongs the recovery period, but without necessarily needing much additional support to wean. Loss or impaired function of myocytes reduces cardiac pump action and oxygen delivery resulting in LCOS [9]. Myocardial stunning refers to reversible areas of post-ischemic myocardial dysfunction after hypoxic injury or reperfusion with normal coronary flow. Stunned myocardium responds to inotropes indicating recruitable ATP stores. Inotropes will not reverse actively ischemic myocardium. The distinction between irreversible cardiogenic shock and transient postoperative cardiac stunning is important as each is associated with different hospital courses and outcomes.

CPB may induce a vasoplegia syndrome that is characterized by profound hypotension from severe peripheral vasodilatation [8]. There is reduced arteriolar reactivity from vascular smooth muscle relaxation that is mediated by nitric oxide, altered K-ATP channels, and vasopressin depletion. Vasoplegia syndrome may be defined as MAP <60 mmHg, CI > 2.5 L/min, and/or catecholamine dependence. Risk factors for this syndrome are listed in Table 21.3. Vasoplegia syndrome occurs in 10–20% of cardiac surgery patients with a higher incidence and mortality rate in ventricular assist device (VAD), heart transplant and septic patients. Management includes increasing intravascular volume and vasopressor therapy with catecholamines, vasopressin or methylene blue.

Diastolic dysfunction (DD) with or without preserved systolic function results in abnormal relaxation and filling from (A) tachycardia; (B) reduced myocardial compliance; and (C) impaired relaxation. DD itself presents as a spectrum of severity from mild (impaired relaxation), moderate (pseudonormal) and severe (restrictive filling). DD occurs in 30% of cardiac surgery patients with a higher incidence in valve, ischemic, hypertensive and elderly patients. The presence of DD may represent an early sign of myocardial ischemia and is predictive of a difficult wean from CPB [10].

Altered preload (volume overload), afterload (high PA pressure), and coronary perfusion (RCA lesion) impairs RV contractility. Pre-existing pulmonary hypertension allows the RV to compensate by increasing wall thickness and displacement of the interventricular septum leftward during the cardiac cycle. Maintenance of diastolic arterial pressure by pharmacologic or MCS prevents decompensation of RV function.

Pharmacotherapy

The choice and dosing of pharmacologic agents depends on the pathophysiology of the patient's pre-existing heart disease and concomitant reperfusion injury. The ideal inotropic drug would increase contractility and ventricular ejection without elevating HR, SVR, and myocardial oxygen consumption (MVO_2). There is no ideal inotrope at present with surprisingly little evidence to support the use of individual agents in weaning or improving important clinical outcomes. Meta-analysis [11] have confirmed that after weaning, goal directed therapy with fluids and inotropes can optimize oxygen consumption and delivery and reduce (A) mortality; (B) vasopressor requirements; (C) duration of inotropic therapy and ventilation; and (D) hospital and ICU length of stay (LOS) in cardiac surgery patients.

Calcium Chloride (CaCl$_2$)

Ionized calcium (Cai) concentrations vary during CPB. Severe ionized hypocalcemia reduces myocardial contractility and SVR, though mild hypocalcemia (Cai > 0.80 mmol/L) has little detrimental effect. In normocalcemic patients calcium chloride ($CaCl_2$) in 5–10 mg/kg (0.5–1.0 g) doses administered by the perfusionist during separation from CPB raises blood Cai concentration, increases MAP (increased SVR), and impairs diastolic function, but without affecting cardiac index. Calcium administration can mitigate hyperkalemia and hypocalcemia and raise MAP but is not advocated if there is ongoing myocardial ischemia.

Adrenergic Agonist

Sympathomimetics are endogenous or synthetic catecholamines and non-catecholamines with specific adrenergic receptor actions that affect both systolic and diastolic function producing variable hemodynamic effects (Table 21.4). Chronic heart failure patients have higher circulating catecholamines, depleted myocardial norepinephrine stores, fewer desensitized β1 receptors and an activated renin-angiotensin system. Indirect acting agents are significantly less effective and a β1 agonist, when used alone, has a plateau effect. Most clinical studies have shown

Table 21.4 Adrenergic Receptors and Catecholamines

Agent	Action	α1 Postsynaptic vasoconstrict	α2 Presynaptic vasoconstrict	β1 ↑ HR + inotropy	β2 Relax smooth muscle	Dopamine receptor
Epinephrine	Direct	+++	+++	++	++	∅
Norepinephrine	Direct	+++	+++	+	∅	∅
Dopamine	Direct	++	+	+	+	+++
Dobutamine	Direct	∅	∅	+++	++	∅
Isoproterenol	Direct	∅	∅	+++	+++	∅
Phenylephrine	Indirect	+++	+++	∅	∅	∅

minimal hemodynamic differences between the various exogenous catecholamines in cardiac surgery patients [12]. Epinephrine, dopamine and dobutamine increase stroke volume at equivalent doses but at the expense of increased HR and MVO_2. Isoproterenol is contraindicated in patients with coronary artery disease, but may be beneficial in heart transplant patients requiring a fast HR and low PVR.

Phosphodiesterase (PDE) Inhibitors

These synthetic non-catecholamine agents inhibit PDE III and elevate intracellular cAMP independent of adrenergic β receptors, and so have synergistic action when combined with β1 agonists. These drugs improve systolic contractility and diastolic lusitropic function by decreasing PCWP, SVR and PVR but without affecting HR or MVO_2. These agents may prevent myocardial ischemia by dilating arterial conduits and inhibiting platelet thrombus formation. Venous and arterial vasodilatation causes significant systemic hypotension mandating an adequate preload and a vasopressor (norepinephrine or vasopressin) to maintain MAP.

Milrinone

Milrinone in RCTs facilitated weaning patients with low LVEF when compared with placebo. In many centers, milrinone is the drug of choice for managing patients with RV failure or high PA pressures. The 30–60 min half-life allows for a loading dose (25–50 μg/kg IV) to be adminis-

tered by the perfusionist on CPB without the need for a maintenance infusion. Alternatively, the anesthesiologist can start an infusion of 0.25–0.5 μg/kg/min without the bolus. Prophylactic inhaled milrinone (5 mg) versus placebo given post-induction of anesthesia in high-risk cardiac surgery patients with pulmonary hypertension increased CO and reduced PA pressure but without impact on the ability to wean from CPB [13]. A meta-analysis of RCTs showed that milrinone given during cardiac surgery may increase mortality [14].

Nitric Oxide

Nitric oxide (NO) is the endogenous endothelial derived relaxing factor responsible for cell relaxation. After CPB impaired endogenous NO synthesis in pulmonary endothelial cells can elevate PVR, inducing RV failure, decreasing CO and resulting in systemic hypotension. Exogenous inhaled NO (iNO) directly delivered via pulmonary alveoli to the pulmonary circulation relaxes vascular smooth muscle cells resulting in vasodilatation (lower PVR) and improves V/Q matching of perfusion to ventilated areas. Local inactivation by hemoglobin (half-life one minute) produces toxic by-products methemoglobin and nitrogen dioxide which should be monitored.

Studies have demonstrated that iNO 20–80 ppm may selectively decrease PVR following mitral valve surgery, CABG, congenital repairs and heart transplantation. To date there has been no large RCT comparing iNO to placebo in cardiac surgery with only a few case reports and small studies showing benefit in weaning. Although iNO can reduce secondary pulmonary hypertension, it may not improve patient survival [15].

Vasopressin

Arginine vasopressin (AVP) is a potent hormonal regulator of blood volume and BP secreted by the posterior pituitary in response to baroreflex or osmotic changes. Specific receptor mediated action in vascular smooth muscle cells (V1) causes vasoconstriction increasing afterload and in renal tubular cells (V2) absorbs free water thereby increasing blood volume.

Hypotension post-CPB is associated with a measured increase in blood AVP levels, but in vasoplegia syndrome these levels are inappropriately low for the degree of arterial hypotension. An exogenous vasopressin infusion has proven valuable in the management of vasoplegia syndrome after CPB, particularly in VAD and heart transplant patients [16]. Prophylactic vasopressin given to patients pre-CPB can reduce post-CPB hypotension, vasoconstrictor requirements and shorten ICU stay [17]. In a prospective single-center RCT, vasopressin when compared to norepinephrine reduced the rates of acute kidney injury, hemodialysis, and atrial fibrillation as well as ICU and hospital LOS in cardiac surgery patients with vasodilatory shock [18].

Methylene Blue

Methylene blue (MB) indirectly blocks the enzyme NO synthetase reducing NO production and facilitating norepinephrine mediated vasoconstriction thereby increasing SVR. The drug may cause cardiac arrhythmias, coronary vasoconstriction, decreased CO, reduced renal and mesenteric blood flow, increased PVR, and deterioration in gas exchange.

There are case reports and small case series supporting the perioperative use of MB to manage vasoplegia syndrome in cardiac surgery, though not specifically to aid weaning. A single bolus dose of 1–2 mg/kg IV effectively treated most patients with vasoplegia (half-life 40 min), with an additional infusion (1 mg/kg/h) for refractory vasoplegic patients. There is a "window of opportunity" to use this drug, after which it is less effective [19]. In patients at high risk for vasoplegia, MB (2 mg/kg) given one hour preoperatively reduced the incidence and severity of the vasoplegia [20].

Levosimendan

Levosimendan is a new class of calcium sensitizing agent that acts independently of cAMP to improve calcium binding to troponin without raising myocardial intracellular calcium concentrations. Inhibition of PDE III opens K-ATP channels producing peripheral and coronary vasodilatation. It is an inodilator that increases contractility without changing MVO_2 or impairing diastolic function.

Levosimendan has improved short-term hemodynamic parameters (increased CO, decreased filling pressures) in decompensated chronic heart failure patients. Early case reports and small trials suggest it may reduce mortality and morbidity (renal failure requiring dialysis, atrial fibrillation, myocardial injury) in cardiac surgery patients with and without systolic dysfunction [21]. European expert consensus recommends that Levosimendan be used preoperatively, rather than specifically for weaning, in high risk cardiac surgery patients [22].

Metabolic Management

In an euthyroid, cold patient, measured free T3 increases with heparin, falls on CPB and for 24 h postoperatively. Thyroid hormone in animals increases myocardial contractility. RCTs do not demonstrate an inotrope sparing effect of exogenous T3 so its routine use is not recommended for cardiac surgery patients. A T3 bolus (0.4 µg/kg) and infusion (0.1 µg/kg) before weaning decreases myocardial ischemia, reducing the need for inotropes and MCS and improving postoperative ventricular function [23].

The metabolic cocktail of glucose (D50W 1 gm/kg) + Insulin 1.5 units/kg + KCl 10 mmol has positive inotropic effects through unclear cellular mechanisms. Glucose Insulin Potassium (GIK) was initially used to provide metabolic support after acute myocardial infarction. Though human studies suggest some benefit in improving contractile function and reducing cardiac arrhythmias, it is not used in weaning [24].

The role of steroids in cardiac surgery patients remains controversial. Despite the theoretical benefits of reducing the inflammatory response RCTs have failed to show any improvement in patient outcome [25]. Steroids increase cardiac index, reduce SVR and reduce the incidence of arrhythmias. There are no studies using steroids as an adjunct to weaning from CPB.

Mechanical Circulatory Support

In addition to inotropic regimens, the early use of MCS can preserve end-organ function while allowing the heart time for recovery [26]. Criteria for considering MCS in a patient on at least two inotropes at high doses includes (A) persistent shock (low CO, high CVP/PAP); (B) evidence of worsening end organ function (lactate, acidosis, low urine); and (C) high probability of death.

Currently available temporary MCS options are the (A) intra-aortic balloon pump (IABP); (B) portable cardiopulmonary pump systems; and (C) VAD. However, all devices have serious complications.

An IABP reduces afterload and augments coronary perfusion, but supplies only a modest 15–20% increase in CO. The balloon catheter is easily inserted percutaneously at the bedside via the femoral artery. There is Class1B evidence a preoperative IABP improves outcomes in patients with a LVEF <25% or ongoing ischemia [27]. IABP use for weaning is well established although the evidence is hard to produce. IABP use in cardiac surgical patients varies from 1.5–17%, but is associated with increased complications in 11–33% of patients.

The simplest portable cardiac pump device is extracorporeal membrane oxygenation (ECMO), a CPB system comprised of centrifugal pump, oxygenator and veno-arterial (VA) cannulation placed either through the femoral or intrathoracic vessels. In the PCCS patient this is a salvage technique with a high mortality [26].

Short term VADs offer temporary continuous or pulsatile flow support to the failing RV, LV or both in patients with adequate ventilation. Intracorporeal devices, extracorporeal devices and cannulae can be inserted percutaneously or during surgery. The pulsatile flow Abiomed BVS 5000 (Abiomed Inc., Denver, COL) and continuous flow CentriMag (Thoratec Corp, Berkley, CA) are two extracorporeal VADs that use existing central cannulation to provide temporary MCS. Continuous flow percutaneous devices such as the extracorporeal TandemHeart (CardiacAssist Inc., Pittsburgh, PA) and the intracorporeal Impella catheter (Abiomed Inc., Denver, COL) can support native cardiac flows up to 5 L/min. The mean time for ventricular support is hours to days and survival from PCCS is 25–46%.

References

1. Lickler M, Diaper J, Cartier V, Ellenberger C, Cikirikcioglu M, Kalangos A, et al. Clinical review: management of weaning from cardiopulmonary bypass after cardiac surgery. Ann Card Anesth. 2012;15:206–23.
2. Engelman R, Baker RA, Likosky DS, Grigore A, Dickinson TA, Shore-Lesserson L, et al. The Society of Thoracic Surgeons, the Society of Cardiovascular Anesthesiologists, and the American Society of Extra Corporeal Technology: clinical practice guidelines for cardiopulmonary bypass-temperature management during cardiopulmonary bypass. Ann Thorac Surg. 2015;100:748–57.
3. Beyersdorf F. The use of controlled reperfusion strategies in cardiac surgery to minimize ischaemia/reperfusion damage. Cardiovasc Res. 2009;83:262–8.
4. Groban L, Butterworth J, Legault C, Rogers AT, Kon ND, Hammon JW. Intraoperative insulin therapy does not reduce the need for inotropic or anti-arrhythmic therapy after cardiopulmonary bypass. J Cardiothorac Vasc Anesth. 2002;16:405–12.
5. Chi D, Chen C, Shi Y, Wang W, Ma Y, Zhou R, et al. Ventilation during cardiopulmonary bypass for prevention of respiratory insufficiency: a meta-analysis of randomized controlled trials. Medicine. 2017;96:e6454.
6. Stern DH, Gerson JI, Allen FB, Parker FB. Can we trust direct radial artery pressure immediately fol-

lowing cardiopulmonary bypass? Anesthesiology. 1985;62:557–61.

7. Rao V, Ivanov J, Weisel RD, Ikonomidis JS, Christakis GT, David TE. Predictors of low cardiac output syndrome after coronary artery bypass. J Thorac Cardiovasc Surg. 1996;112(1):38–51.

8. Fischer GW, Levin MA. Vasoplegia during cardiac surgery: current concepts and management. Semin Thorac Cardiovasc Surg. 2010;22(2):140–4.

9. Bernard F, Denault A, Babin D, Goyer C, Couture P, Couturier A, et al. Diastolic dysfunction is predictive of difficult weaning from cardiopulmonary bypass. Anesth Analg. 2001;92:921–8.

10. Mebazza A, Pitsis AA, Rudiger A, Toller W, Longrois D, Rickstein SE, et al. Clinical review: practical recommendations on the management of perioperative heart failure in cardiac surgery. Crit Care. 2010;14:201.

11. Osawa EA, Rhodes A, Landoni G, Galas FR, Fukushima JT, Park CH, et al. Effect of perioperative goal-directed hemodynamic resuscitation therapy on outcomes following cardiac surgery: a randomized clinical trial and systematic review. Crit Care Med. 2016;44(4):724–33.

12. Gillies M, Bellomo R, Doolan L, Buxton B. Bench to bedside review: inotropic drug therapy after adult cardiac surgery – a systematic literature review. Crit Care. 2005;9:266–79.

13. Denault AY, Bussières JS, Arellano R, Finegan B, Gavra P, Haddad F, et al. A multicentre randomized-controlled trial of inhaled milrinone in high-risk cardiac surgical patients. Can J Anesth. 2016;63(10):1140–53.

14. Zangrillo A, Biondi-Zoccai G, Ponschab M, Greco M, Corno L, Covello RD, et al. Milrinone and mortality in adult cardiac surgery: a meta-analysis. J Cardiothorac Vasc Anesth. 2012;26:70–7.

15. Rodrigues AJ, Evora PM, Evora P. Chapter 6 Use of inhaled nitric oxide in cardiac surgery: what is going on?, in Cardiac surgery – a commitment to science, Technology and Creativity. Intech 2014.

16. Argenziano M, Chen JM, Choudhri AF, Cullinane S, Garfein E, Weinberg AD, et al. Management of vasodilatory shock after cardiac surgery: identification of predisposing factors and use of novel pressor agent. J Thorac Cardiovasc Surg. 1998;116:973–80.

17. Morales D, Garrido MJ, Madigan JD, Helman DN, Faber BA, Williams MR, et al. A double blind randomized trial: prophylactic vasopressin reduces hypotension after cardiopulmonary bypass. Ann Thorac Surg. 2003;75(3):926–30.

18. Hajjar LA, Vincent JL, Barbosa Gomes Galas FR, Rhodes A, Landoni G, Osawa EA, et al. Vasopressin versus norepinephrine in patients with vasoplegic shock after cardiac surgery: the VANCS randomized controlled trial. Anesthesiology. 2017;126(1):85–93.

19. Evora PR, Alves L, Ferreira CA, Menardi AC, Bassetto S, Rodrigues AJ, et al. Twenty years of vasoplegic syndrome treatment in heart surgery. Methylene blue revised. Rev Bras Cir Cardiovasc. 2015;30(1):84–92.

20. Ozal E, Kuralay E, Yildirim V, Killic S, Bolcal C, Kucukarslan N, et al. Preoperative methylene blue administration in patients at high risk for vasoplegic syndrome during cardiac surgery. Ann Thorac Surg. 2005;79:1615–9.

21. Harrison RW, Hasselblad V, Mehta RH, Levin R, Harrington RA, Alexander JH. Effect of levosimendan on survival and adverse events after cardiac surgery: a meta-analysis. J Cardiothorac Vasc Anesth. 2013;27:1224–32.

22. Toller W, Heringlake M, Guarracino F, Algotsson L, Alvarez J, Argyriadou H, et al. Preoperative and perioperative use of levosimendan in cardiac surgery: European expert opinion. Int J Cardiol. 2015;184:323–36.

23. Mullis-Jansson S, Argenziano M, Corwin S, Homma S, Weinberg AD, Williams M, et al. A randomized double blind study of the effect of triiodothyronine on cardiac function and morbidity after coronary bypass surgery. J Cardiovasc Surg. 1999;117:1128–35.

24. Bothe W, Olschewski M, Beyersdorf F, Doenst T. Glucose-insulin-potassium in cardiac surgery: a meta-analysis. Ann Thorac Surg. 2004;78(5):1650–7.

25. Whitlock RP, Devereaux PJ, Teoh KH, Lamy A, Vincent J, Poque J, et al. Methylprednisolone in patients undergoing cardiopulmonary bypass (SIRS): a randomised, double-blind, placebo-controlled trial. Lancet. 2015;386:1243–53.

26. Sylvin EA, Stern DR, Goldstein DJ. Mechanical support for postcardiotomy cardiogenic shock: has progress been made? J Card Surg. 2010;25:442–54.

27. Dietl CA, Berkheimer MD, Woods EL, Gilbert CL, Pharr WF, Benoit CH. Efficacy and cost effectiveness of preoperative IABP in patients with ejection fraction of 0.25 or less. Ann Thorac Surg. 1996;62(2):401–9.

Pulmonary Hypertension and Right Ventricular Dysfunction Post-Cardiopulmonary Bypass

22

Etienne J. Couture, Mahsa Elmi-Sarabi, William Beaubien-Souligny, and André Denault

Main Messages

1. Right ventricular (RV) dysfunction after cardiopulmonary bypass (CPB) is a major complication in cardiac surgery with a mortality rate from 22 to 37%.
2. Six most important causes of PH in cardiac surgery are: (1) left ventricular (LV) dysfunction, (2) lung injury during CPB, (3) protamine administration, (4) aortic or mitral patient prosthesis mismatch, (5) hypoxia, hypercapnia or pulmonary embolism, and (6) pulmonary disease.
3. Echocardiography has a central role in the diagnosis of RVF, but it is important for the clinician to assess the hemodynamic impact of this finding to determine the best course of action.
4. In patients with PH, it has been shown that MAP/MPAP ratio is not influenced by loading conditions and is an independent predictor of hemodynamic complication after cardiac surgery.
5. Pulmonary vasodilators and Phosphodiesterase enzyme (PDE) type 3 inhibitors were strongly recommended to reduce pulmonary pressures and pulmonary vascular resistance (PVR) and improve RV performance.
6. Inhaled therapies commonly used to treat PH in the cardiac surgical setting include inhaled nitric oxide, inhaled prostacyclin (iPGI2), inhaled iloprost, and inhaled PDE inhibitors such as milrinone.

E. J. Couture
Institut Universitaire de Cardiologie et de Pneumologie de Quebec – Universite Laval, Quebec, QC, Canada
e-mail: etienne.couture.3@ulaval.ca

M. Elmi-Sarabi ·W. Beaubien-Souligny
A. Denault (✉)
Montreal Heart Institute, Université de Montréal, Montréal, QC, Canada
e-mail: andre.denault@umontreal.ca

Right ventricular (RV) dysfunction occurring just after cardiopulmonary bypass (CPB) is a major complication in cardiac surgery with a mortality rate from 22 to 37% [1, 2]. One of the major risk factors is preoperative pulmonary hypertension (PH) [3]. In the following chapter, we will define right ventricular failure (RVF) and review the critical role of cardiac and extracardiac ultrasound for its diagnosis and its consequences on extra-cardiac function. We will conclude by briefly describing our approach in managing this condition.

Prevalence and Outcome of Pulmonary Hypertension and Right Ventricular Dysfunction Post-Cardiopulmonary Bypass

Pulmonary hypertension is a hemodynamic problem that can result in RVF. It has a complex pathophysiology and is associated with increased morbidity and mortality. Although the true prevalence of PH in the general population is unknown, the prevalence of pulmonary arterial hypertension (PAH) (group 1 PH) has been estimated to range from five to 15 cases per million and is now believed to affect all age groups and both genders [4].

In the context of cardiac surgery, PH is frequently classified as pre-capillary or post-capillary. Pre-capillary PH is marked by changes limited to the arterial side of the pulmonary circulation, while post-capillary PH reflects changes within the pulmonary venous circulation, between the capillary bed and the left atrium. Since the most common form of PH encountered in the cardiac surgery patient is PH associated with left heart disease [5]; in this context, PH is typically post-capillary.

The PH in cardiac surgery has a complex etiology and may involve several mechanisms acting alone or in combination. We previously identified the six most important causes of PH in cardiac surgery, which may exist before the operation, or appear during or after the procedure: (1) left heart disease or left ventricular (LV) dysfunction; (2) lung injury during CPB; (3) protamine administration; (4) aortic or mitral patient prosthesis mismatch; (5) hypoxia, hypercapnia or pulmonary embolism; and (6) pulmonary disease [3].

Cardiac surgical patients with PH carry a higher risk for surgery than those without PH. Complications such as pneumonia, prolonged mechanical ventilation, renal failure, cardiac arrest, and multiple organ system failure occur more frequently with increasing mean pulmonary artery pressure (MPAP) [6]. In patients with severe PH, the incidence of major postoperative complications was previously reported at 32% [6].

Survival in the postoperative period is determined by the ability of the right heart to deal with the increased pulmonary pressure. Information on pulmonary hemodynamics and RV function is therefore essential to adapt the best approach for management. For this reason, standard hemodynamic monitoring techniques used during anesthesia and in the intensive care unit (ICU) are not sufficient for this high-risk cardiac population. Appropriate perioperative monitoring including, but not limited to, right heart catheterization, transesophageal echocardiography (TEE), and cerebral near-infrared spectroscopy (NIRS) are critical to provide guidance in the management of hemodynamic instability and RVF.

Definition of Right Ventricular Failure After Cardiopulmonary Bypass

There is no specific and uniform definition of RVF in the context of cardiac surgery. In two randomised trials in which prevention of RVF was the primary outcome, different definitions were used (Table 22.1) [1, 2]. Therefore in order to define RVF, hemodynamic, echocardiographic and pharmacologic elements must be present. For instance, similar echocardiographic features can be seen in RV dysfunction and RVF. However, the latter will be associated with reduced oxygen transport and typically reduced brain and systemic NIRS signals.

Cardiac Manifestations: Echocardiographic Evaluation

Guidelines unrelated to cardiac surgery addressing qualitative and quantitative transthoracic echocardiographic (TTE) evaluation and the abnormal RV function criteria in adults are available [7]. Transesophageal echocardiography RV views are similar to those obtained using TTE and a proposition of echocardiographic RV dysfunction for cardiac surgery was published in 2009 [8, 9]. Proposed echocardiographic RV dysfunction criteria are: (A) the presence of RV dila-

Table 22.1 Definition of right ventricular failure

Trial	Right ventricular failure criteria		
	Hemodynamics and cardiopulmonary weaning	Echocardiographic evaluation	Intraoperative direct visual anatomic inspection
TACTICS, Denault et al. 2013 [1]	– Requirement of ≥3 inotropic/vasopressor treatments or 2 at high doses for CPB separation[a] – Return to CPB for hemodynamic instability – Use of rescue therapy for high pulmonary arterial pressure[b] – Use of ventricular assist device – Death (all causes)	> 20% reduction of RV fraction area change	Significant reduction or absence of RV wall motion
Denault et al. 2016 [2]	Difficult or complex separation[c]		

[a]Inotropic/vasopressor treatments at high doses are defined as: dopamine 45 mcg/min; dobutamine 45 mcg/min; norepinephrine >0.05 mcg/min; epinephrine >0.05 mcg/min; milrinone >0.5 mcg/min; phenylephrine >2.5 mcg/min; isoproterenol >0.01 mg/min; vasopressin at a cumulative dose of >10 units or levosimendan ≥0.2 mcg/min
[b]High pulmonary arterial pressure defined as mean pulmonary artery pressure >50 mmHg or systolic pulmonary artery pressure >60 mmHg
[c]Difficult separation defined as the need of at least two different types of pharmacological agents (inotropes and vasopressors). Complex separation (or surgical) is defined as difficult separation plus a surgical intervention (return on CPB, intra-aortic balloon pump (IABP), extracorporeal membrane oxygenation (ECMO)) for weaning or intraoperative death from heart failure. Abbreviations: *CPB* cardiopulmonary bypass, *RV* right ventricular

tation >2/3 of the LV in its transversal diameter; (B) RV fractional area change (RVFAC) <25% or ≥20% reduction compared to the pre-CPB evaluation; (C) a tricuspid annular plane systolic excursion (TAPSE) ≤16 mm, and (D) a systolic speed of the tissue Doppler tricuspid ring (S′) < 10 cm/s [8, 9]. The TEE and TTE RV evaluation is often challenging due to its complex crescent shape geometry that renders imaging of the inflow and outflow in the same two-dimensional (2D) plane difficult. Inward mechanical contraction of the RV is governed by superficial circumferential muscle fibers shortening whereas base-to-apex contraction results from inner longitudinal fibers. In comparison to LV, the base-to-apex shortening assumes a greater role in RV emptying. Views specific to RV should be used to evaluate its dimension and function with a qualitative and quantitative approach [8]. RV function can be evaluated through 2D volumetric and non-volumetric parameters, strain analysis and three-dimensional (3D) parameters.

Echocardiography is useful to characterize the consequences of PH on RV size and function. Specific conditions associated with PH and consequently RV dysfunction can be diagnosed with

this imaging modality. Right ventricular hypertrophy is present if RV free wall exceeds 5 mm. RV remodeling and dilatation will increase the RV sphericity index defined by the ratio of RV end-diastolic mid-papillary diameter on RV end-diastolic longitudinal diameter.

2D Imaging Systolic Function Assessment

Right Ventricle Volumetric Assessment
Qualitative evaluation and estimation of the RV size is made by comparison with the LV. Normal RV is less than two-thirds of the LV; mildly enlarged RV is more than two-thirds but inferior to the LV; moderately enlarged RV is roughly equal to the LV size; and severely enlarged RV is superior to the LV [7]. The RV dysfunction is suspected when RV dilatation from volume overload produce septal flattening in diastole and when RV pressure overload produce septal flattening in both diastole and end-systole. Right ventricular diameter >42 mm at the base and >35 mm at the midlevel is diagnostic of RV dilatation [7]. Volumetric evaluation can be done

with RVFAC defined as (end-diastolic area – end-systolic area)/end-diastolic area × 100. Diagnosis of RV dysfunction is made by RVFAC <35% and its severity can be described as mild, moderate, or severe for values of 25% to 35%, 18% to 25%, and ≤18%, respectively. However, RVFAC does not consider the RV outflow tract volume that corresponds to approximately 20% of the RV volume.

Right Ventricle Non-Volumetric Assessment

Global assessment of RV function can be done by RV myocardial performance index (RVMPI) using pulsed waved Doppler (PWD) or tissue Doppler imaging (TDI) at the lateral tricuspid annulus. It represents an estimate of both RV systolic and diastolic function. It is based on the relationship between ejection and non-ejection work of the heart. The RVMPI is defined as the ratio of isovolumetric time divided by ejection time (ET), or [(isovolumetric relaxation time (IVRT) + isovolumetric contraction time (IVCT))/(ET)]. Presence of RV dysfunction is characterized by a RVMPI >0.43 in PWD and >0.54 in TDI [10]. In valvular surgery, RVMPI is an independent predictor of difficult CPB weaning, mortality, circulatory failure, duration of hospitalization and ICU stay [11]. This parameter is load dependent and unreliable in situations where right atrial pressure is elevated and RR intervals are irregular such as atrial fibrillation because of reduced IVCT.

Regional assessment of RV function corresponds to TDI derived S′, RV acceleration during isovolumic contraction (RVIVA) and TAPSE. Interrogation of S′ by TDI <9.5 cm/s is a sign of RV dysfunction as it represents the basal RV free wall function. The RVIVA is also measured by TDI at the lateral tricuspid annulus. Right ventricular acceleration during isovolumic contraction is defined as the peak isovolumic myocardial velocity divided by time to peak velocity. This parameter is rate dependent and appears to be less load-dependent than RVMPI. Value <2.2 m/s^2 is considered to be related to RV dysfunction. The RV function is commonly assessed by TAPSE as it represents an easily recognizable longitudinal movement on echocardiography. Typically measured in M-Mode and corrected for angulation of interrogation, TAPSE is defined as the total excursion of the tricuspid annulus from end-diastole to end-systole. Tricuspid annular plane systolic excursion <17 mm is suggestive of RV dysfunction. It has been correlated to RV ejection fraction (RVEF). However, it is important to note that TAPSE is angle and load dependent. Also, it reflects the longitudinal displacement of only a single segment of the complex RV 3D structure.

2D Imaging Diastolic Function Assessment

Presence of tricuspid regurgitation or irregular RR intervals renders the analysis of diastolic dysfunction difficult immediately after CPB weaning. However, in the absence of these conditions, gradation of diastolic RV function can be achieved through trans-tricuspid flow (TTF) and hepatic venous flow. Early and late filling waves velocities (E and A wave, respectively) and E deceleration time recorded by pulsed wave Doppler in the TTF and the lateral tricuspid annulus velocity during early filling (E′) recorded by TDI allows diastolic categorization of RV function. A tricuspid E/A ratio < 0.8 suggests impaired relaxation, a tricuspid E/A ratio of 0.8 to 2.1 with an E/E′ ratio > 6 or diastolic flow predominance in the hepatic veins suggests pseudo-normal filling, and a tricuspid E/A ratio > 2.1 with a deceleration time < 120 ms suggests restrictive filling.

Strain Imaging

Right ventricular strain measurements are highly feasible and use an absolute cut-off value of > − 20% (or absolute value <20%) for both RV global longitudinal strain (RVGLS) and RV free wall strain (RVFWS) [12]. The RV strain is worsened after CBP but the clinical significance of that finding is unknown [13]. Preoperative TTE evaluation of the 2D RV longitudinal strain is a better predictor of mortality after cardiac surgery than RVFAC. Abnormal RVFAC (<35%) is associated to the greatest risk of postoperative mortality, probably because abnormal RVFAC reflects a severe and advanced RV dysfunction with both radial and longitudinal RV dysfunction. In patients with preserved RVFAC, RV speckle tracking appears as a sensitive method to identify early RV dysfunction [14]. RV strain imaging can represent an important prognostic value in the PH patient [15] and is associated with mortality after transcatheter aortic valve replacement [16]. Finally, both regional and global RV strain measurements are feasible with TEE during cardiac surgery [17].

3D Imaging

The use of 3D echocardiography to evaluate RV end-diastolic volume by identification of the minimal RV volume frame and end-systolic volume by maximal RV volume frame allows the determination of RVEF. Three-dimensional RVEF <45% is highly suggestive of RV dysfunction. End-diastolic volumes >87 mL/m^2 for men and > 74 mL/m^2 for women are indicative of RV enlargement. Intraoperative RVEF assessment with 3D TEE seems feasible and reproducible in patients with normal RV function and in patients with dilated RV without being excessively time consuming [18].

Echocardiographic Evaluation of Pulmonary Artery Pressure

Pulmonary artery pressure (PAP) can be estimated with the use of a Bernoulli equation when a pulmonary artery catheter is not used. The presence of tricuspid regurgitation makes it possible to estimate systolic pulmonary artery pressure (SPAP) using peak tricuspid regurgitation velocity. Diastolic pulmonary artery pressure (DPAP) can be estimated from the velocity at the end of the pulmonary regurgitation, and MPAP from the maximal velocity of the pulmonary regurgitation. Right atrial pressure must be added to these two previous measurements to obtain an adequate estimate. The MPAP can be estimated by the pulmonary artery acceleration time (AT) (MPAP = 79 − (0.45 × AT) and MPAP = 90 − (0.62 × AT) if AT <120 ms) or derived from the systolic and diastolic pressures (MPAP = (1/3(SPAP) + 2/3(DPAP)).

Extra-Cardiac Manifestations

Hemodynamic Impact of Right Ventricular Dysfunction

The progressive increase in central venous pressure (CVP) in patients with right heart failure has a detrimental impact on organ function. The cardio-renal syndrome, the cardio-intestinal syndrome and the cardio-hepatic syndrome have all been attributed to an inadequate tissue delivery of oxygen and nutriments stemming from a combination of decreased cardiac output and increased venous pressures [19–23]. While autonomic and hormonal autoregulation is able to compensate for a reduced cardiac index to maintain adequate blood flow until it falls below a critical threshold, the presence of elevated venous pressure creates a synergy where interstitial edema and a reduced arterio-venous gradient is providing the "second-hit" resulting in organ dysfunction. Venous congestion appears to be one of the most important factors leading to adverse outcomes in patients with heart failure.

While echocardiography has a central role in the diagnosis of RVF, it is important for the clinician to assess the hemodynamic impact of this finding to determine the best course of action. While a critical decrease in cardiac output resulting in hypotension is immediately clinically evident from the use of traditional monitoring techniques, the impact of venous congestion on organ function is very covert in its presentation. Novel tools are being investigated to provide insight about the hemodynamic impact of RVF.

Venous Pressures Monitoring

Absolute CVP measurements are routinely performed in the perioperative period. The elevation of CVP is associated with an increase in renal dysfunction in broad populations of patients with cardiovascular diseases and is associated with adverse outcomes in critically ill patients [24]. In the setting of cardiac surgery, absolute CVP measurements, six hours after surgery is associated with mortality and renal failure [25]. However, despite multiple sources reporting the association between CVP and outcomes, an absolute cut-off or "target value" to prevent complications has not been determined. In a study by Williams et al. in a large cohort of coronary artery bypass graft surgery patients, the elevation of risk with CVP was present even for values under 9 mmHg [25]. Consequently, other indices should be sought in order to better risk stratify patients. Perfusion pressure (mean arterial pressure (MAP)-CVP, or diastolic arterial pressure (DAP)-CVP) as a surrogate for the arterio-venous pressure gradients in end organs is also associated with renal failure in cardiac surgery patients, and may be a better predictor than absolute CVP values [26].

Additional pressure monitoring to be considered includes the appearance of the CVP and the RV pressure waveform during the cardiac cycle. This information is often readily available and could be used to detect RV dysfunction at the bedside. In the patient with a normal diastolic RV function, pressure inside the RV will remain low during the ventricular systole manifesting as a plateau on RV pressure monitoring (Fig. 22.1a). With increasing diastolic RV dysfunction, ventricular compliance during diastolic decrease and the waveform will have an oblique appearance (Fig. 22.1f) and, in very severe cases, a square-root pattern (Fig. 22.1k). During RV systole, the tricuspid annulus moves downward (TAPSE)

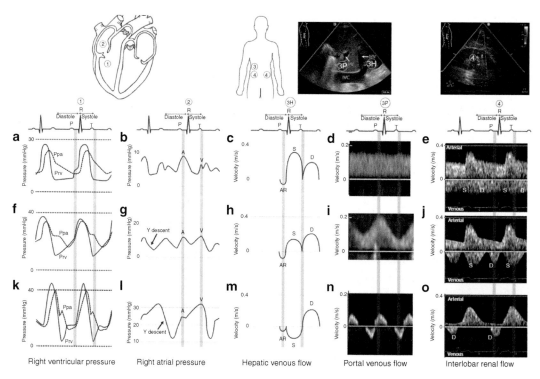

Fig. 22.1 Features of acute right ventricular (RV) failure on (1) RV pressure monitoring (2) right atrial pressure monitoring (3) hepatic vein (HV) and portal vein (PV) transthoracic Doppler ultrasound and (4) renal arterio-venous Doppler ultrasound. Patterns in patients with normal RV function (**a, b, c, d, e**) and typical patterns commonly observed in patients with mild (**f, g, h, i, j**) and severe (**k, l, m, n, o**) RV dysfunction. Abbreviations: AR, atrial reversal; D, diastole; IVC, inferior vena cava; Ppa, pulmonary artery pressure; Prv, right ventricular pressure, S, systole. The numbers on the images correspond to the location of the images: 1, right ventricle; 2, right atrium; 3, liver; 3H, hepatic venous flow; 3P, portal venous flow; 4, renal venous flow. (Adapted from Amsalem et al. [27] and Beaubien-Souligny et al. [28])

which is partially responsible for the decrease in right atrial pressure indicated by the X descent (Fig. 22.1b). With systolic RV dysfunction, the reduction in the TAPSE leads to the disappearance of the X descent (Fig. 22.1g and l) and a prominent Y descent during diastole. Recognition of these patterns could be used by the astute clinician as possible warning signs of RVF in an unstable patient.

Continuous RV pressure monitoring makes it possible to assess the hemodynamic effect of the pharmacological agent on RV function and is also a useful tool in the diagnosis of RV outflow tract obstruction (RVOTO). Excessive inotropic stimulation and afterload reduction may lead to RVOTO that can be instantaneously diagnosed with continuous pulmonary artery and RV pressure monitoring (Fig. 22.2). This condition is

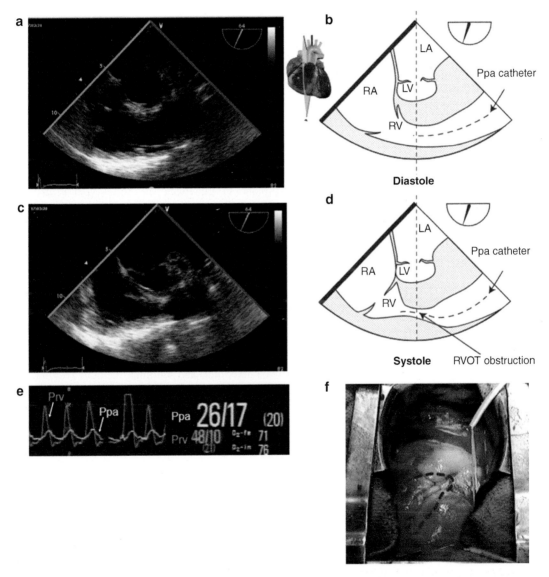

Fig. 22.2 Right ventricular outflow tract (RVOT) obstruction. Mid-esophageal inflow-outflow views in (**a–b**) diastole and (**c–d**) systole show significant collapse of the RVOT during systole. (**e**) A 22 mmHg pressure gradient is present using combined right ventricular pressure (Prv) and pulmonary artery pressure (Ppa) waveforms. (**f**) The intraoperative aspect of the right ventricle (RV) shows a dimpling on the RVOT. Abbreviations: *LA* left atrium, *LV* left ventricle, *RA* right atrium. (With permission of Denault et al. [29])

seen when the RV systolic pressure is at least 6 mmHg above the SPAP. Right ventricular outflow tract obstruction can be dynamic or mechanical and can be the source of important hemodynamic instability [30]. In this situation, similar to dynamic LV outflow tract obstruction associated with systolic anterior motion of the mitral valve, inotropic agents would be contraindicated. If the RVOTO is non-mechanical, volume and beta-blocking agents can be used. Hemodynamic instability from RVOTO can occur in presence of an anterior pneumothorax, during sternal closure and after lung transplantation. This condition is likely to be underdiagnosed in the perioperative period.

The MAP/MPAP ratio helps the clinician to appreciate the importance of PH related to the cardiac condition. In a situation where there is rapid variation of loading conditions, MPAP can be underestimated as it can be reduced proportionally to the decrease in systemic pressures. In patients with PH, it has been shown that MAP/MPAP ratio is not influenced by loading conditions and is an independent predictor of hemodynamic complication after cardiac surgery [31–35]. Also, MAP/MPAP ratio correlates with the TTE interventricular septal curvature and is correlated to five-year mortality after aortic valve replacement [36].

Extra-Cardiac Ultrasound Assessment

By using point-of-care ultrasound, the clinician can investigate the hemodynamic impact of right heart failure in end-organs. Doppler ultrasound of the liver offers the possibility to assess flow in the portal and hepatic veins. These can provide an important insight into the severity of RVF and hepatic congestion and require only basic training in Doppler ultrasound. Hepatic venous flow can be used to evaluate RV systolic function based on the aspect of the Doppler signal pattern. Hepatic vein flow can be obtained using a phased array probe or a curved array probe in the subxiphoid or lateral chest regions. Normal hepatic flow is directed away from the liver and fluctuates during the cardiac cycle as shown in Fig. 22.1c. Systolic flow is usually of higher velocity than diastolic flow. This is due to downward motion of the tricuspid annulus during ventricular systole resulting in a rapid filling of the right atria. In patients with right heart failure, decreased TAPSE and/or tricuspid regurgitation during ventricular systole lead to a reduction of the velocity in systole and to a systolic-to-diastolic ratio less than one as shown in Fig. 22.1h [37]. In severe right heart failure or tricuspid regurgitation, the systolic wave (S) appears to be completely reversed with backward flow in the hepatic veins during systole (Fig. 22.1m).

Flow in the portal vein can be assessed using a phased array or a curved linear array probe positioned in a right mid-axillary coronal view. Portal vein imaging using TEE is accomplished in the transgastric position. A transverse (short axis) cut of the liver is obtained by turning the probe to the right side of the patient. A multiplane angle rotation of 90 to 110 degrees leads to a craniocaudal plane of the liver. The portal vein is usually within a few centimeters of the transducer and the inferior vena cava (IVC) is usually not included in the same 2D view. Venous flow through the portal vein is of low velocity (20 cm/s) because this circulation is isolated from the systemic circulation by the liver sinusoids and splanchnic capillary bed. Therefore, portal venous flow presents minimal variations through the cardiac cycle (Fig. 22.1d). Portal vein pulsatility index (PVPI) can be calculated as the ratio of maximal and minimal velocity [(Vmax – Vmin)/Vmax]. A PVPI of more than 50% can be considered abnormal and is called pulsatile portal flow (Fig. 22.1i and n).

An alternative approach to the portal vein flow evaluation is to assess splenic vein flow. The splenic vein is a direct tributary of the portal vein and thus its assessment could provide the same information. Assessment of splenic vein flow can also be done with TEE via the transgastric approach. This view can be obtained by turning the probe to the left side of the body and by performing a multiplane angle rotation of 90 degrees. This will bring the view close to the splenic hilum. In this view, venous blood will travel in the direction of the probe and the velocities measured during Doppler examination will be positive. An alternative view can be obtained. With the probe toward the posterior aspect of the body, the electronic rotation angle is maintained at 0 degree. From this position, the splenic vein is located anterior to the descending aorta. From this view, the venous flow will be travelling away from the probe and the Doppler signal produced will exhibit negative velocities. An association has been observed between PVPI values greater than 50 % and high right atrial pressure, moderate or greater tricuspid regurgitation, and RV dysfunction [38, 39]. More recently, PVPI has been linked to cardiorenal syndrome and acute kidney injury after cardiac surgery [40, 41]. Intraoperative PVPI ≥ 0.5 has been previously reported to be the most important predictor of postoperative complications after cardiac surgery by being superior to any hemodynamic, 2D and Doppler cardiac measurement [39]. An international multicenter study (NCT03656263) is currently exploring the clinical significance of portal hypertension after cardiac surgery.

Pulsatile blood flow is a sign of post-hepatic portal hypertension and has been studied as a sign of severity in patients with congestive heart failure. The presence of an abnormal portal pulsatility predicts increased CVP and worse functional class in heart failure patients. Venous congestion resulting from congestive heart failure begins with an elevation of the CVP and dilatation of the IVC and its main tributaries such as the hepatic veins. When the dilatation becomes severe, the venous compliance of the IVC is decreased and pressure is transduced through the hepatic sinusoids to the portal system. This results in a decrease in velocities in the portal system or, when severe, in a complete absence or reversal of portal flow. Doppler evaluation of the portal flow could be used as a marker of end-organ venous congestion. For the portal flow to be representative of central venous congestion, other causes of portal hypertension such as cirrhosis and portal thrombosis must be absent. A PF of more than 50% has also been reported in some individuals with low body mass index and normal cardiac function. However, other signs of elevated CVP such as IVC dilatation/non-

collapsibility and abnormal hepatic vein flow waveform should support this finding.

The impact of elevated CVP on intra-renal hemodynamics can be assessed by Doppler ultrasound. In physiological conditions, blood flow in the interlobar veins is continuous during the cardiac cycle (Fig. 22.1e). With high CVP, venous flow transforms into a discontinuous biphasic pattern like the Doppler pattern seen in the hepatic veins (Fig. 22.1j). With severe right heart failure, venous flow transforms into a monophasic discontinuous pattern with flow being present only during diastole (Fig. 22.1o). Discontinuous flow in the interlobar renal veins can be linked to the CVP waveform during the cardiac cycle. As CVP increases and the IVC becomes non-compliant, the CVP waveform is transmitted deep into the renal parenchyma. Flow in the interlobar vein can be observed during the systolic and diastolic filling of the right atria (during the X and Y descent on CVP waveform). As right heart failure worsens, intra-renal venous flow becomes monophasic reflecting the predominance of the Y descent of the CVP waveform analogous to the variation in the S/D ratio in the hepatic vein waveform (decrease filling of the right atria during systole).

In Iida et al., the intra-renal venous flow pattern strongly correlated with death from cardiovascular disease and unplanned hospitalization for heart failure independent of renal resistance index, CVP and hemodynamic status including echocardiographic parameters [42]. In this study, patients with the monophasic discontinuous flow pattern also had lower estimated glomerular filtration rate (55 mL/min/1.73 m²) compared with continuous and biphasic flow (67 mL/min/1.73 m²) (p = 0.005). The biphasic and monophasic patterns have been associated with increased mortality in heart failure [43, 44] and postoperative renal failure in cardiac surgery [41, 45].

Integrating Ultrasound Assessment into Practice

Clinical assessment of RV function during surgery relies on the integration of multiple parameters, each having their own advantages and caveats. As such, patient management should not be based solely on findings from ultrasound assessment. Use of bedside ultrasound and venous waveform interpretation to enhance physical examination would rather provide the opportunity for early detection of the effects of venous congestion on end-organs. This assessment can be repeated to monitor the response to therapy.

Integrating the understanding of the pathophysiology of a clinical syndrome and ultrasonographic assessment, as described in this chapter, may help individualize the management of patients with acute or chronic right heart failure in order to avoid the adverse effects of venous congestion.

Treatment and Management

Treatment of patients with PH and RVF is particularly challenging. The choice of appropriate therapy depends on identifying the underlying cause and the hemodynamic effects of PH (Fig. 22.3). Despite the fact that the treatment of PAH has undergone an extraordinary evolution in recent years, there is currently no specific treatment for PH associated with lung disease and/or hypoxemia or secondary to left heart disease. As a result, drugs with proven efficacy in PAH are increasingly being used, in spite of the absence of clinical trials in support of this approach. Therefore, when managing a patient with PH in the ICU, treatment should primarily target the specific cause of PH and the resolution of RVF.

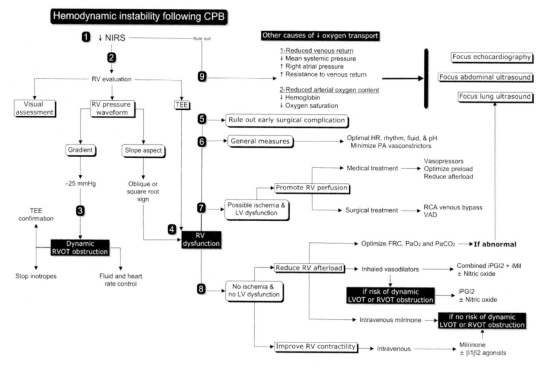

Fig. 22.3 Bedside approach to acute right ventricular (RV) dysfunction in cardiac surgery. Abbreviations: *CPB* cardiopulmonary bypass, *FRC* functional residual capacity, *HR* heart rate, *iPGI2* inhaled prostacyclin (epoprostenol), *iMil* inhaled milrinone, *LV* left ventricle, *LVOT* left ventricular outflow tract, *NIRS* near-infrared spectroscopy, *PA* pulmonary artery, *RCA* right coronary artery, *RVOT* right ventricular outflow tract, *TEE* transesophageal echocardiography, *VAD* ventricular assist device. (Adapted from Denault et al. [46])

Intravenous vasodilators have traditionally been used in managing PH in heart surgery, but they lack specificity for the pulmonary circulation and their systemic hypotensive effects necessitating additional vasopressor support often limit their use. This limitation highlights the need for selective pulmonary vasodilators for this cohort of patients, whereby nebulization of drugs could provide such localized effect with no hypotension.

Following a systematic review of the literature covering the period between 1980 and 2010, Price et al. [47] made recommendations regarding the management of pulmonary vascular and RV dysfunction in intensive care patients. Phosphodiesterase enzyme (PDE) type 3 inhibitors were strongly recommended to reduce pulmonary pressures and pulmonary vascular resistance (PVR) and improve RV performance. Furthermore, the use of pulmonary vasodilators was strongly recommended for reduction of PVR, improvement of cardiac output and oxygenation, and following cardiac surgery when PH and RV dysfunction are present. In addition, a strong recommendation was made for the administration of pulmonary vasodilators by inhalation rather than by intravenous route when systemic hypotension is expected.

Inhalation Therapy in Cardiac Surgery

Several PH-specific therapies have been approved for the treatment of PH. Although not currently approved for this indication, administration by nebulization of some of these agents is being increasingly investigated in adults and in cardiac surgery. Therefore, most of our understanding on the use of inhaled therapy is derived from small observational or single centre trials reported in the literature, and offers little clarity on the best therapeutic option for cardiac surgical patients with PH. Further larger randomized clinical studies are warranted in this field to provide much needed clinical practice guidelines. Inhaled ther-

apies commonly used to treat PH in the cardiac surgical setting include inhaled nitric oxide, inhaled prostacyclin (iPGI2), inhaled iloprost, and inhaled PDE inhibitors such as milrinone.

When to Administer Inhaled Agents in Cardiac Surgery

Owing to their selective pulmonary vasodilator effect, inhaled agents are being increasingly used in high-risk patients during cardiac surgery for management of acute PH or RVF and to facilitate weaning from CPB. However, there is still no consensus on the appropriate timing of drug administration. Review of the literature reveals that inhaled agents are administered at different times throughout the perioperative period. In a study by Groves et al. [48] the impact of early versus late initiation of $iPGI_2$ therapy was retrospectively investigated in 37 consecutive patients undergoing LV assist device placement. Inhaled prostacyclin was initiated at weaning from CPB in group I, whereas it was started shortly after induction of anesthesia and continued throughout and post-CPB in group II. Results show that $iPGI_2$ reduces SPAP and MPAP in the postoperative period regardless of the timing of initiation. Early initiation of therapy reduced SPAP and MPAP more effectively during weaning from CPB, but this was associated with an increased blood loss in the immediate postoperative period. Similarly, Lamarche et al. [49] evaluated the impact and timing of administration of inhaled milrinone (iMil) on retrospective data from 73 high-risk patients undergoing cardiac surgery with CPB. Patients receiving iMil prior to CPB initiation had greater reduction in PAP after CPB and less emergency re-initiation of CPB after weaning compared to those with administration after CPB. No detectable side effects were linked to administration of the drug. These data suggest that administration of $iPGI_2$ and iMil before CPB initiation may help weaning from CPB.

Systematic Review and Meta-Analysis of Inhaled Agents in Cardiac Surgery

In recent years, there has been a growing interest for using inhaled agents for the treatment of PH in cardiac surgery. The efficacy of these inhaled strategies, however, continues to be shown only through a limited number of small trials, case reports and series. We recently published a systematic review and meta-analysis comparing the efficacy of inhaled aerosolized agents with intravenously administered agents or placebo for the treatment and management of PH in patients undergoing cardiac surgery [50]. The purpose of this review was to summarize the state of the art in this field. Databases such as MEDLINE, CENTRAL, EMBASE, Web of Science, and clinicaltrials.gov were searched, which identified 2897 relevant citations. From those, 10 studies were included in the review and meta-analysis, comprising a total of 434 patients.

The primary outcome of the study was the incidence of mortality. Secondary outcomes were length of stay in hospital and in the ICU and evaluation of the hemodynamic profile. The meta-analysis revealed that inhaled aerosolized agents were associated with a significant decrease in PVR and a significant increase in MAP and RVEF when compared to intravenously administered agents. No significant hemodynamically meaningful differences were observed between inhaled agents and placebo. However, an increase in length of stay in the ICU was shown with the use of inhaled aerosolized agents compared to placebo.

This systematic review and meta-analysis showed that the administration of inhaled aerosolized vasodilators is associated with improved RV performance when compared to intravenously administered agents for the treatment of PH during cardiac surgery. This study, however, did not show any benefit on mortality, nor did it support any benefit compared to placebo on major outcomes. The limitations of this review were the limited number of studies published on this topic and the small size of the trials. This review shows that more studies are required in this area of research and that these should focus on clinically significant outcomes.

Intratracheal Milrinone

In acute RVF, the administration of inhaled agents is limited by the availability of a nebuliser and also their time-consuming administration. In such a situation when immediate treatment has to be initiated to avoid further cardiac deterioration and hemodynamic compromise, at the Montreal Heart Institute, we use intratracheal bolus administration of milrinone. Our experience over 12 years has been reported in patients with acute RVF. The success rate in avoiding the use of inotropic agents or return on CPB was 61.9% when intratracheal milrinone was given during CPB separation. Severely decreased left ventricular ejection fraction (<35% vs >50%), longer CPB duration and elevated postoperative fluid balance were found to be significant predictors of persistent RV failure despite intratracheal milrinone [51, 52]. Thus, direct intratracheal bolus administration of milrinone might offer a rapid and easily applicable alternative delivery mode for milrinone in acute RVF.

References

1. Denault AY, Pearl RG, Michler RE, Rao V, Tsui SS, Seitelberger R, et al. Tezosentan and right ventricular failure in patients with pulmonary hypertension undergoing cardiac surgery: the TACTICS trial. J Cardiothorac Vasc Anesth. 2013;27(6):1212–7.
2. Denault AY, Bussieres JS, Arellano R, Finegan B, Gavra P, Haddad F, et al. A multicentre randomized-controlled trial of inhaled milrinone in high-risk cardiac surgical patients. Can J Anesth. 2016;63(10):1140–53.
3. Denault A, Deschamps A, Tardif JC, Lambert J, Perrault L. Pulmonary hypertension in cardiac surgery. Curr Cardiol Rev. 2010;6(1):1–14.
4. Orem C. Epidemiology of pulmonary hypertension in the elderly. J Geriatric Cardiol. 2017;14(1):11–6.
5. Thunberg CA, Gaitan BD, Grewal A, Ramakrishna H, Stansbury LG, Grigore AM. Pulmonary hypertension in patients undergoing cardiac surgery: pathophysiology, perioperative management, and outcomes. J Cardiothorac Vasc Anesth. 2013;27(3):551–72.
6. Kennedy JL, LaPar DJ, Kern JA, Kron IL, Bergin JD, Kamath S, et al. Does the Society of Thoracic Surgeons risk score accurately predict operative mortality for patients with pulmonary hypertension? J Thorac Cardiovasc Surg. 2013;146(3):631–7.
7. Rudski LG, Lai WW, Afilalo J, Hua L, Handschumacher MD, Chandrasekaran K, et al.

Guidelines for the echocardiographic assessment of the right heart in adults: a report from the American Society of Echocardiography endorsed by the European Association of Echocardiography, a registered branch of the European Society of Cardiology, and the Canadian Society of Echocardiography. J Am Soc Echocardiogr. 2010;23(7):685–713; quiz 86–8.

8. Haddad F, Couture P, Tousignant C, Denault AY. The right ventricle in cardiac surgery, a perioperative perspective: I. Anatomy, physiology, and assessment. Anesth Analg. 2009;108(2):407–21.

9. Haddad F, Couture P, Tousignant C, Denault AY. The right ventricle in cardiac surgery, a perioperative perspective: II. Pathophysiology, clinical importance, and management. Anesth Analg. 2009;108(2):422–33.

10. Lang RM, Badano LP, Mor-Avi V, Afilalo J, Armstrong A, Ernande L, et al. Recommendations for cardiac chamber quantification by echocardiography in adults: an update from the American Society of Echocardiography and the European Association of Cardiovascular Imaging. J Am Soc Echocardiogr. 2015;28(1):1–39.e14.

11. Haddad F, Denault AY, Couture P, Cartier R, Pellerin M, Levesque S, et al. Right ventricular myocardial performance index predicts perioperative mortality or circulatory failure in high-risk valvular surgery. J Am Soc Echocardiogr. 2007;20(9):1065–72.

12. Silverton N, Meineri M. Speckle tracking strain of the right ventricle: an emerging tool for intraoperative echocardiography. Anesth Analg. 2017;125(5):1475–8.

13. Duncan AE, Sarwar S, Kateby Kashy B, Sonny A, Sale S, Alfirevic A, et al. Early left and right ventricular response to aortic valve replacement. Anesth Analg. 2017;124(2):406–18.

14. Ternacle J, Berry M, Cognet T, Kloeckner M, Damy T, Monin JL, et al. Prognostic value of right ventricular two-dimensional global strain in patients referred for cardiac surgery. J Am Soc Echocardiogr. 2013;26(7):721–6.

15. Shukla M, Park JH, Thomas JD, Delgado V, Bax JJ, Kane GC, et al. Prognostic Value of Right Ventricular Strain Using Speckle-Tracking Echocardiography in Pulmonary Hypertension: A Systematic Review and Meta-analysis. Can J Cardiol. 2018;34(8):1069–78.

16. Medvedofsky D, Koifman E, Jarrett H, Miyoshi T, Rogers T, Ben-Dor I, et al. Association of Right Ventricular Longitudinal Strain with Mortality in Patients Undergoing Transcatheter Aortic Valve Replacement. J Am Soc Echocardiogr. 2020;33(4):452–60.

17. Silverton NA, Lee JP, Morrissey CK, Tanner C, Zimmerman J. Regional Versus Global Measurements of Right Ventricular Strain Performed in the Operating Room With Transesophageal Echocardiography. J Cardiothorac Vasc Anesth. 2020;34(1):48–57.

18. Fusini L, Tamborini G, Gripari P, Maffessanti F, Mazzanti V, Muratori M, et al. Feasibility of intraoperative three-dimensional transesophageal echocardiography in the evaluation of right ventricular volumes and function in patients undergoing cardiac surgery. J Am Soc Echocardiogr. 2011;24(8):868–77.

19. Verbrugge FH, Dupont M, Steels P, Grieten L, Malbrain M, Tang WH, et al. Abdominal contributions to cardiorenal dysfunction in congestive heart failure. J Am Coll Cardiol. 2013;62(6):485–95.

20. Hassan MO, Duarte R, Dix-Peek T, Vachiat A, Naidoo S, Dickens C, et al. Correlation between volume overload, chronic inflammation, and left ventricular dysfunction in chronic kidney disease patients. Clin Nephrol. 2016;86 (2016)(13):131–5.

21. Sundaram V, Fang JC. Gastrointestinal and Liver Issues in Heart Failure. Circulation. 2016;133(17):1696–703.

22. Valentova M, von Haehling S, Bauditz J, Doehner W, Ebner N, Bekfani T, et al. Intestinal congestion and right ventricular dysfunction: a link with appetite loss, inflammation, and cachexia in chronic heart failure. Eur Heart J. 2016;37(21):1684–91.

23. Fudim M, Hernandez AF, Felker GM. Role of Volume Redistribution in the Congestion of Heart Failure. J Am Heart Assoc. 2017;6(8).

24. Li DK, Wang XT, Liu DW. Association between elevated central venous pressure and outcomes in critically ill patients. Ann Intensive Care. 2017;7(1):83.

25. Williams JB, Peterson ED, Wojdyla D, Harskamp R, Southerland KW, Ferguson TB, et al. Central venous pressure after coronary artery bypass surgery: does it predict postoperative mortality or renal failure? J Crit Care. 2014;29(6):1006–10.

26. Saito S, Uchino S, Takinami M, Uezono S, Bellomo R. Postoperative blood pressure deficit and acute kidney injury progression in vasopressor-dependent cardiovascular surgery patients. Crit Care. 2016;20(1):74.

27. Amsallem M, Kuznetsova T, Hanneman K, Denault A, Haddad F. Right heart imaging in patients with heart failure: a tale of two ventricles. Curr Opin Cardiol. 2016;31(5):469–82.

28. Beaubien-Souligny W, Bouchard J, Desjardins G, Lamarche Y, Liszkowski M, Robillard P, et al. Extracardiac signs of fluid overload in the critically ill cardiac patient: a focused evaluation using bedside ultrasound. Can J Cardiol. 2017;33(1):88–100.

29. Denault A, Lamarche Y, Rochon A, Cogan J, Liszkowski M, Lebon JS, et al. Innovative approaches in the perioperative care of the cardiac surgical patient in the operating room and intensive care unit. Can J Cardiol. 2014;30(12 Suppl):S459–77.

30. Denault AY, Chaput M, Couture P, Hébert Y, Haddad F, Tardif JC. Dynamic right ventricular outflow tract obstruction in cardiac surgery. J Thorac Cardiovasc Surg. 2006;132(1):43–9.

31. Robitaille A, Denault AY, Couture P, Belisle S, Fortier A, Guertin MC, et al. Importance of relative pulmonary hypertension in cardiac surgery: the mean systemic-to-pulmonary artery pressure ratio. J Cardiothorac Vasc Anesth. 2006;20(3):331–9.

32. Bianco JC, Qizilbash B, Carrier M, Couture P, Fortier A, Tardif JC, et al. Is patient-prosthesis mismatch a perioperative predictor of long-term mortality after

aortic valve replacement? J Cardiothorac Vasc Anesth. 2013;27(4):647–53.

33. Haddad F, Guihaire J, Skhiri M, Denault AY, Mercier O, Al-Halabi S, et al. Septal curvature is marker of hemodynamic, anatomical, and electromechanical ventricular interdependence in patients with pulmonary arterial hypertension. Echocardiography. 2014;31(6):699–707.

34. Rebel A, Nguyen D, Bauer B, Sloan PA, DiLorenzo A, Hassan ZU. Systemic-to-pulmonary artery pressure ratio as a predictor of patient outcome following liver transplantation. World J Hepatol. 2016;8(32):1384–91.

35. Bianco JC, Mc Loughlin S, Denault AY, Marenchino RG, Rojas JI, Bonofiglio FC. Heart Transplantation in Patients >60 Years: Importance of Relative Pulmonary Hypertension and Right Ventricular Failure on Midterm Survival. J Cardiothorac Vasc Anesth. 2018;32(1):32–40.

36. Haddad F, Elmi-Sarabi M, Fadel E, Mercier O, Denault AY. Pearls and pitfalls in managing right heart failure in cardiac surgery. Curr Opin Anaesthesiol. 2016;29(1):68–79.

37. Scheinfeld MH, Bilali A, Koenigsberg M. Understanding the spectral Doppler waveform of the hepatic veins in health and disease. Radiographics. 2009;29(7):2081–98.

38. Styczynski G, Milewska A, Marczewska M, Sobieraj P, Sobczynska M, Dabrowski M, et al. Echocardiographic Correlates of Abnormal Liver Tests in Patients with Exacerbation of Chronic Heart Failure. J Am Soc Echocardiog. 2016;29(2):132–9.

39. Eljaiek R, Cavayas YA, Rodrigue E, Desjardins G, Lamarche Y, Toupin F, et al. High postoperative portal venous flow pulsatility indicates right ventricular dysfunction and predicts complications in cardiac surgery patients. Br J Anaesth. 2019;122(2):206–14.

40. Beaubien-Souligny W, Eljaiek R, Fortier A, Lamarche Y, Liszkowski M, Bouchard J, et al. The Association Between Pulsatile Portal Flow and Acute Kidney Injury after Cardiac Surgery: A Retrospective Cohort Study. J Cardiothorac Vasc Anesth. 2018;32(4):1780–7.

41. Beaubien-Souligny W, Benkreira A, Robillard P, Bouabdallaoui N, Chasse M, Desjardins G, et al. Alterations in Portal Vein Flow and Intrarenal Venous Flow Are Associated With Acute Kidney Injury After Cardiac Surgery: A Prospective Observational Cohort Study. J Am Heart Assoc. 2018;7(19):e009961.

42. Iida N, Seo Y, Sai S, Machino-Ohtsuka T, Yamamoto M, Ishizu T, et al. Clinical implications of intrarenal hemodynamic evaluation by Doppler ultrasonography in heart failure. JACC Heart Fail. 2016;4(8):674–82.

43. Iida N, Seo Y, Sai S, Machino-Ohtsuka T, Yamamoto M, Ishizu T, et al. Clinical Implications of Intrarenal Hemodynamic Evaluation by Doppler Ultrasonography in Heart Failure. JACC Heart Fail. 2016;4(8):674–82.

44. Puzzovivo A, Monitillo F, Guida P, Leone M, Rizzo C, Grande D, et al. Renal Venous Pattern: A New Parameter for Predicting Prognosis in Heart Failure Outpatients. J Cardiovasc Dev Dis. 2018;5(4):52.

45. Beaubien-Souligny W, Denault AY. Real-Time Assessment of Renal Venous Flow by Transesophageal Echography During Cardiac Surgery. A&A practice. 2019;12(1):30–2.

46. Denault AY, Haddad F, Jacobsohn E, Deschamps A. Perioperative right ventricular dysfunction. Curr Opin Anaesthesiol. 2013;26(1):71–81.

47. Price LC, Wort SJ, Finney SJ, Marino PS, Brett SJ. Pulmonary vascular and right ventricular dysfunction in adult critical care: current and emerging options for management: a systematic literature review. Crit Care. 2010;14(5):R169.

48. Groves DS, Blum FE, Huffmyer JL, Kennedy JL, Ahmad HB, Durieux ME, et al. Effects of early inhaled epoprostenol therapy on pulmonary artery pressure and blood loss during LVAD placement. J Cardiothorac Vasc Anesth. 2014;28(3):652–60.

49. Lamarche Y, Perrault LP, Maltais S, Tetreault K, Lambert J, Denault AY. Preliminary experience with inhaled milrinone in cardiac surgery. Eur J Cardiothorac Surg. 2007;31(6):1081–7.

50. Elmi-Sarabi M, Deschamps A, Delisle S, Ased H, Haddad F, Lamarche Y, et al. Aerosolized vasodilators for the treatment of pulmonary hypertension in cardiac surgical patients: a systematic review and meta-analysis. Anesth Analg. 2017;125(2):393–402.

51. Gebhard CE, Desjardins G, Gebhard C, Gavra P, Denault AY. Intratracheal Milrinone Bolus Administration During Acute Right Ventricular Dysfunction After Cardiopulmonary Bypass. J Cardiothorac Vasc Anesth. 2017;31(2):489–96.

52. Gebhard CE, Rochon A, Cogan J, Ased H, Desjardins G, Deschamps A, et al. Acute Right Ventricular Failure in Cardiac Surgery During Cardiopulmonary Bypass Separation: A Retrospective Case Series of 12 Years' Experience With Intratracheal Milrinone Administration. J Cardiothor Vasc An. 2019;33(3):651–60.

Perioperative Blood Management in Cardiac Surgery

23

Nadia B. Hensley, Megan P. Kostibas,
Colleen G. Koch, and Steven M. Frank

Main Messages

1. Among cardiac surgery centers, transfusion rates vary widely, while overall transfusion risks remain considerable.
2. Transfusion-related lung injury is the number one most frequent cause of transfusion-related death, with transfusion-associated circulatory overload being second.
3. Considerations in perioperative blood management include preoperative blood conservation; intraoperative blood conservation; blood conservation during cardiopulmonary bypass; postoperative blood conservation; intraoperative and postoperative transfusion triggers; and the impact of blood storage duration.

Although cardiac surgery constitutes less than 2% of all surgeries in the United States, patients who undergo cardiac surgery receive approximately 10–15% of the nation's blood each year [1]. Despite the known risks and costs associated

with allogeneic transfusions, transfusion rates continue to vary widely among centers that perform cardiac surgery [2]. Recently completed, large, high-quality randomized trials have provided new information that addresses longstanding questions about transfusion in cardiac surgery patients. Two such questions include the ideal hemoglobin trigger for initiating transfusions [3–5] and whether longer duration of blood storage negatively affects outcomes [6]. Furthermore, various methods of blood conservation have been described and refined that dramatically reduce transfusion rates for cardiac surgery. The aim of this chapter is to review evidence-based best practices concerning patient blood management and transfusion therapy in cardiac surgery patients.

Closed cardiac surgery in the early days began with the "blue-baby" operation by Blalock in 1944; however, modern cardiac surgery with a heart-lung machine was first described in the mid-1950s. Transfusion medicine and blood banking also began in the 1940s when methods were discovered that enabled blood to be stored rather than transfused immediately. In the 1970s, when cardiac surgery volumes were increasing, it was recognized that transfusion incurred substantial risks, especially for viral hepatitis. In the early 1980s, the risk of transfusion was compounded by the newly discovered human immunodeficiency (HIV) virus. The years 1983–1984 marked the peak incidence of HIV and viral hep-

N. B. Hensley · M. P. Kostibas · C. G. Koch
S. M. Frank (✉)
Department of Anesthesiology/Critical Care Medicine, Johns Hopkins Medicine, Baltimore, MD, USA
e-mail: sfrank3@jhmi.edu

atitis transmission by transfusion. What followed was the era of restrictive transfusion practice, partly related to viral risk, but also supported by several large randomized trials that compared restrictive to liberal transfusion strategies and demonstrated similar outcomes when less blood was transfused [3, 4].

Although improved testing has made the current risk of transfusion-related viral transmission exceedingly low, the overall transfusion risks remain substantial. Transfusion-associated circulatory overload (TACO) and transfusion-related acute lung injury (TRALI) represent the number one and number two most frequent causes of transfusion-related death, respectively. Infections (primarily bacterial sepsis from platelets) and hemolytic transfusion reactions were the third and fourth most common causes of fatality according cases reported to the US Food and Drug Administration in 2016 (FDA) (Fig. 23.1) [7]. Over the past decade, primarily driven by patient safety and quality concerns, but also cost effectiveness efforts, we have witnessed the growth of patient blood management programs. Such programs aim to optimize blood utilization in a way that will reduce risks and costs while maintaining or improving outcomes, using methods reviewed

in this chapter and described in recent publications [8].

Evidence-Based Methods of Blood Conservation

Preoperative Blood Conservation

The various methods of blood management used for patients undergoing cardiac surgery are listed in Table 23.1. Preoperatively, if time allows, it is important to wait for anticoagulant medication effects to abate before the day of surgery. The advent of direct oral anticoagulant medications and the widespread use of the thienopyridines (e.g. clopidogrel) have challenged cardiac surgeons, as these are widely prescribed by cardiologists for acute coronary events as well as newly inserted coronary stents. The typical patient needs to be off of direct oral anticoagulants for 2–5 days, depending on the medication and the patient's renal function. Patients need between 3 and 5 days for thienopyridines, although both the response to these drugs and the time required for drug-effect resolution are highly variable [9]. Although not yet widespread, preliminary evidence suggests P2Y12 testing to assess recovery

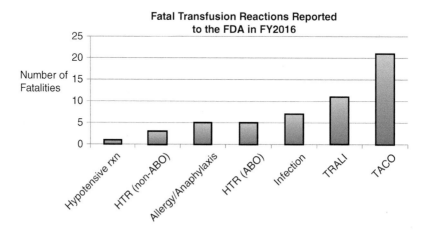

Fig. 23.1 Fatal transfusion reactions reported to the FDA in FY2016. In a report from the Food and Drug Administration (FDA) [9], transfusion-associated circulatory overload (TACO) was the most frequently reported cause of transfusion-related mortality, and transfusion-related acute lung injury (TRALI) was the second most

common cause. Infections (bacterial, viral, parasitic), hemolytic transfusion reactions (HTR) from ABO incompatibility, and allergic/anaphylactic reactions were the next most common causes of death; FY16, Fiscal Year 2016

Table 23.1 Methods of blood conservation for cardiac surgery

1. Education (with emphasis on the RCTs supporting restrictive transfusion)
2. Creation of transfusion guidelines for all blood components
3. Decision support for computerized provider order entry (with best practice advisories)
4. Transfusion guideline compliance audits w/ feedback (reports) to providers
5. Methods to achieve perioperative blood conservation
   (a) Preoperative anemia management
   (b) Discontinuation of anticoagulants and anti-platelet medications before surgery
   (c) Antifibrinolytics (e.g. aminocaproic acid, tranexamic acid)
   (d) Anesthetic management (autologous normovolemic hemodilution, controlled hypotension, normothermia)
   (e) Point-of-care testing (e.g. viscoelastic testing—TEG or ROTEM)
   (f) Surgical methods (newer cautery methods, topical hemostatics and sealants)
   (g) Hemoconcentrators for pump reservoir blood (MUF, ZBUF)
   (h) Autologous cell salvage
   (i) Evidence-based transfusion triggers
   (j) "Why give 2 when 1 will do" Choosing Wisely® campaign for RBCs
   (k) Reduce phlebotomy blood loss (smaller tubes, eliminate unnecessary testing)

MUF modified ultrafiltration, *RBC* red blood cell, *RCT* randomized controlled trial, *ROTEM* rotational thromboelastometry, *TEG* thromboelastography, *ZBUF* zero-balance ultrafiltration
Reprinted in modified format from Frank SM, et al *Anesthesiology*, 2017 [8]

of normal platelet function may be useful to determine patient readiness for surgery after discontinuation of these drugs.

Preoperative anemia diagnosis and treatment represents an opportunity to reduce unnecessary transfusions. Iron deficiency anemia is common, and recent studies have shown that patients with heart failure are particularly susceptible [10]. Anemia of chronic disease—recently renamed anemia of inflammation—is also common in elderly patients with chronic conditions. Both of these conditions are treatable, given enough time before surgery, assuming the surgery is not urgent or emergent. Intravenous iron and/or erythropoietin have been used to increase the hemoglobin at

a rate of about 1 g per week [11]. Ensuring that patients are diagnosed and treated early enough before scheduled surgery can be challenging even when surgery is non-emergent.

Intraoperative Blood Conservation

Multiple methods of intraoperative blood conservation are available. Autologous blood salvage (cell salvage or autotransfusion) has been an important method of blood conservation for cardiac surgery since the late 1970s when the technology was first introduced. In this procedure, shed blood is collected and washed in a conical-shaped centrifuge bowl to remove debris and concentrate the cells. The final product returned to the patient consists of red blood cells (RBCs) and saline, devoid of any plasma, clotting factors, and platelets. The efficacy of cell salvage for reducing transfusion requirements in cardiac surgery was shown in a meta-analysis by Carless et al. [12] who reported the relative risk of exposure to allogeneic RBCs to be 0.77 and the RBC savings to be 0.68 units per patient. A longstanding belief that cell salvage promotes coagulopathy is based on two premises: residual heparin and dilutional coagulopathy. However, little evidence supports these assertions. First, the amount of residual heparin in salvaged, washed blood is negligible, especially in relation to the amount of heparin administered during cardiopulmonary bypass (CPB). In addition, protamine reversal should neutralize any leftover heparin. Second, the dilutional coagulopathy after salvaged blood should be no different than that which occurs with banked RBCs. The need for plasma and platelets should be considered when approximately 50% or more of the total blood volume has been replaced. Ideally, coagulation testing with a point-of-care, rapid-turnaround result will guide the decision to transfuse plasma and/or platelets, as well as the need for fibrinogen replacement with cryoprecipitate.

Acute normovolemic hemodilution (ANH) has been used despite ongoing debate regarding its effectiveness [13]. This method involves phlebotomy at the beginning of surgery, storage of the fresh whole blood in citrated anticoagulant, and then dilution of the patient's blood so that when bleeding occurs, fewer red blood cells are lost from the circulation. Based on a recent meta-analysis, ANH does appear to be effective at reducing exposure to allogeneic blood, providing that (1) patients have a high enough starting hemoglobin level; (2) enough blood is removed to allow substantial hemodilution; and (3) enough blood is shed during surgery to make ANH worthwhile. Given the use of cell salvage and hemoconcentration of pump blood, the main benefit of ANH may be the fresh clotting factors and platelets that are given back to the patient at the end of surgery, as the ANH blood is fresh whole blood.

One common cause of excess bleeding during and after cardiac surgery is hypothermia, which impairs coagulation at the level of the clotting cascade and decreases platelet function. Furthermore, coagulation tests such as the INR and the thromboelastogram are routinely run at 37 °C and will come back normal in hypothermic patients, giving a false picture of normal clotting function. Prevention of hypothermia-related bleeding includes use of milder hypothermia during surgery with more local (topical) cardiac cooling rather than systemic cooling, and also more complete rewarming before separation from bypass. However, rewarming at too high a temperature can adversely impact neurologic outcomes by overheating the brain at a time when it is most susceptible to ischemic insults. The completeness of rewarming is typically assessed using a peripheral (bladder or rectal) temperature rather than a true core (blood, esophageal, or nasopharyngeal) temperature. Slower rewarming at a lower blood temperature can result in more complete warming and prevent overheating the vital organs.

Antifibrinolytics such as epsilon aminocaproic acid and tranexamic acid (the lysine analogs) have become almost universally administered during cardiac surgery. Until 2008, aprotinin was the antifibrinolytic of choice, but it was removed from the US market after a randomized trial (the BART trial) [14] reported increased

mortality. A longstanding question over effectiveness of antifibrinolytics was addressed in the recent large randomized trial by Myles et al. [15], which showed that tranexamic acid was effective compared to placebo at reducing transfusion requirements (46% reduction) and reoperation for bleeding (1.4% vs. 2.8%); however the incidence of postoperative seizures was increased (0.7% vs. 0.1%). Because seizures appeared to be a dose-related side effect, the dose was reduced by 50% partway through the study. Importantly, the incidence of thrombotic events was not increased by tranexamic acid. Aminocaproic acid is sometimes used to avoid the risk of seizures with tranexamic acid.

Topical hemostatic agents and sealants are efficacious for reducing bleeding during cardiac surgery. Achneck et al. [16] comprehensively reviewed the numerous products that are available, including those most often used in cardiac surgery. Thrombin and gelatin are often mixed together and are also sold as a combination product. Fibrin sealants are also used in cardiac surgery and have shown effectiveness in re-operative cases. Because patients undergoing revision cardiac surgery can require two- to three-fold the amount of transfused blood products, every method of blood conservation becomes critically important [17].

The delicate balance between clotting and bleeding is sometimes a challenge, especially during cardiac surgery. Adding to this challenge is the turnaround time for lab tests, which ideally is short enough to make important clinical decisions on therapy. Typically, the activated clotting time (ACT) is used to determine dosing of heparin and its reversal for patients who require CPB. Since the test result is measured in seconds, and the typical target during extracorporeal support is 400–480, meaningful results take 7–8 min.

Residual coagulation abnormalities occur commonly after reversal of heparin. In such patients, viscoelastic testing can be helpful for diagnosing and treating the bleeding. Thromboelastography (TEG) and rotational thromboelastometry (ROTEM) are the two primary tests available. These are whole blood clotting tests that yield useful information within 5–10 min (for initiation of clot) or 10–30 min (for clot strength and stability). These tests can help the clinician determine if the coagulopathy is due to clotting factor or fibrinogen deficiency, and they offer quantitative and qualitative information about platelet dysfunction. New variations of these tests that include addition of tissue factor yield more rapid results (1–2 min), especially for clot initiation, which is used to diagnose clotting factor deficiencies.

Clinical studies showing utility for viscoelastic testing in cardiac surgery are limited in number, but in general they support the use of this testing to reduce transfusion requirements, and perhaps even to improve outcomes. A 1999 study by Shore-Lesserson et al. [18] in patients undergoing complex cardiac surgery (e.g. combined coronary artery bypass graft valve, multiple valve, reoperation, or thoracic aortic procedure) used a TEG-based algorithm to determine treatment for microvascular bleeding. The decision to give protamine, plasma, platelets, cryoprecipitate, or antifibrinolytics was determined by TEG results and an algorithm. Use of this algorithm led to decreases in the percentage of patients who required plasma (7.5% vs. 30.8%) and platelets (13.2% vs. 28.8%). The conclusion was that earlier diagnosis and treatment of coagulation abnormalities resulted in earlier hemostasis and a decreased transfusion requirement. In a recent meta-analysis [19] of 15 trials, viscoelastic testing (TEG or ROTEM) reduced overall mortality (RR, 0.52; 95% CI, 0.28 to 0.95), but only eight trials provided data on mortality, and the studies included had a high risk of bias. The viscoelastic testing group had a reduced chance of receiving RBCs (RR, 0.86), plasma (RR, 0.57), and platelets (RR, 0.73), but the risk of reoperation did not decrease. In summary, viscoelastic testing seems to play a valuable role in cardiac surgery and may be useful for more accurately targeting blood component therapy. A TEG-based algorithm that we have been using at Johns Hopkins Hospital to manage post-CPB microvascular bleeding is shown in Fig. 23.2.

Blood Conservation During Cardiopulmonary Bypass

Membrane oxygenators activate the coagulation cascade, dilute platelets and clotting factors, and induce fibrinolysis and systemic inflammatory response syndrome. Various studies have attempted to mitigate these risks with a technique known as modified ultrafiltration (MUF), which has been shown to reduce postoperative blood loss and blood product utilization. MUF involves use of a hydrostatic pressure gradient to remove water and some low-molecular-weight substances from plasma, producing protein-rich whole blood to be returned to the patient after the cessation of CPB. When this technique is used during CPB, it is considered conventional ultrafiltration, or zero-balance ultrafiltration. The ultrafiltration occurs on the arterial side of the pump after blood has been pressurized by the roller pump and gone through the oxygenator membrane. The outlet is connected to the patient's venous line as blood reenters the patient's right atrium after passing through the hemofilter. MUF was created by pediatric cardiac surgeons who were attempting to reduce the hemodilutional effects of CPB, which are particularly pronounced in children but also occur in adults. In a meta-analysis that compared MUF to no ultrafiltration, Boodhwani et al. [20] showed that MUF significantly reduced transfusion requirements. In a prospective randomized trial of 573 patients, Luciani et al. [21] found not only that the mean volume of RBCs transfused for each patient was lower when MUF was used, but also that the proportion of patients who did not receive any blood products was higher (51.8% vs. 38.1%, P = 0.001). MUF is a blood conservation strategy that is likely underutilized in adults but has become the standard of care for pediatric cardiac surgical patients.

For zero-balance or conventional ultrafiltration during CPB, and the ultrafiltrate is replaced with an equal volume of balanced electrolyte solution. The zero-balance ultrafiltration filter unit is connected to the CPB pump, takes blood

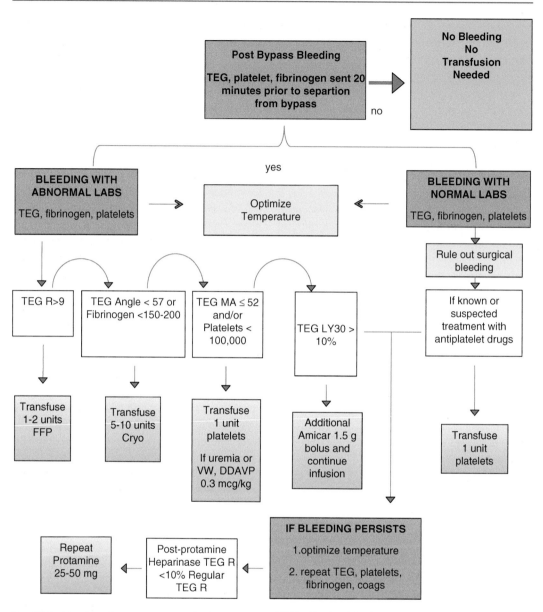

Fig. 23.2 Algorithm for management of microvascular bleeding and transfusion. The Johns Hopkins Hospital TEG-based algorithm for microvascular bleeding. Given the more rapid turnaround time for thromboelastography (TEG) than for traditional coagulation tests (PT, PTT, INR), this algorithm is used to determine therapy for cardiac surgery patients when bleeding persists after cardiopulmonary bypass. It requires a kaolin TEG, heparinase TEG, platelet count, and fibrinogen level

from a pre-membrane port, and runs in parallel to the main cardiopulmonary circuit. To prevent patient blood flow from dropping, the arterial pump rate is increased to compensate for the blood flow through the hemofilter. The main theoretical advantage is that zero-balance ultrafiltra-

tion can be used to reduce the inflammatory mediators that are activated when blood contacts a foreign surface. Thus, this technique might decrease lung injury, neurologic inflammation, bleeding, and acute kidney injury, as well as other indicators of morbidity. A recent meta-analysis showed no significant difference in intensive care unit length of stay, duration of ventilation, chest tube output, or other parameters between patients who received zero-balance ultrafiltration and those who received no hemofiltration [22].

Smaller diameter tubing, shorter tubing length, and low-volume oxygenators can reduce the hemodilution that occurs when patients are placed on CPB. Such low-volume circuits conserve blood and can reduce transfusion requirements. One result, however, is that the pump is moved closer to the surgical field, resulting in less physical space between the operating surgeons and the bypass pump.

Another commonly used perfusion-driven method of blood conservation is retrograde autologous prime (RAP). By using the patient's own venous blood to prime the cardiopulmonary bypass circuit by retrograde flow, hemodilution can be reduced, thereby reducing anemia and transfusion requirements. Typically, the crystalloid used to prime the circuit is pushed out and discarded during the RAP. RAP has been shown to reduce hemodilution and transfusion requirements in both adult and pediatric patients. In one study of adults, RAP reduced hemodilution by 10% (by nadir hematocrit), decreased the percentage of patients who required intraoperative transfusion (from 3% to 23%), and decreased the percentage of patients requiring transfusion during the entire hospitalization (from 27% to 53%) [22].

Postoperative Blood Conservation

Some patients who undergo cardiac surgery require as much transfusion in the postoperative period as they do during surgery. The primary goal postoperatively is to reduce bleeding, which is typically measured by the chest tube output. Excessive or massive bleeding is defined as blood loss of 100–200 mL per hour, on average, for the first 4 h, or more than 2 L in 24 h after surgery. Return to the operating room should be considered when this level of bleeding occurs. Viscoelastic testing often can be used to accurately diagnose the cause of postoperative bleed-

ing; however it will not detect bleeding that results from residual hypothermia as the test is run at 37 °C. Patients are more at risk for bleeding at core temperatures ≤35 °C.

Some centers collect the shed blood from chest and mediastinal drains, which can be transfused with or without cell washing. The transfusion of unwashed blood, however, may incur risk, because such blood is laden with various inflammatory mediators [23]. Furthermore this practice has not been clearly shown to reduce transfusion requirements and has been shown to induce fever, perhaps from an inflammatory reaction.

A particularly concerning problem is the large amount of blood removed from patients for lab testing. Such blood loss from phlebotomy can be substantial, especially for patients in intensive care units, where it can account for more than 60 mL/day. The blood lost includes not only that sent to the laboratory, but also the blood discarded when saline is cleared from the indwelling catheter tubing through which the blood is drawn. In a recent study, it was shown that the average cardiac surgery patient loses 500 mL of blood for lab testing after 10 days in the hospital, and 1000 mL of blood after 20 days [24]. These investigators "were astonished by the extent of bloodletting," with some patients losing a volume of blood equivalent to one to two RBC units [24]. At least three methods can be offered as potential solutions to this problem. First, reduce lab test ordering to those tests that are truly essential, rather than ordering daily blood draws just because the patient is in the hospital. Second, use an in-line blood return device so that the blood drawn to clear the saline from the lines can be returned in a sterile fashion back to the patient. And third, use smaller phlebotomy tubes. Tube volumes vary from 0.5 to 10 mL, or a 20-fold difference. We have switched to pediatric-size tubes throughout most of our hospital (2–4 mL size), rather than adult-size tubes (6–10 mL). The neonatal tubes (0.5 mL) are challenging to use because they do not run through the automated lab machines and must be manually run. Also, because their caps cannot be punctured by a needle, they must be uncapped, which poses a small risk of splash.

The concept of postoperative hemoglobin drift is well recognized. Hemoglobin levels nearly always decrease while patients are hospitalized. This phenomenon is especially true acutely after surgery for four reasons: (1) bleeding continues at varied rates after a patient leaves the operating room; (2) blood is lost through phlebotomy, as described above; (3) hemodilution occurs as a result of intravenous fluid given or fluids that are redistributed into the vascular compartment; and (4) erythropoiesis becomes impaired as a result of surgical stress, which elevates the hepcidin level, a substance critical for mobilizing iron stores for erythropoiesis. Since the body routinely creates and destroys 1% of the red cell mass daily, impaired erythropoiesis predisposes patients to hospital-acquired anemia. After cardiac surgery, hemoglobin levels typically decrease by an average of 1.8 g/dL. The nadir is usually seen on postoperative day three to four, followed by an average increase of 0.7 g/dL over postoperative days 4–10, likely due to hemoconcentration from diuresis [25]. This small but significant upward trend should be considered when using the hemoglobin level to determine need for transfusion.

Transfusion Triggers

Intraoperative Transfusion Triggers

In contrast to the postoperative setting, the ideal intraoperative hemoglobin transfusion trigger for cardiac surgical patients has not been rigorously studied. The Society of Thoracic Surgeons and Society of Cardiovascular Anesthesiologists Blood Conservation Clinical Practice Guidelines [1] suggest a lower limit of 6 g/dL for patients on CPB with moderate hypothermia, although they recognize that high-risk patients may need higher hemoglobin levels. This recommendation is supported by relatively weak evidence in the guideline. Some centers have begun monitoring cerebral tissue oxygen content with near-infrared spectroscopy technology; however no conclusive evidence shows that this type of monitoring can reliably guide transfusion therapy. By lowering

metabolic rate, hypothermic bypass reduces oxygen demands for all vital organs, meaning that lower hemoglobin levels will be tolerated. However, some groups now use either very mild or no systemic hypothermia. Instead they use selective regional cooling of the chest cavity, leaving the brain and kidneys at normal temperature. Additional studies are needed to determine the ideal hemoglobin levels during CPB.

Postoperative Transfusion Triggers

In the past decade, practice has moved toward transfusing less blood to patients, including those undergoing cardiac surgery. This change in practice is supported by one small and three large randomized trials that showed non-inferiority when a restrictive transfusion strategy was compared to a liberal strategy. The three large studies carried out in cardiac surgical patients were the Transfusion Requirements after Cardiac Surgery (TRACS) Trial in 2010 [3], the Transfusion Indication Threshold Reduction (TITRe2) in 2015 [4], and the Transfusion Requirements in Cardiac Surgery (TRICS III) in 2017 [5]. These studies each included postoperative transfusion triggers, and neither demonstrated a difference in the primary outcomes between a liberal and a restrictive transfusion strategy (Fig. 23.3).

TRACS Trial [3]
The TRACS trial enrolled 502 patients and compared restrictive and liberal transfusion triggers (hematocrit 24% vs. 30%, respectively). The primary outcome was a composite of morbidity and mortality, which occurred with similar frequency in the liberal (10%) and restrictive (11%) groups (P = 0.85) (Fig. 23.3).

TITRe2 Trial [4]
The TITRe2 trial compared hemoglobin triggers of 7.5 g/dL (restrictive) and 9.0 g/dL (liberal) in 2007 postoperative cardiac surgery patients. The primary outcome was a serious infection or ischemic event, which occurred with similar frequency in the liberal (33.0%) and restrictive (35.1%) groups (P = 0.30) (Fig. 23.3). The fact

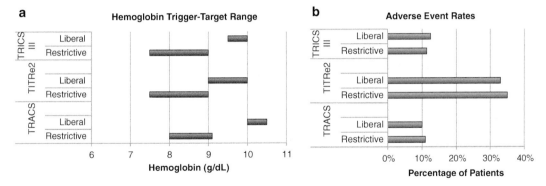

Fig. 23.3 Hemoglobin and primary outcome data are shown for the liberal and restrictive transfusion groups of the TRACS [3], TITRe2 [4], and TRICS III [5] trials. Panel A: The left edge of the red bars represents the hemoglobin trigger (prior to transfusion) for each group, and the right edge represents the hemoglobin target (daily average hemoglobin). Panel B: Among cardiac surgery patients, adverse event rates for the primary outcome (as defined by these trials) were similar (non-inferior) in those assigned to the lower (restrictive) and higher (liberal) hemoglobin transfusion thresholds

that outcome event rates were similar in the two transfusion groups strongly supports use of a restrictive approach, as we only add risk and cost by administering more blood than is necessary. Although the restrictive group in the TITRe2 trial had higher postoperative mortality at 90 days (4.2 vs. 2.6%, P = 0.045), this was a secondary outcome, with no statistical adjustment for multiple comparisons, making the significance questionable. This finding suggests that we may not fully understand tolerable lower levels of hemoglobin in high-risk patients.

TRICS III Trial [5]

The TRICS III trial is the largest randomized trial ever on transfusion triggers, in which over 5000 cardiac surgery patients were randomized to a lower (restrictive) or higher (liberal) hemoglobin trigger (7.5 vs. 9.5 g/dL), starting with induction of anesthesia and continuing in the intensive care unit. On the post-ICU wards, the two groups were treated with triggers of 7.5 vs. 8.5 g/dL. The primary outcome of death, myocardial infarction, stroke, or renal failure requiring dialysis was no different (non-inferior) between groups (restrictive 11.4%, liberal 12.5%). Of interest, this was the one study of the three large trials that included the intraoperative period for these transfusion strategies. Perhaps most interesting is the finding that patients aged 75 or greater had a worse primary outcome in the liberal compared to the restrictive group (14.1 vs. 10.2%; P = 0.004), and one-half of all patients enrolled were in this age group. This is the first time that elderly patients specifically have been shown to do better when given less blood. The other special aspect of the TRICS III study is the 6-month follow-up report [26] on the same primary outcome which was similar in the restrictive (17.4%) and the liberal (17.1%) groups (non-inferior). Hospital readmissions and emergency department visits were also no different between groups. In summary, the TRICS III trial being so large and with longer follow-up, has shown in a fairly conclusive fashion that giving cardiac surgery patients more blood than needed is either unhelpful, or actually harmful to the older patients.

Cleveland Clinic Trial [27]

This trial included over 700 adult cardiac surgery patients randomized to receive less blood (hematocrit trigger 24%) or more blood (hematocrit trigger 28%) from the start of surgery and throughout the hospital stay. The transfusion rate was decreased by 28% in the lower hematocrit group and no differences in morbidity or mortality were reported. The investigators concluded that the risks of anemia and transfusion were equally balanced within these hematocrit ranges, and that liberal transfusion only added risks and costs without benefit.

A recent meta-analysis [28] of randomized controlled trials involving transfusion triggers reported that restrictive thresholds may place patients at risk for adverse postoperative outcomes. The methods differed from those of other studies in that the authors used a context-specific approach (i.e. they separated groups for analysis according to patient characteristics and clinical settings). Risk ratios (RRs) were calculated for the following 30-day complications: inadequate oxygen supply, mortality, a composite of both, and infections. Thirty-one trials were regrouped into five context-specific risk strata. In patients undergoing cardiac/vascular procedures, restrictive strategies possibly increased the risk of events reflecting inadequate oxygen supply (RR, 1.09; CI, 0.97 to 1.22) and mortality (RR, 1.39; CI, 0.95 to 2.04), and the composite risk of events did reach statistical significance (RR, 1.12; CI, 1.01 to 1.24). Given the limitations of meta-analyses, this finding does not clearly support a liberal transfusion strategy in cardiac surgery patients.

One caveat is that when patients are actively bleeding, they will need to be transfused more liberally because whatever hemoglobin threshold is chosen, transfusion must at least keep pace with the bleeding.

Impact of Blood Storage Duration

RBC storage is an unnatural state during which numerous time-related changes occur, including morphologic and biochemical changes and accumulation of cellular byproducts. Many of these changes are nonlinear [29] and interrelated [30]. The FDA limits storage of RBCs to 42 days based on two requirements: (1) there is less than 1% RBC hemolysis at the end of storage and (2) in vivo RBC survival is >75% at 24 h after transfusion. The 42-day storage limit was not based on RBC product effectiveness or post-transfusion outcomes but has remained unchanged for years.

The Red Blood Cell Storage Lesion

The RBC storage lesion represents changes related to progressive deterioration in the RBC product over storage time. One of the hallmarks of storage lesion relates to changes to RBC morphology. Depending on the duration of storage, RBC units contain varying percentages of normal discocytes, as well as echinocytes and spherocytes. Loss of RBC shape and reduced deformability may contribute to decreased capillary perfusion and increases in aggregation and thrombosis [31]. In response to stress as storage duration increases, RBCs lose membrane integrity secondary to vesiculation processes, with resultant accumulation of microvesicles. Microparticle-encapsulated hemoglobin is of concern clinically because of increased nitric oxide scavenging, potentially leading to reduced tissue oxygenation. Furthermore, older RBC units have a higher free iron content, which may increase non-transferrin-bound iron, predisposing patients to hospital-acquired infections. The storage-related changes in RBCs are outlined in Table 23.2.

Donor phenotypes can contribute to RBCs being more or less susceptible to storage lesion, which may influence RBC survival and the quality of the donor unit. Dumont and Aubuchon [32] reported substantial variability among donors in reference to end-of-storage radiolabeled RBC recovery, which ranged from 35% to 82%. In addition to characteristics of the donor, preservation milieu can influence variability in deterioration of the RBC product. Thus, expiration dates that currently distinguish fresh and old RBC groups may not correspond to metabolic aging patterns during storage. Omics technology could play a future role in better understanding markers for storage-related changes to RBCs.

Clinical Studies on Duration of Storage

Recent controlled trials report similar outcomes in patients randomized to shorter or longer duration of RBC storage in clinical settings of cardiac

Table 23.2 Characteristic changes to red blood cells during storage

Morphologic	Biochemical	Substance accumulation
Loss of shape and membrane integrity	Decreased pH	Increased microvesicles
Membrane loss	Decreased glutathione	Increased inflammatory mediators
Membrane protein and lipid conformational and organizational changes	Decreased S-nitrosohemoglobin (SNO-Hb) bioactivity	Senescent red blood cells
Increased aggregability	Decreased 2,3 diphosphoglycerate	Oxidative stress
Viscoelastic changes	Decreased adenosine triphosphate	Interleukin-8, TNF-alpha, TGF-beta
Oxidative injury to structural proteins, lipids, and carbohydrates	Increased free hemoglobin	Increased reactive oxygen species
Increased population of spherocytes and echinocytes	Increased lactate	Bioactive lipids (activate neutrophils)
Reduced deformability	Increased potassium and sodium	Lipids
Decreased membrane domain	Increased ammonium	Cytokines
Increased band 3 oligomers	Decreased labile proteins: complement, fibronectin, coagulation factors	Complement, anaphylatoxins C3a and C5a
Increased ceramide rafts	Decreased NADH	Membrane attack complexes (MAC)

surgery [33], intensive care [34], and pediatric surgery (Fig. 23.4) [35]. However, it is important to recognize that these trials have different definitions for what constitutes fresh and old RBC units. Furthermore, in vitro aging processes are not necessarily aligned with the fresh and old RBC groupings used in these studies. Bordbar and colleagues [29] identified distinct metabolic states that exhibited nonlinear decay in stored RBCs, suggesting inconsistent cutoffs to define fresh and old RBC units. Of note, these authors asked a more fundamental question: "what is old and what is fresh?"

Mortality was the primary outcome, and results are shown separately for adults and neonates, infants, and children. No significant difference is apparent; however, studies were not allowed to purposefully transfuse blood in the last week or two of the allowed 42-day storage limit (Reprinted from Carson, et al., JAMA 2016;316:2025–35) [6]. Differences in methodology have also been proposed as a reason for inconsistencies in findings between observational and clinical trials on storage duration. For example, RBC units transfused in recent trials were likely not old enough to be used in a proper examination of clinical outcomes after long-term storage (i.e. RBCs at the end of shelf-life, 5–6 weeks storage duration). Other investigators noted that recent clinical trials were underpowered to answer the question of whether prolonged RBC storage (4–6 weeks) is associated with increased mortality [36]. Furthermore, Klein [36] and others at the Clinical Center of the National Institutes of Health now use an upper limit of 35 days for RBC storage, similar to that used in Ireland, Germany, and the UK. The percentage of RBC units transfused after 35 days of storage is reportedly between 9.7% and 20.7%. The most recent recommendations endorsed by the AABB are to continue with current guidelines (i.e. no changes in RBC storage duration limits), or preferentially use fresh RBCs [6].

Extremes of Transfusion

Patient Who Don't Agree to Transfusion

For personal or religious reasons, some patients do not agree to allogeneic blood transfusions. Such patients receive specialized treatment called "bloodless" care [37]. Centers that specialize in

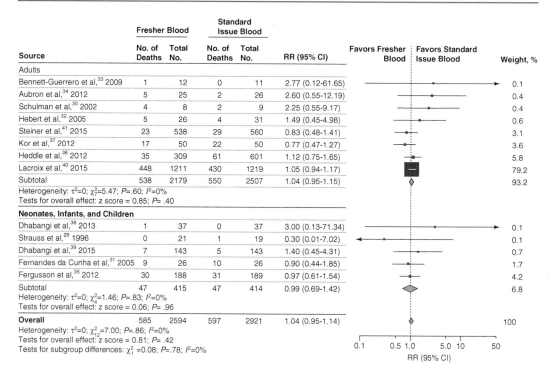

	Fresher Blood		Standard Issue Blood				
Source	No. of Deaths	Total No.	No. of Deaths	Total No.	RR (95% CI)		Weight, %
Adults							
Bennett-Guerrero et al,[33] 2009	1	12	0	11	2.77 (0.12-61.65)		0.1
Aubron et al,[34] 2012	5	25	2	26	2.60 (0.55-12.19)		0.4
Schulman et al,[30] 2002	4	8	2	9	2.25 (0.55-9.17)		0.4
Hebert et al,[32] 2005	5	26	4	31	1.49 (0.45-4.98)		0.6
Steiner et al,[41] 2015	23	538	29	560	0.83 (0.48-1.41)		3.1
Kor et al,[37] 2012	17	50	22	50	0.77 (0.47-1.27)		3.6
Heddle et al,[36] 2012	35	309	61	601	1.12 (0.75-1.65)		5.8
Lacroix et al,[40] 2015	448	1211	430	1219	1.05 (0.94-1.17)		79.2
Subtotal	538	2179	550	2507	1.04 (0.95-1.15)		93.2
Heterogeneity: $\tau^2=0$; $\chi^2_7=5.47$; $P=.60$; $I^2=0\%$							
Tests for overall effect: z score = 0.85; $P=.40$							
Neonates, Infants, and Children							
Dhabangi et al,[38] 2013	1	37	0	37	3.00 (0.13-71.34)		0.1
Strauss et al,[29] 1996	0	21	1	19	0.30 (0.01-7.02)		0.1
Dhabangi et al,[39] 2015	7	143	5	143	1.40 (0.45-4.31)		0.7
Fernandes da Cunha et al,[31] 2005	9	26	10	26	0.90 (0.44-1.85)		1.7
Fergusson et al,[35] 2012	30	188	31	189	0.97 (0.61-1.54)		4.2
Subtotal	47	415	47	414	0.99 (0.69-1.42)		6.8
Heterogeneity: $\tau^2=0$; $\chi^2_4=1.46$; $P=.83$; $I^2=0\%$							
Tests for overall effect: z score = 0.06; $P=.96$							
Overall	585	2594	597	2921	1.04 (0.95-1.14)		100
Heterogeneity: $\tau^2=0$; $\chi^2_{12}=7.00$; $P=.86$; $I^2=0\%$							
Tests for overall effect: z score = 0.81; $P=.42$							
Tests for subgroup differences: $\chi^2_1 =0.08$; $P=.78$; $I^2=0\%$							

Fig. 23.4 Meta-analysis of randomized clinical trials comparing fresher and standard-issue blood

bloodless medicine are well versed with methods used to ensure good outcomes when blood is not an option. All of the above methods of blood conservation are utilized, starting with aggressive preoperative anemia diagnosis and treatment as outlined in a report by Jassar et al. [38]. Often, intravenous iron and/or erythropoietin are administered preoperatively to increase the red cell mass to a target threshold determined by the patient's body mass. Because smaller patients have a lower total blood volume and thus a lower allowable blood loss, a higher preoperative hemoglobin is targeted. A weekly visit to an outpatient infusion clinic may be required for intravenous administration of iron dextran (1000 mg), along with erythropoietin or darbepoetin. Intraoperatively, meticulous surgical technique is used, and perfusionists play a major role in blood conservation as outlined above. When all blood conservation methods are optimized, these patients who do not accept transfusion do just as well, or better, than patients who accept allogeneic transfusion [39, 40].

Patients Who Receive Massive Transfusion

Transfusion for blood loss that approaches or exceeds one blood volume (10 units) is considered to be a massive transfusion, although the true definition usually involves a time period (typically 24 h). Such patients are likely to require not only RBCs but also plasma and platelets, and the ideal ratio of these blood components is important to consider. The only randomized trial that addressed this ratio was carried out in hemorrhaging trauma victims (the PROPPR Trial) [41]. That study showed no difference in the primary outcome (mortality) at 24 h between the higher and lower plasma- and platelet-to-RBC ratio groups. However, the incidence of hemorrhagic death was higher in the group that received less plasma and platelets, and the investigators interpreted this finding to favor a 1:1:1 ratio of RBCs, plasma, and platelets for massive transfusion. Whether or not these findings apply to non-trauma patients or cardiac sur-

Fig. 23.5 Algorithm for massive transfusion protocol. The Johns Hopkins Hospital massive transfusion protocol. The ratio of blood components represents a 1:1:1 ratio for red blood cells (RBCs), plasma (FFP), and platelets. An apheresis unit of platelets contains 1 unit of plasma and the number of platelets present in 6 units of whole blood (thus the 6:5:1 unit ratio for RBCs, FFP, and platelets). Although not shown, viscoelastic coagulation testing (thromboelastography, TEG) is recommended to guide the ratio of blood components transfused, when possible

Massive Transfusion Protocol (When to Initiate)
- Loss of entire blood volume within 24 hrs
- 50% of blood volume in 3 hrs
- Ongoing bleeding at ≥150 ml/min
- Rapid bleeding with circulatory failure despite volume replacement

Massive Transfusion Protocol (Procedure)
- Sample for type and screen to blood bank
- Blood products in containers (coolers)
- 1:1:1 ratio of RBC:FFP:Platelets (6 u RBC, 5 u FFP, 1 apheresis unit platelets)
- 10 u Cryoprecipitate in coolers 3, 6, and 9
- Complete use of 1 cooler before next cooler
- Upon issuing a cooler, blood bank prepares next cooler
- 1 cooler every 20-30 min until protocol discontinued

- Labs upon initiation
  type and screen
  CBC
  PT/PTT/INR
  ABG
  Comp Metabolic panel
  iCa
  Lactate

- Labs to send every one hour
  CBC
  PT/PTT/INR
  Fibrinogen
  ABG
  iCa
  Lactate

gery is unclear. Ideally, point-of-care or rapid-turnaround lab testing should be used to monitor coagulation and guide the ratio of blood components given. See Fig. 23.5 for the Johns Hopkins massive transfusion protocol.

References

1. Society of Thoracic Surgeons Blood Conservation Guideline Task F, Ferraris VA, Brown JR, et al. 2011 update to the Society of Thoracic Surgeons and the Society of Cardiovascular Anesthesiologists blood conservation clinical practice guidelines. Ann Thorac Surg. 2011;91:944–82.
2. Bennett-Guerrero E, Zhao Y, O'Brien SM, et al. Variation in use of blood transfusion in coronary artery bypass graft surgery. JAMA. 2010;304:1568–75.
3. Hajjar LA, Vincent JL, Galas FR, et al. Transfusion requirements after cardiac surgery: the TRACS randomized controlled trial. JAMA. 2010;304:1559–67.
4. Murphy GJ, Pike K, Rogers CA, et al. Liberal or restrictive transfusion after cardiac surgery. N Engl J Med. 2015;372:997–1008.
5. Mazer CD, Whitlock RP, Fergusson DA, Hall J, Belley-Cote E, Connolly K, Khanykin B, Gregory AJ, de Medicis E, McGuinness S, Royse A, Carrier FM, Young PJ, Villar JC, Grocott HP, Seeberger MD, Fremes S, Lellouche F, Syed S, Byrne K, Bagshaw SM, Hwang NC, Mehta C, Painter TW, Royse C, Verma S, Hare GMT, Cohen A, Thorpe KE, Juni P, Shehata N, Investigators T, Perioperative Anesthesia Clinical Trials G. Restrictive or liberal red-cell transfusion for cardiac surgery. N Engl J Med. 2017;377:2133–44.
6. Carson JL, Guyatt G, Heddle NM, et al. Clinical practice guidelines from the AABB: red blood cell transfusion thresholds and storage. JAMA. 2016;316:2025–35.
7. Fatalites reported to the FDA following blood collection and transfusion. 2016. https://www.fda.gov/biologicsbloodvaccines/safetyavailability/reportaproblem/transfusiondonationfatalities/default.htm. Accessed March 2, 2019.
8. Frank SM, Thakkar RN, Podlasek SJ, et al. Implementation of a health system-wide blood management program using a clinical community approach. Anesthesiology. 2017;127(5):754–64.
9. Ferraris VA, Saha SP, Oestreich JH, et al. 2012 update to the Society of Thoracic Surgeons guideline on use of antiplatelet drugs in patients having cardiac and noncardiac operations. Ann Thorac Surg. 2012;94:1761–81.
10. Cohen-Solal A, Leclercq C, Deray G, et al. Iron deficiency: an emerging therapeutic target in heart failure. Heart. 2014;100:1414–20.
11. Resar LM, Wick EC, Almasri TN, et al. Bloodless medicine: current strategies and emerging treatment paradigms. Transfusion. 2016;56:2637–47.
12. Carless PA, Henry DA, Moxey AJ, et al. Cell salvage for minimising perioperative allogeneic blood transfusion. Cochrane Database Syst Rev. 2010:CD001888.
13. Grant MC, Resar LM, Frank SM. The efficacy and utility of acute normovolemic hemodilution. Anesth Analg. 2015;121:1412–4.

14. Fergusson DA, Hebert PC, Mazer CD, et al. A comparison of aprotinin and lysine analogues in high-risk cardiac surgery. N Engl J Med. 2008;358:2319–31.

15. Myles PS, Smith JA, Forbes A, et al. Tranexamic acid in patients undergoing coronary-artery surgery. N Engl J Med. 2017;376:136–48.

16. Achneck HE, Sileshi B, Jamiolkowski RM, et al. A comprehensive review of topical hemostatic agents: efficacy and recommendations for use. Ann Surg. 2010;251:217–28.

17. Hensley NB, Kostibas MP, Gupta PB, et al. Blood utilization in revision vs. first-time cardiac surgery: An update in the era of patient blood management. Transfusion. 2018;58(1):168–75.

18. Shore-Lesserson L, Manspeizer HE, DePerio M, et al. Thromboelastography-guided transfusion algorithm reduces transfusions in complex cardiac surgery. Anesth Analg. 1999;88:312–9.

19. Wikkelso A, Wetterslev J, Moller AM, Afshari A. Thromboelastography (TEG) or thromboelastometry (ROTEM) to monitor haemostatic treatment versus usual care in adults or children with bleeding. Cochrane Database Syst Rev. 2016:CD007871.

20. Boodhwani M, Williams K, Babaev A, et al. Ultrafiltration reduces blood transfusions following cardiac surgery: a meta-analysis. Eur J Cardiothorac Surg. 2006;30:892–7.

21. Luciani GB, Menon T, Vecchi B, et al. Modified ultrafiltration reduces morbidity after adult cardiac operations: a prospective, randomized clinical trial. Circulation. 2001;104:I253–9.

22. Zhu X, Ji B, Wang G, et al. The effects of zero-balance ultrafiltration on postoperative recovery after cardiopulmonary bypass: a meta-analysis of randomized controlled trials. Perfusion. 2012;27:386–92.

23. Liumbruno GM, Waters JH. Unwashed shed blood: should we transfuse it? Blood Transfus. 2011;9:241–5.

24. Koch CG, Reineks EZ, Tang AS, et al. Contemporary bloodletting in cardiac surgical care. Ann Thorac Surg. 2015;99:779–84.

25. George TJ, Beaty CA, Kilic A, et al. Hemoglobin drift after cardiac surgery. Ann Thorac Surg. 2012;94:703–9.

26. Mazer CD, Whitlock RP, Fergusson DA, Belley-Cote E, Connolly K, Khanykin B, Gregory AJ, de Medicis E, Carrier FM, McGuinness S, Young PJ, Byrne K, Villar JC, Royse A, Grocott HP, Seeberger MD, Mehta C, Lellouche F, Hare GMT, Painter TW, Fremes S, Syed S, Bagshaw SM, Hwang NC, Royse C, Hall J, Dai D, Mistry N, Thorpe K, Verma S, Juni P, Shehata N, Investigators T, Perioperative Anesthesia Clinical Trials G. Six-month outcomes after restrictive or liberal transfusion for cardiac surgery. N Engl J Med. 2018;379:1224–33.

27. Koch CG, Sessler DI, Mascha EJ, Sabik JF III, Li L, Duncan AI, Zimmerman NM, Blackstone EH. A randomized clinical trial of red blood cell transfusion triggers in cardiac surgery. Ann Thorac Surg. 2017;104:1243–50.

28. Hovaguimian F, Myles PS. Restrictive versus liberal transfusion strategy in the perioperative and acute care settings: a context-specific systematic review and meta-analysis of randomized controlled trials. Anesthesiology. 2016;125:46–61.

29. Bordbar A, Johansson PI, Paglia G, et al. Identified metabolic signature for assessing red blood cell unit quality is associated with endothelial damage markers and clinical outcomes. Transfusion. 2016;56:852–62.

30. Donadee C, Raat NJ, Kanias T, et al. Nitric oxide scavenging by red blood cell microparticles and cell-free hemoglobin as a mechanism for the red cell storage lesion. Circulation. 2011;124:465–76.

31. Salaria ON, Barodka VM, Hogue CW, et al. Impaired red blood cell deformability after transfusion of stored allogeneic blood but not autologous salvaged blood in cardiac surgery patients. Anesth Analg. 2014;118:1179–87.

32. Dumont LJ, AuBuchon JP. Evaluation of proposed FDA criteria for the evaluation of radiolabeled red cell recovery trials. Transfusion. 2008;48:1053–60.

33. Steiner ME, Ness PM, Assmann SF, et al. Effects of red-cell storage duration on patients undergoing cardiac surgery. N Engl J Med. 2015;372:1419–29.

34. Lacroix J, Hebert PC, Fergusson DA, et al. Age of transfused blood in critically ill adults. N Engl J Med. 2015;372:1410–8.

35. Fergusson DA, Hebert P, Hogan DL, et al. Effect of fresh red blood cell transfusions on clinical outcomes in premature, very low-birth-weight infants: the ARIPI randomized trial. JAMA. 2012;308:1443–51.

36. Klein HG. The red cell storage lesion(s): of dogs and men. Blood Transfus. 2017;15:107–11.

37. Resar LM, Frank SM. Bloodless medicine: what to do when you can't transfuse. Hematology Am Soc Hematol Educ Program. 2014;2014:553–8.

38. Jassar AS, Ford PA, Haber HL, et al. Cardiac surgery in Jehovah's Witness patients: ten-year experience. Ann Thorac Surg. 2012;93:19–25.

39. Frank SM, Wick EC, Dezern AE, et al. Risk-adjusted clinical outcomes in patients enrolled in a bloodless program. Transfusion. 2014;54:2668–77.

40. Pattakos G, Koch CG, Brizzio ME, et al. Outcome of patients who refuse transfusion after cardiac surgery: a natural experiment with severe blood conservation. Arch Intern Med. 2012;172:1154–60.

41. Holcomb JB, Tilley BC, Baraniuk S, et al. Transfusion of plasma, platelets, and red blood cells in a 1:1:1 vs a 1:1:2 ratio and mortality in patients with severe trauma: The PROPPR randomized clinical trial. JAMA. 2015;313:471–82.

Perioperative Antifibrinolytics and Coagulation Management

24

John Fitzgerald, Aidan Sharkey, and Keyvan Karkouti

Main Messages
1. Excessive bleeding is one of the most common cardiac surgery perioperative complications.
2. Postoperative bleeding that requires re-exploration and multiple blood product transfusions is associated with increased risk of morbidity.
3. Point of Care testing has been beneficial in providing clinicians with timely and specific differentiation on factors attributing to coagulopathy, allowing a more targeted blood products transfusion approach.

One of the most common perioperative complications of cardiac surgery is excessive bleeding. Postoperative bleeding requiring transfusion of multiple blood products or re-exploration is associated with an increased risk of morbidity including prolonged mechanical ventilation, acute respiratory distress syndrome and infection, and mortality [1]. While the cause of bleeding may be primarily surgical in many cases, often an impor-

tant contributing factor is a disruption in the complex interactions of the coagulation pathway caused by the conduct of surgery and cardiopulmonary bypass (i.e. cardiac surgery-associated coagulopathy). Although guidelines exist to aid in blood conservation interventions and provide guidance on best transfusion practise [2], it is often difficult in the dynamic setting of surgery to identify the specific factors that contribute to the coagulopathy. Because of this, clinicians often employ an empirical approach to coagulation management. The advent of point of care testing (POCT), however, has proved beneficial in providing more specific and timely information of any deficiencies, allowing for a more targeted approach to transfusion. In this chapter, we provide an introduction to the utility of POCT and address the various defects that can occur in the patient's normal hemostasis mechanisms. By better understanding the different components of cardiac surgery-associated coagulopathy, we can identify the primary defects that contribute to bleeding and thereby devise more effective therapeutic strategies. Although each component is discussed separately below, it is with the understanding of the inherent complexity of the coagulation pathway and the interplay of the different components.

J. Fitzgerald · A. Sharkey · K. Karkouti (✉)
Department of Anesthesia and Pain Management,
Toronto General Hospital, University Health
Network, University of Toronto, Toronto, Canada
e-mail: Keyvan.Karkouti@uhn.ca

© Springer Nature Switzerland AG 2021
D. C. H. Cheng et al. (eds.), *Evidence-Based Practice in Perioperative Cardiac Anesthesia and Surgery*, https://doi.org/10.1007/978-3-030-47887-2_24

Perioperative Considerations

Monitoring Coagulation Using Viscoelastic Point-of-Care Devices

Standard lab tests of coagulation, which typically include platelet count, prothrombin time, partial thromboplastin time, and fibrinogen level, may not be sufficient to adequately describe the complex and multiple interacting components of the coagulation cascade. There are a number of areas where these tests fall short including a lack of information on platelet function and also the interaction between the platelets, clotting factors and red blood cells. POCT (point of care testing) devices emphasize a cell based model of coagulation which places a greater importance on the pivotal role of platelets. Standard lab tests utilise plasma as their sample and thus provide information on the first phase of coagulation up to fibrin formation whereas POCT uses whole blood which produces information on all phases of coagulation from fibrin formation to fibrinolysis. This gives useful information regarding the kinetics of clot formation and the overall tensile strength of the clot. Additionally, standard lab tests can suffer from delays in sample processing and obtaining results leading to prolonged intervals of time before intervention. POCT may be performed in a more time sensitive manner and may allow for protocol driven intervention in the immediate operative period.

As such, viscoelastic coagulation tests have been described in a number of different protocols to help guide transfusion practices (Fig. 24.1). In addition to a more targeted approach to coagula-

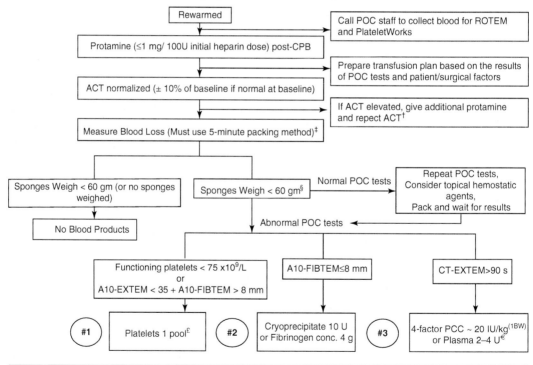

Fig. 24.1 An example of blood transfusion algorithm incorporating ROTEM. Reprinted from Keyvan Karkouti et al.: TACS Investigators. Point-of-Care Hemostatic Testing in Cardiac Surgery A Stepped-Wedge Clustered Randomized Controlled Trial. Circulation. 2016;134:1152–1162

tion management, the overall aim of these algorithms is to reduce inappropriate blood product transfusion. The Society of Thoracic Surgeons and Society of Cardiothoracic Anesthesiologists practice guidelines recommend the use of POC tests in a multimodal transfusion guideline and has been deemed a Class 1 recommendation [2]. Despite this, there are a number of limitations that have been highlighted with regard to these devices. There are no adequate studies comparing the various algorithms or the different devices employed in these algorithms. As such it is difficult to make specific recommendations about their use in the clinical setting, such as which device to use, when, and in what population. Additionally, the values obtained are not interchangeable, meaning an algorithm designed for one particular device will have measurements that are non-applicable to other devices. Also, POCT have yet to definitively show that, when compared to standard laboratory tests, they more consistently predict postoperative bleeding [3]. There is, however, increasing evidence that their use improves management of coagulopathy and reduces transfusions [4].

One of the main motivations to improve POC assessment of platelet reactivity was for monitoring the effects of platelet active medications, particularly those being given during vascular stent placement. In cardiac surgery, these devices are being investigated as a way of determining optimum timing for withdrawal of antiplatelet drugs or determining appropriate thresholds for platelet transfusions in the perioperative period. There are a number of different platelet assays used in clinical or research settings. A comparison of all available devices is beyond the scope if this chapter, however, these methods show similar trends in activity but their overall results correlate poorly and cannot be used interchangeably [5].

Hyperfibrinolysis

Pathophysiology

Within the body, endothelial cells release t-PA (tissue-plasminogen activator), a major activator of plasminogen. As a patient's blood passes through the extracorporeal circuit of CPB, the level of tPA secretion increases five times above normal physiological levels [6]. This increase in active tPA levels is considered to play a major role in the hyperfibrinolysis observed during CPB. Indeed, the extent of fibrinolysis is related to the duration of time spent on bypass and is increased following prolonged procedures. However, it should be noted that increased tPA alone will not result in increased fibrinolytic activity. Fibrin must also be present in order for plasminogen to become activated. In the CPB circuit, fibrin is present in soluble and circuit bound form. The CPB circuit itself provides a large surface area to facilitate the conversion of plasminogen to plasmin. It had been observed that the initiation of CPB is associated with a 10- to 100-fold increase in plasmin generation [7]. Overall the hyperfibrinolytic state promoted by CPB consumes fibrinogen. There is then a paucity of fibrinogen available for normal coagulation after discontinuation of bypass. Plasmin also partially activates platelets which renders them less reactive to further activation by typical physiological pathways involving agonists such as adenosine diphosphate and arachidonic acid. Furthermore, excessive levels of plasmin can damage platelets through cleavage of their glycoprotein IIb receptor [8]. There is a naturally occurring physiological inhibitor of plasmin called α2-antiplasmin or α2-plasmin inhibitor (α2-PI). This acts by rapidly neutralising free plasmin but has little to no effect on bound plasmin. Therefore, it can be seen that α2-PI is a potent inhibitor when it comes to pathological fibrinolysis where the amount of unbound plasmin is increased, but it would have little effect on physiological fibrinolysis where the plasmin is primarily bound to fibrin. This varying effect means that during normal physiological circumstances in the body, normal clot lysis can take place whilst not affecting overall hemostasis.

Therapies

Drugs used to treat hyperfibrinolysis are considered in two categories as there are significant differences between their mechanism of action and how they ultimately effect hemostasis and clot lysis. The lysine analogues such as tranexamic acid and epsilon-aminocaproic acid (EACA) occupy lysine binding sites on plasminogen. This stops the binding of plasminogen to the active lysine residue site on the fibrin molecule, as such plasminogen is not further transformed into its active form via the action of t-PA. Thus, lysine analogues prevent excessive plasmin formation involved in hyperfibrinolysis. Of these two drugs, tranexamic acid is more studied with stronger evidence for its use [9]. It is more potent and has a longer elimination half-life.

Both result in meaningful reductions in blood loss and the need for allogeneic red cell transfusion. They seem to be as effective as aprotinin (see below) for at least low risk cardiac surgery [10]. In one study, patients in the tranexamic acid group received 46% fewer units of blood products than did those in the placebo group [11]. Unfortunately, there is still little agreement on the most effective dose of these agents and there have been concerns regarding high doses being associated with seizures postoperatively [12]. A randomized trial comparing groups of patients undergoing coronary artery bypass operations showed that tranexamic acid at a dose of up to 100 mg/kg was indeed associated with an increased propensity for seizures [11]. In this trial patients who received TXA had a seizure incidence of 0.7% compared to 0.1% in those who didn't receive TXA. There are a number of postulated mechanisms but the most well described involves the c-Aminobutyric acid type A (GABA-A) receptors and glycine receptors. These receptors are the predominant mediators of inhibition in the central nervous system. Glycine and TXA are structurally similar, suggesting that TXA competes with glycine at the agonist binding site of glycine receptors. Therefore, TXA may directly reduce inhibitory neurotransmission. This "disinhibition" increases the excitability of the central nervous system resulting in convulsive activity [13]. Adhering to the recommended dosing of TXA for patients based on their renal function is strongly advised in order to optimize reduction

Table 24.1 Recommended dosing of Tranexamic acid in high risk patients based on renal function to achieve a plasma concentration of 100 mg/L

Kidney function	Glomerular filtration rate (GFR)	Recommended bolus loading dose (mg/kg)	Recommended maintenance infusion dose (mg/kg/h)
Normal	>90	30	16
Mild reduction	60–89	30	11–16
Moderate reduction	30–59	25–30	5–10
Severe reduction	15–29	25–30	3–5
Renal failure	<15	25–30	3–5

in fibrinolysis whilst minimising the risk of seizures (Table 24.1).

It is also postulated that a reduction in fibrinolysis without a similar reduction in thrombin generation would result in the increased potential for thrombotic complications; however, studies have failed to establish increased risk of myocardial infarction, stroke, deep vein thrombosis, or pulmonary embolism from TXA or EACA use in cardiac surgery.

The serine protease inhibitor aprotinin exerts its effect by inhibiting t-PA thereby preventing the conversion of plasminogen to plasmin. In addition to this, unlike the lysine analogues, aprotinin exhibits a variety of other actions including a reduction in platelet activation. The mechanism for this is likely mediated by blocking PAR4 receptors and by blocking thrombin activation of platelet PAR1 receptors [14]. This may help reduce overall platelet dysfunction by inhibiting platelet aggregation and microaggregate formation during CPB.

The efficacy of aprotinin has been shown in multiple clinical trials that have found it to substantially reduce transfusion of blood products during cardiac surgery [15]. In fact, a retrospective analysis involving high risk patients suggested a lower incidence of major hemorrhage and a significant reduction in mortality in those given aprotinin compared to tranexamic acid [16]. Unfortunately, there are bodies of data on aprotinin suggesting that it may be associated with an increased risk of adverse outcomes including mortality [17]. The primary concerning feature was the potential for anaphylactic reactions after a second exposure. This was seen more commonly in the first 6 months following the initial exposure, its clinical picture ranging from rash to full anaphylaxis and cardiovascular collapse.

The BART study was a blinded, randomized controlled trial that concluded aprotinin was not superior to tranexamic acid at preventing the primary end-point of massive bleeding and was associated with an increased mortality. It recommended not using aprotinin in high risk cardiac surgery and ultimately led to a moratorium of its use. However, when this data was revisited, several limitations in the BART data analysis ultimately resulted in the regulatory authorities in Canada and Europe to allow the licence to be re-granted. In fact, a recent Cochrane review of all anti-fibrinolytics reports that in high risk cardiac surgery, where there is a substantial probability of serious blood loss, aprotinin may be preferred over tranexamic acid [18]. It states that aprotinin does not appear to be associated with an increased risk of vascular occlusion and death, but the data does not exclude an increased risk of renal failure. In summary, evidence suggests that the use of either of these three agents in in cardiac surgery reduces red cell transfusion.

Hypofibrinogenemia

Pathophysiology

Fibrinogen, the precursor to fibrin, is a critical component of the coagulation cascade. It binds platelets, supporting platelet aggregation and promotes coagulation. Due to the fact that fibrinogen contributes a major structural component of the clot rather than an enzymatic function, it has by far the highest concentration of any plasma coagulation factor [19]. Unlike other coagulation factors that have a large margin of reserve, only a modest drop in fibrinogen levels will result in abnormalities in coagulation and an increase in bleeding complications. Patients undergoing cardiac surgery with CPB will have a depletion of

their plasma fibrinogen level by up to 50% due to surgical bleeding, hemodilution due to administration of fluids and initiation of CPB, and consumption due to activation of the clotting cascade while on CPB [20].

Our understanding of the relationship between fibrinogen levels and bleeding in cardiac surgical patients has evolved in recent years. Previous guidelines have suggested that therapy should only be considered in bleeding patients with a fibrinogen level less than or equal to 0.8 g/L. Recent studies however have shown that the probability of large volume transfusion is increased when fibrinogen levels are decreased below 2.0 g/L [20]. Current best practice advocates keeping plasma fibrinogen levels above the critical level of 1.5–2.0 g/L to prevent excessive hemorrhage, large-volume transfusion, and associated adverse outcomes. This critical level is reached in approximately 5% of cardiac surgical patients, but the well-established practice of fibrinogen supplementation in bleeding patients with acquired hypofibrinogenemia is primarily based on theoretical principles rather than high-grade clinical evidence.

Therapies

Options for treating acquired hypofibrinogenemia differ between North America and Europe with Cryoprecipitate being the mainstay of treatment in North America and purified human-derived fibrinogen concentrate the treatment of choice in most of Europe. Treating hypofibrinogenemia with plasma is not recommended due to its low fibrinogen concentration. These practice differences were not evidence-based as there was scant data in the literature determining the most appropriate fibrinogen supplementation therapy. The FIBRES randomized controlled non-inferiority trial comparing cryoprecipitate to fibrinogen concentrate showed that fibrinogen concentrate is non-inferior to cryoprecipitate in bleeding patients with acquired hypofibrinogenemia after cardiac surgery [21]. Irrespective of the therapy selected, the overriding aim of therapy should be to maintain fibrinogen levels greater than the critical level of 1.5–2.0 g/L. The characteristics of the two therapies are as follows:

1. Cryoprecipitate is an allogenic blood product (ABP) that is prepared by thawing frozen plasma to 2–4 °C, harvesting the resultant precipitate by centrifugation, and then re-freezing it to −20 °C. Its contents include fibrinogen, Factor VIII, Factor XIII and von Willebrand factor. While it can be potentially used for treating factor deficiencies, its use is typically limited to treating hypofibrinogemia due to its low and variable factor concentration. While currently being the mainstay of treatment in North America for hypofibrinogemia, it has some important limitations [22]. Firstly, the amount of fibrinogen in each unit varies from 120 to 796 mg per unit, and of the transfused fibrinogen only about 50% is recoverable. Consequently, the increase in plasma fibrinogen levels in response to cryoprecipitate is limited and variable, ranging from an increase of 0.05 to 0.1 g/L in fibrinogen levels per unit transfused. Secondly, cryoprecipitate is not a purified product and contains large amounts of contaminants such as fibronectin and platelet micro-particles that may contribute to occurrence of microvascular thrombotic events and subsequent organ dysfunction. Thirdly, rapid administration of cryoprecipitate is precluded by the timely and labour-intensive process of thawing, reconstituting in plasma, and pooling of cryoprecipitate.

2. Fibrinogen concentrates are prepared from pooled human plasma and are available as lyophilized powders that are reconstituted in small volumes. While currently not widely used in North America, they possess potential advantages over cryoprecipitate [22]. Firstly, they have a lower risk of transfusion transmissible disease as they undergo several virus removal and inactivation steps that remove contaminants and inactivate viruses. Secondly, they contain a consistent amount of fibrinogen and thus the response to therapy is more predictable. Lastly, fibrinogen replacement can take part in a timelier fashion since the product can be administered immediately after it is reconstituted with sterile water.

Platelet Dysfunction

Pathophysiology

The cause of platelet dysfunction observed in patients undergoing cardiac surgery is multifactorial. As previously mentioned, many patients may already be taking antiplatelet medication. In non-elective scenarios, insufficient time may have passed to allow their clinical effect to diminish. Similarly, this cohort of patient often suffers from other comorbidities including renal and liver dysfunction which also contribute independently to platelet dysfunction. More specifically, it is the widespread platelet activation that occurs in the cardiopulmonary circuit that ultimately results in much of the platelet dysfunction seen in the immediate postoperative period. Fibrinogen bound to the CPB circuit creates a large surface area for platelet binding through their GPIIb/IIIa receptors. Once these platelets are bound, the typical cascade of activation, release of platelet granules and micro-aggregation occurs. Pro-inflammatory ligands on the platelet surface further promote thrombin formation. Thrombin generated during CPB, in turn, further activates platelets through PAR1 (protease activated receptor 1) [23].

Therapies

Platelet Transfusion

The exact thresholds and effective dose of platelets has yet to be determined. Much of the data in this area is derived from the haematological and oncological settings. It is likely that there may not be a specific value that defines all scenarios and that different threshold must be applied to the specific setting. The liberal use of platelets has been kept in check by some observational studies that suggest excessive platelet administration may be associated with an increased risk of adverse events [24]. However, rather than a direct causal effect, it may be that platelet transfusion is more of a surrogate marker for sicker patients who are more likely to bleed in any case.

Desmopressin

In addition to platelet transfusion, there are other strategies considered to augment existing platelet function. Desmopressin, a synthetic analogue of arginine vasopressin, induces the release of the contents of endothelial cell-associated Weibel–Palade bodies. The resulting increase in factor VIII and von Willebrand factor concentrations is thought to increase platelet function and adhesiveness to the vessel wall with no effect on platelet count. The increased release of factors from storage sites is transient which explains the tachyphylaxis observed clinically after repeat dosing. A recent Cochrane review stated that in adults undergoing cardiac surgery, the observed reduction in total blood loss and volume of red cells transfused was small and unlikely to be of clinical importance [25]. However, it did acknowledge a paucity of evidence and suggested that it is possible that people who are more vulnerable to bleeding, such as those taking antiplatelet agents, may gain more benefit from desmopressin.

Red Cell Mass

It has been recognized that anemic patients have an increased propensity to bleed. Indeed, hematocrit has been shown to correlate inversely with the bleeding time [26]. There have been some suggested theories for this effect including increased red cell mass concentrating platelets near the endothelium whereby they become activated during times of injury or red cells having a direct effect by increasing thromboxane production by platelets. Although a higher transfusion threshold for actively bleeding patients should be considered, more trials are needed before recommending the use of red cell transfusions to correct impaired platelet function [26].

Thrombin Deficiency

Pathophysiology

In describing thrombin generation there are three distinct phases; initiation, amplification and propagation. The primary physiologic event in

initiating thrombin formation is the exposure of tissue factor at the wound site and its interaction with activated factor VII. In a feedback manner, this small initial amount of thrombin generation then activates factors V, VIII and XI as well as platelets resulting in the amplification phase. This phase culminates in the formation of a highly efficient prothrombinase complex on the surface of the activated platelet which is responsible for the propagation phase of thrombin generation. The formed thrombin then converts fibrinogen to fibrin and propagates polymerization to form the hemostatic plug [27].

As a result of thrombin being a common enzymatic step in multiple hemostatic cascades, its reduced formation may be the result of a diverse range of coagulation deficits. Deficiency of thrombin generation after cardiac surgery in which patients undergo CPB is a recognized phenomenon and studies have demonstrated the relationship between reduced indices of thrombin generation and perioperative blood loss [28]. Factors leading to reduced thrombin generation are complex and multifactorial and include heparinization, hypothermia, hemodilution, contact activation within the cardiopulmonary bypass circuit, consumptive coagulopathy and inadequate clot stabilization.

Most of our recent understanding about cardiac surgery-associated defects in thrombin generation comes from experimental assays such as calibrated automated thrombography (CAT). Thus, therapies aimed at improving thrombin generation have to be based on imperfect assays (e.g. INR and clotting time [CT] of viscoelastic assays), or initiated empirically once other causes of coagulopathy have been excluded [29].

Therapies

Since thrombin generation is the key event in propagation of the coagulation cascade, there are multiple upstream targets which indirectly augment thrombin generation, including administration of platelets and solutions containing clotting factors. This is in conjunction with ensuring that the correct environment exists for normal coagulation such as normothermia, normocalcemia and correction of any acidosis if present. Options for replacing thrombin directly include administration of plasma, prothrombin complex concentrates (PCCs), activated prothrombin complex concentrates (aPCCs) or Factor eight inhibitor bypass activity (FEIBA) and Activated Factor VIIa (rFVIIa) [30].

1. Plasma contains all coagulation factors as well as naturally occurring anticoagulant proteins. It is effective as a volume expander and in delivering multiple factors but its drawback is that the quantity of factors in a unit of plasma is small and varies with each unit; thus, it is not ideal for the rapid restoration of low clotting factor levels [31]. A dose of 15 ml/kg is recommended for transfusion when plasma is to be given for factor replacement.

2. Prothrombin complex concentrates (PCCs) are synthetic preparations containing multiple factors including II, VII, IX and X. While they are primarily used for reversal of Vitamin K antagonists, they are being more generally used in the bleeding perioperative patient. Studies in post CPB patients show that PCC administration improves thrombin generation [30]. Potential advantages of PCCs over plasma include a lower volume of injection, more predictable pharmacodynamic profile and lower potential virulence given they are synthetically derived. A dose of 20–25 U/kg is recommended for transfusion when PCCs is to be given for factor replacement.

3. Recombinant factor VIIa (rFVIIa) is a potent pharmacological prohemostatic agent that is currently only licenced for use in hemophilia patients. It acts by binding to the surface of platelets and increases activation of both FIX and FX resulting in increased thrombin generation above normal levels. While initially showing promising results in early trials, a systematic review of its use in cardiac showed no mortality benefit and actually showed an increase in the incidence of adverse events such as death, cerebral infarction or other thromboembolic events [32]. Currently its use is generally reserved for patients in whom other therapies have failed, in which instance it is used off-label. A dose of 45 mcg/kg is recommenced for controlling coagulopathic bleeding.

4. Factor eight inhibitor bypass activity (FEIBA) is another procoagulant agent that has been used in managing refractory bleeding, albeit less than rFVIIa. It is an activated prothrombin complex concentrate, containing prothrombin, nonactivated factors II, IX and X and activated factors II and VII [33]. The mode of action of FEIBA is complex but the end result is induction and facilitation of thrombin generation, a process for which factor V is crucial. Studies have shown that factor Xa and prothrombin play a critical role in the activity of FEIBA [34]. Similar to rFVIIa there are concerns relating to thromboembolic events. Studies into the perioperative use of FEIBA are limited but the few studies that have been undertaken have shown that rFVIIa and FEIBA have similar efficacy and adverse event profiles in managing refractory post-bypass bleeding in cardiac surgery patients [35]. Given that the majority of the literature has focused on the use of rFVIIa in cardiac surgery, the use of FEIBA is limited in the perioperative setting.

References

1. Sellman M, Intonti MA, Ivert T. Reoperations for bleeding after coronary artery bypass procedures during 25 years. Eur J Cardiothorac Surg. 1997;11:521–7.
2. Ferraris VA, Ferraris SP, Saha SP, et al. Perioperative blood transfusion and blood conservation in cardiac surgery: the Society of Thoracic Surgeons and The Society of Cardiovascular Anesthesiologists clinical practice guideline. Ann Thorac Surg. 2007;83(5 Suppl):S27–86.
3. Lee GC, Kicza AM, Liu KY, Nyman CB, Kaufman RM, Body SC. Does rotational thromboelastometry (ROTEM) improve prediction of bleeding after cardiac surgery? Anesth Analg. 2012;115(3):499–506.
4. Karkouti K, Callum J, Wijeysundera DN, Rao V, Crowther M, Grocott HP, Pinto R, Scales DC, TACS investigators. Point-of-Care Hemostatic Testing in Cardiac Surgery: A Stepped-Wedge Clustered Randomized Controlled Trial. Circulation. 2016;134(16)1152–62.

5. Corredor C, Wasowicz M, Karkouti K, Sharma V. The role of point-of-care platelet function testing in predicting postoperative bleeding following cardiac surgery: a systematic review and meta-analysis. Anaesthesia. 2015;70(6):715–31.
6. Valen G, Eriksson E, Risberg B, Vaage J. Fibrinolysis during cardiac surgery: release of tissue plasminogen activator in arterial and coronary sinus blood. Eur J Cardiothorac Surg. 1994;8:324–30.
7. Chandler WL, Velan T. Plasmin generation and D-dimer formation during cardiopulmonary bypass. Blood Coagul Fibrinolysis. 2004;15:583–91.
8. de Haan J, van Oeveren W. Platelets and soluble fibrin promote plasminogen activation causing downregulation of platelet glycoprotein Ib/IX complexes: protection by aprotinin. Thromb Res. 1998;92:171–9.
9. Fears R, Greenwood H, Hearn J, Howard B, Humphreys S, Morrow G, Standring R. Inhibition of the fibrinolytic and fibrinogenolytic activity of plasminogen activators in vitro by the antidotes ε-aminocaproic acid, tranexamic acid and aprotinin. Fibrinolysis. 1992;6:79–86.
10. Henry DA, Carless PA, Moxey AJ, O'Connell D, Stokes BJ, McClelland B, Laupacis A, Fergusson D. Anti-fibrinolytic use for minimising perioperative allogeneic blood transfusion. Cochrane Database Syst Rev. 2007;4:CD001886.
11. Myles PS, Smith JA, Forbes A, Silbert B, Jayarajah M. Tranexamic acid in patients undergoing coronary-artery surgery. N Engl J Med. 2017;376(2):136–48.
12. Martin K, Wiesner G, Breuer T, Lange R, Tassani P. The risks of aprotinin and tranexamic acid in cardiac surgery: a one-year follow-up of 1188 consecutive patients. Anesth Analg. 2008;107(6):1783–90.
13. Lecker I, Wang D-S, Whissell PD, Avramescu S, David Mazer MD, Orser BA. Tranexamic acid–associated seizures: causes and treatment. Ann Neurol. 2016;79:18–26.
14. Day JR, Punjabi PP, Randi AM, Haskard DO, Landis RC, Taylor KM. Clinical inhibition of the seven-transmembrane thrombin receptor (PAR1) by intravenous aprotinin during cardiothoracic surgery. Circulation. 2004;110:2597–600.
15. Ray MJ, Marsh NA. Aprotinin reduces blood loss after cardiopulmonary bypass by direct inhibition of plasmin. Thromb Haemost. 1997;78:1021–6.
16. Sander M, Spies CD, Martiny V, Rosenthal C, Wernecke KD, von Heymann C. Mortality associated with administration of high-dose tranexamic acid and aprotinin in primary open-heart procedures: a retrospective analysis. Crit Care. 2010;14(4):R148.
17. Fergusson DA, Hebert PC, Mazer CD, et al. A comparison of aprotinin and lysine analogues in high-risk cardiac surgery. N Engl J Med. 2008;358(22):2319–31.
18. Henry DA, Carless PA, Moxey AJ, et al. Antifibrinolytic use for minimising perioperative alloge-

neic blood transfusion. Cochrane Database Syst Rev. 2011;3:CD001886.
19. Levy JH, Goodnough LT. How I use fibrinogen replacement therapy in acquired bleeding. Blood. 2015;125(9):1387–93.
20. Karkouti K, Callum J, Crowther MA, McCluskey SA, Pendergrast J, Tait G, Yau TM, Beattie WS. The relationship between fibrinogen levels after cardiopulmonary bypass and large volume red cell transfusion in cardiac surgery: an observational study. Anesth Analg. 2013;117(1):14–22.
21. Callum J, Farkouh ME, Scales DC, et al. Effect of fibrinogen concentrate vs cryoprecipitate on blood component transfusion after cardiac surgery: the FIBRES randomized clinical trial. JAMA 2019;322(20):1–11.
22. Franchini M, Lippi G. Fibrinogen replacement therapy: a critical review of the literature. Blood Transfus. 2012;10(1):23–7.
23. Dalen M, van der Linden J, Lindvall G, Ivert T. Correlation between point-of-care platelet function testing and bleeding after coronary artery surgery. Scand Cardiovasc J. 2012;46(1):32–8.
24. Speiss BD, Royston D, Levy JH, et al. Platelet transfusions during coronary artery bypass graft surgery are associated with serious adverse outcomes. Transfusion. 2004;44:1143–8.
25. Desborough MJ, Oakland K, Brierley C, Bennett S, Doree C, Trivella M, Hopewell S, Stanworth SJ, Estcourt LJ. Desmopressin use for minimising perioperative blood transfusion (Review). Cochrane Database Syst Rev. 2017;7(7):CD001884.
26. Valeri CR, Cassidy G, Pivacek LE, Ragno G, Lieberthal W, Crowley JP, Khuri SF, Loscalzo J. Anemia-induced increase in the bleeding time: implications for treatment of nonsurgical blood loss. Transfusion. 2001;41(8):977–83.
27. Ghadimi K, Levy JH, Welsby IJ. Prothrombin complex concentrates for bleeding in the perioperative setting. Anesth Analg. 2016;122(5): 1287–300.
28. Coakley M, Hall JE, Evans C, Duff E, Billing V, Yang L, et al. Assessment of thrombin generation measured before and after cardiopulmonary bypass surgery and its association with postoperative bleeding. J Thromb Haemost. 2011;9(2):282–92.
29. Baglin T. The measurement and application of thrombin generation. Br J Haematol. 2005;130(5):653–61.
30. Percy CL, Hartmann R, Jones RM, Balachandran S, Mehta D, Dockal M, et al. Correcting thrombin generation ex vivo using different haemostatic agents following cardiac surgery requiring the use of cardiopulmonary bypass. Blood Coagul Fibrinolysis. 2015;26(4):357–67.
31. Sarode R, Milling TJ Jr, Refaai MA, Mangione A, Schneider A, Durn BL, et al. Efficacy and safety of a 4-factor prothrombin complex concentrate in patients

on vitamin K antagonists presenting with major bleeding: a randomized, plasma-controlled, phase IIIb study. Circulation. 2013;128(11):1234–43.

32. Yank V, Tuohy CV, Logan AC, et al. Systematic review: benefits and harms of in-hospital use of recombinant factor VIIa for off-label indications. Ann Intern Med. 2011;154:529.

33. Turecek PL, Varadi K, Gritsch H, et al. FEIBA: mode of action. Haemophilia. 2004;10:3–9.

34. Himmelspach M, Richter G, Muhr E, et al. A fully recombinant partial prothrombin complex effectively bypasses FVIII *in vitro* and *in vivo*. Thromb Haemost. 2002;88:1003–11.

35. Rao VK, Lobato RL, Bartlett B, et al. Factor VIII inhibitor bypass activity and recombinant activated factor VII in cardiac surgery. J Cardiothorac Vasc Anesth. 2014;28(5):1221–6.

Heparin-Induced Thrombocytopenia and Alternatives to Heparin

25

Linda Shore-Lesserson and Alan Finley

Main Messages

1. Heparin-induced thrombocytopenia (HIT) is a clinicopathologic diagnosis that results from immune complex activation of platelets and renders patients hyperaggregable and susceptible to thrombosis
2. The 4T's score can be used to assess the patient likelihood of having HIT
3. Immunologic testing for HIT is sensitive but very non-specific for disease, as many patients will have antibody to the heparin/PF4 complex but will not have activated platelets
4. Evidence of hyperaggregability by HIPA or SRA testing is more specific for HIT; a positive functional test of hyperaggregability suggests that an anticoagulation strategy other than unfractionated heparin be considered

5. Multiple clinical strategies have been successfully used in HIT patients; if cardiac surgery cannot be postponed until antibody levels are undetectable, alternative anticoagulation strategies should be considered
6. Alternative anticoagulation strategies include direct thrombin inhibitors, heparin after plasmapheresis, and heparin plus platelet inhibitors
7. The majority of the evidence-base is in favor of the use of bivalirudin for cardiac surgery in HIT patients

L. Shore-Lesserson (✉)
Department of Anesthesiology, Zucker School of Medicine at Hofstra Northwell, Northwell Health System, Northshore University Hospital, Manhasset, NY, USA
e-mail: Lshoreless@northwell.edu

A. Finley
Anesthesia and Perioperative Medicine, Medical University of South Carolina, Charleston, SC, USA
e-mail: finleya@musc.edu

Heparin-induced thrombocytopenia (HIT) refers to the reduction in platelet count that occurs when patients receive heparin therapy. It can be seen in 35% of patients receiving heparin. There are two common types of thrombocytopenia responses to heparin. HIT Type 1 occurs as a result of heparin's proaggregatory effect on platelets, causing clumping and a reduction in measured platelet count. This reaction is a mild thrombocytopenia, is a benign occurrence, usually occurs during the first few days of heparin therapy, and resolves without discontinuation of heparin. In contrast, HIT Type 2 is an immune response (IgG) to the complex formed when heparin binds to platelet factor 4 (PF4). PF4 binds both heparin and platelet glycosaminoglycans which initiates the

© Springer Nature Switzerland AG 2021
D. C. H. Cheng et al. (eds.), *Evidence-Based Practice in Perioperative Cardiac Anesthesia and Surgery*, https://doi.org/10.1007/978-3-030-47887-2_25

immune response. The immunoglobulin Fc portion then engages the platelet membrane causing activation of the platelet, release of dense granule contents and procoagulant microparticles. The end result is hyperaggregability.

HIT Type 2 (HIT 2) is marked by a dramatic reduction in platelet count (absolute number <50/µL or >50% reduction), occurs later (5–9 days) after initiation of heparin therapy, increases the risk of thrombosis, and will not resolve without cessation of heparin therapy [1]. HIT 2 occurs more rarely (2–5% of patients), but in these patients, thrombosis occurs in up to 20% and is associated with mortality in nearly half of the cases. HIT 2 with thrombosis is referred to as HITT. Often the first appearance of this condition can be limb necrosis, myocardial infarction, other arterial thromboses, and even mortality. Diagnosis of this condition is especially complicated in cardiac surgical patients who already experience varying degrees of thrombocytopenia due to cardiopulmonary bypass (CPB). Despite the more common temporal course, "delayed-onset HIT" can develop without an anamnestic response in patients who have no prior exposure to heparin [2]. Diagnostic testing for HIT and appropriate interpretation of such testing are critical in order to confirm the appropriate anticoagulant treatment strategy. Selection of heparin versus an alternative anticoagulant is based upon the probability that a patient has HIT, and the relative risks of bleeding and thrombosis. If CPB or continued anticoagulation is needed, an evidence-based approach is described.

Perioperative Considerations

Thrombocytopenia is a common occurrence, especially in perioperative cardiac surgery patients. However, since there are many etiologies for a low platelet count, it is critically important to make the correct diagnosis in HIT before embarking on a pathway of procedural cancellations, expensive testing, or use of new and unfamiliar anticoagulants. Lo and colleagues created and validated the 4T's score, based upon clinical presentation, to assess the probably that a patient has

HIT [3]. This score assesses four characteristics of the clinical presentation and assigns a score of 0, 1, or 2 to each category; thus the total score ranges from 0 to 8. The 4T's that are assessed include the **T**hrombocytopenia (platelet count), **T**iming of the platelet count drop, Presence of **T**hrombosis, and presence of other possible causes of **T**hrombocytopenia (Table 25.1).

If the likelihood is high based on clinical assessment (i.e. 4T score 6–8) that a patient has HIT, then serologic testing is recommended. A multidisciplinary guideline on anticoagulation in cardiac surgery co-published by the Society of Thoracic Surgeons, Society of Cardiovascular Anesthesiologists, and American Society of Extracorporeal Technology, recommends best practice based upon the evidence published. This document assigns a Class IIa recommendation to the use of a clinical scoring estimate to guide the use of serologic testing [4].

Table 25.1 4T's score for assessing likelihood of HIT

Thrombocytopenia	Platelet count fall >50% and nadir ≥20	2
	Platelet count fall 30–50% or nadir 10–19/µL	1
	Platelet count fall <30% or nadir<10/µL	0
Timing of platelet count fall	Onset 5–10 days or <1 day w heparin exposure within 30 days	2
	Onset unclear, >10 days, or <1 day w exposure 30–100 days ago	1
	Onset <4 days without recent exposure	0
Thrombosis or other sequelae	New thrombosis or skin necrosis	2
	Progressive or recurrent thrombosis, non-necrotizing skin lesions	1
	None	0
Other causes for Thrombocytopenia	None apparent	2
	Possible	1
	Definite	0
Total Score		

≤3 points: low probability for HIT (<1% in meta-analysis)

4–5 points: intermediate probability (14% probability of HIT)

6–8 points: high probability (64% probability of HIT)

Serologic testing for HIT can be performed either by testing for the presence of the antibody to heparin/platelet factor 4 (termed anti-PF4 antibody), or by testing for the presence of hyperaggregability in the presence of heparin. Antibody testing is typically accomplished using an Enzyme Linked Immunosorbent Assay (ELISA), a highly sensitive test; it is very helpful, if negative, in excluding the possibility of HIT. Threshold optical density (OD) values indicating a positive result are OD > 0.4. This assay is prevalent in many laboratories and has even been modified to be measured as a rapid point-of-care test [5]. Although it is the most common test used for diagnosis of HIT, it is not diagnostic of HIT, and should only serve as a good screen for patients needing further testing. Many patients, upon exposure to heparin, will develop antibodies to PF4; in fact this number can approach 30%. Since the incidence of HIT is not nearly this high, it stands to reason that the presence of antibody does not, in itself, confirm the diagnosis. The true presence of disease is marked by a propensity to hyperaggregability, though large scale studies have even shown an increase in morbidity in patients who are simply antibody positive [6, 7]. The reason for the discrepancy between antibody positivity and presence of disease is that many of the antibodies do not actually bind and activate platelets. In order to more specifically diagnose HIT, a functional assay to detect hyperaggregation in response to heparin, should be performed (Class IIa recommendation) [4].

The two common functional assays include the Heparin Induced Platelet Aggregation Assay (HIPA), and the Serotonin Release Assay (SRA). These tests are more labor intensive, and are not run routinely in most laboratories, an impediment to obtaining an accurate diagnosis of HIT. The implementation of a functional assay for HIT is a branch point in the decision tree when evaluating a patient with moderate to high levels of antibody by ELISA testing (OD > 0.4). A positive HIPA or SRA is strongly suggestive of HIT and directs the practitioner to using an alternative anticoagulation strategy [8]. A negative HIPA or SRA can indicate a lack of hyperaggregability, and can also be used to document efficacy of therapeutic plasmapheresis in removing the hyperaggregation risk of HIT immune globulins. Often the functional assay will become negative despite persistence of a positive ELISA [9].

Management of anticoagulation for the patient with HIT has been the subject of intense investigation. Paramount is the cessation of heparin therapy and the elimination of heparin from the patient's current therapeutic regimen. This means elimination of heparin during dialysis, during cell salvage, non-use of heparin-bonded catheters, and elimination of subcutaneous heparins used for deep venous thrombosis prophylaxis. When deciding on a management strategy for anticoagulation for CPB, there are two basic strategies. One is the complete avoidance of heparin, and the other strategy is *use* of heparin but with removal of its propensity to bind and activate platelets.

Avoidance of heparin includes use of the non-heparin containing anticoagulant agents. Most of these agents have fallen out of favor or are no longer commercially available due to major hemorrhagic complications with their use during CPB. The anticoagulants that remain in clinical use for patients with HIT are the direct thrombin inhibitors (DTI) bivalirudin, hirudin, and argatroban. Argatroban is frequently used in intensive care medicine for HIT patients who have deep vein thrombosis, mechanical heart valves, atrial fibrillation, etc., however its use in CPB has been fraught with excess bleeding and transfusion requirements [10]. Owing to extensive hepatic elimination, and a longer half-life than bivalirudin, argatroban is not recommended for use during CPB. Bivalirudin undergoes auto-digestion and renal elimination and has a more optimal pharmacokinetic profile than its congener hirudin. Bivalirudin is the DTI most extensively studied in cardiovascular surgery and will be further discussed in the Evidence-Based Management section [11].

Heparin use with removal of platelet activation can be accomplished by therapeutic plasmapheresis to remove immune globulin, or by the addition of anti-platelet medications, that will inhibit platelet activation [12]. Large case series have been published using iloprost [13] to inhibit platelet aggregation, noting hypotension as the only significant complication [14]. To accomplish the same goal, Koster and colleagues have used tirofiban with heparin and successfully averted pro-thrombotic complications of HIT, however, bleeding is a common complication of this strategy [15].

Evidence-Based Best Practice Management

Thrombocytopenia is a common occurrence and has many etiologies. A specific diagnosis of HIT in the cardiac surgical patient is important before embarking upon alternative therapeutic pathways that may have risk or be unfamiliar to the practitioner. On clinical grounds, a scoring system should be used to identify patients at high risk for having HIT [16]. In a patient with thrombocytopenia, the 4T's score is very useful as a screening tool for the need for further workup. In a meta-analysis of trials evaluating the 4T's score, a low 4T's score had a very high negative predictive value for excluding HIT. Intermediate or high scores were not very specific for HIT and suggest the need for further ELISA testing [17]. This serologic testing should be performed to determine the presence of and quantification of antibody to heparin/PF4. The ELISA is a highly sensitive assay and is thus an excellent screen for the absence of disease. A positive screen indicates that further testing should be sought with the functional assays that detect platelet hyperaggregability in the presence of heparin. Once a positive HIPA or SRA confirms a diagnosis of HIT, the clinician must embark upon one of three decision management strategies.

The first management option is to postpone surgery. After a period of approximately 90 days, heparin-PF4 antibody levels should have cleared. The temporal course of HIT antibody formation and elimination has been extensively studied by Warkentin and colleagues who have recommended postponement of surgery, when feasible [18]. After 90 days, a reassessment of antibody level using the ELISA should be performed, and in all likelihood will yield a negative result. If so,

surgery can proceed with intraoperative use of heparin (Class IIa) [4], however an alternative anticoagulant should be considered postoperatively if anticoagulation will be required. In the situation where surgery cannot be postponed until the antibody level is undetectable, an alternative anticoagulant strategy should be used.

The second management option includes the use of the alternative anticoagulant DTI bivalirudin (Class IIa) [4]. Bivalirudin dosing has undergone pharmacokinetic study for both percutaneous intervention patients and for CPB. In CPB, patients with normal or mildly reduced renal function are dosed at 1 mg/kg bolus, 50 mg in the CPB prime, followed by 2.5 mg/kg/h. In percutaneous procedures, a lower dose bivalirudin is recommended and further adjustments are made for patients with reduced creatinine clearance. The above recommended CPB dose was the dose used in the EVOLUTION-ON trial that compared bivalirudin to unfractionated heparin in CPB patients in a blinded randomized fashion [19]. Activated clotting time was maintained at 2.5 times baseline. Bivalirudin was shown to be non-inferior to heparin in this trial. Randomized trials in off-pump cardiac surgery have also shown equivalence between bivalirudin and heparin, and perhaps a graft patency benefit when using bivalirudin as the anticoagulant [20, 21].

The third choice for management includes the use of heparin with a strategy for reducing the risk of platelet activation. While this scientific approach is sound, and descriptive literature indicates success in using this technique [4], the evidence supporting these methods is not as robust (Class IIb) as the randomized trials that have studied bivalirudin.

References

1. Warkentin TE, Greinacher A. Heparin-induced thrombocytopenia: recognition, treatment, and prevention: the Seventh ACCP Conference on Antithrombotic and Thrombolytic Therapy. Chest. 2004;126(3 Suppl):311S–37S.
2. Warkentin TE. Clinical picture of heparin-induced thrombocytopenia (HIT) and its differentiation from

non-HIT thrombocytopenia. Thromb Haemost. 2016;116(5):813–22.

3. Lo GK, Juhl D, Warkentin TE, Sigouin CS, Eichler P, Greinacher A. Evaluation of pretest clinical score (4 T's) for the diagnosis of heparin-induced thrombocytopenia in two clinical settings. J Thromb Haemost. 2006;4(4):759–65.

4. Shore-Lesserson L, Baker RA, Ferraris VA, et al. The Society of Thoracic Surgeons, The Society of Cardiovascular Anesthesiologists, and The American Society of ExtraCorporeal Technology: Clinical Practice Guidelines—Anticoagulation During Cardiopulmonary Bypass. Anesth Analg. 2018;126(2):413–24.

5. Sachan D, Gupta N, Chaudhary R. Rapid diagnosis of heparin-induced thrombocytopenia using a particle gel immunoassay in at-risk cardiac surgery patients. Asian J Transfus Sci. 2013;7(1):92–3.

6. Bennett-Guerrero E, Slaughter TF, White WD, Welsby IJ, Greenberg CS, El-Moalem H, et al. Preoperative anti-PF4/heparin antibody level predicts adverse outcome after cardiac surgery. J Thorac Cardiovasc Surg. 2005;130(6):1567–72.

7. Kress DC, Aronson S, McDonald ML, Malik MI, Divgi AB, Tector AJ, et al. Positive heparin-platelet factor 4 antibody complex and cardiac surgical outcomes. Ann Thorac Surg. 2007;83(5):1737–43.

8. Warkentin TE, Arnold DM, Nazi I, Kelton JG. The platelet serotonin-release assay. Am J Hematol. 2015;90(6):564–72.

9. Warkentin TE, Sheppard JA, Chu FV, Kapoor A, Crowther MA, Gangji A. Plasma exchange to remove HIT antibodies: dissociation between enzyme-immunoassay and platelet activation test reactivities. Blood. 2015;125(1):195–8.

10. Agarwal S, Ullom B, Al-Baghdadi Y, Okumura M. Challenges encountered with argatroban anticoagulation during cardiopulmonary bypass. J Anaesthesiol Clin Pharmacol. 2012;28(1):106–10.

11. Anand SX, Viles-Gonzalez JF, Mahboobi SK, Heerdt PM. Bivalirudin utilization in cardiac surgery: shifting anticoagulation from indirect to direct thrombin inhibition. Can J Anaesth. 2011;58(3):296–311.

12. Welsby IJ, Um J, Milano CA, Ortel TL, Arepally G. Plasmapheresis and heparin reexposure as a management strategy for cardiac surgical patients with heparin-induced thrombocytopenia. Anesth Analg. 2010;110(1):30–5.

13. Palatianos GM, Foroulis CN, Vassili MI, Matsouka P, Astras GM, Kantidakis GH, et al. Preoperative detection and management of immune heparin-induced thrombocytopenia in patients undergoing heart surgery with iloprost. J Thorac Cardiovasc Surg. 2004;127(2):548–54.

14. Palatianos G, Michalis A, Alivizatos P, Lacoumenda S, Geroulanos S, Karabinis A, et al. Perioperative use of iloprost in cardiac surgery patients diagnosed with heparin-induced thrombocytopenia-reactive antibodies or with true HIT (HIT-reactive antibodies plus thrombocytopenia): an 11-year experience. Am J Hematol. 2015;90(7):608–17.

15. Koster A, Kukucka M, Bach F, Meyer O, Fischer T, Mertzlufft F, et al. Anticoagulation during cardiopulmonary bypass in patients with heparin-induced thrombocytopenia type II and renal impairment using heparin and the platelet glycoprotein IIb-IIIa antagonist tirofiban. Anesthesiology. 2001;94(2):245–51.

16. Greinacher A. Heparin-induced thrombocytopenia. N Engl J Med. 2015;373(3):252–61.

17. Cuker A, Gimotty PA, Crowther MA, Warkentin TE. Predictive value of the 4Ts scoring system for heparin-induced thrombocytopenia: a systematic review and meta-analysis. Blood. 2012;120(20):4160–7.

18. Warkentin TE, Kelton JG. Temporal aspects of heparin-induced thrombocytopenia. N Engl J Med. 2001;344(17):1286–92.

19. Dyke CM, Smedira NG, Koster A, Aronson S, McCarthy HL 2nd, Kirshner R, et al. A comparison of bivalirudin to heparin with protamine reversal in patients undergoing cardiac surgery with cardiopulmonary bypass: the EVOLUTION-ON study. J Thorac Cardiovasc Surg. 2006;131(3):533–9.

20. Merry AF. Bivalirudin, blood loss, and graft patency in coronary artery bypass surgery. Semin Thromb Hemost. 2004;30(3):337–46.

21. Smedira NG, Dyke CM, Koster A, Jurmann M, Bhatia DS, Hu T, et al. Anticoagulation with bivalirudin for off-pump coronary artery bypass grafting: the results of the EVOLUTION-OFF study. J Thorac Cardiovasc Surg. 2006;131(3):686–92.

Perioperative Management of Cardiac Surgical Emergency

26

Nian Chih Hwang and Priscilla Hui Yi Phoon

Main Messages

1. Cardiac surgical emergencies can be complex; anesthesiologists play an important role in coordinating theatre staff and managing patient's hemodynamics to ensure good outcomes.
2. Diagnosis for aortic dissection can be challenging given the diverse clinical manifestations; the use of transesophageal echocardiography, computed tomography or magnetic resonance imaging in high-risk patients is recommended.
3. In-hospital mortality for patients with Type A aortic dissection is high and is largely influenced by the patient's co-morbidities and dissection related complications; anesthesiologists need to be prepared for intraoperative coagulopathy and take the necessary measures for blood conservation.
4. Patients with acute coronary syndromes presenting for emergency surgery can be challenging to manage especially in the setting of cardiogenic shock and anti-platelet/fibrinolytic therapy; a balance between myocardial oxygen supply and demand is favorable in preventing further myocardial insult.
5. Excessive bleeding is associated with a three- to fourfold increase in mortality and early exploration is key to reducing the severity of bleeding and minimizing blood product usage.

N. C. Hwang (✉) · P. H. Y. Phoon
Department of Cardiothoracic Anaesthesia, National Heart Centre Singapore, Singapore, Singapore

Department of Anaesthesiology, Singapore General Hospital, Singapore, Singapore
e-mail: hwang.nian.chih@singhealth.com.sg;
priscilla.phoon.h.y@singhealth.com.sg

Ascending Aortic Dissection Repair

Aortic dissection occurs when a tear in the tunica intima allows ingress of blood resulting in separation of the aortic wall layers and creating a false lumen with variable proximal and distal margins. It is a rare but potentially fatal condition with a mortality rate of 1–2% per hour if left untreated [1]. Classification is based on anatomical location and duration of onset of symptoms. In general, Stanford Type A dissections involving the ascending aorta (DeBakey Types I and II) require surgical intervention while Stanford Type B dissections involving the descending aorta only (DeBakey Type III) are managed conservatively (Class I, Level of evidence B) [2].

© Springer Nature Switzerland AG 2021
D. C. H. Cheng et al. (eds.), *Evidence-Based Practice in Perioperative Cardiac Anesthesia and Surgery*, https://doi.org/10.1007/978-3-030-47887-2_26

Pathophysiology

Intimal tears usually occur in areas subjected to large fluctuations in aortic wall tension. Factors that increase mechanical wall stress (such as hypertension, atherosclerosis or following deceleration injury) or decrease wall strength and integrity (such as aortic aneurysmal dilation, connective tissue disease or inflammatory vasculitis) can lead to medial wall degeneration which commonly precedes aortic dissection. The presence of an intimal flap in the aorta is pathognomonic. Common sites include along the greater curve of the aorta (within 10 cm of the aortic valve) and descending aorta immediately distal to the origin of the left subclavian artery [3].

Diagnosis

Patients typically present with sudden onset of sharp chest pain which may radiate to the back and abdomen depending on the extent of dissection. Tachycardia and hypertension can result from pain, anxiety and sympathetic stimulation which may lead to worsening dissection or rupture. Complications include:

- Cardiac tamponade
- Aortic rupture
- Acute aortic regurgitation leading to left heart failure
- Acute myocardial ischemia with coronary ostia involvement
- Hemothorax
- Neurological deficits from cerebral malperfusion

Diagnosis can be challenging given the diverse clinical manifestations and the International Registry of Acute Aortic Dissection (IRAD) data suggests that these patients do not present classically [1]. The 2010 American Heart Association (AHA) guidelines on thoracic aortic disease recommend the use of transesophageal echocardiography (TEE), computed tomographic (CT) imaging or magnetic resonance imaging (MRI) to identify or exclude aortic dissection in high-risk patients (Class I, Level of evidence B) [2].

The use of TEE in aortic dissection with possible aortic valve involvement is a Class I recommendation [4]. TEE can provide important information regarding location and extent of dissection, ventricular function, myocardial ischemia and complications such as pericardial effusion, cardiac tamponade, aortic regurgitation and involvement of coronary ostia by the dissection flap. Advantages include real-time imaging, portability and lack of contrast or radiation exposure. Its use, however, is limited by availability, operator skill and experience, sedation requirements, artifact generation and the inability to image the distal ascending aorta and proximal aortic arch well due to interposition of the trachea and left main bronchus.

The European Society of Cardiology task force on the diagnosis and management of aortic dissection [5] recommends the following diagnostic goals:

- Confirm diagnosis
- Identify location of intimal tear and delineate extent of dissection
- Identify true and false lumens and distinguish between communicating and non-communicating dissection
- Assess for involvement of coronary, carotid, subclavian, celiac, mesenteric and renal arteries
- Identify and grade severity of aortic regurgitation
- Detect extravasation resulting in periaortic or mediastinal hematoma, cardiac tamponade and hemothorax

Preoperative Management

Such patients should be transferred to and managed in a specialized cardiothoracic center. Management depends on the initial clinical presentation. Patients with poor neurological status (Glasgow coma scale <8) or hemodynamic instability should be promptly intubated (Table 26.1). The primary goal is to reduce shear forces acting on the aortic wall and halt further propagation of dissection. This involves controlling the systolic blood pressure

Table 26.1 European Society of Cardiology task force recommendations for initial management of aortic dissection [5]

Recommendations	Class I	Class IIa	Class IIb	Class III	Level of evidence
1. Intubation and ventilation in hemodynamically unstable patients	✓				C
2. Transfer to ICU	✓				C
3. Detailed history and physical examination (where possible)	✓				C
4. Documentation of ischemia on ECG	✓				C
* Imaging to exclude aortic dissection before thrombolysis	✓	✓			C
5. Heart rate and blood pressure monitoring	✓				C
6. Analgesia	✓				C
7. Reduction of systolic blood pressure with beta-blockers	✓				C
* Calcium-channel blockers in patients with obstructive pulmonary disease	✓	✓			C
8. Additional vasodilator therapy using GTN, SNP and hydralazine	✓				C

to 100–120 mmHg and heart rate to less than 60 beats/min (Class I, Level of evidence C) [2]. Beta-blockers such as intravenous esmolol, metoprolol or labetalol are commonly used as first-line therapy. However, they should be used cautiously in the presence of acute aortic regurgitation due to blockade of the compensatory tachycardia. Labetalol inhibits both α1 and β1 receptors and offers the advantage of potent heart rate and blood pressure control from a single agent, hence potentially eliminating the need for a direct vasodilator such as nitroglycerin (GTN), sodium nitroprusside (SNP) and hydralazine. Direct vasodilators can be added if further control is required and should only be started after beta-blockade as the reflex tachycardia and increased ventricular contraction can worsen aortic wall tension. Pain should be managed appropriately with intravenous opioids.

Conversely, volume administration titrated to improvement of blood pressure is reasonable in the hypotensive patient. Vasopressors can be added but with the potential risk of causing further false lumen propagation. Inotropic agents are likely to increase the force and rate of ventricular contraction and therefore increase shear stress on the aortic wall [2]. Immediate surgical intervention is usually required.

Preparing the Patient for Surgery

Anesthetic management can be extremely challenging given the need for expeditious surgical intervention. History, physical examination, diagnosis and management of co-existing medical conditions may be limited. Subsequent discussion will be focused on Stanford Type A dissection where surgical repair involves replacing the affected aortic segment with an interposition graft together with an aortic valve resuspension or composite graft replacement depending on the extent of aortic root involvement (Class I, Level of evidence C) [2]. Endovascular stenting is not an appropriate surgical option.

Prior to the start of surgery, it is good practice to conduct team briefings and review checklists to ensure patient safety and decrease surgical errors (Class I, Level of evidence B) [6]. A preoperative briefing involving all operating room (OR) personnel allows exchange of information and identifies potential issues. Effective teamwork and communication has been found to enhance patient care [6].

In addition to the standard invasive and non-invasive monitoring required for cardiac surgery, large-bore peripheral or central venous access catheters should be inserted to allow rapid transfusion of fluids and blood products when necessary. The innominate artery is essential for cerebral blood flow and blood pressure should be invasively monitored via the right radial artery. It has been recommended that arterial blood pressure proximal and distal to the aortic arch be simultaneously monitored to detect differences across the aortic arch [7]. Arterial access for intra-arterial cannulations can be achieved via a combination of bilateral radial, or right radial and femoral arteries. Continuous TEE monitoring can provide real-time assessment of cardiac anatomy and function as well as guide surgical decision making.

The use of near infrared spectroscopy (NIRS) may allow early detection of reduced cerebral perfusion and guide appropriate interventions before irreversible neurological injury occurs [7]; however, the evidence of net positive impact for NIRS remains sparse at this time. The trend and tracing of bispectral index (BIS) monitoring can be used to guide cooling of the patient for aortic arch repairs. During cooling, electroencephalography (EEG) activity decreases until electrocerebral silence occurs, which is usually around temperatures of 15–18 °C or after 45–50 minutes of cooling. Once electrocerebral suppression has been achieved, EEG monitoring cannot provide further guidance on the possibility of ongoing ischemia. Alterations to EEG activity prior to institution of deep hypothermia may indicate interruption to cerebral blood flow and immediate interventions should be instituted [8]. Prolonged EEG recovery during rewarming has been associated with neurological injury [7]. Placement and set up of other cerebral monitoring devices such as transcranial Doppler and measurement of jugular venous oxygen saturation can be time-consuming and may be not be practical in the acute setting.

Intraoperative Management

Surgical access to the ascending aorta is usually performed via a median sternotomy. Anesthetic management depends on the presenting hemodynamic profile prior to induction and various intra-operative phases of surgery. Judicious fluid administration and blood pressure control are important to prevent worsening of the dissection as well as to avoid severe hypotension occurring from a reduction in sympathetic tone and hypovolemia.

Depending on the extent of the dissection, arterial cannulation for antegrade perfusion can be established via the true lumen of the dissected ascending aorta, distal aortic arch, right axillary artery, right subclavian artery or innominate artery. Femoral artery cannulation can provide retrograde perfusion but at the risk of worsening the dissection if arterial flow is directed into the false lumen. Venous cannulation can be right atrial, femoral or bicaval.

Aortic arch repair often involves disrupting the cerebral blood supply and is associated with high neurological complication rates of up to 26% [7]. The aim of cerebral protection is to limit neurological injury and preserve cognitive function (Class I, Level of evidence B) [2]. This may be undertaken in the form of profound hypothermia, continued selective antegrade or retrograde cerebral perfusion or deep hypothermic circulatory arrest (DHCA). Institutional experience influences the selection of technique (Class IIa, Level of evidence B) [2]. For DHCA, the patient is cooled to 18–20 °C via the extracorporeal circulation as soon as CPB is initiated. A head-cooling jacket with circulating iced water or ice packed around the head can further achieve topical cooling. Esophageal and urinary bladder or rectal core temperatures should be measured. Most patients tolerate 30 minutes of DHCA without significant neurological dysfunction though this duration can be extended with the use of continued cerebral perfusion techniques [2]. Hypothermic strategies without cerebral perfusion were found to have a higher operative mortality or neurological complication rate compared to those utilizing antegrade or retrograde cerebral perfusion [9]. Rewarming is usually performed slowly to avoid cerebral ischemia and hyperthermia [2]. The gradient between core and peripheral temperatures should be less than 5 °C [10] with discontinuation of rewarming at 36–37 °C [7].

There is no strong evidence supporting the routine use of neuroprotective adjuncts such as barbiturates or calcium channel blockers [2], though there is some inconclusive evidence pointing towards the use of corticosteroids in decreasing cytokine release and lysosomal breakdown during hypothermia [10].

Intraoperative coagulopathy occurring in aortic dissection repairs is a well-known clinical entity previously thought to be induced by hypothermia and CPB [11]. Whereas CPB induces fibrinolysis, aortic dissection itself has been found to be associated with a consumptive state resembling disseminated intravascular coagulopathy. It has been demonstrated that turbulent blood flow and thrombosis in the false lumen activates the hemostatic system even before surgery [11].

Activation of the coagulation, complement and fibrinolytic systems as well as initiation of a systemic inflammatory response syndrome occur when blood contacts the non-endothelial surfaces of the extra-corporeal circuit. The best studied of the anti-fibrinolytic agents are tranexamic acid, ε-aminocaproic acid and aprotinin. Lysine analogues (tranexamic acid, ε-aminocaproic acid) reduce total blood loss, decrease blood transfusion requirements and are indicated for blood conservation (Class I, Level of evidence A) [12]. While aprotinin administration has been shown to reduce the rate of postoperative re-exploration for bleeding, its routine use is not recommended due to its potential risk for allergic or anaphylactic reactions as well as an increased risk of 30-day mortality, stroke, renal and heart failure compared to lysine analogues (Class III, Level of evidence A) [12, 13].

The average CPB duration for aortic dissection repairs often exceeds 3 h [8]. Higher heparin concentrations should be maintained during CPB to reduce activation of the hemostatic system, reduce platelets and coagulation factors consumption as well as blood transfusion requirements (Class IIb, Level B evidence) [12]. Titrating the dose of protamine to reverse the effect of heparin, starting at approximately 50% of the total heparin dose, is recommended to reduce the risk of bleeding (Class IIb, Level B evidence) [12]. Fibrinogen should also be replaced early [11]. Recombinant factor VIIa concentrate may be considered in the event of severe intractable bleeding unresponsive to routine hemostatic measures (Level IIb, Class B evidence) [12] but this may result in a higher incidence of acute thrombotic complications including stroke.

Cell saver devices should routinely be used after separation from CPB for blood conservation and to reduce the risk of allogeneic blood product transfusion (Class I, Level of evidence A) [12]. Viscoelastic point-of-care (POC) tests for coagulation profiles, using thromboelastography (TEG®) or rotational thromboelastometry (ROTEM®), can guide transfusion decisions and supplement transfusion algorithms in a multidisciplinary approach towards blood conservation (Class I, Level of evidence A) [12]. However, pooled effect estimates show that though viscoelastic POC tests reduced transfusion requirements, they had no effect on mortality, stroke, chest reopening for hemostasis as well as length of ICU and hospital stay [14].

Postoperative Management

Patients should be closely monitored in the ICU for complications such as bleeding, acute kidney injury (AKI), mesenteric ischemia, myocardial infarction and cerebrovascular accident (Table 26.2)

Table 26.2 Complications of Type A aortic dissection repairs [2]

Complications (Causative Factors)	Incidence
1. Myocardial infarction (coronary artery disease (CAD), dissection of coronary artery ostia)	1–5%
2. Heart failure (inadequate myocardial protection, ventricular distension)	1–5%
3. Infections (contamination, inadequate antibiotic coverage, obesity, suboptimal glucose control, immunosuppression)	1–5%
4. Stroke (ischemic, embolic)	2–8%
5. Reopening for bleeding (CPB-induced coagulopathy, inadequate hemostasis)	1–6%
6. Respiratory failure (pulmonary edema, transfusion-related acute lung injury (TRALI))	5–15%
7. Ventricular arrhythmias (myocardial ischemia, inadequate myocardial protection)	1–5%

AKI is relatively common after repair of Type A dissection (40–50%) and is an independent risk factor for 30-day mortality [15]. Severity of AKI influences both short and long-term patient outcomes and should be recognized early and treated promptly [15]. Mesenteric ischemia is another important predictor of mortality with an incidence of approximately 3.7% [1].

In-hospital mortality for patients with Type A aortic dissection has remained high at 17–26% despite advances in surgical techniques and is largely influenced by the patient's co-morbidities and dissection related complications [1, 15]. Measures to mitigate adverse outcomes include correction of anemia, strict perioperative blood glucose control, judicious use of vasoactive drugs to maintain perfusion, as well as avoiding nephrotoxic agents, hemodynamic instability, hypoxia and malperfusion states [7, 15].

Emergency Coronary Artery Bypass Grafting

In this current era where patients with acute coronary syndromes (ACS) are primarily treated with percutaneous coronary intervention (PCI) or thrombolysis to restore coronary perfusion, the role of emergency CABG has been limited to the following situations (Table 26.3).

The incidence of emergency CABG in ST-segment elevation myocardial infarction (STEMI) patients is relatively low (3.2–10.9%) [16] but these patients are at higher risk than those undergoing elective CABG. Lee and colleagues reported a higher in-hospital mortality of

up to 26% in patients presenting with cardiogenic shock compared to 1.2% in those with stable angina [17]. Predictors of operative mortality include advanced age, female gender, presence of mechanical complications or cardiogenic shock, preoperative use of intra-aortic counter-pulsation balloon pump (IABP), pulmonary or renal disease and serum troponin concentration [16].

Emergency CABG within 24 h after PCI is uncommon [16, 18]. This is due to advances in operator techniques as well as antiplatelet and fibrinolytic therapies. Indications include ongoing ischemia, threatened occlusion with substantial myocardium at risk (Class I, Level of evidence B), hemodynamic compromise (Class I, Level of evidence B) or complication of PCI [16, 18].

Preoperative Management

Patients with ACS presenting for emergency CABG can be complex and challenging especially those with cardiogenic shock requiring inotropic and mechanical circulatory support. These patients would often have received antiplatelet or fibrinolytic therapy, making perioperative coagulopathy a significant issue. The urgency of surgery also means inadequate time for fasting and optimization given the small window for myocardial reperfusion before irreversible necrosis. Targeted history and physical examination should be made in the limited time available, determining the presence of co-existing diseases, severity of CAD and management that the patient had already received.

Table 26.3 Recommendations for emergency CABG in AMI [16]

Recommendations	Class I	Class IIa	Class IIb	Class III	Level of Evidence
1. PCI cannot be performed or failed	✓				B
2. Persistent and significant cardiac ischemia at rest	✓				B
3. Mechanical complications such as ruptured ventricular septum, papillary muscle or free wall	✓				B
4. Coronary anatomy unsuitable for PCI	✓				B
5. Cardiogenic shock refractory to medical therapy	✓				B
6. Life-threatening ischemic ventricular arrhythmias with significant left main or triple vessel disease	✓				C

Early administration of antiplatelet and antithrombotic drugs has improved overall survival [18]. The aggressive use of potent antiplatelet agents in addition to aspirin, such as glycoprotein IIb/IIIa receptor inhibitors (abciximab, tirofiban) and adenosine diphosphate (ADP) $P2Y_{12}$ receptor inhibitors (ticlopidine, clopidogrel, prasugrel, ticagrelor), means that platelet function is often substantially impaired at the time of surgery. If possible, emergency CABG should be delayed for at least 12 h in patients who had abciximab and four hours for tirofiban to limit perioperative blood loss and need for transfusion (Class I, Level of evidence B) [16, 19]. Prophylactic platelet transfusion in the presence of glycoprotein IIa/IIIb receptor inhibitors is not advised and should only be considered when there is excessive bleeding after separation from CPB [18].

Exposure to clopidogrel within 5 days of CABG was found to be the strongest predictor of major perioperative bleeding and need for chest reopening [18]. Both clopidogrel and ticlopidine should be stopped for at least 24 h before emergency CABG (Class I, Level of evidence B) [16]. Observational data suggest that an off-pump CABG (OPCAB) technique by an experienced surgeon, meticulous surgical hemostasis, use of topical hemostatic and antifibrinolytic agents as well as judicious platelet and coagulation factors transfusion can reduce bleeding [16]. However, there is insufficient data to prove that the reduced risk of bleeding after discontinuing clopidogrel outweighs the added risk of myocardial ischemic events [18].

Bivalirudin is the only direct thrombin inhibitor recommended for use in patients with ACS. It has a short half-life of 25 minutes and should be stopped for at least 3 h before emergency CABG [18].

Intraoperative Management

Anesthetic management can be challenging as the balance between myocardial oxygen supply and demand needs to be favorable to prevent further myocardial insult and adverse outcomes [16]. Coronary perfusion can be optimized by preventing tachycardia as well as maintaining adequate diastolic and left ventricular end-diastolic pressures (Class I, Level of evidence B) [16]

Invasive monitoring should be established preoperatively. For patients who are critically ill with left main disease or a left ventricular ejection fraction less than 30%, perioperative use of IABP to augment coronary perfusion is considered reasonable to reduce mortality (Class IIa, Level of evidence B) [16]. Pulmonary artery catheter insertion has been recommended in patients with cardiogenic shock undergoing emergency CABG (Class I, Level of evidence C) [16].

The goals of induction and maintenance of anesthesia include avoiding myocardial depression and peripheral vasodilatation as well as obtunding sympathetic responses to intubation and surgical stimulation. Volatile halogenated anesthetic agents and opioids have ischemic preconditioning properties which can mitigate the risk of myocardial ischemia (Class IIa, Level of evidence A) [16]. Intraoperative hypotension is a risk factor for adverse outcomes [16] but may be unavoidable given the circumstance of the patient and nature of surgery. This may occur during vascular cannulation and weaning from CPB. Displacement of the heart and application of cardiac stabilizer devices along the coronary arteries and apex of the heart to facilitate OPCAB can alter the geometry of cardiac chambers and reduce both stroke volume and blood pressure [20]. Preventive measures include placing the patient in a slight Trendelenburg position to aid venous return as well as judicious use of fluids and vasoactive drugs to increase systemic blood pressures prior to any manipulation. While prompt management of hemodynamic instability is essential, the surgeon must be allowed full concentration during graft anastomosis for best outcomes. Intraoperative TEE can assist in monitoring regional wall motion abnormalities as well as ventricular and valvular function (Class IIa, Level of evidence B) [16].

Both on-pump and OPCAB techniques, when performed by experienced teams of surgeons, anesthesiologists and perfusionists adhering to the recommended guidelines, have been found to be equally safe and effective [21]. OPCAB is associated with less perioperative bleeding, renal and neurocognitive dysfunction due to avoidance of aortic manipulation and CPB [22]. In patients with failed PCI presenting for emergency CABG, OPCAB may reduce the risk of renal failure, need for IABP and surgical re-exploration for hemostasis [22]. For patients who are hemodynamically unstable, an on-pump technique is preferred as surgery is less technically challenging with better long-term graft patency [16]. However, emergency conversion to CPB during attempted OPCAB results in significantly higher morbidity and mortality [23].

Recommendations from the various societies on perioperative blood management [12, 16] are summarized in Table 26.4.

Intraoperative hyperglycemia is an independent risk factor for perioperative complications including death [24]. The use of intravenous insulin infusion to maintain postoperative blood glucose concentrations less than 180 mg/dL or 10 mmol/L has been recommended to reduce the incidence of adverse outcomes, including deep sternal wound infections (Class I, Level of evidence B) [16].

Weaning from CPB can be challenging. Patients with preoperative cardiogenic shock or requiring high infusion rates of vasoactive agents may require IABP or extra-corporeal membrane oxygenator (ECMO) to help separation from CPB. The use of IABP or ECMO on long-term patient outcomes remains uncertain [18].

Postoperative Management

Extubation criteria are the same as for patients receiving elective CABG surgery. As per routine, patients are monitored for development of complications such as bleeding, AKI and cerebrovascular ischemic events [16]

A multidisciplinary approach towards ensuring optimal patient analgesia and comfort is recommended (Class I, Level of evidence B) [16]. Adequate pain control allows for early mobilization and reduces the risk of postoperative pulmonary complications. Morphine has been found to be superior than fentanyl in providing postoperative pain relief with similar times to extubation [25]. The routine use of a high thoracic epidural for analgesia is uncertain (Class IIb, Level of evidence B) [16] with concerns over neuraxial

Table 26.4 Recommendations for blood conservation during emergency CABG [12, 16]

Recommendations	Class I	Class IIa	Class IIb	Class III	Level of Evidence
A. Preoperative					
1. Identify high-risk patients (advanced age, anemia, low body mass index, urgent surgery, antithrombotic drugs, coagulopathy) and implement a multimodal approach consisting of transfusion algorithms, POC testing and blood conservation strategies	✓				A
2. Stop ADP P2Y$_{12}$ receptor inhibitors if possible	✓				B
B. Intraoperative					
1. Consider OPCAB to reduce perioperative bleeding and blood transfusion		✓			A
2. Administer lysine analogues (ε-aminocaproic acid and tranexamic acid) during on-pump CABG	✓				A
3. Maintain higher heparin concentrations during long CPB times (>2–3 h) to reduce activation of hemostatic system and consumption of platelets and coagulation factors			✓		B
4. Administer lower doses of protamine starting at 50% of total heparin dose			✓		B
5. Consider topical hemostatic agents as part of a multimodal strategy			✓		C

bleeding in the setting of perioperative antiplatelet and fibrinolytic therapy, heparinization and CPB-induced coagulopathy. Cyclooxygenase-2 inhibitors are not recommended due to the incidence of adverse cardiovascular events (Class III, Level of evidence B) [16].

Mediastinal Re-exploration for Bleeding

Despite improvements in surgical and blood conservation techniques, the incidence of mediastinal re-exploration for hemostasis is approximately 2.2–4.2% [26]. Re-operation for excessive postoperative bleeding is associated with emergency surgery, multiple coronary anastomoses, extensive dissection, prolonged CPB time, low intraoperative core temperature, low body mass index, advanced age and high preoperative serum creatinine concentrations [26].

Management of postoperative bleeding depends on the etiology of blood loss. Excessive postoperative bleeding may be due to deficiency of coagulation factors, anastomotic leak or vascular injury. While blood products may be transfused to correct coagulopathy, the rate of mediastinal blood loss determines the necessity for surgical exploration [27]. No standardized definition for postoperative bleeding exists though a recent study defined active bleeding as blood loss exceeding 1.5 ml/kg/h for 6 consecutive hours within the first 24 hours [27]. As excessive bleeding is associated with a three- to fourfold increase in mortality, early exploration is key to reducing the severity of bleeding and minimizing blood product usage [26].

Intraoperative Management

Coagulation factors can be replaced by transfusing fresh frozen plasma (FFP), cryoprecipitate or factor concentrates. The American Society of Anesthesiologists (ASA) guidelines recommend FFP transfusion for active bleeding related to deficiencies in the coagulation cascade, as defined by a prothrombin time and activated partial thromboplastin time more than 1.5× mean value of a normal reference population [28]. A dose of 15–20 ml/kg of FFP may increase serum factor concentrations by 30% [29]. Cryoprecipitate is usually indicated for dys- or hypo-fibrinogenemia (<1.5–2 g/L) and 10 U will increase fibrinogen levels by 1 g/L [28].

Several plasma-derived and recombinant factor concentrates have been used for the treatment of coagulopathy and bleeding after cardiac surgery. These include prothrombin complex concentrates (PCC) [30], fibrinogen [31] and recombinant factor VIIa [32]. PCC consists of factors II, IX and X and can be administered to rapidly replace vitamin-K dependent coagulation factors. However, concerns over an increased risk of thrombotic complications have limited its use to patients who are bleeding and have been on oral anticoagulant therapy (grade 1B recommendation) or have coagulopathy with increased bleeding tendency (grade 2C recommendation) [33]. In cases of significant bleeding with suspected dys- or hypo-fibrinogenemia, fibrinogen concentrate should be first-line therapy (grade IC recommendation) and cryoprecipitate only given when it is unavailable [33]. Advantages of factor concentrates include quicker administration as there is no need for thawing or warming, greater efficacy and a lower risk of fluid overload. In addition, there is no association with viral infections or TRALI [30].

Platelet function can be impaired from preoperative antiplatelet therapy, exposure to CPB as well as dilutional and consumptive coagulopathy [29]. One unit of apheresis-derived platelet is equivalent to six units of random-donor platelet and transfusion of one such unit should increase platelet count by 30,000–60,000/μL [29]. For patients with uremia or Type I von Willebrand disease, the use of 1-deamino-8-D-arginine vasopressin (DDAVP) or desmopressin may reduce excessive bleeding (Class IIb, Level of evidence B) [12].

While inadequately neutralized heparin or heparin rebound may be treated with titrated doses of 20–60 mg of protamine, excessive doses can aggravate platelet dysfunction and activate the complement pathway [29]. The role of lysine analogues has been previously discussed.

Correction of hypothermia, hypocalcemia and acidosis should occur concurrently. Viscoelastic POC tests are useful in yielding quicker results compared to standard laboratory tests, isolating specific coagulation defects and guiding targeted blood product therapy. Rapid infusion systems facilitate rapid warming and transfusion of blood products. The use of intraoperative cell salvage to process mediastinal shed blood and subsequent reinfusion of washed blood may be considered for blood conservation (Class IIb, Level of evidence B) [12].

Postoperative Management

Correction of coagulopathy and monitoring for further bleeding should continue in the ICU. Following massive transfusion, complications such as fluid overload, fever, infection, sepsis, TRALI, electrolyte imbalances as well as dilutional coagulopathy can occur. Organ ischemia secondary to hypotension may affect postoperative recovery.

Cardiac surgical emergencies can be complex and challenging to manage. Anesthesiologists play an important role in coordinating OR personnel, managing hemodynamics and instituting preventive measures to ensure optimal patient outcomes.

References

1. Berretta P, Patel HJ, Gleason TG, et al. IRAD experience on surgical type A acute dissection patients: results and predictors of mortality. Ann Cardiothorac Surg. 2016;5(4):346–51.
2. Hiratzka LF, Bakris GL, Beckman JA, et al. 2010 ACCF/AHA/AATS/ACR/ASA/SCA/SCAI/SIR/STS/SVM guidelines for the diagnosis and management of patients with Thoracic Aortic Disease: a report of the American College of Cardiology Foundation/American Heart Association Task Force on Practice Guidelines, American Association for Thoracic Surgery, American College of Radiology, American Stroke Association, Society of Cardiovascular Anesthesiologists, Society for Cardiovascular Angiography and Interventions, Society of Interventional Radiology, Society of Thoracic Surgeons, and Society for Vascular Medicine. Circulation. 2010;121(13):e266–369.
3. Hebballi R, Swanevelder J. Diagnosis and management of aortic dissection. Contin Educ Anaesth Crit Care Pain. 2009;9(1):14–8.
4. Cheitlin MD, Armstrong WF, Aurigemma GP, et al. ACC/AHA/ASE 2003 guideline update for the clinical application of echocardiography—summary article: a report of the American College of Cardiology/American Heart Association Task Force on Practice Guidelines (ACC/AHA/ASE Committee to Update the 1997 Guidelines on the Clinical Application of Echocardiography). J Am Coll Cardiol. 2003;42:954–70.
5. Erbel R, Alfonso F, Boileau C, et al. Diagnosis and management of aortic dissection: Task Force on Aortic Dissection, European Society of Cardiology. Eur Heart J. 2001;22(18):1642–81.
6. Wahr JA, Prager RL, Abernathy JH III, et al. Patient safety in the cardiac operating room: human factors and teamwork: a scientific statement from the American Heart Association. Circulation. 2013;128(10):1139–69.
7. Harrington DK, Ranasinghe AM, Shah A, et al. Recommendations for haemodynamic and neurological monitoring in repair of acute type A aortic dissection. Anesthesiol Res Pract. 2011;2011:949034.
8. Bavaria JE, Brinster DR, Gorman RC, et al. Advances in the treatment of acute type A dissection: an integrated approach. Ann Thorac Surg. 2002;74(5):S1848–52.
9. Englum BR, He X, Gulack BC, et al. Hypothermia and cerebral protection strategies in aortic arch surgery: a comparative effectiveness analysis from the STS Adult Cardiac Surgery Database. Eur J Cardiothoracic Surg. 2017;52(3):492–8. https://doi.org/10.1093/ejcts/ezx133.
10. Conolly S, Arrowsmith JE, Klein AA. Deep hypothermic circulatory arrest. Contin Educ Anaesth Crit Care Pain. 2010;10(5):138–42.
11. Guan XL, Wang XL, Liu YY, et al. Changes in the hemostatic system of patients with acute aortic dissection undergoing aortic arch surgery. Ann Thorac Surg. 2016;101(3):945–51.
12. Ferraris VA, Brown JR, Despotis GJ. 2011 update to the Society of Thoracic Surgeons and the Society of Cardiovascular Anesthesiologists blood conservation clinical practice guidelines. Ann Thorac Surg. 2011;91(3):944–82.
13. Fergusson DA, Hébert PC, Mazer CD, et al. A comparison of aprotinin and lysine analogues in high-risk cardiac surgery. N Engl J Med. 2008;358(22):2319–31.
14. Serraino GF, Murphy GJ. Routine use of viscoelastic blood tests for diagnosis and treatment of coagulopathic bleeding in cardiac surgery: updated systematic review and meta-analysis. Br J Anaesth. 2017;118(6):823–33.
15. Ko T, Higashitani M, Sato A, et al. Impact of acute kidney injury on early to long-term outcomes in

patients who underwent surgery for type A acute aortic dissection. Am J Cardiol. 2015;116(3):463–8.
16. Hillis LD, Smith PK, Anderson JL, et al. 2011 ACCF/AHA Guideline for Coronary Artery Bypass Graft Surgery: executive summary: a report of the American College of Cardiology Foundation/American Heart Association Task Force on Practice Guidelines. Circulation. 2011;124(23):2610–42.
17. Lee JH, Murrell HK, Strony J, et al. Risk analysis of coronary bypass surgery after acute myocardial infarction. Surgery. 1997;122:675–80.
18. Brown C, Joshi B, Faraday N, et al. Emergency cardiac surgery in patients with acute coronary syndromes: a review of the evidence and perioperative implications of medical and mechanical therapeutics. Anesth Analg. 2011;112(4):777–99.
19. Cheng DK, Jackevicius CA, Seidelin P, et al. Safety of glycoprotein IIb/IIIa inhibitors in urgent or emergency coronary artery bypass graft surgery. Can J Cardiol. 2004;20(2):223–8.
20. Murkin JM. Hemodynamic changes during cardiac manipulation in off-CPB surgery: relevance in brain perfusion. Heart Surg Forum. 2002;5(3):221–4.
21. Lamy A, Devereaux PJ, Prabhakaran D, et al. Five-year outcomes after off-pump or on-pump coronary-artery bypass grafting. N Engl J Med. 2016;375(24):2359–68.
22. Stamou SC, Hill PC, Haile E, et al. Clinical outcomes of nonelective coronary revascularization with and without cardiopulmonary bypass. J Thorac Cardiovasc Surg. 2006;131:28–33.
23. Patel NC, Patel NU, Loulmet DF, et al. Emergency conversion to cardiopulmonary bypass during attempted off-pump revascularization results in increased morbidity and mortality. J Thorac Cardiovasc Surg. 2004;128:655–61.
24. Doenst T, Wijeysundera D, Karkouti K, et al. Hyperglycemia during cardiopulmonary bypass is an independent risk factor for mortality in patients undergoing cardiac surgery. J Thorac Cardiovasc Surg. 2005;130:1144.
25. Murphy GS, Szokol JW, Marymont JH, et al. Morphine-based cardiac anesthesia provides superior early recovery compared with fentanyl in elective cardiac surgery patients. Anesth Analg. 2009;109:311–9.
26. Kristensen KL, Rauer LJ, Mortensen PE, et al. Reoperation for bleeding in cardiac surgery. Interact Cardiovasc Thorac Surg. 2012;14(6):709–13.
27. Colson PH, Gaudard P, Fellahi JL, et al. Active bleeding after cardiac surgery: A prospective observational multicentre study. PLoS One. 2016;11(9): e0162396.
28. Stehling LC, Donerty DC, Faust RJ, et al. Practice Guidelines for blood component therapy: a report by the American Society of Anesthesiologists Task Force on Blood Component therapy. Anesthesiology. 1996;84:732–47.
29. Despotis G, Avidan M, Eby C. Prediction and management of bleeding in cardiac surgery. J Thromb Haemost. 2009;7(Suppl 1):111–7.
30. Cappabianca G, Mariscalco G, Biancari F, et al. Safety and efficacy of prothrombin complex concentrate as first-line treatment in bleeding after cardiac surgery. Crit Care. 2016;20(5):1172–6.
31. Fassl J, Buse GL, Filipovic M, et al. Perioperative administration of fibrinogen does not increase adverse cardiac and thromboembolic events after cardiac surgery. Br J Anaesth. 2015;114(2):225–34.
32. Warren O, Mandal K, Hadjianastassiou V, et al. Recombinant activated factor VII in cardiac surgery: a systematic review. Ann Thorac Surg. 2007;83:707–14.
33. Kozek-Langenecker SA, Afshari A, Albaladejo P, et al. Management of severe perioperative bleeding: guidelines from the European Society of Anaesthesiology. Eur J Anaesthesiol. 2013;30:270–382.

Regional Anesthesia Techniques and Management in Cardiothoracic Surgery

27

Jodie Beuth and George Djaiani

Main Messages
1. Optimal perioperative pain control can translate into improved patient outcomes and potentially lower incidence of chronic pain.
2. Multimodal approach for perioperative pain management is a common practice in most of the cardiac surgery units.
3. Both acute and transitional pain service teams play an active role and are very effective in perioperative surveillance of patients undergoing cardiac surgery.
4. Benefits of regional techniques in selected groups of patients may lower perioperative morbidity and mortality reaching beyond the benefits of superior pain control.

The most commonly used neuraxial techniques in cardiac surgery include thoracic epidural anesthesia/analgesia (TEA), and spinal anesthesia. TEA is used either in combination with general anesthesia (GA) or as sole source of anesthesia as in the case of 'awake cardiac surgery'. Spinal anesthesia modalities include favourable analgesia profiles following administration of intrathecal opioids [1, 2], as well as deliberate 'total spinal' with high dose local anesthetic in combination with light GA. These techniques are not universally employed, with an international survey of cardiac anaesthesiologists suggesting that 7.6% of respondents used spinal anesthesia and 7% used thoracic epidural techniques for cardiac surgery [3]. The reason for this limited use is associated with balanced consideration of the proposed benefits from these neuraxial techniques weighed against the potential increased risks.

Advantages of Neuraxial Anesthesia for Cardiac Surgery

The benefits of regional anesthesia techniques in cardiac surgery relate predominantly to the sympatholytic effects in patients with severe coronary disease, respiratory benefits associated with minimisation or avoidance of endotracheal intubation and mechanical ventilation, as well as superior analgesia quality [2, 4]. Thoracic neuraxial blockade of the cardiac accelerator fibres can result in optimised hemodynamic stability due to increased myocardial oxygen supply, reduced oxygen demand, improved coronary perfusion, and reduction in the incidence of supraventricular tachyarrhythmias [3, 5, 6]. Improved analgesia can lead to reduced respiratory complication rate, as well

J. Beuth · G. Djaiani (✉)
Department of Anesthesia and Pain Management, Toronto General Hospital, University Health Network, University of Toronto, Toronto, Canada
e-mail: George.Djaiani@uhn.ca

© Springer Nature Switzerland AG 2021
D. C. H. Cheng et al. (eds.), *Evidence-Based Practice in Perioperative Cardiac Anesthesia and Surgery*, https://doi.org/10.1007/978-3-030-47887-2_27

as shortened extubation time, and decreased intensive care unit length of stay [2, 5, 7, 8]. Furthermore, endotracheal intubation may be avoided altogether in patients undergoing awake cardiac surgery [9]. Other reported benefits associated with neuraxial anesthesia include reduction in perioperative stress response, improved glycemic control, reduction in systemic opioid use, and reduced incidence of postoperative delirium [10, 11]. While all of these aforementioned benefits seem advantageous, it needs to be determined if utilization of neuraxial anesthesia is associated with improved long term outcomes.

Multiple meta-analyses have been performed to analyse the efficacy of neuraxial techniques in cardiac surgery [2, 5, 6]. A recent review of 25 studies including a total of 3062 patients showed no difference in perioperative myocardial infarction or cerebrovascular accident between those receiving TEA with or without GA compared to GA alone [5]. However, the authors showed a significant reduction in respiratory complications, lower rates of supraventricular arrhythmias, faster extubation time, reduced intensive care length of stay, decreased postoperative pain [5], and reduction in acute kidney injury [6].

The latest Cochrane review [12] of 3047 patients from 31 studies showed similar findings comparing GA for cardiac surgery with or without TEA. There was significant reduction in respiratory complications and arrhythmia in the group receiving supplemental epidural analgesia whilst no difference related to myocardial infarction, cerebrovascular events, or mortality [12].

A meta-analysis of 1106 patients in 25 randomised controlled trials assessing the effectiveness of addition of intrathecal morphine in combination with GA versus GA alone found no benefit regarding mortality, morbidity associated with myocardial infarction, arrhythmias, time to extubation, or duration of hospitalization [13]. In the subset of 17 randomised controlled trials involving 668 patients, addition of intrathecal morphine was associated with moderate reduction in systemic opioid use and reduced postoperative pain scores, however, this effect was abated after 24 h showing no advantage over analgesia achieved with thoracic epidural [2].

Neurological Complications

There are a number of potentially significant adverse events that can occur with the use of neuraxial techniques in cardiac surgery, hence, appropriate patient selection is crucial. The most feared complication associated with the use of neuraxial techniques in a patient who will be systemically anticoagulated within a short time frame is that of epidural hematoma [4]. Additionally, quite often patients scheduled for cardiac surgery are taking antiplatelet agents which preclude the safe use of neuraxial techniques [14]. The true incidence of spinal cord injury from epidural hematoma is difficult to establish due to a rare occurrence of this complication [2, 15]. Consequently, the risk analysis has been extrapolated from the literature and mathematical modelling [16]. There have been three case reports of patients with confirmed epidural hematomas post epidural catheter insertion for cardiac surgery, and while the incidence may be rare, this is a clinically devastating complication [16–18]. Although it can be speculated that the incidence of epidural hematoma may be increased in patients with subsequent systemic anticoagulation, the analyses by Royce et al. [19] and Hemmerling et al. [20] suggest that the incidence of epidural related hematoma in cardiac surgery is comparable to that of the general surgical population. The estimate of incidence in recent publications from 2015 and 2013 state a risk of 1: 3552 (95% CI; 1: 2552–1:5841) [21] and 1:5493 (95% CI, 1:970–1:31,114) respectively [20].

Neurological surveillance of cardiac surgical patients post neuraxial technique must be meticulous, and concerns of neurological compromise warrant urgent imaging of the spinal cord to rule out hematoma. Subsequently, an urgent neurosurgical consultation may be required with access to neurosurgical facilities if laminectomy is warranted. There is good evidence for complete resolution of neurological symptoms if spinal cord decompression is performed within 8 h [22, 23]. Delayed interventions, particularly beyond 24 h, often result in poor neurological recovery [22, 23].

Recommendations to minimise the incidence of epidural hematoma in the cardiac surgical patient include careful patient selection and adherence to suggested guidelines below [14].

Recommendations for neuraxial blockade for cardiac surgery:

- Neuraxial blockade not recommended within 7 days of clopidogrel or within 14 days of ticlodipine unless normal platelet function can be demonstrated [14]
- Avoidance of neuraxial technique and/or catheter removal with any evidence of coagulopathy
- Consideration for delaying surgery for 24 h if epidural puncture is traumatic (i.e. bloody tap)
- Avoidance of multiple passes with epidural insertion (maximum of three attempts) [7]
- Minimum interval between catheter placement and systemic heparinization of 1 h
- Preference for epidural insertion via midline approach and saline injection into the epidural space to minimise trauma to epidural venous plexus
- Avoidance of anticoagulant[1] or antiplatelet use (except aspirin) until epidural catheter is removed[1]
- Intensive neurological surveillance post neuraxial intervention
- Fast track approach with early awakening to assess neurological function of the spinal cord
- Immediate access to neuroimaging and neurosurgical consult
- Use of minimally required dose of heparin with appropriate monitoring [7]
- Use of lowest doses of local anesthetic for epidural infusion postoperatively to avoid motor block and assess neurological function [7]

The incidence of infective complications from neuraxial techniques is also exceedingly rare. The estimated frequency in non-cardiac surgery is 0–0.05% [3]. Risk factors include a breach of sterility for epidural insertion, duration of catheter in situ, and patient factors such as immunocompromised status, malignancy, diabetes and steroid use [3]. These risk factors can be extrapolated to the cardiac surgical patient, and whilst cardiac surgery would not necessarily predicate a patient to increased risk of epidural abscess, the nature of cardiopulmonary bypass, potential exposure to transfusion of blood products, and prolonged mechanical ventilation may contribute to impaired immunocompetency of the patient [3] Additionally, the hemodynamic perturbations of cardiac surgery can compromise spinal cord perfusion with hemodilutional anemia, relative hypotension, aortic dissection, potential displacement of aortic plaques, and the use of intra-aortic balloon pumps with associated embolic events that are known to have caused spinal cord ischemia after cardiac surgery [3, 24].

Techniques

Thoracic Epidural Anesthesia

Epidural insertion is either done the day before surgery or on the day of surgery. The majority of institutions typically insert epidural catheters the day before surgery to minimise any complications associated with a potentially traumatic puncture [14, 25]. Placement of a high thoracic epidural targets the T1–T5 nerve roots, resulting in a dense sensory and motor blockade, and sympatholysis of the cardiac accelerator fibres. Technique varies and can involve introduction of the epidural needle between the spinous processes from C7 to T5 [7]. A combination of local anesthetic with opioid is administered for an average duration of three to four days postoperatively.

Loading Dose
- Ropivacaine 0.375–0.75% 5–8 ml with or without opioid[2]
- Bupivacaine 0.25–0.5% 5–12 ml with opioid[2]

---

[1]Anticoagulant use for venous thromboembolic prophylaxis or therapeutic anticoagulation with intravenous heparin should adhere to the ASRA guidelines pertaining to timing of administration related to needle puncture and catheter removal [14].

[2]Opioid regime typically includes sufentanil 15–25 mcg or fentanyl 20 mcg.

Maintenance Infusion
- Ropivacaine 0.2% with fentanyl 2mcg/ml @ 5–14 ml/h.
- Bupivacaine 0.5% with morphine 25mcg/ml @ 4–10 ml/h.
- Bupivacaine 0.125% with clonidine 0.0006% @ 10 ml/h.

Spinal Anesthesia

The advantage of the high spinal technique is likely related to attenuation of the stress response to cardiac surgery and the associated cardiovascular stability with improved cardiac indices and lower pulmonary vascular resistance [13, 26]. In addition, some reports have suggested that high spinal anesthesia resulted in less beta-receptor dysfunction, lower stress response, and modified anti-inflammatory and immune systems when compared to general anesthesia alone in the cardiac surgical setting [26, 27]. Careful patient selection is crucial, and Trendelenburg positioning with significant vasoactive support is often required to maintain adequate mean arterial pressure [26, 28]. Commonly, hyperbaric local anesthetic solutions are administered combined with opioids for improved analgesic effect postoperatively, with most of the published data using a combination of hyperbaric local anesthetic solution and intrathecal morphine (e.g. 20–40 mg of 0.75% hyperbaric bupivacaine with 0.3–0.4 mg morphine, and often sufentanil 10–20 mcg) [28].

Awake Cardiac Surgery

With the advances in surgical technologies and technique, there has been interest in the performance of 'awake cardiac surgery' using high thoracic epidural without GA. Since the emergence of awake cardiac surgery in late 90s, there have been a few hundred cases published from India, Turkey, Germany, and Saudi Arabia [25]. The technique involves positing an epidural catheter at the level from C7 to T3, generally the day prior to surgery. A dense block is established slowly to minimise the risk of phrenic nerve block from spread of local anesthetic [10]. Choice of local anesthetic is typically 5–10 ml of bupivacaine or ropivacaine 0.5% with 25 mcg of fentanyl followed by an infusion of 0.5% bupivacaine with fentanyl 4 mcg/ml at 5 ml/h. [25]

The advantages of this technique include excellent analgesia postoperatively and avoidance of GA [9]. The major drawback of this technique is the need for potential conversion to GA with reported incidence of 3.7–12% [10]. The main indications for conversion includes patient distress, respiratory failure, unacceptable patient movement, deterioration of block quality, and cardiovascular instability [10].

Patient and procedure selection is important. Considerations for ACS are discussed below.

Selection Criteria [25]
- Target coronary artery more than 2 mm in size with discrete lesion
- Absence of left ventricular dysfunction
- Absence of aortic regurgitation
- Normal sinus rhythm
- Symptomatic carotid artery disease
- Absence of difficult airway
- Cooperative patient

Contraindications [10]
- Lack of patient consent
- Surgical preference for general anesthesia
- Anticipation of technically difficult surgery
- Recent myocardial infarction
- Requirement for coronary artery endarterectomy
- Any contraindication to epidural anesthesia
- Acute complications of myocardial infarction (i.e. ventricular rupture/ventricular septal defect)

Disadvantages [10]
- Unprotected airway
- Shivering—challenging to avoid hypothermia with limited active warming [25]
- Inability to perform transesophageal echocardiography
- Spontaneously ventilating patient may increase surgical difficulty

- Risk of pneumothorax in spontaneously ventilating patient
- Diaphragmatic paralysis (incidence 0.6%)
- Potential for gastric distension if non-invasive ventilation is used in sedated patients
- Some limitations on team communication
- Epidural related risk of complications
- Epidural block does not cover saphenous graft harvest
- Conversion to GA [10]
  - Deterioration of epidural anesthesia quality
  - Unacceptable amount of patient movement or coughing
  - Respiratory distress or failure
  - Hemodynamic instability or cardiac arrest
  - Patient agitation or distress

Additional Techniques of Regional and Local Anesthesia

Some of the minimally invasive cardiac surgical procedures require thoracotomy incisions to provide optimal surgical exposure. Unilateral paravertebral analgesia provides excellent pain relief after thoracotomy incisions. The two widely used options include either a single shot injection of local anesthetic (slow release liposomal drugs may last up to 72 h) or continuous infusion via the paravertebral catheter. The catheter can be sited either preoperatively with ultrasound guidance or intraoperatively under direct vision by the surgeon [29]

Other regional techniques, such as bilateral sternal blockade, or sternal wound subcutaneous catheters, have shown promise with respect to less pain and reduced opioid requirements [30, 31]; however, caution should be exercised due to potentially higher sternal wound infection rates [32].

References

1. Ng WCJ, Djaiani G. Dose response study of intrathecal morphine for off-pump coronary artery bypass grafting: a pilot prospective randomized double-blinded controlled clinical trial. J Cardiol Cardiovasc Ther. 2017;3:555610.
2. Liu SS, Block BM, Wu CL. Effects of perioperative central neuraxial analgesia on outcome after coronary artery bypass surgery: a meta-analysis. Anesthesiology. 2004;101:153–61.
3. Djaiani G, Fedorko L, Beattie WS. Regional anesthesia in cardiac surgery: a friend or a foe? Semin Cardiothorac Vasc Anesth. 2005;9:87–104.
4. Chaney MA. Intrathecal and epidural anesthesia and analgesia for cardiac surgery. Anesth Analg. 2006;102:45–64.
5. Zhang S, Wu X, Guo H, Ma L. Thoracic epidural anesthesia improves outcomes in patients undergoing cardiac surgery: meta-analysis of randomized controlled trials. Eur J Med Res. 2015;20:25.
6. Svircevic V, van Dijk D, Nierich AP, et al. Meta-analysis of thoracic epidural anesthesia versus general anesthesia for cardiac surgery. Anesthesiology. 2011;114:271–82.
7. Mehta Y, Kulkarni V. Thoracic epidural analgesia in cardiac surgery. Ann Card Anaesth. 2003;6:175–82.
8. Djaiani GN, Ali M, Heinrich L, et al. Ultra-fast-track anesthetic technique facilitates operating room extubation in patients undergoing off-pump coronary revascularization surgery. J Cardiothorac Vasc Anesth. 2001;15:152–7.
9. Chakravarthy M, Jawali V, Patil TA, et al. Conscious cardiac surgery with cardiopulmonary bypass using thoracic epidural anesthesia without endotracheal general anesthesia. J Cardiothorac Vasc Anesth. 2005;19:300–5.
10. Chakravarthy M. Future of awake cardiac surgery. J Cardiothorac Vasc Anesth. 2014;28:771–7.
11. Greisen J, Nielsen DV, Sloth E, Jakobsen CJ. High thoracic epidural analgesia decreases stress hyperglycemia and insulin need in cardiac surgery patients. Acta Anaesthesiol Scand. 2013;57:171–7.
12. Svircevic V, Passier MM, Nierich AP, et al. Epidural analgesia for cardiac surgery. Cochrane Database Syst Rev. 2013:Cd006715.
13. Zangrillo A, Bignami E, Biondi-Zoccai GG, et al. Spinal analgesia in cardiac surgery: a meta-analysis of randomized controlled trials. J Cardiothorac Vasc Anesth. 2009;23:813–21.
14. Horlocker TT, Wedel DJ, Rowlingson JC, et al. Regional anesthesia in the patient receiving antithrombotic or thrombolytic therapy: American Society of Regional Anesthesia and Pain Medicine Evidence-Based Guidelines (Third Edition). Reg Anesth Pain Med. 2010;35:64–101.
15. Jack ES, Scott NB. The risk of vertebral canal complications in 2837 cardiac surgery patients with thoracic epidurals. Acta Anaesthesiol Scand. 2007;51:722–5.
16. Ho AM, Chung DC, Joynt GM. Neuraxial blockade and hematoma in cardiac surgery: estimating the risk of a rare adverse event that has not (yet) occurred. Chest. 2000;117:551–5.
17. Sharma S, Kapoor MC, Sharma VK, Dubey AK. Epidural hematoma complicating high thoracic epidural catheter placement intended for cardiac surgery. J Cardiothorac Vasc Anesth. 2004;18:759–62.

18. Bang J, Kim JU, Lee YM, et al. Spinal epidural hematoma related to an epidural catheter in a cardiac surgery patient – a case report. Korean J Anesthesiol. 2011;61:524–7.

19. Royse CF. High thoracic epidural analgesia for cardiac surgery: time to move from morbidity to quality of recovery indicators. Ann Card Anaesth. 2009;12:168–9. author reply 70–1

20. Hemmerling TM, Cyr S, Terrasini N. Epidural catheterization in cardiac surgery: the 2012 risk assessment. Ann Card Anaesth. 2013;16:169–77.

21. Landoni G, Isella F, Greco M, et al. Benefits and risks of epidural analgesia in cardiac surgery. Br J Anaesth. 2015;115:25–32.

22. Castellano JM, Durbin CG Jr. Epidural analgesia and cardiac surgery: worth the risk? Chest. 2000;117:305–7.

23. Imanaka K, Kyo S, Yokote Y, et al. Paraplegia due to acute spinal epidural hematoma after routine cardiac surgery. Intensive Care Med. 2000;26:826.

24. Sevuk U, Kaya S, Ayaz F, Aktas U. Paraplegia due to spinal cord infarction after coronary artery bypass graft surgery. J Card Surg. 2016;31:51–6.

25. Chakravarthy M. Technique of awake cardiac surgery. Tech Reg Anesth Pain Manag. 2008;12:87–98.

26. Lee TW, Grocott HP, Schwinn D, Jacobsohn E. High spinal anesthesia for cardiac surgery: effects on beta-adrenergic receptor function, stress response, and hemodynamics. Anesthesiology. 2003;98:499–510.

27. Lee TW, Kowalski S, Falk K, et al. High spinal anesthesia enhances anti-inflammatory responses in patients undergoing coronary artery bypass graft surgery and aortic valve replacement: randomized pilot study. PLoS One. 2016;11:e0149942.

28. Kowalewski R, Seal D, Tang T, et al. Neuraxial anesthesia for cardiac surgery: thoracic epidural and high spinal anesthesia – why is it different? HSR Proc Intensive Care Cardiovasc Anesth. 2011;3:25–8.

29. Raveglia F, Rizzi A, Leporati A, et al. Analgesia in patients undergoing thoracotomy: epidural versus paravertebral technique. A randomized, double-blind, prospective study. J Thorac Cardiovasc Surg. 2014;147:469–73.

30. Eljezi V, Duale C, Azarnoush K, et al. The analgesic effects of a bilateral sternal infusion of ropivacaine after cardiac surgery. Reg Anesth Pain Med. 2012;37:166–74.

31. White PF, Rawal S, Latham P, et al. Use of a continuous local anesthetic infusion for pain management after median sternotomy. Anesthesiology. 2003;99:918–23.

32. Agarwal S, Nuttall GA, Johnson ME, et al. A prospective, randomized, blinded study of continuous ropivacaine infusion in the median sternotomy incision following cardiac surgery. Reg Anesth Pain Med. 2013;38:145–50.

Part III

Perioperative Monitoring Technology and Management

Spinal Cord Ischemia Monitoring and Protection

28

Albert T. Cheung and Jaime R. López

Main Messages

1. Spinal cord ischemia is a potential risk of thoracic or thoracoabdominal aorta operations.
2. Thoracoabdominal aortic aneurysm extent and aortic graft length are the most important risk factors for determining the risk of postoperative spinal cord ischemia.
3. Strategies for preventing and treating spinal cord ischemia include; making the spinal cord less vulnerable to ischemia and infarction; minimizing duration of cord ischemia during operation; augmenting spinal cord blood flow; and detection of ischemia while patient is under anesthesia in order to start immediate intervention.
4. Providing immediate treatment after performing neurologic assessment to detect spinal cord ischemia, and main-

taining adequate spinal cord perfusion pressure are the objectives for managing patients at risk for spinal cord ischemia.

Operations on the thoracic or thoracoabdominal aorta pose a risk of spinal cord ischemia and infarction that may lead to permanent paraplegia or paraparesis [1, 2]. Spinal cord ischemia is the direct consequence of temporary or permanent interruption of blood flow through intercostal or segmental arterial collaterals that arise from the diseased segments of the descending thoracic or thoracoabdominal aorta. Open surgical repair to replace a diseased segment of the descending thoracic or thoracoabdominal aorta with an interposition graft for the treatment of aneurysms, dissection, traumatic injury, or atherosclerotic ulcers requires temporary interruption of blood flow through the aorta and the sacrifice or reimplantation of intercostal or segmental arteries that supply blood to the spinal cord. Thoracic and thoracoabdominal aortic endovascular repair does not require interruption of blood flow in the aorta, but requires the obligate exclusion of the intercostal and segmental arteries within the covered segments of the aorta. After open or endovascular repair of the thoracic or thoracoabdominal aorta, spinal cord perfusion becomes

A. T. Cheung (✉)
Department of Anesthesiology, Perioperative and Pain Medicine, Stanford University School of Medicine, Stanford, CA, USA
e-mail: ATCheung@stanford.edu

J. R. López
Department of Neurology and Neurological Sciences, Stanford University, Stanford, CA, USA

© Springer Nature Switzerland AG 2021
D. C. H. Cheng et al. (eds.), *Evidence-Based Practice in Perioperative Cardiac Anesthesia and Surgery*, https://doi.org/10.1007/978-3-030-47887-2_28

more dependent on blood supply from collateral networks arising from the vertebral arteries and from the hypogastric vascular network. An understanding of the pathophysiology of spinal cord ischemia together with strategies to prevent, detect, and treat this complication is a critical part of the surgical, anesthetic, and perioperative care of patients undergoing thoracic and thoracoabdominal aortic repair.

Vascular Anatomy of the Spinal Cord

The spinal cord has a complex blood supply that varies among individual patients that is often described as a collateral network (Fig. 28.1).

In general terms, the anterior region of the spinal cord is supplied by the anterior spinal artery. The anterior spinal artery is formed from the vertebral arteries after they branch off the subclavian arteries. The vertebral arteries join at the level of the foramen magnum to form the anterior spinal artery that descends along the length of the spinal cord in the anterior median fissure (Fig. 28.2).

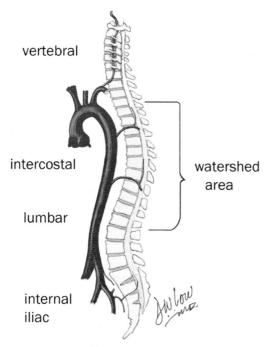

Fig. 28.1 Spinal cord blood supply

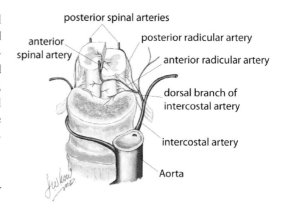

Fig. 28.2 The anterior region of the spinal cord is supplied by the anterior spinal artery and the posterior region of the spinal cord is supplied by a pair of posterior spinal arteries

The anterior spinal artery then gives rise to multiple sulcal arteries, that penetrate the spinal cord via the anterior median fissure and supply the anterior two thirds of the spinal cord (Fig. 28.2) [3, 4]. The posterior region of the spinal cord is supplied by the paired posterior spinal arteries. The posterior spinal arteries are derived either from the vertebral or posterior inferior cerebellar arteries and runs caudally along the posterior surface of the spinal cord just medial to the posterior nerve roots. As the spinal arteries travel distally into the thoracic and lumbar portions of the spinal cord, spinal perfusion becomes increasingly dependent on blood flow from collateral vessels (Fig. 28.3) [5].

Arteries from the thoracic aorta become important collateral sources of regional blood supply to the spinal cord. Dorsal branches of the posterior intercostal arteries give rise to segmental medullary arteries that pass through the intervertebral foramina and divide into anterior and posterior radicular arteries (Fig. 28.2). The radicular arteries course medially and form a series of anastomoses with the anterior and posterior spinal arteries. The posterior spinal arteries have a more consistent segmental anatomy and tend to be continuous, but the anterior spinal artery frequently is attenuated or entirely discontinuous. For this reason, the anterior spinal artery is more dependent on its segmental supply to maintain perfusion [6, 7]. Anterior radicular arteries

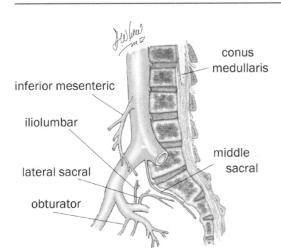

Fig. 28.3 The hypogastric vascular network supplies the caudal end of the spinal cord via the collateral vascular network

inferior mesenteric

iliolumbar

lateral sacral

obturator

conus medullaris

middle sacral

derived from ascending cervical, deep cervical, intercostal, iliolumbar, and sacral segmental arteries also provide contributions to the anterior spinal artery. Detailed anatomic studies have identified a large segmental artery, the arteria radicularis magna, also known as the artery of Adamkiewicz, that is believed to be important for supplying blood to the lower two thirds of the thoracolumbar spinal cord [6, 8]. The arteria radicularis magna has been described to originate from the left side in 63% to 80% of individuals and most commonly arises from the T8-L2 region of the descending thoracic aorta [3, 7–10]. Because of its variable integrity and dependence on collateral circulation, the anterior spinal cord is particularly prone to ischemia during periods of hemodynamic instability [5, 10–12]. Watershed regions exist at the vertebral levels of T1, T5, and T8–T9, where the spinal cord is often smallest (Fig. 28.1) [6, 7, 13].

Blood supply to the spinal cord may be best described as a complex collateral network with contributions from the vertebral arteries, segmental arteries, and hypogastric arteries. The presence of a collateral network explains why spinal cord perfusion can be maintained when one collateral source is compromised. A collateral network may also produce the potential for vascular steal in the event that a low resistant pathway

exists within the system. The presence of a collateral network also explains why hypotension may trigger the onset of spinal cord ischemia and why augmenting arterial pressure, reducing the cerebrospinal fluid pressure and maintaining cardiac output is effective for the treatment of spinal cord ischemia after thoracic and thoracoabdominal aortic repairs.

The Incidence and Risk Factors for Spinal Cord Ischemia

The incidence (Table 28.1) and risk of spinal cord ischemia after thoracic and thoracoabdominal aortic repairs depends primarily on the extent of the repair and whether the procedure was performed as an open surgical repair or a thoracic endovascular aortic repair (TEVAR). In a 30-year clinical series of 1509 patients undergoing open thoracoabdominal aortic repairs described by Svensson and Crawford in 1993, the incidence of spinal cord ischemia was 15% among patients with Crawford extent I aneurysms, 31% for those with Crawford extent II aneurysms, 7% for those with extent III aneurysms, and 4% for those with extent IV aneurysm (Fig. 28.4) [21]. Two additional contemporary series (n = 2286 patients undergoing open surgical repairs described by Coselli

Table 28.1 Incidence of spinal cord ischemia (SCI) and reversible ischemic spinal cord syndrome (RISCS) after thoracic and thoracoabdominal endovascular aortic repair

Study	SCI (% Total)	RISCS (% of SCI)
Ullery BW, et al. J Vasc Surg Surg 2011 [14]	12/424 (2.8%)	11/12 (91.7%)
Scali ST, et al. J Vasc Surg 2014 [15]	68/741 (9.2%)	30/68 (44.1%)
O'Callaghan A, et al. J Vasc Surg 2015 [16]	19/87 (21.8%)	11/19 (58.9%)
Maurel B, et al. Eur J Vasc Endovasc Surg 2015 [17]	8/204 (3.9%)	5/8 (62.5%)
Dias NV, et al. Eur J Vasc Endovasc Surg 2015 [18]	22/72 (31.0%)	15/22 (68.2%)
Bisdas T, et al. J Vasc Surg 2015 [19]	23/142 (16.0%)	20/23 (87.0%)

RISCS reversible ischemic spinal cord syndrome, *SCI* spinal cord ischemia

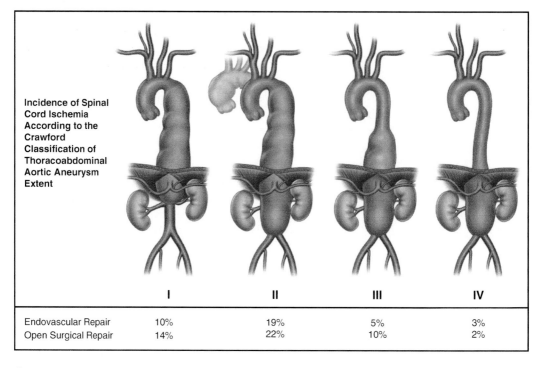

Incidence of Spinal Cord Ischemia According to the Crawford Classification of Thoracoabdominal Aortic Aneurysm Extent				
	I	**II**	**III**	**IV**
Endovascular Repair	10%	19%	5%	3%
Open Surgical Repair	14%	22%	10%	2%

Fig. 28.4 The Crawford classification for characterizing the extent of thoracoabdominal aortic aneurysms (TAAA) is a major factor predicting the risk for spinal cord ischemia for both open surgical and endovascular repair [20]

in 2007; n = 372 patients described by Greenberg in 2008) reported also that the incidence of spinal cord ischemia depended on the Crawford extent of the aneurysm with extent II aneurysm repairs involving the entire descending thoracoabdominal aorta posing the greatest risk for paraplegia [20, 22].

The initial clinical experience with TEVAR suggested that endovascular repair was associated with an overall decreased risk for spinal cord ischemia [23, 24]. TEVAR procedures avoided the need to cross clamp the aorta, the subsequent reperfusion syndrome, and the associated hemodynamic consequences that may have attenuated the physiologic alterations that contribute to spinal cord ischemia. Subsequent studies indicate that the lower incidence of spinal cord ischemia observed among patients undergoing TEVAR was that most TEVAR procedures were for the treatment of isolated descending thoracic aortic aneurysms. When patients undergoing TEVAR procedures were stratified according to aneurysm

extent, the incidence of spinal cord ischemia was comparable to that of open repairs [20]. In several contemporary clinical series of patients with Crawford extent I to IV thoracic and thoracoabdominal aneurysms treated with endovascular procedures, the incidence of spinal cord ischemia was reported to be as great as 31% [15–19].

The most important risk factor (Table 28.2) predicting the risk of postoperative spinal cord ischemia is the aneurysm extent and the length of the aortic graft [20–22]. Other risk factors for predicting the risk of spinal cord ischemia are less well established and vary among individual centers and the patient populations studied. Commonly cited risk factors include location of the aneurysm in the proximity of the arteria magna, extended aortic cross clamp time during open surgical repairs, the number of segmental or intercostal arteries re-implanted during operation, perioperative hypotension, or emergency operations [1, 21].

Among patients undergoing endovascular repair, the aneurysm extent and the length of

Table 28.2 Risk factors for spinal cord ischemia (SCI) after open or endovascular thoracic and thoracoabdominal aortic repair

Category	Risk factors
Demographic	• Age • Male gender • Lower body mass index • Preoperative renal insufficiency • Chronic obstructive pulmonary disease (COPD) • Prior abdominal aortic aneurysm
Anatomic	• Extent of thoracic or thoracoabdominal disease • Aortic pathology • Prior distal or proximal aortic endovascular repair • Number of patent segmental arteries
Perioperative	• Emergency operation • Procedure duration • Aortic cross clamp duration • Fluoroscopy time • Open surgical repair • Total length of endovascular coverage • Coverage of left subclavian artery • Number of endovascular stent grafts implanted • Fenestrated or branched endovascular repair • Hypotension • Access site injury • Bleeding • Perioperative renal failure • Hypogastric artery occlusion • Use of iliac artery conduit

endograft coverage of the aorta has also been consistently identified as a risk factor for postoperative spinal cord ischemia [15, 18–20]. In the study reported by Greenberg, multivariate analysis revealed that the extent of required repair according to the Crawford classification was the primary factor associated with the development of spinal cord ischemia in both groups [20]. Within the endovascular group, the highest incidence of spinal cord ischemia occurred among those patients with Crawford extent II aneurysms (19%), followed by extent I (10%), extent III (5%), and extent IV (3%), respectively [20]. In the The European Collaborators on Stent/Graft Techniques for Aortic Aneurysm Repair (EUROSTAR) registry, the use of three or more stent grafts was an independent risk factor for spinal cord ischemia (OR = 3.5; P = .043)

[24]. In a retrospective study analyzing three-dimensional reconstructions of preoperative and postoperative computed tomographic angiograms of 241 patients who underwent TEVAR, patients who developed postoperative spinal cord ischemia had a greater absolute (260.5 ± 40.9 vs. 195.8 ± 81.6 mm, P = .002) and relative (88.8% ± 12.1% vs 67.6% ± 24.0%, P = .001) length of aortic coverage compared to those without spinal cord ischemia [25]. Other risk factors associated with spinal cord ischemia after TEVAR include left subclavian artery coverage [24], iliac artery injury [26], prior abdominal aortic aneurysm repair, [20, 26–30] thoracic aortic pathology type [28, 31], and hypogastric artery occlusion [31]. Despite the potential for spinal cord malperfusion, TEVAR for the treatment of Stanford type B aortic dissection has not been observed to increase the risk of SCI [24]. A number of demographic and perioperative variables that may represent surrogates for the severity of underlying vascular disease have also been shown to be associated with the development of spinal cord ischemia. The EUROSTAR registry together with three other recent studies have found showed coexisting renal disease to be an independent risk factor for spinal cord ischemia [14, 15, 24, 29]. Other reported risk factors include age, male gender, lower body mass index, hypertension, chronic obstructive pulmonary disease, emergent procedure, duration of procedure, intraoperative fluoroscopy time, estimated blood loss, use of an iliac artery conduit, and perioperative hypotension [15, 25, 26, 28, 32, 33]. It is likely that improvements in neuroprotection, operative techniques, and perioperative management will modify risk factors for spinal cord ischemia as the clinical experience evolves.

Clinical Manifestations of Spinal Cord Ischemia

Spinal cord ischemia should be considered upon the appearance of any new lower-extremity motor or sensory deficit in the postoperative period that cannot be attributed to stroke or a peripheral nerve injury. Neurological deficits caused by spinal cord ischemia can vary widely with regard to severity, onset, and potential for recovery. Serial neurological assessment of lower extremity motor strength in the postoperative period provides an objective means to detect spinal cord ischemia that can be performed by physicians or nursing staff. Various scoring systems have been described to provide a clinical classification of the severity of the neurologic deficits associated with spinal cord ischemia. Crawford, et al. described a functional scoring system ranging from one (near or complete paralysis) to four (able to walk but requires assistance) [34]. The modified Tarlov score grades the severity of the deficit on a scale from zero to five with zero having no lower extremity movement to five being normal) [33, 35]. The American Spinal Injury Association (ASIA) provides a comprehensive and reproducible system for classifying the severity of impairment based on both sensory and motor defects in each lower extremity [36]. The ASIA score is generated by rating motor strength of the hip flexors, knee extensors, ankle dorsiflexors, long toe extensors, and ankle plantar extensors on a scale of zero (flaccid paralysis) to five (normal strength), together with rating whether sensation is absent, impaired, or normal in each of the spinal dermatomes (Table 28.3). In descriptive terms, paraplegia is often used to describe bilateral lower-extremity complete paralysis and paraparesis is used to describe bilateral or asymmetric lower-extremity weakness that can be quantified using a scale of one to five [36].

Existing clinical experience suggests that spinal cord ischemia complicating thoracic and thoracoabdominal aortic repair is a heterogeneous syndrome that may manifest a spectrum of neurologic deficits that vary depending on the location, severity, and extent of the ischemic insult [14, 26]. Patients may exhibit bilateral lower extremity motor weakness that may be either symmetrical or asymmetrical. Sensory deficits are common and may be present in up to 70% of patients, but patients may also manifest isolated motor weakness [26]. Variability in spinal cord perfusion as a consequence of anatomic variations, the patency of collateral networks, the severity of underlying vascular disease, and the extent of the repair among different patients may explain the spectrum of neurologic findings asso-

Table 28.3 Scoring the severity of motor and sensory deficits

Score	Description
Motor	
0	Total paralysis
1	Palpable or visible contraction
2	Active movement, gravity eliminated
3	Active movement against gravity
4	Active movement against some resistance
5	Active movement against full resistance
5*	Normal corrected for pain or disuse
NT	Not testable
Sensory	
0	Absent
1	Altered
2	Normal
NT	Not testable
Lower extremity muscle groups according to vertebral level	
(Designate as right, left, or bilateral)	
L2	Hip flexors
L3	Knee extensors
L4	Ankle dorsiflexors
L5	Long toe extensors
S1	Ankle plantar flexors

Based on the International Standards for Neurological Classification of Spinal Cord Injury [36]

ciated with this condition. Ischemia-reperfusion injury and thromboembolism may be additional mechanisms contributing to spinal cord injury that may further affect the clinical diversity of the neurologic manifestations in this condition.

A neurological deficit noted on awakening from anesthesia, regardless of severity, is regarded as immediate-onset spinal cord ischemia or infarction. Neurological deficits classified as immediate-onset are attributed to an intraoperative event that directly caused or triggered spinal cord ischemia. Because the onset and timing of the intraoperative ischemic events in anesthetized patients cannot always be determined, the condition is typically associated with a spinal cord infarction and interventions in the postoperative period to treat this condition by increasing spinal cord perfusion have been less effective. Immediate-onset spinal cord ischemia or infarction is generally associated with a poor prognosis [14, 26]. In contrast, the new onset development of lower-extremity motor deficits following an initial normal postoperative neurological exam is defined as delayed-onset spinal cord ischemia. Several series have reported that delayed-onset spinal cord ischemia can present within hours or even up to several months after operation [26, 27, 37–39]. In contrast to immediate-onset spinal cord ischemia, delayed-onset spinal cord ischemia often is a manifestation of spinal cord ischemia prior to its evolution to spinal cord infarction and may improve or even resolve in response to interventions directed at improving spinal cord perfusion. For this reason, reversible ischemic spinal cord syndrome (RISCS) is often used to describe patients with delayed-onset spinal cord ischemia who recover in response to treatment. Clinical series have reported that between 37% and 73% of episodes of postoperative spinal cord ischemia after open surgical repairs may be classified as delayed-onset [26, 40]. Among patients undergoing TEVAR procedures, 58% to 83% of postoperative spinal cord ischemic episodes were reported as delayed-onset [17, 19, 26, 41]. Postoperative events that have been linked to the development of delayed-onset SCI include hypotension, thrombosis, hematoma, embolization, and elevated cerebrospinal fluid (CSF) pressures [26, 27, 42, 43].

Table 28.4 Intraoperative strategies to prevent spinal cord ischemia

Goal	Strategy
Decrease the susceptibility to spinal cord ischemia	• Mild to moderate systemic hypothermia • Deep hypothermic circulatory arrest • Selective epidural hypothermia • Avoid hyperthermia • Pharmacologic neuroprotection
Minimize the duration of spinal cord ischemia	• Partial left heart bypass • Sequential aortic clamping and repair • Staged repair
Augment spinal cord perfusion and blood flow	• Lumbar cerebrospinal fluid drainage • Arterial blood pressure augmentation • Oversewing back-bleeding segmental arteries • Left subclavian artery revascularization • Avoid arterial hypotension • Avoid venous hypertension • Avoid anemia
Early detection of spinal cord ischemia	• Intraoperative somatosensory evoked potential (SEP) monitoring • Intraoperative motor evoked potential (MEP) monitoring • Early postoperative serial neurologic examinations • Avoid neuraxial anesthesia

Intraoperative Strategies to Prevent Spinal Cord Ischemia

Spinal cord ischemia after open thoracic aortic operations is caused by aortic cross-clamping or circulatory arrest followed by the sacrifice or exclusion of segmental arterial branches from the native descending aorta. In TEVAR procedures, spinal cord ischemia is a consequence of sacrificing segmental arterial vessels or other arterial collaterals that are in the excluded segments of the aorta after endovascular stent graft deployment. Many strategies have been developed to prevent and treat spinal cord ischemia at the time of operation. Strategies include techniques to make the spinal cord less susceptible to ischemia and infarction, minimize the duration of cord isch-

emia during operation, augment spinal cord blood flow, and detect spinal cord ischemia in the anesthetized patient to permit immediate intervention (Table 28.4). Even though spinal cord ischemia is caused by the anatomic consequences of operation, ischemia can often be treated, and infarction prevented by physiologic interventions.

The original technique used in TAAA repair was to temporarily interrupt blood flow to the descending aorta by placing a clamp across the proximal neck of the aneurysm segment while sewing in the vascular interposition graft. This approach is often referred to the "clamp-and-sew" technique and can still be used successfully. With the "clamp-and-sew" technique, the risk of spinal cord ischemia is related to the duration of time the aorta is cross clamped and may range from 8% for cross clamp times of less than

30 minutes to as great as 27% for cross clamp times exceeding 60 min [21, 43–45]. The most commonly used technique to reduce the duration of spinal cord ischemia during repair is partial left heart bypass. Partial left heart bypass overcomes the limitations of the Gott passive shunt and provides a controlled means to perfuse the distal aorta by directing blood from the left atrium to the distal descending aorta or femoral artery while both the proximal and distal extent of the aneurysmal segment of the aorta is clamped [46, 47]. Both proximal and distal perfusion pressures and flows can be controlled and monitored during partial left heart bypass by manipulating the central venous pressure, left atrial pressure, contralateral femoral artery pressure, cardiac output, and centrifugal pump flow. Avoiding proximal hypertension may attenuate increases in the cerebrospinal fluid pressure during repair. Adding a heat exchanger to the perfusion circuit also facilitates deliberate hypothermia and re-warming. During partial left heart bypass with a proximal aortic cross clamp, the distal aortic cross clamp can be advanced sequentially from the proximal anastomosis to the distal anastomosis as each segment of the descending aorta is reconstructed to minimize end organ ischemia and the length of the descending aorta that is excluded from the circulation. Occluding or over-sewing segmental arteries that back bleed into the open aorta is advocated to prevent vascular steal since the presence of back bleeding indicates that these arteries have adequate collateral flow [1]. Use of a perfusion circuit with systemic anticoagulation during repair also permits the selective perfusion of mesenteric branch vessels through separate balloon-tipped catheters.

Techniques to increase the spinal cord tolerance to temporary ischemia are often necessary or used as a neuroprotective adjunct because of the obligate need to temporarily interrupt collateral blood supply to the spinal cord during operation. Like the brain, the spinal cord has high basal metabolic activity and will manifest neuronal dysfunction within a short time after the interruption of blood flow. Deliberate hypothermia is the only clinically effective intervention that has been proven to consistently protect the central nervous system in conditions of ischemia [48]. The protective effect of hypothermia is believed to be a combination of its actions to reduce metabolic demand, stabilize cell membranes, and attenuate the inflammatory and excitotoxic responses to ischemia during reperfusion. Mild systemic hypothermia is typically employed for spinal cord protection prior to aortic cross clamping for open TAAA repair performed using the "clamp-and-sew" or partial left heart bypass technique. Mild systemic hypothermia in the range of 32–34 °C does not normally complicate circulatory management and can be achieved by allowing the nasopharyngeal temperature to decrease gradually in response to surgical exposure after the induction of general anesthesia. Re-warming can be accomplished with a heat exchanger in the perfusion circuit or irrigating the thorax with warmed saline at the time of operation. Alternatively, rewarming can be delayed or initiated in the postoperative period with a forced-air warming blanket or similar device. Deep or profound systemic hypothermia in the range of 10–18 °C with cardiopulmonary bypass and deep hypothermic circulatory arrest has been reported as a technique for TAAA repair, particularly if the repair involves the distal aortic arch [49]. Techniques for selective spinal cord hypothermia to as low as 26 °C by infusing cold saline into the epidural space have been described for spinal cord protection but have only been used at a limited number of centers [50]. Consensus opinion recommends avoiding hyperthermia during re-warming after deliberate hypothermia because hyperthermia may potentiate reperfusion injury [2].

The effectiveness of pharmacologic neuroprotectants used alone or in combination to prevent or treat spinal cord ischemia has not been proven and evidence to support their efficacy is indeterminate at best. Nevertheless, traditional protocols may include methylprednisolone 1 g i.v. (or 30 mg/kg i.v.), mannitol 12.5 g to 25 g i.v., magnesium 1 g to 2 g i.v., lidocaine 100 mg to 200 mg i.v., thiopental 0.5 g to 1.5 g iv, or propofol 25–75 mcg/kg/min i.v. as adjuncts for spinal cord protection. Small clinical series have also reported the use of naloxone 1 mcg/kg/h. i.v. or intrathecal papaverine at a dose of 30 mg [51, 52].

Spinal cord perfusion can be augmented surgically by reattaching intercostal or segmental arteries individually or as a patch into the vascular interposition graft during operation. Large segmental arteries with little or no back bleeding may be particularly important for spinal cord perfusion. Although re-implanting intercostal or segmental arteries may decrease the risk of spinal cord ischemia, the time and effort required to perform this additional procedure may prolong the period of spinal cord ischemia during repair and the additional vascular anastomoses with the prosthetic graft may compromise the durability of the final repair. Intraoperative neurophysiologic monitoring (IONM) to detect evidence of spinal cord ischemia can be used to guide the decision to surgically re-implant intercostal and segmental arteries. In TEVAR, it is not possible to surgically re-implant or preserve blood flow in the segmental arteries excluded by the stent graft. In TEVAR procedures that require left subclavian artery coverage and exclusion by the endovascular stent graft, it is possible to preserve left subclavian artery flow by surgical transposition of the subclavian artery onto the left carotid artery [53]. Alternatively, left subclavian artery flow can be preserved with a left carotid to subclavian bypass graft and subsequent coil embolization of the proximal left subclavian artery stump prior to TEVAR [53]. Maintaining blood flow in the left subclavian artery may be important for spinal cord perfusion because its branches that include the vertebral artery provide vascular collaterals supplying the anterior spinal artery and the cervical end of the spinal cord.

Spinal cord perfusion can also be augmented physiologically by vasopressor therapy to increase the arterial pressure, lumbar cerebrospinal fluid drainage to decrease the cerebrospinal fluid pressure, and medical interventions to optimize cardiac output and reduce venous pressures. The physiologic basis for lumbar cerebrospinal fluid drainage is that spinal cord perfusion pressure can be estimated by the difference between the mean arterial pressure and the lumbar cerebrospinal fluid pressure. Based on this relationship, increased lumbar cerebrospinal fluid pressure has the potential to decrease spinal cord perfusion pressure. Draining cerebrospinal fluid by percutaneous insertion of a silastic catheter into the subarachnoid space between lumbar spinal processes has the potential to increase spinal cord perfusion pressure by decreasing the cerebrospinal fluid pressure. The technique can be performed prior to operation in patients at risk for spinal cord ischemia or after operation in the event of acute postoperative spinal cord ischemia. Cerebrospinal fluid is drained into a sealed reservoir and the pressure within the subarachnoid space is transduced to achieve a target lumbar cerebrospinal fluid pressure of 10 mm Hg. Two systematic reviews and meta-analyses have been performed to evaluate the efficacy of lumbar cerebrospinal fluid drainage based on 372 published reports that included 3 randomized controlled trials involving 289 patients and 5 cohort studies involving 505 patients [54, 55]. The conclusions from analysis of the pooled data, including an analysis by the Cochrane Collaborative, supported the efficacy of lumbar cerebrospinal fluid drainage as a component of the multi-modality approach for prevention of neurological injury after thoracoabdominal aortic repair. Since the publication of these two meta-analyses, clinical experience on the efficacy of lumbar cerebrospinal fluid drainage has continued to accumulate for patients undergoing both open and endovascular aortic repairs. A class I recommendation for lumbar cerebrospinal fluid drainage for patients at risk for spinal cord ischemia, meaning that the procedure should be performed and that the benefits greatly exceeded the risks was issued by the American College of Cardiology Foundation and American Heart Association 2010 guidelines on the management of patients with thoracic aortic diseases, the 2014 European Society of Cardiology guidelines on the diagnosis and treatment of aortic diseases, and the European Association for Cardio-Thoracic Surgery position paper on spinal cord protection during thoracic and thoracoabdominal aortic surgery and endovascular aortic repair [1, 2].

Augmenting the arterial pressure alone or in combination with lumbar cerebrospinal fluid drainage is another important physiologic intervention to increase spinal cord perfusion [26, 56, 57]. Inconsistent control or insufficient augmentation of the arterial pressure may explain in part the controversy surrounding the effectiveness of lumbar cerebrospinal fluid drainage for treating spinal cord ischemia because decreasing lumbar cerebrospinal fluid pressure alone severely limits the ability to improve spinal cord perfusion pressure based on the equation: spinal cord perfusion pressure = mean arterial pressure – lumbar cerebrospinal fluid pressure. In general, vasopressor agents such as phenylephrine, epinephrine, norepinephrine, or vasopressin are administered to achieve and maintain a mean arterial pressure of 80 mm Hg or greater to ensure a spinal cord perfusion pressure of at least 70 mm Hg. The mean arterial pressure can be augmented further in increments of 5 mm Hg if spinal cord ischemia persists [1, 26, 56, 58]. During augmentation of the arterial pressure it is also important to

assure that cardiac output is satisfactory and that the central venous pressure is not elevated. Venous hypertension in a manner similar to increased cerebrospinal fluid pressure may also compromise spinal cord perfusion [59]. Hypotension from bleeding or other causes is often associated with the onset of spinal cord ischemia after thoracoabdominal aortic aneurysm repair, but clinical observations suggest also that spinal cord ischemia may be the primary cause of hypotension as well. The sympathetic ganglia of the autonomic nervous system resides in the thoracic and lumbar region of the spinal cord and hypotension from neurogenic shock may accompany spinal cord ischemia in many patients. In some patients, hypotension caused by neurogenic shock from autonomic dysfunction may represent an early sign of spinal cord ischemia (Fig. 28.5) [26, 56, 60, 61].

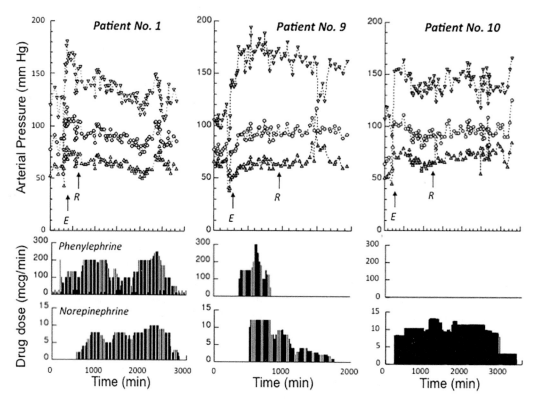

Fig. 28.5 Temporal trends in the systolic, diastolic, and mean arterial pressure among three patients who had delayed-onset spinal cord ischemia after open surgical thoracoabdominal aortic aneurysm repair. In each case, the onset of spinal cord ischemia manifested by paraplegia was preceded by hypotension (E). Recovery from spinal cord ischemia in response to vasopressor therapy to augment the arterial pressure and lumbar cerebrospinal fluid drainage to decrease the cerebrospinal fluid pressure coincided with the recovery of autonomic nervous system function and the restoration of arterial pressure. Adapted from Cheung AT, et al. Ann Thorac Surg 2002; 74:413–419 [56]

In this situation, immediate treatment of hypotension associated with spinal cord ischemia is necessary to prevent infarction.

Finally, arterial pressure should be monitored carefully when antihypertensive therapy is resumed after successful open or endovascular thoracic and thoracoabdominal aortic repairs to avoid unintentional hypotension that may precipitate spinal cord ischemia. The benefits of arterial pressure augmentation must be weighed against the risk of bleeding and the risks associated with temporary elevation in arterial pressure when implementing this technique in the perioperative period. Blood pressure augmentation was recommended for the treatment of spinal cord ischemia in the European Association for Cardio-Thoracic Surgery position paper on spinal cord protection during thoracic and thoracoabdominal aortic surgery and endovascular aortic repair and spinal cord perfusion pressure optimization was assigned a class IIa (benefits exceed risks) recommendation for spinal cord protection from the American College of Cardiology Foundation and American Heart Association 2010 guidelines on the management of patients with thoracic aortic diseases [1, 2].

Early intraoperative detection of spinal cord ischemia is important. Early detection permits early intervention before ischemia evolves to infarction [56, 57, 62]. The challenges of detecting spinal cord ischemia during operation in anesthetized patients may explain in part the poor prognosis and unresponsiveness to treatment among patients with immediate postoperative paraplegia after thoracic and thoracoabdominal aortic repair. Because it is not possible to perform a traditional neurologic examination, somatosensory evoked potential (SSEP) and/or motor evoked potential (TcMEP) monitoring is necessary to detect spinal cord ischemia during operation [63–65] (Fig. 28.6).

The clinical objectives for intraoperative neurophysiologic monitoring is to provide intermittent assessment of spinal cord function during operations to detect intraoperative spinal cord ischemia, identify critical vessels for reimplantation, and to establish the mean arterial pressure adequate for spinal cord perfusion. The

detection of reversible transient spinal cord ischemic changes by IONM may identify also patients who may be at risk for delayed postoperative spinal cord ischemia resulting in paraplegia or paraparesis (Fig. 28.7).

Comparing the amplitude and latency of SSEP or TcMEP signals recorded simultaneously from the upper and lower extremities provides an internal control to distinguish changes caused by anesthetics or artifacts from those caused by spinal cord ischemia. Another benefit of IONM is that it can detect limb ischemia caused by malperfusion and distinguish this condition from spinal cord ischemia (Fig. 28.8). Stimulation of peripheral nerves not affected by limb ischemia, such as the pudendal nerve can assist in quickly determining if the loss of signals is due spinal cord or peripheral nerve ischemia.

Intraoperative SSEP monitoring is performed by placing stimulating electrodes on the skin adjacent to peripheral nerves in the arms or legs. Typically, in the upper extremity the median nerve is electrically stimulated at the wrist and for the lower extremity the posterior tibial nerve is stimulated at the ankle. Electrical stimulation of the peripheral nerves in the limbs generate action potentials that can be measured from recording electrodes placed over various locations along the neural pathways and record electrical potentials corresponding to the peripheral nerves in the limbs, lumbar plexus, brachial plexus, spinal cord, brainstem, thalamus and cerebral cortex. A potential limitation of SSEP monitoring is that this technique only directly monitors the spinal cord dorsal columns and spinal cord ischemia confined to the anterior spinal cord may cause a selective motor deficit without involving the posterior sensory tracts. Nevertheless, sensory deficits are commonly present in patients with spinal cord ischemia and an advantage of SSEP monitoring is that it is relatively easy to perform in anesthetized patients. Although high concentrations of inhaled anesthetics, thiopental, or propofol can attenuate cortical SSEP signals, the fidelity of recorded potentials is improved with neuromuscular blockade. A balanced general anesthetic with inhaled anesthetics maintained at a

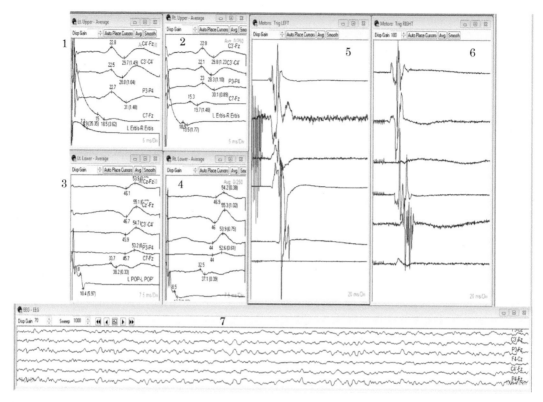

Fig. 28.6 Example of multimodality intraoperative neurophysiologic monitoring (IONM). Panels 1 and 2 show SSEPs after left and right median nerve stimulation, respectively. The first three traces from top to bottom are cortical generated SSEPs; the forth trace is from the cervical spinal cord; and the fifth trace is generated from the brachial plexus. Panels 3 and 4 show left and right lower limb posterior tibial nerve SSEPs, respectively. The first four traces from the top to the bottom are cortical generated SSEPs; the fifth trace is from the cervical spinal cord; and the sixth trace is generated from the peripheral tibial nerve at the popliteal fossa. Panels 5 and 6 show TcMEPs recorded from left and right sides, respectively. Recordings from top to bottom traces are from the following muscles: intrinsic hand muscles, psoas, vastus lateralis, tibialis anterior, abductor halluces, and anal sphincter. Panel 7 shows a six-channel EEG waveform. The top three traces are generated from the left cerebral hemisphere and the bottom three traces from the right hemisphere. The recording montage is as follows: F3, C3, P3, F4, C4, P4, all referenced to Fz

concentration of 0.5 MAC (minimum alveolar concentration) provides consistent conditions for monitoring intraoperative SSEPs.

Transcranial motor evoked potentials are elicited through transcranial electrical stimulation of cortical and subcortical corticospinal (motor) pathways and have also been advocated for the detection of intraoperative spinal cord ischemia. To monitor TcMEPs, myogenic evoked potentials are produced in extremity muscle groups by delivering multipulse, electrical stimulation to the scalp, overlying the motor cortex. The evoked electrical potentials elicited from this stimulation travel from the motor cortex, along the corticospi-

nal tracts, activating the anterior horn cells in the spinal cord, peripheral nerves, and finally to muscles. The muscle generated electrical potential is most commonly recorded using intramuscular needle electrodes. When using TcMEPs, muscle recordings should be obtained from upper extremities, as a control, and from the lower extremities to monitor thoracic and lumbar spinal cord function. An interruption in this pathway will result in the loss or reduction of amplitude in the TcMEPs. Clinical experience suggests that TcMEP monitoring may be more sensitive and detect spinal cord ischemia earlier than SSEPs [66]. TcMEP monitoring has been used to identify critical inter-

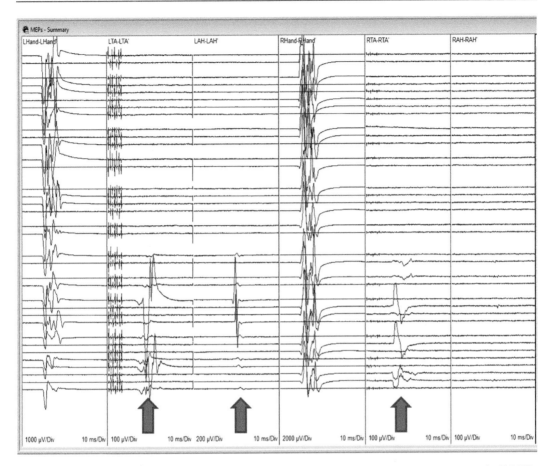

Fig. 28.7 Intraoperative spinal cord ischemia demonstrated in serial transcranial motor evoked potential (TcMEP) recordings over time (top to bottom) from the left (L) and right (R) hands, tibialis anterior (TA), and abductor halluces (AH). Spinal cord ischemia was manifested by the bilateral loss of lower extremity TcMEPs from the tibialis anterior (TA) and abductor halluces (AH) after aortic cross clamping. The lower extremity TcMEPs recovered gradually over time within 30 min after increasing the mean arterial pressure in response to the treatment of intraoperative spinal cord ischemia (arrows). TcMEPs from the right hand (RHand) and left hand (LHand) where unaffected during the episode of spinal cord ischemia

costal arteries for reattachment following the acute loss of lower extremity TcMEP signals during TAAA repair and can detect limb ischemia caused by malperfusion [64, 65]. Intraoperative TcMEP monitoring can be more challenging to perform in anesthetized patients because TcMEPs are attenuated by neuromuscular blocking drugs and many general anesthetic agents. General anesthetic regimens utilizing intravenous infusions of remifentanil, ketamine, propofol, or etomidate without neuromuscular blockade or carefully controlled incomplete neuromuscular blockade are often required to maintain satisfactory TcMEP signals during operation [66].

Clinical observations and physiologic rationale support the ability of SSEP and TcMEPs to detect spinal cord ischemia in anesthetized patients, but the sensitivity and specificity of these techniques remains to be determined. Intraoperative changes or loss of SSEP or TcMEP signals are not always caused by spinal cord ischemia [63, 65]. A functioning peripheral nerve is required to generate both SSEP and TcMEP signals and peripheral nerve ischemia from any cause will affect the associated SSEP or TcMEP. Vascular malperfusion of a lower extremity can cause loss of peripheral SSEP or TcMEP in the absence of spinal cord ischemia if blood

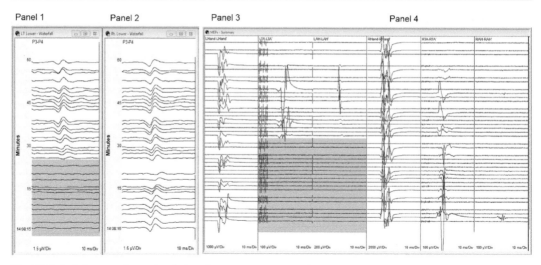

Fig. 28.8 Left leg vascular malperfusion demonstrated by intraoperative somatosensory evoked potential (SSEP) and transcranial motor evoked potential (TcMEP) recordings over time (from top to bottom). Panel I shows left lower extremity SSEPs and Panel 2 shows right lower extremity SSEPs over time. Panel 3 shows left lower extremity TcMEPs and Panel 4 shows right lower extremity TcMEPs recorded simultaneously. Unilateral loss of left lower extremity SSEPs and TcMEPs following surgical cannulation of the left femoral artery indicated ischemia of the left lower extremities caused by malperfusion (highlighted regions in Panel 1 and Panel 3)

flow to the limb is significantly compromised. Malperfusion causes a loss of SSEP or TcMEP from the affected ischemic limb. Lower extremity malperfusion may be caused by aortic dissection, atheroembolism, or most commonly from arterial cannulation of the femoral artery for extracorporeal circulation. Similar to malperfusion, operations performed by cross clamping the aorta without distal aortic perfusion will cause cortical SSEP and TcMEP signals from both lower extremities to diminish in amplitude over time after aortic cross clamping. Acute intraoperative cortical stroke or brain infarct will also produce changes in SSEP or TcMEPs. SSEP or TcMEP changes caused by cortical stroke can be distinguished from changes caused by spinal cord ischemia by comparing signals recorded at different sites along the neural conduction pathway. Cortical stroke is associated with selective loss of cortical signals and if extensive cerebrovascular territories are involved, typically affects both upper and lower extremity evoked potentials.

Several studies have suggested that staging of thoracoabdominal aortic aneurysm repairs using endovascular, open surgical, or combined techniques may decrease the risk of spinal cord isch-emia [16, 67]. In these observational studies, staged repair was either intentionally planned or was unintentional in patients who had prior aortic repairs. Among the patients who had extensive thoracoabdominal aortic aneurysms repaired in two separate stages, there was a decreased incidence of spinal cord ischemia or a decrease severity of spinal cord ischemia compared to patients who had repairs performed as a single procedure [16, 67]. The protective effect of staged repairs can be explained by the ability of the collateral network that provides perfusion to the spinal cord to compensate over time following the loss of segmental artery collaterals. Based on this rationale, two lesser ischemic insults may have less of a physiologic impact than one large ischemic insult. Following this line of reasoning, a technique to condition the collateral network and prevent vascular steal by coil embolizing segmental arteries prior to repair is being investigated to decrease the risk of spinal cord ischemia [1]. The potential advantages of staged repairs must be weighed against the risk of aneurysm rupture between the two procedures or incomplete repair in patients being lost to follow-up after the first procedure. In addition, the optimal time to perform the second stage of the repair has not been determined.

Postoperative Detection, Treatment, and Prevention of Spinal Cord Ischemia

Improvements in surgical, anesthetic, and perfusion techniques have decreased the risk of immediate onset spinal cord ischemia. Recent clinical series indicate that the majority of spinal cord ischemic events occur in the postoperative period, can be classified as delayed onset, and often respond to treatment [14–19, 25, 26, 56]. The objectives for the postoperative management of patients at risk for spinal cord ischemia are to ensure adequate spinal cord perfusion pressure, perform serial neurologic assessment to detect spinal cord ischemia, and provide immediate treatment (Fig. 28.9). A consensus decision should be made between the surgeons, anesthesiologists, and critical care team to establish a target range for the mean arterial pressure and the lumbar cerebrospinal fluid pressure at the time that care is transferred. Typically, the mean arterial pressure is maintained between 85 mm Hg to 95 mm Hg and the lumbar cerebrospinal fluid pressure is kept at 10 mm Hg. The admission orders should include serial neurologic assess-

Fig. 28.9 Clinical algorithm that can be used for the prevention and treatment of spinal cord ischemia in patients undergoing open or endovascular thoracic or thoracoabdominal aneurysm repair

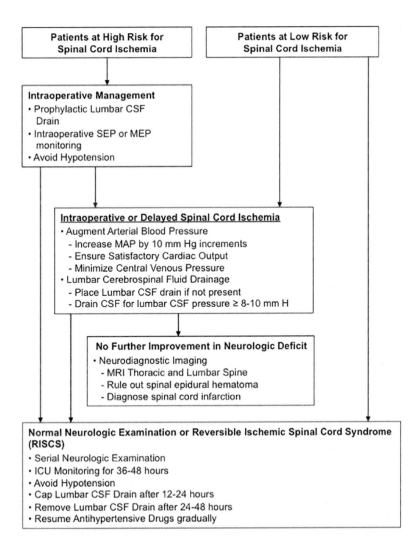

ments of lower extremity strength to be performed on an hourly basis together with instructions on the physician to be notified in the event that lower extremity weakness is detected.

Successes reported in the treatment of delayed postoperative spinal cord ischemia may be attributed to early diagnosis and immediate interventions to increase spinal cord perfusion [17, 18, 26, 56, 57, 60, 62]. One clinical series reported no recovery from spinal cord ischemia when treatment was delayed by 27 or 32 h [57]. Another clinical series reported that patients with spinal cord ischemia treated by lumbar cerebrospinal fluid drainage had full or partial recovery when treatment was initiated within 10 hours but those treated at an average of 19 h after onset had no recovery [62]. For these reasons, treatment should be initiated at the onset of signs or symptoms of spinal cord ischemia and treatment should not be delayed for neurodiagnostic imaging studies. Neurologic assessment of lower extremity motor function should be performed serially as soon as the patient recovers from general anesthesia and efforts should be made to permit early emergence from general anesthesia to permit neurologic assessment. For TEVAR, neurologic examination can be performed immediately after operation upon emergence from general anesthesia. Although epidural anesthesia or analgesia can be used for postoperative pain management in patients undergoing TEVAR or TAAA repairs, it is important to distinguish the effects of central neuroaxial blockade by local anesthetics from spinal cord ischemia. For this reason, it is justified to avoid the use of regional anesthesia or analgesia with local anesthetics until the patient demonstrates normal neurologic function. Any neurologic deficit detected should be considered to be spinal cord ischemia until disproved. Because autonomic dysfunction may be associated with spinal cord ischemia, unexplained hypotension may be an early sign of spinal cord ischemia [26, 56].

The treatment of delayed onset spinal cord ischemia in the postoperative period is directed towards increasing spinal cord perfusion pressure by augmenting the arterial pressure and decreasing the lumbar cerebrospinal fluid pressure.

Clinical algorithms have recommended increasing the arterial pressure serially by increments of 5–10 mm Hg by the administration of vasopressor agents, emergent placement of a lumbar cerebrospinal fluid drainage catheter if the patient does not have one in place, and drainage of lumbar cerebrospinal fluid to achieve a lumbar cerebrospinal fluid pressure of 10 mm Hg (Fig. 28.9) [1, 26, 58]. Reports of full or partial recovery from delayed postoperative paraplegia after TEVAR or TAAA repair support the effectiveness of interventions directed at improving spinal cord perfusion for the treatment of spinal cord ischemia [17, 18, 26, 56, 57, 60, 62, 68]. In addition, postoperative events such as hypotension, heart failure, hemorrhage, or increased cerebrospinal fluid pressure that decrease spinal cord perfusion may also increase the risk of paraplegia after TEVAR or TAAA repair. For these reasons, maintaining spinal cord perfusion by augmenting arterial blood pressure and augmenting cardiac output, together with preventing hypotension, reducing CSF pressure, and reducing central venous pressure is important for the prevention and treatment of spinal cord ischemia. Furthermore, antihypertensive agents should be resumed gradually and cautiously in patients with hypertension who are at risk for spinal cord ischemia after TEVAR or TAAA repair.

Safety Considerations for Lumbar Cerebrospinal Fluid Drainage

Considering the severity of spinal cord ischemia and the potential for paraplegia, prophylactic lumbar cerebrospinal fluid drainage can often be justified in patients at risk for spinal cord ischemia. Because lumbar cerebrospinal fluid drainage has inherent risks, it is important to recognize potential complications of lumbar cerebrospinal fluid drainage to maximize its benefit (Table 28.5). The most important complication associated with lumbar cerebrospinal drainage is subdural hematoma that is caused by injury and bleeding from bridging dural veins as a consequence of intracranial hypotension from cerebrospinal fluid removal (Fig. 28.10 subdural hematoma).

Table 28.5 Complications of lumbar cerebrospinal fluid drainage and strategies to minimize the complications of lumbar cerebrospinal fluid drainage

Complication	Techniques to minimize risk
Epidural Hematoma	Normalize coagulation function at the time of lumbar catheter placement and removal. Avoid anticoagulation therapy or antiplatelet therapy while lumbar cerebrospinal fluid drain is in place.
Catheter Fracture	Catheter placement and removal only by experienced personnel.
Subdural hematoma Post-lumbar puncture headache Cerebellar Hemorrhage Abducens Nerve Palsy	Maintain lumbar CSF pressure greater than 8 mm Hg to 10 mm Hg during CSF drainage. Monitor and limit volume of CSF drainage per hour. Cap lumbar CSF catheter for 12–24 h prior to removal.
Infection Cerebrospinal Fluid Leak	Maintain closed CSF collection system. Minimize duration of CSF drainage. Remove CSF catheter when not in use.

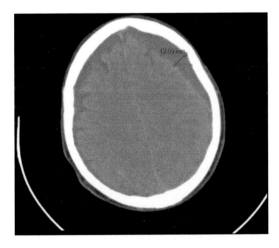

Fig. 28.10 Computed tomographic (CT) scan of the head without contrast demonstrating bilateral subdural hematomas in the frontoparietal regions in a patient with confusion and refractory nausea after removal of a lumbar cerebrospinal fluid drainage catheter placed for thoracic endovascular aortic repair. Subdural hematomas appear on the CT scan as extra-axial, crescent-shaped collections adjacent to the cerebral cortex that may produce a mass effect causing sulcal effacement or midline shift

The risk of subdural hematoma was identified in a retrospective study that found an incidence of 3.5% among 230 patients who had lumbar cere-brospinal fluid drains placed for thoracoabdominal aortic aneurysm repairs [69]. In the clinical series, lumbar cerebrospinal fluid drainage was set to drain for a pressure greater than 5 cm H_2O (3.7 mm Hg), the volume of cerebrospinal fluid drained was a risk factor for subdural hematoma, and the mortality rate among the patients with subdural hematoma was 50%. The incidence of subdural hematoma as a complication of lumbar cerebrospinal fluid drainage in three large contemporary retrospective clinical series ranged from 0.45% to 2.0% [70–72]. Signs and symptoms associated with subdural hematoma are often nonspecific but have reported to include blood in the cerebrospinal fluid, coma, drowsiness, ataxia, headache, nausea, and hemiparesis. There are also several reports of intracerebellar hemorrhage caused by intracranial hypotension as a complication of lumbar cerebrospinal fluid drainage [72–74]. Computed tomographic scan of the head should be performed to check for the presence of subdural hematoma or intracranial hemorrhage in patients with altered mentation or non-focal neurologic deficits undergoing lumbar cerebrospinal fluid drainage. Clinical protocols to continuously monitor the lumbar cerebrospinal fluid pressure, limit the volume of cerebrospinal fluid drained per hour, and to allow the lumbar cerebrospinal fluid pressure to return to normal before removing the drainage catheter may limit the risk of subdural hematoma [1, 69, 70, 72, 75].

Less common complications associated of lumbar cerebrospinal fluid drainage include catheter fracture, cerebrospinal fluid leak, post-dural puncture headache, abducens nerve palsy, and meningitis [70, 72, 75]. Supervised catheter removal by qualified individuals familiar with the material characteristics of the catheters may decrease the risk of catheter fracture. Some patients with catheter fracture required laminectomy for removal of the catheter fragment [70, 72, 75]. The risk of meningitis can be minimized by maintaining a closed system to monitor, drain, and collect the cerebrospinal fluid within a reservoir and to remove the drainage catheter as soon as it is no longer being used [75]. Both conservative management and epidural blood patch has been reported for the treatment of persistent cerebrospinal fluid leakage or postdural puncture headache [72]. Spinal, epidural, or neuraxial hematoma and even direct spinal cord injury complicating lumbar cerebrospinal fluid catheter placement or removal remains an important concern, but these complications have only been reported rarely in the medical literature [76–78]. In the few reports of spinal and epidural hematoma, the complication occurred during drain removal in two of the reported cases, the condition was diagnosed by magnetic resonance imaging, and treatment included both conservative management and open surgical decompression. Systemic anticoagulation with heparin during operation does not appear to increase the risk of hemorrhagic complications of lumbar cerebrospinal fluid drainage if the catheter is inserted prior to operation and removed after coagulation function had been restored [70, 72, 75].

References

1. Etz CD, Weigang E, Hartert M, Lonn L, Mestres CA, Di Bartolomeo R, Bachet JE, Carrel TP, Grabenwoger M, Schepens MA, Czerny M. Contemporary spinal cord protection during thoracic and thoracoabdominal aortic surgery and endovascular aortic repair: a position paper of the vascular domain of the European Association for Cardio-Thoracic Surgery. Eur J Cardiothorac Surg. 2015;47:943–57.
2. Hiratzka LF, Bakris GL, Beckman JA, et al. 2010 ACCF/AHA/AATS/ACR/ASA/SCA/SCAI/SIR/STS/ SVM guidelines for the diagnosis and management of patients with Thoracic Aortic Disease. Circulation. 2010;121:e266–369.
3. Svensson LG, Klepp P, Hinder RA. Spinal cord anatomy of the baboon--comparison with man and implications for spinal cord blood flow during thoracic aortic cross-clamping. S Afr J Surg. 1986; 24:32–4.
4. Sliwa JA, Maclean IC. Ischemic myelopathy: a review of spinal vasculature and related clinical syndromes. Arch Phys Med Rehabil. 1992;73:365–72.
5. Shamji MF, Maziak DE, Shamji FM, Ginsberg RJ, Pon R. Circulation of the spinal cord: an important consideration for thoracic surgeons. Ann Thorac Surg. 2003;76:315–21.
6. Gharagozloo F, Larson J, Dausmann MJ, Neville RF Jr, Gomes MN. Spinal cord protection during surgical procedures on the descending thoracic and thoracoabdominal aorta: review of current techniques. Chest. 1996;109:799–809.
7. Cheshire WP, Santos CC, Massey EW, Howard JF Jr. Spinal cord infarction: etiology and outcome. Neurology. 1996;47:321–30.
8. Dommisse GF. The blood supply of the spinal cord: a critical vascular zone in spinal surgery. J Bone Joint Surg Br. 1974;56:225–35.
9. Biglioli P, Roberto M, Cannata A, et al. Upper and lower spinal cord blood supply: the continuity of the anterior spinal artery and the relevance of the lumbar arteries. J Thorac Cardiovasc Surg. 2004;127:1188–92.
10. Boll DT, Bulow H, Blackham KA, Aschoff AJ, Schmitz BL. MDCT angiography of the spinal vasculature and the artery of Adamkiewicz. AJR Am J Roentgenol. 2006;187:1054–60.
11. Strauch JT, Lauten A, Spielvogel D, et al. Mild hypothermia protects the spinal cord from ischemic injury in a chronic porcine model. Eur J Cardiothorac Surg. 2004;25:708–15.
12. Miyairi T, Kotsuka Y, Morota T, et al. Paraplegia after open surgery using endovascular stent graft for aortic arch aneurysm. J Thorac Cardiovasc Surg. 2001;122:1240–3.
13. Gillilan LA. Veins of the spinal cord: anatomic details; suggested clinical applications. Neurology. 1970;20:860–8.
14. Ullery BW, Cheung AT, Fairman RM, et al. Risk factors, outcomes, and clinical manifestations of spinal cord ischemia following thoracic endovascular aortic repair. J Vasc Surg. 2011;54:677–84.
15. Scali ST, Wang SK, Feezor RJ, Huber TS, Martin TD, Klodell CT, Beaver TM, Beck AW. Preoperative prediction of spinal cord ischemia after thoracic endovascular aortic repair. J Vasc Surg. 2014;60:1481–90.
16. O'Callaghan A, Mastracci TM, Eagleton MJ. Staged endovascular repair of thoracoabdominal aortic aneurysms limits incidence and severity of spinal cord ischemia. J Vasc Surg. 2015;61:347–54.
17. Maurel B, Delclaux N, Sobocinski J, Hertault A, Martin-Gonzalez T, Moussa M, Spear R, Le Roux M, Azzaoui R, Tyrrell M, Haulon S. The impact of early pelvic and lower limb reperfusion and attentive peri-operative management on the incidence of spinal cord ischemia during thoracoabdominal aortic aneurysm endovascular repair. Eur J Vasc Endovasc Surg. 2015;49:248–54.
18. Dias NV, Sonesson B, Kristmundsson T, Holm H, Resch T. Short-term outcome of spinal cord ischemia after endovascular repair of thoracoabdominal aortic aneurysms. Eur J Vasc Endovasc Surg. 2015;49:403–9.
19. Bisdas T, Panuccio G, Sugimoto M, Torsello G, Austermann M. Risk factors for spinal cord ischemia after endovascular repair of thoracoabdominal aortic aneurysms. J Vasc Surg. 2015;61:1408–16.
20. Greenberg RK, Lu Q, Roselli EE, Svensson LG, et al. Contemporary analysis of descending thoracic and thoracoabdominal aneurysm repair. A comparison of endovascular and open techniques. Circulation. 2008;118:808–17.

21. Svensson LG, Crawford ES, Hess KR, Coselli JS, Safi HJ. Experience with 1509 patients undergoing thoracoabdominal aortic operations. J Vascul Surg. 1993;17:357–68.
22. Coselli JS, Bozinovski J, LeMaire SA. Open surgical repair of 2286 thoracoabdominal aortic aneurysms. Ann Thorac Surg. 2007;83:S862–4.
23. Bavaria JE, Appoo JJ, Makaroun MS, Verter J, Yu ZF, Mitchell RS, Gore TAG Investigators. Endovascular stent grafting versus open surgical repair of descending thoracic aortic aneurysms in low-risk patients: a multicenter comparative trial. J Thorac Cardiovasc Surg. 2007;133:369–77.
24. Buth J, Harris PL, Hobo R, et al. Neurologic complications associated with endovascular repair of thoracic aortic pathology: incidence and risk factors. A study from the European Collaborators on Stent/Graft Techniques for Aortic Aneurysm Repair (EUROSTAR) registry. J Vasc Surg. 2007;46:1103–10.
25. Feezor RJ, Martin TD, Hess PJ Jr, et al. Extent of aortic coverage and incidence of spinal cord ischemia after thoracic endovascular aneurysm repair. Ann Thorac Surg. 2008;86:1809–14.
26. Cheung AT, Pochettino A, McGarvey ML, et al. Strategies to manage paraplegia risk after endovascular stent repair of descending thoracic aortic aneurysms. Ann Thorac Surg. 2005;80:1280–8. discussion 1288–1289
27. Gravereaux EC, Faries PL, Burks JA, et al. Risk of spinal cord ischemia after endograft repair of thoracic aortic aneurysms. J Vasc Surg. 2001;34:997–1003.
28. Martin DJ, Martin TD, Hess PJ, Daniels MJ, Feezor RJ, Lee WA. Spinal cord ischemia after TEVAR in patients with abdominal aortic aneurysms. J Vasc Surg. 2009;49:302–6.
29. Schlosser FJ, Verhagen HJ, Lin PH, et al. TEVAR following prior abdominal aortic aneurysm surgery: increased risk of neurological deficit. J Vasc Surg. 2009;49:308–14.
30. Baril DT, Carroccio A, Ellozy SH, et al. Endovascular thoracic aortic repair and previous or concomitant abdominal aortic repair: is the increased risk of spinal cord ischemia real? Ann Vasc Surg. 2006;20:188–94.
31. Khoynezhad A, Donayre CE, Bui H, Kopchok GE, Walot I, White RA. Risk factors of neurologic deficit after thoracic aortic endografting. Ann Thorac Surg. 2007;83:S882–9.
32. Weigang E, Hartert M, Siegenthaler MP, et al. Perioperative management to improve neurologic outcome in thoracic or thoracoabdominal aortic stent-grafting. Ann Thorac Surg. 2006;82:1679–87.
33. Chiesa R, Melissano G, Marrocco-Trischitta MM, Civilini E, Setacci F. Spinal cord ischemia after elective stent-graft repair of the thoracic aorta. J Vasc Surg. 2005;42:11–7.
34. Crawford ES, Svensson LG, Hess KR, et al. A prospective randomized study of cerebrospinal fluid drainage to prevent paraplegia after high-risk surgery on the thoracoabdominal aorta. J Vasc Surg. 1991;13:36–45.
35. Estrera AL, Miller CC III, Huynh TT, et al. Preoperative and operative predictors of delayed neurologic deficit following repair of thoracoabdominal aortic aneurysm. J Thorac Cardiovasc Surg. 2003;126:1288–94.
36. International Standards for Neurological Classification of Spinal Cord Injury. Available at: http://asia-spinalinjury.org/wp content/uploads/2016/02/International_Stds_Diagram_Worksheet.pdf. Accessed on Dec 6, 2017.
37. Doss M, Balzer J, Martens S, et al. Emergent endovascular stent grafting for perforated acute type B dissections and ruptured thoracic aortic aneurysms. Ann Thorac Surg. 2003;76:493–8. discussion 497–498
38. Estrera AL, Sheinbaum R, Miller CC, et al. Cerebrospinal fluid drainage during thoracic aortic repair: safety and current management. Ann Thorac Surg. 2009;88:9–15.
39. Tiesenhausen K, Hessinger M, Tomka M, Portugaller H, Swanidze S, Oberwalder P. Endovascular treatment of mycotic aortic pseudoaneurysms with stent-grafts. Cardiovasc Intervent Radiol. 2008;31:509–13.
40. Wong DR, Coselli JS, Amerman K, Bozinovski J, Carter SA, Vaughn WK, LeMaire SA. Delayed spinal cord deficits after thoracoabdominal aortic aneurysm repair. Ann Thorac Surg. 2007;83:1345–55.
41. Eagleton MJ, Shah S, Petkosevek D, Mastracci TM, Greenberg RK. Hypogastric and subclavian artery patency affects onset and recovery of spinal cord ischemia associated with aortic endografting. J Vasc Surg. 2014;59:89–94.
42. Heller LB, Chaney MA. Paraplegia immediately following removal of a cerebrospinal fluid drainage catheter in a patient after thoracoabdominal aortic aneurysm surgery. Anesthesiology. 2001;95:1285–7.
43. Kasirajan K, Dolmatch B, Ouriel K, Clair D. Delayed onset of ascending paralysis after thoracic aortic stent graft deployment. J Vasc Surg. 2000;31:196–9.
44. Crawford ES. Thoraco-abdominal and abdominal aortic aneurysms involving renal, superior mesenteric, celiac arteries. Ann Surg. 1974;179:763–72.
45. Bicknell CD, Riga CV, Wolfe JH. Prevention of paraplegia during thoracoabdominal aortic aneurysm repair. Eur J Vasc Endovasc Surg. 2009;37:654–60.
46. Read RA, Moore EE, Moore FA, Haenel JB. Partial left heart bypass for thoracic aorta repair. Survival without paraplegia. Arch Surg. 1993;128:746–50.
47. Donahoo JS, Brawley RK, Gott VL. The heparin-coated vascular shunt for thoracic aortic and great vessel procedures: a ten-year experience. Ann Thorac Surg. 1977;23:507–13.
48. Griepp RB, Stinson EB, Hollingsworth JF, et al. Prosthetic replacement of the aortic arch. J Thorac Cardiovasc Surg. 1975;70:1051–63.
49. Kouchoukos NT, Masetti P, Murphy SF. Hypothermic cardiopulmonary bypass and circulatory arrest in the management of extensive thoracic and thoracoabdominal aortic aneurysms. Semin Thorac Cardiovasc Surg. 2003;15:333–9.

50. Davison JK, Cambria RP, Vierra DJ, et al. Epidural cooling for regional spinal cord hypothermia during thoracoabdominal aneurysm repair. J Vasc Surg. 1994;20:304–10.

51. Acher CW, Wynn MM, Hoch JR, et al. Combined use of cerebral spinal fluid drainage and naloxone reduces the risk of paraplegia in thoracoabdominal aneurysm repair. J Vasc Surg. 1994;19:236–46.

52. Svensson LG, Hess KR, D'Agostino RS, et al. Reduction of neurologic injury after high-risk thoracoabdominal aortic operation. Ann Thorac Surg. 1998;66:132–8.

53. Woo EY, Bavaria JE, Pochettino A, et al. Techniques for preserving vertebral artery perfusion during thoracic aortic stent grafting requiring aortic arch landing. Vasc Endovasc Surg. 2006;40:367–73.

54. Cina CS, Abouzahr L, Arena GO, et al. Cerebrospinal fluid drainage to prevent paraplegia during thoracic and thoracoabdominal aortic aneurysm surgery: a systematic review and meta-analysis. J Vasc Surg. 2004;40:36–44.

55. Khan SN, Stansby G. Cerebrospinal fluid drainage for thoracic and thoracoabdominal aortic aneurysm surgery. Cochrane Database Syst Rev. 2004:CD003635.

56. Cheung AT, Weiss SJ, McGarvey ML, et al. Interventions for reversing delayed-onset postoperative paraplegia after thoracic aortic reconstruction. Ann Thorac Surg. 2002;74:413–9.

57. Ackerman LL, Traynelis VC. Treatment of delayed-onset neurological deficit after aortic surgery with lumbar cerebrospinal fluid drainage. Neurosurgery. 2002;51:1414–21.

58. Sinha AC, Cheung AT. Spinal cord protection and thoracic aortic surgery. Curr Opin Anaesthesiol. 2010;23:95–102.

59. Etz CD, Zoli S, Bischoff MS, et al. Measuring the collateral network pressure to minimize paraplegia risk in thoracoabdominal aneurysm resection. J Thorac Cardiovasc Surg. 2010;140:S125–30.

60. Chiesa R, Melissano G, Marrocco-Trischitta MM, Civilini E, Setacci F. Spinal cord ischemia after elective stent-graft repair of the thoracic aorta. J Vasc Surg. 2005;42:11–7.

61. Maniar HS, Sundt TM III, Prasad SM, et al. Delayed paraplegia after thoracic and thoracoabdominal aneurysm repair: a continuing risk. Ann Thorac Surg. 2003;75:113–9.

62. Keith CJ, Passman MA, Carignan MJ, et al. Protocol implementation of selective postoperative lumbar spinal drainage after thoracic aortic endograft. J Vasc Surg. 2012;55:1–9.

63. Guerit JM, Witdoeckt C, Verhelst R, et al. Sensitivity, specificity, and surgical impact of somatosensory evoked potentials in descending aorta surgery. Ann Thorac Surg. 1999;67:1943–6.

64. Jacobs MJ, Elenbaas TW, Schurink GW, et al. Assessment of spinal cord integrity during thoracoab-

dominal aortic aneurysm repair. Ann Thorac Surg. 2002;74:S1864–6.

65. Husain AM, Swaminathan M, McCann RL, Hughes GC. Neurophysiologic intraoperative monitoring during endovascular stent graft repair of the descending thoracic aorta. J Clin Neurophysiol. 2007;24:328.

66. Shine TS, Harrison BA, De Ruyter ML, et al. Motor and somatosensory evoked potentials: their role in predicting spinal cord ischemia in patients undergoing thoracoabdominal aortic aneurysm repair with regional lumbar epidural cooling. Anesthesiology. 2008;108:580–7.

67. Etz CD, Zoli S, Mueller CS, et al. Staged repair significantly reduces paraplegia rate after extensive thoracoabdominal aortic aneurysm repair. J Thor Cardiovasc Surg. 2010;139:1464.

68. Safi HJ, Miller CC III, Azizzadeh A, Iliopoulos DC. Observations on delayed neurologic deficit after thoracoabdominal aortic aneurysm repair. J Vasc Surg. 1997;26:616–22.

69. Dardik A, Perler BA, Roseborough GS, Williams GM. Subdural hematoma after thoracoabdominal aortic aneurysm repair: an underreported complication of spinal fluid drainage? J Vasc Surg. 2002;36:47–50.

70. Youngblood SC, Tolpin DA, LeMaire SA, Coselli JS, Lee VV, Cooper JR Jr. Complications of cerebrospinal fluid drainage after thoracic aortic surgery: a review of 504 patients over 5 years. J Thorac Cardiovasc Surg. 2013;146:166–71.

71. Wynn MM, Mell MW, Tefera G, Hoch JR, Acher CW. Complications of spinal fluid drainage in thoracoabdominal aortic aneurysm repair: a report of 486 patients treated from 1987 to 2008. J Vasc Surg. 2009;49:29–34.

72. Estrera AL, Sheinbaum R, Miller CC, Azizzadeh A, Walkes JC, Lee TY, Kaiser L, Safi HJ. Cerebrospinal fluid drainage during thoracic aortic repair: safety and current management. Ann Thorac Surg. 2009;88:9–15.

73. Leyvi G, Ramachandran S, Wasnick JD, Plestis K, Cheung AT, Drenger B. Case 3--2005 risk and benefits of cerebrospinal fluid drainage during thoracoabdominal aortic aneurysm surgery. J Cardiothorac Vasc Anesth. 2005;19:392–9.

74. Settepani F, van Dongen EP, Schepens MA, Morshuis WJ. Intracerebellar hematoma following thoracoabdominal aortic repair: an unreported complication of cerebrospinal fluid drainage. Eur J Cardiothorac Surg. 2003;24:659–61.

75. Cheung AT, Pochettino A, Guvakov DV, et al. Safety of lumbar drains in thoracic aortic operations performed with extracorporeal circulation. Ann Thorac Surg. 2003;76:1190–6.

76. Mehmedagic I, Resch T, Acosta S. Complications to cerebrospinal fluid drainage and predictors of spinal cord ischemia in patients with aortic disease undergoing advanced endovascular therapy. Vasc Endovasc Surg. 2013;47:415–22.

77. Murakami H, Yoshida K, Hino Y, Matsuda H, Tsukube T, Okita Y. Complications of cerebrospinal fluid drainage in thoracoabdominal aortic aneurysm repair. J Vasc Surg. 2004;39:243–5.

78. Weaver KD, Wiseman DB, Farber M, Ewend MG, Marston W, Keagy BA. Complications of lumbar drainage after thoracoabdominal aortic aneurysm repair. J Vasc Surg. 2001;34:623–7.

Neuromonitoring During Cardiac Surgery

29

Choy Lewis, Suraj D. Parulkar, John Bebawy, and Charles W. Hogue

Main Messages

1. While specific, the routine use of electroencephalography (EEG) for monitoring for cerebral ischemia is limited by its low sensitivity, technical complexity, and influence by many confounding factors.
2. Somatosensory evoked potentials (SSEP) can detect derangements (e.g. physiological, surgical) to the dorsal ascending sensory nervous system, including the sensory cortex.
3. Motor evoked potentials (MEP) are used to detect ischemia or injury to the prefrontal motor cortex and ventral descending motor tracts.
4. Transcranial Doppler (TCD) monitoring can provide important information during surgery confirming bilateral cerebral perfusion and for detection of cerebral embolization, its use, though, is limited due to its susceptibility to motion and electrical artifact; further, insonation of the middle cerebral artery is not possible in over 10% of patients.
5. The adequacy of cerebral oxygen supply in relation to metabolic oxygen demand can be monitored using jugular bulb venous oxygen saturation; widespread use of this technique requires special expertise and the need for confirmation of correct placement usually radiographically—extra-cranial venous contamination can further confound interpretation of the data.
6. Near Infra-red spectroscopy (NIRS) monitoring of $rScO_2$ provides a continuous measure of the adequacy of cerebral oxygen delivery for meeting cerebral O_2 metabolic demand.
7. Prospective, multicenter studies have noted that the frequency of $rScO_2$ desaturations during CPB occur in 60% to 70% of patients depending on definitions.
8. While interventions widely used to reverse regional cerebral oxygen saturation ($rScO_2$) desaturations (e.g. ↑ MAP, ↑F_1O_2, normalizing CPB flow and $PaCO_2$, etc.) are effective, the clinical benefit on patient complications including neurological complications is not yet clearly define.
9. Clinical monitoring of cerebral blood flow autoregulation is now possible using TCD based CBF velocity measurement in conjunction with MAP.

C. Lewis · S. D. Parulkar · J. Bebawy · C. W. Hogue (✉)
Department of Anesthesiology, Northwestern
University Feinberg School of Medicine,
Chicago, IL, USA
e-mail: charles.hogue@northwestern.edu

© Springer Nature Switzerland AG 2021
D. C. H. Cheng et al. (eds.), *Evidence-Based Practice in Perioperative Cardiac Anesthesia and Surgery*, https://doi.org/10.1007/978-3-030-47887-2_29

10. Laboratory and clinical investigations have validated rScO$_2$ as an acceptable surrogate of CBF for bed-side autoregulation monitoring.
11. A growing body of clinical data have shown that deviations of MAP outside the autoregulation limits is associated with patient complications suggesting that basing patient blood pressure management on this physiologic endpoint may have potential for ensuring organ perfusion during surgery.

Neurological complications after cardiac surgery are an important source of patient morbidity, mortality, and altered quality of life that contribute well over $2 billion dollars annually to the cost of care of patients in the US [1]. These complications represent a spectrum of disorders that include clinical stroke, postoperative delirium, and postoperative cognitive dysfunction (POCD). The frequency of all neurological complications varies depending on the patient risk profile, the type of procedure, and importantly, the thoroughness of patient examination. Clinical stroke occurs in roughly 2% of patients after coronary artery bypass graft surgery, but studies that employ sensitive brain MR imaging report clinically asymptomatic acute ischemic injury in up to 50% of patients [1]. Moreover, the frequency of delirium after cardiac surgery varies between ~10% to 50% depending on whether detailed examination is performed by trained individuals using validated instruments such as the confusion assessment method or confusion assessment method for patients in the ICU [2]. Cerebral embolization has largely been embraced as the primary cause of brain injury, the realization that cerebral hypoperfusion is an important source brain injury during cardiac surgery has strengthened the case of neuromonitoring during cardiac surgery [1].

In this chapter we will provide an overview of approaches to central nervous system monitoring during cardiac and major vascular surgery. This will include discussions of the electroencephalography (EEG), somatosensory evoked potentials (SSEP), motor evoked potentials (MEP), transcranial Doppler (TCD) monitoring, and monitors of cerebral oxygenation balance. The use of TCD or processed near infra-red spectroscopy (NIRS), for monitoring cerebral autoregulation will be further reviewed.

Electroencephalography

Monitoring of the EEG entails the acquisition of cortical electrical signals from scalp electrodes which are placed in standardized locations per the "10–20 system". These electrical signals represent micro-voltages which occur at various frequencies and originate from postsynaptic pyramidal neurons in the cerebral cortices. Voltage frequencies are classically divided into particular bandwidths listed in Table 29.1. At any given brain state, given the anesthetic and cerebral milieu present, these waves can and do overlap, and Fourier transformation is needed to parse out the individual components which exist.

Reduced cerebral oxygen supply in relation to cerebral oxygen metabolic demand results in a shift in the EEG to slower theta and delta frequencies. Such acute EEG changes are specific for cerebral ischemia. The sensitivity of EEG monitoring for cerebral ischemia, though, is confounded by several factors including ischemia occurring in non-monitored brain areas including deeper brain areas. Other confounding variables that can affect the EEG limiting its utility for detecting cerebral ischemia include hypothermia, anesthetics, electromyographic artifact, and interference from electro-cautery or the CPB pump itself. Moreover, the EEG only monitors the superficial layers of the cerebral cortex.

Table 29.1 Electroencephalographic bands and frequencies

Band	Frequency (Hz)
Gamma	26–80
Beta	13–25
Alpha	9–12
Theta	5–8
Delta	1–4
Slow-wave	<1

Processed EEG

While monitoring of the raw EEG is not routine in most cardiac centers, monitoring of the processed EEG (pEEG) such as the bispectral index monitor (BIS, Medtronic, Inc., Minneapolis, MN, USA), the SEDline (PSI, Masimo Corporation, Irvine, CA USA), Narcotrend Monitor (MonitorTechnik, Bad Bramstedt, Germany), E-Entropy (GE Healthcare, Chicago, IL), NeuroSENSE (NeuroWave systems, Inc., Cleveland, OH), is more common. Each has its own proprietary algorithm. BIS was initially proposed as a monitor of depth of hypnosis, with the potential to ensure amnesia during general anesthesia of great clinical interest. Several studies have assessed the use of BIS in predicting or preventing awareness under general anesthesia [3–5]. For the most part, these studies have shown potential benefit of BIS monitoring for prevention of intraoperative awareness compared with standard care that does not include special monitoring. In contrast, there appears to be no value in BIS monitoring for this purpose compared with titration of volatile anesthetics based on end-tidal agent concentrations monitoring. There may be some benefit of BIS monitoring to ensure amnesia if TIVA is used.

Other data have suggested that BIS monitoring may decrease anesthetic dose and ensure more rapid recovery although a benefit in cardiac surgical patients is not clearly established [6]. Randomized studies support that titrating seda-tion or anesthetic depth based on BIS monitoring reduces the frequency and/or severity of postoperative delirium. A systematic review and meta-analysis from the Cochrane group supported the use of the use of BIS-guided anesthetic titration for reducing the incidence of postoperative delirium compared with usual care but the quality of evidence was viewed as moderate [7].

Somatosensory Evoked Potential

SSEPs represent a neuromonitoring modality which can detect derangements (e.g. physiological, surgical) to the dorsal ascending sensory nervous system, including the sensory cortex. Technically, SSEPs are performed by stimulation of a mixed peripheral nerve, usually the median or ulnar nerve in the upper extremity or the posterior tibial nerve in the lower extremity, and subsequent recording of the response to that stimulation at Erb's point (near the clavicle), the subcortex (at the inion of the skull), or the contralateral somatosensory cortex. Anesthetics have a profound effect on these low-voltage potentials at the cortical level, and the anesthetic regimen must be clearly delineated, and its effects understood. Because these signals are small in amplitude (median voltage, 1 μvolt), they require signal averaging over a period of time (minutes) and filtration (to reduce EEG, EMG, and ECG contamination) (Fig. 29.1).

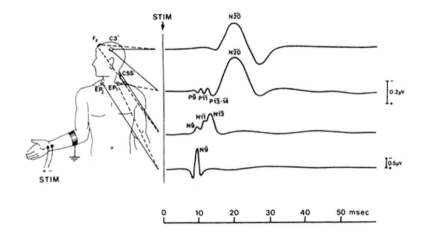

Fig. 29.1 Somatosensory evoked potentials originating from the right median nerve and recorded (in ascending order) at Erb's point on the right, the subcortex at the inion, and the left somatosensory cortex. The x-axis represents latency time (msec) while the y-axis represents voltage amplitude (μVolts) of the potentials

The utility of SSEPs in cardiac surgery is primarily in detecting dysfunction (related to hypoperfusion or embolic-related ischemia) in the somatosensory cortex. SSEPs have been used especially in cases of aortic arch or hemi-arch replacement, where adequate perfusion to the cortex via the carotid arteries is of significant concern. EEG is also used frequently in this setting, and is usually the preferred method of detecting cerebral ischemia, because signal acquisition is faster and more sensitive than that which can be achieved with SSEPs. SSEPs have been used extensively in thoracic and thoracoabdominal aortic surgery as well and have been shown to correlate well with the development of spinal cord ischemia and permanent paralysis when signals are lost [8]. In this clinical context, preservation or return of diminished or absent SSEPs, either by surgical or anesthetic modification, seems to be a positive prognostic indicator for intact spinal cord function and the avoidance of paraplegia at the end of surgery. In this regard, the specificity of SSEP changes is high, approaching 90% in most studies, while the sensitivity seems to be lower (approaching 50%).

Motor Evoked Potential

MEPs have been increasingly utilized over the last two decades, and have gained some popularity in cardiac surgery as well, owing to certain advantages which they possess over the neuromonitoring modalities listed above. MEPs originate from a high voltage (100–500 V) stimulation produced at the cortex (usually transcranially via cathode and anode scalp electrodes) and are recorded in major peripheral muscle groups by quantification of what is known as a compound muscle action potential (CMAP). Unlike SSEPs, these signals are usually robust in amplitude, do not require signal averaging or filtration, and are easily and quickly obtainable (Fig. 29.2).

Whereas SSEPs detect disruption to the ascending dorsal sensory tracts and sensory cor-

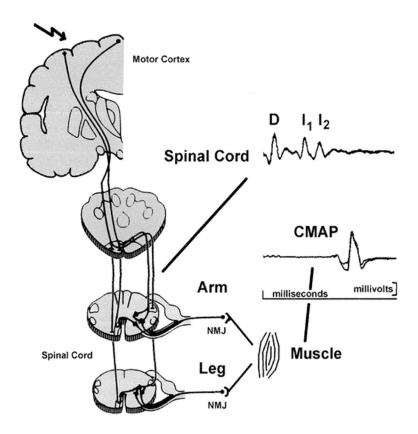

Fig. 29.2 Motor evoked potentials originating from the right motor cortex and recorded from the left hand and foot. The x-axis represents latency time (msec) while the y-axis represents voltage amplitude (μVolts) of the potentials. As shown, motor evoked potentials are elicited only on the contralateral extremities (ipsilateral extremities unaffected)

tex, MEPs are used to detect ischemia or injury to the prefrontal motor cortex and ventral descending motor tracts. Similar to SSEPs, MEPs are exquisitely sensitive to the anesthetic regimen being used, and the avoidance of nondepolarizing neuromuscular blocking agents and elevated concentrations of potent inhaled anesthetics is warranted.

The usefulness of MEPs in cardiac surgery, similar to SSEPs, is in detecting real or impending ischemia to the motor cortex. Their utility in thoracic aortic and aortic arch surgery has been established as well. Similar to SSEPs, MEPs have been studied extensively in thoracoabdominal aortic surgery, with proven benefit in predicting neurologic injury due to spinal cord ischemia [9]. There is evidence to suggest that monitoring of MEPs during thoracic and thoracoabdominal aneurysm repair is of value in predicting the absence of paraplegia postoperatively when MEPs are maintained during surgery [10].

Transcranial Doppler

TCD monitoring of cerebral blood flow (CBF) velocity can provide important information during surgery such as confirming directional blood flow during antegrade cerebral perfusion as is used often for aortic arch surgery. Even during routine surgery, TCD monitoring can provide an early warning of reduced CBF due to arterial cannula malposition or aortic dissection. The early detection of these potentially catastrophic events may allow for corrective surgical interventions preventing cerebral ischemic injury. Monitoring of middle cerebral artery with TCD has been advocated as a means for detecting cerebral embolization manifest as high-intensity signals ("HITS"). A sudden increase in HITS can alert clinicians to search for a source of embolization including entrained air.

Despite the above potential utility, TCD monitoring has several limitations. First, this type of monitoring requires specialized skills. Further, in up to 10% to 15% of patients, a trans-temporal insonating window of the middle cerebral artery is not present. Other limitations of TCD monitor-

ing include its susceptibility to motion and electrical artifact. The former often requires frequent repositioning of the TCD probe. Regardless, a recent systematic review concluded that TCD has limited use for reducing postoperative cognitive dysfunction due to microembolization [11]. Guidelines for monitoring during cardiovascular surgery lists TCD as a class III indication for detecting cerebral embolization or hypoperfusion [12].

Regional Cerebral Oxygen Saturation

In the past, measurement of jugular bulb venous oxygen saturation (SjvO$_2$) was the only clinical tool available for monitoring the adequacy of cerebral oxygen balance. This method has several limitations including technical challenges associated with placement of an oximetric catheter retrograde via internal vein cannulation, the need to radiographically confirm its position, and extracranial contamination of venous drainage.

The clinical introduction of NIRS monitoring of regional cerebral oxygen saturation (rScO$_2$) was met with enthusiasm as it provided clinicians for the first time the ability to non-invasively and continuously assess the adequacy of cerebral oxygen delivery for meeting cerebral O$_2$ metabolic demand, This method capitalizes on the physical fact that light in the near infrared spectrum (700 to 900 nm) penetrates bone, muscle, and other tissue. The distinct peak absorption spectra of oxyhemoglobin and deoxyhemoglobin can be compared with light absorption of total hemoglobin. Thus, rScO$_2$ is determined as the relative concentrations of oxyhemoglobin versus total hemoglobin. This conceptually simple model, though, must acknowledge several potential sources of error including the potential reflection and scattering of light due to varying tissue interfaces and composition.

Differential NIRS is another algorithm to enhance spatial resolution of NIRS while accounting for light scatter. This approach involves placement of a sensor near the light source to account for extracranial light absorption in addition to a distal sensor [13].

Clinically, NIRS monitoring provides an assessment of the balance between cerebral oxygen supply versus demand. This is because NIRS does not include plethysmography as for pulse oximetry. Thus, light absorption occurs from arterial, capillary, and venous blood and from any chromophore. The majority of blood in the brain is venous blood. While variability exists between manufacturers, monitoring algorithms assume a fixed distribution between venous and arterial blood (~70% to 75% venous to 25% to 30% arterial). Variability in this the venous arterial blood distribution can alter the accuracy of $rScO_2$ under conditions of reduced SaO_2 and hypocapnia [14].

Several clinical studies have questioned the accuracy of subtraction algorithms for accounting for light absorption from superficial tissue in calculating $rScO_2$. Decrements in $rScO_2$ correlated with ipsilateral reduction in TCD cerebral blood flow velocity ($r = 0.56$) but not laser Doppler flow velocity of the scalp ($r = 0.13$). There were no decrements in $rScO_2$ during cross-clamping of the ipsilateral external carotid artery except when accompanied by systemic hypotension or in the presence of extracranial-to-intracranial shunting. The sensitivity of $rScO_2$ to detect reduction in cerebral blood flow was 87.5% and specificity 100% [15].

Is there Patient Benefit from $rScO_2$ Monitoring?

Multiple investigations have reported a benefit for patient outcome with the use of NIRS monitoring during cardiac surgery. In a systematic review, several small uncontrolled observational studies suggest that NIRS monitoring could provide the detection of CPB cannula malposition in a time frame that would allow for early correction. Others have suggested that the use of $rScO_2$ monitoring during surgery reduce the risk of stroke. Six of nine studies that evaluated cognitive outcomes reported that acute $rScO_2$ decrements during CPB led to cognitive impairment after surgery. These studies, though, have many limitations including the limited psychometric

testing batteries in some studies, and performing the evaluations prior to hospital discharge but not at later time points after surgery [16].

There have since been two prospective, multicenter studies evaluating the frequency of $rScO_2$ desaturations during CPB and the effectiveness of an intervention algorithm. Our group enrolled 235 patients undergoing CABG and/or valve surgery at eight US centers [17]. We observed that $rScO_2$ desaturations (>20% decrease from room air baseline) occurred in 61% of patients. Of 340 identified $rScO_2$ events, 34% resolved with usual clinical care and 66% with treatment with the intervention algorithm. In a study of 201 patients undergoing cardiac surgery at eight Canadian centers, $rScO_2$ desaturations (>10% decrement from baseline) occurred in 71 (70%) of the 102 intervention group patients and 56 (57%) of the 99 control group patients ($P = 0.04$) [18]. Reversal was successful in 69 (97%) of the intervention group patients. There were no differences in adverse events between the groups failing to confirm the earlier findings by Murkin et al. [19]

The potential benefits of $rScO_2$ monitoring during CABG and/or cardiac valvular surgery have been evaluated in several prospectively randomized controlled studies that are summarized in Table 29.2 [18–24]. These studies evaluated a variety of outcomes that included cognitive and postoperative complications.

Most of the studies that included cognitive end-points used insensitive methods that did not include detailed psychometric testing. Other issues included non-blinding of clinicians caring for the patients, poor adherence with the intervention algorithm for addressing $rScO_2$ desaturations, not continuing the $rScO_2$ intervention in the ICU early after surgery, and insufficient study sample size. Serraino and Murphy [25] recently performed a systematic review and meta-analysis testing the hypothesis that goal-directed optimization of $rScO_2$ during cardiac surgery leads to reduction in neurological complications (neurocognitive function, biomarkers), organ injury, red blood cell transfusion, mortality, or health-care costs. Of ten prospectively randomized, controlled trials of an intervention algorithm for reversing $rScO_2$ desaturations identified, only

Table 29.2 Prospectively randomized studies that have evaluated whether interventions to reverse acute decrements in regional cerebral oxygen saturation ($rScO_2$) lead to improved patient outcomes after CABG surgery

Study	Year	N	Definition of $rScO_2$ desaturation	Primary outcome	Main findings	Limitations
Murkin et al. [19]	2007	200	>30% ↓ from baseline for > 1 min	Postoperative complications	Compared with intervention group, control patients had prolonged $rScO_2$ desaturation ($p = 0.014$) and longer hospitalization in ICU ($p = 0.029$). Controls had more major organ morbidity and mortality[a] than intervention arm ($p = 0.048$)	Insufficient power to address neurological end-points or overall complications. No risk adjustments
Slater et al. [20]	2009	240	>20% ↓ from baseline	Cognitive decline	No difference in cognitive decline between groups. Prolonged $rScO_2$ desaturation associated with prolonged hospitalization and risk for cognitive decline at hospital discharge, but not at 3 months after surgery. No difference in major complications between groups	Poor adherence to intraoperative intervention for reversing $rScO_2$ desaturation. Prolonged $rScO_2$ desaturation was defined post hoc based on collected data
Mohandas et al. [21]	2013	100	Absolute value <50% or > 20% ↓ from baseline (intervention started at >15% ↓ of baseline)	>20% decline on mini-mental state exam after surgery or antisaccadic eye movement test 1 week and 3 months after surgery	Intervention group had lower frequency of cognitive impairment 1 week and 3 months after surgery	No power calculation in the study; insensitive methods for assessing cognitive function; no assessment of adherence to study protocol
Colak et al. [22]	2015	200	>20% ↓from baseline	↓ ≥ 3 points mini-mental state exam and ↓of ≥1 SD Color Trail or Grooved Peg Board Tests 7 days after surgery	Cognitive decline less in intervention than controls (28% versus 58%)	Limited psychometric testing battery; non-standard definition of cognitive decline Clinicians not blinded to $rScO_2$ data Adherence to intervention protocol not quantified
Kara et al. [23]	2015	79	>20% ↓from baseline	Cognitive function assessed with Montreal cognitive assessment test.	Intervention group had higher cognitive performance than controls	Insufficient power to exclude type I error. Insensitive method for assessing cognitive function. No specific protocol for reversing $rScO_2$ decrements

(continued)

Table 29.2 (continued)

Study	Year	N	Definition of rScO₂ desaturation	Primary outcome	Main findings	Limitations
Deschamps et al. [18]	2016	201	>10% ↓from baseline lasting >15 s	Success rate of reversing rScO₂ decrement from baseline >10% from baseline	rScO₂ desaturation load less in intervention than control group. No difference between intervention and controls in the frequency of clinical delirium, the duration of mechanical lung ventilation, ICU length of stay, and major organ morbidity or mortality[a]	Insufficient sample size for excluding benefit of intervention on postoperative complications (a secondary study aim)
Rogers et al. [24]	2017	204	Absolute value <50% or >30% ↓ from baseline	Cognitive function 3 months after surgery	No difference between intervention and controls in postoperative cognitive function. Intervention group had higher scores on verbal fluency than controls. No difference between groups in red blood cell transfusion, biomarker of brain, kidney injury, or myocardial injury, adverse events, or health-care costs	Limited blinding of health-care personnel to rScO₂ data. High rate of non-adherence with protocol (18%) in the intervention group

[a]Stroke, renal failure requiring dialysis, lung ventilation >48 h, deep sternal wound infection, reoperation, or death

two were considered at low risk for bias. Meta-analysis found that, compared with controls, optimization of rScO₂ during surgery had no effect on mortality (risk ratio [RR], 0.76, 95% confidence interval [CI], 0.30 to 1.96), major morbidity including stroke (RR, 1.08, 95% CI, 0.40 to 2.91), red cell transfusion, or health-care resource utilization. The quality of the available evidence for assessing these outcomes, though, was rated as low or very low. Further, the combined sample size of the studies assessing these outcomes ranged from 958 to 1138 patients. In the study by Deschamps et al. [18] the authors estimate that a future randomized study to assess whether rScO₂ monitoring leads to patient benefit versus the current standard of care would require 3080 patients to detect a difference in mortality, 4638 to detect difference in stroke, and 1610 to detect a difference in delirium.

Thus, the available data has shown a link between rScO₂ desaturations during surgery and adverse postoperative events. The data further supports the effectiveness of an intervention algorithm for reversing rScO₂ desaturations.

Nonetheless, whether reversal of rScO₂ desaturations leads to improved patient outcomes has not been clearly shown or refuted. The latter question of whether a monitoring device can lead to interventions that improve patient outcomes, though, is not the standard for their regulatory approval and has not been the metric for adoption of other monitors in the operating room or ICU (e.g. ECG monitoring, end-tidal CO₂ monitoring, transesophageal echocardiography, etc.). Moreover, many of the outcomes evaluated in prior investigations have multifactorial etiologies making isolating the effect of manipulation of only one variable such as rScO₂ difficult.

Cerebral Autoregulation Monitoring

Computer processing of hemodynamic data information can be used for monitoring CBF autoregulation at the patient's bedside. Several surrogates of CBF have been used for this purpose including intracranial pressure data and

TCD [26]. Early advocacy for CBF autoregulation monitoring was mostly limited to neurocritical care. In patients with traumatic brain injury, optimizing cerebral perfusion pressure based on autoregulation metrics was shown to be associated with improved patient outcomes [27].

One approach for monitoring CBF autoregulation involves the continuous calculation of a Pearson correlation coefficient between TCD measured CBF velocity and MAP using filtered signals that focus on low frequencies (0.2 s to 2 min) associated with autoregulatory vasomotor regulation. The variable mean velocity index (Mx) is generated. With intact autoregulation, Mx is near zero since there is no correlation between CBF velocity and MAP. When MAP is outside the autoregulation range, however, Mx approaches one since CBF velocity and MAP are now correlated or flow is pressure-dependent.

There are many limitations with TCD monitoring including its susceptibility to motion and electrical interference as stated earlier. In a series of laboratory and clinical investigations, our group has validated that $rScO_2$ can serve as a surrogate of CBF for clinical autoregulation monitoring [28]. The basis of this approach relies on the fact that $rScO_2$ provides an indication of the adequacy of O_2 supply versus demand and the fact that factors determining $rScO_2$ other than CBF (i.e. hemoglobin concentration, oxygen saturation, cerebral metabolic rate for O_2) are stable over short periods of time in the low, autoregulatory frequencies. Analogous to Mx, the variable COx is generated representing the correlation coefficient between cerebral perfusion pressure and $rScO_2$. When MAP is in the autoregulation range, COx thus approaches zero but when MAP is below or above the limits of autoregulation, COx approaches one as changes in CBF and MAP are correlated. An example of Mx and COx obtained during CPB in an adult patient are shown in Figs. 29.3 and 29.4.

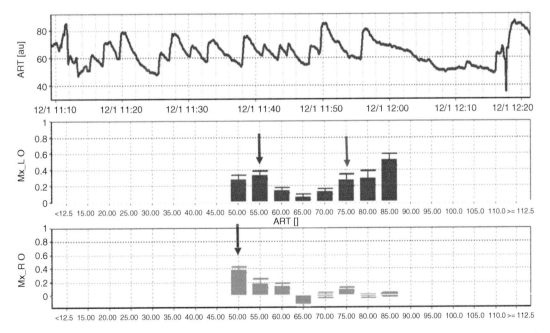

Fig. 29.3 An example of mean velocity index (Mx) derived as the correlation coefficient between transcranial Doppler measured cerebral blood flow velocity and arterial pressure during cardiopulmonary bypass. Values for Mx from the left and right middle cerebral artery measurements are displayed. The top graph is a time line series of blood pressure. Mx is averaged and placed in 5 mmHg blood pressure bins. When blood pressure is in the autoregulation range, Mx is near zero. When blood pressure is below or above the limits of autoregulation, Mx approaches 1. The red arrow represents the likely lower limit of autoregulation while the blue arrow the upper limit of autoregulation. Note that an upper limit of autoregulation is not observed in the right side and that the lower limit of autoregulation varies between the right and left side

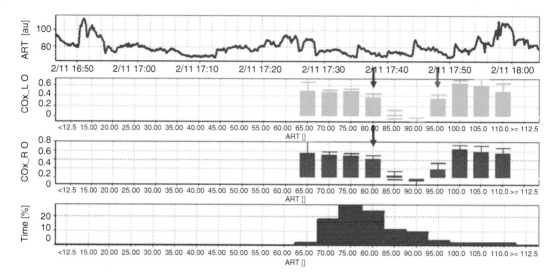

Fig. 29.4 An example of cerebral oximetry index (COx) derived as the correlation coefficient between filtered regional cerebral oximetry signals and arterial pressure during cardiopulmonary bypass. Values for COx from the left and right sides are shown. The top graph is a time line series of blood pressure. COx is averaged and placed in 5 mmHg blood pressure bins. The bottom graph is the percent of the recording at each 5 mmHg bin. When blood pressure is in the autoregulation range, COx is near zero. When blood pressure is below or above the limits of autoregulation, COx approaches one. The red arrow represents the likely lower limit of autoregulation while the blue arrow the upper limit of autoregulation. Note, this patient spent the majority of time during cardiopulmonary bypass with their blood pressure below the lower limit of autoregulation (approximately 80 mmHg)

In our on-going clinical investigations, we have observed a wide range of MAPs at the lower limit of autoregulation (LLA) during CPB (40 to 90 mmHg). The implication of this finding is that when blood pressure targets are chosen empirically, many patients have their MAP below the LLA. We have reported that this situation is associated with postoperative morbidity including acute kidney injury and major organ morbidity and mortality including stroke [29]. At the same time, we have further observed that MAP above the upper limit of autoregulation is associated with clinical delirium [30]. Thus, systematically raising MAP targets during CPB could result in cerebral hyperperfusion in some patients, increasing cerebral embolic load and possibly contributing to cerebral edema since capillary integrity may be compromised from the inflammatory response to surgery. Regardless, there is a growing body of evidence that suggests that individualizing MAP targets during CPB based on CBF autoregulation data may provide a means for reducing perioperative complications.

References

1. Hogue CW Jr, Palin CA, Arrowsmith JE. Cardiopulmonary bypass management and neurologic outcomes: an evidence-based appraisal of current practices. Anesth Analg. 2006;103:21–37.
2. Inouye SK. Delirium in older persons. N Engl J Med. 2006;354:1157–65.
3. Myles PS, Leslie K, McNeil J, et al. Bispectral index monitoring to prevent awareness during anaesthesia: the B-aware randomised controlled trial. Lancet. 2004;363:1757–63.
4. Messina AG, Wang M, Ward MJ, et al. Anaesthetic interventions for prevention of awareness during surgery. Cochrane Database Syst Rev. 2016;10:CD007272.
5. Avidan MS, Jacobsohn E, Glick D, Group B-RR, et al. Prevention of intraoperative awareness in a high-risk surgical population. N Engl J Med. 2011;365:591–600.
6. Villafranca A, Thomson IA, Grocott HP, et al. The impact of bispectral index versus end-tidal anesthetic concentration-guided anesthesia on time to tracheal extubation in fast-track cardiac surgery. Anesth Analg. 2013;116:541–8.
7. Siddiqi N, Harrison JK, Clegg A, et al. Interventions for preventing delirium in hospitalised non-ICU patients. Cochrane Database Syst Rev. 2016;3:CD005563.

8. Keyhani K, Miller CC, Estrera AL, et al. Analysis of motor and somatosensory evoked potentials during thoracic and thoracoabdominal aortic aneurysm repair. J Vasc Surg. 2009;49:36–41.

9. Liu LY, Callahan B, Peterss S, et al. Neuromonitoring using motor and somatosensory evoked potentials in aortic surgery. J Card Surg. 2016;31:383–9.

10. Yoshitani K, Masui K, Kawaguchi M, et al. Clinical utility of intraoperative motor-evoked potential monitoring to prevent postoperative spinal cord injury in thoracic and thoracoabdominal aneurysm repair: an audit of the Japanese Association of Spinal Cord Protection in aortic surgery database. Anesth Analg. 2018 Mar;126(3):763–8.

11. Martin KK, Wigginton JB, Babikian VL, et al. Intraoperative cerebral high-intensity transient signals and postoperative cognitive function: a systematic review. Am J Surg. 2009;197:55–63.

12. Alexandrov AV, Sloan MA, Tegeler CH, American Society of Neuroimaging Practice Guidelines Committee, et al. Practice standards for transcranial Doppler (TCD) ultrasound. Part II. Clinical indications and expected outcomes. J Neuroimaging. 2012;22:215–24.

13. Murkin J, Arango M. Near-infrared spectroscopy as an index of brain and tissue oxygenation. Br J Anaesth. 2009;103(Suppl 1):i3–i13.

14. Schober A, Feiner JR, Bickler PE, Rollins MD. Effects of changes in arterial carbon dioxide and oxygen partial pressures on cerebral oximeter performance. Anesthesiology. 2018;128:97–108.

15. Davie SN, Grocott HP. Impact of extracranial contamination on regional cerebral oxygen saturation: a comparison of three cerebral oximetry technologies. Anesthesiology. 2012;116:834–40.

16. Zheng F, Sheinberg R, Yee MS, Ono M, et al. Cerebral near-infrared spectroscopy monitoring and neurologic outcomes in adult cardiac surgery patients: a systematic review. Anesth Analg. 2013;116:663–76.

17. Subramanian B, Nyman C, Fritock M, et al. A multicenter pilot study assessing regional cerebral oxygen desaturation frequency during cardiopulmonary bypass and responsiveness to an intervention algorithm. Anesth Analg. 2016;122:1786–93.

18. Deschamps A, Hall R, Grocott H, Canadian Perioperative Anesthesia Clinical Trials Group, et al. Cerebral oximetry monitoring to maintain normal cerebral oxygen saturation during high-risk cardiac surgery: a randomized controlled feasibility trial. Anesthesiology. 2016;124:826–36.

19. Murkin JM, Adams SJ, Novick RJ, et al. Monitoring brain oxygen saturation during coronary bypass surgery: a randomized, prospective study. Anesth Analg. 2007;104:51–8.

20. Slater JP, Guarino T, Stack J, et al. Cerebral oxygen desaturation predicts cognitive decline and longer hospital stay after cardiac surgery. Ann Thorac Surg. 2009;87:36–44. discussion 44-5

21. Mohandas BS, Jagadeesh AM, Vikram SB. Impact of monitoring cerebral oxygen saturation on the outcome of patients undergoing open heart surgery. Ann Card Anaesth. 2013;16:102–6.

22. Colak Z, Borojevic M, Bogovic A, et al. Influence of intraoperative cerebral oximetry monitoring on neurocognitive function after coronary artery bypass surgery: a randomized, prospective study. Eur J Cardiothorac Surg. 2015;47:447–54.

23. Kara I, Erkin A, Sacli H, et al. The effects of near-infrared spectroscopy on the neurocognitive functions in the patients undergoing coronary artery bypass grafting with asymptomatic carotid artery disease: a randomized prospective study. Ann Thorac Cardiovasc Surg. 2015;21:544–50.

24. Rogers C, Stoica S, Ellis L, et al. A randomised trial of near infra-red spectroscopy for the personalised optimisation of cerebral tissue oxygenation during cardiac surgery. Br J Anaesth. 2017;119(3):384–93.

25. Serraino GF, Murphy GJ. Effects of cerebral near-infrared spectroscopy on the outcome of patients undergoing cardiac surgery: a systematic review of randomised trials. BMJ Open. 2017;7:e016613.

26. Czosnyka M, Brady K, Reinhard M, et al. Monitoring of cerebrovascular autoregulation: facts, myths, and missing links. Neurocrit Care. 2009;10:373–86.

27. Aries MJ, Czosnyka M, Budohoski KP, et al. Continuous determination of optimal cerebral perfusion pressure in traumatic brain injury. Crit Care Med. 2012;40:2456–63.

28. Brady K, Joshi B, Zweifel C, et al. Real-time continuous monitoring of cerebral blood flow autoregulation using near-infrared spectroscopy in patients undergoing cardiopulmonary bypass. Stroke. 2010;41:1951–6.

29. Ono M, Brady K, Easley RB, et al. Duration and magnitude of blood pressure below cerebral autoregulation threshold during cardiopulmonary bypass is associated with major morbidity and operative mortality. J Thorac Cardiovasc Surg. 2014;147:483–9.

30. Hori D, Brown C, Ono M, et al. Arterial pressure above the upper cerebral autoregulation limit during cardiopulmonary bypass is associated with postoperative delirium. Br J Anaesth. 2014;113:1009–17.

Perioperative Monitoring Technology and Management: Coagulation Monitoring Technologies and Techniques

30

Pascal Colson, Seema Agarwal, Aamer Ahmed, and On behalf of Haemostasis and Transfusion EACTA Subcommittee

Main Messages
1. Perioperative coagulation monitoring plays a pivotal role in the concept of patient blood management.
2. Preoperative use of Standard Laboratory Tests (SLT) should be preceded by a comprehensive clinical investigation.
3. Point-of-Care Testing (POCT) may be useful in screening for undiagnosed bleeding tendencies or to check compliance with antiplatelet therapy.
4. POCT are strongly recommended to monitor coagulation during and after cardiac surgery.
5. POCT should be part of treatment algorithms, integrated in a comprehensive blood-conservative strategy.

Blood conservation in the perioperative period has been shown to be beneficial in terms of long term patient outcomes. Despite this, 20% of all blood products are used in cardiac surgery [1]. Massive blood loss, which can occur in cardiac surgery, may be linked to the development of acquired coagulation defects. It is the successful management of these defects using technologies both in the laboratory and point of care that results in control of hemostasis [2], and a reduction in allogeneic blood and blood product transfusion [3] ultimately leading to better patient outcomes [2].

In recent years the importance of managing the entire patient pathway from initial referral to surgery from the family physician, through the perioperative period to postsurgical discharge back to primary care has become a subject of great interest. The concept of patient blood management and its benefit to patient outcomes has been established [4], in the US, by the Australian National Blood Authority [5] and within Europe,

On behalf of Haemostasis and Transfusion EACTA Subcommittee

P. Colson (✉)
Département d'Anesthésie-Réanimation Armaud de Villeneuve, Centre Hospitalier Universitaire de Montpellier, Montpellier, France
e-mail: p-colson@chu-montpellier.fr

S. Agarwal
Department of Anaesthesia and Critical Care, Liverpool Heart and Chest Hospital, Liverpool, UK
e-mail: Seema.Agarwal@lhch.nhs.uk

A. Ahmed
Department of Anaesthesia and Critical Care, Glenfield Hospital, University Hospitals of Leicester NHS Trust, Leicester, UK
e-mail: aamer.ahmed@uhl-tr.nhs.uk

© Springer Nature Switzerland AG 2021
D. C. H. Cheng et al. (eds.), *Evidence-Based Practice in Perioperative Cardiac Anesthesia and Surgery*, https://doi.org/10.1007/978-3-030-47887-2_30

led by the European Association of Cardiothoracic Anaesthesiologists (EACTA) and European Society of Anaesthesiology (ESA) [6]. Within these pathways the role of perioperative coagulation management is key.

The Society for the Advancement of Blood Management in the USA defines patient blood management as "the timely application of evidence-based medical and surgical concepts designed to maintain hemoglobin concentration, optimize hemostasis and minimize blood loss in an effort to improve patient outcome." This has been shown to improve patient outcomes [2]. Point of care testing (POCT) to dynamically manage perioperative bleeding is an integral part of this.

Standard Laboratory Test

Definition: Standard laboratory tests of coagulation generally consist of

- Platelet count.
- Prothrombin time (performed by adding a thromboplastin reagent containing a tissue factor, calcium, and phospholipids) initiating coagulation via the extrinsic coagulation pathway.
- Activated partial thromboplastin time (performed by adding silica and phospholipid extract free of tissue factor to the plasma) initiating coagulation via the intrinsic coagulation pathway.
- Fibrinogen assay.

Limits in Real-Time Monitoring

While these laboratory tests may be helpful in elucidating the cause of bleeding, they have numerous disadvantages. They measure one specific part of the coagulation system at one point in time. With turnaround time in some laboratories exceeding 30 min, the results are often of little use in the dynamic situation of acute hemorrhage. The tests are done mainly in the plasma rather than whole blood and at a standard temperature of 37 °C rather than the patient's temperature. Platelet function tests are generally only available in specialist hematology laboratories and have a turnaround time of hours. In light of these limitations, clinicians have sought to use POCT.

Point of Care Testing: POCT

Whole Blood: TEG™/ROTEM™

By their nature, POCT devices are situated close to the patient and so allow the clinician to see the results quickly, as they develop. They consistently detect changes in coagulation. There are two main devices used: the TEG™ (TEG Haemonetics Corporation) and the ROTEM™ (Rotational Thromboelastometer, TEM International); both these devices offer a global view of hemostasis with a visual representation of clot development. They are performed on citrated whole blood, although both may also be performed on fresh whole blood.

Principles

The devices work in a similar fashion to assess the viscoelastic properties of blood under low shear conditions. In the TEG™ there is a cylindrical cup holding the blood which oscillates for 10 s at a time. A pin is suspended in the blood sample via a torsion wire and is monitored for motion. After fibrin- platelet bonding has occurred, linking the pin and the cup together, the torque of the rotation is transmitted to the pin which is then converted by an electromagnetic signal into an electrical signal—the TEG™ trace [7]. The strength of the bonds affects the magnitude of the pin motion so output is directly related to the strength of the formed clot. With clot retraction and lysis the fibrin platelet bonds are broken. The same principles apply in ROTEM™; the main technical difference being that it is the pin which rotates whilst the cup remains stationary. The ROTEM system also uses a different activator—Ellagic acid rather than kaolin, which may make it less sensitive to residual heparin. Both devices suffer from a lack of robust quality control and are operator dependent [8]. The results of the two systems are closely related but they are not completely interchangeable [3].

The manufacturers of TEG™ or ROTEM™ have worked on a new generation of apparatus, to make them easier to use with automated measurement (TEG 6 s, and ROTEM Sigma). Both have introduced a cartridge-based device with more robust quality control and offer the advantages of a reduction in operator dependent error and technical faults. For the TEG 6 s, whole blood is inserted into the cartridge and delivered to a microcell which is excited with a multi-frequency signal from a piezoelectric actuator. The resulting harmonic motion of the sample is measured optically; as the sample clots and moves from liquid to gel and solid phase the harmonic motion changes, this is represented as the familiar TEG™ trace. It does not measure the viscoelasticity of the clot directly [9]. TEG6s is capable of performing four tests simultaneously from one citrated blood sample. ROTEM Sigma uses the same basic concept of rotating the pin in smaller cups than the former device.

Uses

A number of tests can be performed to assess various parts of the coagulation system (Tables 30.1 and 30.2). The addition of heparinase to the test reveals the underlying coagulation status when heparin is present. The commonly measured variables are shown in Fig. 30.1 and Table 30.2. ROTEM™ provides an additional test with aprotinin to inhibit fibrinolysis (APTEM), although the added information on fibrinolysis is small.

The tests have limitations and this must be borne in mind. The tests are run at 37 degrees Centigrade so cannot reflect the effects of hypothermia. They are not sensitive to the effects of platelet adhesion so cannot detect Von Willebrand factor deficiency. Hemodilution and low platelet count as well as the usage of HES solutions influence the results of most POC devices. They are dependent on quality control and regular calibration to generate valid results.

Table 30.1 The common TEG™/ROTEM™ tests

TEG™ Test	ROTEM™ Test	Function
Kaolin	INTEM	Activated test of global hemostasis via intrinsic pathway—usually performed as a baseline
Functional fibrinogen	FIBTEM	Assessment of fibrinogen
RapidTEG®	EXTEM	Tissue factor activated test of extrinsic pathway—assessment of clot strength quickly
Heparinase	HEPTEM	Test of global hemostasis via intrinsic pathway with the effect of heparin removed

Table 30.2 Meaning of TEG™/ROTEM™ test abnormality

TEG	ROTEM	What does it measure?	Abnormality
R time	CT	Time to first significant clot formation—clot initiation	Increased in factor deficiency or excess heparin
K α angle	CFT α angle	Clot kinetics Clot strengthening	Decreased in fibrinogen-platelet linkage deficiency
MA (maximal amplitude)	MCF (maximal clot firmness)	Maximum strength of clot	Decreased in fibrinogen or platelet deficiency (not in platelet inhibition)
LY30	CL 30	Percent lysis 30 min after maximal clot strength	Increased in fibrinolysis

Anticoagulation Monitoring: Activated Clotting Time (ACT)

The ACT is a POCT of coagulation that is used to monitor the anticoagulant effect of unfractionated heparin in patients on cardiopulmonary bypass (CPB), ECMO or undergoing percutaneous transluminal coronary angioplasty. In most cases of CPB a dose of heparin is administered to maintain the ACT >400–480 s.

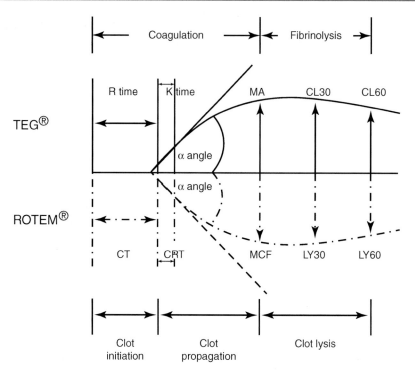

Fig. 30.1 The commonly measured variables obtained with TEG™ or ROTEM™ devices. *R time* time elapsing between initiation of the test and the point where clotting provides enough resistance to produce a 2 mm amplitude reading on the tracing, *CT* coagulation time (same as R time), *K time and CFT (clot formation time)* time from 2 min to 20 mm amplitude, *α angle* slope between R and K for TEG, angle of tangent at 2-mm amplitude for ROTEM, *MA* maximal amplitude, *MCF* maximal clot firmness, *CL and LY, clot lysis* percentage reduction in amplitude 30 min after reaching MA (TEG) or 30 min after CT (ROTEM)

The most commonly used ACT devices are the Hemochron (International Technidyne Inc., Edison, New Jersey) with Celite activator and the Hemotec (Medtronic Hemotec, Parker, Colorado) device with kaolin activator.

Principles

Fresh, whole blood is added to a tube containing a surface activator. This result in the activation of coagulation via the intrinsic pathway, using an automated technique; the time to clot formation is recorded.

Uses

Clotting times vary between ACT analysers, depending on the source and the formula of the activator, the amount of activator relative to the sample volume, or the method of clot detection.

In a non-anticoagulated patient, using celite activation, the ACT is in the region of 107 s ± 13 s.

During CPB, heparin is titrated to maintain an ACT of between 400 and 600 s. During ECMO, heparin is titrated to maintain the ACT between 200 and 260 s.

The ACT is influenced by a number of variables including aprotinin which prolongs the time to clot formation thus overestimating the concentration of heparin (i.e. gives a longer ACT); aprotinin has a lesser effect upon kaolin-based ACTs. Other causes of a prolonged ACT include hypothermia, hemodilution and clotting factor deficiencies.

Anticoagulation Monitoring: Hemostasis Management System (HMS)

The HMS is a POCT device which provides a heparin dose response and protamine dose response as an alternative or addition to the ACT for monitoring heparin and protamine. Hemochron PRT (Protamine Response Test) and Hepcon instrument (Medtronic Hemotec, Parker, Colorado) provide a protamine dose-response test.

Principles

The HMS is a cartridge-based test of hemostasis, performed on whole blood. First the heparin dose-response test is performed to determine an individual's response to heparin. The HDR (Heparin Dose Response) cartridge consists of six chambers containing various amounts of heparin; unheparinised whole blood from the patient is added and the clotting time measured. These results are plotted and the slope of the graph is used to predict the dose of heparin required to reach an ACT of 480secs.

The Hemochron PRT test is an ACT based measurement on a heparinized blood sample that contains a known quantity of protamine. The Hepcon instrument has a protamine dose-response test, the protamine titration assay.

Uses

During bypass, the heparin assay cartridge is used to determine the patient's heparin blood concentration. Results of this assay also include the predicted dose of protamine required to reverse the heparin fully. After the protamine has been given, the heparin assay and ACT can be repeated to check there is no residual heparin and the ACT has returned to baseline. Studies using HMS have demonstrated that patients may receive higher doses of heparin and lower doses of protamine with this system.

Platelet Function Testing

There are many platelet function testing devices which have been shown to be possibly useful in cardiac surgery, among them: Multiplate™, TEG™, VerifyNow™ and Plateletworks™. All four work by the same principle; that is, by adding a platelet agonist to cause the uninhibited (reactive) platelets to aggregate; those which are inhibited will not aggregate. The commonly used

agonists are Arachidonic acid (AA) to assess aspirin induced inhibition and ADP to assess inhibition via ADP antagonists.

The Multiplate™ is a multiple electrode aggregometer which uses impedance based aggregometry in whole anticoagulated blood to measure platelet function. After the addition of the platelet agonist, the platelets aggregate and accumulate on the electrode surface changing the electrical resistance between them. This resistance is continuously measured and produces an impedance curve. In addition to AA and ADP there is a TRAP test (Thrombin Receptor Activating Peptide) used to monitor Gp2b3a antagonists.

The standard TEG™ or ROTEM™ are not able to measure the effects of antiplatelet medication due to overwhelming thrombin generation in the plastic cup. An adaption—TEG™ PlateletMapping™ (TEG™ PM) can show the effects of aspirin and ADP antagonists. TEG™ PM uses heparinized whole blood so that thrombin production is eliminated. The heparinized blood is used to run two concurrent traces; one which measures the contribution of fibrinogen to the clot strength, the second which measures the clot strength due to fibrinogen and the platelets which are not inhibited. By comparing these two traces with the patient's non heparinised TEG™, a measurement of the relative clot strength due to remaining platelet function can be ascertained. A dedicated cartridge has been designed to be used with TEG 6 s with an automated, simplified technique. ROTEM™ have added a platelet function test which does not use thromboelastography to one of their devices. The ROTEM platelet has two aggregometry channels (working by the same principle as the Multiplate) offering tests aimed at the detection of anti-platelet medications. The VerifyNow™ uses the principle of light transmission aggregometry. The equipment consists of an instrument and disposable single use cartridges containing fibrin coated beads and a platelet aggregant. Citrated blood is drawn into the cartridge; when the platelets are reactive they bind to the fibrin coated beads, aggregate and allow an increase in light transmittance. Where the platelets are inhibited, they do not bind to the beads but remain in solution and there is little change in light transmission.

The Plateletworks™ provides an assessment of platelet function based on full blood count measurements with and without platelet agonist. The agonist leads to aggregation of uninhibited, reactive platelets; with more aggregation there is a lower the platelet count on the second tube.

When to do it?

Preoperative Assessment

Standard Laboratory Test
Preoperative use of Standard Laboratory Tests (SLT) should always be preceded by a comprehensive investigation of clinical and family bleeding history, and detailed information of a patient's medication. This investigation alone may unmask signs of bleeding or diseases which may cause hemostatic failure [10].

Preoperative SLTs are not recommended routinely in elective surgery [9]. However, in cardiac surgery the effects of CPB on the coagulation pathway justify preoperative tests. Nevertheless POCT may replace the need for SLT [11].

Point of Care Testing: POCT

The exact timing of the POCT remains open to debate as the evidence is not clear. If there is a coagulopathy present as surgery starts it becomes apparent early after skin incision. Most algorithms indicate that TEG or ROTEM tests should be performed as baselines before the administration of heparin and subsequently at the end of protamine administration in the operating room. However, there is a poor correlation between baseline tests results and the prediction of subsequent bleeding. The TEG has a high negative predictive value, so it is more useful in screening for exclusion of surgical bleeding postoperatively.

Platelet Monitoring

Many patients take antiplatelet medication prior to cardiac surgery. Since most of the oral formulations have long half-lives, discontinuation 24 to 48 h before surgery is not sufficient to eliminate their antiaggregant effect. Platelet function tests may be used to determine the extent of platelet dysfunction present, to determine the optimal time for surgery and whether platelet transfusion is necessary.

Platelet function tests have been incorporated into transfusion algorithms using POCT, although the correlation between platelet function tests and perioperative bleeding may be poor [12, 13].

Anticoagulation Treatment

Heparin Therapy
The most common drug used to anticoagulate patients during CPB is unfractionated heparin. Conventional anti-factor Xa tests are unsuitable for on-site heparin monitoring in CPB patients where POCT are mandatory.

The Activated Clotting Time (ACT) The initial ACT measurement should be performed prior to the administration of any heparin to get a reference value. Measurements have to be repeated regularly, usually every 30 min during CPB, with repeated doses of heparin as required. However, ACT measurement correlates poorly with actual heparin plasma levels during CPB due to a wide range in heparin sensitivity.

Heparin Concentration Due to the uncertainty of ACT results, a quantitative heparin test could be preferred such as the Hepcon HMS system. However, the precision and bias of the Hepcon test suggest that both ACT and heparin concentration measurement limitations should be taken into consideration in the anticoagulation management during CPB [14]. The current recommendation from the European Association of Cardiothoracic Surgery is routine use of Hepcon monitoring (Class IIb recommendation. Level of Evidence B).

POCT Monitoring Towards the end of CPB, tests may be performed to assess the extent of coagulopathy present. A baseline trace is usually performed together with an assessment of

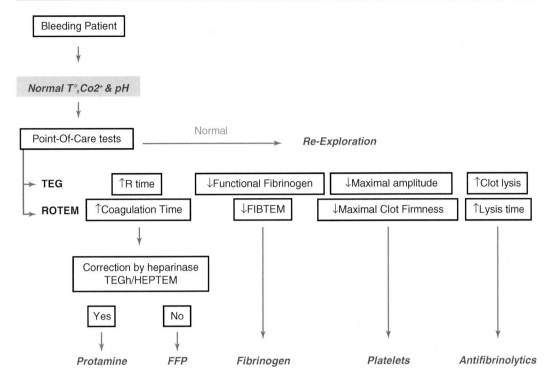

Fig. 30.2 Decision algorithm according to TEG™ or ROTEM™ main results. *FFP* Fresh Frozen Plasma

fibrinogen, both with the addition of heparinase to negate the effect of the systemic heparinisation of the patient. These then allow blood products to be requested.

On separation from CPB, protamine is administered to reverse residual heparinisation and the any pre-ordered blood products are administered. Further transfusions are then guided by further use of the POCT devices. At this point the four common tests may be performed to assess whether there is any residual heparin, assess fibrinogen and obtain a quick assessment of clot strength (Fig. 30.2).

Others (Bivalirudin, Argatroban, Etc)

When an alternative to HNF is required during CPB, direct thrombin inhibitors are used to safely perform cardiac procedures. These agents include mainly bivalirudin and argatroban which are preferred because of their short half-lives. However, argatroban is not licensed for use in CPB.

The only available method to measure therapeutic levels of these agents is the ecarin clotting time and recent modifications of this test allow POCT for cardiac surgery patients [15]. However, ACT can also be used. A baseline ACT value is checked before giving bivalirudin, aiming for a target of ACT for CPB of 2.5 times the baseline during CPB. There are developments going on to measure thrombin inhibitors with POCT devices [16].

Protamine

Heparin reversal: Most centers utilize a formula based on the initial HNF dose given, and ACT is performed then to assess heparin reversal. However, ACT level is too insensitive to accurately diagnose incomplete heparin neutralization.

The use of individualized protamine dose-response curves has been shown to result in a reduction in total protamine dose to reduce postoperative bleeding [17].

Heparin rebound: Residual low levels of heparin can be detected by sensitive heparin concentration monitoring in the first hour after protamine reversal and can be present for up to six hours postoperatively.

Tests that can assess residual heparin after protamine neutralization include heparin neutralized thrombin time (HNTT) which measures TT after addition of protamine. A normal HNTT and elevated TT indicate residual heparin while prolonged HNTT and TT suggest a fibrinogen problem or that the heparin level was too high and was not neutralized by the HNTT.

POCT Monitoring

The TEG™ and ROTEM™ are exquisitely sensitive to heparin and a comparison of the kaolin trace with the heparinase traces (or ROTEM™ equivalent) may show differences (generally with a prolonged R time and/or a reduced MA on the kaolin which corrects with heparinase) when the ACT is normal. This is generally easily corrected with additional protamine.

In Case of Bleeding

During Surgery If there is bleeding after reversal of heparin then the TEG/ROTEM allows one to tease out some of the causes—e.g. inadequate reversal of protamine, rebound from tissue bound heparin, clotting factor deficiency, hypofibrinogenemia, fibrinolysis and to a lesser extent platelet dysfunction. Using combinations of activators, it is possible to determine levels of platelet inhibition as well. By separating the maximum amplitude generated due to platelet activity and the contribution due to fibrinogen it is possible to ascertain the degree of inhibition of platelet function.

Postoperative Care (ICU) In the intensive care unit, common causes of bleeding include surgical bleeding, postoperative anemia due to hemodilution, acid/base disturbances, hypocalcemia, temperature drop as well as residual heparin effect (heparin rebound) and post bypass platelet dysfunction that may be exacerbated by uremia. Anticoagulation required in the case of venovenous (VV) and venoarterial (VA) ECMO circuits may complicate the picture.

POCT should be used in the case of all patients undergoing ongoing postoperative blood loss to selectively guide transfusion. Tests should be performed in those patients that are bleeding, followed by repeat tests each time after a clinical intervention has taken place such as administration of further protamine for heparin rebound, or blood products or fibrinogen for coagulopathy. This can then guide the indications and timing for surgical re-exploration. Decision algorithms can be designed with TEG™ or ROTEM (Fig. 30.2), keeping in mind that the results of each technique are not interchangeable [3].

Coagulation Monitoring as an Integral Part of Blood Management Strategy

The concept of patient blood management comprises three pillars grouped as optimizing hematopoiesis, minimizing blood loss and bleeding, and harnessing and optimization of physiological reserve of anemia. Each pillar has pre, peri and postoperative recommendations or suggestions for patient blood management (Fig. 30.3) [18].

Within each of these pillars there is an area where coagulation management may be considered. Coagulation monitoring should include laboratory tests as well as access to POCT. The lab based tests are still considered to be the most accurate, however the time taken to return results has led to the increasing use of validated POCT such as TEG™ or ROTEM™.

Before Surgery

Some patients may have disturbances such as iatrogenic antiplatelet therapy or hypercoagulable states. Scoring systems such as TRUST, and TRACK [19, 20] have identified anemia as a risk factor. However, no study has identified preoperative treatment as a risk factor for bleeding or transfusion.

In recent years the effect of antiplatelet therapies has come to the fore as increasing use amongst cardiologists has led to greater numbers of patients presenting for elective and emergent cardiac surgery whilst under platelet inhibition. POCT may be useful in screening for undiag-

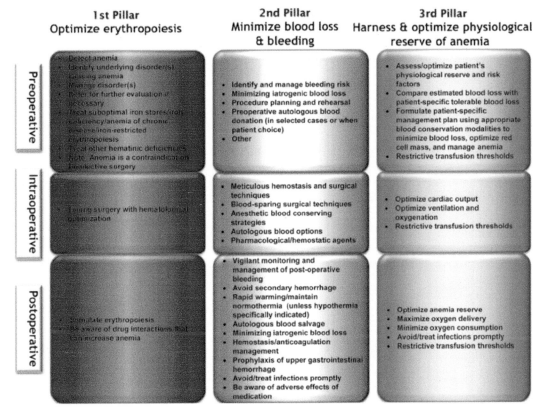

| 1st Pillar Optimize erythropoiesis | 2nd Pillar Minimize blood loss & bleeding | 3rd Pillar Harness & optimize physiological reserve of anemia |

Preoperative
- Detect anemia
- Identify underlying disorder(s) causing anemia
- Manage disorder(s)
- Refer for further evaluation if necessary
- Treat suboptimal iron stores/iron deficiency/anemia of chronic disease/iron-restricted erythropoiesis
- Treat other hematinic deficiencies
- Note: Anemia is a contraindication for elective surgery

- Identify and manage bleeding risk
- Minimizing iatrogenic blood loss
- Procedure planning and rehearsal
- Preoperative autologous blood donation (in selected cases or when patient choice)
- Other

- Assess/optimize patient's physiological reserve and risk factors
- Compare estimated blood loss with patient-specific tolerable blood loss
- Formulate patient-specific management plan using appropriate blood conservation modalities to minimize blood loss, optimize red cell mass, and manage anemia
- Restrictive transfusion thresholds

Intraoperative
- Timing surgery with hematological optimization

- Meticulous hemostasis and surgical techniques
- Blood-sparing surgical techniques
- Anesthetic blood conserving strategies
- Autologous blood options
- Pharmacological/hemostatic agents

- Optimize cardiac output
- Optimize ventilation and oxygenation
- Restrictive transfusion thresholds

Postoperative
- Stimulate erythropoiesis
- Be aware of drug interactions that can increase anemia

- Vigilant monitoring and management of post-operative bleeding
- Avoid secondary hemorrhage
- Rapid warming/maintain normothermia (unless hypothermia specifically indicated)
- Autologous blood salvage
- Minimizing iatrogenic blood loss
- Hemostasis/anticoagulation management
- Prophylaxis of upper gastrointestinal hemorrhage
- Avoid/treat infections promptly
- Be aware of adverse effects of medication

- Optimize anemia reserve
- Maximize oxygen delivery
- Minimize oxygen consumption
- Avoid/treat infections promptly
- Restrictive transfusion thresholds

Fig. 30.3 Concept of patient blood management. The three pillars are grouped as optimizing hematopoiesis, minimizing blood loss and bleeding, and harnessing and optimization of physiological reserve of anemia. The three pillars have pre-, peri- and post-operative inputs in patient blood management. Adapted with permission from Hoffman A. et al. [18]

nosed bleeding tendencies or to check compliance with antiplatelet therapy.

During Surgery

During CPB, dilutional hypofibrinogenemia and non-pulsatile flow can lead to disturbances in the microcirculation causing changes in oxygen delivery to end organs. This can lead to clotting factor deficiencies, in particular for liver-derived factors, VII, IX and X.

POCT are used as part of treatment algorithms to guide factor replacement and autologous blood product therapy. An example of a clinical algorithm with TEG™ is shown Fig. 30.4. This allows a systematic approach to be adopted to each aspect of the coagulopathic process. Equally it has been shown that the timely use of protocol driven algorithms leads to considerable reductions in transfusion of autologous blood and blood products [1, 2].

After Surgery

In the postoperative phase, coagulopathy that is acquired can worsen bleeding volumes and hence outcomes. In the ICU patients may suffer a temperature drop after hypothermic CPB, and low cardiac output states lead to acidemia and lactic acidosis and electrolyte imbalance such as hypocalcemia can contribute to coagulopathy worsening. Here we would suggest the use of POCT to

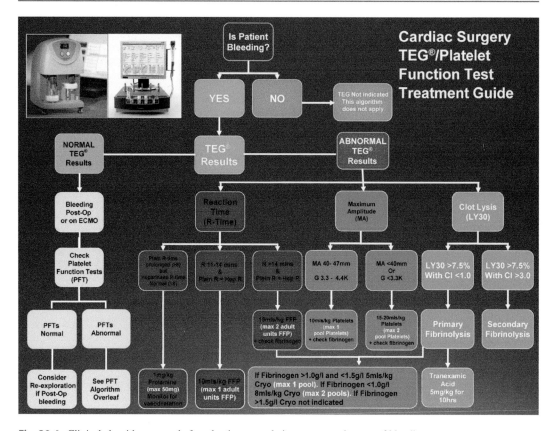

Fig. 30.4 Clinical algorithm example for adapting coagulation treatment in case of bleeding

screen for surgical bleeding vs. coagulopathy before treatment is initiated with blood product replacement or surgical intervention such as resternotomy.

In conclusion, patient blood management requires an integrated and multidisciplinary approach to the surgical pathway. Accurate coagulation management guided by TEG/ROTEM and lab results is key to reducing transfusion and bleeding.

References

1. Ferraris VA, Ferraris SP, Saha SP, Hessel EA 2nd, Haan CK, et al. Perioperative blood transfusion and blood conservation in cardiac surgery: the Society of Thoracic Surgeons and The Society of Cardiovascular Anesthesiologists clinical practice guideline. Ann Thorac Surg. 2007;83(5 Suppl):S27–86.
2. Clevenger B, Mallett SV, Klein AA, Richards T. Patient blood management to reduce surgical risk. Br J Surg. 2015;102(11):1325–37.
3. Bolliger D, Tanaka KA. Roles of thrombelastography and thromboelastometry for patient blood management in cardiac surgery. Transfus Med Rev. 2013;27(4):213–20.
4. Shander A, Van Aken H, Colomina MJ, Gombotz H, Hofmann A, et al. Patient blood management in Europe. Br J Anaesth. 2012;109(1):55–68.
5. Farmer SL, Towler SC, Leahy MF, Hofmann A. Drivers for change: Western Australia Patient Blood Management Program (WA PBMP), World Health Assembly (WHA) and Advisory Committee on Blood Safety and Availability (ACBSA). Best Pract Res Clin Anaesthesiol. 2013;27:43–58.
6. Kozek-Langenecker SA, Ahmed AB, Afshari A, Albaladejo P, Aldecoa C, et al. Management of severe perioperative bleeding: guidelines from the European Society of Anaesthesiology: first update 2016. Eur J Anaesthesiol. 2017;34(6):332–95.
7. Mallett SV, Cox DJ. Thromboelastography. Br J Anaesth. 1992;69(3):307–13.
8. Whiting D, DiNardo JA. TEG and ROTEM: technology and clinical applications. Am J Hematol. 2014;89(2):228–32.
9. Gurbel PA, Bliden KP, Tantry US, Monroe AL, Muresan AA, et al. First report of the point-of-care

TEG: a technical validation study of the TEG-6S system. Platelets. 2016;27(7):642–9.

10. American Society of Anesthesiologists Task Force on Preanesthesia Evaluation. Practice advisory for preanesthesia evaluation: a report by the American Society of Anesthesiologists Task Force on Preanesthesia evaluation. Anesthesiology. 2002;96:485–96.

11. Weber CF, Gorlinger K, Meininger M, Herrmann E, Bingold T, et al. Point-of-care testing. A prospective, randomized clinical trial of efficacy in coagulopathic cardiac surgery patients. Anesthesiology. 2012;117:531–47.

12. Agarwal S, Johnson RI, Shaw M. Preoperative point-of-care platelet function testing in cardiac surgery. J Cardiothorac Vasc Anesth. 2015;29(2):333–41.

13. Karkouti K, Callum J, Wijeysundera DN, Rao V, Crowther M, et al. TACS investigators point-of-care hemostatic testing in cardiac surgery: a stepped-wedge clustered randomized controlled trial. Circulation. 2016;134(16):1152–62.

14. Garvin S, FitzGerald DC, Despotis G, Shekar P, Body SC. Heparin concentration–based anticoagulation for cardiac surgery fails to reliably predict heparin bolus dose requirements. Anesth Analg. 2010;111:849–55.

15. Nowak G. The ecarin clotting time: a universal method to quantify direct thrombin inhibitors. Pathophysiology of haemostasis and thrombosis. Pathophysiol Haemost Thromb. 2003;33:173–83.

16. Körber MK, Langer E, Köhr M, Wernecke KD, Korte W, von Heymann C. In vitro and ex vivo measurement of prophylactic Dabigatran concentrations with a new Ecarin-based thromboelastometry test. Transfus Med Hemother. 2017;44(2):100–5.

17. LaDuca FM, Zucker ML, Walker CE. Assessing heparin neutralization following cardiac surgery: sensitivity of thrombin time-based assays versus protamine titration methods. Perfusion. 1999;14:181–7.

18. Hoffmann A, Farmer S, Shander A. Five drivers shifting the paradigm from product-focused transfusion practice to patient blood management. Oncologist. 2011;16(Suppl 3):3–11.

19. Alghamdi AA, Davis A, Brister S, Corey P, Logan A. Development and validation of transfusion risk understanding scoring tool (TRUST) to stratify cardiac surgery patients according to their blood transfusion needs. Transfusion. 2006 Jul;46(7):1120–9.

20. Kim TS, Lee JH, An H, Na CY. Transfusion risk and clinical knowledge (TRACK) score and cardiac surgery in patients refusing transfusion. J Cardiothorac Vasc Anesth. 2016;30(2):373–8.

Perioperative Transesophageal Echocardiography in Cardiac Surgery Procedures

31

Annette Vegas

Main Messages
1. TEE is a valuable diagnostic and monitoring modality that can be used in the operating room to guide interventions and assess the result of surgery.
2. Parameters used to assess LV function and valve lesion severity are dynamic and change under anesthesia and with loading conditions.
3. Significant operator experience and a thorough knowledge of anatomy and pathology are required to establish the correct diagnosis.

Technology

Transesophageal echocardiography (TEE) technology has advanced over decades from rudimentary origins as m-mode imaging (1979), monoplane probes (1982), biplane probes (late 1980s) to multiplane probes (1990s) that provide two-dimensional (2D) images, Doppler and other modes. Matrix array TEE probes (2007) now enable volume scanning of the heart for the dis-

play of three-dimensional (3D) images in real-time [1]. Evolving ultrasound machine software makes it feasible to rapidly analyze returning ultrasound data on-cart affording quantitative assessment of ventricular function and valve structure.

The TEE probe resembles a gastroscope, roughly 90 cm in length and 1 cm in diameter with a tip, shaft and handle. The TEE probe tip houses the transducer which is comprised of piezo-electric crystals, 256 for 2D imaging and over 2000 for 3D imaging. The high frequency (5.0 MHz) TEE probe is positioned in the esophagus near the heart thus reducing the tissue penetration required to display high resolution ultrasound images. The heart is imaged from posterior to anterior by TEE in contrast to the anterior to posterior approach used with transthoracic echocardiography (TTE).

Each ultrasound mode interprets and displays returning sound waves differently. The 2D mode shows structural anatomy to allow for the quantification of size and assessment of myocardial and valvular function. The color Doppler mode displays blood flow within the heart and great vessels using different color maps. Normal flow is unidirectional and smooth (laminar). Regurgitant or stenotic valvular flow or flow through abnormal connections typically appears as turbulent flow due to variations in blood velocities. The pulsed and continuous wave Doppler modes present information in a spectral trace of velocity

A. Vegas (✉)
University Health Network, Toronto General Hospital, Toronto, ON, Canada
e-mail: annette.vegas@uhn.ca

© Springer Nature Switzerland AG 2021
D. C. H. Cheng et al. (eds.), *Evidence-Based Practice in Perioperative Cardiac Anesthesia and Surgery*, https://doi.org/10.1007/978-3-030-47887-2_31

versus time that reveals details about timing, direction and amount of flow. Quantification of blood flow velocity permits calculation of pressure gradients, and the derivation of hemodynamic information. Integration of different Doppler parameters determines valve lesion severity. Tissue Doppler Imaging (TDI) and speckle tracking echocardiography (STE) are new ultrasound modes that examine low velocity myocardial motion to better assess cardiac mechanics.

TEE Views

The 2D TEE probe generates a sector plane to scan the heart, while the 3D TEE probe acquires a 3D dataset that after instantaneous processing displays a volume of the heart. TEE probe manipulation consists of probe shaft (A) advancing/withdrawing or (B) turning right (clockwise)/left (counterclockwise), probe tip (C) right/left lateral flexion or (D) anteflexion (anterior)/retroflexion (posterior) and (E) changing the transducer angle (0–180°). Slight probe manipulation and transducer angle changes can dramatically alter the TEE image displayed. The complex interaction of the probe and image plane intersection of the heart is best appreciated by using a high-fidelity mannequin or online simulator with a 3D augmented reality heart model [2].

Guidelines for performing comprehensive 2D and 3D cardiac imaging involve customary imaging planes which standardize nomenclature and generate sufficient information for complete cardiac assessment [3–5]. Current ASE/SCA guidelines suggest acquiring 28 different 2D TEE views (Fig. 31.1). Each imaging view is named by the probe position, major anatomic structure, orientation of the imaging plane (either long axis [LAX] or short axis [SAX]) and imaging angle. The reader is referred to excellent guideline papers for detailed descriptions of how to obtain and identify the content of each view.

Role and Indications

In the perioperative setting, TTE provides sufficient information in many patients such that TEE may be unnecessary. However TEE offers high resolution images and may be indicated when poor quality TTE images are unable to satisfactorily resolve a clinical question particularly in the evaluation of native valve disease, prosthetic valve function, ventricular function, and congenital heart disease [6]. TEE is superior to TTE for the diagnosis of aortic dissection, complications of endocarditis and cardiac source of embolism. TEE is an essential adjunct for guidance during percutaneous and many open cardiac procedures. TEE is a valuable diagnostic modality to determine the etiology of hemodynamic instability in the immediate postoperative setting. TEE is an expensive perioperative program to start and maintain as it requires special equipment and operator expertise.

Current SCA and ASA practice guidelines for perioperative TEE endorse the use of TEE for all cardiac or thoracic aorta surgery patients [7]. These recommendations are based on scientific evidence for clinical decision-making and the effectiveness of echocardiography to influence patient outcome (Table 31.1).

Intraoperative TEE is used for a well-defined indication. By performing a complete study and examining all cardiac structures during the precardiopulmonary bypass (CPB) period the echocardiographer confirms known pathology and identifies any new pathology that may alter the operative procedure. A more limited study in the post-CPB period assesses the adequacy of surgery, ventricular function and the absence of complications that may require further surgical intervention (Table 31.2). The goal of the echocardiographer is to contribute timely information on which the surgeon and anesthesiologist can make informed decisions. TEE is a superior monitor compared to a pulmonary artery catheter to evaluate myocardial ischemia, biventricular func-

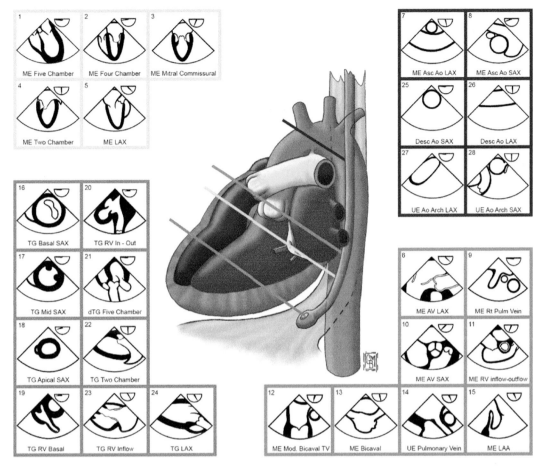

Fig. 31.1 Diagram of ASE 28 Standard TEE Views. Cardiac structures can be grouped together and imaged at three levels: (1) upper esophageal (UE), (2) mid esophageal (ME) and (3) transgastric (TG). In the six UE/ME views the aorta is examined for the presence of aortic pathology such as aneurysms, dissections or atheroma. The 13 ME views can be divided into groups to evaluate (1) the left ventricle (LV) and mitral valve (MV), and (2) the aortic, pulmonic and tricuspid valves and (3) the intra-atrial septum, left atrial appendage and pulmonary veins. Advancing the probe into the stomach attains the nine TG views. The classic doughnut view of the LV is obtained at the base, mid and apical portions of the heart to assess ventricular function. The TG views are also critical for spectral Doppler alignment to measure pressure gradients across the aortic valve and left ventricular outflow tract (LVOT). The right heart is assessed from different ME and TG views. [With permissions from Willa Bradshaw and Gian-Marco Busato]

Table 31.1 Role for perioperative TEE

Preoperative [5]	Intraoperative [6]	Postoperative [6]
• Evaluate	Strongest evidence, TEE useful	• Hemodynamic instability
– Native valve disease	• Valve repairs	• Cardiac tamponade (local)
– Prosthetic valve function	• Congenital heart	• Endocarditis
– Ventricular function	• Obstructive cardiomyopathy	
– Congenital heart disease	• Endocarditis	
• Diagnose	• Aortic dissection	
– Aortic dissection	• Ventricular assist device	
– Endocarditis complications	• Hemodynamic instability	
– Etiology of stroke	• Heart transplantation	

Table 31.2 Intraoperative TEE findings

Procedure	Pre-CPB	Post-CPB
Coronary artery bypass graft	• Ventricular function (regional, global) • Aneurysm • Thrombus • MR	• Ventricular function (regional, global) • Residual MR • Remodel LV
Valve repair	• Valve anatomy • Calcification leaflets, annulus • Regurgitation severity • Chamber size	• Repaired anatomy • Residual regurgitation • New valve stenosis, pressure gradient • Ventricular function • Complications
Valve replacement	• Annulus size • Annular calcification • Lesion severity • Chamber size	• Prosthetic valve function • Pressure gradients • Paravalvular leak • Ventricular function
Congenital heart	• Cardiac anatomy • Shunts • Chamber size • RVSP • Associated anomalies	• Repair anatomy • Residual shunt • Obstructions • Valve insufficiency • Ventricular function
Hypertrophic obstructive cardiomyopathy	• Turbulent LVOT flow • Septal measurements • SAM of anterior leaflet • MR • Pressure gradients (LVOT, intracavitary)	• Laminar LVOT flow • Septal thickness • Residual SAM • Residual MR • Pressure gradients • No VSD, AI
Endocarditis	• Multiple valves • Vegetations • Regurgitation, stenosis • Abscess • Pseudoaneurysm • Fistula	• Repair or replacement • Valve function • Ventricular function • No shunt flow
Aortic pathology	• Atheroma (location, mobility) • Aneurysm (size, location, AI) • Dissection (flap, true/false lumens, AI, pericardial effusion, hemothorax) • Ventricular function	• Atheroma presence • Valve sparing • Valve replacement • Residual flow in lumens • Ventricular function
Ventricular assist device	• RV function • LV thrombus • AI • PFO/ASD	• Cannula location • Cannula flow • Decompression chambers • Residual AI, PFO
Heart transplant	• RVSP • IVC, SVC size	• Ventricular function • Anastomosis sites • PFO
Percutaneous procedures	• Confirm anatomy • Guide wire • Device deployment	• Device function • Ventricular function • Complications
Hemodynamic instability	• Ventricular function • Valve function • Pericardial effusion • Pulmonary embolism • Volume status	

AI aortic insufficiency, *ASD* atrial septal defect, *IVC* inferior vena cava, *LV* left ventricle, *LVOT* left ventricular outflow tract, *MR* mitral regurgitation, *PFO* patent foramen ovale, *RV* right ventricle, *RVSP* right ventricular systolic pressure, *SVC* superior vena cava, *VSD* ventricular septal defect

tion and determine volume status. Despite ubiquitous use neither technology has yet proven to change patient outcome in any large studies.

Contraindications and Complications

Absolute contraindications to TEE include significant pathology of the oropharynx, esophagus or stomach. Epicardial scanning [8] using a standard transthoracic ultrasound probe in a sterile sheath placed directly on the heart permits imaging when the risk of TEE exceeds the benefit. When properly used TEE is safe without serious complications, as reported following 7200 intraoperative TEEs [9].The commonest complication is a sore throat and the most serious is esophageal perforation. Echocardiography requires focused attention to acquire and interpret the images. Distraction from patient care to provide a TEE study during the vulnerable immediate post-CPB period can compromise the patient. Errors of interpretation can expose the patient to the additional risk of too much or not enough surgery or treatments.

Technical limitations to the use of intraoperative TEE include unfavorable lighting conditions, electrical cautery interference and surgical manipulations of the heart. In addition anesthesia alters cardiac loading conditions that affect determination of valvular lesion severity.

Specific Perioperative TEE Applications

Monitoring Myocardial Function

TEE is mainly used during coronary artery bypass grafting (CABG) surgery to examine biventricular function. The right ventricle (RV) and left ventricle (LV) differ in structure and function, as the RV acts as a low pressure reservoir for the LV. For ease of communication the ASE and SCA recommend a 16-segment model [10] to describe the LV, dividing the basal and mid levels each into six segments and the apex

into four. All 16 segments are examined in multiple views of the LV with assessment of overall size, global function, and regional wall motion abnormality (RWMA).

In current clinical practice, analysis of LV segmental function is based on visualization of endocardial motion and/or myocardial thickening of each segment during systole. A qualitative grading scale for wall motion is used: (A) normal segment thickens and moves inward, (B) hypokinetic segment thickens and moves inward less, (C) an akinetic segment does not thicken or move inward and (D) a dyskinetic segment fails to thicken and moves paradoxically outward during systole. Global longitudinal strain as determined by STE can provide a semi-quantitative assessment of RWMA [10].

Visual inspection of wall motion affords a simple expeditious appraisal of global ventricular function but it is imprecise. Quantitative parameters of RV and LV systolic function can be derived from 2D and Doppler images (Table 31.3 and Fig. 31.2).

Most normal values relate to TTE and are assumed to be similar for TEE [10]. Unfortunately most parameters are dynamic and continually change under the influence of anesthesia, load dependency, heart rate and rhythm. Fractional area change (FAC) and fractional shortening (FS) are measures of systolic performance. These are simple convenient techniques that offer semiquantitative information about global ventricular function in the absence of RWMA. Though feasible the calculation of right and left ventricular cardiac output and ejection fraction (EF) is time consuming as it is based on measurements of cardiac volumes. End-diastolic and end-systolic ventricular volumes obtained from 3D datasets or by STE can more accurately determine EF.

Valve Repairs and Replacement

TEE can precisely define valve anatomy (leaflet number, thickening, and calcification), determine the mechanism of valve dysfunction (leaflet mobility) and quantify the severity of the valvular lesion. Significant operator experience and a

Table 31.3 Ventricular systolic indices

Systolic index	Method	Left ventricle		Right ventricle	
		Normal	Abnormal	Normal	Abnormal
Fractional shortening (FS) (m-mode)	$FS = 100 \times \dfrac{(LVIDd - LVIDs)}{LVIDd}$	>26–45% (33 ± 7)	<25%	NA	NA
Fractional area change (FAC) (2D)	$FAC = 100 \times \dfrac{(EDA - ESA)}{EDA}$	>40–60% (57 ± 20)	<40%	>42–56% (49 ± 7)	<35%
Ejection fraction (EF)	$EF = 100 \times \dfrac{(EDV - ESV)}{EDV}$	>55% (62 ± 7)	<55%	>51.5–64.5% (58 ± 6.5)	<45%
Annular plane systolic excursion (MAPSE/TAPSE)	Movement lateral annulus of the TV, MV by m-mode	12 ± 2 mm	<8 mm	21–27 mm (24 ± 3.5)	<17 mm
S′ (TDI)	S′ velocity lateral annulus of the TV, MV	>8 cm/s	<5 cm/s	>9.8–16.4 (14.1 ± 2.3)	<9.5 cm/s
Myocardial performance index (MPI) (by pulsed wave* or TDI**)	$MPI = \dfrac{(ICT \pm IRT)}{ET}$	0.39 ± 0.05	>0.50	0.26 ± 0.085* 0.38 ± 0.08**	> 0.43* >0.54**
dP/dt	MR = 32 mmHg/time TR = 12 mmHg/time	>1200 mmHg/sec	<800 mmHg/sec	>400 mmHg/sec	<400 mmHg/sec
Global longitudinal peak systolic strain (GLPSS)	Speckle tracking echocardiography	> −20 (more negative)	< −20 (more positive)	> −29 ± 4.5 (more negative)	< −20 (more positive)

LVID left ventricle internal diameter in d (diastole) or s (systole), *EDA* end diastolic area, *ESA* end-systolic area, *EDV* end-diastolic volume, *ESV* end systolic volume, *ICF* isovolumic contraction time, *IRT* isovolumic relaxation time, *ET* ejection time, *MR* mitral regurgitation; *MV* mitral valve, *TDI* tissue Doppler imaging, *TR* tricuspid regurgitation, *TV* tricuspid valve
Asterisks relate to the different values depend on method of interrogation pulsed wave or TDI

thorough knowledge of anatomy and pathology are required to establish the correct diagnosis. Detailed anatomic information obtained from 2D and 3D imaging guides the surgeon's choice of valve repair or replacement. Benefits to valvular repair include reduced perioperative morbidity and mortality, no anticoagulation requirement, long-term durability and freedom from reoperation. Determination of valve lesion severity uses multiple parameters and is best done preoperatively under optimal loading conditions [11, 12]. TEE also examines the response of the cardiac chambers to volume or pressure overload, presence of intracardiac thrombus and sites for cannulation.

Mitral Valve (MV)

The MV apparatus is an intricate anatomic structure that for normal function requires the interaction of all the components; leaflets, annulus, chordae, papillary muscles and LV walls. Abnormalities can occur in each portion so precise evaluation directs the surgeon in the options for MV repair or replacement. The use of 3D TEE permits a real-time assessment of dynamic leaflet function in a single screen (Fig. 31.3). Processing of 3D datasets can generate a static or dynamic 3D MV model with a multitude of measurements [13].

Structural (primary) disease of the leaflets and functional (secondary) disease of the MV subvalvular portions can cause varying degrees of valvular stenosis, regurgitation or mixed lesions. Mitral stenosis may occur from rheumatic or calcific disease and typically requires mitral valve replacement (MVR). The mechanism of mitral regurgitation (MR), as classified by Carpentier, is based on mitral leaflet motion with several possible underlying etiologies [12].

- Type 1: Normal motion: dilated cardiomyopathy, perforated leaflet
- Type 2: Excessive motion (prolapse, flail): fibro-elastic, Barlow's
- Type 3: Restrictive motion: (systole and diastole) rheumatic, (systole) ischemic

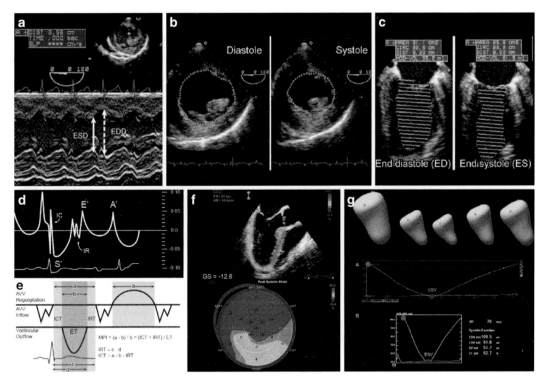

Fig. 31.2 Assessment of LV Function. Left ventricular function can be assessed using different techniques. (**a**) Shortening Fraction estimates systolic function using linear measurements of end-diastolic and end-systolic LV chamber diameters from a TG mid SAX view. (**b**) Fractional Area Change (FAC) measures end-diastolic and end-systolic LV chamber areas from a TG mid SAX view. (**c**) Simpson's Method of *Discs* (MOD) uses mid-esophageal 2 Chamber or 4 Chamber views to trace the endocardium at end-systole and end diastole. Integrated machine software divides the LV into slices to calculate the volume. (**d**) Tissue Doppler Imaging (TDI) of the lateral mitral valve annulus obtained in a mid-esophageal 4 Chamber view is shown, with systolic function related to the S′ wave. (**e**) Myocardial Performance Index (MPI) is measured using spectral Doppler of the aortic outflow and mitral inflow. (**f**) Strain and strain rate can now be easily measured using speckle tracking shown here for a mid-esophageal 2 Chamber view as well as peak systolic strain in a bull's eye format. (**g**) An endocardial cast from a 3D dataset can be analyzed to estimate LV volumes and ejection fraction

Degenerative MV disease from fibroelastic deficiency or myxoid infiltration (Barlow's Disease) is a spectrum of disorders with excessive MV leaflet motion that ranges from billowing, prolapse to flail. The pre-CPB TEE exam determines the scallops involved (single, multiple), mitral annulus size and MR jet direction and severity. The post-CPB TEE exam evaluates residual MR, presence of systolic anterior motion of the anterior mitral valve leaflet and LV function.

Functional MR occurs with structurally normal MV leaflets and often results from incomplete leaflet closure due to annular dilatation from left atrial or LV enlargement or altered LV geometry from RWMA. The fixed leaflet and chordal length restricts leaflet motion causing eccentric MR in the same direction as the tethered leaflet or central MR if both leaflets are affected. Surgery for functional MR is less beneficial and indicated only in the presence of severe MR and/or symptoms refractory to medical management [14].

Aortic Valve (AV)

The aortic root describes the apparatus that supports the AV and comprises the aortic annulus, valve cusps, sinuses of Valsalva, sino-tubular junction (STJ), and the proximal ascending aorta. The left ventricular outflow tract (LVOT) is just

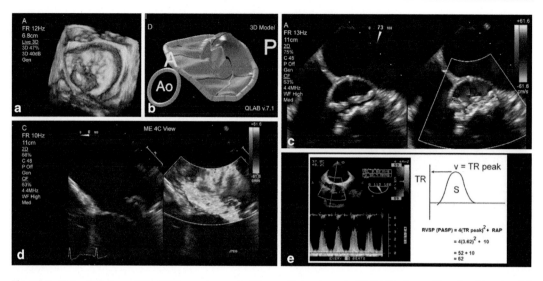

Fig. 31.3 Valve Pathology. Mitral Valve prolapse of a P2 segment from fibro-elastic disease is shown using (**a**) 3D TEE enface view, (**b**) static *MV* model and (**c**) 2D image with color Doppler. (**d**) Bicuspid aortic valve with thickened cusps and minimal systolic flow is shown in a 2D mid-esophageal AV SAX view with color Doppler. (**e**) Tricuspid regurgitation spectral Doppler trace can be used to estimate right ventricular systolic pressure (RVSP) or pulmonary artery systolic pressure (PASP) from the peak velocity and estimate of right atrial pressure (RAP)

inferior to the AV and supports the AV annulus. Analogous to the MV, coordinated interplay of all these components is necessary for optimal valve function.

Aortic stenosis (AS) is the commonest single valve lesion in North America presenting for surgery. The etiology of AS is often from progressive calcification of the AV, a bicuspid valve or less often rheumatic valve disease (Fig. 31.3). Assessment of AS severity is made preoperatively using TTE [11]. The choice of surgical aortic valve replacement (SAVR) or transcatheter aortic valve replacement (TAVR) is based on patient comorbidities, structure of the diseased valve, peripheral vascular access and the amount of coronary artery disease.

The mechanism of aortic insufficiency (AI) can be classified, similar to the MV, according to cusp mobility and guides the surgical intervention [15]:

- Normal: perforation, aortic root (aneurysm, dissection)
- Excessive: prolapse, flail
- Restricted: calcified, rheumatic

The severity of AI is difficult to quantify particularly if an eccentric jet is present [12]. The pre-CPB TEE exam evaluates aortic cusp number and mobility, AI jet direction and severity, and measures the aortic root size. This information helps determine whether the AV can be spared or needs replacement. The post AV sparing TEE exam evaluates aortic root morphology, residual AI, and LV function.

Tricuspid Valve (TV)

The TV is the largest cardiac valve with a structure similar to the MV comprising leaflets, annulus, chordae, papillary muscles and RV walls. Functional (secondary) tricuspid regurgitation (TR) from annular dilatation is much more common than structural (primary) TV disease. Severe TR and/or annular dilatation are indications for TV repair in the setting of left-sided valvular disease [14]. In the absence of RVOT obstruction or pulmonic stenosis, the peak TR pressure when added to the right atrial pressure is an easy non-invasive method to estimate pulmonary artery systolic pressure (Fig. 31.3).

Valve Replacement

Pre-CPB annulus size measurements, presence and location of calcification and involvement of multiple valves guides the surgical management during valve replacement surgery. Post-CPB the prosthetic valve is assessed for adequacy of function, pressure gradients and the presence of paravalvular leak. TEE color Doppler has a high sensitivity for paravalvular leak which must be distinguished from physiologic washing jets present with normally functioning mechanical valves [16]. Small paravalvular leaks frequently improve after protamine administration, while large leaks require re-intervention. High valvular gradients often occur immediately post-CPB from the altered load conditions. Other complications related to valve replacement should be excluded such as worsening of other valve function, ventricular dysfunction (global or regional) and LVOT obstruction. Significant LVOT obstruction can occur with septal hypertrophy and hypovolemia post AVR for AS. Preservation of mitral subvalvular structures and valve struts may obstruct the LVOT post MVR.

Congenital Heart

Practical constraints of TEE probe size limited the early introduction of intraoperative TEE in pediatric congenital cardiac surgery. Smaller TEE probes and epicardial scanning have increased the role of echocardiography during pediatric procedures. Echocardiography can define the congenital lesion, associated anomalies, and the adequacy of corrective or palliative procedures. These are challenging patients to image so combined expertise in echocardiography and congenital heart disease is essential for an accurate assessment.

Simple congenital lesions such as atrial septal defect (ASD), ventricular septal defect (VSD), patent ductus arteriosus, and coarctation can be easily imaged using 2D and color Doppler modes. Complex congenital heart lesions (transposition of the great vessels, tetralogy of Fallot, and uni-chamber hearts) may be uncorrected, palliated or completely corrected and imaging relies on a sequential-segmental approach to look at the arrangement of the atria, ventricles and great vessels. Intraoperative TEE assesses lesion type, shunt direction, chamber size, RV pressures, ventricular function and associated anomalies. Post-

CPB TEE exam determines the adequacy of repair of septal defects and identifies residual shunts, obstructions and valvular insufficiency.

Hypertrophic Obstructive Cardiomyopathy (HOCM)

HOCM is an uncommon but lethal genetic cardiac pathology. Surgical septal myectomy is indicated for severe drug-refractory symptoms or if the mean LVOT pressure gradient is >50 mmHg at rest or with provocation. The echocardiographic findings reveal a dynamic obstruction of the LVOT. The thickened septal ventricular muscle contracts during systole drawing the anterior mitral valve leaflet into the LVOT, referred to as systolic anterior motion (SAM), resulting in turbulent flow in the LVOT and an eccentric posterior directed MR jet.

The pre-CPB TEE exam measures the maximal septal thickness and depth into the LV, SAM-septal contact point and distance from the right coronary cusp, presence of MR and peak LVOT gradient from a dagger shaped continuous wave spectral Doppler trace. Following myectomy the post-CPB TEE exam establishes absence of SAM, presence of laminar LVOT flow, reduction in MR, provoked (post premature ventricular contraction) LVOT peak gradient <20 mmHg and absence of an iatrogenic VSD.

Endocarditis

Based on the Duke criteria, echocardiography is the imaging technique of choice for the diagnosis of endocarditis. Major findings include the presence of vegetations, abscess, new partial dehiscence of a prosthetic valve and new valvular regurgitation, with minor findings of new nodular valve thickening, valve perforations and non-oscillating mass.

TEE has proven sensitive and specific for detecting vegetations on native and prosthetic valves and complications of perivalvular extension such as abscess, pseudoaneurysm or fistula. Echocardiography identifies vegetations as irregular echo dense independently mobile masses and documents the location, number and size. All valves should be examined as multiple valves may be involved. Perivalvular abscess is common in prosthetic valve endocarditis since the sewing ring is the primary site of infection. Prosthetic valve rocking occurs with >40% circumferential ring dehiscence. Intraoperative TEE defines the etiology of valve regurgitation from leaflet/cusp malcoaptation, leaflet perforation, torn chordae, flail cusp or perivalvular leak and evaluates the adequacy of valvular repair or replacement.

Aortic Atheroma

Stroke is one of the most devastating complications of cardiac surgery. While the etiology of stroke in this setting is multi-factorial a major factor is plaque at the site of aortic cannulation. TEE is useful in examining the proximal ascending aorta, arch and descending aorta, though the trachea creates a blind spot in the distal ascending aorta where aortic cannulation commonly occurs. This region is well examined using an epiaortic probe in a sterile sheath placed directly on the ascending aorta to image the aorta in both short axis and long axis [17].

Epiaortic scanning permits precise localization and characterization of plaque within the aorta. An epiaortic study is better than TEE and surgical palpation for identifying aortic plaque. The presence of aortic atheroma allows the surgeon to consider alternative strategies for aortic cannulation. Whether the identification of ascending aortic atheroma and altered surgical technique reduces stroke is yet to be proven.

Aortic Aneurysms and Dissection

Aortic aneurysms are a permanent, localized dilatation of the aorta having a diameter of at least 1.5 times that of the expected normal diameter of a given segment. Determination of aortic size can be made by echocardiography, computerized tomography (CT) or magnetic resonance imaging

(MRI) [18]. Pre-emptive surgery is indicated to prevent rupture of the dilated segment when the size reaches >50 mm.

Acute aortic syndromes occurring from different pathologies such as aortic dissection, intramural hematoma and penetrating ulcer require urgent surgery to prevent lethal consequences. Aortic dissection involves a tear in the intima that allows blood to flow between the intimal and medial/advential layers creating a false lumen. As blood separates these layers, the intima is compressed creating a smaller true lumen.

TEE has evolved to become a diagnostic modality of choice for aortic dissection with a high sensitivity (97%) and specificity (100%). It is widely available and has the advantage of being performed at the patient's bedside without interfering with intensive monitoring or treatment. TEE evaluation of dissection includes identification of the intimal tear origin, dissection extent, perfusion adequacy in the lumens, LV function and the presence of complications. Complications that may be detected using TEE include pericardial effusion, presence and severity of AI and RWMA from coronary artery dissection. The presence of a structurally normal AV may permit a valve sparing procedure with documentation post-CPB of residual AI.

Devices

TEE has become invaluable in the guidance of percutaneous procedures such as device closures (ASD, VSD, left atrial appendage), transcatheter valves and valve repairs. Real-time 3D TEE allows better spatial orientation for positioning of the guide wires and catheters used to safely deploy the device. Adequacy of device function and complications associated with deployment are key ongoing features of TEE assessment.

TEE is also important during implantation of ventricular assist devices (VADs) to identify inter-atrial shunts (PFO, ASD), AI and ventricular thrombus in the pre-CPB period. Cannula position, de-airing, chamber decompression and RV function are examined for in the post-CPB TEE exam.

Hemodynamic Instability

TEE provides essential information in hemodynamically unstable patients in the ICU, recovery room and during noncardiac surgery. While small in sample size most studies show an overall positive impact. Echocardiography can differentiate severe ventricular dysfunction from other life-threatening causes of hypotension related to valvular pathology, pericardial effusion/tamponade and pulmonary embolism. The result of an urgent TEE in the unstable post-cardiac surgery patient is unpredictable but can modify clinical management.

Qualitative TEE estimates ventricular filling and function and directs the administration of fluids, inotropes, and vasopressors. Severe hypovolemia is recognized as a marked decrease in the ventricular end-diastolic area with an increased ejection fraction. Arterial vasodilatation, severe AI or MR and VSD can manifest the same LV filling and ejection pattern but are differentiated by using color Doppler.

References

1. Vegas A, Meineri M. Core review: three-dimensional transesophageal echocardiography is a major advance for intraoperative clinical management of patients undergoing cardiac surgery: a core review. Anesth Analg. 2010;110(6):1548–73.
2. Jerath A, Vegas A, Meineri M, Silversides C, Feindel C, Beattie S, et al. An interactive online 3D model of the heart to assist in learning the 20 standard TEE views. Can J Anesth. 2011;58(1):14–21.
3. Shanewise JS, Cheung AT, Aronson S, Stewart WJ, Weiss RI, Mark JB, et al. ASE/SCA guidelines for performing a comprehensive intraoperative multiplane transesophageal echocardiographic examination: recommendations of the American Society of Echocardiography Council on Intraoperative Echocardiography Board and the Society of Cardiovascular Anesthesiologists Task Force for certification in perioperative transesophageal echocardiography. Anesth Analg. 1999;89:870–84.
4. Hahn R, Abraham T, Adams MS, Bruce CJ, Glas KE, Lang RM, et al. Guidelines for performing a comprehensive transesophageal echocardiographic examination: recommendations from the American Society of Echocardiography and the Society of Cardiovascular Anesthesia. J Am Soc Echocardiogr. 2013;26:921–64.
5. Lang RM, Badano LP, Tsang W, Adams DH, Agricola E, Buck T, et al. EAE/ASE recommendations for image acquisition and display using three-dimensional echocardiography. J Am Soc Echocardiogr. 2012;25(1):3–46.
6. Douglas PS, Garcia MJ, Haines DE, Lai WW, Manning WJ, Patel AR, et al. ACCF/ASE/AHA/ASNC/HFSA/HRS/SCAI/SCCM/SCCT/SCMR 2011 appropriate use criteria for echocardiography. J Am Soc Echocardiogr. 2011;24:229–67.
7. American Society of Anesthesiologists and the Society of Cardiovascular Anesthesiologists. Practice guidelines for perioperative transesophageal echocardiography. An updated report by the American Society of Anesthesiologists and the Society of Cardiovascular Anesthesiologists Task Force on Transesophageal Echocardiography. Anesthesiology. 2010;112:1084–96.
8. Reeves ST, Glas KE, Eltzschig H, Mathew JP, Rubenson DS, Hartman GS, et al. Guidelines for performing a comprehensive epicardial echocardiography examination: recommendations of the American Society of Echocardiography and the Society of Cardiovascular Anesthesiologists. J Am Soc Echocardiogr. 2007;20(4):427–37.
9. Kallmeyer IJ, Collard CD, Fox JA, Body SC, Sherman SK. The safety of intraoperative transesophageal echocardiography: a case series of 7200 cardiac surgical patients. Anesth Analg. 2001;92:1126–30.
10. Lang RM, Badano LP, Mor-Avi V, Afilalo J, Armstrong A, Ernande L, et al. Recommendations for cardiac chamber quantification by echocardiography in adults: an update from the American Society of Echocardiography and the European Association of Cardiovascular Imaging. J Am Soc Echocardiogr. 2015;28:1–39.
11. Baumgartner H, Hung J, Bermejo J, Chambers JG, Evangelista A, Griffin BP, et al. Echocardiographic assessment of valve stenosis: EAE/ASE recommendations for clinical practice. J Am Soc Echocardiogr. 2009;22:1–23.
12. Zoghbi WA, Adams D, Bonow RO, Enriquez-Sarano M, Foster E, Grayburn PA, et al. Recommendations for noninvasive evaluation native valvular regurgitation: a report from the American Society of Echocardiography developed in collaboration with the Society Cardiovascular Magnetic Resonance. J Am Soc Echocardiogr. 2017;30:303–71.
13. Mahmood F, Matyal R. A quantitative approach to the intraoperative echocardiographic assessment of the mitral valve for repair. Anesth Analg. 2015;121:34–58.
14. Nishimura RA, Otto CM, Bonow RO, Carabello BA, Erwin JP, Guyton RA, et al. AHA/ACC guideline for the management of patients with valvular heart disease: executive summary: a report of the American College of Cardiology/American Heart Association Task Force on Practice Guidelines. Circulation. 2014;63(22):e57–188.

15. El Khoury G, Glineur D, Rubay J, Verhelst R, d'Acoz Y, Poncelet A, et al. Functional classification of aortic root/valve abnormalities and their correlation with etiologies and surgical procedures. Curr Opin Cardiol. 2005;20(2):115–21.
16. Zoghbi WA, Chambers JB, Dumesnil JG, Foster E, Gottdiener JS, Grayburn PA, et al. Recommendations for evaluation of prosthetic valves with echocardiography and Doppler ultrasound: a report from the ASE Guidelines and Standards Committee and the Task Force on Prosthetic Valves. J Am Soc Echocardiogr. 2009;22(9):975–1014.
17. Glas KE, Swaminathan M, Reeves ST, Shanewise JS, Rubenson D, Smith PK, et al. Guidelines for the performance of a comprehensive intraoperative epiaortic ultrasonographic examination. Recommendations of the American Society of Echocardiography and the Society of Cardiovascular Anesthesiologists; Endorsed by the Society of Thoracic Surgeons. J Am Soc Echocardiogr. 2007;20:1227–35.
18. Goldstein SA, Evangelista A, Abbara S, Arai A, Asch FM, Badano LP, et al. Multimodality imaging of diseases of the thoracic aorta in adults: from the American Society of Echocardiography and the European Association of Cardiovascular Imaging Endorsed by the Society of Cardiovascular Computed Tomography and Society for Cardiovascular Magnetic Resonance. J Am Soc Echocardiogr. 2015;28:119–82.

Echocardiography for Structural Heart Disease Procedures

32

Stanton K. Shernan

Main Messages

1. In patients undergoing transcatheter aortic valve replacement (TAVR), the use of three-dimensional echocardiography may enable a more accurate estimation of calculated native and prosthetic aortic area when relying on the commonly used continuity equation. Measuring the heights of both coronary ostia, determining positioning the TAVR within the landing zone, evaluating the extent of calcification in the vicinity of valve deployment area and diagnosing post-deployment complications including residual aortic insufficiency, are all important objectives for the comprehensive periprocedural echocardiographic examination.

2. In patients undergoing MitraClip procedures, the optimal morphological characterizations of the mitral valve (MV) include mitral regurgitation originating from the mid-portion (A2–P2 region); minimal calcification within the intended grasping area of the leaflet; MV area > 4 cm^2; a posterior leaflet length > 10 mm; flail width < 15 mm; flail gap <10 mm; gap between leaflets <2 mm; leaflet coaptation depth < 11 mm and leaflet coaptation length > 2 mm.

3. Following MitraClip placement, an echocardiographic examination should be performed to determine the degree of residual mitral regurgitation which should not greater than 1–2+; the absence of significant mitral stenosis usually defined by a mean trans-mitral gradient >5 mmHG, and the anatomical and functional combined area from both orifices, which should be no less than 1.5 cm^2 but ideally >2–2.5 cm^2.

4. For patients undergoing percutaneous approaches towards perivalvular leak (PVL) occlusion, cut off values for mild, moderate, and severe PVL are $<10\%$, 10% -20%, and $> 20\%$ of the sewing ring circumference respectively. However, this technique may result in an underestimation of PVL when a jet does not occupy a large circumferential extent, but has a greater radial width. Furthermore, while the summation of the circumferential extent of multiple

S. K. Shernan (✉)
Brigham and Women's Hospital, Harvard Medical School, Boston, MA, USA
e-mail: sshernan@partners.org

simultaneous non-contiguous regurgitant jets to obtain a single PVL severity grade may be intuitive, this approach has not been formally validated.

5. For patients undergoing left atrial appendage (LAA) occlusion, periprocedural echocardiography should be used to ensure accurate device sizing and ostial occlusion by determining the general shape of the LAA using multiplane transesophageal echocardiography imaging at 0°, 45°, 90° and 135° rotational angles. For the Watchman LAA occluder device, the landing zone measurement is obtained from the inferior rim of the LAA ostium at the level of the circumflex coronary artery, to a point 1–2 cm distal to the tip of the left upper pulmonary vein rim. The LAA depth is measured orthogonal to this measurement.

The evolutionary trajectory of echocardiography technology from its initial description by Edler and Hertz in 1953 to current three-dimensional (3D) matrix array displays, has been extraordinary [1]. Along with technical complexity, the diversity of clinical application for the use of echocardiography has also continued to expand. Once used primarily as a diagnostic tool for ambulatory populations, echocardiography has become a fundamental monitor of cardiac performance in the intraoperative environment for surgical patients with cardiovascular disease. In addition TEE and transthoracic echocardiography (TTE) are currently used preoperatively to risk-stratify and triage patients for optimal perioperative care, as well as postoperatively in hemodynamically unstable patients in the critical care setting. While fluoroscopy remains the traditional imaging technique for interventional cardiology procedures, significant radiation exposure and the requirement for intravenous contrast to visualize soft tissue structures remain limiting features. Consequently, echocardiography has also become at least a complimentary, if not a

standard imaging modality to guide interventional cardiology procedures for structural heart disease, thus elevating the role of the echo-anesthesiologist as a co-proceduralist and an even more critical member of the structural heart disease team. The number of structural heart disease procedures in which echocardiography may have clinical utility has been expanding exponentially. This chapter will focus specifically on the primary principles and practical applications of echocardiographic imaging in patients undergoing transcatheter aortic valve replacement (TAVR), the MitraClip, perivalvular leaks and the Watchman as a left atrial appendage occlusion device.

TAVR

The percutaneous placement of a bovine pericardial bioprosthesis mounted within a stainless steel balloon-expandable stent was first described in 2002 by Cribier et al., following successful implantation in a patient with severe aortic stenosis (AS), who presented in cardiogenic shock [1–3]. Since this historic event, the transcatheter aortic valve replacement (TAVR) approach has revolutionized the treatment of severe AS. Over 26,000 TAVRs in more than 350 centers were performed in the US between 2012 and 2014, and well over 200,000 have been performed worldwide [4]. While this interventional approach was initially introduced as an alternative to conventional surgical AVR (SAVR) for management of inoperable patients, the number of TAVRs is expected to grow in the US and Europe as indications expand [5–7]. The American Heart Association/American College of Cardiology recommended TAVR as a Class I indication for inoperable patients, and as a Class IIa indication in patients who are operative candidates, but are at high-risk for mortality and complications after SAVR [8]. Recent data from the PARTNER-2A randomized clinical trial has demonstrated lower stroke and mortality rates for TAVR leading to FDA approval for even intermediate-risk patients [5]. Thus, the technical development and familiarity with the TAVR approach has enabled this technique to become safe and cost effective, and in several studies an equivalent, if not better option compared to SAVR for high risk, intermediate risk and perhaps even low risk patients with AS [9]. This may be especially relevant since complications are declining and outcomes are improving following TAVR, whereas medically managed patients have a one year mortality of 51% and an average survival of only 1.8 years [5].

While the number of patients who have received TAVR globally has increased significantly over the past several years, a number of changes in valve and transcatheter delivery system technology along with increasing familiarity of the patient population has enabled significant changes in both the interventional technique and periprocedural management. Initially established as a transfemoral technique, higher risk patients may require novel approaches via trans-subclavian, trans-apical and even trans-caval techniques. In addition, while general anesthesia and invasive monitoring was used primarily during the early introductory phases of TAVR, monitored anesthetic techniques using short acting intravenous agents have become routine for this procedure in Europe, and are gradually becoming more popular in the US. Similarly while intraprocedural fluoroscopy remains the standard imaging device for TAVR, the use of TEE as a diagnostic tool for cardiac disease and complications, as a monitor of cardiac performance and as an imaging device to help navigate valve deployment, is rapidly becoming replaced by preoperative CT scan screening and post deployment transthoracic echocardiography (TTE). Nonetheless, some patients in whom CT imagery is inadequate, and in those with chronic renal insufficiency who cannot tolerate large volumes of contrast, and even many high-risk patients may still benefit from intraprocedural TEE. Furthermore, the use of general anesthesia and TEE are still used routinely in the majority of US sites [10]. Thus, it is still important for the anesthesiologist who is responsible for the care of TAVR patients to have a fundamental understanding of the utility of TEE for this procedure.

The intra-procedural use of TEE for patients undergoing TAVR procedures primarily focuses on assessing aortic valve (AV) pathology and collateral structures to either validate pre-procedural CT and echocardiography findings, or as the initial comprehensive imaging modality if this information is incomplete or not available. Determining the severity of AS and any concurrent aortic insufficiency is important. The anatomy of the AV should also be defined including the number of cusps as well as the presence and location of any calcium, which has been shown to correlate with post-TAVR deployment and perivalvular leaks (PVL). The measurement of the AV annulus, along with the Sinus of Valsalva and sinotubular junction diameters may be valuable for determining TAVR sizing. Furthermore, the identification of significant atheroma in the thoracic aorta, arch and ascending aorta may also be important as its presence may complicate a transfemoral catheter-based technique, and therefore warrant consideration for a different approach for TAVR delivery. While all of this information is now almost routinely determined by the pre-procedure CT scan, TEE may be required if this data is not available.

The rapid expansion of TAVR procedures along with the use of TEE for these interventions has enabled an increased understanding of aortic root geometry. Once thought of as a symmetrical circle, 3D echocardiography has demonstrated that the surgical aortic annulus is often elliptical in shape (Fig. 32.1) thus enabling more accurate sizing of the native annular and prosthetic valve [11].

Similarly, the left ventricular outflow tract has been shown with 3D echocardiography to often be a larger elliptical, rather than a smaller circular shape. Thus, compared to 2D echocardiography, the use of 3D echocardiography may enable a more accurate estimation of calculated native and prosthetic AV area when relying on the commonly used continuity equation [12]. It may also be important to determine the heights of both coronary ostia, which should ideally be at least 11–14 mm relative to the basilar attachment of the leaflet at the annulus, to avoid obstruction by the native leaflets following prosthetic valve deployment. Concern for this potential complica-

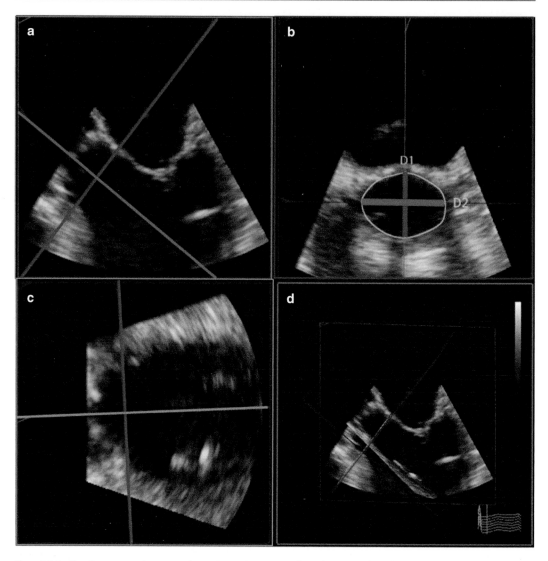

Fig. 32.1 Quad screen demonstrating three two-dimensional (*2D*) image planes (**a**, **b**, **c**) obtained from an original 3D data set (D) of the aortic valve (AV) and the base of the heart. (**a**) Sagittal multiplanar transection representing a long axis view. (**b**) Coronal multiplanar transection demonstrating the elliptical shape of the AV annulus. (**c**) Long axis multiplanar transection orthogonally oriented to the image plane shown in the (**a**) quadrant. (**d**). Three-dimensional composite of the three multiplanar transections shown in quadrants **a**, **b** and **c**

tion even when determined by pre-procedure CT scan may warrant the use of TEE during the procedure to assist both with TAVR deployment and the diagnosis of an obstructed coronary ostium. In rare circumstances, the placement of a prophylactic stent may be required to protect the coronary ostia from obstruction. Furthermore, the initial intra-procedural TEE exam should include a comprehensive evaluation of commonly observed concurrent pathology including mitral or tricuspid regurgitation and any global or regional impairment of either ventricle. Finally, a comprehensive TEE exam should include an investigation of the cardiac apex for visibility and pathology if an alternative transapical access site is being considered.

Continuation of the intraprocedural TEE examination follows the sequence of procedural

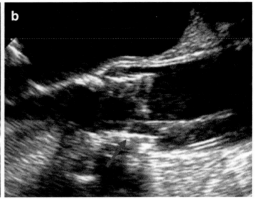

Fig. 32.2 Transesophageal echocardiographic mid-esophageal aortic valve long axis views during TAVR. (**a**) Intravalvular balloon inflation (yellow arrow) during TAVR deployment. (**b**) Deployed TAVR (red arrow) positioned within the native aortic valve apparatus

steps. A thorough evaluation of the guide wire, introduction of the delivery catheter and device placement is important to rule out initial injury to the thoracic aorta and aortic root structures. In addition, transapical TAVR approaches may result in injury to the mitral subvalvular apparatus. The use of TEE may also serve as a useful complimentary tool to fluoroscopic guidance for facilitating the positioning and orientation of the prosthetic valve prior to final deployment. (Fig. 32.2).

Familiarity with the normal echocardiographic appearance of different prosthetic devices and deployment techniques is important. The two most common generation valve systems approved for use in the US are the Sapien 3 (Edwards Lifescience, Irvine, CA) and the CoreValve Evolut-R (Medtronic, Minneapolis, MN). Both valve systems have been associated with favorable outcomes, however their design differences have clinical implications [13]. The Sapien valve is a *balloon-expandable* device which requires rapid ventricular pacing at the time of deployment to minimize arterial pulse pressure and transaortic flow, thus helping to reduce antero-grade or retrograde migration or even embolization. The CoreValve is *self-expanding* and does not require pacing since it is gradually released and deployed into position. However, its longer profile has been associated with a greater

risk of requiring at least temporary periproce-dural pacing. While the intention during rapid pacing is to reduce the blood pressure to mini-mize cardiac stress during valvuloplasty, some patients with ventricular dysfunction may remain hypotensive during the recovery phase. In addi-tion, emboli may be released into the coronaries or systemically during valvuloplasty or deploy-ment resulting in significant hemodynamic and/ or neurological instability. Consequently, resus-citative medications, pacing and even cardiopul-monary bypass (CPB) may be necessary. The etiology of diminished cardiac performance asso-ciated with a persistent need for pharmacological hemodynamic support following valve deploy-ment should be evaluated with TEE or TTE and communicated to the remainder of the structural heart team members to coordinate the most effec-tive treatment.

Following TAVR deployment, a comprehen-sive assessment of persistent complications is critical including documenting the abnormal movement or actual anterograde or retrograde embolization of the prosthetic valve emboliza-tion, the presence of a pericardial effusion, and both regional and global ventricular function. Persistent regurgitation following TAVR is not uncommon. Central leaks are frequently observed at least initially and are often benign (Fig. 32.3).

Fig. 32.3
Transesophageal echocardiographic mid-esophageal aortic valve long axis views demonstrating a mild central leak (red arrow) following TAVR deployment

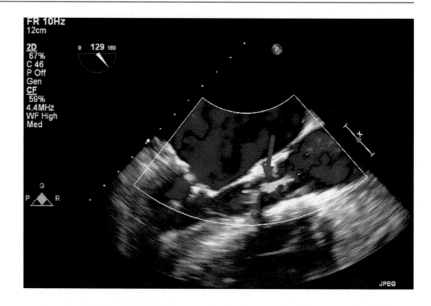

Fig. 32.4
Transesophageal echocardiographic mid-esophageal aortic valve long axis views demonstrating a mild-moderate perivalvular leak (white arrow) following TAVR deployment

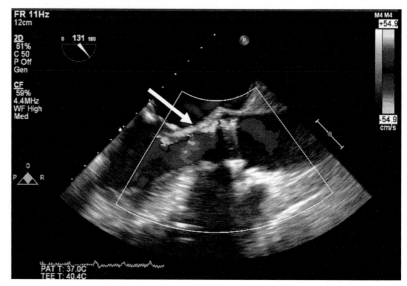

However, prosthetic leaflet injury may occur and require additional ballooning or even the placement of a second prosthetic valve. Perivalvular leaks (PVL) have also received significant attention since larger ones have been associated with increased post-procedural morbidity [14] (Fig. 32.4). The diagnosis should therefore include both the location and sizing for severity. Treatment may also include attempts to reduce the size of larger leaks either by additional balloon expansion of the device or the use of TEE-guided placement of an occluder [15].

MitraClip

Degenerative mitral valve disease (DMVD) is the most common form of organic mitral valve (MV) pathology in the US with an estimated incidence of 2–4% impacting over 150 million people worldwide [16]. Most afflicted patients remain asymptomatic, however 5–10% progress to severe mitral regurgitation (MR) with a one year mortality of 6–7% [16]. While annuloplasty repair and valve replacement have remained the mainstay surgical approaches for the invasive management of DMVD over the last several decades, a large number and variety of transcatheter devices for the minimally invasive management of MV disease are currently under investigation [17]. However, the only transcatheter device currently approved for this indication in the US is the Mitraclip (Abbott) which enables an edge-to-edge leaflet approximation and repair via a trans-atrial septum approach (Fig. 32.4). The outcomes in patients with DMVD who have received this device worldwide appear to be favorable for improved MR severity grade, LV geometry, NYHA classification and hospital readmission [18]. Experience with the MitraClip in patients with functional MR (FMR) has been less extensive.

The role of periprocedural echocardiography for the MitraClip can be divided into three main categories: 1) patient selection; 2) interventional guidance and 3) post-MitraClip deployment evaluation. The initial echocardiographic evaluation for patient selection involves the identification and confirmation of MR etiology, mechanism, severity grading and overall suitability for MitraClip placement. The MitraClip has been used worldwide for patients with DMVD and more recently for FMR [19]. Echocardiographic grading of MR severity for MitraClip patients can be achieved using current guidelines recommendations [20]. The optimal morphological characterization of the MV which is most responsive to MitraClip intervention displays several important characteristics [21, 22]. While it should be understood that all ideal characteristics of the MV are unlikely to be encountered in every case, the optimal patient displays MR originating from the mid-portion (A2–P2 region) where primary chordae tendinae usually do not exist, thus minimizing the chances of entanglement and potential

interference with MitraClip placement. Calcification in the intended grasping area of the leaflet should also be minimal to non-existent. Consequently, patients with rheumatic heart disease, endocarditis, and perforations of clefts are generally not optimal MitralClip candidates. Ideally, the MV area should be >4 cm^2; a posterior leaflet length > 10 mm to enable closure with minimal leaflet stress; flail width < 15 mm; flail gap <10 mm; gap between leaflets <2 mm; leaflet coaptation depth < 11 mm and leaflet coaptation length > 2 mm [21]. Patients with FMR and significant pulmonary hypertension may also experience increased post-procedural morbidity [23]. With increased experience of the procedural team, these criteria may be less restrictive as commissural lesions, tethered leaflets characteristic of FMR valves, small amounts of calcium, and even clefts may be manageable using the MitralClip technique.

Although fluoroscopy remains an important imaging tool for the MitraClip procedure, complimentary interventional guidance by 2D and 3D TEE is still a standard. However, the use of echocardiography during a MitraClip procedure can be extremely challenging, and requires advanced 2D and 3D technical skills for acquiring images as well as a comprehensive understanding of MV anatomy, dynamic geometry and physiology. In addition, a thorough understanding of the MitralClip technology and procedure steps, as well as vigilance and excellent communication skills are essential assets for the anesthesiologist and echocardiographer. Following the initial exam to confirm patient eligibility, collateral pathology including the presence of other valve lesions (i.e. tricuspid regurgitation, AS), any changes from pre-procedural imaging data, measures of regional and global ventricular performance and the presence of any pericardial effusions, the next step is to delineate the inter-atrial septum (IAS) and to identify an optimal transseptal puncture site. (Fig. 32.5).

The usual desired transseptal crossing site is at a superior-posterior entry, but will depend on

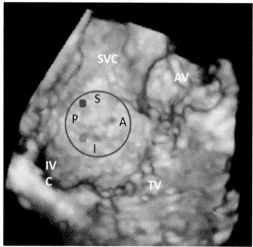 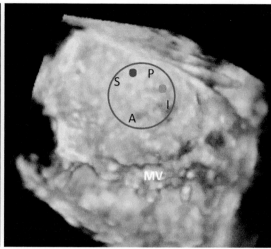

Fig. 32.5 Three-dimensional transesophageal echocardiographic views of the intra-atrial septum (IAS). Left Panel. Three-dimensional transesophageal echocardiographic (TEE) view from the right atrial perspective demonstrating the superior (S), Inferior (I), Anterior (A) and Posterior (P) rims of the IAS. Right Panel. Three-dimensional TEE view from the left atrial perspective demonstrating the superior (S), Inferior (I), Anterior (A) and Posterior (P) rims of the IAS. The RED DOT represents the ideal transseptal atriotomy access site (Superior-Posterior) for a MitraClip procedure. The GREEN DOT represents the ideal transseptal atriotomy access site (Inferior-Posterior) for a Watchman left atrial appendage occlusion procedure. *AV* Aortic valve, *TV* tricuspid valve, *MV* Mitral valve, *IVC* Inferior vena cava, *SVC* Superior vena cava

Fig. 32.6 Orthogonal 2D x-plane images of the intra-atrial septum (IAS) showing the ideal Superior(S)-Posterior(P) trans-septal atriotomy access site demonstrated by the yellow arrows for a MitraClip procedure. Left Panel: Superior and inferior (I) rims of the IAS shown in the bicaval view. Right Panel: IAS shown from an orthogonal perspective to the plane in the Left Panel. *AoR* Aortic root, *LA* Left atrium, *RA* Right atrium, *SVC* Superior vena cava, *A* Anterior

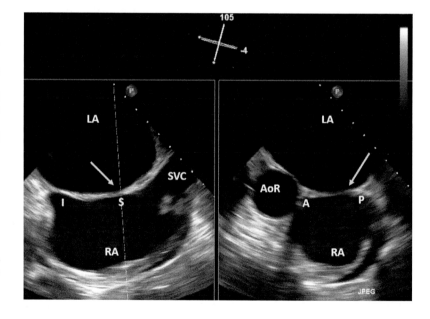

the site of MV pathology as more medial lesions require a more inferior transseptal crossing site to obtain greater height. Slight adjustments in the superior-posterior direction may be necessary depending upon the intended corresponding medial or lateral position of the first clip [21, 24]. An anterior entry site should be avoided in order to enable an ideal parallel orientation of the catheter delivery system to the MV coaptation line. In addition, the IAS puncture site should be targeted approximately 4–5 cm above the annular plane for DMVD patients but slightly more posteriorly, and only 3–4 cm for FMR patients to account for the apical tethering of the coaptation point below the annular plane [21]. Insertion through an atrial septal aneurysm, patient foramen ovale, or atrial septal defect should be avoided. An x-plane TEE view demonstrating both a mid-esophageal bicaval view to display a superior-inferior plane, and a simultaneous orthogonal anterior-posterior plane is often used to establish the optimal site of IAS crossing (Fig. 32.6).

Following needle puncture and dilation, the steerable guide catheter is inserted across the IAS and advanced towards the direction of the left pulmonary veins. The clip delivery system is then advanced under TEE and fluoroscopic guidance taking care not to perforate the left atrium while the clip is steered toward a position hovering in the left atrium above the site of the greatest excessive leaflet motion and MR severity. The clip is then rotated usually under 3D TEE guidance to an orientation which is perpendicular to the coaptation line to minimize engagement with any chordae tendinae in the vicinity (Fig. 32.7).

Confirmation should be pursued using an x-plane format displaying both a mid-esophageal mitral commissural view in which the clip arms should not be visible, and a simultaneous orthogonal long axis view in which the clips arms should be demonstrated at equal lengths if the clip is truly perpendicular to the coaptation line (Fig. 32.8).

While the most eligible DMVD patients present with A2/P2 disease and therefore the absence of chords or decreased chordal density in this area, experienced interventionalists can successfully place clips at more lateral and medial positions, although greater degrees of TEE expertise and guidance may be required to prevent clip entanglement. Visualizing the clip as it is subsequently advanced into the left ventricle may require lowering the gain of the 3D TEE en face image of the MV to enable the best visualization and guidance. Once initially positioned, it is very important to confirm with TEE that both the anterior and posterior leaflet tips at the site of malcoaptation are directly interfacing with the landing zone of each clip arm. A grasping trial can then be performed followed by an evaluation with 2D and 3D grey scale for clip placement, leaflet insertion and motion followed by 2D and 3D color flow Doppler to assess for residual MR which should not greater than 1–2+. Mitral stenosis usually defined by a mean trans-mitral gradient >5 mmHG, should also be assessed by spectral Doppler [25, 26]. Either orifice of the

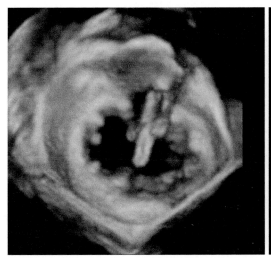
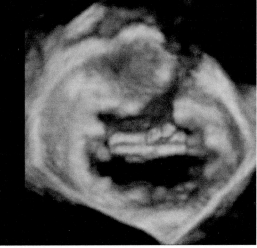

Fig. 32.7 Three-dimensional transesophageal echocardiographic image from the left atrial perspective. Left Panel: Correct positioning of the MitralClip which is perpendicular to the mitral valve coaptation line. Right Panel: Incorrect orientation of the MitraClip when it is oriented parallel to the mitral valve coaptation line

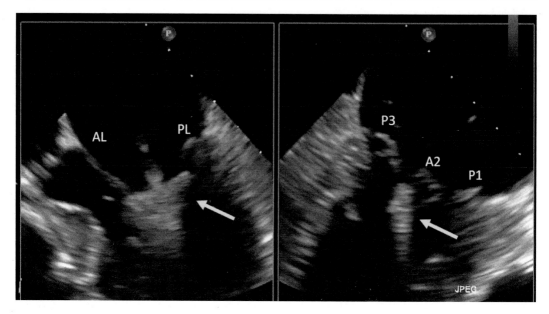

Fig. 32.8 Orthogonal two-dimensional x-plane images of a correctly oriented MitraClip advanced below the mitral leaflet tips. Left Panel: Anterior-posterior orientation demonstrating both arms of the MitraClip below the anterior (AL) and posterior (PL) mitral valve leaflets. Right Panel: Orthogonal view to the image in the Left Panel showing the MitraClip just below the mitral leaflet coaptation line. P1: Lateral scallop of the posterior mitral valve leaflet; P3: Medial scallop of the posterior mitral valve leaflet; A2: Middel scallop of the anterior mitral valve leaflet

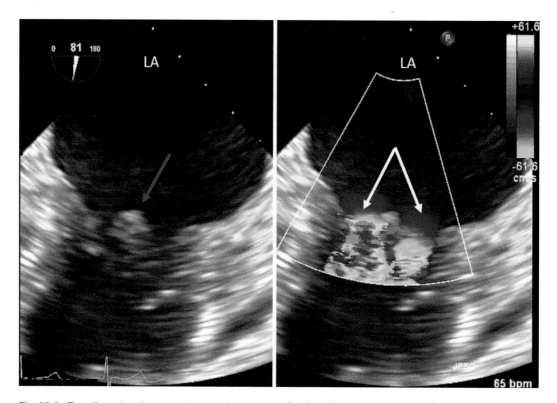

Fig. 32.9 Two-dimensional transesophageal echocardiographic mid-esophageal mid-commissural images of the mitral valve following a MitraClip (red arrow) procedure showing the grey-scale (Left Panel) and color flow Doppler images (Right Panel) of the double orifice (white arrows) during diastole

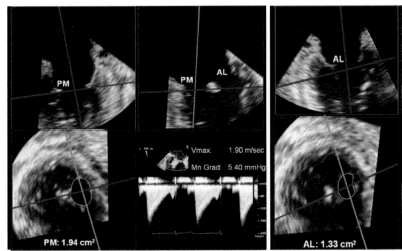

Fig. 32.10 Mitral valve double orifices created after a MitraClip procedure shown in quad screen displays acquired from *3D* data sets. Left Panel: Measurements of the posterior medial (PM) orifice area (lower left) and transvalvular pressure gradient (lower right). Right Panel: Measurements of the anterior lateral (AL) orifice area (lower left) and transvalvular pressure gradient (lower right). Note that despite the asymmetry, the PM and AL orifice areas (1.94 cm^2 vs. 1.33 cm^2) and the difference between mean pressure gradients (Mn Grad: 5.4 mmHg vs. 4.90 mmHg) are not clinically significant. Vmax: maximum trans-orifice velocity

resulting double-orifice can be evaluated by continuous wave Doppler since the actual pressure gradient should be independent of orifice size even if asymmetric (Fig. 32.9) [27].

Anatomical and functional combined area from both orifices should be measured using 3D TEE using a target of no less than 1.5 cm^2 [28] but ideally >2–2.5 cm^2 [29] (Fig. 32.10).

If the results are not acceptable, the arms of the MitraClip can be re-opened and the clip repositioned before it is released. Alternatively, unless there is evidence of mitral stenosis (MS), a second or even third clip can be placed at the site of residual regurgitation and the process is repeated until an acceptable result is achieved. Re-evaluation for residual regurgitation or stenosis should also be performed after each clip is deployed as the tension created by the delivery system can distort the functional geometry of the mitral apparatus prior to release. Finally, a focused TEE exam should include a comprehensive evaluation for any complications including regional or global changes in ventricular function, injury to left atrial or collateral structures including a pericardial effusion associated with delivery system penetration, and significant inter-atrial shunt due to the iatrogenic IAS puncture which may present as refractory hypoxemia and require closure.

Perivalvular Leaks

Perivalvular leaks represent pathological regurgitation originating outside of a prosthetic valve ring usually due to incomplete apposition against the native annulus. The incidence of PVLs range from 2–17% and are more common following MV replacement (7–17%) compared to AV replacement (2–10%) [30]. The longer term postoperative incidence may be even higher [31]. The mechanism of PVL can vary depending upon the timing of presentation. Early PVLs often present in the operating room and are usually directly related to the surgical technique. PVLs which manifest later following surgery may result from suture dehiscence or infection. Risk factors for the development of PVLs include use of biological valves, prolonged CPB time, preoperative atrial fibrillation, significant annular calcification, re-operation and the use of a TAVR technique [32, 33]. Although most PVLs do not have to be repaired, approximately 1.5% present with significant signs or symptoms of significant congestive heart failure or concerns for actual dehiscence usually require an interventional procedure [34, 35]. Early intervention may be required in up to 6% of patients experiencing an inadequate valve repair or greater than mild PVL, although most smaller PVLs with a vena contracta width < 0.3 cm are usually hemodynamically insignificant and present with minimal to no additional risk [34, 35]. PVLs may also be associated with atrial fibrillation, sepsis, increased transfusion requirements in the presence of hemolytic anemia due to turbulence, and increased ICU and overall hospital length of stay [31, 36]. The decision to return to CPB should take into consideration the risk of a prolonged aortic cross clamping and surgery. In higher risk patients, a consideration for percutaneous closure may be warranted. Percutaneous closure of PVL has been reported to be successful in 60–90% of cases, which may be desirable given a reported 16% mortality incidence in patients requiring re-operations for PVL [37].

The intraoperative TEE examination for a patient undergoing a PVL closure should initially be targeted towards determining the location and severity of the regurgitant jet(s). Regarding the former, it is critical to differentiate a central leak within the prosthetic ring from a true PVL (Fig. 32.11).

Trace or mild regurgitant jets are commonly visualized emanating from the central point of leaflet coaptation or occasionally at the commissures of prosthetic valves. Alternatively, mechanical valves often exhibit normal closing jets which represent transient transvalvular flow just prior to valve closure. Mechanical valves may also display washing jets at the juncture of the valve occluders or between an occluder and the valve housing. Washing jets are enabled by the mechanical valve manufacturers to attenuate thrombus formation on the underside of the valve, and are usually centrally directed although the number and jet direction can vary significantly depending upon the flow dynamics of the prosthetic valve. Abnormal intravalvular jets may also occur at the site of sutures and usually resolve following protamine administration, while more serious central leaks may be generated by obstruction of the valve due to sutures, debris, calcium, and the subvalvular apparatus. [38] Determining the specific location of the jet is also important especially if a surgical repair is anticipated as the surgeon may not be able to visualize a physiological hole during CPB in the absence of normal transvalvular pressures in the unloaded ventricle. The location of MVR PVLs can be described according to its position relative to native anterior and posterior leaflet scallops using CFD in multiple mid-esophageal 2D views. Attempting to image AVR PVLs in a mid-

Fig. 32.11 Mid-esophageal short axis view of a TAVR showing a central leak (red arrow) and a perivalvular leak (white arrow)

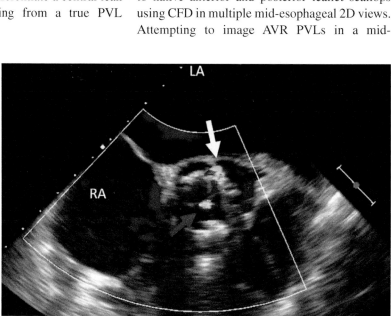

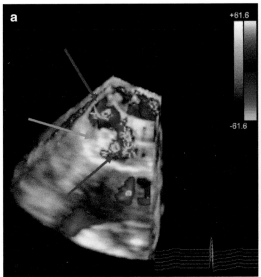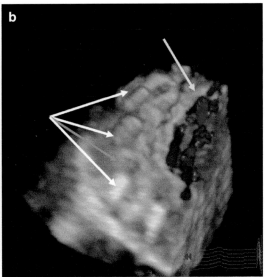

Fig. 32.12 Three dimensional transesophageal echocardiographic views of a transcatheter approach to occluding a perivalvular leak of a bi-leaflet mechanical prosthetic mitral valve. Left Panel: Perivalvular leak (red arrows) on either side of a single occluder device (green arrow).

Right Panel: Following the placement of three additional occluder devices (white arrows), the perivalvular leak is eliminated. Normal washing jets of a bi-leaflet mechanical valve are also demonstrated (yellow arrow)

esophageal AV long axis view may be difficult due to jets being obscured by drop out associated with the prosthetic ring. Thus, the location of AVR PVLs may be best determined from the mid-esophageal AV short axis and deep transgastric long-axis view, and should be described according to its position relative to the native right, left and non-coronary cusps. During an attempt at PVL occlusion using a percutaneous approach in a beating heart, 2D with and without CFD may be adequate, although continuous real-time 3D CFD imaging remains a critical imaging tool to compliment fluoroscopic guidance and may provide a more efficient way of both locating PVLs and effectively communicating this important information to the surgeon or interventionalist (Fig. 32.12).

Following TAVR, PVLs may occur in up to 70% of cases. More severe leaks have been associated with increased 30-day and one year mortality [39, 40]. Thus, expertise determining the presence and location of PVLs remains an important skill.

Accurate grading of PVL severity is necessary since trace and even mild regurgitation often does not have to be addressed. Doppler techniques may be used to evaluate regurgitant volumes, orifice areas and fractions. The vena contracta width (VCW) has also been shown to correlate reasonably well with angiographic grading of PVL severity, however similar to a native mitral regurgitation eccentric, jet areas measured from wall hugging jets may underestimate overall severity [14, 33]. In addition, regurgitant jets are sensitive to transvalvular pressure gradients and therefore may appear smaller when the left ventricular pressure is diminished. Perhaps most importantly, VCW and jet area are single dimension measures of potentially complex and asymmetric effective regurgitant orifices and therefore may represent an over-simplified technique for determining PVL severity. However, multiplanar reconstruction of PVLs using 3D CFD echocardiography may be more effective for determining the actual VCA of the effective regurgitant orifice with a value of $>/= 0.13$ cm^2 indicating greater than a mild MVR PVL (EROA) (Fig. 32.13) [33, 41].

Similar techniques are used for measuring PVL severity following AVR. However, jet

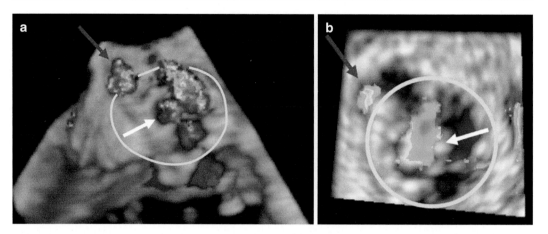

Fig. 32.13 Three dimensional transesophageal echocardiographic (TEE) views of a bioprosthetic mitral valve with both and anteromedial perivalvular (red arrow) and pathological central (white arrow) leaks. (**a**) Three dimen- sional TEE full volume image. (**b**) Short axis view at the plane of the vena contracta area (red arrow) of the perival- vular leak. Yellow circles: Bioprosthetic annular ring

width and VCW displayed in the TEE mid-esophageal long axis view may be limited by acoustic shadowing or the presence of either eccentric jets or multiple jets. 3D TEE with multiplanar reconstruction may enable the creation of a more accurate short axis plane to grade the AVR PVL by measuring the VCA. Techniques for grading AVR PVLs have evolved recently especially with the growth of TAVR and now include the circumferential extent of the neck of the PVL jet compared to the total circumference of the sewing ring as displayed in the TEE mid-esophageal short axis view. [14, 30] Cut off values for mild, moderate, and severe PVL are <10%, 10% −20%, and > 20% of the sewing ring circumference respectively [33]. However, this technique may result in an underestimation of PVL when a jet does not occupy a large circumferential extent but has a greater radial width [14]. Furthermore, while the summation of the circumferential extent of multiple simultaneous non-contiguous regurgitant jets to obtain a single PVL severity grade may be intuitive, this approach has not been formally validated [14, 30]. A multiwindow, multiparametric approach using up to a seven-class grading scheme may be worthwhile to limit variability is assessing PVL severity especially in patients with multiple jets [42].

Left Atrial Appendage Occlusion

Atrial fibrillation (AF) is prevalent in approximately 1–2% of the US population, and is responsible for 15–20% of all strokes [43–45]. Over 90% of strokes in patients with AF are caused by emboli from the left atrial appendage (LAA). While coumadin remains a mainstay treatment for patients with AF who are at risk of thrombus formation and embolic stroke, up to 50% of these patients do not receive anticoagulants and therefore may be eligible for an LAA occlusion device to prevent embolization [43–45]. Among the variety of LAA occlusion devices that have been evaluated, the Watchman device (Boston Scientific) has been FDA approved since 2015 and remains among the most extensively studied [46]. In a meta-analysis of 2400 patients who received a Watchman device, the incidence of hemorrhagic stroke, cardiovascular and unexplained death, and non-procedural bleeding was significantly lower compared to patients receiving coumadin [47].

Periprocedural echocardiography is an important compliment to fluoroscopy to determine patient eligibility, procedural guidance and diagnosing complications for the Watchman LAA occlusion device. Following induction of general anesthesia and endotracheal intubation, an initial

TEE survey should include the diagnosis of any baseline pericardial effusion, the location of pulmonary veins and the circumflex coronary artery, and ruling out the presence of LAA thrombus. Most of the remainder of the TEE exam should be devoted to determining TEE evaluation of the LAA anatomy and geometry including its shape, length, number of lobes, and orifice dimensions. The LAA shape is exceptionally variable and can present with multiple lobes. Several shape variations have been described including cone-shaped, cactus, windsock, and cauliflower [48]. While controversial, the "chicken wing" formation of the LAA is thought by some to be associated with the most challenging success rates for closure due to its inherent significant asymmetry and acute angle [46]. The identification of multiple lobes including those which are shallow and near the coumadin ridge, may also pose a challenge for optimal closure. Once the general shape is determined, a comprehensive echocardiographic examination of LAA anatomic parameters should be obtained to ensure accurate device sizing and ostial occlusion. While under-sizing may enable device leakage or embolization, over-sizing may promote cardiac injury. Optimal sizing requires multiplane TEE examination at $0°$, $45°$, $90°$ and $135°$ rotational angles (Fig. 32.14).

For the Watchman LAA occluder device, the landing zone measurement is obtained from the inferior rim of the LAA ostium at the level of the circumflex coronary artery, to a point 1–2 cm distal to the tip of the LUPV rim. Larger diameters are usually found at $120°$–$135°$ [46, 47]. The LAA depth is measured orthogonal to this measurement. 3D TEE measurements of the LAA have been shown to correlate more closely than 2D TEE with CT results and can be used to obtain an enface view and both circumference and maximal LAA diameter [48–50].

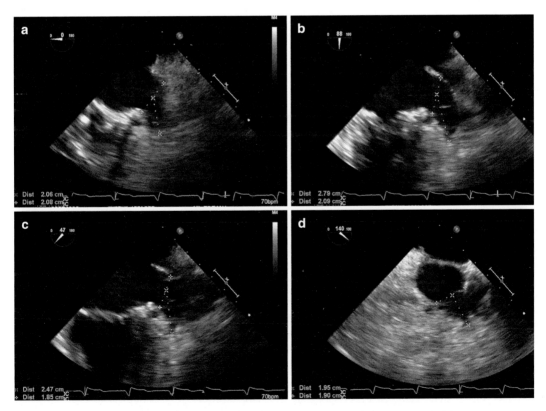

Fig. 32.14 Two-dimensional transesophageal image planes of the left atrial appendage (LAA) created by multiplane rotation (**a, b, c, d**). Both the short axis diameter and the length of the LAA should be measured to obtain the largest dimensions for LAA and to assure accurate occluder device sizing

Fig. 32.15 Color flow Doppler x-plane orthogonal images of a recently deployed Watchman, left atrial appendage occluder (arrows)

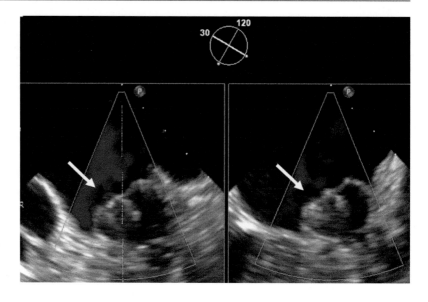

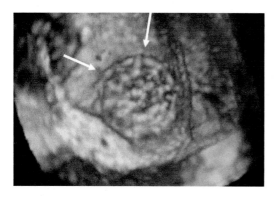

Fig. 32.16 Three-dimensional echocardiographic short axis image of a recently deployed Watchman left atrial appendage occluder device (arrows)

(jet size </= to 5 mm by 2D and 3D CFD and the lack of device protrusion >4–7 mm beyond the LAA ostium [46, 51] (Fig. 32.15).

Stability of the device is optimal when fixation barbs are in contact with the LAA wall; 8–20% device compression compared to pre-deployment diameter can be confirmed, and gentle traction of the catheter (i.e. "tug test") does not result in movement of the device relative to the surrounding structures (Fig. 32.16).

Following deployment of the device, it is important to rule out complications including a new pericardial effusion, device embolization or a symptomatic iatrogenic ASD.

Echocardiography imaging compliments fluoroscopy during the procedural steps for guiding placement of a LAA occlusion device. The initial transatrial septal puncture should be targeted at a posterior and inferior location guided by x-plane and 3D TEE imaging of the inter-atrial septum (Fig. 32.5). The next step involves the introduction of the delivery sheath into the LAA followed by device deployment. The ideal position of the deployed device includes avoidance of collateral structure injury (i.e. pulmonary vein; MV; circumflex artery), the absence of a peri-device leak

References

1. Singh S, Goyal A. The origin of echocardiography. Tex Heat Inst J. 2007;34(4):431–8.
2. Vahl TP, Kodali SK, Leon MB. Transcatheter aortic valve replacement 2016: a modern-day "through the looking glass" adventure. J Am Coll Cardiol. 2016;67:1472–87.
3. Zamorano J, Badano L, Bruce C, et al. EAE/ASE Recommendations for the use of echocardiography in new transcatheter interventions for valvular heart disease. J Am Soc Echocardiogr. 2011;24:937–65.

4. Holmes D, Nishimura R, et al. for the STS/ACC TVT Registry. Annual outcomes with transcatheter valve therapy: from the STS/ACC TVT Registry. Ann Thorac Surg. 2016;101:789–800.

5. Leon M, Smith C, Mack M, et al. Transcatheter aortic-valve implantation for aortic stenosis in patients who cannot undergo surgery. N Engl J Med. 2010;363:1597–607.

6. Smith C, Leon M, Mack M, et al. Transcatheter versus surgical aortic-valve replacement in high-risk patients. N Engl J Med. 2011;364:2187–98.

7. Thourani V, Kodali S, Makkar R, et al. Transcatheter aortic valve replacement versus surgical valve replacement in intermediate-risk patients: a propensity score analysis. Lancet. 2016;387:2218–25.

8. Nishimura R, Otto C, Bonow R, et al. 2014 AHA/ACC guideline for the management of patients with valvular heart disease: a report of the American College of Cardiology/American Heart Association Task Force on Practice Guidelines. J Am Coll Cardiol. 2014;63:e57–e185.

9. Arora S, Vavalle J. Transcatheter aortic valve replacement in intermediate and low risk patients-clinical evidence. Ann Cardiothorac Surg. 2017;6(5):493–7.

10. Bufton K, Augoustides J, Cobey F. Anesthesia for transfemoral aortic valve replacement in North America and Europe. J Cardiothorac Vasc Anesth. 2013;27(1):46–9.

11. Doddamani S, Bello R, Friedman MA, et al. Demonstration of left ventricular outflow tract eccentricity by real time 3D echocardiography: implications for the determination of aortic valve area. Echocardiography. 2007;24(8):860–6.

12. Khalique O, Hamid N, Kodali S, et al. Improving the accuracy of effective orifice area assessment after transcatheter aortic valve replacement: validation of left ventricular outflow tract diameter and pulsed-wave Doppler location and impact of three-dimensional measurements. J Am Soc Echocardiogr. 2015;28(11):1283–93.

13. Abdel-Wahab M, Mehilli J, Frerker C, et al. Comparison of balloon-expandable vs self-expandable valves in patients undergoing transcatheter aortic valve replacement: the CHOICE randomized clinical trial. JAMA. 2014;311:1503–14.

14. Pibarot P, Hahn R, Weissman N, Monaghan M. Assessment of paravalvular regurgitation following TAVR: a proposal of unifying grading scheme. J Am Coll Cardiol Img. 2015;8:340–60.

15. Perk G, Lang R, Garcia-Fernandez M, et al. Use of real-time three-dimensional transesophageal echocardiography in intracardiac catheter based interventions. J Am Soc Echocardiogr. 2009;22:865–82.

16. Freed L, Levy D, Levine R, et al. Prevalence and clinical outcome of mitral-valve prolapse. N Engl J Med. 1999;341(1):1–7.

17. Maisano F, Alfieri O, Banai S, et al. The future of transcatheter mitral valve interventions: competitive or complimentary rile of repair vs replacement? Eur Heart J. 2015;36(26):1651–9.

18. Whitlow PL, Feldman T, Pedersen WR, et al. Acute and 12-month results with catheter-based mitral valve leaflet repair: the EVEREST II (Endovascular Valve Edge-to-Edge Repair) High Risk Study. J Am Coll Cardiol. 2012;59(2):130–9.

19. Feldman T, Mehta A, Guerrero M, Levisay JP, Salinger MH. Mitraclip therapy for mitral regurgitation: secondary mitral regurgitation. Interv Cardiol Clin. 2016;5(1):83–91.

20. Zoghbi WA, Adams D, Bonow RO, et al. Recommendations for noninvasive evaluation of native valvular regurgitation: a report from the American Society of Echocardiography developed in collaboration with the Society of Cardiovascular Magnetic Resonance. J Am Soc Echocardiogr. 2001;30(4):303–71.

21. Wunderlich NC, Siegel RJ. Peri-interventional echo assessment fro the MitraClip procedure. Eur Heart J Cardiovasc Imaging. 2013 Oct;14(10):935–49.

22. Lubos E, Schlüter M, Vettorazzi E, et al. MitraClip therapy in surgical high-risk patients: identification of echocardiographic variables affecting acute procedural outcome. JACC Cardiovasc Interv. 2014;7(4):394–402.

23. Taramasso M, Denti P, Latib A, et al. Clinical and anatomical predictors of MitraCLip therapy failure for functional mitral regurgitation: single central clip strategy in asymmetric tethering. Int J Cardiol. 2015;186:286–98.

24. Alkhouli M, Charanjit S, Rihal C, Holmes D. Trans-septal techniques for emerging structural heart interventions. J Am Coll Cardiol Interv. 2016;9:2465–80.

25. Neuss M, Schau T, Isotani A, Pilz M, Schopp M, Butter C. Elevated mitral valve pressure gradient after mitraclip implantation deteriorates long-term outcome in patients with severe mitral regurgitation and severe heart failure. J Am Coll Cardiol Img. 2017;10(9):931–9.

26. Biaggi P, Felix C, Gruner C, et al. Assessment of mitral valve repair using the mitraclip system: comparison of different echocardiographic methods. Circ Cardiovasc Imaging. 2013;6:1032–40.

27. Trzcinka A, Fox J, Shook D, et al. Echocardiographic evaluation of mitral inflow hemodynamics after asymmetric double orifice repair. Anesth Analg. 2014;119(6):1259–66.

28. Feldman T, Wasserman H, Herrmann H, et al. Percutaneous mitral valve repair using the edge-to-edge technique: six-month results of the EVEREST phase I clinical trial. J Am Coll Cardiol. 2005;46:2134–40.

29. Altiok E, Hamada S, Brehmer K, et al. Analysis of procedural effects of percutaneous edge-to-edge mitral valve repair by 2D and 3D echocardiography. Circ Cardiovasc Imaging. 2012;5:748–55.

30. Konokse R, Whitener G, Nicoara A. Intraoperative evaluation of paravalvular regurgitation by transesophageal echocardiography. Anesth Analg. 2015;121:329–36.

31. Kliger C, Eiros R, Isasti G, et al. Review of surgical prosthetic parvalvular leaks diagnosis and catheter-based closure. Eur Heart J. 2013;34:638–49.

32. Sponga S, Perron J, Dagenais F, et al. Impact of residual regurgitation after aortic valve replacement. Eur J Cardiothorac Surg. 2012;42:486–92.

33. Zogbhi W, Chambers J, Dumesnil J, et al. Recommendation for evaluation of prosthetic valves with echocardiography and Doppler ultrasound: a report from the American Society of Echocardiography's Guidelines and Standards Committee and the Task Force on Prosthetic Valves. J Am Soc Echocardiogr. 2009;22:975–1014.

34. Bach DS. Transesophageal echocardiographic (TEE) evaluation of prosthetic valves. Cardiol Clin. 2000;18:751–71.

35. Lau W, Carroll J, Deeb G, Tait A, Back D. Intraoperative transesophageal echocardiographic assessment of the effect of protamine on paraprosthetic aortic insufficiency immediately after stentless tissue aortic valve replacement. J Am Soc Echocardiogr. 2002;15:1175–80.

36. Wasowiwicz M, Meineri M, Djaiani G, et al. Early complciations and immediate postoperative outcomes of paravalvular leaks after valve replacement surgery. J Cardiothorac Vasc Anesth. 2011;25:610–4.

37. Kim M, Casserly I, Garcia J, et al. Percutaneous trasncatheter closure of prosthetic mitral paravalvular leaks: are we there yet? JACC Cardiovasc Interv. 2009;2:81–90.

38. Morehead A, Firstenberg M, Shiota T, et al. Intraoperative echocardiographic detection of regurgitant jets after valve replacement. Ann Thorac Surg. 2000;69(1):135–9.

39. Sinning J, Vasa-Nicotera M, Chin D, et al. Evaluaiton and management of paravavular aortic regurgitation after transcatheter aortic valve replacement. J Am Coll Cardiol. 2013;62:11–20.

40. Athhappan G, Patvardhan E, Tuzcu E, et al. Incidence, predictors and outcomes of aortic regurgitation after transcatheter aortic valve replacement: meta-analysis and systematic review of literature. J Am Coll Cardiol. 2013;61:1585–95.

41. Franco E, Almeria C, de Augustin J, et al. Three-dimensional color Doppler transesophageal echocardiography for mitral paravalvular leak quantification and evaluation of percutaneous closure success. J Am Soc Echocardiogr. 2014;27:1153–63.

42. Hahn R, Pibarot P, Weissman N, Rodriguez L, Jaber W. Assessment of paravalvular aortic regurgitation after transcatheter aortic valve replacement: intracore laboratory variability. J Am Soc Echocardiogr. 2015;28:415–22.

43. Wunderlich N, Beigel R, Swaans M, Ho S, Siegel R. Percutaneous interventions for left atrial appendage exclusion. JACC Cardiovasc Interv. 2015;8:472–88.

44. Holmes D, Doshi S, Kar S, et al. Left atrial appendage closure as an alternative to warfarin for stroke prevention in atrial fibrillation: a patient-level meta-analysis. J Am Coll Cardiol. 2015;65:2614–23.

45. Cabrera J, Saremi F, Sanchez-Quintana D. Left atrial appendage: anatomy and imaging landmarks pertinent to percutaneous transcatheter occlusion. Heart. 2014;100:1636–50.

46. Fastner C, Behnes M, Sartorius B, et al. Procedural success and intra-hospital outcome related to left atrial appendage morphology in patients that receive an interventional left atrial appendage closure. Clin Cardiol. 2017;40(8):566–74.

47. Chan S, Kannam J, Douglas P, Manning W. Multiplane transesophageal echocardiographic assessment of left atrial appendage anatomy and function. Am J Cardiol. 1995;76:528–30.

48. Shah S, Bardo D, Sugeng L, et al. Real-time three-dimensional echocardiography of the left atrial appendage: initial experience in the clinical setting. J Am Soc Echocardiogr. 2008;21:1362–8.

49. Nakajima H, Seo Y, Ishizu T, et al. Analysis of the left atrial appendage by three-dimensional transesophageal echocardiography. Am J Cardiol. 2010;106:885–92.

50. Unsworth B, Sutaria N, Davies D, Kanagaratnam P. Successful placement if left atrial appendage closure device is heavily dependent on 3-dimensional transesophageal imaging. J A Coll Cardiol. 2011;58:1283.

51. Holmes D, Reddy V, Turi Z, et al. Percutaneous closure of the left atrial appendage versus warfarin therapy for prevention of stroke in patients with atrial fibrillation: a randomized non-inferiority trial. Lancet. 2009;374:534–42.

Perioperative Transthoracic Echocardiography

33

Y. E. Chee and H. B. Song

Main Messages

1. Transthoracic echocardiography (TTE) is a non-invasive alternative to widely used transesophageal echocardiography in cardiac surgery, with comparable diagnostic and monitoring capabilities.
2. Undifferentiated murmurs, unexplained dyspnea or hypoxemia; unexplained hypotension; altered functional capacity; and PEA cardiac arrest are the commonest indications for TTE in the perioperative setting.
3. Etiologies commonly requiring TTE assessment perioperatively include valvulopathy, hypovolemia, RV dysfunction or failure, impaired LV systolic function, and pulmonary embolism.
4. Adoption of a perioperative FoCUS protocol is highly recommended to encourage systematic approach, efficient scanning and diagnostic accuracy.

Cardiac ultrasound has gone through an unprecedented growth since its introduction into clinical practice in the 70s [1]. This state-of-the-art technology today is capable of providing useful information on cardiac morphology, physiology and functionality in a standard comprehensive echocardiographic examination. The advent of portable ultrasound machines has transformed echocardiography into a point-of-care imaging modality (POCUS, point-of-care cardiac ultrasound) that can be performed at the patient bedside. Cardiac ultrasound has since emerged as a bedside real-time diagnostic tool complimenting standard physical examination in many acute care settings such as emergency departments (ED) and critical care units (CCU), and recently the perioperative period.

Despite the fact that transesophageal echocardiography (TEE) has become an indispensable tool in cardiac surgery [2–4] and cardiac anesthesiologists have embraced the skill in TEE for more than 35 years, the semi-invasive nature of TEE with rare but potentially fatal complications has prohibited its widespread use beyond cardiac surgery and outside the operating theater [5]. To this end, transthoracic echocardiography (TTE) offers a non-invasive alternative with equal diagnostic and monitoring capabilities, particularly in the postoperative setting in the cardiac surgical ICU.

Y. E. Chee (✉)
Department of Anesthesia, Queen Mary Hospital,
The University of Hong Kong,
Hong Kong SAR, China

H. B. Song
Department of Anesthesia, West China Hospital,
Sichuan University, Chengdu, Sichuan, China

© Springer Nature Switzerland AG 2021
D. C. H. Cheng et al. (eds.), *Evidence-Based Practice in Perioperative Cardiac Anesthesia and Surgery*, https://doi.org/10.1007/978-3-030-47887-2_33

Feasibility and Impact

Bedside diagnostic use of TTE by non-cardiologists has been well validated across disciplines including perioperative settings [6–20]. Studies have demonstrated the feasibility of non-cardiologist novices identifying major pathologies on echocardiography after limited training with good agreement (90 to 99%) to that judged by cardiologists [21–23].

Canty et al. [19] studied the feasibility and impact of anesthesiologist-performed TTE at the preoperative assessment clinic (PAC) on the subsequent anesthetic management plans in 100 elective surgical patients who were either older than 65 years of age or suspected of cardiac disease. Results revealed a 54% change in anesthetic plans with 20% involving escalation and 34% involving de-escalation of treatment plans. These changes included decision to defer surgery for cardiac referral, adoption of different surgical technique or alternative mode of anesthesia, use of invasive hemodynamic monitoring, choice of intraoperative vasopressors, and postoperative admission to a high-dependency unit.

Cowie [24] investigated the feasibility and impact of perioperative anesthesiologist-led TTE services on anesthetic management. Referrals were initiated by case-anesthesiologists when needs arose and spanned the entire spectrum of perioperative period. Results demonstrated that 84% of the cases had their perioperative care plans modified based on the TTE findings performed and reported by anesthesiologists.

Song et al. [25] developed a custom-made TTE transducer holder for continuous intraoperative TTE monitoring (cTTE) (Fig. 33.1) via the parasternal approach.

To date, this is the first intraoperative continuous noninvasive echocardiographic monitoring device for cardiac function assessment ever reported. This novel application of TTE has been successfully applied in adult patients during circulatory failure and cardiac arrest respectively, and pediatric patients upon completion of percutaneous closure of ventricular septal defects.

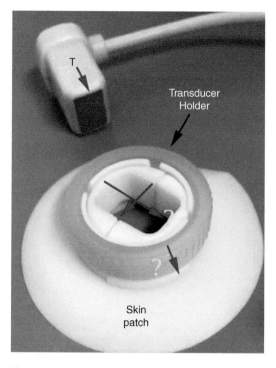

Fig. 33.1 TTE holder that allows continuous TTE monitoring at the parasternal long axis view

Similar feasibility results with significant clinical impact were demonstrated by several other studies on anesthesiologist-led TTE during perioperative patient care. This applies to both elective and emergency settings, with greater influence in emergency surgery [14–18].

Scope of Perioperative TTE

Anesthesiologists are often confronted with cardiac condition of uncertain clinical significance, and hence the dilemma in deciding whether to defer surgery for proper cardiac workup or simply proceed to surgery with caution. Conventionally, patients with a suspected or symptomatic cardiac condition discovered at the PAC are referred to cardiologists for cardiac assessment prior to elective surgery. This invariably results in undue delay in surgery due to the high demand and long waitlist for cardiology consultation in many centers. Much effort has been spent to ascertain the feasibility and impact of anesthesiologist-performed TTE at the preoperative assessment clinic (PAC) and to define the scope of POCUS that would adequately cover the spectrum of diverse etiologies requiring echocardiographic assessment.

In Canty's study [19] on anesthetist-performed TTE at PAC, reasons that commonly triggered echocardiographic examinations were: signs and symptoms that raised the suspicion of undiagnosed cardiac disease or deterioration of know cardiac condition; undifferentiated systolic ejection murmur (SEM); impaired function state; abnormal cardiac investigation; and suspected pulmonary hypertension (PHT) or right ventricular dysfunction. The significant TTE findings that impacted subsequent anesthetic management were: left ventricular (LV) dysfunction; PHT; significant aortic stenosis (AS); mitral regurgitation (MR); aortic regurgitation (AR); and tricuspid regurgitation (TR), in order of decreasing frequencies.

In Cowie's study [24] on perioperative anesthesiologist-led TTE service, common reasons for echocardiographic referrals were undifferentiated murmurs (56%), hemodynamic instability (26%) and suspected ventricular dysfunction (10%), with undifferentiated systolic ejection murmur (38%) being the commonest indication for perioperative TTE referral. The most frequent site of referral was PAC (68%), followed by PACU (16%) and operating room (OR) (12%).

Jasudavisius et al. [26] conducted a systematic review on the perioperative use of TTE and TEE in high-risk or hemodynamically unstable patients. Thirteen studies were included with a total of 968 patients analyzed, of which 568 were high-risk patients referred for preoperative assessment and the remaining 400 were intraoperative consultations at the time of major hemodynamic compromise or cardiac arrest. Accordingly, the most common etiologies in the preoperative group were valvulopathy (24.4% was aortic valve disease and 20% was mitral valve disease), low LV ejection fraction (25.4%), RV failure (6.6%), and hypovolemia (6.3%). The most common diagnoses in the intraoperative group were hypovolemia (33.2%), low ejection fraction (20.5%), RV failure (13.1%), RWMA (10.1%) and pulmonary embolism (PE) (5.8%). All other diagnoses accounted for less than 10% of diagnoses.

The review highlighted several salient points:

1. Pathologies encountered in the perioperative environment are somewhat different from and much more diverse than those commonly encountered in the ED or ICU;
2. Etiologies needing echocardiographic assessment at the PAC are again somewhat different from those encountered intraoperatively or postoperatively;
3. TTE is likely to be useful in the preoperative and postoperative periods where patients are not intubated and mechanically ventilated.

Based on the evidence from limited studies, the indications for perioperative TTE can be conveniently summarized into (but are not limited to) the following five aspects:

1. Undifferentiated murmurs
2. Unexplained hypotension
3. Undifferentiated dyspnea or hypoxemia
4. Altered functional capacity
5. Non-Shockable cardiac arrest

To strike a balance between the diversity in the perioperative environment and the echocardiographic competency of non-cardiologists operators (i.e. anesthesiologists in this instance), the diagnostic targets of perioperative TTE have been practically devised as follow:

1. LV dimensions and systolic function
2. RV dimension and systolic function
3. Volume status
4. Pericardial effusion & tamponade physiology
5. Qualitative or semi-quantitative valvular assessment
6. Spontaneous cardiac movements (SCM) in PEA/asystole cardiac arrest

These diagnostic targets are in line with the recommendations for Focused Cardiac Ultrasound (FoCUS) by WINFOCUS [27].

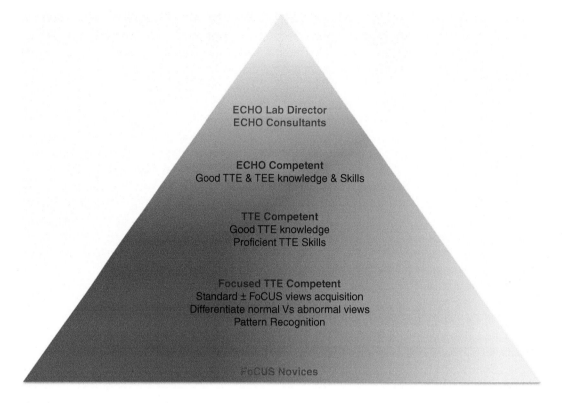

ECHO Lab Director
ECHO Consultants

ECHO Competent
Good TTE & TEE knowledge & Skills

TTE Competent
Good TTE knowledge
Proficient TTE Skills

Focused TTE Competent
Standard ± FoCUS views acquisition
Differentiate normal Vs abnormal views
Pattern Recognition

FoCUS Novices

Fig. 33.2 The expertise pyramid

Limited, Focused or Pattern Recognition: The Expertise Pyramid

Despite widespread application of TTE in many disciplines including emergency and critical care medicine, [7–10, 21, 27, 28] adoption by anesthesiologists and incorporation into training curriculum have lagged [29]. Regrettably, evidence-based curriculum for perioperative TTE has not been fully developed, and competency requirements remain somewhat undefined.

Perioperative TTE performed by anesthesiologists is not intended to replace standard comprehensive echocardiographic assessment by cardiologists. Rather, it is meant to serve as a bedside real-time diagnostic tool complementing physical examination and to gather sufficient information to assess physiologic status. Its ultimate aim is to provide essential information to guide specific interventions (e.g. fluid loading or inotropes) or the decision-making process (e.g. acute tamponade) in a timely manner [30–35]. Therefore, only echocardiographic modalities

that are in accord with the FoCUS [27] examination will be described in this writing, with the exception of 3DE and myocardial deformation imaging (due to their potential to be incorporated into FoCUS after undergoing an automation technology transformation).

Perioperative TTE is likely to evolve into an expertise pyramid as described by Royce CF (Fig. 33.2) [36] with the broad base of the pyramid representing rudimentary cardiac ultrasound scanning mastered by most acute care clinicians, and the top of the pyramid representing highly trained and qualified experts in TTE. The middle of the pyramid is clinicians with a spectrum of moderately advanced skill and knowledge in TTE [37–41].

Features of FoCUS

As stated in the "International Evidence-Based Recommendations for Focused Cardiac Ultrasound" published by WINFOCUS in 2014, FoCUS entails the following features: [27].

Fig. 33.3 Parasternal long axis view (PLAX) in diastole as the mitral valve is opened   . RV: right ventricle; LV: left ventricle; LVOT: left ventricular outflow tract; MV: Mitral valves; AV: aortic valves; LA: left atrium; DA: descending aorta

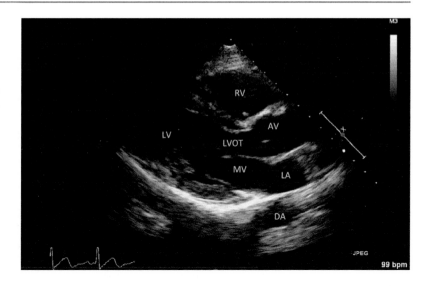

- Problem-oriented
- Goal-directed
- Time sensitive
- Simplified with limited echocardiographic views
- Qualitative or semi-quantitative
- Repeatable
- Performed at the point of care
- Clinician-performed

In the context of FoCUS, not all cardiac pathologies need to be identified and not every pathology detected needs to be addressed immediately. Should FoCUS fail to elucidate etiology that is clinically suspected, cardiac referral for formal comprehensive echocardiographic evaluation should be contemplated [27, 42–45].

Echocardiographic Windows

FoCUS examination does not require the execution of all the views of a standard comprehensive echocardiographic assessment. A limited number of views, such as parasternal long axis, parasternal short axis (mid papillary level), subcostal long axis, subcostal inferior vena cava (IVC) and apical four chambers are sufficient to establish the likely diagnosis in most circumstances. More than one view should however be obtained if clinical situation allows.

Parasternal Views

The transducer is placed on a line joining the apex beat to the mid-point of the right clavicle, immediately adjacent to the left lateral sternal margin. This is normally at the third or fourth intercostal space. By pointing the orientation marker (OM) on the transducer toward the patient's right shoulder, the parasternal long-axis (PLAX) view (Fig. 33.3) is displayed. Rotation of the transducer 90° clockwise will display the parasternal short-axis (PSAX) view (Fig. 33.4). Image quality often improves by turning the patient to the left side.

From the PLAX view, classical M-mode can be applied for quantitative measurements of wall thickness and chamber dimensions. In addition, the PLAX view is used to measure the diameter of the left ventricular outflow tract (LVOT), to look for hypertrophic obstructive cardiomyopathy (HOCM) or systolic anterior movement (SAM) of mitral valve anterior leaflet.

The PSAX view is a convenient echocardiographic window for rapid diagnosis of multiple cardiac pathologies, including hypovolemia or hyperdynamic state, left ventricular systolic dysfunction, regional wall motion abnormality (RWMA), left ventricular hypertrophy, right ventricular dilatation, and pericardial effusion.

Fig. 33.4 Parasternal short axis view. RV: right ventricle; LV: left ventricle; PM: posteromedial papillary muscle

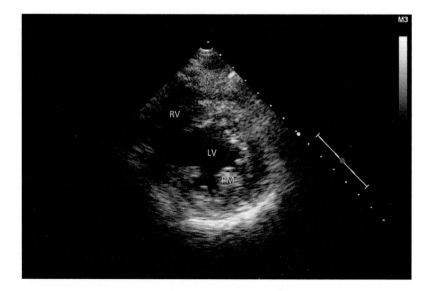

Fig. 33.5 Apical 4 chamber view. TV: tricuspid valves; LPV: left pulmonary vein; RPV: right pulmonary vein

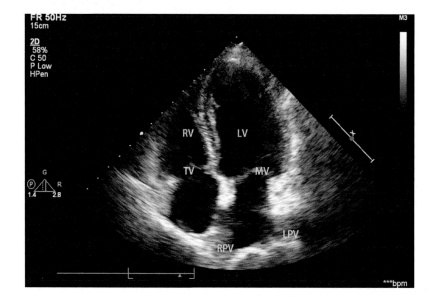

Apical 4 Chamber View

The transducer is placed over the apex beat with the OM pointed towards the patient's left and tilted cranially so the ultrasound beam is directed parallel to the long axis of the heart. Small adjustments are made until all four chambers are presented in middle of the screen.

The apical 4-chamber view (A4C) (Fig. 33.5) allows qualitative evaluation of LV and RV systolic function, left atrial size, and right ventricular size. The RV size should not exceed two-thirds of the LV, provided the LV is normal.

Subcostal Long Axis View

To obtain the long axis view (SC LAX) (Fig. 33.6), the transducer is placed inferior to the right costal curvature pointing toward the patient's left shoulder. The OM is orientated toward the patient's left side and caudally until all four cardiac chambers

Fig. 33.6 Subcostal 4 chamber view (SC 4Ch). RA: right atrium; RV right ventricle; LV: left ventricle

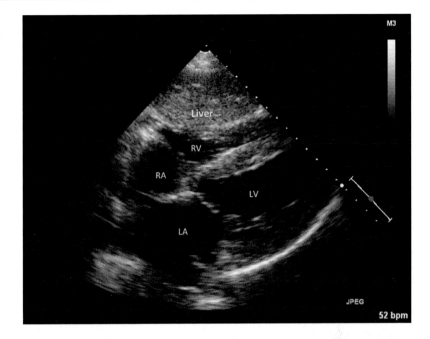

Fig. 33.7 Subcostal IVC long axis view (SC IVC). RA: right atrium; HV: hepatic vein; IVC: inferior vena cava; M-Mode interrogation: red dotted arrow

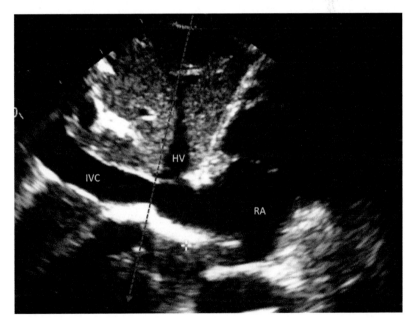

appear on the screen. By counterclockwise rotation, the subcostal short-axis view can be obtained, displaying the short axis of the LV and part of the RV. The subcostal long axis view is the ideal window for diagnosing inter-atrial septal (IAS) defects, and for viewing tamponade physiology and systolic functions of both ventricles.

Subcostal IVC View

To obtain the subcostal IVC view (SC IVC) (Fig. 33.7), the probe is placed medially from the SC LAX view to display the RA on the right of the screen, bringing a large part of the liver into view. The probe is then rotated 90° counterclockwise until the long axis of the IVC is through the liver and merges into the RA.

It is very important to merge the IVC with the RA as this is the most reliable way to differentiate IVC from the abdominal aorta, which has a similar appearance and dimensions. Visualizing this merge on the display allows certainty that the IVC, not the aorta, is being viewed.

The Perioperative TTE Toolbox

In the absence of authoritative guidelines on what echocardiographic modalities should be included in the perioperative TTE toolbox, the authors of this writing have taken the liberty to construct one.

General Principles

Under most circumstances in the perioperative period, qualitative assessment is sufficient to reach a diagnosis that allows timely intervention [7–10, 21, 22, 27] [28, 46]. Nevertheless, quantitative assessment provides objective and measureable data that serves as the baseline for serial comparisons subsequently, [47] and should be attempted if time and situation permit.

In the context of FoCUS, 2D and M-mode imaging are the basic cardiac ultrasound techniques sufficient in most acute settings [14, 27–29] [31, 48, 49]. Color Flow Doppler (CFD) serves as the roadmap for flow hence a useful screening tool if valvular lesion is suspected [27]. The role of other Doppler modalities in FoCUS remains undefined.

For standardization, end-diastole is defined as the first frame after mitral valve closure or the frame in which LV dimension measurement is the largest. End-systole is defined as the frame immediately after aortic valve closure or the frame in which the LV dimension is the smallest [50].

All measurements should be performed on more than one cardiac cycle to account for beat-to-beat variability. An average of three beats for patients in normal sinus rhythm and a minimum

of five beats in those with atrial fibrillation are recommended [50]. All values reported should be indexed to BSA to allow valid comparison among individuals with different body sizes.

Real time three-dimensional echocardiography (RT 3DE) and myocardial deformation imaging (i.e. strain & strain rate) are rapidly becoming the new standards in chamber quantification and LV systolic function assessment, supported by technology development and a growing body of knowledge [51]. The major drawback is the lengthy analytic process, which will soon be overcome by the automated adaptive analytic technology [51]. For this reasons, they are described in this writing, although briefly.

Left Ventricle

LV function can be assessed by both qualitative and quantitative means. Two-dimensional echocardiographic examination at the parasternal windows is often sufficient to obtain an overall appreciation of the LV systolic function, make crude estimation of LV EF, and identify regional wall motion abnormality (RWMA).

LV Size

LV size should be routinely measured as part of the LV function assessment. LV wall thickness and internal dimensions should be obtained from the PLAX view (Fig. 33.8), using either 2D-guided M-mode interrogation or the 2D image. LV diameter should be measured with the caliper or interrogating beam positioned at the tip of mitral valve leaflets and perpendicular to the LV long axis. Measurement should be taken from leading edge to leading edge in M-mode, and from trailing edge to leading edge in 2DE [50].

Biplane method of disks summation technique (modified Simpson's rule) is the current recommended method for echocardiographic volume quantifications. LV endocardial borders in both A4C and A2C views are traced after image optimization. Papillary muscles are excluded, and the

Fig. 33.8 LV end-diastole internal dimension. LV long axis: blue long arrow; LV end diastole internal diameter: red double arrow; Antero-septal wall & Inferno-lateral wall thickness: blue double arrows

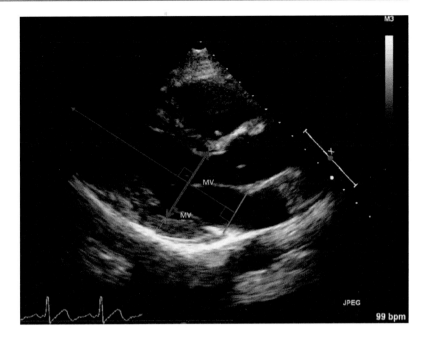

loop closes with a straight line connecting the two ends of mitral annulus. LV length is defined as the distance from the midpoint of this connecting line to the farthest point in the apex. The longer of the two measurements taken from A4C and A2C views should be used. Efforts should be made to avoid LV apex foreshortening, and to optimize gain for better endocardial border delineation.

Contrast agents have been implicated to improve endocardial delineation when multiple endocardial segments are poorly visualized, but are impractical in the perioperative settings and seldom used.

3DE volume quantification technology is not affected by LV apex foreshortening and is the preferred technique when expertise is available. However, the technology is still not available on many small portable machines and may not be practical in most perioperative settings.

For general reference, 2DE LV EDVs of 74 mL/m^2 for men and 61 mL/m^2 for women and LV ESVs of 31 mL/m^2 for men and 24 mL/m^2 for women should be used as the upper limits of the corresponding normal range.

LV Global Systolic Function

Fractional shortening (FS) can be derived from linear measurements obtained from 2D images or 2D-guided M-mode imaging using the equation FS = (LVIDd − LVIDs) ÷ LVIDd × 100%, where LVIDd and LVIDs are the LV internal diameter at the end-diastole and end-systole respectively.

Fractional area change (FAC) is derived from the end-diastolic (EDA) and end-systolic areas (ESA) obtained by tracing the LV endocardial border in the PSAX view during end-diastole and end-systole respectively. The formula used is FAC = [(EDA − ESA) ÷ EDA] × 100%.

Both the FS and FAC techniques are simple and easily repeatable. FAC shows a good correlation with EF measured by radionuclide angiography and scintigraphy methods. However, these techniques are load-dependent, and clinical correlation is severely compromised by RWMA due to coronary artery disease or conduction abnormalities.

Ejection fraction (EF) is derived from EDV and ESV using the formula EF = (EDV − ESV) ÷ EDV, where EDV and ESV can be derived from 2DE or 3DE as described above. The biplane method of disks (modified Simpson's rule) is the currently recommended 2D method to assess LV EF. 3DE-based EF measurements are accurate and reproducible and should be used when available and feasible [52, 53]. In general, EF in the range of 53% to 73% is considered normal in adults >20 years old. EF indexed to BSA reduces variability across genders and age groups and is thus preferred.

Global longitudinal strain (GLS) is a measure of the LV longitudinal deformation throughout the cardiac cycle using speckle-tracking technology (STE) [54–56]. It is the most commonly used strain-based measurement of LV global systolic function. Images from the apical four-chamber, two-chamber and three-chamber views are required for the measurement of LV longitudinal strain whereas short-axis views at basal, mid and apical levels are needed for the measurement of radial and circumferential strain. Peak GLS describes the relative length change of LV myocardium between end-diastole and end-systole and is calculated as GLS% = (MLs − MLd) ÷ MLd, where MLs and MLd are myocardial lengths at end-systole and end-diastole respectively. As myocardial length is shorter during systole, GLS is expected to be a negative number. Normal values for GLS vary with the sampling site, vendor and software version, resulting in considerable heterogeneity in the published literature [57–59]. Peak GLS in healthy subjects is usually approximately −20%. Peak GLS below this value corresponds with an increased likelihood of an abnormal systolic function. GLS is a valuable and sensitive tool for follow-up examinations provided the same vendor and software version are used (relevant formulas are tabulated in Table 33.1; normal values of LV dimensions and function that are relevant to the context of perioperative TTE are summarized in Table 33.2).

Segmentation and regional wall motion abnormality (RWMA): Visual appreciation of endocardial thickening or endocardial excursion is a semi-qualitative method for regional myocardial function assessment. The LV has been divided into segments to facilitate regional function

Table 33.1 GLS formulas

Formulae
FS = (LVIDd − LVIDs) ÷ LVIDd × 100%
FAC = [(EDA − ESA) ÷ EDA] × 100%
EF = (EDV − ESV) ÷ EDV
GLS% = (MLs − MLd) ÷ MLd
CI = [IVC$_{max}$ − IVC$_{min}$] ÷ IVC$_{mean}$
DI = [IVC$_{max}$ − IVC$_{min}$] ÷ IVC$_{min}$

FS Fractional shortening, *LVIDd*, LV end-diastole internal dimension, *LVIDs* LV end-systole internal dimension, *EF* Ejection fraction, *EDV* End diastolic volume, *ESV* End systolic volume, *FAC* Fractional area change, *EDA* End diastolic area, *ESA* End systolic area, *GLS* Global longitudinal strain, *MLs* Myocardial length at end systole, *MLd* Myocardial length at end diastole, *CI* Collapsibility index, *DI* Distensibility index, *IVC max* Maximum IVC diameter, *IVC min* Minimum IVC diameter, *IVC mean* Mean IVC diameter

Table 33.2 Normal values for 2DE parameters of LV size and function according to gender

	Male	Female
Relative wall thickness (cm)	0.24–0.42	0.22–0.42
Septal wall thickness (cm)	0.6–1.0	0.6–0.9
LVIDd (mm)	50.2 ± 4.1	45.0 ± 3.6
LVIDs (mm)	32.4 ± 3.7	28.2 ± 3.3
EDV (biplane) (ml)	106 ± 22	76 ± 15
ESV (biplane)(ml)	41 ± 10	28 ± 7
Indexed EDV (ml/m^2)	54 ± 10	45 ± 8
Indexed ESV (ml/m^2)	21 ± 5	16 ± 4
LV EF (biplane)	62 ± 5	64 ± 5
GLS (%)	> −20	> −20

LVIDd LV end-diastole internal dimension, *LVIDs* LV end-systole internal dimension, *EF* Ejection fraction, *EDV* End diastolic volume, *ESV* End systolic volume, *FAC* Fractional area change, *EDA* End diastolic area, *ESA* End systolic area, *GLS* Global longitudinal strain

assessment and the segmentation schemes (Fig. 33.9a, b) reflect the coronary perfusion territories.

Three LV segmentation models (16-, 17- and 18-segment models), have been designed to accommodate different needs in various clinical practices. The 16-segment model is recommended for RWMA assessment as endocardial thickening or excursion at the apical cap is generally imperceptible. Each segment should be evaluated in multiple views and a four-grade scoring system should be applied as follows: (1) normal or hyperkinetic, (2) hypokinetic or reduced thickening, (3)

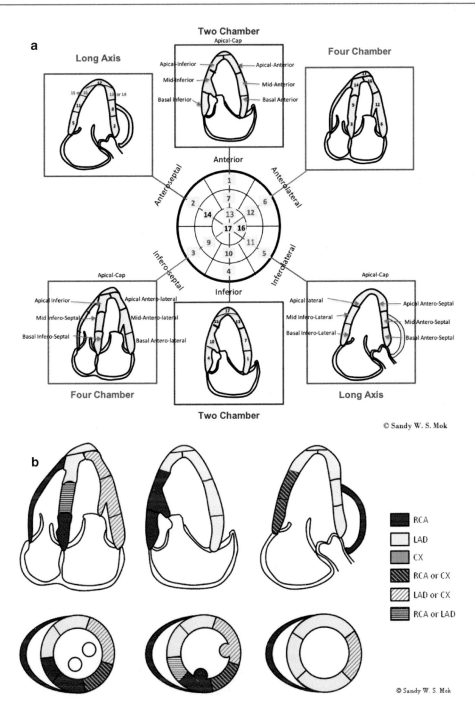

Fig. 33.9 (a) Orientation of A4C, A2C and ALX views in relation to the Bull's-eye display of the LV segments (center). Top panels show actual images and bottom panels schematically depict the LV wall segments in each view. Diagram taken from Lang RM et al. Recommendations for cardiac chamber quantification by echocardiography in adults: an update from the American Society of Echocardiography and the European Association of Cardiovascular Imaging. J Am Soc Echocardiogr. 2015; 28:1–39. (b) Typical distribution of right coronary artery (RCA), left anterior descending artery (LAD), and left circumflex artery (LCx). The arterial distribution varies among patients. Some segments have variable coronary perfusion. Diagram taken from Lang RM et al. Recommendations for cardiac chamber quantification by echocardiography in adults: an update from the American Society of Echocardiography and the European Association of Cardiovascular Imaging. J Am Soc Echocardiogr. 2015; 28:1–39

akinetic or negligible thickening, (4) dyskinetic or systolic thinning or bulging (Table 33.3).

Appreciation of regional wall motion abnormalities can be challenging to FoCUS providers who are not equipped with the trained eyes, especially in the presence of tethering, conduction abnormality or paced rhythms.

Right Ventricle (RV)

The complex geometry (crescent shape) of the RV poses a challenge to its echocardiographic imaging and quantifications. This is now overcome by advancement in technology such as Doppler tissue imaging (DTI), strain imaging and 3D technology, where DTI and strain imaging are useful for RV regional function assessment, and 3D imaging quantitates RV volumes and ejection fraction [60, 61].

RV Size

Qualitative assessment of RV size in relation to that of LV in either PSAX or A4C views is com-

Table 33.3 Grade scoring system of regional wall motion abnormality

1	Normal or hyperkinetic
2	Hypokinetic or reduced thickening
3	Akinetic or negligible thickening
4	Dyskinetic or systolic thinning or bulging

monly used in acute perioperative settings. A RV/LV ratio of 0.6 or more usually signifies RV dilation (Fig. 33.10) [47, 62].

For quantitative assessment, RV dimensions are best estimated from a RV-focused apical four-chamber view with care taken to ensure a center position of the LV apex in the scanning sector and the largest basal RV diameter is measured. In general, diameter > 41 mm at the base and > 35 mm at the midlevel in the RV-focused view indicates RV dilatation [47, 62–65].

The unique crescent shape of the RV renders most 2DE methods used for LV volume quantification invalid for this purpose. Efforts to derive RV volumes from 2DE views have had little success. Most of these methods are cumbersome, require views that are not easily obtainable in many patients, yield only modest accuracy at best, and lack validation in substantial patient populations. Therefore, RV volume determination by 2D echocardiography remains largely a research entity and echocardiographically derived RV ejection fraction remains impractical to assess RV function.

RV Systolic Function

Tricuspid Annular Plane Systolic Excursion (TAPSE) is a widely adopted surrogate of RV systolic function that is easily obtainable by 2D guided M-mode registration of the cyclic apico-basal (longitudinal) excursion of the tricuspid

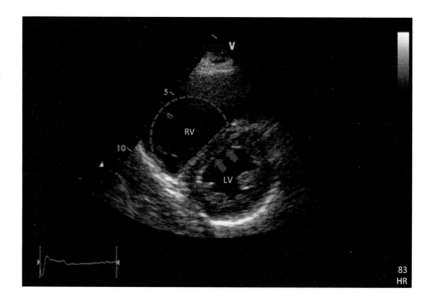

Fig. 33.10 Parasternal short axis view. Dilated RV: RV/LV ratio > 0.6; flattened interventricular septum: thick red arrows; and D-shape LV

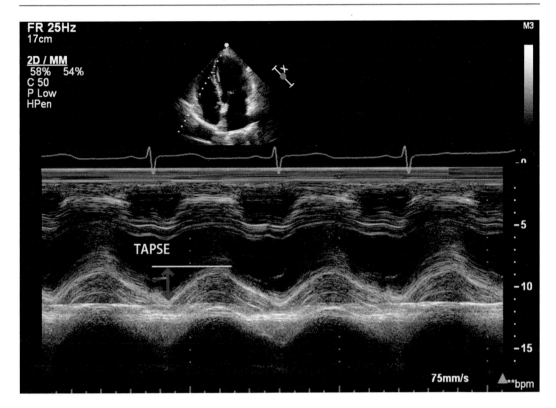

Fig. 33.11 TAPSE tricuspid annular plane systolic excursion

lateral annulus in the apical four-chamber view [47, 62]. (Fig. 33.11) The value has been shown to correlate well with RV systolic function predicted by radionuclide-derived RV EF, albeit a mere one-directional measurement.

TAPSE may however over- or underestimate RV function in the presence of translational motion [47, 62, 66]. In general, TAPSE <17 mm is highly suggestive of RV systolic dysfunction, with slight variation across genders. (Table 33.4).

2D FAC: FAC measured from the A4C view provides an estimate of global RV systolic function. It is important to ensure that the entire RV is contained in the imaging sector, including its apex and free wall, during both systole and diastole. While tracing the RV area, care must be taken to include the trabeculae and moderator band. RV FAC < 35% is indicative of RV systolic dysfunction [47, 62, 63].

DTI-derived tricuspid lateral annular systolic velocity (S′): There was debate concerning the inclusion of this modality, as Doppler interroga-

tion is not usually recommended in FoCUS. However, in the absence of well validated modalities for RV systolic function assessment, DTI-derived S′-wave velocity (from A4C view) is easy to measure, reliable, and reproducible, and has been shown to correlate well with other measures of global RV systolic function [67]. It is important to keep the basal segment and the annulus aligned with the Doppler cursor to avoid velocity underestimation. Similar to TAPSE, S′ is a one-directional measurement and hence influenced by cardiac translational motion. In general, S′ velocity < 9.5 cm/sec measured on the free-wall side is indicative of RV systolic dysfunction.

Strain and Strain Rate: The large body of currently available evidence on RV GLS is mainly derived from single-center studies with a limited number of subjects, involving equipment and software supplied by only two vendors, and using software designed for LV measurements and extrapolated to the RV. As a result, no normal reference ranges are currently recommended for either global or regional RV strain and strain rate. Abovementioned limitations aside, strain and strain rate of RV free wall have been shown to be useful parameters for assessing global and regional RV systolic function in general clinical settings. For reference, pooled data has suggested that an absolute value of global longitudinal strain (GLS) < 20% for the RV free wall may indicate abnormal RV systolic function, though this is largely based on data from one vendor and should be interpreted accordingly [62, 66]. (Tables 33.4 and 33.5).

Volume Status and Fluid Responsiveness

Qualitative Assessment of LV
Qualitative assessment of LV via the parasternal long-axis (PLAX) and short-axis (PSAX) views allow gross assessment of volume status. End systolic LV cavity obliteration, or "kissing papillary" sign (Fig. 33.12), is highly suggestive of intravascular volume depletion [68].

LV End Diastolic Area (EDA)
LV end diastolic area (EDA) measured from the PSAX view at the mid papillary level (papillary

Table 33.4 Normal values for 2DE parameters of RV size

	Mean ± SD	Normal range
RV basal diameter (mm)	33 ± 4	25–41
RV mid diameter (mm)	27 ± 4	19–35
RV longitudinal diameter (mm)	71 ± 6	59–83
RV wall thickness (mm)	3 ± 1	1–5

Table 33.5 Normal values for 2DE parameters of RV function

	Mean ± SD	Standard Cutoff
TAPSE (mm)	24 ± 3.5	<17
RV FAC (%)	49 ± 7	<35
Pulsed Doppler S wave (cm/sec)	14.1 ± 2.3	<9.5
RV free wall 2D strain (%)	−29 ± 4.5	> −20

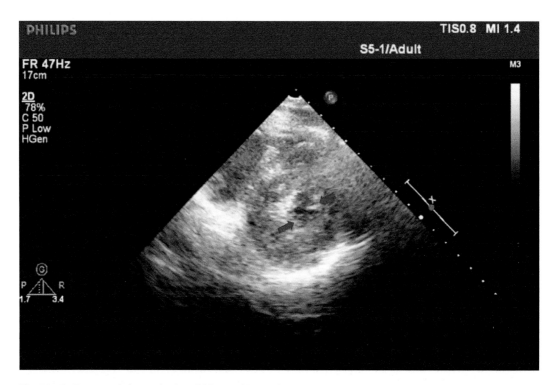

Fig. 33.12 Parasternal short axis view. Obliterated LV cavity at end-systole in profound hypovolemia, also named the "kissing papillary" sign

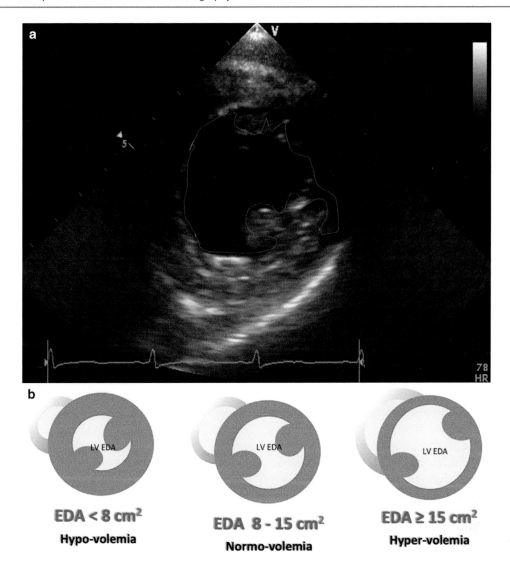

Fig. 33.13 (**a**) Parasternal short axis view. LV EDA tracing with papillary muscles excluded. (**b**) LV EDA measurements and volume status estimations

muscles excluded) is commonly used to estimate volume status, with EDA between eight to 15 cm^2 indicating normovolemia, less than eight cm^2 indicating hypovolemia, and higher than 15cm^2 indicating volume overload, either relative or absolute [68]. (Fig. 33.13a, b).

Inferior Vena Cava (IVC)

Combination of IVC dimension and its phasic variation throughout the respiratory cycle have been shown to correlate with the central venous pressure (CVP) or right atrial pressure (RAP), both of which are commonly used surrogates for filling pressure and volume status [69, 70]. As recommended by the American Society of Echocardiography (ASE) Guidelines 2015, the maximum IVC diameter should be measured with the patient in supine position, from the subcostal IVC long axis view, at a point immediately caudal to the IVC-hepatic vein junction using

M-Mode (Fig. 33.7) and leading edge technique (inner edge to inner edge of the vessel wall). This point ranges from one to three cm distal to the IVC-RA junction [69–75].

An IVC diameter of <1.1 cm implies the likelihood of volume depletion, whereas IVC diameter > 2.1 cm implies the likelihood of relative or absolute volume overload [69–75]. End of expiration was previously the preferred phase of the respiratory cycle to measure IVC parameters, but this has been refuted by recent studies that demonstrated similar strength in predicting CVP irrespective of the respiratory phase measurement was taken. Therefore, there are no specific recommendations on the optimal phase of respiratory cycle for IVC measurements in the latest ASE guidelines [50].

Mechanical ventilation increases intrathoracic pressure and reduces venous return, which in turn influences the caval dimension and collapsibility. Thus the correlations between IVC dimension and CVP in mechanically ventilated patients are generally inconsistent and unreliable, especially when positive end expiratory pressure (PEEP) is applied [69–75]. This is reflected in the latest guidelines from the ASE, which recommend against routine application in this setting. Nevertheless, a small IVC (<1.2 cm) in mechanically ventilated patients should point toward reduced right-sided filling pressure and depleted volume status, with a stronger correlation in the absence of PEEP.

Low CVP does not necessarily correlate with fluid responsiveness. IVC dimension does not predict fluid responsiveness in both spontaneously breathing and mechanically ventilated patients. In general, fluid responsiveness can be accurately predicted in both spontaneously breathing and mechanically ventilated patients by a more than 20% change in velocity time integral (VTI) or stroke volume (SV) during passive leg raising (PLR) [76–78]. This requires pulsed-wave Doppler (PWD) interrogation.

IVC respiratory variation, Collapsibility Index (CI) and Distensibility Index (DI): During spontaneous respiration, cyclic variation in pleural pressure is transmitted to the right atrium (RA) causing cyclic variation in venous return and IVC dimension. This intra-thoracic pressure is lowest at the end of inspiration and reaches its peak at the

Table 33.6 IVC diameter, respiratory variation and RAP/CVP

IVC diameter (cm)	Respiratory variation (%)	RAP/CVP (mmHg)
<1.1	Spontaneously collapse	0–5
1.1–2.1	> 50%	5–10
1.1–2.1	< 50%	10–15
>2.1	< 50%	15–20
>2.1	Minimal/no variation	>20

IVC Inferior vena cava, *RAP* Right atrial pressure, *CVP* Central venous pressure

end of expiration, resulting in 50% or more variation in IVC dimension throughout the respiratory cycle in normovolemic patients. Respiratory variation of IVC is expressed as the difference between maximum and minimum diameters of the IVC divided by its maximum diameter.

In spontaneously breathing patients, IVC diameter < 1.1 cm with complete inspiratory collapse correlates to CVP of 5 mmHg or less and volume depletion, whereas distended IVC (diameter > 2.1 cm) that lacks respiratory variation is predictive of CVP > 20 mmHg. The approximate correlation between these IVC parameters and CVP readings are shown in Table 33.6.

In positive pressure ventilation, IVC Collapsibility Index (CI) is defined as the difference between maximum and minimum IVC diameters divided by its mean diameter (Table 33.1), with the CI > 12% implying volume depletion and predicting fluid responsiveness [71–73]. Conversely, IVC Distensibility Index (DI) is expressed as the difference between maximum and minimum IVC diameters divided by its minimum diameter (Table 33.1), with the DI > 18% indicating volume depletion and being predictive of fluid responsiveness in mechanically ventilated patients [68, 79].

Pericardium

Pericardial effusion appears as echo-free space between the visceral and parietal pericardium. Echocardiographic assessment should be aimed to (1) differentiate between global or loculated effusion; (2) quantify the effusion; (3) describe fluid appearance; and (4) rule in or rule out tamponade physiology [80]. (Fig 33.14a, b).

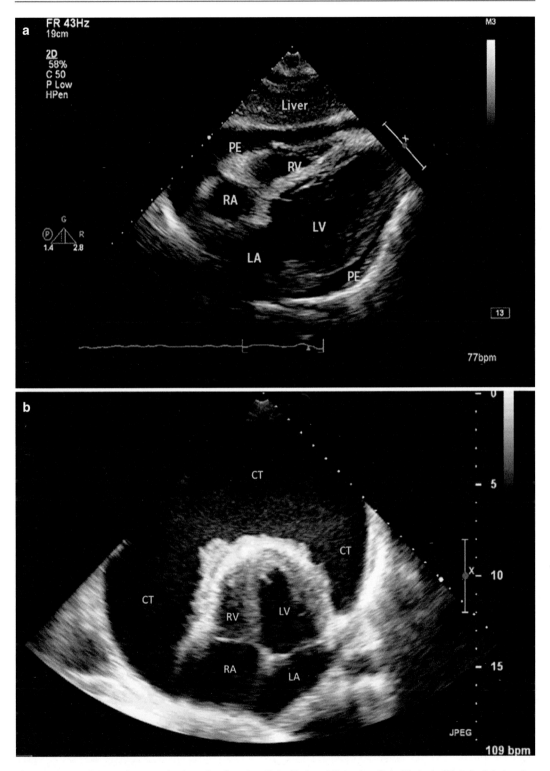

Fig. 33.14 (**a**) Subcostal long axis view. Small pericardial effusion: PE (pericardial effusion). (**b**) Apical 4 chamber view. CT: cardiac tamponade

Four standard views (PLAX, PSAX, SC LAX, and A4C) are commonly used to assess pericardial effusion and to differentiate between global or loculated collection. A single view (usually SC LAX) should suffice to diagnose significant pleural effusion in emergent situations, but one should be aware of the risk of overestimation with the SC LAX view that can be angle-dependent. Pleural effusions in adults are classified according to the AP dimension measured at end-diastole as trivial (seen only in systole), mild (<10 mm), moderate (10–20 mm), and severe (>20 mm) [81–83]. Clinical symptoms may not necessarily be in proportion to the amount of pleural collection detected.

Echocardiography should be obtained immediately if cardiac tamponade is suspected. Common 2D and M-mode features of tamponade physiology include large pericardial effusion, systolic RA free wall collapse, diastolic RV free wall collapse, septal "bouncing" and IVC plethora.

Valvular Assessment

Ejection systolic murmur is common and has been reported to present in up to 50% of unselected patients aged over 60 years, making detection of ejection systolic murmur of uncertain clinical significance one of the common occurrences at the preoperative assessment clinic (PAC) [48, 84–88]. It has been shown that untreated valvular lesions of moderate or above in severity are associated with increased perioperative cardiac morbidity and mortality in noncardiac surgery, especially when impaired LV function is present [89–93]. Echocardiographic valvular assessment is complex, entailing Doppler interrogation techniques [92–96] that require extensive echocardiography training and thus is well beyond the scope of FoCUS. However, appreciation of the potential role of severe valvular dysfunction in shock and heart failure can undoubtedly be lifesaving [97].

In the context of perioperative TTE performed by non-cardiologist, the general sentiment is to stay with the 2D and M-mode imaging for "Pattern recognition", such as thickened and calcified leaflets with markedly reduced mobility in severe aortic stenosis (Fig. 33.15). The simplified approach is supported by results of many feasibility studies demonstrating recognition of major valve disease on the basis of simple morphologic findings by non-cardiologists with limited training using pocket-sized devices [23, 98–100]. Undiagnosed murmurs detected at the PAC, be it

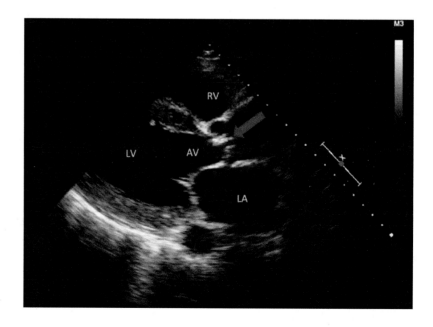

Fig. 33.15 Parasternal long axis view. Severe aortic stenosis with thickened & calcified aortic valves: red arrow

symptomatic or asymptomatic, should ideally be referred for formal cardiology assessment prior to elective surgery.

Cardiac Arrest

Current utility of TTE during cardiac arrest is to determine the presence of myocardial mechanical activity (MMA) and to detect reversible causes including profound hypovolemia, [101, 102] cardiac tamponade, [103–105] pulmonary embolism [60, 61] and tension pneumothorax. Presence of MMA predicts better survival [106–108] on an otherwise undifferentiated population of arrested patients, whereas detection of reversible causes expedites intervention. However outcome benefit has not been demonstrated in the use of TTE in cardiac arrest [27, 35, 109–111].

PEARLS for ACLS-compliant FoCUS evaluation:

1. Provide high quality BCLS/ACLS per AHA/ERC/ILCOR guidelines without delay for at least five cycles of chest compression/ventilation before considering echocardiographic examination [112]
2. Preparation for FoCUS evaluation should parallel the CPR effort
3. Perform echocardiographic evaluation in non-shockable cardiac arrest
4. Sonographer should not be one of the essential BCLS/ACLS providers
5. Echocardiography should only be performed during the 10-second No Flow Interval (NFI) for pulse check [111, 113]
6. SC LAX view is usually preferred to minimize delay in resumption of CPR at the end of no flow interval [103, 114].
7. If diagnosis cannot be made within the 10-second NFI, stop scanning and resume CPR immediately for another five cycles before another attempt. Consider parasternal approach if the initial subcostal approach was inconclusive.
8. Communicate clearly with the resuscitation team regarding the echocardiographic findings.
9. Good documentation is essential.

Table 33.7 Focused TTE Protocols

FAST	Focused abdominal sonography for TRAUMA
UHP	Undifferentiated hypotensive patient ultrasound protocol
FATE	Focused assessment with transthoracic echocardiography
FEER	Focused Echo evaluation in resuscitation
CAUSE	Cardiac arrest UltraSound exam
RUSH	Rapid ultrasound in shock
FEELS	Focused echocardiographic evaluation in life support
EGLS	Echo guided life support
CORE	Concentrated overview of resuscitative efforts
BEAT	Bedside echocardiographic assessment in trauma/critical care
BLEEP	Bedside limited Echo' by emergency physicians

Focused TTE Protocols

A systematic approach using a pre-determined scanning sequence increases screening capability and diagnostic accuracy. Various focused TTE protocols have been described in emergency and critical care medicine literature (Table 33.7) [6–10] many of which have been proven useful to guide clinical management of patients who are hemodynamically unstable or critically ill [6]. However, these protocols have either incorporated imaging that is irrelevant in the perioperative setting, or excluded scanning that is important during or after surgery [14, 31, 91, 115, 116]. Evident by the protocol-based approaches described in literature, [6, 7, 10–13, 29, 109] adopting a well thought out perioperative FoCUS protocol is highly recommended [27].

Despite the well-established diagnostic value of the point-of-care transthoracic echocardiography by many disciplines, adoption by anesthesiologists and incorporation into the perioperative use has lagged. Multiple studies have demonstrated the feasibility of anesthesiologist-led TTE in the perioperative period and its impact on patient management. A diverse range of indications (undifferentiated murmurs, unexplained hypotension, altered functional capacity, undifferentiated dyspnea or hypoxemia and PEA cardiac arrest) and etiologies (valvulopathy, impaired LV systolic function, hypovolemia, RV dysfunction or failure and pulmonary embolism) that needed perioperative TTE assessment have been described. To meet the clinical needs of such diversity, residency program with structured perioperative TTE curriculum and TTE protocols specifically designed for perioperative use are warranted.

References

1. Oka Y. The evolution of intraoperative transesophageal echocardiography. MT Sinai J Med. 2002;69(1–2):18–20.
2. Reeves ST, Finley AC, Skubas NJ, Swaminathan M, Whitley WS, Glas KE, et al. Special article: basic perioperative transesophageal echocardiography examination: a consensus statement of the American Society of Echocardiography and the Society of Cardiovascular Anesthesiologists. Anesth Analg. 2013;117(3):543–58.
3. Kremer P, Cahalan M, Beaupre P, Schroder E, Hanrath P, Heinrich H, et al. Intraoperative monitoring using transesophageal 2-dimensional echocardiography. Anaesthesist. 1985;34(3):111–7.
4. Beaupre PN, Kremer PF, Cahalan MK, Lurz FW, Schiller NB, Hamilton WK. Intraoperative detection of changes in left ventricular segmental wall motion by transesophageal two-dimensional echocardiography. Am Heart J. 1984;107(5 Pt 1):1021–3.
5. Piercy M, McNicol L, Dinh DT, Story DA, Smith JA. Major complications related to the use of transesophageal echocardiography in cardiac surgery. J Cardiothorac Vasc Anesth. 2009;23(1):62–5.
6. Kimura BJ, Shaw DJ, Agan DL, Amundson SA, Ping AC, DeMaria AN. Value of a cardiovascular limited ultrasound examination using a hand-carried ultrasound device on clinical management in an outpatient medical clinic. Am J Cardiol. 2007;100(2):321–5.
7. Rose JS, Bair AE, Mandavia D, Kinser DJ. The UHP ultrasound protocol: a novel ultrasound approach to the empiric evaluation of the undifferentiated hypotensive patient. Am J Emerg Med. 2001;19(4):299–302.
8. Jensen MB, Sloth E, Larsen KM, Schmidt MB. Transthoracic echocardiography for cardiopulmonary monitoring in intensive care. Eur J Anaesthesiol. 2004;21(9):700–7.
9. Carr BG, Dean AJ, Everett WW, Ku BS, Mark DG, Okusanya O, et al. Intensivist bedside ultrasound (INBU) for volume assessment in the intensive care unit: a pilot study. J Trauma. 2007;63(3):495–500. discussion-2
10. Perera P, Mailhot T, Riley D, Mandavia D. The RUSH exam: rapid ultrasound in SHock in the evaluation of the critically Ill. Emerg Med Clin North Am. 2010;28(1):29–56. vii
11. Atkinson PR, McAuley DJ, Kendall RJ, Abeyakoon O, Reid CG, Connolly J, et al. Abdominal and cardiac evaluation with sonography in shock (ACES): an approach by emergency physicians for the use of ultrasound in patients with undifferentiated hypotension. EMJ. 2009;26(2):87–91.
12. Lanctot FVM, Beaulieau Y. EGLS: echo-guided life support. An algorithmic approach to undifferentiated shock. Crit Ultrasound J. 2011;3:123–9.
13. Holm JH, Frederiksen CA, Juhl-Olsen P, Sloth E. Perioperative use of focus assessed transthoracic echocardiography (FATE). Anesth Analg. 2012;115(5):1029–32.
14. Pershad J, Myers S, Plouman C, Rosson C, Elam K, Wan J, et al. Bedside limited echocardiography by the emergency physician is accurate during evaluation of the critically ill patient. Pediatrics. 2004;114(6):e667–71.
15. Gerlach RM, Saha TK, Allard RV, Tanzola RC. Unrecognized tamponade diagnosed preinduction by focused echocardiography. Can J Anaesth. 2013;60(8):803–7.
16. Canty DJ, Royse CF. Audit of anaesthetist-performed echocardiography on perioperative management decisions for non-cardiac surgery. Br J Anaesth. 2009;103(3):352–8.
17. Faris JG, Veltman MG, Royse CF. Limited transthoracic echocardiography assessment in anaesthesia and critical care. Best Pract Res Clin Anaesthesiol. 2009;23(3):285–98.
18. Ramsingh D, Fox JC, Wilson WC. Perioperative point-of-care ultrasonography: an emerging technology to be embraced by anesthesiologists. Anesth Analg. 2015;120(5):990–2.
19. Canty DJ, Royse CF, Kilpatrick D, Bowman L, Royse AG. The impact of focused transthoracic echocardiography in the pre-operative clinic. Anaesthesia. 2012;67(6):618–25.
20. Griffee MJ, Merkel MJ, Wei KS. The role of echocardiography in hemodynamic assessment of septic shock. Crit Care Clin. 2010;26(2):365–82. table of contents
21. Chalumeau-Lemoine L, Baudel JL, Das V, Arrive L, Noblinski B, Guidet B, et al. Results of short-term training of naive physicians in focused general ultrasonography in an intensive-care unit. Intensive Care Med. 2009;35(10):1767–71.
22. Diaz-Gomez JL, Perez-Protto S, Hargrave J, Builes A, Capdeville M, Festic E, et al. Impact of a focused transthoracic echocardiography training course for rescue applications among anesthesiology and critical care medicine practitioners: a prospective study. J Cardiothorac Vasc Anesth. 2015;29(3):576–81.
23. Shmueli H, Burstein Y, Sagy I, Perry ZH, Ilia R, Henkin Y, et al. Briefly trained medical students can effectively identify rheumatic mitral valve injury using a hand-carried ultrasound. Echocardiography. 2013;30(6):621–6.
24. Cowie B. Focused cardiovascular ultrasound performed by anesthesiologists in the perioperative

period: feasible and alters patient management. J Cardiothorac Vasc Anesth. 2009;23(4):450–6.

25. Song H, Tsai SK, Liu J. Tailored holder for continuous echocardiographic monitoring. Anesth Analg. 2018;126(2):435–7.

26. Jasudavisius A, Arellano R, Martin J, McConnell B, Bainbridge D. A systematic review of transthoracic and transesophageal echocardiography in non-cardiac surgery: implications for point-of-care ultrasound education in the operating room. Can J Anaesth. 2016;63(4):480–7.

27. Via G, Hussain A, Wells M, Reardon R, ElBarbary M, Noble VE, et al. International evidence-based recommendations for focused cardiac ultrasound. J Am Soc Echocardiogr. 2014;27(7):683.e1–e33.

28. Kimura BJ, Yogo N, O'Connell CW, Phan JN, Showalter BK, Wolfson T. Cardiopulmonary limited ultrasound examination for "quick-look" bedside application. Am J Cardiol. 2011;108(4):586–90.

29. Mizubuti GB, Allard RV, Tanzola RC, Ho AM. Pro: focused cardiac ultrasound should be an integral component of anesthesiology residency training. J Cardiothorac Vasc Anesth. 2015;29(4):1081–5.

30. Moore CL, Copel JA. Point-of-care ultrasonography. N Engl J Med. 2011;364(8):749–57.

31. Manasia AR, Nagaraj HM, Kodali RB, Croft LB, Oropello JM, Kohli-Seth R, et al. Feasibility and potential clinical utility of goal-directed transthoracic echocardiography performed by noncardiologist intensivists using a small hand-carried device (SonoHeart) in critically ill patients. J Cardiothorac Vasc Anesth. 2005;19(2):155–9.

32. Jones AE, Tayal VS, Sullivan DM, Kline JA. Randomized, controlled trial of immediate versus delayed goal-directed ultrasound to identify the cause of nontraumatic hypotension in emergency department patients. Crit Care Med. 2004;32(8):1703–8.

33. Levitt MA, Jan BA. The effect of real time 2-D-echocardiography on medical decision-making in the emergency department. J Emerg Med. 2002;22(3):229–33.

34. Yanagawa Y, Nishi K, Sakamoto T, Okada Y. Early diagnosis of hypovolemic shock by sonographic measurement of inferior vena cava in trauma patients. J Trauma. 2005;58(4):825–9.

35. Breitkreutz R, Price S, Steiger HV, Seeger FH, Ilper H, Ackermann H, et al. Focused echocardiographic evaluation in life support and peri-resuscitation of emergency patients: a prospective trial. Resuscitation. 2010;81(11):1527–33.

36. Royse CF, Canty DJ, Faris J, Haji DL, Veltman M, Royse A. Core review: physician-performed ultrasound: the time has come for routine use in acute care medicine. Anesth Analg. 2012;115(5):1007–28.

37. Hadi A, Vloka JD, Koorn R, Thys DM. Transthoracic echocardiography in perioperative medicine. Can J Anaesth. 1999;46(6):616.

38. Lau G, Swanevelder J. Echocardiography in intensive care--where we are heading? Anaesthesia. 2011;66(8):649–52.

39. Orme RM, Oram MP, McKinstry CE. Impact of echocardiography on patient management in the intensive care unit: an audit of district general hospital practice. Br J Anaesth. 2009;102(3):340–4.

40. Labovitz AJ, Noble VE, Bierig M, Goldstein SA, Jones R, Kort S, et al. Focused cardiac ultrasound in the emergent setting: a consensus statement of the American Society of Echocardiography and American College of Emergency Physicians. J Am Soc Echocardiogr. 2010;23(12):1225–30.

41. van Klei WA, Kalkman CJ, Tolsma M, Rutten CL, Moons KG. Pre-operative detection of valvular heart disease by anaesthetists. Anaesthesia. 2006;61(2):127–32.

42. Price S, Via G, Sloth E, Guarracino F, Breitkreutz R, Catena E, et al. Echocardiography practice, training and accreditation in the intensive care: document for the world interactive network focused on critical ultrasound (WINFOCUS). Cardiovasc Ultrasound. 2008;6:49.

43. Fox K. A position statement: echocardiography in the critically ill. Acute Med. 2008;7(2):95–6.

44. Wright J, Jarman R, Connolly J, Dissmann P. Echocardiography in the emergency department. EMJ. 2009;26(2):82–6.

45. Hahn RT. Should echocardiographers embrace the FOCUS examination? J Am Soc Echocardiogr. 2013;26(4):A32–3.

46. Canty DJ, Royse CF, Kilpatrick D, Williams DL, Royse AG. The impact of pre-operative focused transthoracic echocardiography in emergency non-cardiac surgery patients with known or risk of cardiac disease. Anaesthesia. 2012;67(7):714–20.

47. Ling LF, Obuchowski NA, Rodriguez L, Popovic Z, Kwon D, Marwick TH. Accuracy and interobserver concordance of echocardiographic assessment of right ventricular size and systolic function: a quality control exercise. J Am Soc Echocardiogr. 2012;25(7):709–13.

48. Das P, Pocock C, Chambers J. The patient with a systolic murmur: severe aortic stenosis may be missed during cardiovascular examination. QJM. 2000;93(10):685–8.

49. Kimura BJ, Gilcrease GW 3rd, Showalter BK, Phan JN, Wolfson T. Diagnostic performance of a pocket-sized ultrasound device for quick-look cardiac imaging. Am J Emerg Med. 2012;30(1):32–6.

50. Lang RM, Badano LP, Mor-Avi V, Afilalo J, Armstrong A, Ernande L, et al. Recommendations for cardiac chamber quantification by echocardiography in adults: an update from the American Society of Echocardiography and the European Association of Cardiovascular Imaging. J Am Soc Echocardiogr. 2015;28(1):1–39.e14.

51. Medvedofsky D, Mor-Avi V, Amzulescu M, et al. Three-dimensional echocardiographic quantification of the left-heart chambers using an automated adaptive analytics algorithm: multi-center validation study. Eur Heart J Cardiovasc Imaging. 2017;19:1–12.

52. Dorosz JL, Lezotte DC, Weitzenkamp DA, Allen LA, Salcedo EE. Performance of 3-dimensional echo-

cardiography in measuring left ventricular volumes and ejection fraction: a systematic review and meta-analysis. J Am Coll Cardiol. 2012;59(20):1799–808.

53. Muraru D, Badano LP, Peluso D, Dal Bianco L, Casablanca S, Kocabay G, et al. Comprehensive analysis of left ventricular geometry and function by three-dimensional echocardiography in healthy adults. J Am Soc Echocardiogr. 2013;26(6):618–28.

54. Reisner SA, Lysyansky P, Agmon Y, Mutlak D, Lessick J, Friedman Z. Global longitudinal strain: a novel index of left ventricular systolic function. J Am Soc Echocardiogr. 2004;17(6):630–3.

55. Dalen H, Thorstensen A, Aase SA, Ingul CB, Torp H, Vatten LJ, et al. Segmental and global longitudinal strain and strain rate based on echocardiography of 1266 healthy individuals: the HUNT study in Norway. Eur J Echocardiogr. 2010;11(2):176–83.

56. Voigt JU, Pedrizzetti G, Lysyansky P, Marwick TH, Houle H, Baumann R, et al. Definitions for a common standard for 2D speckle tracking echocardiography: consensus document of the EACVI/ASE/Industry Task Force to standardize deformation imaging. Eur Heart J Cardiovasc Imaging. 2015;16(1):1–11.

57. Yingchoncharoen T, Agarwal S, Popovic ZB, Marwick TH. Normal ranges of left ventricular strain: a meta-analysis. J Am Soc Echocardiogr. 2013;26(2):185–91.

58. Kocabay G, Muraru D, Peluso D, Cucchini U, Mihaila S, Padayattil-Jose S, et al. Normal left ventricular mechanics by two-dimensional speckle-tracking echocardiography. Reference values in healthy adults. Rev Esp Cardiol. 2014;67(8):651–8.

59. Takigiku K, Takeuchi M, Izumi C, Yuda S, Sakata K, Ohte N, et al. Normal range of left ventricular 2-dimensional strain: Japanese ultrasound speckle tracking of the left ventricle (JUSTICE) study. Circ J. 2012;76(11):2623–32.

60. Kurkciyan I, Meron G, Sterz F, Janata K, Domanovits H, Holzer M, et al. Pulmonary embolism as a cause of cardiac arrest: presentation and outcome. Arch Intern Med. 2000;160(10):1529–35.

61. Comess KA, DeRook FA, Russell ML, Tognazzi-Evans TA, Beach KW. The incidence of pulmonary embolism in unexplained sudden cardiac arrest with pulseless electrical activity. Am J Med. 2000;109(5):351–6.

62. Mor-Avi V, Lang RM, Badano LP, Belohlavek M, Cardim NM, Derumeaux G, et al. Current and evolving echocardiographic techniques for the quantitative evaluation of cardiac mechanics: ASE/EAE consensus statement on methodology and indications endorsed by the Japanese Society of Echocardiography. J Am Soc Echocardiogr. 2011;24(3):277–313.

63. Shimada YJ, Shiota M, Siegel RJ, Shiota T. Accuracy of right ventricular volumes and function determined by three-dimensional echocardiography in comparison with magnetic resonance imaging: a meta-analysis study. J Am Soc Echocardiogr. 2010;23(9):943–53.

64. D'Oronzio U, Senn O, Biaggi P, Gruner C, Jenni R, Tanner FC, et al. Right heart assessment by echocar-diography: gender and body size matters. J Am Soc Echocardiogr. 2012;25(12):1251–8.

65. Willis J, Augustine D, Shah R, Stevens C, Easaw J. Right ventricular normal measurements: time to index? J Am Soc Echocardiogr. 2012;25(12):1259–67.

66. Giusca S, Dambrauskaite V, Scheurwegs C, D'Hooge J, Claus P, Herbots L, et al. Deformation imaging describes right ventricular function better than longitudinal displacement of the tricuspid ring. Heart. 2010;96(4):281–8.

67. Innelli P, Esposito R, Olibet M, Nistri S, Galderisi M. The impact of ageing on right ventricular longitudinal function in healthy subjects: a pulsed tissue Doppler study. Eur J Echocardiogr. 2009;10(4):491–8.

68. Varas JL, Diaz CM, Blancas R, et al. Inferior vena cava Distensibility index predicting fluid responsiveness in ventilated patients. Intensive Care Med Exp. 2015;3(Suppl):A600.

69. Dipti A, Soucy Z, Surana A, Chandra S. Role of inferior vena cava diameter in assessment of volume status: a meta-analysis. Am J Emerg Med. 2012;30(8):1414–9.e1.

70. Zengin S, Al B, Genc S, Yildirim C, Ercan S, Dogan M, et al. Role of inferior vena cava and right ventricular diameter in assessment of volume status: a comparative study: ultrasound and hypovolemia. Am J Emerg Med. 2013;31(5):763–7.

71. Kircher BJ, Himelman RB, Schiller NB. Noninvasive estimation of right atrial pressure from the inspiratory collapse of the inferior vena cava. Am J Cardiol. 1990;66(4):493–6.

72. Bodson L, Vieillard-Baron A. Respiratory variation in inferior vena cava diameter: surrogate of central venous pressure or parameter of fluid responsiveness? Let the physiology reply. Crit Care. 2012;16(6):181.

73. Ciozda W, Kedan I, Kehl DW, Zimmer R, Khandwalla R, Kimchi A. The efficacy of sonographic measurement of inferior vena cava diameter as an estimate of central venous pressure. Cardiovasc Ultrasound. 2016;14(1):33.

74. Feissel M, Michard F, Faller JP, Teboul JL. The respiratory variation in inferior vena cava diameter as a guide to fluid therapy. Intensive Care Med. 2004;30(9):1834–7.

75. Barbier C, Loubieres Y, Schmit C, Hayon J, Ricome JL, Jardin F, et al. Respiratory changes in inferior vena cava diameter are helpful in predicting fluid responsiveness in ventilated septic patients. Intensive Care Med. 2004;30(9):1740–6.

76. Monnet X, Rienzo M, Osman D, Anguel N, Richard C, Pinsky MR, et al. Passive leg raising predicts fluid responsiveness in the critically ill. Crit Care Med. 2006;34(5):1402–7.

77. Preau S, Saulnier F, Dewavrin F, Durocher A, Chagnon JL. Passive leg raising is predictive of fluid responsiveness in spontaneously breathing patients with severe sepsis or acute pancreatitis. Crit Care Med. 2010;38(3):819–25.

78. Maizel J, Airapetian N, Lorne E, Tribouilloy C, Massy Z, Slama M. Diagnosis of central hypovole-

mia by using passive leg raising. Intensive Care Med. 2007;33(7):1133–8.

79. Moretti R, Pizzi B. Inferior vena cava distensibility as a predictor of fluid responsiveness in patients with subarachnoid hemorrhage. Neurocrit Care. 2010;13(1):3–9.

80. Oh JK, Seward JB, Tajik AJ. The echo manual. 3rd ed. New York: Lippincott Williams & Wilkins; 2006.

81. Perez-Casares A, Cesar S, Brunet-Garcia L, Sanchez-de-Toledo J. Echocardiographic evaluation of pericardial effusion and cardiac tamponade. Front Pediatr. 2017;5:79.

82. Weitzman LB, Tinker WP, Kronzon I, Cohen ML, Glassman E, Spencer FC. The incidence and natural history of pericardial effusion after cardiac surgery--an echocardiographic study. Circulation. 1984;69(3):506–11.

83. Maisch B, Seferovic PM, Ristic AD, Erbel R, Rienmuller R, Adler Y, et al. Guidelines on the diagnosis and management of pericardial diseases executive summary; the task force on the diagnosis and management of pericardial diseases of the European society of cardiology. Eur Heart J. 2004;25(7):587–610.

84. Aronow WS, Schwartz KS, Koenigsberg M. Correlation of aortic cuspal and aortic root disease with aortic systolic ejection murmurs and with mitral anular calcium in persons older than 62 years in a long-term health care facility. Am J Cardiol. 1986;58(7):651–2.

85. Aronow WS, Kronzon I. Correlation of prevalence and severity of valvular aortic stenosis determined by continuous-wave Doppler echocardiography with physical signs of aortic stenosis in patients aged 62 to 100 years with aortic systolic ejection murmurs. Am J Cardiol. 1987;60(4):399–401.

86. Lindroos M, Kupari M, Heikkila J, Tilvis R. Prevalence of aortic valve abnormalities in the elderly: an echocardiographic study of a random population sample. J Am Coll Cardiol. 1993;21(5):1220–5.

87. Stewart BF, Siscovick D, Lind BK, Gardin JM, Gottdiener JS, Smith VE, et al. Clinical factors associated with calcific aortic valve disease. Cardiovascular health study. J Am Coll Cardiol. 1997;29(3):630–4.

88. Freed LA, Levy D, Levine RA, Larson MG, Evans JC, Fuller DL, et al. Prevalence and clinical outcome of mitral-valve prolapse. N Engl J Med. 1999;341(1):1–7.

89. Goldman L, Caldera DL, Nussbaum SR, Southwick FS, Krogstad D, Murray B, et al. Multifactorial index of cardiac risk in noncardiac surgical procedures. N Engl J Med. 1977;297(16):845–50.

90. Kertai MD, Bountioukos M, Boersma E, Bax JJ, Thomson IR, Sozzi F, et al. Aortic stenosis: an underestimated risk factor for perioperative complications in patients undergoing noncardiac surgery. Am J Med. 2004;116(1):8–13.

91. Rohde LE, Polanczyk CA, Goldman L, Cook EF, Lee RT, Lee TH. Usefulness of transthoracic echocardiography as a tool for risk stratification of patients undergoing major noncardiac surgery. Am J Cardiol. 2001;87(5):505–9.

92. Nishimura RA, Otto CM, Bonow RO, Carabello BA, Erwin JP 3rd, Guyton RA, et al. 2014 AHA/ACC guideline for the management of patients with valvular heart disease: a report of the American College of Cardiology/American Heart Association Task Force on Practice Guidelines. J Thorac Cardiovasc Surg. 2014;148(1):e1–e132.

93. Nishimura RA, Otto CM, Bonow RO, Carabello BA, Erwin JP 3rd, Fleisher LA, et al. 2017 AHA/ACC focused update of the 2014 AHA/ACC Guideline for the Management of Patients with Valvular Heart Disease: a report of the American College of Cardiology/American Heart Association Task Force on Clinical Practice Guidelines. J Am Coll Cardiol. 2017;70(2):252–89.

94. Lancellotti P, Moura L, Pierard LA, Agricola E, Popescu BA, Tribouilloy C, et al. European Association of Echocardiography recommendations for the assessment of valvular regurgitation. Part 2: mitral and tricuspid regurgitation (native valve disease). Eur J Echocardiogr. 2010;11(4):307–32.

95. Lancellotti P, Tribouilloy C, Hagendorff A, Moura L, Popescu BA, Agricola E, et al. European Association of Echocardiography recommendations for the assessment of valvular regurgitation. Part 1: aortic and pulmonary regurgitation (native valve disease). Eur J Echocardiogr. 2010;11(3):223–44.

96. Baumgartner H, Hung J, Bermejo J, Chambers JB, Evangelista A, Griffin BP, et al. Echocardiographic assessment of valve stenosis: EAE/ASE recommendations for clinical practice. J Am Soc Echocardiogr. 2009;22(1):1–23. quiz 101-2

97. Vahanian A, Ducrocq G. Emergencies in valve disease. Curr Opin Crit Care. 2008;14(5):555–60.

98. Andersen GN, Haugen BO, Graven T, Salvesen O, Mjolstad OC, Dalen H. Feasibility and reliability of point-of-care pocket-sized echocardiography. Eur J Echocardiogr. 2011;12(9):665–70.

99. Giusca S, Jurcut R, Ticulescu R, Dumitru D, Vladaia A, Savu O, et al. Accuracy of handheld echocardiography for bedside diagnostic evaluation in a tertiary cardiology center: comparison with standard echocardiography. Echocardiography. 2011;28(2):136–41.

100. Manno E, Navarra M, Faccio L, Motevallian M, Bertolaccini L, Mfochive A, et al. Deep impact of ultrasound in the intensive care unit: the "ICU-sound" protocol. Anesthesiology. 2012;117(4):801–9.

101. Hernandez C, Shuler K, Hannan H, Sonyika C, Likourezos A, Marshall J. C.A.U.S.E.: cardiac arrest ultra-sound exam--a better approach to managing patients in primary non-arrhythmogenic cardiac arrest. Resuscitation. 2008;76(2):198–206.

102. Price S, Uddin S, Quinn T. Echocardiography in cardiac arrest. Curr Opin Crit Care. 2010;16(3):211–5.

103. Hayhurst C, Lebus C, Atkinson PR, Kendall R, Madan R, Talbot J, et al. An evaluation of echo in life support (ELS): is it feasible? What does it add? Emerg Med J. 2011;28(2):119–21.

104. Pepi M, Muratori M. Echocardiography in the diagnosis and management of pericardial disease. J Cardiovasc Med. 2006;7(7):533–44.

105. Tayal VS, Kline JA. Emergency echocardiography to detect pericardial effusion in patients in PEA and near-PEA states. Resuscitation. 2003;59(3):315–8.

106. Blaivas M, Fox JC. Outcome in cardiac arrest patients found to have cardiac standstill on the bedside emergency department echocardiogram. Acad Emerg Med. 2001;8(6):616–21.

107. Salen P, O'Connor R, Sierzenski P, Passarello B, Pancu D, Melanson S, et al. Can cardiac sonography and capnography be used independently and in combination to predict resuscitation outcomes? Acad Emerg Med. 2001;8(6):610–5.

108. Salen P, Melniker L, Chooljian C, Rose JS, Alteveer J, Reed J, et al. Does the presence or absence of sonographically identified cardiac activity predict resuscitation outcomes of cardiac arrest patients? Am J Emerg Med. 2005;23(4):459–62.

109. Breitkreutz R, Walcher F, Seeger FH. Focused echocardiographic evaluation in resuscitation management: concept of an advanced life support-conformed algorithm. Crit Care Med. 2007;35(5 Suppl):S150–61.

110. Breitkreutz R, Walcher F, Seeger FH. ALS conformed use of echocardiography or ultrasound in resuscitation management. Resuscitation. 2008;77(2):270–2. author reply 2–3

111. Niendorff DF, Rassias AJ, Palac R, Beach ML, Costa S, Greenberg M. Rapid cardiac ultrasound of inpatients suffering PEA arrest performed by nonexpert sonographers. Resuscitation. 2005;67(1):81–7.

112. Christenson J, Andrusiek D, Everson-Stewart S, Kudenchuk P, Hostler D, Powell J, et al. Chest compression fraction determines survival in patients with out-of-hospital ventricular fibrillation. Circulation. 2009;120(13):1241–7.

113. Hazinski MF, Nolan JP, Billi JE, Bottiger BW, Bossaert L, de Caen AR, et al. Part 1: executive summary: 2010 international consensus on cardiopulmonary resuscitation and emergency cardiovascular care science with treatment recommendations. Circulation. 2010;122(16 Suppl 2):S250–75.

114. Volpicelli G. Usefulness of emergency ultrasound in nontraumatic cardiac arrest. Am J Emerg Med. 2011;29(2):216–23.

115. Cowie BS. Focused transthoracic echocardiography in the perioperative period. Anaesth Intensive Care. 2010;38(5):823–36.

116. Conlin F, Roy Connelly N, Raghunathan K, Friderici J, Schwabauer A. Focused transthoracic cardiac ultrasound: a survey of training practices. J Cardiothorac Vasc Anesth. 2016;30(1):102–6.

Myocardial Protection During Cardiac Surgery

34

Amine Mazine, Myunghyun M. Lee,
and Terrence M. Yau

Main Messages

1. The two main types of cardioplegic solutions in use are crystalloid (acellular) cardioplegia and blood cardioplegia.
2. Blood cardioplegia has a number of theoretical metabolic advantages and has been shown to reduce postoperative low cardiac output syndrome and enzyme release but has not been conclusively demonstrated to have an effect on mortality when compared with crystalloid cardioplegia.
3. Cardioplegia can be cold, warm or tepid. Each of these temperatures has advantages and drawbacks. While normothermic cardioplegia reduces low cardiac output syndrome and enzyme release, no effect of cardioplegic temperature on mortality has yet been demonstrated.
4. Cardioplegia can be delivered antegrade, retrograde, or by a combined approach of antegrade and retrograde. The optimal delivery method should be tailored to the individual patient's clinical and anatomic details.
5. In recent years, the use of modified crystalloid cardioplegic solutions—often administered as a single dose granting an extended period of protection—has garnered increasing interest, particularly for valvular surgery. While initial results have been encouraging, further studies are required to confirm the safety of these approaches and to compare their efficacy with established methods of myocardial protection in various subgroups of patients, particularly those with coronary artery disease or pre-existing ventricular dysfunction.

A. Mazine · M. M. Lee
Division of Cardiac Surgery, Department of Surgery, University of Toronto, Toronto, ON, Canada

T. M. Yau (✉)
Division of Cardiac Surgery, Department of Surgery, University of Toronto, Toronto, ON, Canada

Peter Munk Cardiac Centre, Division of Cardiovascular Surgery, Toronto General Hospital, University Health Network, Toronto, ON, Canada
e-mail: terry.yau@uhn.ca

The goal of myocardial protection in the setting of cardiac surgery is to minimize myocardial ischemia/reperfusion injury during cardiopulmonary bypass, primarily by reducing myocardial oxygen consumption and requirements. This is usually achieved with the use of cardioplegic solutions which induce rapid diastolic arrest, produce mild to moderate hypo-

© Springer Nature Switzerland AG 2021
D. C. H. Cheng et al. (eds.), *Evidence-Based Practice in Perioperative Cardiac Anesthesia and Surgery*, https://doi.org/10.1007/978-3-030-47887-2_34

thermia, buffer ischemic acidosis, mitigate substrate depletion and ionic disturbances, and prevent intracellular edema. While there exists a number of non-cardioplegic methods of myocardial protection—e.g. intermittent cross-clamp fibrillation, fibrillation on bypass without aortic clamping, beating heart on bypass, deep hypothermic circulatory arrest—these fall beyond the scope of the present chapter, which focuses on the various aspects of cardioplegia administration during cardiac surgery.

Historical Background

In 1883, Sydney Ringer described the antagonistic effects of potassium on myocardial contractility [1]. This pioneering work provided the scientific basis for current approaches to induction of cardiac arrest with potassium cardioplegia. With the advent of open heart surgery using cardiopulmonary bypass, strategies to create a quiescent, bloodless field and to protect the heart from ischemic injury were needed. One of the first methods used was hypothermic arrest, pioneered by Bigelow and colleagues in Toronto in the 1950s [2]. A few years later, Melrose and colleagues introduced the concept of reversible chemical cardiac arrest using potassium citrate injected in the aortic root [3]. After an initial wave of enthusiasm, the Melrose approach was largely abandoned following the publication of several studies demonstrating an association between potassium citrate arrest and severe myocardial necrosis. It was not until a number of years later that the poor outcomes associated with the original Melrose solution were attributed to the high potassium concentrations [4]. In the ensuing years, many surgeons shifted from the use of potassium-induced arrest to normothermic cardiac ischemia, intermittent aortic occlusion, or continuous coronary perfusion with a beating heart. These techniques were adopted with some success in the United States, despite clinical evidence linking normothermic cardiac ischemia to the development of ischemic myocardial contracture—the so-called "stone heart" [5]—in a subset of patients.

Whereas in North America cardioplegia had been largely abandoned in favor of alternative techniques, in Germany, Bretschneider and colleagues continued studying chemically induced cardiac arrest and eventually introduced a histidine protein buffered, low-sodium, calcium-free, procaine-containing solution (Bretschneider solution) [6]. Shortly after, Hearse and colleagues introduced a crystalloid solution based on Ringer's solution with its normal concentration of sodium and calcium, with the addition of potassium chloride and magnesium chloride to arrest the heart rapidly and provide additional cardioprotective benefit [7]. This solution was first introduced to clinical practice in 1975 by Braimbridge and colleagues at St. Thomas' Hospital, hence its appellation, the St. Thomas' solution [8].

On the basis of improved clinical outcomes, the use of cardioplegia for myocardial protection was progressively reintroduced in North America in the 1980s and gradually replaced normothermic aortic occlusion. Controversy persisted, however, regarding the ideal composition of crystalloid cardioplegic solutions. Concomitant to this controversy was the introduction of a new variant of cardioplegia, namely potassium-enriched blood cardioplegia [9]. Despite further refinements and innovations over the last three decades, hypothermia and potassium-mediated cardiac arrest remain the cornerstones of myocardial protection to this day.

Types of Cardioplegic Solutions: Crystalloid Versus Blood

Cardioplegic solutions are designed to arrest the heart rapidly in diastole, create a flaccid heart, provide the operator with a quiescent, bloodless field, protect the heart against ischemia-reperfusion injury, and, importantly, allow the heart to regain adequate electromechanical function to support the systemic circulation rapidly after the ischemic interval. Currently, the two main types of cardioplegic solutions in use are *crystalloid (acellular) cardioplegia* and *blood cardioplegia*.

Crystalloid Cardioplegia

Crystalloid cardioplegic solutions were introduced several decades ago, and over the years, a number of different formulations have been developed. Despite differences in composition, these formulations all feature relatively high concentrations of potassium to induce hyperkalemic diastolic arrest and at least mild degrees of hypothermia. Broadly speaking, crystalloid cardioplegia can be divided in two types: the *intracellular* type, characterized by low or absent concentrations of sodium and calcium (e.g. Bretschneider solution), and the *extracellular* type, containing relatively higher concentrations of sodium and calcium (e.g. St. Thomas' solution).

The various ingredients that compose crystalloid solutions serve different purposes, including:

1. Induction of rapid cardiac arrest using potassium.
2. Stabilization of pH using buffers such as bicarbonate, phosphate, histidine or THAM (tris-hydroxymethyl-aminomethane).
3. Maintenance of intracellular ionic and metabolic homeostasis (e.g. avoidance of intracellular calcium overload by providing a hypocalcemic solution and adding magnesium).
4. Stabilization of cellular membranes with steroids, calcium antagonists, procaine and/or oxygen free radical scavengers (e.g. glutathione).
5. Prevention of cell edema with the addition of colloids such as mannitol to maintain normal oncotic pressures.
6. Avoidance of substrate depletion with the addition of glucose, insulin, nucleosides and L-arginine to stimulate NO production.
7. Reduction of myocardial oxygen consumption, decrease in energy demand, and conservation of ATP reserves achieved by cooling the solution.

The main disadvantage of crystalloid cardioplegia is its limited oxygen-carrying capacity. The use of oxygenated crystalloid cardioplegia has been proposed to overcome the oxygen deficit issue, but has never achieved significant clinical use [10].

Blood Cardioplegia

In order to avoid the oxygen deficits associated with crystalloid cardioplegia, blood was introduced in the late 1970s as a more effective vehicle for the delivery of potassium-induced cardiac arrest. Blood cardioplegia has since become the most commonly used cardioplegic solution in North America.

The physiologic advantages of blood cardioplegia include:

1. Enhanced oxygen and carbon dioxide exchanging ability, which allows for intermittent re-oxygenation of the heart during arrest.
2. Excellent buffering and reducing capacity.
3. Presence of colloid, which avoids deleterious oncotic pressure gradients.
4. Presence of endogenous antioxidants and oxygen free radical scavengers.
5. Limited hemodilution compared to crystalloid cardioplegia, especially when large volumes of cardioplegic solutions are used.
6. Physiologic electrolyte composition and pH.
7. Better preservation of microvascular responses compared with crystalloid cardioplegia [11].

Although several different formulations of blood cardioplegia had been proposed, previously the solution was prepared by mixing autologous blood from the perfusion circuit with a crystalloid solution that consisted of citrate-phosphate-dextrose (to lower ionic calcium), tris-hydroxymethyl aminomethane (THAM, for buffering), and potassium chloride (to induce diastolic arrest). Nowadays, THAM is no longer commonly added (as its buffering capacity is exceeded by the endogenous buffering capacity of the blood component of cardioplegia) and magnesium is usually added for membrane stabilization. The final concentration of potassium used to arrest the heart is approximately 20–30 mEq/L. After the initial *induction* dose, subsequent *maintenance* doses—which may be intermittent or continuous—frequently use a potassium concentration of 8–10 mEq/L, but this concentration can be varied continuously in order to maintain cardiac arrest with the minimum dose of potassium. Over time, the ratio of blood to crystalloid has generally increased from 2:1 to 4:1 to 8:1 and ultimately, with the goal of minimizing hemodilution, the use of undiluted blood cardioplegia with minimal amounts of crystalloid additives—the so-called *miniplegia*—was introduced [12].

Table 34.1 Major advantages and limitations of warm versus cold cardioplegia

Temperature	Advantages	Limitations
Cold	Low myocardial metabolism, allowing the safe conduct of complex surgical interventions	Delayed recovery of cardiomyocyte mitochondrial metabolism and ventricular function
Warm	Rapid recovery of myocardial metabolism	Potentially increased risk of neurological injury; requires near continuous delivery

Comparative Studies

Despite its proposed physiological advantages, the superiority of blood cardioplegia over crystalloid cardioplegia remains a matter of controversy, with certain studies demonstrating superior outcomes, while others show no difference. Importantly, most of the evidence surrounding this question is derived from single-center studies with significant limitations, such as the inclusion of only a small number of patients, heterogeneity in the subset of patients studied, and lack of detail regarding clinical management.

In 2006, Guru and colleagues reported results of a meta-analysis of 34 randomized controlled trials comparing blood and crystalloid cardioplegia in adult patients [13]. The authors demonstrated a lower incidence of low output syndrome and lesser degrees of creatine kinase MB increase with the use of blood cardioplegia, but found no differences in the incidence of hard clinical endpoints such as death or myocardial infarction [13].

Temperature of Cardioplegia

The ideal temperature of cardioplegic solutions is a controversial issue which has been widely studied (Table 34.1). The standard method of delivering either blood or crystalloid cardioplegia is with intermittent hypothermic infusion at 8–12 °C, with variations in the temperature and ratio of the systemic blood and crystalloid components of the cardioplegic formulation.

Hypothermia decreases myocardial metabolism and therefore allows for prolonged cardioplegic interruptions, thereby facilitating surgical exposure. This strategy allows for excellent myocardial protection, even when homogeneous delivery of the cardioplegic solution is not entirely feasible. While it produces reliable protection—including in high-risk patients—hypothermic cardioplegia infusion has the disadvantage of reducing myocardial metabolism not only during cardioplegic arrest, but also during reperfusion after cross-clamp removal. As a result, this delayed recovery of aerobic myocardial metabolism results in delayed recovery of ventricular function, because of inadequate mitochondrial energy production.

In an attempt to reduce the duration of metabolic and functional dysfunction after cross-clamp removal, Teoh and colleagues introduced the concept of a terminal infusion of warm blood cardioplegia before removing the cross-clamp (the "hot shot") to accelerate recovery of temperature-dependent mitochondrial respiration [14]. A few years later, with the advent of continuous cardioplegia delivery systems, the technique of warm blood cardioplegia—whereby the heart is electromechanically arrested but continuously perfused with warm blood cardioplegia—was introduced. The principle underlying this approach is that if warm cardioplegia can be given continuously during the cross-clamp period, then the temperature-dependent mitochondrial enzymatic function of the myocardium can be preserved during cardioplegic arrest, leading to improved early ventricular function [15].

This is especially useful for patients who are actively ischemic upon presentation to the operating room, in order to permit cellular repair while the heart is arrested but perfused. Other advantages of this approach include:

1. Near elimination of anaerobic ischemic injury.
2. Early resumption of normal sinus rhythm after removal of the aortic cross-clamp.
3. Avoidance of prolonged durations of rewarming and reperfusion, thus decreasing total cardiopulmonary bypass time.
4. Elimination of systemic hypothermia, and its associated vasoconstriction.

Despite these advantages, warm blood cardioplegia is associated with certain major caveats:

1. Difficulties in visualization of the operative field—e.g. when performing distal coronary anastomoses—frequently mandate temporary discontinuation of the cardioplegic infusion. This can result in increased ischemic injury if cardioplegia administration is interrupted for more than 13 minutes [16].
2. If warm blood cardioplegia cannot be delivered homogeneously (e.g. in the presence of aortic insufficiency or left main stenosis, or when delivered retrograde with shunting of cardioplegia into non-nutritive perfusion via Thebesian and sinusoidal veins), surgeons run the risk of normothermic ischemia of the under-perfused regions.
3. Warm blood cardioplegia is often associated with difficulties in maintaining complete electromechanical arrest.
4. Warm blood cardioplegia is often associated with systemic vasodilation during cardiopulmonary bypass, which mandates the use of vasoconstrictive alpha agonists to maintain adequate perfusion pressures.
5. The combination of warm cardioplegia with systemic warming to 37 °C results in increased rates of adverse neurologic events [17]. Therefore, when using warm cardioplegia, the systemic perfusion temperature should be allowed to drift down to 34 °C, with slow rewarming to avoid hyperthermic brain injury.

The Warm Heart Trial randomized 1732 patients undergoing isolated coronary artery bypass grafting (CABG) to warm or cold blood cardioplegia and normothermic versus mildly hypothermic systemic perfusion. The trial showed no statistically significant difference in rates of early mortality, myocardial infarction or stroke. However, warm blood cardioplegia was associated with significantly lower rates of low output syndrome and with lesser degrees of perioperative creatine kinase MB increase [18]. Late results of this trial showed no statistically significant difference in long-term survival, and further demonstrated that in both groups, patients who experienced non-fatal perioperative events had decreased late survival [19].

In an effort to overcome the deficits of warm blood cardioplegia, without the disadvantages of cold cardioplegia, tepid (29 °C) cardioplegia was introduced. Hayashida and colleagues demonstrated reduced anaerobic lactate and acid release during arrest with the use of tepid cardioplegia compared to warm and cold cardioplegia [20]. However, the superiority of tepid cardioplegia with regards to clinical endpoints has not been established.

Methods of Delivery

Cardioplegia can be delivered antegrade (via the aortic root, directly into the coronary ostia, or through a saphenous vein graft), retrograde (into the coronary sinus) or by a combined approach of antegrade and retrograde. The optimal delivery method should be tailored to the individual patient (Table 34.2).

Antegrade delivery into the aortic root while the aorta is cross-clamped is the most commonly used technique for cardioplegia delivery when the aorta does not need to be opened. Induction of cardioplegic arrest is typically achieved with the administration of 10–15 mL/kg body weight of cardioplegic solution (more in patients with hypertrophied ventricles), delivered at a rate of 250 mL to 300 mL per minute to ensure aortic valve closure. The rate of administration is adjusted to maintain an aortic root perfusion

Table 34.2 Major advantages and limitations of various cardioplegia delivery methods

Delivery method	Advantages	Limitations
Antegrade	Simple, reproducible technique Predictable myocardial protection	• May require frequent interruptions (*unless cardioplegia cannulae are snared into the coronaries*) • Ventricular distention with aortic valve incompetence • Cumbersome during aortic valve surgery • Risk of coronary embolization in redo CABG • Risk of selective cannulation in patients with short left main • Decreased perfusion distal to coronary stenosis/occlusion
Retrograde	May allow for more continuous delivery	• Requires cannulation of coronary sinus • Not feasible in the presence of persistent left SVC • Unreliable perfusion to right ventricle and posterior septum
Combined	Potentially optimized myocardial protection	• Complex and cumbersome delivery system

pressure of 60–80 mmHg. During induction, the left ventricle is continuously monitored to ensure that dilatation—secondary to aortic valve incompetence—does not occur. Direct cannulation of the coronary ostia is frequently used in cases requiring opening of the ascending aorta (e.g. aortic valve replacement, replacement of the aortic root or of the ascending aorta), or in the presence of moderate or more aortic insufficiency. After the initial induction dose of antegrade cardioplegia, intermittent maintenance doses of 300 to 500 mL of low-potassium cardioplegia are administered throughout the procedure in order to maintain cardiac arrest. For CABG cases, maintenance doses are typically given after one to two anastomoses. For valvular surgery, maintenance doses are given every 15 to 20 min, or

earlier if there is evidence of resumption of electrical activity. Careful de-airing of the aortic root is performed before each maintenance dose.

Delivery of antegrade cardioplegia using the approach described above is simple, reproducible and provides predictable myocardial protection. However, it has several limitations:

1. Potential for disruption of an atherosclerotic plaque at the catheter insertion site, resulting in either embolization or dissection of the ascending aorta or the coronary arteries if cannulated directly.
2. In patients with total occlusion or severe coronary stenosis, distal perfusion and adequate myocardial protection may be difficult to achieve. This is less of an issue in patients with well-collateralized chronic lesions.
3. Antegrade cardioplegia delivery may lead to ventricular distention in patients with incompetent aortic valves (either from pre-existing aortic insufficiency, or from aortic incompetence triggered by retraction of the heart during surgery). Ventricular distention decreases the transmyocardial perfusion pressure gradient, thus decreasing cardioplegia delivery and compromising myocardial protection.
4. Antegrade cardioplegia may be cumbersome during aortic valve surgery, which frequently requires individual cannulation of the coronary ostia. This approach is associated with a small but potentially fatal risk of iatrogenic coronary artery dissection or stenosis related to an unrecognized cannulation injury.
5. In the presence of a short left main, ostial cannulation is associated with a risk of unintentional selective delivery into the left anterior descending or circumflex coronary artery, which severely compromises protection of the lateral and anterior wall, respectively.
6. Antegrade cardioplegia delivery must be used with caution in the setting of redo CABG operations, as older patent saphenous vein grafts typically exhibit diffuse and friable atherosclerosis, which may embolize during manipulation of the heart—an issue that is compounded by the use of antegrade cardioplegia.

To overcome the limitations of antegrade cardioplegia delivery, the technique of retrograde cardioplegia administration through the coronary sinus was developed. This approach finds its conceptual origins in the work of Pratt who, in 1898, demonstrated that oxygenated blood could be delivered to the ischemic heart via the coronary venous system [21]. It was only sixty years later, however, that this approach was first introduced clinically, when Lillehei and colleagues used retrograde coronary sinus perfusion to protect the heart during aortic valve surgery [22]. The technique of retrograde cardioplegia delivery entails insertion of a catheter—with or without a self-inflating balloon cuff—into the coronary sinus, either prior to the initiation of cardiopulmonary bypass, or with partial interruption of venous return during cardiopulmonary bypass (to allow distention of the right atrium and to facilitate positioning of the catheter in the coronary sinus). Retrograde cardioplegia can be used for both induction and maintenance of cardioplegic arrest. It allows for continuous administration of cardioplegia throughout the procedure, typically at a rate of 200 mL/min, ensuring that the coronary sinus perfusion pressure does not exceed 40 mmHg to avoid endothelial damage and coronary sinus rupture, a rare but potentially serious complication.

Other advantages of retrograde cardioplegia over the antegrade approach include:

1. Distribution of the cardioplegic solution to areas of myocardium supplied by severely stenotic or occluded coronary arteries.
2. Enhanced distribution to the subendocardium.
3. The potential to both prevent embolization and wash out previously embolized debris in saphenous vein grafts during reoperative coronary surgery.

The limitations of retrograde cardioplegia delivery include:

1. Occasional technical issues, such as difficulty inserting the catheter into the coronary sinus, or easy dislocation of the catheter into the right atrium, particularly during manipulation of the heart for lateral wall grafts.
2. Potentially inhomogeneous protection of the heart, particularly the posterior septum, due to the variability in the venous anatomy of the heart or occlusion of the orifice of the posterior interventricular vein by the catheter balloon.
3. Suboptimal protection of the right ventricle because of shunting into Thebesian and sinusoidal channels.
4. Because coronary sinus pressures >40 mmHg may cause coronary sinus rupture, the protection of hypertrophied hearts—which require higher coronary perfusion pressure to achieve satisfactory transmyocardial pressure gradients—is difficult with the use of retrograde cardioplegia only.
5. Increased risk of inadequate right ventricle myocardial protection in patients with pulmonary hypertension and hypertrophied right ventricles.

The advantages of both antegrade and retrograde delivery systems can be combined with the concomitant use of both strategies. While most routine on-pump cardiac procedures can be carried out safely with the use of antegrade cardioplegia only, a dual approach combining both antegrade and retrograde techniques may be beneficial in patients with poor left ventricular function, those in whom a long cross-clamp time is anticipated, and those with occlusive coronary artery disease. While this approach has some theoretical benefits, its clinical superiority has not been established.

While numerous studies have documented the safety and efficacy of various cardioplegia delivery systems, there is a paucity of prospective head-to-head comparisons in large cohorts of patients. As a result of this lack of high-quality data, there is considerable variability in clinical practice. However, the most important route to achieving good myocardial protection is having a surgeon who pays careful attention to this aspect of the operation.

Novel Strategies for Myocardial Protection

In general, single-dose cardioplegia strategies have been utilized more commonly in neonatal and pediatric surgery. However, in recent years, the use of single-dose cardioplegia in adults has garnered increasing interest, particularly for valvular surgery. As result, there has been renewed interest in the use of crystalloid cardioplegia. In this section, we briefly discuss recent evidence surrounding the use of Custodiol cardioplegia and Del Nido cardioplegia.

Custodiol Cardioplegia

Custodiol—also known as histidine-tryptophan-ketoglutarate (HTK) cardioplegia—is an intracellular crystalloid cardioplegia used in some centers for myocardial protection during complex cardiac procedures, and for organ preservation in the setting of transplantation [23]. Notable ingredients of Custodiol cardioplegia include:

1. Histidine, as a buffer.
2. Ketoglutarate, which enhances adenosine triphosphate production during reperfusion.
3. Tryptophan, which stabilizes the cell membrane.
4. Mannitol, which decreases cellular edema and serves as a free-radical scavenger.

The full composition of Custodiol cardioplegia is detailed in Table 34.3. The main advantage of this cardioplegic solution is its administration as a single dose, which can offer myocardial protection for up to three hours, thus allowing the conduct of complex procedures without interruption. This approach is particularly attractive in the setting of minimally invasive cardiac surgery, where frequent re-dosing of cardioplegia may lead to significant increases in aortic cross-clamp times.

While there is a paucity of data comparing Custodiol cardioplegia to conventional myocardial protection techniques, limited evidence suggests that Custodiol may offer myocardial protection that is equivalent to that of conventional cardioplegia. In a systematic review and meta-analysis of 2114 patients, Edelman and colleagues demonstrated similar rates of early mortality, myocardial infarction, low output syndrome, as well as comparable increases in creatine kinase MB between patients receiving Custodiol cardioplegia and those receiving conventional cardioplegia [23]. Importantly, all studies included in this meta-analysis were either observational, or randomized a small number of patients, highlighting the need for a prospective, adequately powered randomized controlled trial in this area.

Del Nido Cardioplegia

Del Nido solution is a calcium-free, potassium-rich, non-glucose based solution, and has an electrolyte composition similar to that of extracellular fluid (Table 34.4). It is mixed with fully oxygenated blood in a 4:1 ratio. Its mechanism of action involves potassium-based myocyte depolarization, with concomitant lidocaine sodium channel blockade. It also contains additives that act as free radical scavengers, buffers and calcium channel blockers.

Table 34.3 Composition of Custodiol solution [23]

Sodium (Na^+)	15 mmol/L
Potassium (K^+)	9 mmol/L
Magnesium (Mg^{2+})	4 mmol/L
Calcium (Ca^{2+})	0.015 mmol/L
Histidine	198 mmol/L
Tryptophan	2 mmol/L
Ketoglutarate	1 mmol/L
Mannitol	30 mmol/L
pH	7.02–7.20 at 25 °C

Table 34.4 Composition of del Nido solution [24]

Plasma-Lyte A	1000 mL
Mannitol [20%]	16 mL
Magnesium sulfate ($MgSO_4$) [50%]	4 mL/L
Sodium bicarbonate ($NaHCO_3$) [1 mEq/mL]	13 mL/L
Potassium chloride (KCl) [2 mEq/mL]	13 mL/L
Lidocaine 1%	13 mL

Del Nido cardioplegia is administered as a single dose (20 mL/kg body weight, up to 1000 mL), providing up to 180 min of myocardial protection. It has been used for over two decades at some institutions, primarily for pediatric cardiac surgery [25]. As is the case for Custodiol, however, there is a paucity of published data regarding the use of del Nido cardioplegia in adults, and no randomized controlled trial comparing this solution to conventional cardioplegia has been published to date.

In a propensity-matched analysis, which included 220 patients undergoing mitral valve surgery and 170 undergoing aortic valve surgery, Mick and colleagues demonstrated similar outcomes between del Nido cardioplegia and blood cardioplegia with regards to operative mortality and perioperative complications [24]. Measures of myocardial injury, such as troponin T levels, postoperative left ventricular ejection fraction, and postoperative inotropic/pressor support were also similar between the two groups. However, del Nido cardioplegia was associated with decreased perturbations of intraoperative glucose levels, decreased need for postoperative insulin drips, decreased surgical times and lower costs. Despite these encouraging results, the authors of this study state that in the absence of any randomized data—and given the excellent and time-tested results provided by blood cardioplegia—caution is still warranted in adopting del Nido cardioplegia for adult cardiac surgery, and further studies are required to refine its indications in this setting. One of the main concerns surrounding the use of del Nido or Custodiol cardioplegia in adults is the lack of evidence supporting its use in ischemic hearts, where significant coronary artery disease may result in inhomogeneous or incomplete delivery.

Conclusion

Despite the considerable progress that has been made in the field of myocardial protection for cardiac surgery, the ideal cardioplegic solution and optimal delivery method remain elusive. Due to a number of theoretical physiological advantages, blood cardioplegia is favored over crystalloid cardioplegia in the majority of North American centers despite the absence of any compelling evidence of its superiority with regards to clinical endpoints. There also remains equipoise surrounding the optimal temperature of cardioplegic solutions, with a gradual shift in recent years towards the use of tepid (29 °C) or mildly hypothermic solutions. Both the antegrade and retrograde routes of administration remain valuable options, and their use must be tailored to the individual patient based on a number of anatomical and physiological factors. Finally, novel strategies using modified crystalloid solutions—administered as a single dose granting an extended period of protection —offer the promise of facilitating minimally invasive and complex valvular operations. Incorporation of these novel strategies into routine practice must, however, be preceded by rigorous evaluation of their safety and efficacy in comparison with established methods of myocardial protection in various subgroups of patients.

References

1. Ringer S. A further contribution regarding the influence of the different constituents of the blood on the contraction of the heart. J Physiol. 1883;4(1):29–42.
2. Bigelow WG, Lindsay WK, Greenwood WF. Hypothermia; its possible role in cardiac surgery: an investigation of factors governing survival in dogs at low body temperatures. Ann Surg. 1950;132(5):849–66.
3. Melrose DG, Dreyer B, Bentall HH, Baker JB. Elective cardiac arrest. Lancet. 1955;269(6879):21–2.
4. Tyers GF, Todd GJ, Niebauer IM, Manley NJ, Waldhausen JA. The mechanism of myocardial damage following potassium citrate (Melrose) cardioplegia. Surgery. 1975;78(1):45–53.
5. Cooley DA, Reul GJ, Wukasch DC. Ischemic contracture of the heart: "stone heart". Am J Cardiol. 1972;29(4):575–7.
6. Reidemeister JC, Heberer G, Bretschneider HJ. Induced cardiac arrest by sodium and calcium depletion and application of procaine. Int Surg. 1967;47(6):535–40.
7. Hearse DJ, Stewart DA, Braimbridge MV. Cellular protection during myocardial ischemia: the development and characterization of a procedure for the induction of reversible ischemic arrest. Circulation. 1976;54(2):193–202.

8. Braimbridge MV, Chayen J, Bitensky L, Hearse DJ, Jynge P, Cankovic-Darracott S. Cold cardioplegia or continuous coronary perfusion? Report on preliminary clinical experience as assessed cytochemically. J Thorac Cardiovasc Surg. 1977;74(6):900–6.

9. Buckberg GD. A proposed "solution" to the cardioplegic controversy. J Thorac Cardiovasc Surg. 1979;77(6):803–15.

10. Guyton RA, Dorsey LM, Craver JM, Bone DK, Jones EL, Murphy DA, et al. Improved myocardial recovery after cardioplegic arrest with an oxygenated crystalloid solution. J Thorac Cardiovasc Surg. 1985;89(6):877–87.

11. Sellke FW, Shafique T, Johnson RG, Dai HB, Banitt PF, Schoen FJ, et al. Blood and albumin cardioplegia preserve endothelium-dependent microvascular responses. Ann Thorac Surg. 1993;55(4):977–85.

12. Hayashida N, Isomura T, Sato T, Maruyama H, Higashi T, Arinaga K, et al. Minimally diluted tepid blood cardioplegia. Ann Thorac Surg. 1998;65(3):615–21.

13. Guru V, Omura J, Alghamdi AA, Weisel R, Fremes SE. Is blood superior to crystalloid cardioplegia? A meta-analysis of randomized clinical trials. Circulation. 2006;114(1 Suppl):I331–8.

14. Teoh KH, Christakis GT, Weisel RD, Fremes SE, Mickle DA, Romaschin AD, et al. Accelerated myocardial metabolic recovery with terminal warm blood cardioplegia. J Thorac Cardiovasc Surg. 1986;91(6):888–95.

15. Yau TM, Ikonomidis JS, Weisel RD, Mickle DA, Ivanov J, Mohabeer MK, et al. Ventricular function after normothermic versus hypothermic cardioplegia. J Thorac Cardiovasc Surg. 1993;105(5):833–43. discussion 43–4

16. Lichtenstein SV, Naylor CD, Feindel CM, Sykora K, Abel JG, Slutsky AS, Warm Heart Investigators, et al. Intermittent warm blood cardioplegia. Circulation. 1995;92(9 Suppl):II341–6.

17. Martin TD, Craver JM, Gott JP, Weintraub WS, Ramsay J, Mora CT, et al. Prospective, randomized trial of retrograde warm blood cardioplegia: myocardial benefit and neurologic threat. Ann Thorac Surg. 1994;57(2):298–302. discussion–4

18. The Warm Heart Investigators. Randomised trial of normothermic versus hypothermic coronary bypass surgery. Lancet. 1994;343(8897):559–63.

19. Fremes SE, Tamariz MG, Abramov D, Christakis GT, Sever JY, Sykora K, et al. Late results of the warm heart trial: the influence of nonfatal cardiac events on late survival. Circulation. 2000;102(19 Suppl 3):III339–45.

20. Hayashida N, Ikonomidis JS, Weisel RD, Shirai T, Ivanov J, Carson SM, et al. The optimal cardioplegic temperature. Ann Thorac Surg. 1994;58(4):961–71.

21. Pratt FH. The nutrition of the heart through the vessels of Thebesius and the coronary veins. Am J Phys. 1898;1:86–103.

22. Lillehei CW, Dewall RA, Gott VL, Varco RL. The direct vision correction of calcific aortic stenosis by means of a pump-oxygenator and retrograde coronary sinus perfusion. Dis Chest. 1956;30(2):123–32.

23. Edelman JJ, Seco M, Dunne B, Matzelle SJ, Murphy M, Joshi P, et al. Custodiol for myocardial protection and preservation: a systematic review. Ann Cardiothorac Surg. 2013;2(6):717–28.

24. Mick SL, Robich MP, Houghtaling PL, Gillinov AM, Soltesz EG, Johnston DR, et al. del Nido versus Buckberg cardioplegia in adult isolated valve surgery. J Thorac Cardiovasc Surg. 2015;149(2):626–34. discussion 34–6

25. Matte GS, del Nido PJ. History and use of del Nido cardioplegia solution at Boston Children's Hospital. J Extra Corpor Technol. 2012;44(3):98–103.

On-Pump and Off-Pump Coronary Revascularization Surgery

35

Louay M. Habbab and André Lamy

Main Messages

1. Off-pump coronary-artery bypass grafting (OPCAB) surgery was established to avoid complications related to cardiopulmonary bypass and aortic manipulation that accompany ON-PUMP coronary-artery bypass grafting (CABG); nevertheless, only 20% of myocardial revascularization procedures worldwide are performed off-pump.

2. Several large-scale RCTs did not demonstrate differences in major adverse cardiovascular and cerebrovascular outcomes and some studies showed more frequent incomplete revascularization, reduced long term graft patency and mortality in OPCAB surgery. However, these RCTs did consistently show lower ventilation times, ICU stay and transfusion rates with OPCAB, with significant variability in experience with OPCAB techniques.

3. Until multivariable analysis of patients from these large-scale RCTs identify subgroups of patients who will benefit from OPCAB or on-pump CABG, and until the current guidelines are updated, the single absolute indication for OPCAB is severely atherosclerotic aorta.

4. Retrospective data from specific high-risk subpopulations suggest significant benefit from an OPCAB approach in females, in patients 75 years of age or older, and in patients with elevated Society of Thoracic Surgeons (STS) predicted risk score (>3%).

5. Absolute contraindications for OPCAB include cardiogenic shock, ischemic arrhythmia, anatomic factors preventing rotation of the heart, and urgent/emergent cases of left main coronary artery disease.

6. Balanced general anesthesia with narcotic and inhalation agent with or without regional anesthesia block is commonly used in OPCAB surgery, and the goal of early extubation and fast track recovery.

L. M. Habbab (✉)
Hamilton General Hospital, McMaster University,
McMaster Clinic, Hamilton, ON, Canada
e-mail: louay@habbab.com

A. Lamy
Division of Cardiac Surgery, Hamilton General
Hospital, McMaster University,
Hamilton, ON, Canada

© Springer Nature Switzerland AG 2021
D. C. H. Cheng et al. (eds.), *Evidence-Based Practice in Perioperative Cardiac Anesthesia and Surgery*, https://doi.org/10.1007/978-3-030-47887-2_35

7. OPCAB can be very challenging in patients with cardiomegaly and severe left ventricular dysfunction, deep intramyocardial coronary artery targets, and anticipated need for endarterectomy or plasty.

Coronary artery disease (CAD) is the leading cause of hospital admissions and mortality worldwide. Coronary-artery bypass grafting (CABG) reduces mortality among patients with extensive coronary artery disease [1]. The first milestones in CABG development were without cardiopulmonary bypass (CPB) support (Table 35.1).

Soon after the introduction of off-pump CABG (OPCAB), the need for a clean, still, and bloodless field was very noticeable, resulting in the introduction of on-pump CABG in 1967. This resulted in more ideal and reproducible results, with considerably better operating conditions, and was performed by a broad group of surgeons. The enthusiasm for on-pump gradually gave way to concerns about its safety, especially regarding complications arising from CPB (not specifically CABG). These concerns included micro-embolic showering during manipulation of the aorta and neurocognitive dysfunction, and CPB triggered whole-body inflammatory response due to contact activation of the complement cascade, leading to multiple organ dysfunction affecting the kidneys, liver, lungs, brain and heart itself. With on-pump, perioperative mortality is about 2%, and myocardial infarction, stroke, or renal failure requiring dialysis develop in an additional 5–7% of patients. The proportion of patients recovering without any complication was found to be only 64.3%. These and other observations, with the development of mechanical and pharmacological organ stabilizers and intracoronary shunts, revived OPCAB in the early 1990s.

Table 35.1 History of the development of coronary artery bypass surgery (CABG)

Year	Main event
1876	First establishment that coronary blood supply interruption can cause angina pain and myocardial infarction (MI).
1910	First attempted CABG in animals.
1916	Discovery of heparin.
1926	First development of a CPB machine for total body perfusion used in animals.
1950	First implant of the internal mammary artery (IMA) into the myocardium.
1953	First successful open-heart procedure (ASD closure) on a human utilizing a CPB machine.
1953	First placement of arterial grafts in the coronary circulation.
1955	First saphenous vein harvest and use as a graft from aorta into the myocardium.
1958	First open coronary artery endarterectomy without CPB (off-pump).
1960	First off-pump coronary artery bypass (OPCAB) of IMA using a specially designed metal ring.
1962	First practical cardiac angiography visualizing the coronary arteries.
1964	First successful off-pump IMA-coronary artery anastomosis using a suture technique.
1967	First CABG of autogenous saphenous vein grafts on CPB (on-pump).
1967	First published series of off-pump left IMA to LAD anastomosis.
1968	First published series of on-pump saphenous vein grafts to restore coronary artery blood flow.
1971	First use of radial artery conduit.
1973	First successful complete anastomoses on a beating heart.
1975	First myocardial protection by means of cold cardioplegia with safe perfusion techniques.
1980s	Increased prevalence and improved safety of on-pump CABG.
1986	First report on improved clinical outcomes with the use of the IMA vs. vein grafting alone.
1990s	Interest emerged in performing OPCAB grafting to avoid preoperative comorbidities of CAB.
1998	First thoracoscopic harvesting of the left IMA.
2000	First minimally invasive and robotic surgical approach.

CABG coronary artery bypass grafting, *CPB* coronary artery bypass, *IMA* internal mammary artery, *MI* myocardial infarction, *OPCAB* off-pump coronary artery bypass

General Features

Full median sternotomy is performed in both on-pump and OPCAB surgery. The type of harvested conduits used, and the technique for the actual suture anastomosis of the vessels are the same for both procedures. Both on-pump and OPCAB surgery differ in terms of: method of perfusion and pump-related complications; stabilization of operative field; cannulation; type of cross-clamp; and heparinization. In addition, OPCAB surgery requires specialized anesthetic management that focuses on short-acting medications, preservation of normothermia, aggressive hemodynamic support, early extubation and postoperative analgesia. A comparison of on-pump and OPCAB surgery is provided in Table 35.2.

Surgical Techniques of OPCAB Compared to On-Pump CABG

Preoperative Assessment

Preoperative assessment of patients undergoing OPCAB surgery requires the following:

- Careful history taking and thorough physical examination to investigate for the presence of risk factors associated with increased perioperative morbidity and mortality and to calculate the risk score to stratify and inform patients of their individual risk.
- Reviewing patient's coronary anatomy and the extent of cardiac ischemia to choose the appropriate anesthetic approach.

Table 35.2 Comparison of features of on-pump and OPCAB coronary artery bypass surgery

Feature	On-pump	Off-pump (OPCAB)
Perfusion	Aerobic perfusion by pump oxygenator	Aerobic perfusion by Beating heart
Pump-related complications	SIR with possible CNS, cardiac, pulmonary, renal, and GI complications	No pump-related complications
Stabilization	Heart is arrested by cardioplegia solution	Movement of operative field is minimized by epicardial-wall stabilizer
Cannulation	Requires aortic and venous cannulation	Does not require invasive cannulation
Cross-clamp	Complete aortic cross-clamp for distal anastomoses	Partial cross-clamp for proximal anastomoses or no-touch technique
Heparinization	Requires systemic heparinization to allow CPB and antifibrinolytic use is common	Requires lower heparin dose
Anesthetic medications	Long acting	Short-acting
Temperature management	Hypothermia	Normothermia, needs active heating measures throughout operation
Hemodynamic disturbances	Minimal	Major due to heart manipulations and require aggressive hemodynamic support
Use of inotropic support	For separation from CPB	For hemodynamic support and often is weaned following completion of distal revascularization
IV fluid administration	Usually restricted to minimize hemodilution	Fluid loading is often required to ensure adequate for hemodynamic support
Extubation	Extubation and recovery are relatively delayed compared to OPCAB	Extubation is early and recovery is faster

CNS central nervous system, *CPB* cardiopulmonary bypass, *GI* gastrointestinal, *OPCAB* on-pump coronary artery bypass, *OPCAB* off-pump coronary artery bypass, *SIR* systemic inflammatory response

- Discussion with the team regarding the surgical plan, the anesthesia management and sequencing of coronary revascularization in order to improve blood flow and myocardial oxygenation during subsequent anastomoses and cardiac displacement.

Premedication

Premedication includes:

- An intermediate-acting benzodiazepine (e.g. temazepam or lorazepam), administered orally 1 h before surgery, to reduce the patient's anxiety.
- A β-blocker such as oral atenolol or metoprolol, at the time of premedication in order to prevent arrhythmia.

Operating Room Readiness

Operating room set-up procedures include:

- CPB machine ready for quick setup with a perfusionist in attendance.
- Temperature up to 24 °C, warming pad or mattress placed on the operating table, and use of air warming device.
- External pads connected to a defibrillator (internal pads and a pacemaker should also be available).

Monitoring

Monitoring include:

- A five-lead surface ECG (basic standard involves lead II and V5) with automated ST segment analysis.
- Oxygen saturation monitoring (pulse oximetry).
- Continuous urinary output (Foley catheter).
- End tidal carbon dioxide monitoring.
- Esophageal and rectal temperature.

- Arterial blood pressure by cannulating radial and/or femoral artery.
- Central venous pressure (CVP) catheter.
- Swan-Ganz catheters with continuous cardiac output and central venous oxygen saturation monitoring capability only used in very high-risk patients with poor ventricular function.
- Pacing pulmonary artery catheter can allow atrial or ventricular pacing if needed.
- Transesophageal echocardiography (TEE).
- Depth of unconsciousness in patients operated under general anesthesia (GA).
- Neuromuscular monitoring.
- Coagulation profile monitoring.

Pre-procedure Planning

Pre-procedural considerations include:

- Meticulous attention to details; this is critical to success, as the safety margin with OPCAB is reduced compared to traditional on-pump CABG.
- Every member the cardiac surgery team, including the surgeon, anesthesiologist, surgical assistant, nurse and perfusionist, should be educated in OPCAB protocols and the difference between conventional CABG and OPCAB. They should be prepared to go on cardiopulmonary bypass, if needed.
- Unlike on-pump where the anesthesiologist plays a passive role during the performance of bypass grafting, involvement of the anesthesia team is essential for successful OPCAB.
- The anesthesiologist should plan to inform the surgeon when administering vasopressors or inotropes, if there are ST segment or rhythm disturbances, and if the blood pressure is not responding to pharmacologic interventions.
- The surgeon should plan to communicate with the anesthesiologist prior to displacing the heart, occluding a coronary artery, inserting or removing a shunt, and especially when reperfusing the heart, since each of these procedures can be associated with significant hemodynamic disturbances during surgery.

Procedural Considerations

Anesthetic Considerations

In addition to providing safe induction and maintenance of anesthesia using a technique that minimizes myocardial ischemia, (the primary goal for any other coronary artery surgery), the anesthetic goals of management of OPCAB surgery should include: considering fast-track anesthesia; maintaining normothermia; and providing hemodynamic stability [2, 3].

Considering Fast-Track Anesthesia

Fast track anesthesia includes a balanced opioids and inhalational general anesthesia, rapid emergence and appropriate plan for postoperative care, which includes early extubation and ambulation along with excellent postoperative analgesia [4].

- It is currently the most commonly employed practice for OPCAB surgery.
- Research suggests that it is safe with no evidence of increased cardiopulmonary morbidity
- It is cost effective, and has many potential benefits including:
  - Improved postoperative hemodynamic performance
  - Earlier patient mobilization
  - Reduced risk of ventilator-associated pneumonia
  - Reduced ventilator-related costs
  - Shorter ICU time
  - Decreased hospital length of stay.

The three anesthetic approaches in OPCAB surgery [3] are:

1. General anesthesia (GA) with controlled ventilation, with balanced opioids and inhalation anesthesia or total intravenous anesthesia (TIVA).
2. Combined GA and regional analgesia with controlled ventilation using high thoracic epidural analgesia (TEA) or combined GA/intrathecal morphine (ITM). This approach can be beneficial, but further studies are required to verify the effectiveness of this technique and

to determine the optimal dose of morphine, which provides adequate analgesia with minimal risk of respiratory depression (an impactful side effect during the postoperative period).

3. Awake regional anesthesia with spontaneous ventilation using TEA alone. The feasibility of this technique has been confirmed, but not the safety and effectiveness.

Anesthesia induction and maintenance commonly employs an induction dose of propofol with low dose of narcotic and balanced concentration of neuromuscular blocker and inhalational agent.

- Narcotics:
  - Remifentanil, sufentanil and fentanyl [5]. No benefit has been shown with the use of one agent over the other.
- Neuromuscular blockers:
  - Short acting neuromuscular blockers (cisatracurium, rocuronium or vecuronium) are recommended.
  - If a long-acting neuromuscular blocking agent such as pancuronium is used, care should be taken to avoid intermittent rebolus, and neuromuscular blockade should be reversed before extubation.
- Inhalational agents:
  - Shorter acting agents, such as sevoflurane and desflurane, are beneficial with operating room extubation as a goal in applicable patients.

Management of postoperative analgesia options include:

- Most commonly titrating intravenous morphine with or without nonsteroidal antiinflammatory drugs (NSAIDs) prior to the end of surgery.
- Prolonging the infusion of remifentanil (expensive) using higher doses to achieve an adequate level of analgesia.
- The use of dexmedetomidine (an ideal anesthetic adjuvant with no antiemetic effects) might lead to a better postoperative pain control by reducing intra-and postoperative consumption of opioids and better hemodynamic stability in some centers.

- Single shot spinal morphine prior to anesthesia induction or continuous epidural catheter have been used for postoperative analgesia.

Maintaining Normothermia

Maintaining normothermia (34–36 °C) is extremely important in optimizing patient outcomes and hemodynamic stability during OPCAB.

Postoperative hypothermia can increase the risk of:

1. Myocardial infarction
2. Wound infection
3. Blood loss
4. Extended anesthesia care
5. Prolonged recovery and hospitalization

Passive and active warming techniques to prevent unintentional hypothermia include:

1. Blankets and a hypothermia prevention cap.
2. Preheating the OR to 24 °C before set-up begins; the room temperature can then be cooled to a comfortable level for the surgical team.
3. Applying a Cath Lab blanket around the patient's head and sides before starting the procedure.
4. Using warmed irrigation fluids intraoperatively.
5. Using warmed IV fluids.
6. Using a blood warmer.
7. Warming and humidifying ventilator gases by an airway heat/moisture exchanger.

Providing Hemodynamic Stability

It is vitally important that the anesthesiologist continually observes and treats the hemodynamic and rhythm responses throughout OPCAB surgery, but especially during cardiac manipulation and regional ischemia. Three critical events associated with hemodynamic instability—vertical displacement of heart; cardiac compression from myocardial stabilizer; myocardial ischemia during coronary

artery occlusion for anastomosis. Prior to heart manipulation and positioning, the blood pressure should be elevated at least 20% above baseline using IV vasopressor bolus and Trendelenberg positioning.

Hemodynamic goals can be achieved through:

1. Fluid management
2. The use of table positioning. Using Trendelenburg positioning will fill the heart maximally and increase blood pressure. Rolling the table to the right allows gravity to pull the heart over and provides access to the back wall when the surgeon works on the diagonal and circumflex vessels.
3. The use of small boluses of nor-epinephrine or levophed to support blood pressure and cardiac output, but all efforts should be made to avoid significant inotropic or vasopressor support.

A simplified approach to the diagnosis and management of different causes of hemodynamic instability during OPCAB [6] is shown in Fig. 35.1.

Surgical Considerations

Initial Stage Considerations

- A traditional sternotomy is performed.
- The left IMA should be made as long as possible in order to avoid excessive tension when the heart is elevated after the graft until the LAD is performed. Skeletonization of LIMA is preferable as maximal length is achieved in shortest time.
- Total arterial revascularization is feasible with OPCAB and the use of composite conduits (Y or T graft) with the left and right IMA and the radial artery is preferred.
- The heparin dose (1–1.5 mg/kg) is 1/3 of the standard dose for cardiopulmonary bypass. The target ACT is greater than 300 s. The ACT should be checked every 30 min with heparin supplemented as needed.

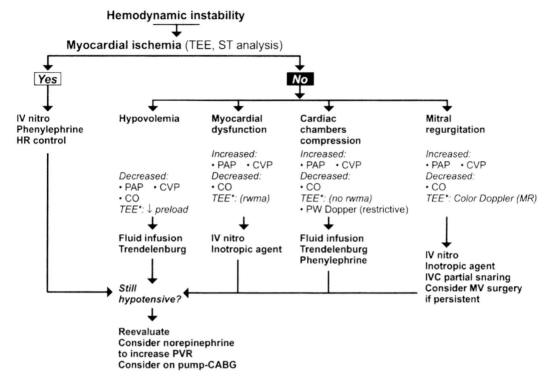

Fig. 35.1 Diagnosis and management of hemodynamic instability during OPCAB surgery. (Reprinted with permission from Couture et al. Mechanisms of hemodynamic changes during off-pump coronary artery bypass surgery. Can J Anesth. 2002;49:835–859). *CABG* coronary artery bypass grafting, *CVP* central venous pressure, *CO* cardiac output, *HR* heart rate, *IV* intravenous, *IVC* inferior vena cava, *MR* mitral regurgitation, *MV* mitral valve, *NTG* nitroglycerin, *AP* pulmonary artery pressure, *RWMA* regional wall motion abnormality, *SVR* systemic vascular resistance, *TEE* transesophageal echocardiography

Exposure of the coronary arteries:

- During OPCAB, the surgeon needs good coronary artery exposure in order to be able to position the heart without affecting its natural ability to pump; therefore, extra time should be allowed to obtain the best presentation and stabilization.
- If adequate exposure cannot be obtained, the anastomosis should not be compromised and the traditional approach should be used.
- Anatomic structures in the chest cavity, including the sternum, pleura and pericardial edge should be assessed first prior to positioning the heart, as they can compress the heart and lead to decreased cardiac output and hemodynamic instability during OPCAB.

Positioning the Heart

Positioning the heart for OPCAB surgery is a balance between achieving good exposure and maintaining hemodynamic stability. Communication between surgeon and anesthesiologist is a critical component of successful surgery.

Proper positioning and stabilization are critical for the success of OPCAB and can be achieved by many available dedicated instruments:

1. Suction devices: These devices have a flexible arm that can be adjusted and tightened to make rigid, as well as clips by that can be attached to the sternal retractor. There are two types of suction devices:

(a) A cup-shaped device that is placed on the apex of the heart to position and stabilize.

(b) A two-pronged foot, where the prongs are placed on either side of the segment of artery being grafted to stabilize that region of the heart.

2. Tape and snare: A broad tape (or a small pack) is fixed to the posterior pericardium between the right and left superior pulmonary, which is then snared. Traction on the tape and the snare serves to lift the apex of the heart.

3. Direct pressure stabilizers: These are simple rigid systems that use metal plates to stabilize the area being grafted by pressing down on it. They do not stabilize as effectively as the suction devices, and tend to cause more hemodynamic compromise. These devices are used more in mini-thoracotomy coronary surgery, because they are less bulky than suction stabilizers and are reusable.

Drawbacks of using stabilizers:

1. Myocardial bruising can be caused when suction is too high.
2. The phrenic nerve can be injured when widely opening the pleura.
3. The descending aorta and esophagus can be damaged if stay sutures are placed too deep in the pericardium.
4. Cardiac output can be reduced by compressing and distorting the heart.

Sequence of Anastomoses

The coronary arteries should be grafted in order of increasing cardiac displacement: the anterior wall vessels followed by inferior wall vessels, and finally, lateral wall vessels. Therefore, the LIMA to LAD graft is usually first, followed by the inferior wall grafts (PDA, RCA), and the lateral wall grafts (OM) are usually last. The guiding principle is that more cardiac displacement is tolerated with increasingly complete revascularization. Although the proximal anastomoses can be performed before or after the distal anastomoses, completing the proximal anastomosis first has the advantage of immediate perfusion through the graft after the completion of the distal anastomosis. Proximal occlusion of the target vessel is accomplished with an encircling suture or silastic tape passed widely around the vessel proximal to the site chosen for anastomosis (no distal occlusion is necessary). Anastomosis of the obtuse marginal vessels is easier from the left side of the table. Temporary pacing wires should be placed before occluding the right coronary artery proximal to the bifurcation to manage possible A-V block. A CO_2 blower is crucial for beating heart surgery but must be used very carefully at a flow rate not >5 L/min, to prevent damage to the coronary endothelium. Directing the gas jet directly into the vessel lumen must be avoided to prevent gas embolization or intimal dissection.

Managing Myocardial Ischemia

Reducing myocardial ischemia during OPCAB can be achieved by:

1. Increasing oxygen delivery by:
   (a) Maintaining an adequate mean arterial pressure (MAP): This is the most important maneuver to decrease myocardial ischemia.
   (b) Using intra-coronary shunts: Inserting a small shunt into the coronary artery is extremely useful in minimizing the amount of ischemia and improving the safety of the operation as it can provide:
      (i) Distal perfusion,
      (ii) A bloodless field
      (iii) A guide for the placement of anastomotic sutures.
   (c) Nitrates: Nitroglycerin (NTG) has been used to treat active ischemia; however, it decreases preload and can be detrimental when higher filling pressures are needed to ensure optimal ventricular filling.
2. Reducing the oxygen consumption through a decrease in HR and contractility as well as

decreasing the occurrence of arrhythmias. The following pharmacological prophylaxis can be used:

(a) Perioperative use of β-blocking agents such as esmolol or metoprolol.
(b) Calcium antagonists such as diltiazem.

3. Increasing tolerance to ischemia (preconditioning), which could be:

(a) Mechanical: Though on the decline, ischemic preconditioning, by coronary occlusion followed by a period of reperfusion, can also increase the tolerance to ischemia and can be used as a technique of myocardial protection.
(b) Pharmacological: Using isoflurane and sevoflurane can activate a preconditioning mechanism when administered at minimum alveolar concentration at least 30 min before ischemic insult.

Total Arterial Grafting Without Aortic Manipulation (No-Touch Strategy)

- An extension of OPCAB designed to optimize graft patency of arterial grafts and minimize stroke risk.
- This technique is associated with the lowest stroke rate.
- It is accomplished by using single or double IMA with sequential grafting.
- Depending on the coronary anatomy and available conduits, there are several potential graft–target arrangements:
  - Bilateral IMAs with radial arterial/saphenous vein T/Y-graft(s)
  - Bilateral IMAs with radial artery/saphenous vein extension(s)
  - K-grafts IMAs with arterial graft(s)

Heparin Reversal

- Although heparin reversal is not mandatory, one-half of the calculated protamine dose can be administered.

On-Pump Versus OPCAB in the Literature

OPCAB surgery was established to avoid complications related to CPB and aortic manipulation that accompany OPCAB. Nevertheless, despite the initial enthusiasm on this technique, only 20% of myocardial revascularization procedures worldwide are performed off-pump. In large retrospective studies of surgical revascularization, OPCAB has outperformed on-pump for major outcomes including risk-adjusted operative mortality [7, 8]; however, these studies were challenged by selection bias that led to several large-scale randomized controlled trials (RCTs) [9–17]. Several large-scale RCTs did not demonstrate differences in major adverse cardiovascular and cerebrovascular outcomes and some showed increased death, more frequent incomplete revascularization and reduced long term graft patency for OPCAB [18]. However, these RCTs did consistently show lower ventilation times, ICU stay and transfusion rates with OPCAB and importantly, there was significant variability in experience with OPCAB techniques. Retrospective data from specific high-risk subpopulations suggest significant benefit from an OPCAB approach in females, patients 75 years of age or older and patients with elevated STS predicted risk score (>3%). The details of these RCTs and their follow-up data are summarized in Table 35.3.

Table 35.3 Major randomized controlled trials comparing on-pump with OPCAB revascularization

Study	Publication year	On-pump/ OPCAB (n/n)	F/U (year)	Notes	Major conclusions
Octopus (van Dijk D. et al. [9])	2007	(139/142)	(5)	Low-risk patient population only	No difference in cognitive function or cardiac outcome
BHACAS I & II (Angelini G.D. et al. [10])	2009	(201/200)	(6–8)	Significant improvement in OPCAB between trials I and II	No difference in graft patency or perceived QOL

(continued)

Table 35.3 (continued)

Study	Publication year	On-pump/ OPCAB (n/n)	F/U (year)	Notes	Major conclusions
ROOBY (Shroyer A.L. et al. [11])	2009	(1099/1104)	(1)	Low-to-moderate risk (relatively young and healthy) males only; insufficient surgeon experience with OPCAB; very high OPCAB to CPB conversion rate	No difference in neuropsychological outcomes Lower graft patency and higher mortality in OPCAB
SMART (Angelini G.D. et al. [12])	2011	(99/98)	(6–8)	Single center; highly experienced surgeons in OPCAB	No difference in mortality or graft patency, lower costs in OPCAB
CORONARY (Lamy A. et al. [13, 14])	2013	(2377/2375)	(1)	Largest multicenter RCT to date; highly experienced surgeons in OPCAB, included a somewhat higher risk group of patients	No significant difference in death, MI, stroke, renal failure requiring dialysis, QOL, cognitive function or repeat coronary revascularization
GOPCABE (Diegeler A. et al. [15])	2013	(11,797/1191)	(1)	Patients >75 years (median age 78.5 years)	No difference in early death, stroke or MI
CORONARY (Lamy A. et al. [16])	2016	(2377/2375)	(5)	Same as at 1-year follow up	No significant difference in death, stroke, MI, renal failure, or repeat coronary revascularization
ROOBY-FS (Shroyer A.L. et al. [17])	2017	(1099/1104)	(5)	Same as at 1-year follow up	Significantly higher death rate and significantly lower rates of event-free survival in the OPCAB group

BHACAS beating heart against cardioplegic arrest studies, *CORONARY* the CABG off or on pump revascularization study, *GOPCABE* German off-pump CABG in elderly, *ROOBY* randomized on/off bypass trial, *SMART* surgical management of arterial revascularization therapies

Current Recommendations

Recommendations for On-Pump CABG in the Practice Guidelines

Clinical guidelines on on-pump CABG have been issued by the American College of Cardiology (ACC)/American Heart Association (AHA), the European Society of Cardiology (ESC)/European Association for Cardio-Thoracic Surgery (EACTS) and the Society of Thoracic Surgeons (STS) [19–23]. A summary of the recommendations provided by these guidelines is shown in Table 35.4.

Recommendations for the preoperative and postoperative management of antiplatelet therapy in patients undergoing CABG have been pro-

vided by the same organizations [24, 25] and are summarized in Table 35.5.

Recommendations for OPCAB in the Practice Guidelines

The issue of off- versus on-pump approaches to CABG surgery was only addressed by the 2011 ACC/AHA Guidelines for CABG Surgery and the 2014 ESC/EACTS Guidelines on Myocardial Revascularization.

In the ACCF/AHA Guidelines, no formal recommendation was given, but the concluding remarks focused on the avoidance of aortic manipulation, regardless of an on- versus off-pump approach in patients with evidence of aor-

Table 35.4 Indications for on-pump CABG in the guidelines

Indication	2011 ACC/AHA	2014 ACC/AHA	2017 ACC/AHA	2014 ESC/EACT
Left main disease	Class I		Class I	Class I
Three-vessel disease with or without proximal LAD artery disease	Class I		Class I	Class I
Two-vessel disease with proximal LAD artery disease	Class I		Class I	Class I
Two-vessel disease without proximal LAD artery disease	Class IIa with extensive ischemia		Class IIa with extensive ischemia	Class IIb
Single-vessel disease with proximal LAD artery disease	Class IIa with LIMA for long-term benefit		Class IIa with LIMA for long-term benefit	Class I
Single-vessel disease without proximal LAD artery disease	Class III: Harmful		Class III: Harmful	Class IIb
LV dysfunction	Class IIa EF 35–50% Class IIb EF < 35%		Class IIa EF 35–50% Class IIb EF < 35%	Class I EF < 40%
Survivors of sudden cardiac death with presumed ischemia-mediated VT	Class I		Class I	Class I
Diabetic patients with multi-vessel disease	Class IIa, particularly if LIMA used to LAD	Class I with three-vessel or complex two-vessel disease involving proximal LAD, particularly if LIMA can be used to LAD and provided a good candidate for surgery	Class IIa reasonable with LIMA	Class I with acceptable surgical risk

EF ejection fraction, *LAD* left anterior descending artery, *LV* left ventricle, *LIMA* left internal mammary artery, *VT* ventricular tachycardia

Table 35.5 Antiplatelet therapy in patients undergoing CABG

Recommendation	2011 ACC/AHA	2012 ACC/AHA	2012 STS	2014 ACC/AHA	2014 ESC/EACT
Preoperative management					
In patients referred for CABG, administer of aspirin preoperatively	Class I (100–325 mg daily)	Class I		Class I (81–325 mg daily	Class I (75–160 mg daily)
In patients at increased risk for bleeding and those who refuse blood transfusion, discontinue aspirin 3–5 days prior to surgery			Class IIa		Class I
In patients referred for non-urgent CABG, discontinue clopidogrel and ticagrelor for at least 5 days and prasugrel for at least 7 days before surgery to limit blood transfusions	Class I	Class I		Class I	Class I

(continued)

Table 35.5 (continued)

Recommendation	2011 ACC/ AHA	2012 ACC/ AHA	2012 STS	2014 ACC/ AHA	2014 ESC/ EACT
In patients referred for urgent CABG, discontinue clopidogrel and ticagrelor for at least 24 h to reduce major bleeding complications	Class I			Class I	
In patients referred for urgent CABG, discontinue eptifibatide and tirofiban for at least 2–4 h and abciximab for at 12 h	Class I	Class I (discontinue eptifibatide and tirofiban 4 h)		Class I	
Postoperative management					
Administer aspirin to CABG patients indefinitely	Class I (100–325 mg daily)		Class I	Class I (81–325 mg daily)	Class I (75–160 mg daily)
Administer clopidogrel and ticagrelor, in addition to aspirin, for 12 months				Class I	Class IIb
In patients intolerant or allergic to aspirin, clopidogrel (75 mg daily) is a reasonable alternative	Class IIa			Class I	Class I
In CABG after acute coronary syndromes, restart dual antiplatelet therapy when bleeding risk is diminished			Class I		
Once postoperative bleeding risk is decreased, consider testing response to antiplatelet drugs, either with genetic testing or with point-of-care platelet function testing, to optimize antiplatelet drug effect and minimize thrombotic risk to vein grafts			Class IIb		

tic atherosclerotic disease, acknowledging that this may be more readily achieved with an off-pump approach.

The European Task Force in 2014 had the benefit of more robust data to make the following recommendations:

1. OPCAB and/or no-touch on-pump techniques on the ascending aorta are recommended in patients with significant atherosclerotic disease of the ascending aorta in order to prevent perioperative stroke as a Class I.
2. OPCAB surgery can be 'considered' for subgroups of high risk patients in high-volume off-pump centers as a Class IIa.

Subsequent controlled trials and a large volume of retrospective database evidence suggest that complexity of the debate between off- versus on-pump approaches may revolve around surgical expertise and patient, with major points of argument are generally summed up as follows:

Pro-OPCAB Arguments:

1. Reduction of neurocognitive dysfunction by avoiding cannulation and aortic cross-clamping.
2. Avoidance of the systemic inflammatory response and its postoperative sequelae.
3. Decreased blood product use with better postoperative pulmonary and renal function.

Pro ON-PUMP Arguments:

1. Incomplete revascularization with OPCAB, which translates into poorer long-term graft patency.

2. Emergency conversion of OPCAB into on-pump resulting in higher mortality.
3. Higher degree of technical difficulty of OPCAB, with no proven advantage for clinically-important outcomes.

Multivariable analysis involving thousands of patients in the reported large RCTs will likely identify subgroups of patients who will benefit from on-pump or OPCAB CABG. When this occurs, the procedure that is best for the patient can be selected. Until this occurs, and until the current guidelines are updated, the following recommendations can be made:

1. The single absolute indication for OPCAB, which can be used to accomplish a completely no-touch aorta technique, is severely atherosclerotic aorta.
2. OPCAB surgery might be associated with more favorable outcomes in patients presenting with the following risk factors:
   (a) Elevated STS predicted risk score (>3%).
   (b) Patients 75 years of age or older.
   (c) Female.
   (d) Acute/subacute STEMI.
   (e) Repeat revascularization.
   (f) Renal failure.
   (g) Previous stroke/cerebrovascular disease.
3. Absolute contraindications for OPCAB include:
   (a) Cardiogenic shock.
   (b) Ischemic arrhythmia.
   (c) Anatomic factors preventing rotation of the heart.
      (i) Previous left pneumonectomy.
      (ii) Severe pectus excavatum.
   (d) Urgent/emergent classes left main coronary artery disease.
4. Factors that can make OPCAB very challenging:
   (a) Cardiomegaly Severe left ventricular dysfunction.
   (b) Deep intramyocardial coronary artery targets.
   (c) Anticipated need for endarterectomy or plasty.

References

1. Buxton BF, Galvin SD. The history of arterial revascularization: from Kolesov to Tector and beyond. Ann Cardiothorac Surg. 2013;2:419–26.
2. Hammering TM, Romano G, Terrasini N, Noiseux N. Anesthesia for off-pump coronary artery bypass surgery. Ann Card Anaesth. 2013;16:28–39.
3. Sun J, Peng YG. On- or off-pump coronary artery bypass: what is the evidence? J Anesth Perioper Med. 2016;3:35–41.
4. Cheng DC, Karski J, Peniston C, et al. Morbidity outcome in early versus conventional tracheal extubation after coronary artery bypass grafting: a prospective randomized controlled trial. J Thorac Cardiovasc Surg. 1996;112(3):755–64.
5. Cheng DC, Newman M, Duke P, et al. The efficacy and resource utilization of remifentanil and fentanyl in fast track CABG surgery: a prospective randomized double-blind controlled multicenter trial. Anesth Analg. 2001;92(5):1094–102.
6. Couture P, Denault A, Limoges P, et al. Mechanisms of hemodynamic changes during off-pump coronary artery bypass surgery. Can J Anesth. 2002;49:835–59.
7. Cheng DC, Bainbridge D, Martin JE, Novick RJ. Does off pump coronary artery bypass reduce mortality, morbidity, and resource utilization when compared with conventional coronary artery bypass? A meta-analysis of randomized trials. Anesthesiology. 2005;102:188–203.
8. Polomsky M, He X, O'Brien SM, et al. Outcomes of offpump versus on-pump coronaryartery bypass grafting: impact of preoperative risk. J Thorac Cardiovasc Surg. 2013;145:1193–48.
9. van Dijk D, Spoor M, Hijman R, et al. Octopus Study Group. Cognitive and cardiac outcomes 5 years after off-pump vs on-pump coronary artery bypass graft surgery. JAMA. 2007;297:701–8.
10. Angelini GD, Culliford L, Smith DK, et al. Effects of on- and off-pump coronary artery surgery on graft patency, survival, and health-related quality of life: long-term follow-up of 2 randomized controlled trials. J Thorac Cardiovasc Surg. 2009;137:295–303.
11. Shroyer AL, Grover FL, Hattler B, et al. On-pump versus off-pump coronary-artery bypass surgery. N Engl J Med. 2009;361:1827–37.
12. Puskas JD, Williams WH, O'Donnell R, et al. Off-pump and on-pump coronary artery bypass grafting are associated with similar graft patency, myocardial ischemia, and freedom from reintervention: long-term follow-up of a randomized trial. Ann Thorac Surg. 2011;91:1836–42.
13. Lamy A, Devereaux PJ, Prabhakaran D, et al. Off-pump or on-pump coronary-artery bypass grafting at 30 days. N Engl J Med. 2012;366:1489–97.
14. Lamy A, Devereaux PJ, Prabhakaran D, et al. Effects of off-pump and on-pump coronary-artery bypass grafting at 1 year. N Engl J Med. 2013;368:1179–88.

15. Diegeler A, Börgermann J, Kappert U, et al. Off-pump versus on-pump coronary-artery bypass grafting in elderly patients. N Engl J Med. 2013;368:1189–98.

16. Lamy A, Devereaux PJ, Prabhakaran D, et al. Five-year outcomes after off-pump or on-pump coronary-artery bypass grafting. N Engl J Med. 2016;375:2359–68.

17. Shroyer AL, Hattler B, Wagner TH, et al. Five-year outcomes after on-pump and off-pump coronary-artery bypass. N Engl J Med. 2017;377:623–32.

18. Puskas J, Martin J, Cheng DC, et al. ISMICS consensus conference and statements of randomized controlled trials of off-pump versus conventional coronary artery bypass surgery. Innovations. 2015;10(4):219–29.

19. Kolh P, Windecker S, Alfonso F, et al. 2014 ESC/ EACTS guidelines on myocardial revascularization: the task force on myocardial revascularization of the European Society of Cardiology (ESC) and the European Association for Cardio-Thoracic Surgery (EACTS). Developed with the special contribution of the European Association of Percutaneous Cardiovascular Interventions (EAPCI). Eur J Cardiothorac Surg. 2014;46:517–92.

20. Hillis LD, Smith PK, Anderson JL, et al. 2011 ACCF/ AHA guideline for coronary artery bypass graft surgery. A report of the American College of Cardiology Foundation/American Heart Association Task Force on Practice Guidelines. Developed in collaboration with the American Association for Thoracic Surgery, Society of Cardiovascular Anesthesiologists, and Society of Thoracic Surgeons. J Am Coll Cardiol. 2011;58:e123–210.

21. Fihn SD, Gardin JM, Abrams J, et al. 2012 CCF/AHA/ ACP/AATS/PCNA/SCAI/STS guideline for the diagnosis and management of patients with stable ischemic heart disease: a report of the American College of Cardiology Foundation/American Heart Association Task Force on Practice Guidelines, and the American College of Physicians, American Association for Thoracic Surgery, Preventive Cardiovascular Nurses Association, Society for Cardiovascular Angiography and Interventions, and Society of Thoracic Surgeons. J Am Coll Cardiol. 2012;60:e44–164.

22. Fihn SD, Blankenship JC, Alexander KP, et al. 2014 ACC/AHA/AATS/PCNA/SCAI/STS focused update of the guideline for the diagnosis and management of patients with stable ischemic heart disease: a report of the American College of Cardiology/ American Heart Association Task Force on Practice Guidelines, and the American Association for Thoracic Surgery, Preventive Cardiovascular Nurses Association, Society for Cardiovascular Angiography and Interventions, and Society of Thoracic Surgeons. J Thorac Cardiovasc Surg. 2015;149:e5–23.

23. Patel MR, Calhoon JH, Dehmer GJ, et al. ACC/ AATS/AHA/ASE/ASNC/SCAI/SCCT/STS 2017 appropriate use criteria for coronary revascularization in patients with stable ischemic heart disease: a report of the American College of Cardiology Appropriate Use Criteria Task Force, American Association for Thoracic Surgery, American Heart Association, American Society of Echocardiography, American Society of Nuclear Cardiology, Society for Cardiovascular Angiography and Interventions, Society of Cardiovascular Computed Tomography, and Society of Thoracic Surgeons. J Am Coll Cardiol. 2017;69:2212–41.

24. Sousa-Uva M, Storey R, Huber K, et al. Expert position paper on the management of antiplatelet therapy in patients undergoing coronary artery bypass graft surgery. Eur Heart J. 2014;35:1510–4.

25. Ferraris VA, Saha SP, Oestreich JH, et al. 2012 update to the Society of Thoracic Surgeons guideline on use of antiplatelet drugs in patients having cardiac and noncardiac operations. Ann Thorac Surg. 2012;94:1761–81.

Robotic Coronary Artery Revascularization

36

Bob Kiaii

Main Messages

1. Robotic surgery provides an interface that enhances dexterity, allows scaling of motions, provides tremor filtering, and allows endoscopic microsurgery. This interface exists between the surgeon's hands and the surgical instruments.
2. The three levels of robotic coronary surgery in practice are: a) Telerobotic conduit harvesting and manual anastomosis; b) Arrested heart totally endoscopic coronary artery bypass; and c) Totally endoscopic coronary artery bypass.
3. Indications for robotic revascularization are: single or double vessel coronary artery disease with Grade I-II LV function; high risk for open sternotomy approach; multi-vessel disease utilizing hybrid technique; and coronary arteries, left anterior descending coronary artery, with ostial stenosis not amenable to PCI.

Until 1995, cardiac surgery was far behind other surgical specialties in the field of minimal access surgery [1]. With modification of cardiopulmonary bypass techniques and reduction in incision size, several cardiac surgical procedures were able to be performed safely and effectively. Unfortunately, despite early enthusiasm in minimal access cardiac surgery, most surgeons were skeptical and very critical of cardiac surgical procedures performed through small incisions owing to possibilities of unsafe operations and inferior results. Despite this reluctance of accepting a new approach, significant advances occurred in a short time with encouraging results. Concurrent advances in cardiopulmonary perfusion, intracardiac endoscopic visualization, instrumentation, and robotic telemanipulation resulted in a dramatic shift toward efficient and safe cardiac procedures through minimal access. Today, performing a variety of different cardiac procedures through small incisions has become standard practice for many surgeons and patients are becoming aware of the increasing availability.

Evolution

The term minimal access or minimally invasive cardiac surgery has referred to the size of the incision, the avoidance of sternotomy, and in some cases avoidance of cardiopulmonary bypass. Thus far, the incisions used in minimal

B. Kiaii (✉)
Department of Surgery, Western University,
London, ON, Canada
e-mail: bkiaii@ucdavis.edu

access cardiac surgical procedures include: small sternal incisions, parasternal incisions, minithoracotomies, and endoscopic/totally port access.

In order to perform an ideal minimal access cardiac operation, surgeons must become familiar with operating in restricted spaces through tiny incisions with assisted endoscopic vision and enhanced instrumentation [1].

Criteria for Ideal Cardiac Operation

- Tiny incisions
- Endoscopic ports
- Central antegrade perfusion
- Tactile feedback
- Eye-brain-like, three-dimensional (3D) visualization
- Adequate intracardiac access
- No instrument conflicts

Adapted from Franco, KL, Verrier ED, Advanced Therapy in Cardiac Surgery. 2003 Randolph Chitwood, Robot-assisted Mitral Valve Surgery

Endoscopic approaches remain challenging in cardiac surgery [1] with only a small number of surgeons using these techniques regularly due to the limitations of conventional endoscopic instruments. Many of these limitations with conventional endoscopic approaches have been overcome with the development of robotic surgical systems or computer-assisted surgical systems.

Robotic surgery allows a digital interface between the surgeon's hands and the instruments. This interface enhances dexterity, allows scaling of motions, provides tremor filtering, and enables the performance of endoscopic microsurgery [1]. Therefore, the use of robotic surgical systems over the last few years has enabled cardiac surgeons to perform minimally invasive endoscopic coronary artery bypass grafting (CABG) on the beating heart and open heart procedures with improvement in cardiopulmonary bypass (CPB) systems. This eliminates the need for sternotomy, and reduces tissue trauma, translating into decreased patient morbidity, increased patient satisfaction, shorter hospital stays, and potentially reduced healthcare costs.

Telemanipulation Systems

Initially two telemanipulation systems were available; the ZEUS™ (Computer Motion®, Goleta, CA) and the da Vinci™ surgical system (Intuitive Surgical®, Sunnyvale, CA). However, these two companies merged and only the da Vinci system is commercially available. It is presently the only robotic surgical system used by the majority of healthcare centers worldwide.

The da Vinci™ Surgical System (Intuitive Surgical®, Sunnyvale, CA) has evolved through numerous generations, starting with the original generation, followed by the S, Si, and most recently the Xi.

The da Vinci system is comprised of a surgeon console, a surgical cart, and the vision system. The surgeon console includes the display system, master handles, user interface, and the electronic controller. The surgeon at the console is able to view the transmitted image of the surgical field through a high-resolution 3D display. The system provides natural hand-eye coordination. Motion scaling allows for various ratios for mastering instrument motions. The tremor filter minimizes the involuntary tremors.

The surgical cart is stationed at the side of the operating table and consists of four robotic arms. One central arm is for the endoscope and the other three arms are for the surgical instruments. The instruments (end effectors) are attached to the three instrument arms and are recognized automatically by the system. The instruments can easily be interchanged. Because of the endowrist feature of the instruments, a total of 6 degrees of freedom are possible.

Evolution of Minimally Invasive Robot-Assisted Coronary Bypass Surgery

Over the last 15 years, cardiac surgeons have recognized the importance of achieving video dexterity and are adopting video-assisted techniques in increasing numbers. The early work by Drs. Nataf in Paris, Mayfield in Atlanta, and Wolf in Cincinnati [1, 2], laid the groundwork for an endoscopic minimally invasive revolution. The development of video-assisted techniques and the use of new equipment in cardiac procedures represented a paradigm shift and quantum leap in our efforts to provide a less traumatic coronary revascularization procedure. In parallel to these developments, new robotic technology was emerging and demonstrating efficacy in endoscopic surgery in other disciplines.

There are presently three levels of robotic coronary surgery currently being practiced:

1) Telerobotic conduit harvesting and manual anastomosis, referred to as endoscopic atraumatic coronary artery bypass (endoACAB). In this procedure, the surgeon harvests the internal thoracic artery (ITA) from the master console and performs a manual anastomosis through a mini-thoracotomy.
2) Arrested heart totally endoscopic coronary artery bypass. In this procedure, the surgeon harvests the ITA from the master console and performs anastomosis robotically and remotely from the master console via port-access on the arrested heart.
3) Totally endoscopic coronary artery bypass (TECAB). In this procedure, conduit harvesting, preparation, target vessel preparation, control and anastomosis are all performed by the surgeon remotely from the master console via port-access on the beating heart.

Indications for Robotic Revascularization

- Single or double vessel coronary artery disease with grade I-II left ventricular function
- Coronary arteries: left anterior descending coronary artery (LAD), with ostial stenosis not amenable to percutaneous coronary intervention (PCI)
- Multi-vessel disease utilizing hybrid technique (single or bilateral ITA grafting with PCI of other diseased vessels)

- High risk for open sternotomy approach
  - Ascending aortic atheroma or calcified aorta
  - Patients with poor ventricular function
  - Co-morbid conditions making a conventional surgery high risk

Patient Selection

Aside from understanding the standard contraindications to surgical coronary artery revascularization, patient selection for robotic coronary artery revascularization involves a history and physical exam heavily weighted on uncovering factors affecting external and internal thoracic structures. Anatomy hindering preoperative port placement, limiting robotic arm movement (working space), or reducing the already limited field of view inside the thorax, will cause significantly increased chances of surgical error and expose the patient to unnecessary risk. Although it seems intuitive that intrathoracic working space and general chest conditions (i.e. adiposity) can be estimated based upon external anatomy, this is not necessarily the case and this assumption can lead to a higher rate of conversion to sternotomy. Preoperative computed tomography (CT) can greatly assist with estimating intrathoracic working space and in some cases, predict intrathoracic adiposity.

Patient Selection for Robotic Coronary Artery Surgical Revascularization
- Absolute contraindications:
  - Extensive pleural symphysis
  - Previous left lung surgery
- Relative contraindications:
  - Morbid obesity
  - Significant cardiac enlargement (insufficient space in thoracic cavity)
  - Thick chest wall
  - Previous history of coronary artery bypass surgery
  - Diffuse distal coronary disease
  - Intramyocardial coronary arteries
  - Severe pulmonary disease (intolerance to single lung ventilation)

Operative Technique

Anesthesia Considerations

- Para vertebral block or intrathecal block for postoperative pain control
- Double lumen endotracheal tube or bronchial blocker
- Central venous pressure/Swan Ganz Catheter
- CO_2 insufflations of the thoracic cavity during the procedure
  - Intrathoracic pressures 5–15 mmHg
- Maintaining normothermia with warming and forced air blankets

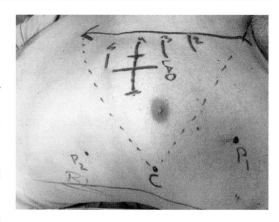

Fig. 36.1 Proper patient positioning

Preparation, Positioning and Draping

Initial positioning of the patient can have a considerable effect on the operative procedure, as proper positioning minimizes interference from internal and external body structures with the robotic equipment. Judicious care at this stage ensures the necessary landmarks for port placement in order to maximize robotic arm maneuverability intraoperatively.

The patient is positioned at the left edge of the operating room table. A comfortable support is placed under the distal two-thirds of the left side of the patient's thorax. This support usually takes the form of a rolled up towel and should elevate the patient thorax 6–8 inches superiorly. The left arm is positioned at the side of the OR table to allow the left shoulder to drop posteriorly. The table is rotated 30° up so the patient is in the partial left lateral position (Fig. 36.1).

Leads and external defibrillator pads are positioned on the patient's chest away from the left lateral and midclavicular areas of the thorax, so as not to interfere with port placement. One pad is placed on the right anterior lateral thorax and the other on the left posterior thorax. The patient is prepped in a routine manner for conventional CABG. The only variation in prep is exposure of the patient's thorax and axilla on the one-side for port placement.

Port Placement

Proper port placement is fundamental to the success of the operation. Placement of each port is centered on constructing an ideal configuration that ensures mobilization of the ITAs from the first rib to the sixth rib with the least amount of impedance to the robotic arms. It is imperative that the surgeon be meticulous with each individual patient, taking the necessary time needed to ensure proper completion of port placement prior to moving forward with the operation. Suboptimal port placement can frequently result in dangerous internal and/or external robotic arm collisions.

The lack of intrathoracic visualization is the premiere challenge to determining port placement. Careful review of the coronary angiogram, chest radiographs, and computed tomography (CT) of the heart with contrast preoperatively, along with direct examination of the anatomical structures of the individual patient in the operating room, help to alleviate this problem.

- Chest radiograph:
  - The chest radiograph is evaluated in an orderly manner. The following thoracic landmarks are identified and marked:
    - Supra-sternal notch
    - Angle of Louis
    - Xiphoid

- Second, third, fourth, fifth intercostal spaces (ICS)
- Left internal thoracic artery (LITA) and right internal thoracic artery (RITA) locations—1–3 cm lateral to the sternum
  - The position of the heart in the mediastinum is noted.
  - The size of the heart in relation to the pleural space on the port access side of the chest is noted.

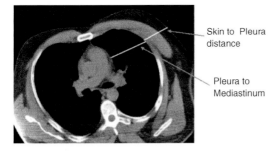

Fig. 36.2 Computed tomography showing the distance from pleura to mediastinum

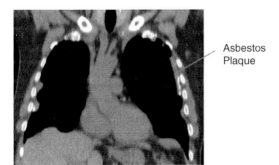

Fig. 36.3 Presence of asbestos plaques, important in identifying safe location for port placement

- Lateral view: the degree of space between the anterior surface of heart and underside of thorax is observed.

- Computed tomography of heart:
  - The intrathoracic space is assessed. The distance from the pleural surface to the mediastinum cannot be less than 1.7 cm at the camera port space (which is usually the fifth ICS: Fig. 36.2). A distance less than 1.7 cm will not provide adequate intrathoracic space for adequate degrees of freedom of the robotic instrument.
  - Other anatomical abnormalities such as asbestos plaques are ruled out (Fig. 36.3).
  - The anteroposterior (AP) measurement and the transverse (Trv) distance of the chest cavity are determined. If the AP/Trv ratio is less than 45%, it reduces the success of robotic–assisted coronary artery revascularization [3]. The vertical distance from the LAD to the chest wall is also a factor in the success of the operation. If this distance is less than 15 mm, there is less chance of being able to perform the operation robotically [3] (Fig. 36.4).
  - Location of the coronary arteries if intramyocardial is assessed. Access to intramyocardial vessels for revascularization is challenging and can result in conversion (Fig. 36.5).

- Direct Examination of Patient's Thorax:
  - The external anatomical characteristics of the patient's thorax are evaluated, and the internal anatomical characteristics are conceptualized based on the previously viewed

Fig. 36.4 Antero-posterior (AP), transverse measurement (TRV), and left anterior descending (LAD) to chest wall distance

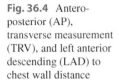
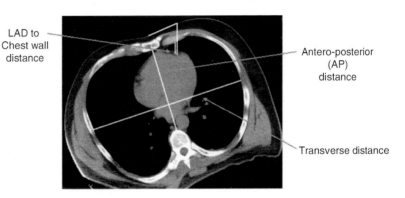

chest radiograph, computed tomography and preoperative coronary angiogram.

- Where each port is to enter the thoracic cavity is outlined using a felt marker, using the standardized guidelines discussed below (Fig. 36.1). Necessary adjustments are made for individual patients based on information acquired from diagnostic imaging and patient examination.

Standardized Guidelines for Port Placement

- Triangle Model of Configuration [2]
  - Proximal to distal end of LITA is one side of the triangle (surgical area).

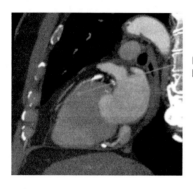

Intramyocardial LAD

Fig. 36.5 Intramyocardial location of LAD (left anterior descending) coronary artery

- Endoscope is positioned at the fifth ICS in axillary line (one vertex of triangle).
- Lines from endoscope port extend to both proximal and distal ends of the LITA (triangle formed).
- 'Camera Cone' created (Fig. 36.6)
- Instrument ports are placed outside the camera cone (Figs. 36.1 and 36.7).
- Ports are placed a few centimeters off the line of the defined triangle.
- 7–10 cm are allowed between ports to ensure robotic arms have full range of motion without collision.
- A circle is created from the camera port (7–10 cm) and placing ports inside this circle is avoided.

- Common Port Locations
  - Port site will vary based on body habitus. A larger thorax would require more obtuse angles in order to visualize the entire anatomy whereas as a small thorax would require more acute angles for the same reason.
  - Endoscope Port: fifth ICS anterior axillary line (AAL) or slightly medial to this point depending on body habitus.
  - Right and Left Instrument Ports: third and seventh ICS respectively. Two to three cm

Fig. 36.6 Triangle model of configuration (Adapted from Falk et al. 2001 [2])

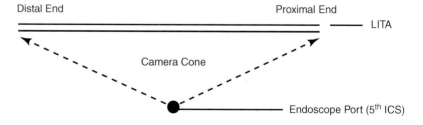

Fig. 36.7 Port placement positioning based on triangle model (Adapted from Falk et al. 2001 [2])

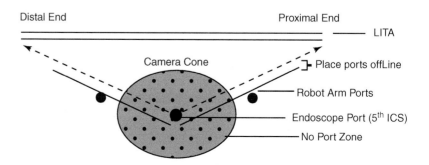

medial to the AAL or midway between AAL and midclavicular line (MCL).

Takedown of Left Internal Thoracic Artery (LITA)

Once the robotic instruments are adequately positioned within the thoracic cavity, the surgical workspace for harvesting the LITA is maximized using single lung ventilation and continuous CO_2 insufflation to keep intrathoracic cavity pressure between 5–10 mm Hg [4, 5]. The surgeon must be overly sensitive to visual cues throughout the surgical procedure compensating for a lack of haptic feedback with robotic assistance. This prevents unnecessary tension or trauma to the arterial conduit during mobilization. Using a 30° endoscope angled up inserted into the camera port, an initial inspection of the internal mammary artery and its relation to surrounding anatomical structures within the thorax is performed.

The procedure:

- Single lung ventilation is requested and the anaesthesia team is informed of insufflation initiation.
- The endoscope port is inserted. There must be no adhesions, as these can preclude the possibility of performing the procedure endoscopically. Occasionally adhesions can be taken down safely; if not, conversion to conventional surgery is necessary. The thoracic cavity is insufflated with CO_2 through the insufflation port on the endoscope cannula keeping insufflation pressures between 5–10 mmHg, while ensuring the blood pressure does not drop.
- The endoscope is inserted and moved freely through its full range of motion by the surgeon's hands. The distal and proximal ends of the LITA are located and care is taken to ensure the endoscope does not collide with external body parts such as the hip or shoulder (occasionally to reach the lower third aspect of the ITA through the same port incision, the port is "punched down" to the fourth ICS).

- The inner cavity is inspected with the endoscope to be certain there is a clear path for insertion of instrument ports.
- Insertion of instrument ports is observed with a direct view from the endoscope.
- The robot is docked and the robotic arms adapted to the appropriate endoscopic ports.
- The instruments are inserted through the ports and attached to the instrument arms.
- A verres needle is inserted at around the sixth ICS MCL and attached to low suction for venting.

Initial inspection of the LITA:

- The LITA is located (most visible at second rib)
- The LITA is followed proximally to its origin at the subclavian artery and distally to the sixth ICS. Arterial pulsation is a beneficial guide. Adipose tissue and muscle obscure the artery at the mid and lower 1/3 respectively
- The phrenic nerve is located. It should be clearly visible traversing the pericardium. It is followed proximally towards the origin of the ITA.

Key points to remember for successful robotic assisted takedown of the ITA:

- The ITA can be harvested using skeletonizing technique or as a pedicle.
- Progress must be in a slow and controlled manner maintaining hemostasis.
- Identify ITA and vein and work from the known to the unknown.
- Keep ITA and robotic instruments in view at all times.
- Use a 'no-touch' technique to mobilize ITA to reduce trauma.
- The cautery/spatula blade is held in the right arm and a DeBakey in the left arm.
- The DeBakey instrument can be alternated with a robotic bipolar forceps. The parietal pleura is incised at the most visible point. This is 1 cm medial to the artery at the second rib. A low monopolar electrocautery setting at 10–15 W is used.

- Dissection is started by scoring the fascia with the spatula 1 cm lateral and medial to the LITA
- Dissection is continued with a lateral to medial technique, and the LITA is slowly taken down with a combination of spatula blade blunt dissection and electrocautery.
- Move proximal to the top of the first rib and then distal to the sixth ICS. Care must be given not to put undue tension on the pedicle during mobilization. Mobilization to the top of the first rib provides an additional 3–4 cm of length to the pedicle and makes distal anastomosis easier.
- Small branches off the LITA are cauterized a safe distance from the vascular pedicle. Larger branches require instrument interchange and clips to be applied.
- Once adequate length of LITA has been harvested, the vessel is skeletonized distally.
- Heparin is given and distal LITA is clipped and left attached to the chest wall.
- For bilateral ITA harvesting, the right pleural space is entered and the RITA is harvested first using exactly similar technique. There may be the occasional need to switch to zero-degree endoscope.
- The anesthesiology team will need to be aware of managing the bilateral pneumothorax during the ITA harvest.

Hemostasis Management

To maintain hemostasis when bleeding occurs, the severity of the bleed in relation to the increased magnification of the image projected by the endoscope is evaluated. When small venous or arterial branches are responsible, gentle pressure is applied to the area for 2–3 min with the tip of the robotic instruments. This is often all that is required. If bleeding continues and the site of concern is in clear view, a clip is applied to the vessel and the distal end cauterized. A robotic bipolar instrument may be helpful. Surgicel™ hemostasis gauze is also effective if needed.

If bleeding is felt to be of a high severity or the patient shows signs of hemodynamic instability,

robotic instrumentation is removed immediately and the procedure is converted to a conventional CABG via sternotomy.

LITA to LAD Anastomosis

If the anastomosis is to be performed manually through a small incision, then the endoscopic Octopus Nuvo stabilizer (Medtronic, Minneapolis, MN) (Fig. 36.8) is utilized through the same port incisions. However, if the anastomosis is to be performed robotically, a fourth endoscopic port is inserted in the subxiphoid area slightly to the left side of the costal margin and adapted to the fourth robotic arm. The da Vinci endowrist stabilizer (Fig. 36.9) is placed in this port.

Pericardiotomy

- 2–3 cm anterior to the phrenic nerve.
- Using the fourth arm the pericardial fat is first removed.
- Pericardium is opened.

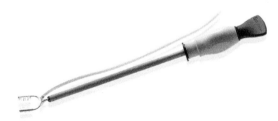

Fig. 36.8 Octopus Nuvo Stabilizer (Medtronic, Minneapolis, MN)

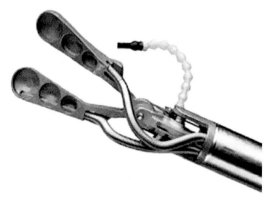

Fig. 36.9 da Vinci endowrist stabilizer

- LAD artery is identified based on its location on the ventricular septum and to the apex.

Anastomosis

- If performed totally endoscopically, the ITA pedicle is not detached from the chest wall until anastomosis is performed to avoid torsion of graft.
- If performed through mini-anterior thoracotomy, ITA pedicle is transected and to avoid torsion, using a clip, it is attached to the edge of the pericardium in the normal anatomical orientation at the site where the anastomosis is to be performed.

Mini-Anterior Thoracotomy Approach or Atraumatic Coronary Artery Bypass (ACAB) [5, 6]

- A long needle is inserted under the direct visualization of the endoscope to identify the optimal ICS to perform thoracotomy for best exposure of LAD.
- Insufflation can be momentarily stopped to take away the shift in the mediastinum.
- The intercostal space is marked from inside using electrocautery.
- The robot is undocked and instrument ports removed.
- Mini-anterior thoracotomy is performed.
- The pericardiotomy site and the ITA pedicle are identified.
- The ITA is detached and delivered through incision and two suspension sutures are immediately placed to prevent the pedicle from twisting.
- ITA length and flow are assessed and anastomosis prepared for.
- Port site is selected for the endoscopic Octopus Nuvo stabilizer (Medtronic, Minneapolis, MN) (Fig. 36.8).
- Stabilization is achieved.
- Proximal and distal occlusion snares or intravascular shunt are applied, depending on patient's hemodynamics
- Anastomosis is performed in the usual fashion.

- Graft flow is checked using an intraoperative flow measuring device.
- ITA patency and PCI of other coronary vessels at the same time are checked via intraoperative angiography in the specialized hybrid operating room (Fig. 36.10).

Totally Endoscopic Coronary Artery Bypass (TECAB) can be performed on an arrested heart (AHTECAB) or beating heart (BHTECAB). In AHTECAB, the patient is placed on cardiopulmonary bypass (CPB) usually peripherally and cardiac arrest is usually achieved using the endoaortic balloon clamp. The anastomosis is then performed [7].

- Once site of anastomosis on the LAD identified, occlusion silastic snares are placed proximally and distally.
- The suture to be used for anastomosis is placed in the thoracic cavity to avoid CO_2 leaks during the procedure.
- The da Vinci endowrist stabilizer (Fig. 36.9) is inserted through a subxiphoid port and stabilization of the selected area is achieved.
- The anastomosis begins in the usual fashion by inserting the first stitch in the ITA while still attached to the chest wall.
- After this stitch, the ITA is detached and anastomosis completed in the usual fashion.
- If anastomotic connectors are available, the anastomosis can be achieved with the help of connectors such as the Cardica C-port distal anastomosis system [8] (Cardica Inc., Redwood City, CA).
- Irrigation or a blower is used during the anastomosis to keep the vessel clear of blood and provide adequate visualization of the LAD.
- ITA patency and PCI are checked at the same time as the other vessels via intraoperative angiography if needed in the hybrid operating room [9, 10] (Fig. 36.10).

Follow-Up

The long-term patient follow-up at a mean of 8 years demonstrated an excellent level of satisfac-

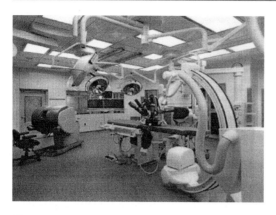

Fig. 36.10 Hybrid cardiac operating room at the London Health Sciences Centre and Canadian Surgical Technologies & Advance Robotics (CSTAR). The room is fully equipped for robotic surgery, angiography, and percutaneous coronary intervention

tion based on Seattle Angina Questionnaire and patency rate of 93% on CT angiography [11].

Future Directions

The continued advancements in robotic technology, imaging and anastomotic connectors has the potential to revolutionize coronary artery revascularization. Minimal access robotic-assisted coronary revascularization preserves chest cavity stability and provides an excellent cosmetic result. Smaller incisions are translated into reduced wound pain and infection, reduced blood loss and transfusion requirements, earlier discharge from hospital, faster recovery times, and earlier return to routine activities. With the development of more refined robotic systems and better instrumentation, robotic-assisted coronary revascularization will further excel. In the future, the optimal revascularization strategy will most likely involve a heart team approach with a combination of endoscopic robotic-assisted grafting

with arterial grafts and catheter-based intervention, allowing the patient to undergo an ultra-fast track [12] recovery with reduction in length of hospital stay.

References

1. Franco KL, Verrier ED. Advanced therapy in cardiac surgery. BC Decker Inc: Hamilton, ON; 2003.
2. Falk V, Loulmet D, Wolf RK. Procedural guide. Robotically assisted IMA harvest. Mountain View, CA: Intuitive Surgical; 2001.
3. Escoto A, Trejos AL, Patel RV, Goela A, Kiaii B. Innovations (Phila). 2014;9(5):349–53.
4. Ohtuska T, Wolf RK, Hiratzka LF, Wurning P, Flege JB. Thoracoscopic internal mammary artery harvest for MICABG using the harmonic scalpel. Ann Thorac Surg. 1997;63:s107–9.
5. Boyd WD, Kiaii B, Novick RJ, et al. RAVECAB: improving outcome in off-pump/minimal access surgery with robotic assistance and video enhancement. Can J Surg. 2001;44:45–50.
6. Kiaii B, McClure RS, Stitt L, et al. Prospective angiographic comparison of direct, endoscopic, and tele-surgical approaches to harvesting the internal thoracic artery. Ann Thorac Surg. 2006;82(2):624–8.
7. Bonaros N, Schachner T, Lehr E, et al. Five hundred cases of robotic endoscopic coronary artery bypass grafting: predictors of success and safety. Ann Thorac Surg. 2013;95(3):803–12.
8. Balkhy HH, Wann LS, Krienbring D, et al. Integrating coronary anastomotic connectors and robotics toward a totally endoscopic beating heart approach: review of 120 cases. Ann Thorac Surg. 2011;92(3):821–7.
9. Kiaii B, McClure RS, Stewart P, et al. Simultaneous integrated coronary artery revascularization with long-term angiographic follow-up. J Thorac Cardiovasc Surg. 2008;136(3):702–8.
10. Adams C, Burns DJ, Chu MW, et al. Single-stage hybrid coronary revascularization with long-term follow-up. Eur J Cardiothorac Surg. 2014;45(3):438–42.
11. Currie ME, Romsa J, Fox SA, et al. Long-term angiographic follow-up of robotic-assisted coronary artery revascularization. Ann Thorac Surg. 2012;93(5):1426–31.
12. Tarola CL, Al-Amodi HA, Balasubramanian S, et al. Ultrafast track robotic-assisted minimally invasive coronary artery surgical revascularization. Innovations. 2017;12(5):346–50.

Surgery of the Aortic Valve and Root

37

Tirone David

Main Messages
1. Pathologies of the aortic valve and root include a calcified anatomically normal triscuspid valve leading to aortic stenosis; congenital bicuspid aortic valve; unicuspid and quadricuspid aortic valves; dilatation of the aortic root with or without associated genetic syndromes such as Marfan and Loeys-Dietz syndromes.
2. Bicuspid aortic valve and dilatation of the aortic root are the most common causes of aortic insufficiency in the Western world.
3. The majority of aortic valve disease patients require aortic valve replacement, and patients with aortic insufficiency and normal or minimally diseased aortic cusps are candidates for aortic valve repair.
4. Patient age and cardiac/non-cardiac comorbidities impact operative mortality for aortic valve diseases

This chapter is an updated version of Chap. 25, Surgery of the Aortic Valve. In: Perioperative Care in Cardiac Anesthesia and Surgery by Cheng & David (eds.), published by Lippincott Williams & Wilkins, Philadelphia, PA; 2006. p. 227–40.

T. David (✉)
The University Health Network,
Toronto, ON, Canada
e-mail: Tirone.David@uhn.ca

Functional Anatomy

The aortic valve is better described as an aortic root because its function depends on more than just the aortic cusps. The aortic root has four anatomic components: aortic annulus, aortic cusps, aortic sinuses or sinuses of Valsalva, and sinotubular junction (Fig. 37.1). The aortic annulus or aorto-ventricular junction attaches the aortic root to the left ventricle, and has a scalloped shape that serves for insertion of the aortic cusps, which are semilunar in shape. The aortic annulus is attached to the interventricular septum in approximately 45% of its circumference and to fibrous tissue in 55% of its circumference. The segment of arterial wall delineated by the annulus proximally and the sinotubular junction distally is the aortic sinus. There are three aortic sinuses and three cusps: right, left, and non-coronary. The left coronary artery arises from the left aortic sinus and the right coronary artery arises from the right aortic sinus.

The highest point of the aortic cusps where two of them come in proximity is called the *commissure*. There are three commissures, and the triangular spaces underneath them are called *sub-commissural triangles*. These triangular spaces are also important for aortic valve function. The sub-commissural triangle between the left and right cusps is made of myocardium, whereas the other two are made of fibrous tissue.

The sinotubular junction is a ridge that demarcates the end of the aortic sinuses and the beginning

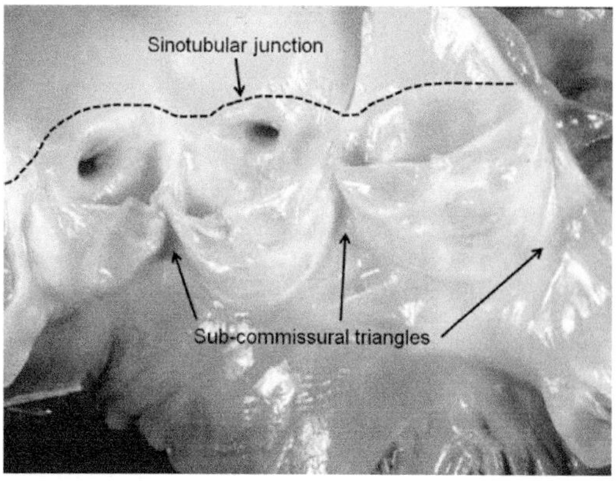

Fig. 37.1 A photograph of an aortic root displaying the sub-commissural triangles, aorto-ventricular junction, aortic cusps, aortic sinuses, coronary artery orifices and sinotubular junction

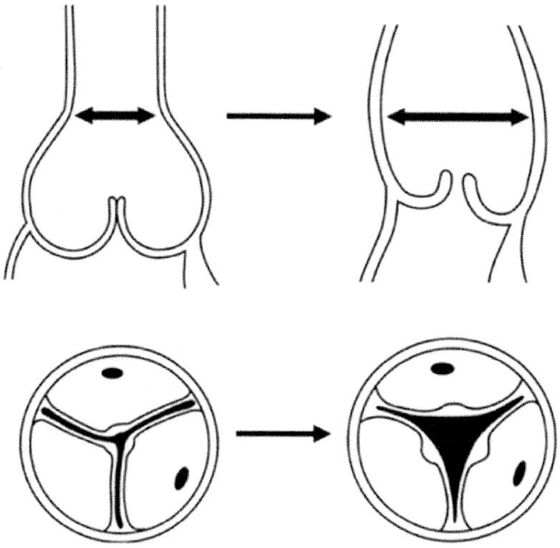

Fig. 37.2 Dilatation of the sinotubular junction causes aortic insufficiency

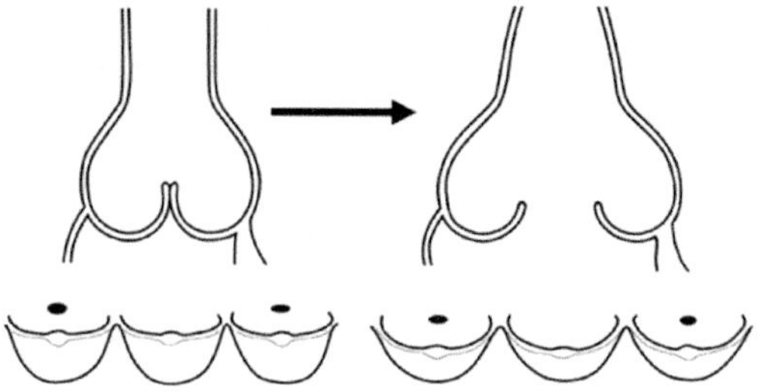

Fig. 37.3 Dilatation of the aortic annulus shortens the commissural heights and causes aortic insufficiency

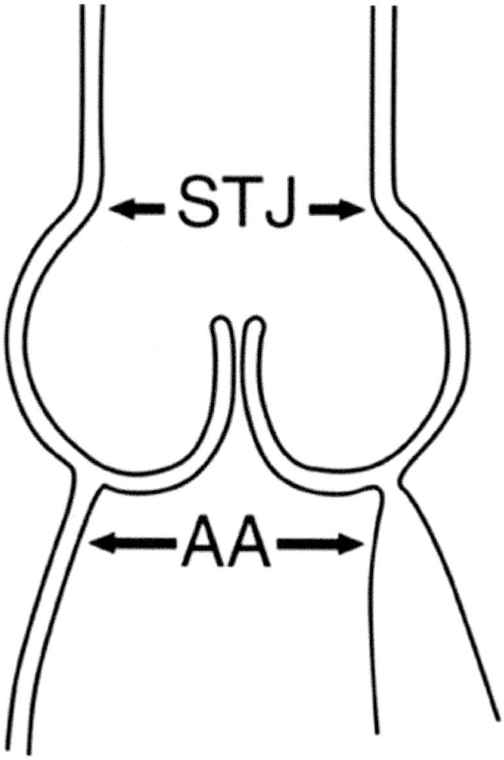

Fig. 37.4 The diameter of the aortic annulus is 15–20% larger than the diameter of the sinotubular junction in children, but it tends to equalize or even become smaller with aging

of the ascending aorta. The commissures of the aortic valve are located immediately below the sinotubular junction. Dilatation of the sinotubular junction pulls the leaflets apart and prevents them from coating centrally with resulting aortic insufficiency (AI) as illustrated in Fig. 37.2. Dilatation of the aortic annulus can also cause AI by displacing the base of the cusp and reducing the heights of the sub-commissural triangles as illustrated in Fig. 37.3.

The aortic sinuses are important to facilitate opening and closure of aortic cusps and minimize the mechanical stress during the cardiac cycle, but isolated anatomic abnormalities of the aortic sinuses do not cause AI. This is why children with rupture of an aortic sinus into another cardiac chamber may have an entirely competent aortic valve.

The aortic root and the ascending aorta are structures that contain a large amount of elastic fibers in young patients. Consequently, these structures expand and shorten during the cardiac cycle. The number of elastic fibers decreases with aging, and the aortic root and ascending aorta become progressively less compliant and larger. The transverse diameter of the aortic annulus at the nadir of the cusps is 15–20% larger than the diameter of the sinotubular junction in children. In adults, these two diameters tend to equalize and sometimes even reverse (Fig. 37.4).

Pathology

An anatomically normal tricuspid aortic valve may become calcified later in life and may cause aortic stenosis (AS). This lesion is called dystrophic calcification, senile calcification, or degenerative calcification. This type of degenerative process is the most common heart valve lesion in the Western World. It is characterized by progressive aortic valve narrowing. There is no therapy that prevents its progression. The pathophysiology of this disease is not completely clear but it is similar to atherosclerosis with endothelial damage, lipid infiltration, inflammation, fibrosis and calcification of the aortic cusps and sometimes the aortic sinuses.

Congenital bicuspid aortic valve (BAV) occurs in approximately 1% of the general population. Males are affected more than females at a ratio of 4:1. There is a relatively high incidence of familial clustering, which suggests an autosomal dominant inheritance with reduced penetrance. Extensive research in the genetics of bicuspid aortic valve is presently being conducted; this disorder is likely heritable. Most patients with BAV have three aortic sinuses and two cusps of different sizes. The larger cusp often contains a raphe instead of a commissure. The raphe extends from the mid portion of the cusp to the aortic annulus, and its insertion in the aortic root is at a lower level than the other two commissures. The morphology of the BAV is often described by Sievers' classification: BAV with two aortic sinuses and no raphe are uncommon and called "Type 0"; the most common occurs with one raphe and is called "Type 1"; and finally, two raphes is referred to as "Type 2" (unicuspid valve). Types 1 and 2 can be sub-classified according to the fused cusps: L-R is the most common form (a raphe in between the left and right cusps). Most patients with BAV have a dominant circumflex artery and a small right coronary artery. BAV may function satisfactorily until late in life when it may become calcified and stenotic. It may also become incompetent, particularly in younger patients, and is often associated with dilated aortic annulus and cusp prolapse.

Unicuspid and quadricuspid aortic valves are uncommon. A unicuspid valve usually causes AS and quadricuspid aortic insufficiency (AI). Patients with unicuspid and BAV frequently have premature degenerative changes of the media of the aortic root and ascending aorta and are at risk of developing an aneurysm of the aortic root, ascending aorta and arch.

A subaortic ventricular septal defect can cause AI because of the distortion of the aortic annulus and cusp prolapse. Another congenital anomaly of the aortic root is supra-aortic stenosis, which consists of a very narrow sinotubular junction, dilated aortic sinuses, and redundant cusps. The cusps may be thickened in some patients, thereby causing restriction. The coronary artery orifices may also be stenotic.

Dilatation of the aortic root and BAV are the most common cause of AI in the Western World. Aortic root aneurysms are usually caused by degenerative diseases of the media and may affect individuals of all ages. A broad spectrum of pathological and clinical entities are grouped under degenerative disorders, ranging from severe degeneration of the media, which can become clinically important early in life in cases such as Loeys-Dietz syndrome or Marfan syndrome, to clinically irrelevant mild dilatation in elderly patients. Patients with aortic root aneurysms are usually in their second or third decade of life when the diagnosis is made. These patients develop AI because of dilation of the sinotubular junction and/or aortic annulus. Annuloaortic ectasia is a term used to describe dilation of the aortic annulus. However, these patients often require surgery before valve dysfunction ensues because the aneurysm can cause aortic dissection and/or rupture.

There are several genetic abnormalities associated with aortic root aneurysm. Marfan syndrome and Loeys-Dietz syndrome are among the most common ones. Marfan syndrome is an autosomal dominant variably penetrant inherited disorder of the connective tissue in which the cardiovascular, skeletal, ocular, and other systems may be involved. The prevalence is estimated to be in 1:5000 people. The clinical features are the result of weakening of the supporting tissues owing to defects in fibrillin 1, a glycoprotein and an important component of the microfibril. The gene for fibrillin 1 (FBN1) is in chromosome 15. Several hundred mutations have been documented. The diagnosis of Marfan syndrome is made on clinical grounds. These patients often develop aortic root aneurysm, which may cause rupture or aortic dissection. Myxomatous degeneration of the mitral valve with consequent annular enlargement and mitral regurgitation may also be present, or be the initial presentation. The prognosis of patients with Marfan syndrome is largely determined by the aortic root aneurysm, which, if left untreated, will rupture, dissect, or cause AI and consequent heart failure. Loeys-Dietz syndrome is a genetic disorder with more severe connective tissue abnormalities than Marfan syndrome. It is caused by a genetic mutation in one of five genes that encode the transforming growth factor-beta (TGF-β) pathway and it is classified in type 1, 2, 3, 4, and 5. This alteration causes problems in the heart, arteries, bones, joints, skin, and internal organs. The prognosis is more serious than Marfan syndrome, with aortic dissection occurring earlier in life despite minimally dilated aortic root.

Aortic dissection involving the ascending aorta can cause AI due to detachment of one or more commissures of the aortic valve.

Rheumatic aortic valve is still seen in North America, but largely in immigrants. This disease causes fibrosis, commissural fusion, thickening, and contraction of the aortic cusps; it may also calcify in later stages. This disease can cause AS and AI.

Infective endocarditis of the aortic valve usually occurs in patients with pre-existing aortic valve disease, particularly BAV, but may also occur in patients with normal valves. The infection destroys one or more cusps and causes AI.

There are also several connective tissue disorders that can cause AI: ankylosing spondylitis, Reiter syndrome, osteogenesis imperfecta, rheumatoid arthritis, systemic lupus erythematosus, and others.

An increasingly more frequent cause of aortic valve disease is prosthetic and biologic valve disease. Mechanical heart valves may become stenotic because of pannus or thrombosis, and bioprosthetic valves and aortic valve homograft may become stenotic or incompetent because of tissue generation, which is frequently associated with calcification and/or cusp tear. Finally, the pulmonary autograft (Ross procedure) may become incompetent because of cusp prolapse and/or dilation of the root, and tissue degeneration with consequent AI.

Pathophysiology

Acquired AS develops gradually and the left ventricle adapts itself by replication of sarcomeres and concentric hypertrophy. As the ventricular mass increases, compliance decreases with consequent increase in left ventricular end-diastolic pressure and left atrial pressure. The degree of AS is considered severe when the aortic valve area is <0.5 cm^2/m^2 of body surface area or the peak systolic gradient exceeds 50 mm Hg with normal cardiac output.

The hemodynamic consequences of AI in the left ventricle depend on its severity and chronicity. Acute severe AI is poorly tolerated by the left ventricle, and heart failure and shock are usually inevitable. Chronic progressive AI results in a gradual increase in left ventricular end-diastolic volume with consequent rise in end-diastolic pressure. These changes in volume and pressure promote replication of the sarcomeres in series with consequent eccentric left ventricular hypertrophy. Because of this hypertrophy, left ventricular ejection fraction is maintained despite a large left ventricular end-diastolic volume, but eventually the ventricle will fail.

Natural History

Asymptomatic patients with AS have a good prognosis. Sudden death is rare among asymptomatic patients. The prognosis becomes poor once symptoms develop, and approximately one-half of patients die within a couple of years. Patients with chronic AI remain asymptomatic for many years but also have a poor prognosis when symptoms develop. Patients with aortic root aneurysm may develop AI but as the dilatation progresses, the risk of aortic dissection and/or rupture increases.

Diagnosis

The classic symptoms of AS (i.e. congestive heart failure, angina pectoris, and syncope) usually occur late in the evolution of the disease. Most patients are diagnosed during a routine physical examination before symptoms develop. On auscultation, there is a harsh systolic murmur, sometimes with a thrill along the left sternal border; often radiating to the neck. The second heart sound is soft, absent, or paradoxically split. The carotid pluses are diminished and delayed. The electrocardiogram may show signs of left ventricular hypertrophy. Echocardiography establishes the diagnosis and provides information regarding its severity, ventricular size and thickness, and pulmonary hypertension. Coronary angiography should be performed in patients older than 45 years, or even in younger patients if they have coronary artery disease risk factors.

AI is not readily diagnosed, and many patients escape clinical detection before it becomes symptomatic. Palpitations and head pounding may occur during exertion. Angina pectoris may occur, but less commonly than in AS. Syncope is rare. Symptoms of congestive heart failure are usually an indication of left ventricular dysfunction. On examination, there is a wide pulse pressure. Echocardiography establishes the diagnosis and provides other important information about the mechanism of AI and left ventricular function. The severity of AI decreases as the left ventricular end-diastolic pressure increases because of a lower pressure gradient between the aorta and left ventricle during diastole.

The diagnosis of aortic root aneurysm is made by imaging of the aorta with echocardiography, CT scan, MR imaging or contrast angiography.

Indications for Surgery

Surgery should be considered in all symptomatic patients and in asymptomatic patients with aortic valve area <0.50 cm^2/m^2, particularly if there is left ventricle is hypertrophy. Coexistent hypertension may be the principal cause of left ventricular hypertrophy.

Patients with symptomatic AI, and asymptomatic patients in whom systolic left ventricular function begins to deteriorate should be considered for surgery.

The indications for surgery in patients with prosthetic aortic valve dysfunction are the same as in native aortic valve disease, but the clinical presentation is broader and more complex. Patients with small paravalvular dehiscence that causes hemolysis and anemia should be considered for re-operation. Mechanical valve stenosis by pannus or thrombus is also an indication for re-operation. Bioprosthetic and biological valves should be re-replaced when there is echocardiography evidence of moderate or severe valve dysfunction.

Surgery should be considered in patients with aortic root aneurysm when its diameter reaches 55 mm. When associated with Marfan syndrome the threshold is 50 mm, and with Loeys-Dietz syndrome, 40 mm. Surgery is recommended even with smaller diameters when there is family history of aortic dissection. Surgery for aortic root aneurysm with BAV is recommended when the diameter exceeds 50 mm.

Aortic Valve Surgery

Most patients with aortic valve disease require aortic valve replacement (AVR). Mechanical valves are durable but require lifelong anticoagulation with warfarin sodium to prevent valve thrombosis and thromboembolism. There are several tissue valves: aortic valve homograft, pulmonary autograft (Ross procedure) and commercially available bioprosthetic valves. Bioprosthetic valves are usually made from porcine aortic valves or constructed from bovine pericardium. In either case, the xenograft tissue is chemically treated with glutaraldehyde to render it less antigenic and more resistant to fatigue. Aortic valve homograft and bioprosthetic valves have limited durability, but they do not require anticoagulation with warfarin sodium.

Patients with AI and normal or minimally diseased aortic cusps are candidates for aortic valve repair. This is where functional anatomy of the aortic valve plays an important role in the selection of operative procedure. Preoperative transesophageal echocardiography is the best diagnostic tool to identify suitable cases for aortic valve reconstruction. Since dilatation of the aortic root is the most common cause of AI, the aortic root may also have to be replaced at the time of aortic valve repair; these operations are referred to as aortic valve sparing operations.

Matching the Patient to the Prosthesis

It is not always simple to match the patient to the type and size of heart valve. Mechanical valves are durable, but because oral anticoagulation with warfarin sodium is mandatory, patients have a constant risk of bleeding. Tissue valves do not require anticoagulation but have limited durability. Therefore, patients who are likely to outlive their tissue valves may require reintervention (open surgical or trans-catheter valve-in-valve procedure). Bioprosthetic valves are ideal for patients 70 years of age or older because the probability of reintervention for valve failure is low. An aortic valve homograft is ideal for patients with active infective endocarditis, particularly if they have an aortic root abscess. The Ross procedure is ideally suited for children and young adults, especially women during childbearing years.

Another important aspect of AVR is the effective orifice area of the implanted valve. Prosthetic valves are obstructive and may be associated with high transvalvular gradient, and cause "patient-prosthesis mismatch." Ideally, the effective orifice areas of a prosthetic valve should be ≥ 0.85 cm^2/m^2 (aortic orifice area/body surface area). If the aortic annulus is too small, it is possible to implant a larger valve by enlarging the aortic annulus with a patch. There are basically two techniques to enlarge the aortic annulus. In the first, the aortic annulus is incised along its fibrous portion, usually along the sub-commissural triangle between the left and non-coronary sinuses and into the base of the anterior leaflet of the mitral valve. This technique allows for implantation of a valve one size larger than the original diameter of the aortic annulus without causing distortion of the mitral valve. Another technique, the Konno procedure, consists of incising the aortic annulus along the sub-commissural triangle between the left and right aortic sinuses. In this procedure, the right ventricle has to be opened just beneath the pulmonary valve and the interventricular septum for a length of 2–4 cm, depending on how much enlargement is desirable. Two separate patches are needed to reconstruct the interventricular septum and the right ventricle. The Konno procedure allows the implantation of a valve two or three sizes larger than the original size of the annulus, but it is a more complicated procedure and is often associated with higher operative mortality and morbidity.

Patient-prosthesis mismatch has become more important since the advent of TAVI and the widespread use of bioprosthetic valves in older patients. Valve-in-valve can be problematic in patients with failed bioprosthetic valves size 21 and smaller because they leave unacceptably high gradients. Thus, the implantation of a larger bioprosthesis at the initial AVR guarantees better long-term outcome particularly if a valve-in-valve becomes necessary.

Operative Techniques

Aortic valve operations can be performed through a midline sternotomy (full or partial) or through a small right anterior thoracotomy. Cardiopulmonary bypass, aortic clamping, opening the ascending aorta, and protection of the myocardium with cardioplegia are necessary to perform aortic valve surgery.

Aortic Valve Replacement

The aorta can be opened through a transverse incision 1 cm above the sinotubular junction or through a hockey-stick incision extended into the non-coronary sinus; we prefer the first method. The diseased aortic cusps are completely excised and the aortic annulus is debrided to remove all calcified tissue. The aortic annulus is measured with specific manufacturer's valve sizers. The prosthetic valve is secured to the aortic annulus according to the type of valve implanted. We prefer to secure mechanical valves with 20–30 simple interrupted sutures of 2-0 polyester. Currently used stented bioprosthetic valves are designed to be implanted on a supra-annular position and, for this reason, 10–12 horizontal mattress polyester sutures with pledgets on the ventricular side of the annulus are used.

During the past decade, transcatheter aortic valve implantation (TAVI) has become an alternative to surgical AVR for the treatment of AS, and it is particularly useful in high and medium risk patients. TAVI is also useful in patients with failed bioprosthetic aortic valves; however, the failed bioprosthesis has to be large enough to allow the deployment of a valve of reasonable size.

Aortic Root Replacement

Patients with aortic root aneurysm and calcified or fibrotic aortic cusps or other abnormality of the root such as extensive dissection, calcification or endocarditis require replacement of the entire aortic root and sometimes the ascending aorta. Combined replacement of the aortic valve and aortic sinuses and part of the ascending aorta is called the Bentall procedure. Replacement of the aortic root can be performed with mechanical or tissue valves. There are commercially available Dacron conduits containing a mechanical valve in one of its ends. Aortic root replacement is done by transecting the ascending aorta immediately above the sinotubular junction and excising the diseased aortic cusps. The coronary arteries are detached from the aortic root leaving 3–5 mm of aortic sinus wall around their orifices. The sewing ring of the mechanical valve is secured to the aortic annulus either using interrupted sutures as described for AVR with mechanical valves; or, with inverting horizontal mattress polyester sutures with pledgets, which are left on the aortic side of the annulus, as illustrated in Fig. 37.5. This technique of suturing should be used only when the aortic annulus is dilated and can accommodate a valve of adequate size. The coronary arteries are re-implanted into this graft, and its distal part is anastomosed to the ascending aorta.

If a bioprosthetic valve is used, it should be sutured to the Dacron graft 5–10 mm from one of its ends, with the graft secured to the aortic annulus as illustrated in Fig. 37.6. This approach facilitates re-operation if required for bioprosthetic valve degeneration.

Aortic root replacement with aortic valve homograft or pulmonary autograft is performed using similar techniques, but the proximal anastomosis is usually performed with running 4-0

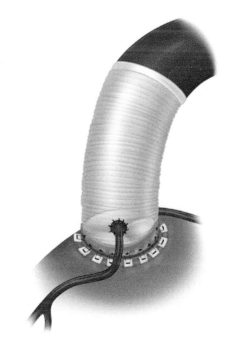

Fig. 37.5 Bentall procedure with a mechanical valve

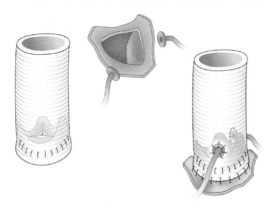

Fig. 37.6 Bentall procedure with a bioprosthetic valve

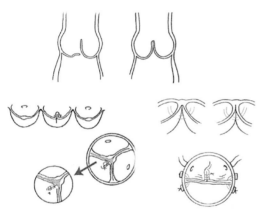

Fig. 37.7 Techniques of cusp repair: plication of the central portion and sub-commissural plication

polypropylene sutures or interrupted 4-0 polyester sutures.

Re-implantation of the coronary arteries is the Achilles heel of aortic root replacement. In addition to performing a hemostatic anastomosis between the coronary arteries and the aortic root graft, it is also extremely important to align them correctly to prevent kinking or torsion with consequent myocardial ischemia. The latter is more common with the right coronary artery.

Aortic Valve Repair and Aortic Valve Sparing Operations

There are several techniques that can be used to repair abnormal aortic cusps:

Cusp Perforation: Occasionally, a cusp perforation is the sole reason for AI. The perforation may be iatrogenic, sequelae of endocarditis, or the result of a papillary fibroelastoma resection. A simple patch of fresh or glutaraldehyde fixed autologous pericardium is adequate to correct the problem. Fresh autologous pericardium can also be used to repair small holes (<6 mm), but the patch should be larger than the defect as it retracts during healing. The patch is sutured on the aortic side of the cusp with a fine polypropylene suture.

Cusp Extension: Cusp augmentation has been used to repair incompetent aortic valves due to rheumatic and congenital disease. Glutaraldehyde-fixed bovine or autologous pericardium has been used for this purpose.

Cusp Prolapse: Cusp prolapse is due to elongation of the free margin. This is corrected by plication along the nodule of Arantius with fine polypropylene sutures. The degree of shortening is determined by examining the other cusps and bringing the prolapsing cusp to the same level of coaptation as the normal ones.

Sub-commissural Plication: Aortic annulus dilatation is associated with broadening of the base of the cusp sub-commissural triangles. It is possible to reduce the degree of dilatation by plication of the triangles with horizontal mattress sutures from the supra-annular sides of the cusps. Figure 37.7 illustrates cusp plication to correct prolapse in tricuspid and bicuspid aortic valves and sub-commissural plication.

Cusp with Stress Fenestration: Dilation of the sinotubular junction increases the mechanical stress along the free margin of the cusp near the commissures and may cause a stress fenestration with thinning and sometimes even detachment from the commissure. This type of lesion has been successfully corrected by weaving a double layer of 7-0 or 6-0 expanded polytetrafluoroethylene sutures along the free margin of the cusp from commissure to commissure or to the nodule of Arantius (Fig. 37.8).

Patients with ascending aorta and/or aortic root aneurysm may have normal or near normal cusps, and reconstruction of the aortic root with preservation of the aortic cusps is often feasible.

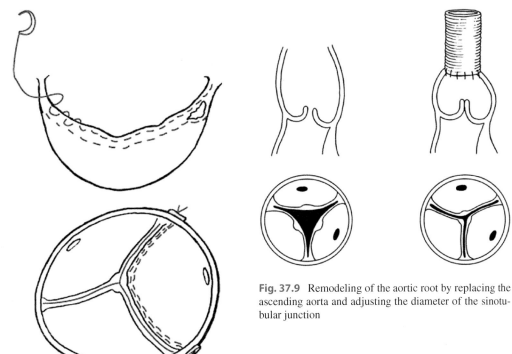

Fig. 37.8 Reinforcement of the free margin of a cusp with a fine Gore-Tex suture

Fig. 37.9 Remodeling of the aortic root by replacing the ascending aorta and adjusting the diameter of the sinotubular junction

There are basically two types of aortic valve sparing operations: remodeling of the aortic root and re-implantation of the aortic valve. Remodeling of the aortic root is done in patients with ascending aortic aneurysm, normal aortic sinuses and AI due to dilatation of the sinotubular junction. Replacement of the ascending aorta with a Dacron graft and correction of the diameter of the sinotubular junction can restore valve function (Fig. 37.9).

If one aortic sinus is dilated it can be replaced with an appropriately tailored tubular Dacron graft (Fig. 37.10), and the same if all three sinuses are aneurysmal (Fig. 37.11). The aortic cusps may also need repair during these procedures.

The technique of re-implantation of the aortic valve is used in patients in whom the aortic root aneurysm is associated with genetic syndromes, incompetent BAV or any other condition associated with annuloaortic ectasia (dilated aortic annulus as illustrated in Fig. 37.3). In this operation, the sinuses are excised and the aorto-

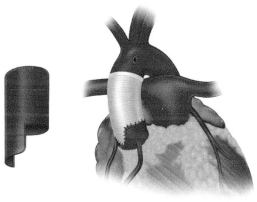

Fig. 37.10 Remodeling of the aortic root with replacement of one aortic sinus and adjustment of the sinotubular junction diameter

ventricular junction freed from surrounding tissues down to just beneath its lower level. A Dacron graft of diameter that corresponds to the appropriate sinotubular junction diameter (or approximately twice the height of the cusps) is sutured to the left ventricular outflow tract along a horizontal plane immediately below the lowest level of the aorto-ventricular junction (except in the commissural area between the left and right cusps to prevent damage to the Bundle of His).

Fig. 37.11 Remodeling of the aortic root with replacement of all three aortic sinuses

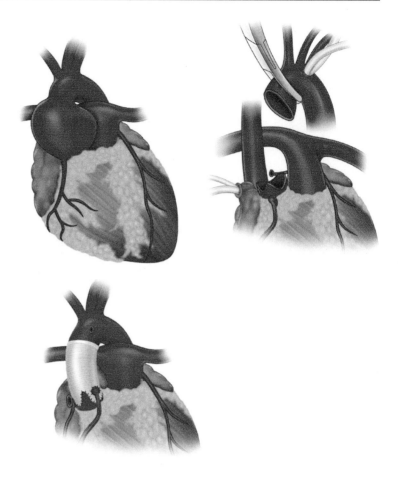

The three commissures are suspended inside the graft and the aortic annulus, and remnants of the aortic sinuses are sutured to the graft. The coronary arteries are re-implanted into their respective sinuses. If neo-aortic sinuses are desired, a graft one size larger than needed is used and darts may be placed in between commissures to create neo-aortic sinuses (Fig. 37.12). Some surgeons prefer to use commercially available Dacron graft with aortic sinuses. The cusps are repaired if necessary. It is important that they co-apt within the Dacron, with a co-aptation height of at least 8 mm.

AI due to BAV can also be corrected by means of aortic valve repair when the cusps are of good quality and the AI is largely due to cusp prolapse. The cusps may require repair as described above.

Most patients with BAV and AI have dilated aortic annulus and re-implantation of the aortic valve may be the best procedure.

Operative Mortality and Morbidity

The operative mortality for AVR varies with the patient's age and cardiac and non-cardiac comorbidities. First-time isolated elective AVR in otherwise healthy patients is associated with an operative mortality of <1%. The risk increases in patients with coronary artery disease, in elderly patients, in active infective endocarditis (particularly if there is a paravalvular abscess), and in patients with other systemic diseases such as peripheral vascular disease, renal failure, and

Fig. 37.12
Re-implantation of the
aortic valve with a
cylindrical graft
(left panel) and
recreation of aortic
sinuses (right panel)

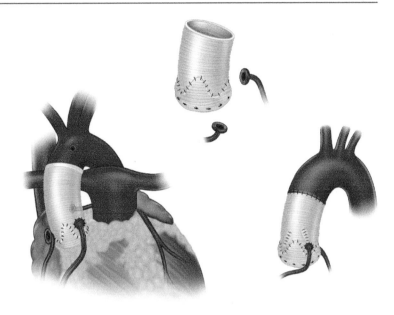

severe chronic obstructive lung disease. The operative risk can be estimated by using the STS Risk Score (*riskcalc.sts.org/*). The operative mortality associated with aortic valve repair and reconstruction of the aortic root is reportedly low at 1–3%, depending on the patient's clinical presentation.

Excessive postoperative bleeding may require re-exploration of the mediastinum in 2–5% of the patients. Perioperative myocardial infarction occurs in 1–2% of patients, particularly if coronary artery disease is present. Myocardial infarction can cause life-threatening ventricular dysrhythmias and/or heart failure. The risk of perioperative stroke varies with a patient's age, the presence of coronary artery disease, and ascending aorta and arch atherosclerosis. It is rare in young patients, but can occur in up to 10% or more of elderly patients. Other complications such as renal and respiratory failure are uncommon and usually predictable. Sternal wound infection is rare if meticulous aseptic operative and intensive care unit techniques are exercised. Patients with prosthetic aortic valves have a constant risk of developing prosthetic valve endocarditis, which is highest during the few months after surgery, occurring in 1–2% of patients. For

this reason, prophylactic antibiotics should be given during the first 2 days after surgery or longer if the patient has a lung or wound infection.

Patients with mechanical valves should be started on heparin or low-molecular weight heparin a couple of hours after removal of the chest drains and on warfarin sodium as soon as they can swallow. There is evidence that patients with bioprosthetic aortic valves may benefit by anticoagulation during the first 6 months after surgery. We continue to give these patients only aspirin and we have not documented an increased risk of death or adverse events during the first year in our patients.

Although aortic valve surgery is performed with intraoperative echocardiography, a postoperative echocardiogram should be obtained before discharge to rule out pericardial effusion and assess valve and ventricular function.

Late Outcomes

Patients who have had aortic valve surgery must remain under surveillance by a cardiologist and have an ECG and echocardiogram annually. Prosthetic valve dysfunction is best treated while ventricular function is normal. Therefore, patients with a failing bioprosthetic valve should have elective re-operations while they are well, instead of waiting until severe heart failure or cardiogenic shock ensues.

Long-term survival after AVR depends on the patient's age, functional class at the time of surgery, left ventricular function, coronary artery disease, and other systemic diseases. The type of valve implanted does not seem to affect long-term survival. Adults who have AVR have a mean age of 65 years, and the 10-year survival is approximately 60% (ranging from 40% to 80% depending on comorbidities).

The risk of thromboembolic events, usually transient ischemic attacks or strokes, is approximately 1–2% per year, but it varies with the patient's age and associated diseases. Therefore, in young patients with tissue valves, the risk of thromboembolism is practically nil, whereas in older patients the risk is approximately 3% per year. The same is true for mechanical valves. Atherosclerosis increases the risk of thromboembolic stroke.

The risk of hemorrhage caused by oral anticoagulants varies with international normalized ratio (INR) level and by patient. The recommended level of anticoagulation for mechanical valves in the aortic position is an INR of 2.0–3.0. At this level of anticoagulation, the risk of major bleeding is less than 1% per year. The risk of bleeding increases with a higher INR.

The risk of developing prosthetic infective endocarditis is approximately 0.3–1.0% per year. Patients with prosthetic valves need antibiotic prophylaxis when exposed to bacteremia. Other valve-related problems are bioprosthetic valve failure, prosthetic valve dehiscence, hemolysis, prosthetic valve stenosis due to pannus, or thrombosis. Most of these complications need surgical re-intervention.

There has been a renewed interest on the Ross procedure for young adults because of its durability and freedom from adverse valve-related events after 20 years of follow-up. Several centers reported freedom from Ross-related reinterventions of 85% at 20 years and freedom from reoperations in excess of 90% in the pulmonary autograft, making this procedure ideal for woman during child bearing years.

The long-term results of aortic valve repair with reconstruction of the aortic root have been excellent in experienced centers. Late development of AI is the main problem with these operations. In our experience with more than 500 patients operated on during the past 25 years, the need for re-operation in the aortic valve was only 5% at 15 years. Other valve-related complications were rare among these patients.

Further Reading

1. Nishimura RA, et al. 2014 AHA/ACC Guideline for the management of patient with valvular heart disease. J Am Coll Cardiol. 2014;63(22):57–185.
2. Baumgartner H, et al. 2017 ESC/EACTS Guidelines for the management of valvular heart disease: the Task Force for the Management of Valvular Heart Disease of the European Society of Cardiology (ESC) and the European Association for Cardio-Thoracic Surgery (EACTS). Eur Heart J. 2017. [Epub ahead of print]
3. David TE. Aortic valve sparing in different aortic valve and aortic root conditions. J Am Coll Cardiol. 2016;68(6):654–64.
4. David TE. Surgical treatment of aortic valve disease. Nat Cardiol Rev. 2013;10(7):375–86.

Surgery of the Mitral Valve

38

Tirone David

Main Messages

1. Common pathologies of mitral valve dysfunction are rheumatic fever, degenerative diseases of the mitral valve, and cardiomyopathies.
2. The most common cause of mitral regurgitation in the Western world is mitral valve prolapse due to degenerative diseases.
3. Mitral valve repair provides better long-term outcomes than mitral valve replacement in patients with degenerative diseases.
4. Patient age, left ventricular function, and coronary artery disease are variables that affect long-term survival after mitral valve surgery.

This chapter is an updated version of Chap. 26, Surgery of the Mitral Valve. In: Perioperative Care in Cardiac Anesthesia and Surgery by Cheng & David (eds.), published by Lippincott Williams & Wilkins, Philadelphia, PA; 2006. p. 241–51.

T. David (✉)
The University Health Network,
Toronto, ON, Canada
e-mail: Tirone.David@uhn.ca

Functional Anatomy

The mitral valve is a complex structure with the following components: left atrium, mitral annulus, leaflets, chordae tendineae, papillary muscles and left ventricular wall (Fig. 38.1). The mitral annulus is an extension of the central fibrous body of the heart from the lateral to the medial fibrous trigones. The posterior leaflet is attached to the posterior wall of the left ventricle, and the anterior leaflet is attached to the intervalvular fibrous body that separates the mitral from the aortic valve. The mitral annulus has a sphincter-like function, because the posterior leaflet is attached to the basoconstrictor muscles (bulbo and sinospiral muscle bundles). The area of the mitral valve is reduced by approximately 25% during systole. The mitral annulus is circular in late diastole and becomes flatter in systole.

The mitral valve leaflets are a single structure but function as two; the anterior and posterior leaflets. The length of the anterior leaflet base corresponds to approximately one-third of the mitral annulus circumference and the base of the posterior leaflet to the remaining two-thirds. The anterior leaflet is narrower and longer than the posterior leaflet, but the areas of the two leaflets are similar.

The areas where the two leaflets join each other are called commissures. There are two commissures; an anterior and a posterior. The posterior leaflet also has two false commissures

© Springer Nature Switzerland AG 2021
D. C. H. Cheng et al. (eds.), *Evidence-Based Practice in Perioperative Cardiac Anesthesia and Surgery*, https://doi.org/10.1007/978-3-030-47887-2_38

471

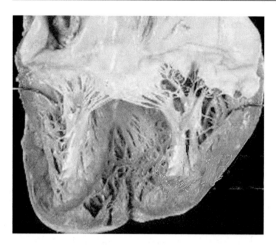

Fig. 38.1 Photograph of a mitral valve. Each papillary muscle anchors one half of the anterior and posterior leaflets

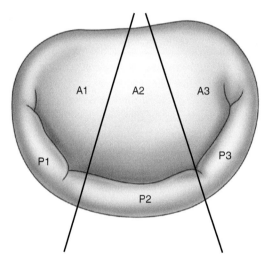

Fig. 38.2 Carpentier's classification of the various segments of the mitral valve

that divide it into three segments; lateral, central and medial scallops. Carpentier's classification of the various mitral valve leaflet segments are universally used (Fig. 38.2).

The chordae tendineae are extensions of the leaflets that reach the papillary muscles. They originate from the free margins of the leaflets as well as from the ventricular surface. The chordae tendineae in the free margins of the leaflets are primary chordae, those in the ventricular surface of the leaflets are secondary chordae, and chor-

dae that attaches the leaflets to the ventricular wall directly are tertiary chordae.

There are two papillary muscles; anterior and posterior. The anterior papillary muscle anchors the lateral half of the mitral valve and the posterior papillary muscle anchors the medial half. The anterior papillary muscle receives its blood supply from branches of the left anterior descending and circumflex arteries, whereas the posterior papillary muscle has a single blood vessel that comes from the posterolateral branch of the right coronary artery. The papillary muscles are an extension of the ventricular wall.

An imaginary line divides the mitral valve in two halves: the medial and lateral halves. The medial half is anchored by the posterior papillary muscle and the lateral half by the anterior papillary muscle. The central segments of both leaflets (A2 and P2) are anchored by both papillary muscles.

Pathology of the Mitral Valve

Rheumatic fever remains a common problem in developing countries. It can cause severe mitral valve dysfunction. During its acute phase, it causes mitral regurgitation (MR) and later may cause mitral stenosis (MS), MR or both. Fibrosis of all components of the mitral valve is the principal pathologic feature of chronic rheumatic valve disease. The leaflets become thickened; the commissures fuse; and the chordae tendineae thicken, fuse, and shorten. The commissures and other parts of the valve may become calcified. The papillary muscles become bulky and hypertrophic. The left atrium is often dilated and the appendage may be filled with clots in cases of MS.

Degenerative diseases of the mitral valve include various entities that range from ruptured chordae tendineae of a grossly normal valve (the so-called fibroelastic deficiency); to various degrees of myxomatous degeneration; to heavy calcification of the mitral annulus, chordae tendineae and sometimes even the papillary muscle heads. Myxomatous degeneration is the most common form of degenerative disease of the mitral valve. The mitral annulus dilates, the leaflets become voluminous and billowing, and the chordae tendineae may thicken, elongate or rupture. These abnormalities can cause leaflet prolapse with consequent MR. Mitral valve prolapse is the most common cause of MR in the Western World.

Dystrophic calcification of the mitral annulus may occur in isolation but may also be present in patients with mitral valve disease such as myxomatous disease and less commonly rheumatic disease. It occurs more often in older patients, and more often in women than men.

Functional mitral regurgitation is defined as a disorder of regional or global left ventricular function in which anatomically intact leaflets fail to coapt, usually because of tethering. Functional MR occurs in patients with ischemic and non-ischemic cardiomyopathy. In ischemic MR, the valve dysfunction can be acute due to a myocardial infarction, or chronic due to remodeling of the necrotic muscle. Papillary muscle rupture can cause massive MR and cardiogenic shock requiring immediate surgical intervention. Congenital mitral valve disease is far less common than acquired diseases (discussed elsewhere in this book).

Pathophysiology of Mitral Valve Disease

Mitral Stenosis

MS is usually caused by rheumatic fever. The normal mitral valve orifice ranges from 4 to 6 cm^2. MS occurs when the mitral valve area is less than 2 cm^2, and it becomes critical when the orifice is reduced to 1 cm^2. Reduction in the mitral valve orifice causes a rise in the left atrial pressure, which in turn raises pulmonary venous and capillary pressure with consequent dyspnea. This problem is aggravated by exercise, stress and atrial fibrillation. The left ventricle is small in patients with MS.

Mitral Regurgitation

The pathophysiology of this lesion is complicated because the regurgitant mitral valve orifice is functionally in competition with the aortic valve orifice. A regurgitant orifice larger than the aortic orifice is not compatible with life. The regurgitant mitral flow depends on the combination of the instantaneous size of the regurgitant orifice and the pressure gradient between the left ventricle and left atrium. MR may be acute or chronic. In acute MR the left ventricle compensates by emptying more completely with consequent reduction in wall tension and by increasing preload. As the regurgitant volume becomes chronic, the ventricle dilates, and according to Laplace principle, wall tension eventually increases to supra-normal levels. Dilation of the left ventricles causes dilation of the mitral annulus with consequent increase in the regurgitant orifice, creating a vicious circle in which "MR begets more MR". The compliance of the left atrium and pulmonary venous bed is an important determinant of hemodynamic and clinical presentation of MR.

Natural History

The onset of MS symptoms is insidious and patients tend to modify their activities to minimize them. Most patients are in advanced functional classes when they seek medical assistance, particularly in countries where rheumatic fever is still a major health problem. In the pre-surgical era, the 5-year survival of patients with MS in New York Heart Association (NYHA) functional classes III and IV was 62% and 15% respectively.

The natural history of MR depends on the severity of regurgitant volume, left ventricular function and the cause of mitral valve dysfunction. Patients with severe MR and impaired ventricular function do not live long whether symptomatic or not. Chronic MR due to mitral valve prolapse is usually well tolerated for many years before left ventricular function becomes impaired; however, most patients are operated on before reaching that point if the valve is repairable. Ischemic MR has a poor prognosis and surgery may only alter the symptoms, with no effect on survival if left ventricular ejection fraction is low. The same can be said for MR due to cardiomyopathy.

Clinical Manifestations and Diagnosis

The principal symptom of MS is dyspnea. Other symptoms are fatigue, decreased exercise tolerance, hemoptysis, and chest pain. Depending on the stage of the disease, these patients may develop pulmonary hypertension and tricuspid regurgitation with symptoms and signs of venous hypertension such as hepatomegaly, peripheral edema, ascites and pleural effusion.

Patients with chronic MR remain asymptomatic for a long time, and by the time symptoms become apparent, left ventricular dysfunction may already be present. Decreased exercise tolerance and fatigue are the early symptoms. Acute MR causes pulmonary congestion and dyspnea, and depending on the severity it may cause cardiogenic shock.

The diagnosis of mitral valve disease can be made by a careful physical examination and confirmed by echocardiography. If the images obtained by a trans-thoracic echocardiogram are inadequate to establish the diagnosis, a trans-esophageal echocardiogram (TEE) can be done and will certainly establish the diagnosis and provide information regarding the mechanism of valve dysfunction. If surgical treatment is indicated, coronary angiography should be performed in patients older than 45 years of age to rule out presence of coronary artery disease.

Treatment

Mitral Stenosis

Symptomatic patients experience significant improvement with diuretics and restriction of sodium intake. Digitalis glycosides are only valuable in patients with atrial fibrillation. Beta blockers may increase exercise tolerance by reducing heart rate. Patients in atrial fibrillation should be anticoagulated with warfarin sodium to reduce the risk of thromboembolism. Newer oral anticoagulants are not as effective as warfarin sodium in rheumatic patients. Symptomatic patients should be investigated, and if appropri-ate, percutaneous balloon valvotomy or mitral valve repair performed.

The feasibility of mitral valve repair as well as of percutaneous balloon valvotomy usually can be determined by preoperative TEE. Stenotic valves with thin and pliable leaflets and chordae tendineae that are at least 1 cm long are usually suitable for percutaneous balloon valvotomy or surgical repair. Surgical repair consists of performing a commissurotomy, and maneuvers to increase mobilization of the leaflets and fused chordae tendineae (such as removal of a fibrous layer from the leaflets, chordal resection and papillary muscle splitting).

Stenotic valves with more advanced fibrotic changes are best managed by valve replacement. The valve should be completely excised and a prosthetic valve secured to the mitral annulus. We believe that resuspension of the papillary muscles with 4-0 Gore-Tex sutures reduces the risk of atrioventricular separation after mitral valve replacement, and may preserve left ventricular systolic function.

Mitral Insufficiency

Afterload reduction is beneficial in patients with both acute and chronic MR. Afterload reduction with nitroprusside is lifesaving in patients with acute MR and cardiogenic shock. Intra-aortic balloon pump is also of value to stabilize patients for angiography and surgery. Symptomatic patients with chronic MR also experience improvement with afterload reduction with an angiotensin inhibitor or oral hydralazine. The cause of MR should be established and symptomatic patients should be treated surgically. If mitral valve repair is feasible, even asymptomatic patients with severe MR should be considered for surgery if they are young and the operative risk is very low (<1%). Mitral valve replacement is reserved for patients in NYHA functional classes III and IV in whom repair is not feasible.

The feasibility of mitral valve repair for MR depends on the pathology of the mitral valve and the surgeon's experience. Although rheumatic MR can be corrected by means of valvuloplasty (by performing maneuvers to increase mobility of the leaflets) and a ring annuloplasty, the long-term results are sub-optimal and repair should be reserved only to young patients with thin and pliable leaflets. MR due to mitral valve prolapse secondary to ruptured chordae tendineae or myxomatous degeneration is ideal for mitral valve repair. TEE can determine the segment(s) of prolapse, the thickness of the leaflets, and the presence or absence of calcium in the annulus and in other parts of the valve. In experienced hands, mitral valve repair is feasible in more than 95% of these patients. Repair consists of segmental leaflet resection, chordal transfer or chordal replacement with Gore-Tex sutures, edge-to-edge suturing, and ring annuloplasty.

Functional MR remains a challenging surgical problem. The pathophysiology is complex and is best studied by TEE in the echo lab. The most common mechanism of MR is tethering of the mitral valve leaflets due to ventricular dysfunction. In ischemic MR, usually only the medial half of the mitral valve is affected because of inferior wall myocardial infarction. Posterior papillary muscle elongation with consequent prolapse of a segment of the leaflets may also be a cause of MR. Other times a combination of these two main mechanisms is responsible for ischemic MR, further complicating its surgical treatment. The mitral annulus may also be dilated. Valve repair should be tailored to correct the abnormal pathophysiology. For patients with functional MR, a simple restrictive annuloplasty has been advocated; however, it is associated with high recurrent rate. Some surgeons propose severance of the secondary chordae tendineae in combination with a restrictive annuloplasty. Others suggest a sling of a prosthetic material around both papillary muscles to approximate them. If repair is not feasible, mitral valve replacement should be performed with preservation of the attachments between the mitral annulus and papillary muscles.

Prosthetic Mitral Valves

If the mitral valve cannot be repaired, replacement with a mechanical or bioprosthetic valve is necessary. Mechanical valves are very durable but require lifelong anticoagulation with warfarin sodium. Bioprosthetic valves have limited durability but do not require anticoagulation in patients in sinus rhythm. The durability of bioprosthetic valves in the mitral position is not as good as in the aortic position. Age plays a role in bioprosthetic valve durability: the freedom from failure at 10 years is around 80% in patients older than 65 years and 60% in younger.

The choice of valve is not always simple and the patient should be consulted before surgery. If a patient is in chronic atrial fibrillation and already taking warfarin sodium, a mechanical valve may be more appropriate. However, if the patient's expected life span is lower than that of the bioprosthetic valve, the use of a bioprosthesis is justifiable even if the patient is in atrial fibrillation because anticoagulation can be maintained at a lower level. Moreover, there is now an operative procedure to treat atrial fibrillation.

Operative Techniques

Mitral valve surgery can be performed through a midline sternotomy (full or partial) or through a right thoracotomy (under direct vision or endoscopically with manual or robotic assisted instruments). Cardiopulmonary bypass, aortic clamping, opening the left atrium, and protection of the myocardium with cardioplegia are necessary.

Mitral Valve Repair for Degenerative Mitral Valve Disease

Prolapse of the posterior leaflet central scallop (P2 of Carpentier's classification) is the most common cause of MR. It may present in isolation or combined with prolapse of other segments. P2 often becomes elongated before prolapsing. A quadrangular, rectangular or triangular resection of the prolapsing segment may be performed (Fig. 38.3).

When resection of the base is necessary it may be preferable to detach part of the remaining posterior leaflet and perform a sliding plasty as illus-

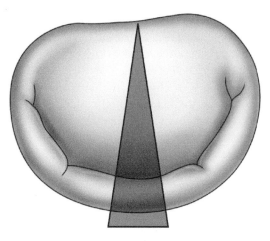

Fig. 38.3 Carpentier's principle of leaflet resection: triangular for the anterior and rectangular or quadrangular for the posterior. A triangular resection can also be used for the posterior leaflet depending on the abnormality of the segment

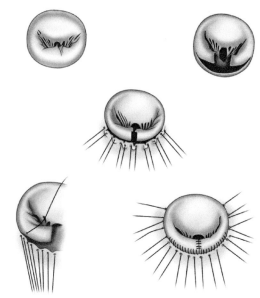

Fig. 38.4 Carpentier's sliding plasty technique for resection of part of the posterior leaflet

trated in Fig. 38.4 to avoid plication of the annulus in a single area.

If the posterior leaflet is small it is best not to resect any segment and correct the prolapse by anchoring the prolapsing segments with neo-chord of 5-0 Gore-Tex sutures as illustrated in Figs. 38.5 and 38.6.

Although prolapse of the anterior leaflet can be corrected by a triangular leaflet resection (Fig. 38.3), it is better not to resect, as this may adversely affect the durability of the repair. The prolapse should be corrected by chordal transfer or creation of neo-chords with Gore-Tex sutures (Figs. 38.5 and 38.6). Instead of transferring a chorda from the posterior leaflet to the anterior (Fig. 38.5), some surgeons have used the Alfieri's technique of edge-to-edge repair (Fig. 38.7), creating a double orifice mitral valve. A mitral annuloplasty is necessary because patients with MR almost invariably have dilated mitral annulus (Fig. 38.8). A posterior band suffices when left ventricular function is normal but a complete rigid ring may be more appropriate for patients with impaired systolic function.

Mitral Valve Replacement

If the posterior leaflet is normal, it should be preserved during mitral valve replacement as shown in Fig. 38.9. Preserving the attachments between the mitral valve and papillary muscles may preserve left ventricular function and prevent spontaneous rupture of the posterior wall of the left ventricle (a rare but dreadful complication of mitral valve replacement). If the leaflets are excessively diseased, as usually is the case in those requiring mitral valve replacement, the valve is completely excised and the papillary muscles are re-suspended with Gore-Tex sutures as shown in Fig. 38.10.

Patients with dystrophic calcification of the mitral annulus and valve dysfunction present a formidable problem. Over two decades ago, we introduced an operative procedure whereby the calcium bar was resected, the mitral annulus reconstructed with autologous or glutaraldehyde fixed bovine pericardium, and the valve repaired or replaced depending on the quality of the leaf-

Fig. 38.5 Prolapse
of the anterior leaflet
can be corrected by
chordal transfer or
creation of new chords
with Gore-Tex sutures

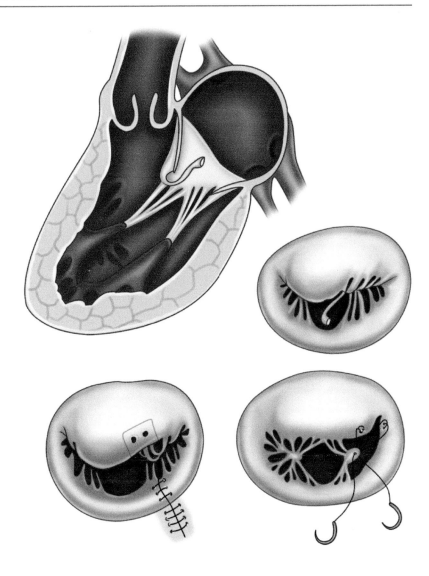

Fig. 38.6 Prolapse of
any segment of the
leaflets can be corrected
by creating new chords
out of Gore-Tex suture.
Multiple inter-dependent
chords can be created
with a single suture by
passing sequentially
through fibrous portions
of the papillary muscle
and free margin of the
prolapsing leaflet

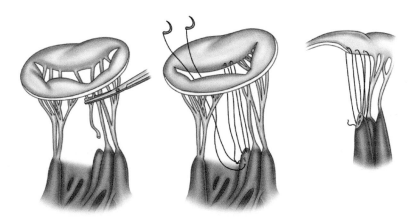

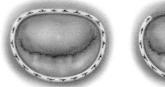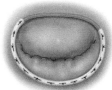

Fig. 38.8 A mitral annuloplasty is necessary during repair for mitral regurgitation. A ring or a posterior band is effective

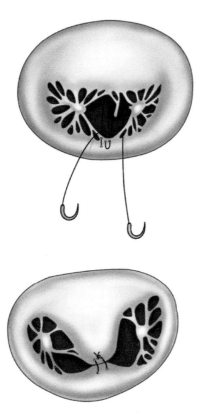

Fig. 38.7 Prolapse of the anterior leaflet: Alfieri's edge-to-edge repair

lets. However, few surgeons have mastered this technique, and when operating on these patients they prefer to implant a bioprosthetic valve without resection of the calcium bar, which is not always feasible. The left atrial appendage should be excised or its orifice closed during mitral valve repair or replacement.

Catheter-based mitral valve interventions have been very successful for rheumatic MS and balloon valvotomy has practically replaced open surgical repair for MS. Techniques and devices to correct MR have not been as successful as TAVI, largely because of the complicated functional anatomy of the mitral valve. Numerous devices have been developed, tested, and abandoned. MitraClip is a device that uses Alfieri's principle of edge-to-edge repair. It was first implanted in 2003 and is now approved by the FDA as an alternative to surgery to treat MR, mostly in inoperable patients. Correction of segmental prolapse of the leaflet can now be

accomplished without cardiopulmonary bypass by introducing a delivery device through the apex of the left ventricle, grasping the prolapsing segment, and deploying a Gore-Tex suture and exteriorizing and tying the ends on the surface of the heart under echocardiographic control. At the time of this writing there were two devices under investigation: Neochord and Harpoon.

Postoperative Care

Patients are initially managed in an intensive care unit soon after surgery. All patients should be anticoagulated with warfarin sodium if any prosthetic device was placed in the mitral valve (artificial valve or annuloplasty ring/band). The INR should be maintained between 2 and 3 for patients who had valve repair or bioprosthetic valves, and between 2.5 and 3.5 for those who received mechanical valves. Anticoagulation is discontinued after 6 months in patients who had valve repair or replacement with bioprosthetic valves if they are in sinus rhythm. Diuretic, angiotensin inhibitor, and anti-dysrhythmic drugs are prescribed as needed. An echocardiogram should be obtained 5 or 6 days postoperatively to assess valve and ventricular function as well as to rule out pericardial effusion.

Clinical Outcomes

The operative mortality for isolated mitral valve repair for MS or MR due to rheumatic or degenerative disease is low and usually around 1% at experienced centers. It is slightly higher for func-

Fig. 38.9 Mitral valve replacement with preservation of the chordae tendineae

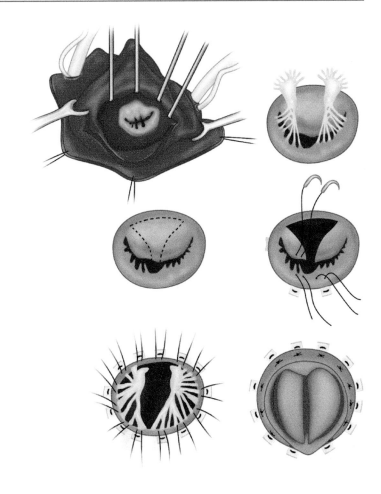

Fig. 38.10 Mitral valve replacement with re-suspension of the papillary muscles with Gore-Tex sutures

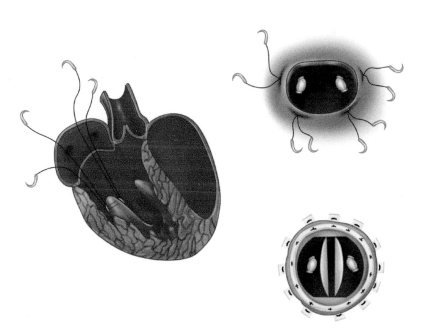

tional MR and in patients with coronary artery disease. The operative mortality for mitral valve replacement is usually much higher than for mitral valve repair, and it depends on the patient's clinical presentation, ventricular function, coronary artery disease and comorbid conditions. Elective procedures in stable patients can be performed with operative mortality of 3–10%, depending if it is an isolated problem or concomitant with others such as tricuspid valve repair and coronary artery disease. In the Society of Thoracic Surgeons Database, the operative mortality for isolated mitral valve replacement is 6%, and combined with coronary artery bypass is twice as high. Patients in cardiogenic shock due to acute MR secondary to myocardial infarction have a high operative mortality, ranging from 25 to 50%.

The long-term survival after mitral valve surgery depends on patient age, left ventricular function, and coronary artery disease. The 10-year survival after mitral valve repair for degenerative disease is around 70–80%. After mitral valve replacement for all pathologies, 10-year survival is around 50% in patients with an average age of 60 years. The long-term survival after mitral valve repair or replacement for functional MR is much lower.

Patients who have mitral valve surgery must see a cardiologist annually and have a complete physical examination as well as an electrocardiogram and echocardiogram. As with all patients with heart valve disease, in additional to atrial fibrillation, they are at risk of developing valve-related complications such as endocarditis, thromboembolism, valve dehiscence with MR, valve stenosis due to thrombus or pannus, and valve degeneration of bioprosthetic valves.

Maze Procedure for Atrial Fibrillation

The maze procedure was developed to treat atrial fibrillation (AF). The operation evolved over a couple of decades and is currently performed in isolation to treat patients with lone AF or, more commonly, is combined with mitral valve surgery in patients with paroxysmal or chronic AF. The original operation is described as "cut-and-sew" maze whereby a set of incisions is made in both atria, and cryolesions in areas that cannot be cut to ablate the atrial tissue in order to prevent re-entry of the abnormal currents in the atria. Since the pulmonary veins are the most common foci of AF, most surgeons perform the maze only in the left atrium.

Several newer techniques of tissue ablation were introduced into surgery during the past two decades as an alternative to the "cut-and-sew" maze. Radiofrequency and cryoablation are the most common methods used for tissue ablation. Other methods such as microwave, laser, and ultrasound are seldom used.

The AF elimination rate with the "cut-and-sew" maze is higher than with other techniques. Most surgeons report at least an 80% freedom of AF at 1 year. The results are better for paroxysmal AF than for permanent AF. The long-term efficacy of newer methods of tissue ablation to perform the maze is satisfactory, but there is steady rate of recurrence with time.

Further Reading

1. Nishimura RA, et al. 2014 AHA/ACC Guideline for the management of patient with valvular heart disease. J Am Coll Cardiol. 2014;63(22):57–185.
2. Baumgartner H, et al. 2017 ESC/EACTS Guidelines for the management of valvular heart disease: the Task Force for the Management of Valvular Heart Disease of the European Society of Cardiology (ESC) and the European Association for Cardio-Thoracic Surgery (EACTS). Eur Heart J. 2017;38:2739–91.
3. Badhwar V. The Society of Thoracic Surgeons 2017 Clinical Practice Guidelines for the Surgical Treatment of Atrial Fibrillation. Ann Thorac Surg. 2017;103:329–41.
4. Levine RA, et al. Mitral valve disease–morphology and mechanisms. Nat Rev Cardiol. 2015;12:689–710.
5. David TE, Armstrong S, Ivanov J. Chordal replacement with polytetrafluoroethylene sutures for mitral valve repair: a 25-year experience. J Thorac Cardiovasc Surg. 2013;145(6):1563–9.
6. David TE, Armstrong S, McCrindle BW, Manlhiot C. Late outcomes of mitral valve repair for mitral regurgitation due to degenerative disease. Circulation. 2013;127(14):1485–92.

Tricuspid Valve Surgery

39

Tirone David

Main Messages
1. Pathologies of the tricuspid valve include dilation of the right ventricle and tethering of the anterior and posterior leaflets, leading to tricuspid regurgitation (TR); congenital anomalies; myxomatous degeneration; trauma; tumours; ischemia; and rheumatic fever.
2. Tricuspid valve surgery is uncommonly performed as an isolated operation.
3. To prevent severe TR, moderate TR should be corrected at the time of mitral/aortic valve surgery.

Functional Anatomy

The functional anatomy of the tricuspid valve is complex and not well understood. This atrioventricular valve has three leaflets: septal, anterior and posterior. The base of the septal leaflet is

This chapter is an updated version of Chap. 27, Tricuspid Valve Surgery. In: Perioperative Care in Cardiac Anesthesia and Surgery by Cheng & David (eds.), published by Lippincott Williams & Wilkins, Philadelphia, PA; 2006. p. 253–56.

T. David (✉)
The University Health Network,
Toronto, ON, Canada
e-mail: Tirone.David@uhn.ca

attached to interventricular septum though fibrous strands (annulus), and its free margin is attached directly to the interventricular septum through chordae tendineae. The base of the anterior leaflet is attached to the anterior wall of the right ventricle by a fibrous annulus and its free margin is anchored by chordae tendineae, which are attached mostly to the anterior papillary muscle and in the area adjacent to the septal leaflet, to the septal band of the interventricular septum. The base of the posterior leaflet is attached to the posterior (diaphragmatic) wall of the right ventricle by a fibrous annulus and to the posterior and anterior papillary muscles through chordae tendineae. This anatomic configuration of the three leaflets makes the function of the tricuspid valve even more complex than that of the mitral valve. The orifice of the tricuspid valve is around 8 cm² and the perimeter of the annulus 11–14 cm in adults.

Pathology

Tricuspid regurgitation (TR) due to dilation of the right ventricle with tethering of the anterior and posterior leaflets is the most common functional abnormality of this valve. The dilation is asymmetric due to the anatomy of the leaflets and it involves mostly the commissural area between the anterior and posterior leaflets (Fig. 39.1). This type of lesion is referred to as "functional

© Springer Nature Switzerland AG 2021
D. C. H. Cheng et al. (eds.), *Evidence-Based Practice in Perioperative Cardiac Anesthesia and Surgery*, https://doi.org/10.1007/978-3-030-47887-2_39

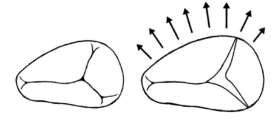

Fig. 39.1 Functional tricuspid regurgitation is due to dilation of the right ventricle with tethering of the anterior and posterior leaflets

TR" because the leaflets and chordae tendineae are normal. It is often associated with left side heart valve disease and other conditions that cause pulmonary hypertension.

An increasingly more commonly recognized problem is functional TR in elderly patients without significant left side heart valve dysfunction or pulmonary hypertension. Its mechanism remains elusive because the right ventricle is not dilated nor is the tricuspid annulus.

Congenital anomalies, rheumatic fever, myxomatous degeneration, endocarditis, ischemia, trauma, and tumors are the usual causes of organic tricuspid valve disease. Rheumatic involvement of the tricuspid valve never occurs in isolation and is often associated with rheumatic mitral valve disease. It causes fibrosis of the leaflets with fusion of the commissures and shortening and fibrosis of the chordae tendineae. It usually causes a mixed lesion with stenosis and regurgitation. Myxomatous degeneration causes billowing of the leaflets and elongation of the chordae tendineae with consequent TR. Endocarditis of the tricuspid valve is commonly seen in intravenous drug users. Papillary muscle infarction/rupture is a rare cause of TR. Papillary muscle rupture may also occur as consequence of trauma. The tricuspid valve becomes stenotic and regurgitant in patients with carcinoid syndrome due to fibrosis of the leaflets and chordae tendineae.

Pathophysiology

TR causes dilation of the right cardiac chambers and eventually impairs right ventricular contractility. Venous hypertension is the hallmark of severe tricuspid valve disease. In addition to the damage to the heart, it causes hepatomegaly, peripheral edema and ascites. If left untreated, cardiac cirrhosis may ensue. Tricuspid stenosis causes venous hypertension and its sequelae.

Diagnosis

Since isolated tricuspid valve disease is rare, symptoms of left side heart failure may prevail. However, patients may also complain of peripheral edema, increased abdominal girth, and sensation of fullness, all consequent to venous hypertension. The diagnosis is confirmed by echocardiography. Most patients with tricuspid valve disease also have mitral valve disease and pulmonary hypertension. If surgery is indicated, coronary angiography should be performed in patients older than 45 years of age.

Treatment

Diuretics and restriction of sodium intake are the principal means to reduce peripheral edema and ascites. Patients with severe TR and pulmonary hypertension should be treated surgically. If the TR is functional, tricuspid valve annuloplasty should be done at the time of the left side valve operation (e.g. mitral valve surgery). If it is due to rheumatic disease, repair is more difficult and involves mobilization of the leaflets by commissurotomy and chordal resection, and ring annuloplasty. If the leaflets are excessively fibrotic, tricuspid valve replacement is necessary.

Infective endocarditis of the tricuspid valve usually responds to appropriate antibiotic therapy. Staphylococcus aureus and fungi are more difficult to eradicate with antibiotics alone and there may also be lung abscesses in these patients. Surgery of the tricuspid valve may be necessary. Repair or replacement is performed depending on how extensive the leaflets destruction is. Valvulectomy alone is not a good alternative in our experience because most patients develop low cardiac output syndrome and ascites.

Isolated TR after trauma is usually well tolerated for many years but right ventricular function must be carefully monitored. Valve repair should be performed before the right ventricle dilates excessively. Once the right ventricle becomes hypokinetic, valve repair does not change the symptoms or prognosis.

Tricuspid Valve Annuloplasty

Functional TR can be corrected by simple reduction of the annulus along the anterior and posterior leaflets, mostly along the commissural area of these two leaflets. There are various commercially available annuloplasty rings, some rigid and others flexible. Rigid rings are probably more appropriate for functional TR. Sizing of the annuloplasty ring and distribution of the sutures are crucial to correct the deformity caused by dilation. A simple rule is to have an orifice no larger than the area of the anterior leaflet of the tricuspid valve and the reduction on the annulus is mostly along the commissures and false commissures.

The De Vega annuloplasty consists of reducing the length of the annulus of the anterior and posterior leaflets with a double layer of non-absorbable suture material. Some surgeons buttress the suture with Teflon felt pledgets to prevent cutting through the annulus and leaflets in patients with increased right ventricular pressure (Fig. 39.2).

Annuloplasty rings are believed to provide more stable repairs than the De Vega annuloplasty (Fig. 39.3).

Tricuspid Valve Replacement

Both mechanical and bioprosthetic valves can be used for tricuspid valve replacement. There is no proof that one type of valve is better than the other in the tricuspid position. Both types of valves are associated with more trouble in the right side of the circulation than in the left, likely because of the anatomy and blood flow characteristics of the right side of the heart. Mechanical valves are associated with risk of valve thrombosis and tissue valve with

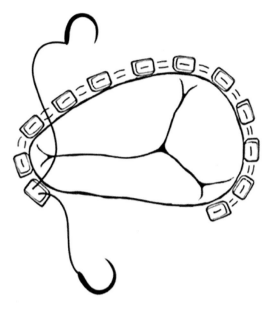

Fig. 39.2 Modified De Vega annuloplasty

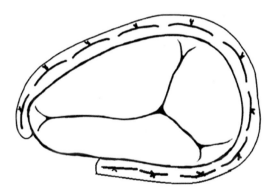

Fig. 39.3 Annuloplasty with Carpentier ring

pannus and stenosis. Permanent epicardial pacemaker leads should be inserted at the time of surgery after tricuspid valve replacement because of the risk of heart block or the future need for an implantable pacemaker.

Clinical Outcomes

Patients who have had tricuspid valve surgery have a tendency to retain fluids for several months and even years requiring diuretic therapy. Mechanical valves in the tricuspid position require higher levels of anticoagulation with warfarin sodium than in the mitral position. The INR should be maintained between 3 and 4.

Tricuspid valve surgery is seldom performed in isolation. It is sometimes done late after correction of left side heart valve lesions and the operative mortality is usually in the double digits because of the preoperative status of the patients. TR after correction of mitral valve dysfunction is usually managed conservatively for many years, and by the time the patients are referred to surgery they are in an advanced New York Heart Functional class, with the right ventricle is already impaired. For this reason alone, even moderate TR should be corrected at the time of mitral/aortic valve surgery to prevent the development of severe TR and eventual deterioration of right ventricular function. Tricuspid valve repair has no effect on long-term survival after mitral valve surgery but if TR is not corrected at the time of the mitral/aortic surgery it may adversely affect functional class and survival. On the other hand, if the tricuspid valve is replaced, long-term survival is reduced. Indications for tricuspid annuloplasty in patients without significant TR at the time of left side heart valve operations are evolving, and hopefully will be better defined in the near future.

Finally, tricuspid annuloplasty for functional TR is associated with high rates of recurrent TR during late follow-up.

Further Reading

1. Nishimura RA, et al. 2014 AHA/ACC Guideline for the management of patient with valvular heart disease. J Am Coll Cardiol. 2014;63(22):57–185.
2. Baumgartner H, et al. ESC/EACTS Guidelines for the management of valvular heart disease: the Task Force for the Management of Valvular Heart Disease of the European Society of Cardiology (ESC) and the European Association for Cardio-Thoracic Surgery (EACTS). Eur Heart J. 2017. [Epub ahead of print]
3. Topilsky Y, et al. Clinical outcome of isolated tricuspid regurgitation. JACC Cardiovasc Imaging. 2014;7:1185–94.
4. Navia JL, et al. Surgical management of secondary tricuspid valve regurgitation: annulus, commissure, or leaflet procedure? J Thorac Cardiovasc Surg. 2010;139:1473–82.
5. Chikwe J, et al. Impact of concomitant tricuspid annuloplasty on tricuspid regurgitation, right ventricular function, and pulmonary Artery hypertension after repair of mitral valve prolapse. J Am Coll Cardiol. 2015;65:1931–8.
6. David TE, et al. Tricuspid regurgitation is uncommon after mitral valve repair for degenerative diseases. J Thorac Cardiovasc Surg. 2017;154:110–22.

Robotic Cardiac Valvular Surgery

40

Bob Kiaii

Main Messages

1. The best surgical outcomes result from best patient selection, and preoperative imaging to assess the thoracic cavity and intercostal space.
2. Robotic surgery has become possible due to advances in computer telemanipulation systems, advances in minimally invasive surgical techniques and instruments, and advances in cardiac anesthesia and perfusion technology.
3. Benefits of smaller incisions include reduced blood loss and transfusion requirements, less wound pain and infection, earlier hospital discharge, and faster recovery times.

Evolution of Minimally Invasive Robotic-Assisted Mitral Valve Surgery

The first minimally invasive valve operations were reported in 1996 [1–4]. Minimally invasive valve surgery began as video-assisted operations.

As robotic technology evolved (Fig. 40.1) [4], the application of robotics in valvular surgery, specifically mitral valve surgery, became more widely accepted [5–14]. With the availability of the left atrial endowrist da Vinci retractor [12], more centres began to adopt robotic-assisted mitral valve surgery. As the experience of numerous centres continued to expand, it became evident that robotic-assisted mitral surgery is safe, produces excellent results, and results in less transfusion rates [8–14].

Patient Selection

Patient selection for the success of robotic mitral valve operation is of utmost important. This results in the best surgical outcome [15]. Preoperative imaging such as chest x-ray and computed tomography is very helpful to assess the thoracic cavity and the intercostal space to provide the best access to the mitral valve. In addition, the ascending aorta and femoral and iliac arteries are assessed for atherosclerosis and suitability for aortic cross-clamping and cannulation.

Patient selection for robotic valve operation [15]

Unsuitable candidates:

- Heavily calcified mitral annulus
- Severe pulmonary hypertension >2/3 systemic pressures

B. Kiaii (✉)
Department of Surgery, Western University,
London, ON, Canada
e-mail: bkiaii@ucdavis.edu

© Springer Nature Switzerland AG 2021
D. C. H. Cheng et al. (eds.), *Evidence-Based Practice in Perioperative Cardiac Anesthesia and Surgery*, https://doi.org/10.1007/978-3-030-47887-2_40

- Significant coronary artery disease requiring concomitant revascularization
- Severe peripheral arterial disease
- Prior right chest surgery

Suitable candidates:

- Primary mitral valve disease
- Re-operative mitral valve patients
- Repairable mitral valve
- Combined tricuspid and mitral operations
- Atrial septal defect repair
- Atrial tumor resection

- Mild annular calcification
- Obese or larger patients
- Elderly patients

Operative Technique

Preparation, Positioning and Draping

The patient is positioned at the right edge of the operating room table. A comfortable support is placed under the distal two-thirds of the right side of the patient's thorax. This support usually takes the form of a rolled up towel and should elevate the patient thorax 6–8 in. superiorly. The right arm is positioned at the side of the OR table to elevate the right shoulder allowing the right axilla to open and become accessible. The table is rotated 30° up (Figs. 40.2 and 40.3).

Perfusion Technology:

The combination of modified traditional perfusion methods with new technology resulted in the development of:

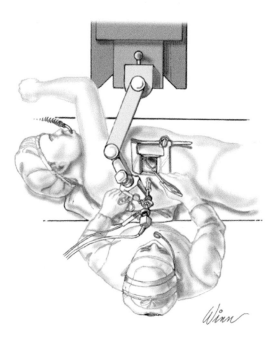

Fig. 40.1 Early experience with robotic assisted Mitral surgery (adapted from Franco, KL, Verrier ED, Advanced Therapy in Cardiac Surgery. 2003 Randolph Chitwood, Robot-assisted Mitral Valve Surgery)

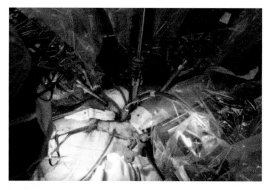

Fig. 40.3 Endoscopic ports adapted to the robotic arms

Fig. 40.2 Patient positioning and port spaces

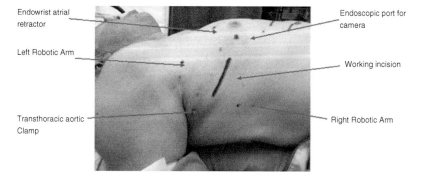

Endowrist atrial retractor

Left Robotic Arm

Transthoracic aortic Clamp

Endoscopic port for camera

Working incision

Right Robotic Arm

- Thin-walled arterial and venous cannulas
- Transthoracic aortic cannulas
- Endoaortic balloon occluders
- Modified aortic clamping devices
- Percutaneous coronary sinus cardioplegia catheters
- Vacuum-assisted venous drainage

Arterial Access:

- Antegrade central aortic cannulation
- Retrograde femoral perfusion

Venous Access:

- Right atrium directly through same incision or separate skin incision
- Bicaval venous cannula
  - To the right atrium using Seldinger technique and echocardiographic guidance combined with 17F percutaneous internal jugular cannula (Fig. 40.4a)
  - Percutaneous femoral venous cannula with multi drainage ports advanced under echocardiographic guidance into the superior vena cava (Fig. 40.4b)

Assisted Venous drainage

- Bio-medicus centrifugal vortex pump to create negative pressure
- Kinetic assisted drainage, no reservoir, as in mini-circuits (Fig. 40.5)

- Vacuum-assisted venous drainage with hard-shell cardiotomy reservoir

Myocardial preservation:

- Antegrade approach
- Retrograde approach
  - Direct insertion
  - Percutaneous retrograde insertion with port-access technology

Aortic occlusion:

- Flexible handle aortic clamps
- Percutaneous transthoracic (Chitwood) aortic cross-clamp
- Intra-aortic balloon occluders
  - Introduced in retrograde fashion

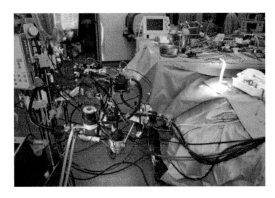

Fig. 40.5 Mini-circuit with Kinetic assist

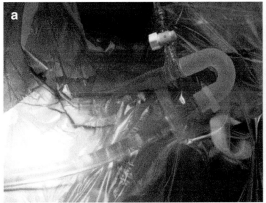
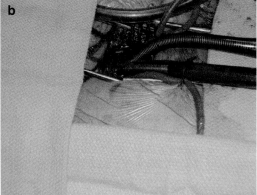

Fig. 40.4 (**a**) Internal jugular cannula. (**b**) Femoral arterial and venous cannula

- Echocardiographic guidance and monitoring very important
- Dislodgement can cause significant problems

Cardiac air removal:

- Continuous CO_2 insufflation
- Prior to removal of x-clamp, ventilate lungs/aortic root vent on suction

Operating Room Set-Up

The operating room arrangement should be modified to accommodate the docking of the robot with cardiopulmonary bypass pump adapted to the cannulas [15] (Fig. 40.6).

Surgical Procedure for Mitral and Tricuspid Procedures

Once the robotic ports are inserted, the pericardium is opened about 2–3 cm anterior to the right phrenic nerve and the pericardium is anchored with pledgetted sutures to the chest wall, bringing the sutures in between designated intercostal spaces. This enables better exposure of the interatrial groove. The cardioplegic cannula is then

inserted in the ascending aorta. The ascending thoracic aorta is cross-clamped with a transthoracic aortic cross-clamp. If the endoaortic balloon clamp is being utilized, myocardial protection is delivered through the endoaortic balloon. The right or left atrium is opened and a drop vent is inserted in the atrial chamber. The atrial wall is retracted with the atrial endowrist retractor placed in the fourth arm (Fig. 40.7). The mitral or tricuspid valves are exposed and appro-

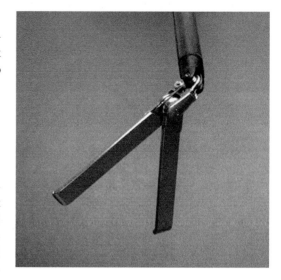

Fig. 40.7 The atrial endowrist retractor

Fig. 40.6 Operating room arrangement in robotic-assisted mitral surgery (adapted from Franco, KL, Verrier ED, Advanced Therapy in Cardiac Surgery. 2003. W. Randolph Chitwood, Robot-assisted Mitral Valve Surgery)

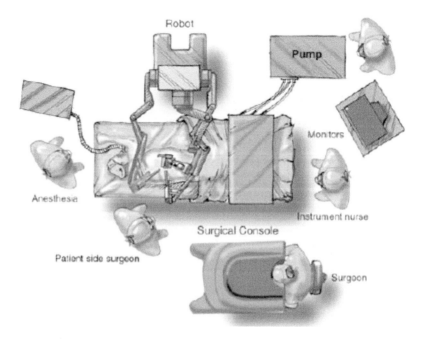

priate valvular intervention (repair or replacement) is performed. The atrium is then closed with a proper de-airing technique along with continuous CO_2 insufflation.

Other Miscellaneous Robotic-Assisted Procedures

At our institution, we have performed numerous other robotic-assisted procedures including closure of simple and complex atrial septal defect [15], CryoMaze atrial ablation for atrial fibrillation [16], insertion of epicardial pacer wires, removal of intracardiac and pericardial masses with pericardiectomy, and removal of iatrogenically placed right atrial foreign bodies [17]. For aortic valve surgery, there is ongoing work for further development of a robotic-assisted aortic valve procedure with preliminary work completed [18–20]. After the description of the first in human totally endoscopic aortic valve replacement [21], there is significant interest in further development of the application of robotic-assistance in aortic valve surgery.

References

1. Cosgrove DM, Sabik JF. Minimally invasive approach for aortic valve operations. Ann Thorac Surg. 1996;62:596–7.
2. Arom KV, Emery RW. Minimally invasive mitral operations. Ann Thorac Surg. 1996;62:1542–4.
3. Cohn LH, Adams DH, Couper GS, et al. Minimally invasive aortic valve replacement. Semin Thorac Cardiovasc Surg. 1997;9:331–6.
4. Chitwood WR. Robot-assisted mitral valve surgery. In: Franco KL, Verrier ED, editors. Advanced therapy in cardiac surgery. Hamilton, ON: BC Decker Inc; 2003. p. 220–9.
5. Chitwood WR, Nifong LW. Minimally invasive videoscopic mitral valve surgery: the current role of surgical robotics. J Card Surg. 2000;15:61–75.
6. Nifong LW, Chu VF, Bailey M, et al. Robotic mitral valve repair: experience with the da Vinci system. Ann Thorac Surg. 2003;75:438–43.
7. Nifong LW, Chitwood WR, Pappas PS, et al. Robotic mitral valve surgery: a United States multicenter trial. J Thorac Cardiovasc Surg. 2005;129:1395–404.
8. McClure RS, Kiaii B, Novick RJ, et al. Computer-enhanced telemanipulation in mitral valve repair: preliminary experience in Canada with the da Vinci robotic system. Can J Surg. 2006;49:193–6.
9. Rodriguez E, Krypson AP, Moten SC, et al. Robotic mitral surgery at East Carolina University: a 6 year experience. Int J Med Robotics Comput Assist Surg. 2006;2:211–5.
10. Woo VJ, Nacke EA. Robotic minimally invasive mitral valve reconstruction yields less blood product transfusion and shorter length of stay. J Surg. 2006;140(2):263–7.
11. Murphy DA, Miller JS, Langford DA, et al. Endoscopic robotic mitral valve surgery. J Thorac Cardiovasc Surg. 2006;132:776–81.
12. Smith JM, Stein H, Engel AM, et al. Totally endoscopic mitral valve repair using a robotic-controlled atrial retractor. Ann Thorac Surg. 2007;84:633–7.
13. Chitwood WR, Rodriguez E, Chu MWA, et al. Robotic mitral valve repairs in 300 patients: a single-center experience. J Thorac Cardiovasc Surg. 2008;136:436–41.
14. Murphy DA, Moss E, Jose B, et al. The expanding role of endoscopic robotics in mitral valve surgery: 1,257 consecutive procedures. Ann Thorac Surg. 2015;100:1675–82.
15. Chu MW, Losenno KL, Fox SA, et al. Clinical outcomes of minimally invasive endoscopic and conventional sternotomy approaches for atrial septal defect repair. Can J Surg. 2014;57(3):E75–81.
16. Rodriguez E, Cook RC, Chu MWA, et al. Minimally invasive biatrial cryomaze operation for atrial fibrillation. Oper Tech Thorac Cardiovasc Surg. 2009;14(3):208–23.
17. Hussain S, Adams C, Mechulan A, et al. Minimally invasive robotically assisted repair of atrial perforaon from a pacemaker lead. Int J Med Robot. 2012;8(2):243–6.
18. Folliguet TA, Vanhuyse F, Magnano D, et al. Robotic aortic valve replacement: case report. Heart Surg Forum. 2004;7(6):E551–3.
19. Folliguet TA, Vanhuyse F, Konstantinos Z, et al. Early experience with robotic aortic valve replacement. Eur J Cardiothorac Surg. 2005;28(1):172–3. Epub 2005 Apr 18
20. Suri RM, Burkhart HM, Schaff HV. Robot-assisted aortic valve replacement using a novel sutureless bovine pericardial prosthesis: proof of concept as an alternative to percutaneous implantation. Innovations (Phila). 2010;5(6):419–23.
21. Vola M, Fuzellier JF, Chavent B, Duprey A. First human totally endoscopic aortic valve replacement: an early report. J Thorac Cardiovasc Surg. 2014;147(3):1091–3.

Circulatory Arrest and Cerebral Protection Strategies

41

Christopher L. Tarola and Michael W. A. Chu

Main Messages
1. Cerebral protection is of upmost importance during aortic arch surgery, as the brain is the organ most susceptible to ischemic injury.
2. A number of cerebral protection strategies have been developed, including hypothermia, selective antegrade cerebral perfusion, and retrograde cerebral perfusion.
3. Monitoring considerations during circulatory arrest include temperature, metabolic status, cerebral and systemic near infrared spectroscopy and other cerebral monitoring.

The brain remains the most susceptible organ to ischemic injury, and optimizing cerebral protection is therefore paramount during aortic arch surgery. At normothermia, cerebral autoregulation varies cerebral perfusion pressure to match cerebral blood flow and metabolic activity. However, the brain's tolerance of ischemia at normothermic temperatures is limited to less than 5 min. This is critically important during cardiac surgery requiring circulatory arrest, particularly hemiarch and total arch replacement for aortic dissection, porcelain aorta, and aortic aneurysms. A number of perfusion and anesthetic strategies have been developed to ameliorate cerebral injury during circulatory arrest by augmenting the brain's tolerance to ischemia, with hypothermia being the most notable.

Hypothermic circulatory arrest (HCA) was first conceptualized in the 1950s in the work of Bigelow and colleagues, through the application of deep hypothermia to extend circulatory arrest up to 10 min in a canine model [1]. In the 1970s, the metabolic effects of deep hypothermia were investigated and applied to aortic surgery by Griepp and colleagues [2]. These investigations demonstrated that a hypothermia-induced reduction in cerebral metabolic rate translated into a transient "clinical safety period" during circulatory arrest, lengthening the brain's tolerance for ischemia and enabling contemporary arch repair.

The intraoperative conduct of HCA has significant surgeon and institution variability, and decisions are further influenced by the complexity of the surgical repair, patient age, and the overall medical status of the patient. The goal of this chapter is therefore to summarize the available cerebral protection strategies, which can be

C. L. Tarola · M. W. A. Chu (✉)
Division of Cardiac Surgery, Department of Surgery, Western University, London Health Sciences Centre, London, ON, Canada

© Springer Nature Switzerland AG 2021
D. C. H. Cheng et al. (eds.), *Evidence-Based Practice in Perioperative Cardiac Anesthesia and Surgery*, https://doi.org/10.1007/978-3-030-47887-2_41

divided across two general concepts: the degree of systemic hypothermia, and the method of adjuvant cerebral perfusion.

Systemic Hypothermia, Deep Hypothermic Circulatory Arrest, and Its Limitations

Systemic hypothermia has been categorized into the following four categories: (1) mild, 28–34 °C; (2) moderate, 20–28 °C; (3) deep, 14–20 °C; and (4) profound, <14 °C [3]. Isolated deep hypothermic circulatory arrest (DHCA) was the first method of cerebral protection used in aortic arch surgery and has demonstrated efficacy in reducing the risk of neurological insults during periods of prolonged cerebral ischemia. Several large, institutional series have demonstrated rates of permanent neurological deficit between 1.3–7%, with hypoperfusion injury believed to cause 30–40% of these insults. However, deep hypothermia is limited by transient neurologic dysfunction (TND) and fine motor deficits, particularly in elderly patients, for durations of circulatory arrest >30 min, resulting in prolonged hospital stay [4–7]. In some instances, TND has demonstrated association with decline in cognitive function at 6 weeks postoperatively [7, 8].

Notably, the duration of the brain's ischemic tolerance under DHCA remains uncertain, though generally a period of 25–30 min is thought to be acceptable. Though this remains a topic of debate, the relationship between decreasing metabolic demand at reduced body temperature has been well described, and periods of DHCA > 60 min are associated with greater postoperative mortality [9]. With respect to cerebral metabolism, McCullough and colleagues estimated cerebral metabolic rate by oxygen consumption during circulatory arrest in 1999 using blood samples harvested from the left carotid artery and jugular venous bulb. By utilizing the Q10 temperature coefficient (the ratio of metabolic rate at temperatures differing by 10 °C), they estimated the safe duration of

circulatory arrest at various temperatures [9]. This research was supported by Fischer and colleagues, who reported that after 30 min of profound circulatory arrest at 15 °C, the oxygen saturation of the frontal cortex falls below a threshold of 60%, resulting in prolonged length of stay by 4 days (3 days longer in ICU) and an increased risk of severe adverse outcomes including death, stroke, and persistent neurological deficits [10].

Although deep hypothermia alone does provide cerebral protection during circulatory arrest, adverse effects on the coagulation cascade causing significant postoperative bleeding, organ dysfunction (renal impairment, visceral ischemia), and prolonged cardiopulmonary bypass time due to long rewarming periods limit this technique. However, institutional series describing aortic arch surgery using straight DHCA have demonstrated favorable 5-year outcomes [11]. The introduction of selective antegrade cerebral perfusion (SACP) by Bachet, Kazui, and others, has resulted in aortic arch surgery being performed more frequently under lesser degrees of hypothermia with equivalent and in some respects, potentially superior outcomes [12, 13].

Selective Cerebral Perfusion with Moderate Hypothermic Circulatory Arrest

Antegrade and retrograde cerebral perfusion strategies were developed as adjuncts to hypothermia to improve cerebral protection during aortic arch surgery by prolonging the period of safety during circulatory arrest. Conceptually, SACP maintains cerebral perfusion for the duration of the surgical repair, though flow remains non-pulsatile and hypothermic. The utilization of moderate hypothermic circulatory arrest (MHCA) with SACP rather than DHCA alone was driven by the aforementioned complications associated with DHCA. Institutional series have demonstrated an up to twofold reduction in renal impairment with MHCA +

SACP compared to DHCA [14, 15]. A 2017 review of the STS Database by Englum and colleagues demonstrated a significantly higher risk of mortality and neurologic impairment when cerebral perfusion was not used as a perfusion adjunct to hypothermia [16]. Furthermore, a 2013 meta-analysis by Tian and colleagues comparing straight DHCA with MHCA + SACP demonstrated a significant reduction in the rate of permanent neurological deficit in the MHCA+ACP group, 12.8% vs. 7.3%, respectively, though there was no difference in TND, reoperation for bleeding, and death [17].

A number of factors should be considered when developing a strategy for continuous cerebral perfusion during aortic arch surgery, including unilateral vs. bilateral cerebral perfusion, direct head vessel cannulation vs. side graft, and axillary vs. innominate artery cannulation. Historically, it had been suggested that the majority of strokes after aortic arch surgery are related to embolic phenomena. The use of SACP using direct arch vessel cannulation in contemporary series has not resulted in worse neurologic outcomes in comparison to straight DHCA. This may suggest that careful direct head vessel cannulation combined with maintaining intraoperative cerebral perfusion reduces neurologic damage due to hypoperfusion, though strategies including alternative cannulation sites (axillary artery) and cannulation distant from atherosclerotic plaques may further reduce this risk.

Cannulation Strategies for Antegrade Cerebral Perfusion

A number of strategies are used to provide SACP during aortic arch surgery, including direct vessel cannulation and prosthetic grafts anastomosed to target vessels, with most institutions favoring either an axillary or innominate artery cannulation technique [18, 19]. Whether axillary or innominate artery cannulation confers improved postoperative outcomes remains undetermined,

and the ongoing Aortic Surgery Cerebral Protection Evaluation ACE randomized trial (randomized trial of axillary versus innominate artery cannulation for antegrade cerebral perfusion) seeks to answer this question. Currently, SACP via a dacron graft anastomosed to the axillary artery is the preferred approach for cerebral protection during aortic arch surgery, however, the delivery of SACP via the innominate artery (either direct or through a side graft) has recently emerged as an alternative (Fig. 41.1).

A number of adverse events have been described with axillary artery cannulation, including seromas, brachial plexus injuries, arm hyper-perfusion, arm ischemia, axillary artery injury and an additional surgical site at risk for infection [19, 20]. As such, many surgeons have adopted an innominate artery approach to SACP. In 2016, we reported our two center series of 140 consecutive patients undergoing aortic arch repair with axillary or innominate artery cannulation and identified a significant reduction in operating room time and mechanical ventilation when an innominate artery cannulation strategy was employed [20]. These findings have been confirmed by others who have also reported a paucity of cannulation-related complications using an innominate artery compared to axillary artery cannulation strategy, despite a theoretical risk of increased cerebral embolic load using an innominate strategy [20, 21]. Both strategies confer favorable results for aortic arch surgery when combined with moderate hypothermia and compared to DHCA alone, and either offers a "reasonable" choice that should be tailored to each individual case, potentially on the basis of preoperative computed tomography findings. For example, in instances of aortic dissection extending to the innominate artery or heavy innominate calcification, an axillary strategy might be chosen. In cases of total arch replacement, we prefer an axillary approach to allow full mobility of the innominate artery during head vessel reconstruction.

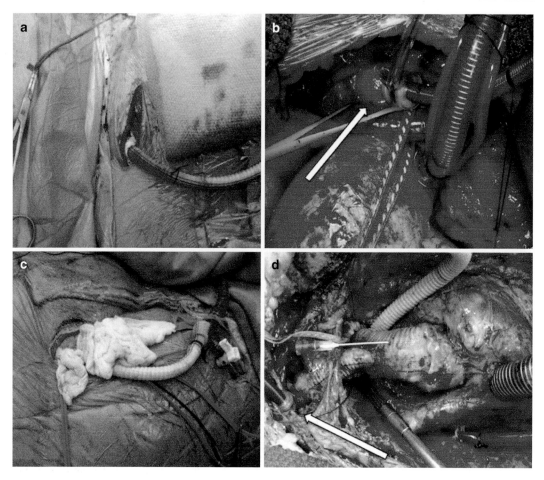

Fig. 41.1 Cannulation strategies during aortic arch repair. (**a**) Right axillary cannulation with an 8-mm dacron side graft. (**b**) Cannulation of right femoral artery. (**c**) Direct innominate artery cannulation with a 16 Fr arterial cannulae placed percutaneously into the innominate artery after initiating cardiopulmonary bypass. (**d**) Direct innominate cannulation during total aortic arch replacement

Unilateral Versus Bilateral Cerebral Perfusion

Significant controversy exists around the application of unilateral (U-SACP) or bilateral antegrade cerebral perfusion (B-SACP) during aortic arch surgery with circulatory arrest, where provider-practice variation is often institution and surgeon dependent. Theoretically, U-SACP relies upon an intact collateral system, Circle of Willis and/or extracranial collaterals, to perfuse the contralateral side, and anatomic anomalies or ipsilateral carotid stenosis pose significant concerns [18, 19]. Proponents of a U-SACP strategy argue that

this strategy avoids excess manipulation of the arch vessels (left carotid and innominate if using an axillary cannulation technique). Previous anatomic investigations have demonstrated significant variability in Circle of Willis anatomy, despite original thoughts that deficiencies were rare, and deficiency estimates that could threaten hypoperfusion during unilateral SACP range up to 60%. These estimates are based upon the expected arterial diameter that would constitute adequate flow, and 15% of patients are estimated to have an incomplete Circle of Willis [22, 23]. However, axillary and innominate cannulation strategies still permit perfusion of the right vertebral artery and extracranial collaterals, which likely affords the excellent results with unilateral SCP in hemiarch and total arch replacements that have been demonstrated by several groups. Studies by Leshnower, Urbanski, and others have demonstrated overall mortality of 1.2–7%, and TND and PND rates of 2.3–5.1% and 0.9–3.6%, respectively [24, 25].

There is support for the routine use of B-SACP over U-SACP. A 5400 patient meta-analysis demonstrated lower rates of TND, despite equal rates of PND and overall mortality, in patients receiving B-SACP [26]. Furthermore, a 3500 patient review demonstrated equivalent neurologic outcomes using the two strategies, but that B-SACP should be considered when circulatory arrest times are expected to be prolonged [27].

Despite the equipoise surrounding this issue, many surgeons opt to utilize a U-SACP during hemiarch repair and B-SACP during total arch repair or when anticipated circulatory arrest times are beyond 30 min. However, the key factor associated with PND and mortality seems to be the total circulatory arrest time, irrespective of the SACP strategy selected, and intraoperative brain perfusion monitoring strategies may ultimately guide the need for B-SACP versus U-SACP. We prefer employing U-SACP as a primary technique; however, when the contralateral brain oximetry decreases greater than 20% from baseline, we will place a retrograde coronary perfusion cannulae directly into the left carotid artery to enable B-SACP.

Antegrade and Retrograde Cerebral Perfusion

Antegrade perfusion is generally the preferred technique of cerebral perfusion during circulatory arrest in most centers, however significant investigation has been completed and is worth brief review. Both strategies are associated with advantages and disadvantages: ACP offers independent cerebral temperature and flow control but manipulation of head vessels and antegrade perfusion can result in plaque fragmentation and embolization. Retrograde perfusion avoids the

need to manipulate arch vessels, but may be compromised by venous valves and may result in cerebral edema (particularly with perfusion pressure >25 mmHg). Retrograde cerebral perfusion (RCP) is performed via the superior vena cava following the initiation of circulatory arrest, requiring isolation and selective cannulation of the SVC. The system is pressurized to 20–25 mmHg to allow flow into the upper extremities and cerebral system.

A meta-analysis including 5060 patients, which investigated the protective effect of SACP and RCP, demonstrated no difference in mortality, PND or TND between the two perfusion strategies [28]. A further 7023 patient review demonstrated that the postoperative incidence of TND was significantly lower in a DHCA+ACP group compared to DHCA+RCP, though there was no significant difference in PND, stroke, or early mortality [29]. It is generally accepted that retrograde cerebral perfusion can maintain cerebral hypothermia, however, some studies have demonstrated a reduced ability of RCP to sustain cerebral metabolism [20]. Retrograde cerebral perfusion is therefore typically used as an adjunct during deep hypothermic circulatory arrest when less than 30 min of circulatory arrest are anticipated. When using warmer systemic temperatures, the protective effect of RCP is unknown.

Monitoring During Circulatory Arrest

Temperature and Flow

It is well accepted that temperature monitoring during HCA is critical to cerebral protection. We therefore rely on peripheral temperature measurement, and most centers typically utilize nasopharyngeal and bladder or rectal temperature probes. Nasopharyngeal temperature is regarded as the best estimate of brain temperature, whereas bladder temperature is more reflective of systemic temperature. However, nasopharyngeal temperature measurement tends to underestimate (by 2–3 °C) cerebral temperatures during re-warming, and therefore caution should be exercised during re-warming to avoid hyperthermia [30].

Although historical studies suggested SACP flows of 5–10 mL/kg/min to target a right radial artery pressure of 50–70 mmHg [20], we prefer higher flows of 10–15 mL/kg/min as we routinely use warmer temperatures for circulatory arrest ranging from 25 to 28 °C.

Glycemic Control

Intraoperative hyperglycemia promotes anaerobic metabolism resulting in intracellular acidosis. The benefits of strict glycemic control during cardiac surgical procedures are well documented in cardiac surgery literature and should be extended to HCA and aortic arch surgery. Given intraoperative hyperglycemia correlates with adverse postoperative outcomes, it is suggested that aggressive management of hyperglycemia during HCA be prioritized, as the risk of adverse neurological events increases at blood glucose levels >10 mmol/L.

pH

The optimal pH of physiologic enzymatic reactions varies with temperature, and pH management during circulatory arrest is an important intraoperative consideration. Arterial CO_2 tension is a major regulator of cerebral flow during HCA, and two main strategies for intraoperative blood gas monitoring are used: alpha-stat and pH-stat [19]. Alpha-stat monitoring has been demonstrated to preserve cerebral autoregulation, and aims to maintain a normal pH and $PaCO_2$ at normothermia, resulting in blood becoming alkaline and hypocapneic under hypothermic conditions. Conversely, pH-stat aims to restore pH and $PaCO_2$ to 7.4 and 40 mmHg, respectively, under hypothermic conditions, resulting in acidosis and hypercapnia when the patient is re-warmed, and eliminating cerebral autoregulation due to sustained cerebral vasodilation of cerebral vessels. Though we prefer alpha-stat monitoring at our center, the optimal

pH monitoring strategy remains unclear. Some investigations have demonstrated improved neurological outcomes with alpha-stat monitoring, believed to result from the physiologic coupling of cerebral autoregulation and metabolism, though pH-stat monitoring appears to be beneficial in neonates and infants [19].

Cerebral Perfusion Monitoring Strategies

A number of strategies utilized during routine cardiac surgery procedures can be utilized to monitor cerebral perfusion and oxygenation during HCA for aortic arch surgery, including near-infrared spectroscopy (NIRS) or cerebral oximetry, electroencephalography (EEG), and bispectral index monitoring (BIS).

NIRS utilizes near-infrared light to measure the hemoglobin saturation of arterial, capillary, and venous blood in the superficial frontal lobe, and should be maintained between 50 and 80 with no greater than a 10-point difference. We utilize cerebral oximetry on all cases and will tailor SACP directly to changes based upon the cerebral oximetry readings. We also place NIRS monitoring pads on the lower limbs bilaterally to monitor distal limb perfusion on all aortic arch cases, especially during acute aortic dissection repairs. This can be particularly helpful when concerned about cannulation strategies and identifying dynamic malperfusion (Fig. 41.2). Electroencephalography is commonly used to measure neuronal activity in the operating room, however requires operation by specialized personnel. BIS simplifies the EEG interface to a single number as opposed to the usual 4–16 channels with EEG, and ranges between 0 (flat line) and 100 (awake patient).

Transcranial doppler ultrasound to measure flow through the middle cerebral artery is an alternative potential strategy, though can be influenced by head or cannula position, or CPB perfusion pressure. Initially utilized in thoracoabdominal aortic surgery, motor and sensory evoked potentials are utilized to detect spinal cord ischemia after cross-clamping the aorta.

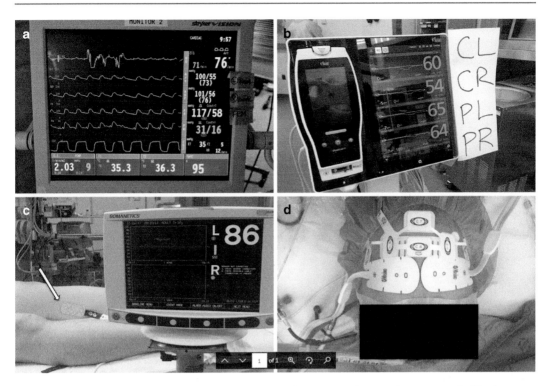

Fig. 41.2 Monitoring strategies during aortic arch surgery. (**a**) Simultaneous lower and upper extremity blood pressure monitoring. (**b**) Cerebral and lower body NIRS monitoring. (**c**) Lower body NIRS. (**d**) Cerebral NIRS sensors

Their usefulness may extend to circulatory arrest, though readings are limited during hypothermia.

Establishing Hypothermic Circulatory Arrest: Pump Setup

Cardiopulmonary bypass set-up generally varies by institution. When performing MHCA with SACP at our center, we utilize a customized circuit (Fig. 41.3a) on a 5-base heart/lung machine (one main pump, one cardioplegia pump, two pump suckers, two vents), an HCU30 heater/cooler (Maquet, Rastatt, Germany) and a Capiox SX 25 membrane oxygenator (Terumo, Ann Arbor, MI) with a Quart arterial filter (Maquet, Rastatt, Germany) and Quest microplegia delivery system (Quest, Allen, Tx) [30]. When utilizing a whole body perfusion technique (combining SACP with lower body perfusion as described later in this chapter), we use a second pump with a Cardiotherm cardioplegia device (Medtronic,

Minneapolis, MN) connected to a second HCU30 heater/cooler for lower body perfusion with independent temperature control [31].

Metabolic Debt and Whole Body Perfusion

Despite the strong belief in optimizing cerebral perfusion during circulatory arrest, there remains a general acceptance of the ischemic load on the spinal cord, mesenteric organs, lower body, and the resultant metabolic debt incurred, particularly as warmer temperatures are used for circulatory arrest. Investigation of spinal ischemia using animal models has demonstrated remarkable increases in ischemic tolerance with modest reductions in temperature, however, the threat of spinal ischemia during circulatory arrest with warmer temperatures should not be discounted [19]. In 2007, Kamiya and colleagues investigated the effect of deep versus moderate hypo-

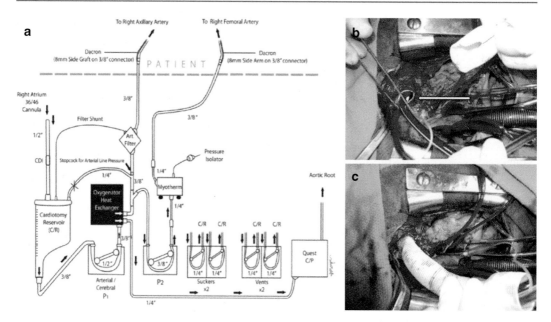

Fig. 41.3 (**a**) Cardiopulmonary bypass circuit used for whole body perfusion with separate roller pumps used for lower body and cerebral perfusion. (**b**) Endotracheal tube placed through the aortic arch into the distal aorta to pro-vide continuous lower body perfusion during circulatory arrest. (**c**) Distal aortic anastomosis sewn around the endotracheal tube to provide ongoing lower body perfusion

thermia, and identified an 18.2% rate of paraplegia in patients with lower-body circulatory arrest at 28 °C for >60 min [32].

Postoperative hyperlactatemia has been demonstrated to be an independent predictor of major complications and mortality after cardiac surgery, and several investigators have demonstrated the negative effects of lower body ischemia during aortic arch surgery [33]. We have previously described our strategy of using simultaneous lower body perfusion, termed "whole body perfusion" (WBP), in addition to SACP during MHCA. We found that use of this novel perfusion strategy resulted in reduced ICU and hospital length of stay, more rapid normalization of postoperative lactate levels, reduced rates of renal dysfunction, and shorter durations of mechanical ventilation [34–36]. At our institution, we employ a whole body perfusion strategy by using right axillary cannulation and one of three options for simultaneous lower body perfusion: (1) a 5.5-mm endotracheal tube placed antegrade through the aortic arch into the descending thoracic aorta (Fig. 41.3b, c); (2) a femoral arterial 8-mm Dacron side graft anastomosed to the femoral artery; or (3) the distal limb of a Thoraflex hybrid graft (Vascutek Terumo, Scotland, UK) during hybrid arch and frozen elephant trunk procedures [30, 34]. We perfuse the lower body at a rate of 1–3 L/min at 25–30 °C, and target a lower limb NIRS within 20% of baseline and a lower limb MAP > 50 mmHg. Della Corte and colleagues utilized 1–1.5 L/min flow in their institutional series utilizing lower body perfusion, and Song and colleagues utilized 1–2 min of intermittent lower body perfusion at 1–1.5 L/min flow [35, 36]. We additionally utilize bilateral leg NIRS for monitoring of lower limb ischemia during circulatory arrest with lower body perfusion.

Results from investigations using a WBP strategy suggest that the use of lower body perfusion in addition to SACP may reduce the incidence of ischemia-induced complications to the visceral organs and spinal cord, especially in extensive aortic-arch operations. Further investigation to determine whether this strategy confers a morbidity and/or mortality benefit is required.

References

1. Bigelow WG, Lindsay WK, Greenwood WF. Hypothermia: its possible role in cardiac surgery: an investigation governing survival in dogs at low body temperatures. Ann Surg. 1950;132:849–66.
2. Griepp RB, Stinson EB, Hollingsworth JF, Buehler D. Prosthetic replacement of the aortic arch. J Thorac Cardiovasc Surg. 1975;70:1051–63.
3. Marx JA. Rosen's emergency medicine: concepts and clinical practice. 7th ed. Philadelphia, PA: Mosby Elsevier; 2010.
4. Gega A, Rizzo JA, Johnson MH, Tranquilli M, Farkas EA, Elefteriades JA. Straight deep hypothermic arrest: experience in 394 patients supports its effectiveness as a sole means of brain preservation. Ann Thorac Surg. 2007;84:759–66.
5. Svensson LG, Crawford ED, Hess KR, Coselli JS, Baskin S, Shenaq SA, et al. Deep hypothermia with circulatory arrest. Determinants of stroke and early mortality in 656 patients. J Thorac Cardiovasc Surg. 1993;106:19–28.
6. Ziganshin BA, Rajbanshi BG, Tranquilli M, Fang H, Rizzo JA, Elefteriades JA. Straight deep hypothermic circulatory arrest for cerebral protection during aortic arch surgery: safe and effective. J Thorac Cardiovasc Surg. 2014;148:888–98.
7. Reich DL, Uysal S, Sliwinski M, Ergin MA, Kahn RA, Konstadt SN, et al. Neuropsychologic outcome after deep hypothermic circulatory arrest in adults. J Thorac Cardiovasc Surg. 1999;117:156–63.
8. Ergin MA, Uysal S, Reich DL, Apaydin A, Lansman SL, McCullough JN, et al. Temporary neurological dysfunction after deep hypothermic circulatory arrest: a clinical marker of long-term functional deficit. Ann Thorac Surg. 1999;67:1887–90.
9. McCullough JN, Zhang N, Reich DL, Juvonen TS, Klein JJ, Spielvogel D, et al. Cerebral metabolic suppression during hypothermic circulatory arrest in humans. Ann Thorac Surg. 1999;67:1895–9.
10. Fischer GW, Lin HM, Krol M, Galati MF, Di Luozzo G, Griepp RB, et al. Noninvasive cerebral oxygenation my predict outcome in patients undergoing aortic arch surgery. J Thorac Cardiovasc Surg. 2011;141:815–21.
11. Damberg A, Carino D, Charilaou P, Peterss S, Tranquilli M, Ziganshin BA, Rizzo JA, Elefteriades JA. Favorable late survival after aortic surgery under straight deep hypothermic circulatory arrest. J Thorac Cardiovasc Surg. 2017; In Press.
12. Kazui T. Update in surgical management of aneurysms of the thoracic aorta. Rinsho Kyobu Geka. 1986;6:7–15.
13. Guilmet D, Roux PM, Bachet J, Goudot B, Tawil N, Diaz F. A new technique of cerebral protection. Surgery of the aortic arch. Presse Med. 1986;15:1096–8.
14. Halkos ME, Kerendi F, Myung R, Kilgo P, Puskas JD, Chen EP. Selective antegrade cerebral perfusion via right axillary artery cannulation reduces morbidity and mortality after proximal aortic surgery. J Thorac Cardiovasc Surg. 2009;138:1081–9.
15. Di Eusanio M, Wesselink RMJ, Morshuis WJ, Dossche KM, Schepens MAAM. Deep hypothermic circulatory arrest and antegrade selective cerebral perfusion during ascending aorta-hemiarch replacement: a retrospective comparative study. J Thorac Cardiovasc Surg. 2003;125:849–54.
16. Englum BR, He X, Gulack BC, Mathew JP, Brennan JM, Reece TB, et al. Hypothermia and cerebral protection strategies in aortic arch surgery: a comparative effectiveness analysis from the STS Adult Cardiac Surgery Database. Eur J Cardiothorac Surg. 2017; https://doi.org/10.1093/ejcts/ezx133.
17. Tian DH, Wan B, Bannon PG, Misfeld M, LeMaire SA, Kazui T, et al. A meta-analysis of deep hypothermic circulatory arrest versus moderate hypothermic circulatory arrest with selective antegrade cerebral perfusion. Ann Cardiothorac Surg. 2013;2:148–58.
18. Luehr M, Bachet J, Mohr FW, Etz CD. Modern temperature management in aortic arch surgery: the dilemma of moderate hypothermia. Eur J Cardiothorac Surg. 2014;45:27–39.
19. Appoo JJ, Bozinovski J, Chu MWA, El-Hamamsy I, Forbes TL, Moon M, et al. Canadian Cardiovascular Society/Canadian Society of Cardiac Surgeons/Canadian Society for Vascular Surgery Joint Position statement on Open and endovascular surgery for thoracic aortic disease. Can J Cardiol. 2016;32:703–13.
20. Chu MWA, Losenno KL, Gelinas JJ, Garg V, Dickson J, Harrington A, et al. Innominate and axillary cannulation in aortic arch surgery provide similar neuroprotection. Can J Cardiol. 2016;32:117–23.
21. Di Eusanio M, Petridis FD, Folesani G, Berretta P, Zardei D, Di Bartolomeo R. Axillary and innominate artery cannulation during surgery of the thoracic aorta: a comparative study. J Cardiovasc Surg. 2014;55:841–7.
22. Merkkola P, Tulla H, Ronkainen A, Soppi V, Oksala A, Koivisto T, et al. Incomplete circle of Willis and right axillary artery perfusion. Ann Thorac Surg. 2006;82:74–9.
23. Papantchev V, Hristov S, Todorova D, Naydenov E, Paloff A, Nikolov D, et al. Some variations of the circle of Willias, important for cerebral protection in aortic surgery – a study in Eastern Europeans. Eur J Cardiothorac Surg. 2007;31:982–9.
24. Leshnower BG, Myung RJ, Kilgo PD, Vassiliades TA, Vega JD, Thourani VH, et al. Moderate hypothermia and unilateral selective antegrade cerebral perfusion: a contemporary cerebral protection strategy for aortic arch surgery. Ann Thorac Surg. 2010;90:547–54.
25. Urbanski PP, Lenos A, Bougioukakis P, Neophytou I, Zacher M, Diegeler A. Mild-to-moderate hypothermia in aortic arch surgery using circulatory arrest: a change of paradigm? Eur J Cardiothorac Surg. 2012;41:185–91.
26. Angeloni E, Benedetto U, Takkenberg JJM, Stigliano I, Roscitano A, Melina G, et al. Unilateral versus bilateral antegrade cerebral protection during circula-

tory arrest in aortic surgery: a meta-analysis of 5100 patients. J Thorac Cardiovasc Surg. 2014;147:60–7.

27. Malvindi PG, Scrascia G, Vitale N. Is unilateral antegrade cerebral perfusion equivalent to bilateral cerebral perfusion for patients undergoing aortic arch surgery? Interact CardioVasc Thorac Surg. 2008;7:891–7.

28. Hu Z, Wang Z, Ren Z, Wu H, Zhang M, Zhang H, et al. Similar cerebral protective effectiveness of antegrade and retrograde cerebral perfusion combined with deep hypothermia circulatory arrest in aortic arch surgery: a meta-analysis and systematic review of 5060 patients. J Thorac Cardiovasc Surg. 2014;248:544–60.

29. Guo S, Sun Y, Liu J, Wang G, Zheng Z. Similar cerebral protective effectiveness of antegrade and retrograde cerebral perfusion during deep hypothermic circulatory arrest in aortic surgery: a meta-analysis of 7023 patients. Artif Organs. 2015;39:300–8.

30. Kakuntla H, Harrington D, Bilkoo I, Clutton-Brock T, Jones T, Bonser RS. Temperature monitoring during cardiopulmonary bypass – do we undercool or overheat the brain? Eur J Cardiothorac Surg. 2004;26:580–5.

31. Fernandes P, Cleland A, Adams C, Chu MWA. Clinical and biochemical outcomes for additive mesenteric lower body perfusion during hypothermic circulatory arrest for complex total aortic arch replacement surgery. Perfusion. 2012;27:493–501.

32. Kamiya H, Hagl C, Kropivnitskaya I, Bothig D, Kallenbach K, Khaladj N, et al. The safety of moderate hypothermic lower body circulatory arrest with selective cerebral perfusion: a propensity score analysis. J Thorac Cardiovasc Surg. 2007;133:501–9.

33. Hajjar LA, Almeida JP, Fukushima JT, Rhodes A, Vincent JL, Osawa EA, et al. High lactate levels are predictors of major complications after cardiac surgery. J Thorac Cardiovasc Surg. 2013;146:455–60.

34. Tarola CL, Losenno KL, Gelinas JJ, Jones PM, Fernandes P, Fox SA, et al. Whole body perfusion for aortic arch repair under moderate hypothermia. Perfusion. 2018;33:254–63.

35. Song SW, Yoo KJ, Shin YR, Lim SH, Cho BK. Effects of intermittent lower body perfusion on end-organ function during repair of acute DeBakey type I aortic dissection under moderate hypothermic circulatory arrest. Eur J Cardiothorac Surg. 2013;44:1070–5.

36. Della Corte A, Scardone M, Romano G, Amarelli C, Biondi A, De Santo L, et al. Aortic arch surgery: thoracoabdominal perfusion during antegrade cerebral perfusion may reduce postoperative morbidity. Ann Thorac Surg. 2006;81:1358–64.

Aortic Arch Reconstructive Surgery

42

Matthew Valdis, Olivia Ginty,
and Michael W. A. Chu

Main Messages

1. Aortic arch reconstruction is required for diameters of greater than 55 mm in aneurysmal disease.
2. Surgical techniques available include hemiarch reconstruction, total arch reconstruction with conventional elephant trunk, and hybrid arch repair with frozen elephant trunk.
3. Management options for difficult left subclavian artery include preoperative carotid-subclavian transposition or bypass with ligation, intraoperative anatomic/extra-anatomic reconstruction, direct cannulation of the SCL ostium from within the aorta with hybrid vascular graft, and intraoperative ligation with postoperative repair/bypass.

M. Valdis · M. W. A. Chu (✉)
Division of Cardiac Surgery, Department of Surgery, Western University, London Health Sciences Centre, London, ON, Canada
e-mail: Michael.Chu@lhsc.on.ca

O. Ginty
Department of Anatomy and Cell Biology, Western University, London, ON, Canada

Surgical Indications

Surgical reconstruction of the aortic arch is indicated for aneurysmal disease when the diameter reaches between 55 mm and 60 mm, depending on the etiology according to the 2014 Canadian Cardiovascular Society (CCS) Thoracic Aortic Disease Guidelines [1]. Similarly, the 2010 American College of Cardiology and American Heart Association (ACC/AHA) Thoracic Aortic Guidelines, as well as the 2014 European Society of Cardiology (ESC) guidelines on the diagnosis and treatment of aortic disease, also recommend the repair of isolated aneurysm of the aortic arch in an asymptomatic patient with diameter greater than 55 mm, who are deemed to be at low-operative risk [2, 3]. Additionally, the guidelines do suggest that a lower threshold for intervention may be considered in patients with specific conditions, such as a diagnosed connective tissue disorders, significant family history, rapid expansion of the aneurysm, and previous aortic dissection or rupture; particularly in centres with expertise in aortic repair [3]. The presence of these conditions helps identify patients at highest risk for an impending catastrophic event even when they do not meet recommended guidelines for early surgical intervention based on aortic diameters alone. Individuals with genetic disorders such as Marfan syndrome, Ehlers-Danlos syndrome (Vascular type), Turner's syndrome and, in particular,

© Springer Nature Switzerland AG 2021
D. C. H. Cheng et al. (eds.), *Evidence-Based Practice in Perioperative Cardiac Anesthesia and Surgery*, https://doi.org/10.1007/978-3-030-47887-2_42

Loeys-Dietz Syndrome all carry a lower size threshold for invention based on significant increase in risk of rupture or dissection.

In addition to this, attention must be paid to females and patients at extremes of body size. Aortic measurements may be indexed over height to give an indication of relative aortic dilation. This technique may be particularly helpful in patients with Marfan and Turner's Syndrome who may have aneurysmal aortic dimensions masked by their tall or short stature, respectively.

All of these factors are taken into consideration with the patient's age, comorbidities and the risks of surgical repair. Unfortunately, many patients still go undiagnosed and their first presentation occurs at the time of acute aortic rupture or dissection. This obviously complicates the care and surgical techniques required to treat such patients; however, this chapter will focus on general principles and technical aspects of aortic arch surgery for aneurysmal disease as well as aortic dissection.

Hemiarch Reconstruction

Repair of the aneurysmal ascending aorta and proximal arch is approached through a conventional midline sternotomy. The innominate vein is mobilized to allow dissection, exposure and circumferential control of the epiaortic vessels and superior aspect of the aortic arch prior to systemic heparinization. However, in patients with fragile aortic tissue or contained ruptured dissections, aortic preparatory work can be completed after initiation of cardiopulmonary bypass or in some cases, under circulatory arrest. The aortopulmonary window is opened and the pericardial reflection is detached from the distal ascending aorta, allowing circumferential mobilization of the ascending aorta and proximal aortic arch. Care is taken to sweep the recurrent laryngeal nerve laterally and away from the distal arch to avoid injury. The pericardium is elevated anteriorly, to bring the aorta into optimal surgical view. Arterial cannulation options include direct cannulation or Dacron

side grafts within the right axillary artery, innominate artery, distal arch or distal ascending aorta within the aneurysm itself. We prefer employing techniques that allow uninterrupted flow when transitioning to antegrade cerebral perfusion during circulatory arrest, such as an 8 mm Dacron side graft sewn on to the right axillary artery or simultaneous aortic cannulation and a 16Fr innominate artery cannula.

Cardiopulmonary bypass is initiated and the remaining aorta is skeletonized. The patient is cooled to target temperature (25–28 °C), which is determined by the amount of aortic reconstructive work anticipated. If safe (most cases), the ascending aorta is clamped and the aortic root work is initiated. Once the target temperature is reached, antegrade cerebral perfusion (ACP) is initiated without any interruption to cerebral flow and the base of the innominate and carotid arteries are controlled with clamps or double-looped vessel loops. The ascending aorta is opened and the aorta is resected obliquely across the aortic arch under the innominate and carotid arteries along the lesser curve of the arch, leaving a slightly longer shelf of aortic tissue on the posterior aspect of the arch. We usually tailor a 26–28 mm woven Dacron graft to preserve the greater/lesser curve of the ascending aorta and telescope the graft into the residual arch for hemostasis, sewing it with 5-0 prolene sutures to minimize needle hole bleeding. After the initial posterior sutures are completed and the graft is parachuted into the posterior wall of the arch, we commonly place a 5.5 mm endotracheal tube into the descending aorta to reinitiate lower body flow (described in previous chapter).

After completion of the arch anastomosis, the clamp is re-applied and central re-warming is initiated. The proximal root work is now completed and the aortic root graft is transected at the neo-sinotubular junction. The root graft is then sewn in a telescoping fashion into the arch graft, taking large suture bites on the medial aspect to shorten and reconstruct the normal anatomic lesser curve of the aorta (Fig. 42.1). The ascending aorta is vented through a small 18g needle placed in the ascending aorta, which can be closed without suture, after removing the needle and re-aligning the Dacron fibres by rubbing the graft together on either side of the needle hole.

Special considerations need to be made for hemiarch reconstruction in the setting of Acute Type A Aortic Dissection (ATAAD). Although controversy exists about clamping the dissected ascending aorta, we still find most patients with dissected ascending aortas safe to clamp with low risk of rupture. This optimizes surgical efficiency by beginning the proximal root repair during cooling. When the aortic dissection extends into either the left or right coronary sinus or a significant proportion of the non-coronary sinus, we prefer using an aortic root replacement strategy as we believe this provides superior hemostasis

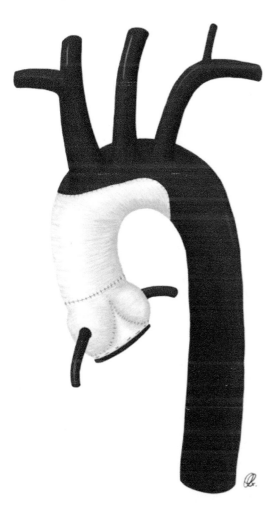

Fig. 42.1 A valve sparing root reconstruction (re-implantation) and hemi-arch reconstruction

and improved late patient outcomes. We use a valve sparing aortic root reconstruction with reimplantation technique if the base of the sinuses has good quality tissue. Alternatively, a root replacement with a mechanical valved conduit or bio-bentall procedure, based on patient factors and patient preference, would suffice. We prefer to minimize the use of felt for aortic reconstruction; however, in very elderly patients with fragile aortic tissue, an external anastomotic felt buttress can improve hemostasis.

Total Arch Reconstruction and Conventional Elephant Trunk

Initial preparation of the aortic arch and isolation of the epiaortic vessels is similar to the hemiarch repair technique described previously. Two strategies for arch reconstruction are commonly employed: (1) the epiaortic vessels are reconstructed first with a trifurcated graft, which can be performed after initiating circulatory arrest or during central cooling (Fig. 42.2a); or (2) the distal arch is reconstructed first on initiating circulatory arrest and then the head vessels are re-attached to the arch graft either directly through an island technique or with separate head vessel graft configurations. We prefer using the first technique on patients requiring standard arch replacements and the second technique in patients who are undergoing hybrid arch repair with novel frozen elephant trunk (FET) grafts (discussed later in this chapter).

Although the distal arch and proximal descending aorta can be dissected out through the mediastinum, this is associated with high rates of recurrent laryngeal nerve injury. We prefer to perform zone 2 arch anastomosis between the base of the carotid and left subclavian artery, which brings the anastomosis much more anterior and preserves the recurrent laryngeal nerve. Management of the subclavian artery is discussed later in this chapter. After circulatory arrest and uninterrupted ACP are initiated, the arch is opened and resected back to identify the optimal place (non-calcified, without penetrating aortic ulcer) for suturing the arch anastomosis. This

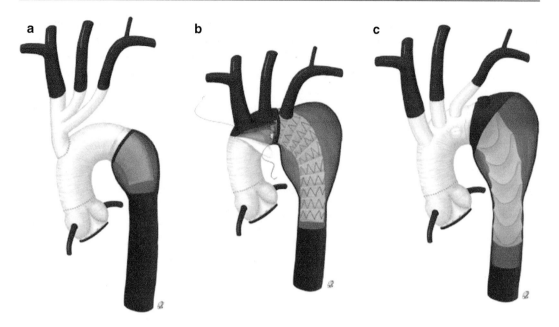

Fig. 42.2 (**a**) A conventional aortic arch and elephant trunk reconstruction. The head vessels are reconstructed with a trifurcated graft. (**b**) Drawing of a hybrid aortic arch repair with an antegrade conventional thoracic endograft deployed through the aortic arch with the proximal end sutured to the native aorta and a hemiarch reconstruction. (**c**) Drawing of a hybrid aortic arch (Zone 2) and frozen elephant trunk reconstruction with a four-branched graft

anastamotic 'zone' is trimmed to create a circular anastomosis. We prefer placing everting, pledgeted 2-0 Ethibond sutures radially around the distal arch to elevate it and parachute down the arch graft or place the elephant trunk in situ. Then, a second layer of running 2-0 or 3-0 prolene is placed to secure the arch anastomosis. We then initiate lower body perfusion, either through a side limb in the arch graft or via previous femoral artery cannulation. The head vessels are then re-attached to the arch graft epiaortic branches or via the previously sewn trifurcated graft. Then, the proximal aortic root work is completed and the arch graft is attached to the root graft at the neo-sinotubular junction. When using a branched arch graft, bilateral antegrade cerebral perfusion can be re-initiated after completing the carotid anastomosis when using lower body perfusion. This allows the arch graft to be anastomosed to the root graft and allow earlier cardiac re-perfusion with the innominate artery reconnected last. We do not prefer the island technique as we have concerns about arch calcification, inadequate hemostasis and leaving residual aortic disease.

When considering ATAAD, we will perform total aortic arch replacement and elephant trunk reconstruction when: (1) the primary tear is in the aortic arch; (2) rupture of the arch occurs; (3) there is malperfusion in critical epiaortic vessels; or (4) the aortic arch is aneurysmal.

Conventional Elephant Trunk Technique

Elephant trunk procedures are performed when the aneurysmal disease extends beyond the aortic arch into the proximal descending thoracic aorta, anticipating a second stage operation (Fig. 42.2a). We also utilize a short elephant trunk in patients with a very fragile aortic arch, such as those with penetrating aortic ulcers or acute type A aortic dissection, to improve distal anastomotic hemostasis. We find it helpful to place four everting, pledgeted 2-0 Ethibond sutures at the corners of the distal arch 'anastomotic zone' to elevate it anteriorly and provide counter-traction. Then, we telescope a 24–26 mm Dacron graft on itself, sewing a radio-opaque umbilical tape circumferentially to mark the distal end of the graft and place this into the descending aorta. The Ethibond sutures are passed through the Dacron graft and four more everting, pledgeted 2-0 Ethibond sutures are passed between the previous sutures through the distal anastomosis and elephant trunk. These sutures are tied and a second layer of 2-0 or 3-0 prolene is run around the anastomosis to secure hemostasis. The arch portion of the elephant trunk graft is then pulled back into the mediastinum and the head vessels are reconstructed in a sequence similar to the one previously described. Arch and elephant trunk grafts that provide thicker sewing cuffs are commercially available as well. In patients with smaller arch aneurysms, or acute aortic dissection, it can be challenging to place an elephant trunk deep into the descending aorta. In these cases, we always prefer using the horizontal mattress Ethibond sutures to close the false lumen and reconstruct the aortic wall layers, and choose a smaller graft to place within the true lumen for the elephant trunk.

Hybrid Aortic Arch and Frozen Elephant Trunk Reconstruction

The 2016 CCS Joint Position Statement on Open and Endovascular Surgery for Thoracic Aortic Disease suggests that hybrid arch techniques "might be considered for single-stage repair in patients with diffuse aneurysms involving the ascending, arch and descending aorta" [4]. Initially, off-label use of conventional thoracic endovascular repair (TEVAR) grafts was deployed in an antegrade fashion through the aortic arch into the descending thoracic aorta. A conventional arch graft would then be sewn to the TEVAR graft or a small segment of native arch would be left in situ with a hemiarch reconstruction (Fig. 42.2b). Although feasible, using off-label TEVAR grafts has several challenges including awkward antegrade deployment, using grafts never designed to negotiate the curve of the arch, sewing directly to TEVAR grafts with proximal open stent, and lack of TEVAR graft preclotting. Several groups have also described

hybrid arch repair with complete arch debranching and zone 0 stent grafting; however, we have avoided this approach as we have concerns about the conformability and stability of zone 0 stent grafting with currently available devices. Currently, there are two commercially available hybrid frozen elephant trunk grafts with prefabricated perfusion limb: (1) the E-vita OPEN PLUS graft (JOTEC, Hechingen, Germany); and (2) the four-branched Thoraflex Hybrid Graft (Vascutek Terumo, Scotland UK) (Fig. 42.3).

Since we have the most experience with the Thoraflex Hybrid graft, we will describe our

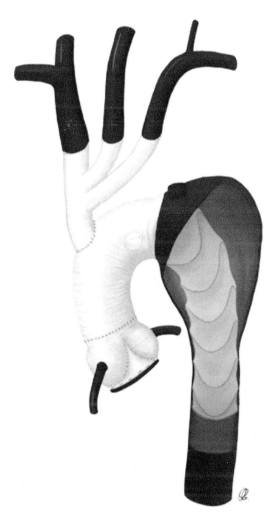

Fig. 42.3 A hybrid aortic arch (Zone 2) and frozen elephant trunk reconstruction with the Ante-flow Thoraflex Hybrid Graft (Vascutek Terumo, Scotland, UK) and reconstruction of the head vessels with a trifurcated graft

technique of hybrid aortic arch and frozen elephant reconstruction with this device (Fig. 42.2c).

Using a three-dimensional (3D) computed tomography (CT) reconstructive program, the hybrid arch FET graft is sized to the descending aortic landing zone to allow at least a 2–3 cm overlap, 20% oversizing for patients with aneurysms and 0% oversizing for patients with aortic dissections (measuring the long axis of the true lumen) or connective tissue disorders. We employ right axillary cannulation with an 8 mm Dacron side graft on all patients undergoing hybrid arch and FET reconstruction. Exposure and preparation of the aortic arch and epiaortic vessels is similar to previously described for conventional arch replacement.

After heparinization, a 6Fr femoral arterial sheath is placed and a guide wire and subsequent catheter are placed up the descending aorta into the aortic arch with transesophageal echocardiographic ± fluoroscopic guidance to ensure the catheter is within the true lumen. During cooling to 25 °C, we complete the aortic root work or replacement of the ascending aorta with a 26 mm graft. After circulatory arrest and initiation of ACP, the arch is resected and a 260 cm Amplatz extra-stiff wire (Cook Medical, Bloomington, USA) is passed through the catheter out the aortic arch into the mediastinum. We then identify and prepare the optimal anastamotic site, ideally zone 2, with everting, pledgeted 2-0 Ethibond sutures placed radially around the distal arch. The Thoraflex Hybrid graft is passed over the wire through the distal arch into the descending aorta. Orientation of the head vessel branches is maintained towards the head with the perfusion limb aiming towards the patient's left arm. The FET cuff is positioned within the anastamotic zone, the guide wire is pulled back and the FET graft is deployed. The 2-0 Ethibond sutures are passed through the Dacron cuff of the FET graft and tied followed by a second layer of running 2-0 prolene to secure hemostasis. An arterial cannula is placed within the perfusion limb, and simultaneous lower body perfusion and re-warming is initiated with a clamp on the hybrid arch graft proximal to the perfusion limb. The subclavian limb is often too close to the arch anastomosis, and as such, we usually address this either before sewing the arch anastomosis with a separate 8 mm graft or preoperatively with a carotid-subclavian transposition. The carotid limb is anastamosed and bilateral antegrade perfusion is initiated. We then attach the proximal end of the hybrid arch graft to the aortic root graft or the ascending aortic graft to allow myocardial reperfusion.

Lastly, we attach the most proximal graft limb to the innominate artery to complete the operation (Fig. 42.2c). The FET should be assessed for complete deployment and distal seal by TEE ± fluoroscopy before leaving the operating room. Final assessment should be deferred until complete re-warming because of the nitinol stent design. We address FET stent underdeployment with antegrade ballooning under fluoroscopic guidance and distal type 1 endoleaks with secondary distal TEVAR stent graft deployment.

Management of Difficult Left Subclavian Artery

Dealing with the left subclavian (SCL) artery during aortic arch repair can be extremely challenging. Many complex arch aneurysms push the subclavian origin high into the left chest, rendering it difficult to reach through a sternotomy. Additionally, direct reconstruction of the SCL origin is associated with a high risk of recurrent laryngeal injury. We believe that thoughtful planning prior to surgery can often help to mitigate the difficult subclavian artery. There are several pre-, intra- and postoperative techniques to address the difficult subclavian artery (Fig. 42.4).

Preoperative Carotid-Subclavian Transposition or Bypass with Ligation (Fig. 42.4)

Ideal for elective cases, this option simplifies the arch reconstruction, with no need to expose the distal arch beyond the carotid, and allows a more proximal zone 2 arch anastomosis. Care must be taken to examine the subclavian ostium from within the aorta to ensure no subclavian back

Fig. 42.4 A carotid subclavian transposition (left) and carotid-subclavian bypass with proximal subclavian occlusion with an Amplatzer Vascular Occluder device (St. Jude Medical Inc, St. Paul, USA)

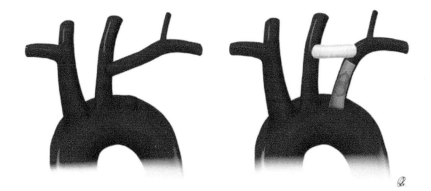

bleeding from inadequate ligation or collateral vessel filling, which would result in a type II endoleak. If back bleeding is identified, then the subclavian origin must be ligated.

Intraoperative Anatomic/Extra-Anatomic Reconstruction

When reachable, direct anastomosis with the subclavian ostium likely remains the optimal solution. Because of the proximity of the SCL and arch anastomosis, sometimes it is easier to sew a separate 8 mm graft to the SCL prior to constructing the arch and re-attaching the proximal end to the proximal arch graft during re-warming (Fig. 42.5). When the SCL origin is deep, we prefer ligation of the origin and extra-anatomic bypass to the left axillary artery through an infraclavicular approach, with an 8 mm graft passed through the second intercostal space across the apex of the left lung, and anastomosed to the proximal arch in the mediastinum (Fig. 42.6).

Direct Cannulation of the SCL Ostium from Within the Aorta with Hybrid Vascular Graft

When the SCL artery is calcified or fragile, a Gore Hybrid Vascular or Viabahn graft (Gore

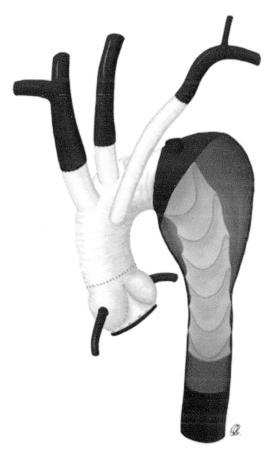

Fig. 42.5 A separate 8-mm Dacron graft anastomosed to the 'hard to reach' subclavian artery, performed as the first step after arch resection under circulatory arrest. The proximal limb is then sewn to the proximal arch graft after all of the other anastomosis have been completed

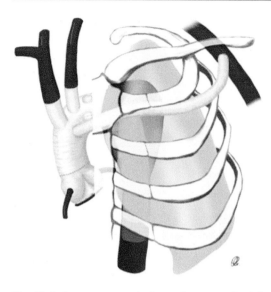

Fig. 42.6 An extra-anatomic 8 mm bypass to the left axillary artery through the first or second intercostal space, over the apex of the left lung. This technique is useful when the subclavian stump is difficult to reach through the mediastinum

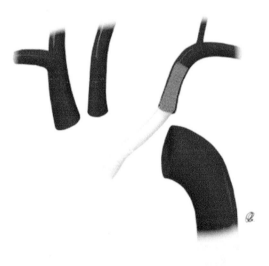

Fig. 42.7 Drawing of a Gore Hybrid Vascular Graft (Gore Medical AZ, USA) deployed within the left subclavian to facilitate easier reconstruction when the distal subclavian is deep and difficult to reach through the mediastinum

Medical AZ, USA) can be inserted antegrade and deployed within the origin of the SCL and the proximal end anastomosed to the arch graft (Fig. 42.7).

Intraoperative Ligation with Postoperative Repair/Bypass

Lastly, the SCL origin can be ligated intraoperatively and the left arm re-assessed postoperatively for ischemia or claudication. This technique requires careful preoperative assessment of vertebral dominance to avoid catastrophic posterior circulation stroke.

Outcomes

Outcomes of elective aortic arch replacement with elephant trunk series for aneurysmal disease are favourable with excellent clinical results. A 2013 paper from Svensson et al. reported an in-hospital mortality of 7.6% and a stroke risk of 8% in a series of 526 patients [5]. Furthermore, elephant trunk procedures have proven to be safe with good outcomes even when employed in the setting of an acute type A dissection. A 2015 systematic review and meta-analysis looking at elephant trunk procedures for the treatment of acute type A aortic dissections, looked at 11 studies encompassing 881 patients ranging in ages between 45 and 67 years of age and found an in-hospital mortality of only 8% [6]. Although there may be obvious selection bias to perform an elephant trunk only on patients presenting with acute dissections that are physically able to undergo such a large and invasive procedure, this mortality rate is more than acceptable when compared to the International Registry of Acute Aortic Dissection database (IRAD) that reports mortality rates between 16.2 and 27.4% [7, 8].

Hybrid arch and FET procedures have reported similar outcomes with in-hospital mortality ranging between 1.8 and 17.2% [9]. The greatest risk to patients appears to be spinal cord ischemia which is likely multifactorial, but risk increases greatly with obstruction of the thoracic intercostal arteries, specifically below T7-T8. In a review of several small studies, the risk of spinal cord injury ranged from 0 to 6% and the incidence of stroke with the hybrid FET ranged between 5 and 10% [10]. Larger studies do exist for the E-Vita hybrid prosthesis, with an open registry created in 2005 with over 575 patients enrolled to date from 10 different European centers. The registry reports an incidence of in-hospital mortality between 12% and 18%, with rates of spinal cord injury and stroke of 3–4% and 0–6% respectively, depending on the presenting clinical situation (aneurysm vs. acute dissection) [10].

References

1. Boodhwani M, et al. Canadian Cardiovascular Society position statement on the management of thoracic aortic disease. Can J Cardiol. 2014;30(6):577–89.
2. Hiratza LF, et al. 2010 ACCF/AHA/AATS/ACR/ASA/SCA/SCAI/SIR/STS/SVM Guidelines for the diagnosis and management of patients with thoracic aortic disease. JACC. 2010;55(14):27–129.
3. Erbul R, et al. 2014 ESC Guidelines on the diagnosis and treatment of aortic diseases. EHJ. 2014;35(41):2873–292.
4. Appoo JJ, et al. Canadian Cardiovascular Society/Canadian Society of Cardiac Surgeons/Canadian Society for Vascular Surgery Joint position statement on open and endovascular surgery for thoracic aortic disease. Can J Cardiol. 2016;32(6):703–13.
5. Svensson LG, Rushing GD, Valenzuela ES, Rafael AE, Batizy LH, Blackstone EH, Roselli EE, Gillinov AM, Sabik JF III, Lytle BW. Modifications, classification, and outcomes of elephant-trunk procedures. Ann Thorac Surg. 2013;96(2):548–58.
6. Lin H-H, Liao S-F, Wu C-F, Li P-C, Li M-L. Outcome of frozen elephant trunk technique for acute type A aortic dissection: as systematic review and meta-analysis. Medicine. 2015;94(16):e694.
7. Hagan P, Nienaber C, Isselbacher E, Bruckman D, Karavite D, Russman P, Evangelista A, Fattori R, Suz T, Oh J, Moore A, Malouf J, Pape L, Gaca C, Sechtem U, Lenferink S, Deutsch H, Diedrichs H, Robles J, Llovet A, Gilon D, Das S, Armstrong W, Deeb G, Eagle K. The International Registry of Acute Aortic Dissection (IRAD): new insights into an old disease. JAMA. 2000;283(7):897–903.
8. Tsai T, Nienaber CA, Isselbacher EM, Trimarchi S, Bossone E, Evangelista A, Oh JK, O'Gara P, Suzuki T, Hutchison S, Cooper JV, Meinhardt G, Myrmel T, Eagle KA, Froehlich J. Acute type A aortic dissection: does a primary tear in the aortic arch affect management and outcomes? Insights from the International Registry of Acute Aortic Dissection (IRAD). Circulation. 2006;114:432–8.
9. Marco L, Pantaleo A, Leone A, Murana G, Di Bartolomeo R, Pacini D. The frozen elephant trunk technique: European Association for cardio-thoracic surgery position and bologna experience. Kor J Thorac Cardiovasc Surg. 2017;50(1):1–7.
10. Ma W-G, Zheng J, Sun L-Z, Elefteriades JA. Open stented grafts for frozen elephant trunk technique: technical aspects and current outcomes. AORTA J. 2015;3(4):122–35.

Surgery of Descending Thoracic Aorta

43

Martin Misfeld, Khalil Jawad,
and Michael A. Borger

Main Messages

1. The pathology involving the descending thoracic aorta includes aneurysm, dissection, atherosclerotic ulcers, intramural hematoma and traumatic injury.
2. Indications for surgical treatment of descending aortic disease have been drastically altered by the successful introduction of TEVAR.
3. Many descending thoracic aortic patients are poor surgical candidates due to comorbidity and age, and TEVAR can minimize surgical trauma and physiologic stresses in such patients.

The descending thoracic aorta begins distal to the left subclavian artery and ends at the level of the diaphragm. The pathology involving this area includes aneurysm, dissection, atherosclerotic ulcers, intramural hematoma and traumatic injury.

M. Misfeld · K. Jawad · M. A. Borger (✉)
Department of Cardiac Surgery, Heart Center,
University of Leipzig, Leipzig, Germany
e-mail: michael.borger@helios-gesundheit.de

Descending Thoracic Aortic Aneurysm (DTAA)

Aortic aneurysms are abnormal dilatations of the aorta (i.e. more than 1.5 times the normal size). The formation of aortic aneurysms is the second most common aortic disease after atherosclerosis. The diagnosis of a DTAA does not exclude the presence of another aortic aneurysm, and screening of the entire aorta is always necessary in such patients. The incidence of all thoracic aortic aneurysms, including DTAA, is approximately 5–10 per 100,000 person-years, with men predominating over women. Although associated with aneurysms, atherosclerosis is not a direct cause of aneurysm formation and growth. There is evidence suggesting a genetic predilection. Other risk factors include hypertension, chronic obstructive lung disease, chronic aortic dissection and infections of the aortic wall.

Patients are usually asymptomatic, but may present with signs and symptoms secondary to compression of surrounding structures. Hoarseness, stridor, dyspnea, dysphagia and plethora may occur due to encroachment upon the left recurrent laryngeal nerve, trachea, esophagus and superior vena cava.

The natural history of DTAA varies with the rate of growth. Aneurysms of the descending aorta grow faster than those of the ascending aorta (3 mm/year versus 1 mm/year) [1]. DTAAs greater

© Springer Nature Switzerland AG 2021
D. C. H. Cheng et al. (eds.), *Evidence-Based Practice in Perioperative Cardiac Anesthesia and Surgery*, https://doi.org/10.1007/978-3-030-47887-2_43

than 6 cm have a twofold risk of rupture when compared to aneurysms with a diameter less than 6 cm over a time of 5 years (16% vs. 31%) [2].

Descending Thoracic Aortic Dissection

Aortic dissection is when an intimal disruption results in the entry of blood into the aortic media, separating it from the adventitia and creating a true and false lumen. When the intimal tear and subsequent dissection occurs in the descending aorta, it is classified as Stanford type B. Stanford type B aortic dissection is less common than type A (i.e. ascending aorta) dissection, which has an incidence of approximately 3 per 100,000 patient-years. Males are more commonly affected by type B aortic dissection than females. Hypertension is the most important risk factor, but other contributing factors include connective tissue disorders (e.g. Marfan syndrome, Loyes-Dietz syndrome), bicuspid aortic valve, aortic coarctation, pregnancy, and surgical manipulation of the aorta. The culprit intimal tear usually occurs just distal to the ligamentum arteriosum, the greatest point of hemodynamic stress. If untreated, visceral and peripheral tissue malperfusion may occur. Aneurysmal dilation and rupture are late complications.

Penetrating Atherosclerotic Ulcer (PAU)

PAU was described for the first time in 1934 by Shennan [3]. PAUs are most often found in the middle and lower descending thoracic aorta. They are caused by large atherosclerotic plaques that penetrate through the intima into the media, resulting in a hematoma within the wall of the aorta. Clinical presentation of PAU is similar to that of classic aortic dissection, although many patients are asymptomatic. The natural history is less well understood but is thought to have a slow progression. PAU is associated with a low but definite incidence of acute rupture. If left untreated, PAU may result in pseudoaneurysm,

intramural thrombus formation, or acute aortic dissection.

Intramural Hematoma (IMH)

The descending thoracic aorta is involved in 60–70% of patients with IMH. IMH is thought to be the result of vasa vasorum rupture within the wall of the aorta, leading to aortic wall disintegration and hematoma formation. The absence of an intimal tear is what distinguishes IMH from PAU. Regional thickening of the aortic wall with the absence of an intimal flap and no enhancement after contrast injection is considered diagnostic. Approximately one third of IMHs enlarge and rupture, one third have no change in size and do not rupture, and one third regress with no sequelae.

Traumatic Injury of the Descending Thoracic Aorta

Traumatic injury of the aorta is infrequent but devastating, accounting for 10–25% of motor vehicle fatalities. More than 90% of cases occur just distal to the ligamentum arteriosum, secondary to acceleration-deceleration injury. Mid-descending thoracic aortic trauma is uncommon, usually caused by compression over the spine. Immediate death occurs in 80% of victims. Of those who survive, 25% die in the first 24 h, another 40% die in the first 4 days, and the remaining have a 2% per year risk of late rupture secondary to pseudoaneurysm formation [4]. Traumatic aortic injuries are classified as type I if confined to an intimal tear, type II if IMH is present, type III if resulting in pseudoaneurysm, and type IV if aortic rupture occurs.

Diagnosis

Physical examination of patients with descending aortic disease is usually non-specific. Numerous chest x-ray findings have been described but are also non-specific. Computed tomography (CT) and magnetic resonance imaging (MRI) have replaced aortography as the diagnostic tests of choice. Echocardiography and intravascular ultrasound may be helpful in select cases.

Aortography is able to provide information regarding intimal tears, dissection and aneurysm location, greatly aiding operative strategy. Aortography may be particularly helpful for defining endoleaks post-thoracic endovascular aortic repair (TEVAR). The disadvantages include lack of detail regarding surrounding structures, and contrast-induced renal failure or allergic reaction.

CT requires radiation exposure and nephrotoxic contrast material, but is more readily available than MRI. CT examinations of the descending aorta do not need to be EKG-gated, as opposed to examinations of the ascending aorta. MRI may be the imaging method of choice for the descending aorta, but its use is limited in the acute situation. It can accurately identify false lumen entries and can distinguish false lumen thrombus from periaortic hematoma. TEE allows precise imaging of aortic wall pathology and flow between true lumen and other areas of interest, while supplying valuable cardiac information [5]. The disadvantages of TEE are requirement of sedation, limited availability, and operator-dependence.

Indications for Surgery

The indications for surgical treatment of descending aortic disease have been drastically altered by the successful introduction of TEVAR [6]. For patients with aneurysms of a degenerative or chronic nature, elective surgical resection is advised when the diameter is > 6 cm or if symptoms are present, and the anatomy is unsuitable for TEVAR therapy. A lower threshold (i.e. 5.5 cm) may be applied for patients with suitable anatomy for TEVAR therapy, because of the lower risk of perioperative complications. For patients with Marfan syndrome or other connective tissue disease disorders, surgical therapy is indicated when the diameter exceeds 5.5 cm because of the increased risk of aortic rupture. TEVAR is contraindicated in such patients.

Most patients with type B aortic dissection are uncomplicated, and should be managed with medical therapy as a bridge to decision. TEVAR therapy is indicated for signs of impending rupture (persisting pain, hypotension and left-sided hemothorax), malperfusion (peripheral or visceral ischemia, renal failure, paraparesis or paraplegia), or failure of medical management (uncontrolled hypertension or rapid growth of descending aorta) in patients with appropriate anatomy. In patients without appropriate anatomy (usually lack of proximal landing zone), conventional open surgery may be considered.

PAU and IMH of the descending thoracic aorta are primarily treated with medical therapy. In patients with symptomatic or rapidly growing PAU, TEVAR is indicated and conventional surgery is reserved for those without appropriate anatomy for TEVAR therapy.

Special Situations

Care should be taken to distinguish PAU from mycotic aneurysm, which can be done based on symptoms and signs of systemic infection. Mycotic aneurysms, although rare, are an indication for conventional open surgery and should not be treated with TEVAR.

Patients who present with gastrointestinal bleeding post-TEVAR should be carefully investigated for an aorto-esophageal fistula. The diagnosis is confirmed by CT and treatment is staged and multi-disciplinary. As the first stage, a cervical esophageal diversion is created and a percutaneous endoscopic gastrostomy performed. The descending aorta is then resected during cardiopulmonary bypass (either in the same procedure or on the following day), and the intra-thoracic esophagus closed proximally and distally. A gastric pull-up is then performed several weeks later.

Treatment

Medical Management

Acute patients should be admitted to the ICU for invasive blood pressure monitoring and to monitor end-organ function. Pharmacologic therapy is instituted to minimize shear forces against the aortic wall and cardiac contractility by lowering systolic blood pressure and minimizing the rises in aortic pressure. Target systolic blood pressure is 100–120 mmHg. Short acting intravenous beta-adrenergic blockers and sodium nitroprusside are used. Beta-blockade should be performed prior to giving nitroprusside to avoid reflex tachycardia. Prophylactic use of beta-blockers, angiotensin-converting enzyme inhibitor, and angiotensin II receptor blocker can be helpful in Marfan patients, since some studies have shown that the use of these drugs could reduce the progression of the aneurysm or the occurrence of complications. Patients should be advised to immediately stop smoking. Studies have shown that smokers have a 0.4 mm/year faster growth of the aortic aneurysm than non-smokers. Although moderate sport could prevent atherosclerosis, competitive sports should be avoided in patients with aortic aneurysm. Patients who do not undergo surgery should have repeat imaging studies, with the frequency determined by the size of the aneurysm.

Surgical Treatment

The principle of surgical management is to excise the diseased segment of descending aorta and restore flow in the true lumen (in the case of aortic dissection) and relevant branches. Various surgical approaches and methods of circulatory support can be performed. The standard approach is to use partial left heart bypass with moderate systemic hypothermia (30 °C). Arterial cannulation is performed in the distal thoracic aorta for operations on the proximal descending aorta, or in the femoral artery for operations extending into the abdomen. Venous cannulation is via the left inferior pulmonary vein or the left atrial appendage. Left heart bypass has the advantage of requiring lower doses of heparinization when compared to full cardiopulmonary bypass (CPB), but the disadvantage of being less able to cope with large, sudden blood volume changes.

A left posterolateral thoracotomy is performed with single lung ventilation. The minimal amount

of aorta is excised in order to preserve intercostal arterial supply of the spinal cord, to circumvent paraplegia. Paraplegia occurs in 2–5% [7] of cases with modern operative techniques and spinal protection.

After commencing circulatory bypass, the aortic arch is usually clamped between the left common carotid and the left subclavian arteries. If proximal disease precludes crossclamping, CPB with deep hypothermic circulatory arrest is required. The aorta is transected distal to the left subclavian and a collagen-impregnated graft is anastomosed to it. The occluding clamp is then removed and placed on the graft. The distal descending thoracic aorta is opened longitudinally. Intercostal arteries above T6 are oversewn, while arteries below this level are individually inspected. Intercostal arteries with poor back bleeding should be reimplanted, while those with very good back bleeding can be sacrificed. The aortic clamp is sequentially moved down the graft as each branch is reattached, allowing early spinal perfusion. The distal anastomosis is made last and the cross-clamp is then removed.

The incidence of spinal cord ischemia varies with surgical technique. Operations performed with left heart bypass are associated with the lowest incidence (2%). However, this is partly due to the fact that less extensive aortic resection procedures are performed with this technique. Paraplegia rates associated with alternative methods such as CPB, heparinized shunts, and 'clamp-and-sew' technique are higher. The latter technique is most detrimental when ischemic time exceeds 30 min. Use of moderate hypothermia, drainage of CSF fluid, regional spinal cooling via epidural, preoperative identification and intraoperative implantation of the anterior spinal artery, and pharmacologic agents such as steroids may also lower the risk of spinal cord injury.

Thoracic Endovascular Aortic Repair (TEVAR)

Many descending thoracic aortic patients are poor surgical candidates due to comorbidity and age. TEVAR minimizes surgical trauma and physiologic stresses in such patients. PAU's are ideal for TEVAR therapy because such patients usually have associated comorbidities and surgical manipulation carries high risk of distal embolic events. TEVAR is the therapy of choice for patients with complicated type B aortic dissection. TEVAR is not indicated for IMH as there is no primary intimal defect. Technical limitations for endovascular stenting include the requirement of radiographic guidance, a minimum of 2 cm of normal proximal and distal aorta for adequate fixation, and a relatively large peripheral vessel for insertion. The most common complication post-TEVAR is endoleak, which oftentimes requires open surgical therapy.

Outcomes

Descending Thoracic Aortic Aneurysm

Long-term survival in untreated descending DTAA is approximately 80% at 1 year and 40% at 5 years. Survival after elective surgical repair is 90% at 30 days and 60% at 5 years. Major morbidity consists of paraplegia, paraparesis and acute renal failure. Hemodialysis is required in 5% of previously healthy individuals and 17% of patients with preoperative renal dysfunction [8, 9].

Descending Thoracic Aortic Dissection

Despite major advancements in aortic surgery over the past several years, the results for acute type B aortic dissection remain unsatisfactory with in-hospital mortality ranging from 25 to 50% [10]. TEVAR is therefore the treatment of choice for complicated acute type B aortic dissection.

Actuarial survival for all patients with type B dissections is 65% at 1 year and 50% at 5 years. Medically managed patients have a survival of 73% at 1 year and 58% at 5 years. Patients requiring surgery for failed medical management have survival rates of 47% at 1 year and 28% at 5 years [11].

Patients requiring intervention for chronic type B aortic dissection with aneurysm formation are generally better treated with conventional surgery than with TEVAR. The results for TEVAR in this patient population have been generally disappointing because of several anatomic and technical issues including inappropriate landing zones, small true lumens as "working spaces," non-pliable dissection membranes, and multiple re-entry sites.

PAU and IMH

Evidence in the literature is lacking on long-term survival with or without surgery in patients with descending thoracic aorta PAU and IMH [12]. TEVAR is a good option for patients with descending aortic PAU, since it is associated with lower morbidity and mortality than conventional open surgery and because such patients frequently have satisfactory landing zones.

Traumatic Injury of the Descending Thoracic Aorta

Traumatic descending aortic injury is associated with a relatively high incidence of major complications such as paraplegia, sepsis, renal failure, hemorrhage and acute respiratory distress syndrome. If patients survive the initial events, however, long-term outcomes are favourable. Because of co-existing injuries, traumatic aortic injury patients are poor candidates for conventional surgical repair requiring full heparinization. TEVAR is therefore the treatment of choice for such patients, and is associated with a significantly lower mortality rate than open surgery (9 vs. 19%) [13].

References

1. Erbel R, Aboyans V, Boileau C, et al. 2014 ESC Guidelines on the diagnosis and treatment of aortic diseases. Eur Heart J. 2014;35:2873–926.
2. Clouse WD, Hallett JW Jr, Schaff HV, et al. Improved prognosis of thoracic aortic aneurysms: a population-based study. JAMA. 1998;280:1926–9.
3. Shennan T. Dissecting aneurysms. Medical Research Council, Special Report Series, No. 193. London: His Majesty's Stationery Office; 1934.

4. Tatou E, Steinmetz E, Jazveri S, et al. Surgical outcomes of traumatic rupture of the thoracic aorta. Ann Thorac Surg. 2000;69:70–3.

5. Vignon P, Gueret P, Vedrinne J, et al. Role of transesophageal echocardiography in the diagnosis and management of traumatic aortic disruption. Circulation. 1995;92:2959–68.

6. Fattori R, Tsai TT, Myrmel T, et al. Complicated acute type B dissection: is surgery still the best option? A report from the International Registry of Acute Aortic Dissection. JACC Cardiovasc Interv. 2008;1:395–402.

7. Wong DR, Coselli JS, Amerman K, et al. Delayed spinal cord deficits after thoracoabdominal aortic aneurysm repair. Ann Thorac Surg. 2007;83:1345–55.

8. Turina MI, Shennib H, Dunning J, et al. EACTS/ESCVS Best practice guidelines for reporting treatment results in the thoracic aorta. Eur J Cardiothorac Surg. 2009;35:927–30.

9. Cohn LH, Adams DH, editors. Cardiac surgery in the adult. New York: McGraw-Hill; 2018.

10. Lansman SL, Hagl C, Fink D, et al. Acute type B aortic dissection: surgical therapy. Ann Thorac Surg. 2002;74:S1833–5.

11. Kouchoukos NT, Dugenis D. Surgery of the thoracic aorta. N Engl J Med. 1997;336:1876–87.

12. von Kodolitsch Y, Csosz SK, Koschyk DH, et al. Intramural hematoma of the aorta: predictors of progression to dissection and rupture. Circulation. 2003;107:1158–63.

13. Murad MH, Rizvi AZ, Malgor R, et al. Comparative effectiveness of the treatments for thoracic aortic transection. J Vasc Surg. 2011;53:p193–9.

Combined Cardiac and Vascular Surgery

Piroze Davierwala, Alexandro Hoyer,
and Michael A. Borger

Main Messages

1. A thorough preoperative evaluation and a carefully devised surgical plan are of utmost importance for patients requiring a combined surgical approach.
2. CABG patients often have associated cerebrovascular disease; options for these patients undergoing CABG and CEA include a combined technique, a staged approach, and a reverse-staged approach.
3. Although less common, CABG patients may have abdominal aortic aneurysm, and simultaneous CABG and AAA repair may be performed in select patients.

Atherosclerosis is a systemic disease and patients with coronary artery disease (CAD) or other atherosclerotic lesions are at an increased risk of other segments of the vascular tree being involved, thereby making them vulnerable to other cardiovascular events. For those patients with indications for cardiac surgery, a combined approach that addresses both the cardiac and vas-

P. Davierwala · A. Hoyer · M. A. Borger (✉)
Department of Cardiac Surgery, Leipzig Heart
Center, Leipzig, Germany
e-mail: michael.borger@helios-gesundheit.de

cular pathology is an option. The chief objective of a combined surgical approach in such patients, who are already prone to increased perioperative morbidity and mortality, is to prevent the occurrence of devastating complications caused by the coexisting vascular disease. Patients who require combined procedures should undergo a thorough preoperative evaluation and careful surgical planning in order to achieve the best possible outcome. The increasing use of endovascular procedures in the treatment of atherosclerotic vascular disorders has to also be considered for such patients.

Carotid Artery Stenosis and Cardiac Surgery

Patients presenting for coronary artery bypass grafting (CABG) frequently have associated cerebrovascular disease. Approximately 25–30% of patients with symptomatic carotid artery stenosis (CAS) have accompanying significant CAD, whereas the estimated prevalence of significant CAS (i.e. >50%) in patients undergoing CABG is 6–10% [1]. Besides aortic atherosclerotic disease, CAS is one of the main risk factors for development of perioperative stroke during or following cardiac surgery [2]. The primary aim of a combined procedure is to prevent the development of a perioperative stroke and / or myocardial infarction. However, a combined procedure should only be considered when the indications for both procedures exist. More definitive evidence for a beneficial outcome following a combined procedure exists for symptomatic as compared to asymptomatic CAS [3, 4].

The options for patients undergoing CABG and carotid endarterectomy (CEA) include a combined technique, a staged approach, and a reverse-staged technique. However, a lack of evidence from randomized controlled trials comparing a combined to a staged approach has left the issue of timing debatable. Additionally, the advent of interventional therapy in the form of carotid artery angioplasty and stenting has broadened the therapeutic options in patients with CAS.

Evaluation of Carotid Artery Stenosis Prior to Cardiac Surgery

There is no clear consensus regarding the use of routine carotid screening for all patients undergoing cardiac surgery. The ACCF/AHA guidelines on the management of patients with extracranial carotid and vertebral artery disease recommend a carotid duplex ultrasound for patients older than 65 years of age, for those with left main CAD, peripheral arterial disease, history of cigarette smoking, stroke or transient ischemic attacks, and/or those with a carotid bruit on physical examination [5]. Preoperative screening should consist of:

1. History: Patients should be actively questioned regarding the history of stroke, reversible ischemic neurological deficit (RIND) or transient ischemic attack (TIA).
2. Physical examination: Auscultation of the neck should be performed to check for bruit over the carotid arteries.
3. Non-invasive testing:
   (A) Duplex scanning combines Doppler scanning and ultrasonography and is the preferred investigation of choice.
   (B) Magnetic resonance angiography (MRA) and/or computed tomography (CT) angiography should be performed in patients with abnormal Duplex scanning results.

(C) CT or MR Imaging of the brain should be performed if there is a history of stroke.
4. Invasive testing: Carotid angiography should be performed when there is concern about the caliber or quality of distal vessels or disease in the aortic arch.

Indications for Carotid Artery Endarterectomy (CEA)

- Symptomatic CAS—ipsilateral retinal or hemispheric cerebral ischemic symptoms within the last 6 months with >80% stenosis (Class IIa, Level of evidence: C) [5]
- Asymptomatic CAS—very controversial (Class IIb, Level of Evidence C). The Asymptomatic Carotid Atherosclerosis Study (ACAS) demonstrated that patients with asymptomatic CAS of 60% or greater will have a reduced 5-year risk of ipsilateral stroke if CEA can be performed with less than 3% risk of perioperative morbidity and mortality [3]. The Asymptomatic Carotid Surgery Trial (ACST) study revealed that patients with severe asymptomatic CAS younger than 75 years of age have a reduced 10-year stroke risk following CEA, half of which is in disabling or fatal strokes [4]. However, these trials excluded patients with significant cardiac disease and the benefit of CEA was lost if perioperative stroke and / or mortality rates exceeded 3%. Such a low perioperative stroke and mortality rate is difficult to achieve in patients undergoing combined CEA and CABG. This view is supported by the recently published results of the Coronary Artery Bypass Grafting and Carotid Endarterectomy Versus Isolated Coronary Artery Bypass Grafting trial (CABACS), which demonstrated that superiority of the combined CEA and CABG approach seems unlikely [6]. Unfortunately, the trial had to be stopped due to curtailment of funds following a slow enrollment rate. The five-year follow-up of patients is still ongoing.

Surgical Revascularization Strategies

Three surgical strategies can be used in patients who undergo both CABG and CEA:

1. A combined approach in which CABG and CEA are performed simultaneously.
2. A staged approach in which CEA is performed prior to CABG as a separate procedure.
3. A reverse-staged approach in which CABG is performed prior to CEA.

Another option for patients with CAS and CAD is to perform only an isolated CABG procedure without intervening on the carotid artery [7, 8], which may be the best option in asymptomatic patients without severe bilateral CAS. The CABG procedure can be performed off-pump without the use of cardiopulmonary bypass (CPB), but it is extremely important to avoid any hypotension that may occur during the operation, especially while positioning the heart for grafting the posterolateral wall.

Operative Technique for Combined Approach

The following is a description of our technique for combined CABG / CEA surgery. We prefer to perform the CEA prior to onset of CPB in order to minimize CPB time and its associated complications, except in specific situations (see below). The surgical steps are:

1. Simultaneous exposure of the heart and carotid artery.
2. Perform CEA while harvesting the saphenous vein.
3. Optional use of carotid shunts while performing CEA. It is useful to check the amount of retrograde flow or pressure (preferably greater than 25 mmHg) distal to the clamped internal carotid artery when deciding whether or not to use a shunt.
4. Fix the distal intima to the arterial wall with 2–3 interrupted sutures if it is thick, in order to reduce the possibility of a dissection.
5. Saphenous vein patch of the endarterectomised carotid artery, particularly if it is not large in caliber.
6. Proceed with CABG.
7. Maintain elevated perfusion pressures (>70 mmHg) during CPB with mild to moderate hypothermia (28–34 °C).
8. Do not close neck incision until patient has received protamine.

CEA can also be performed during CPB, especially in patients with bilateral high grade lesions. Moderate or deep hypothermia during CEA may provide additional cerebral protection, but will increase the length of the procedure, CPB time, and the risk of coagulopathy [9]. However, a benefit for CEA performed on CPB with hypothermia has not been proven [10].

Intraoperative Concerns

The majority of strokes that occur during CABG are secondary to ascending aortic atherosclerosis, and not chiefly due to carotid disease [2]. Patients with carotid disease are at a particularly high risk for ascending aortic atherosclerosis and therefore epiaortic scanning should be performed in all such patients. If significant disease is present, cannulation of the aortic arch beyond the origins of the carotid arteries to minimize cerebral embolization should be considered; or, cannulation of the innominate artery if it is free of disease. Off-pump CABG without aortic manipulation may be the best option, which can be achieved with the use of in-situ or composite arterial grafts. Proximal anastomoses can be performed with minimal aortic manipulation with automated proximal anastomotic devices. As noted above, hypotension must be avoided during subluxation of the heart.

Key Points of Postoperative Care

Maintain adequate perfusion pressure, oxygenation and cardiac output. Watch for bleeding / hematoma in neck region. Re-intubate the patient immediately if an expanding neck hematoma is detected.

An attempt to wake up the patient early after arrival in the intensive care unit should be made to assess the neurological status. Three possibilities exist after the patient is awake irrespective of whether he/she is extubated or not. The patient may be:

1. Awake and oriented: routine postoperative management should be continued.
2. Confused without localizing signs: other causes for confusion should be ruled out and imaging with Doppler should be considered if carotid artery patency is a concern.
3. Hemiplegic or hemiparetic: an emergent angiogram and possible re-exploration of the carotid artery should be considered.

Outcomes After Combined CABG and CEA

Prospective randomized trials have shown that CEA is superior to optimal medical therapy in patients with high-grade CAS [3, 4]. Additionally, there is evidence that carotid artery stenting is non-inferior to CEA in standard and high-risk patients [11, 12]. However, synchronous CEA and CABG procedures are associated with higher morbidity, especially stroke, and mortality rates as compared to isolated CABG. A meta-analysis revealed that the incidence of stroke, myocardial infarction (MI) and mortality following combined surgery is 6%, 5%, and 5% respectively [13]. On the other hand, a staged approach involving CEA or carotid stenting followed later by CABG is associated with the risk of periprocedural (CEA/stenting) or inter-stage MI, which is known to negatively impact survival [14]. The above-mentioned outcomes obviously raise the question as to which strategy provides the best results in patients presenting with high-grade CAS at the time of CABG. In this regard, much more data—preferably from randomized clinical trials (RCTs)—is required.

The CABACS trial was a RCT of asymptomatic patients with severe CAS and showed that combined CABG and CEA was not superior to isolated CABG alone, with isolated CABG patients having a trend towards better results for nearly all primary and secondary outcomes [6]. Moreover, medical therapy with contemporary antiplatelet, lipid lowering, and antihypertensive medications might further diminish the advantages of CEA over medical therapy in patients with severe CAS [15].

For those patients with clear indications for CABG and CEA (see below), no clear recommendations exist with respect to surgical strategy. Each approach carries a risk of stroke and/or MI. A propensity-matched analysis comparing patients undergoing staged carotid artery stenting or CEA followed by open heart surgery (OHS) to those undergoing synchronous CEA and OHS revealed that staged stenting-OHS and combined CEA-OHS are associated with a similar risk of death, stroke, or MI in the short term, with both being better than staged CEA-OHS chiefly due to a greater risk of inter-stage MI. However, stenting-OHS was associated with significantly better outcomes after the first year [14]. A combined approach of CEA and CABG should only be considered in specialized medical centers with experienced surgeons in vascular surgery.

We recommend isolated CABG without intervention (i.e. surgery or stenting) on the carotid artery for asymptomatic patients with unilateral carotid artery disease, irrespective of the severity of CAS. We perform a combined procedure only in patients with severe bilateral asymptomatic disease (e.g. complete occlusion of one carotid artery and >70% stenosis of the other carotid artery or bilateral filiform lesions) or those with unilateral severe symptomatic CAS with an urgent indication for CABG. For all other symptomatic patients with unilateral severe CAS, in whom CABG can be safely postponed for 4–6 weeks, carotid stenting followed by a staged CABG procedure is probably the best option.

Combined Cardiac and Abdominal Aortic Surgery

The incidence of abdominal aortic aneurysm (AAA) in patients undergoing routine CABG is less than 5%, but increases to 10–20% in patients with aneurysms of the ascending aorta. Patients with symptomatic AAA disease often have subclinical coronary disease, with an incidence of almost 50% [16, 17]. However, symptomatic AAAs (i.e. rupture or threatened rupture) usually require emergent treatment before coronary anatomy can be delineated. Simultaneous CABG and AAA repair is therefore an uncommon procedure, but may be considered in very select patients.

A potential advantage of combined CABG / AAA is the ability to scavenge shed blood while the aneurysm is being repaired, assuming that the CABG procedure is performed with CPB. It is also possible to place the abdominal aortic clamp across a depressurized aorta, simply by temporarily decreasing CPB flow. Performing the aortic procedure during CPB support also avoids the rise in left ventricular afterload caused by aortic clamping. Although combined CABG / AAA procedures have been described in the literature over many years, percutaneous stent-graft treatment is becoming increasingly common in such high-risk patients. Currently there is not enough data to support evidence-based recommendations for a combined intervention. Furthermore, prophylactic coronary revascularization prior to major vascular surgery has not been shown to be beneficial in a prospective randomized trial [18]. We currently recommend endovascular repair of AAA prior to CABG surgery in most patients with synchronous disease, reserving combined surgery only for those patients with unsuitable anatomy for endovascular repair.

Diagnosis of AAA

1. History: usually asymptomatic, but patients may have back or abdominal pain.
2. Physical examination: palpation of a pulsatile abdominal mass, signs of peripheral ischemia in presence of additional aortoiliac occlusive disease.
3. Imaging: ultrasound, CT, MR, or conventional angiography. CT angiography is becoming the method of choice because it demonstrates the size and location of the aneurysm (e.g. infra-

renal vs. suprarenal) and the status of major branches (e.g. inferior mesenteric artery). Conventional angiography is considered when CT angiography is inconclusive.

Indications for Combined AAA Repair and CABG

1. Otherwise healthy patient with low perioperative risk.
2. AAA > 5 cm which can be repaired with either a straight tube graft or aorto-bi-iliac graft replacement.
3. Significant CAD requiring surgical intervention (e.g. severe left main stenosis).
4. AAA not anatomically suitable for endovascular repair.

Operative Technique

1. Use antifibrinolytic agents to minimize postoperative bleeding.
2. Perform CABG first. Maintain high perfusion pressures (>70 mmHg) during CPB in order to minimize end-organ ischemia.
3. Following coronary artery grafting, the abdomen is opened and aneurysm is repaired while the patient is on CPB, but with the heart beating.

Postoperative Care

1. Maintain blood pressure between 100 and 120 mmHg for the first 6 h. Consider higher pressures if there is evidence of renal hypoperfusion.
2. The nasogastric tube should be maintained at least for 2 or 3 days, or until there is evidence of normal gastrointestinal peristalsis.
3. Optimize fluid administration as significant amounts are lost to the intra-abdominal third space.
4. Observe respiratory function closely after extubation as there may be some degree of compromise due to intra-abdominal swelling and pain.

5. Maintain adequate urine output.
6. Beware of excessive fluid requirements or falling hematocrit, suggestive of occult intra-abdominal or retroperitoneal bleeding.

Outcomes

Combined CABG and AAA resection is an uncommon procedure, even more so in the current era of increasing endovascular repairs. Therefore, most studies in the literature contain small numbers of patients. Operative mortality is significantly elevated, approximately 10%. Causes of mortality include MI, low cardiac output syndrome, and coagulopathy. Prolonged ventilatory support (>48 h) is also very common, occurring in approximately one-third of patients. Four-year survival is acceptable at 75% [18].

References

1. Van der Heyden J, Suttorp MJ, Bal ET, et al. Staged carotid angioplasty and stenting followed by cardiac surgery in patients with severe asymptomatic carotid artery stenosis: early and long-term results. Circulation. 2007;116:2036–43.
2. Tarakji KG, Sabik JF III, Bhudia SK, et al. Temporal onset, risk factors, and outcomes associated with stroke after coronary artery bypass grafting. JAMA. 2011;305:381–90.
3. Walker MD, Marler JR, Goldstein M, Grady PA, et al. Endarterectomy for asymptomatic carotid artery stenosis. JAMA. 1995;273(18):1421–8.
4. Halliday A, Harrison M, Hayter E, et al. Asymptomatic Carotid Surgery Trial (ACST) Collaborative Group 10-year stroke prevention after successful carotid endarterectomy for asymptomatic stenosis (ACST-1): a multicentre randomised trial. Lancet. 2010;376(9746):1074–84.
5. Brott TG, et al. 2011 ASA/ACCF/AHA/AANN/ AANS/ACR/ASNR/CNS/   SAIP/SCAI/SIR/SNIS/ SVM/SVS guideline on the management of patients with extracranial carotid and vertebral artery disease: a report of the American College of Cardiology Foundation/American Heart Association Task Force on practice guidelines, and the American Stroke Association, American Association of Neuroscience Nurses, American Association of Neurological Surgeons, American College of Radiology, American Society of Neuroradiology, Congress of Neurological Surgeons ... . J Am Coll Cardiol. 2011;57.8:e16–94.
6. Weimar C, Bilbilis K, Rekowski J, et al. Safety of simultaneous coronary artery bypass grafting and carotid endarterectomy versus isolated coronary artery bypass grafting: a randomized clinical trial. Stroke. 2017;48(10):2769–75.
7. Ghosh J, Murray D, Khwaja N, et al. The influence of asymptomatic significant carotid disease on mortality and morbidity in patients undergoing coronary artery bypass surgery. Eur J Vasc Endovasc Surg. 2005;29:88–90.
8. Mahmoudi M, Hill PC, Xue Z, et al. Patients with severe asymptomatic carotid artery stenosis do not have a higher risk of stroke and mortality after coronary artery bypass surgery. Stroke. 2011;42:2801–5.
9. Minami K, Fukahara K, Boethig D, et al. Long-term results of simultaneous carotid endarterectomy and myocardial revascularization with cardiopulmonary bypass used for both procedures. J Thorac Cardiovasc Surg. 2000;119:764–73.
10. Bonacchi M, Prifti E, Frati G, et al. Concomitant carotid endarterectomy and coronary bypass surgery: should cardiopulmonary bypass be used for the carotid procedure? J Cardiac Surg. 2002;17:51–9.
11. Yadav JS, Wholey MH, Kuntz RE, et al. Protected carotid-artery stenting versus endarterectomy in high-risk patients. N Engl J Med. 2004;351:1493–501.
12. Brott TG, Hobson RW 2nd, Howard G, et al. Stenting versus endarterectomy for treatment of carotid-artery stenosis. N Engl J Med. 2010;363:11–23.
13. Borger MA, Fremes SE, Weisel RD, et al. Coronary bypass and carotid endarterectomy: does combined approach increase risk? A meta-analysis. Ann Thorac Surg. 1999;68:14–21.
14. Shishehbor MH, Venkatachalam S, Sun Z, et al. A direct comparison of early and late outcomes with three approaches to carotid revascularization and open heart surgery. J Am Coll Cardiol. 2013;62(21):1948–56.
15. Mahmud E, Reeves R. Carotid revascularization before open heart surgery. J Am Coll Cardiol. 2013;62(21):1957–9.
16. Kioka Y, Tanabe A, Kotani Y, et al. Review of coronary artery disease in patients with infrarenal abdominal aortic aneurysm. Circ J. 2002;66:1110–2.
17. Garofalo M, Nardi P, Borioni R, et al. The impact of coronary revascularization on long-term outcomes after surgical repair of abdominal aortic aneurysm. Ital Heart J. 2005;6(Suppl):369–74.
18. McFalls EO, Ward HB, Moritz TE, et al. Coronary artery revascularization before elective major vascular surgery. N Engl J Med. 2004;351:2795–804.

Surgery for Mechanical Complications of Myocardial Infarction

45

Tirone David

Main Messages

1. Mechanical complications of myocardial infarction include cardiac rupture, mitral regurgitation, and left ventricular aneurysm.
2. The most common site of a cardiac rupture is the free wall of the left ventricle, followed by the interventricular septum (rupture of the interventricular septum causes ventricular septal defect).
3. Surgical options include myocardial revascularization and mitral valve replacement and patch repair.

Cardiac rupture, mitral regurgitation (MR) and left ventricular aneurysm (LVA) are mechanical complications of myocardial infarction (MI). The natural history of acute myocardial infarction has changed dramatically in hospitalized patients over the past several decades because of pharma-

cological and catheter-based interventions. Cardiac rupture and left ventricular aneurysm were common problems in the early days of cardiac surgery, but they are now rare complications of acute transmural myocardial infarction. Left ventricular aneurysms and ischemic MR are discussed elsewhere in this book.

Rupture of the Free Wall of the Ventricle

The free wall of the left ventricle is the most common site of cardiac rupture following acute transmural MI. It usually occurs 4–5 days after the infarct, but it ranges from hours to several weeks. The lateral ventricular wall is the most common site of rupture and it is more likely to occur in women than men, and in older than younger patients.

The pathogenesis of cardiac ruptures remains unclear. The problem likely begins with infarct expansion, which increases wall tension with further dilation and ultimately rupture. The outcome is determined by the rapidity with which the tear extends through the necrotic muscle, and by the size of the rupture. Large and acute ruptures of the left ventricle free wall cause sudden hemodynamic collapse, profound hypotension, electromechanical dissociation and death within minutes. Small and subacute ruptures may be temporarily sealed by clot or fibrinous pericardial

This chapter is an updated version of Chapter 33, Surgery for Mechanical Complications of Myocardial Infarction. In: Perioperative Care in Cardiac Anesthesia and Surgery by Cheng & David (eds.), published by Lippincott Williams & Wilkins, Philadelphia, PA; 2006. p. 285–88.

T. David (✉)
The University Health Network, Toronto, ON, Canada
e-mail: Tirone.David@uhn.ca

adhesions and may be compatible with life for several hours, days, or even longer. On rare occasion a false aneurysm develops.

Acute rupture of the free wall is invariably fatal. Subacute rupture causes hemopericardium and symptoms and signs of acute tamponade. Unless surgically treated, patients with subacute rupture die within hours or days. Surgical treatment consists of patching the necrotic area with Dacron fabric, bovine or autologous pericardium. Chronic false aneurysms may be treated like true aneurysms if the margins of the infarcted muscle are scarred; however, they also often require a patch to restore left ventricular geometry.

Most reports on myocardial rupture involve a few cases to determine the real operative mortality with these operations. We described 12 patients with acute or chronic false aneurysms who underwent surgical repair and three died. Ten patients had posterior false aneurysm (three had severe mitral regurgitation) and two anterior false aneurysms in 1993.

Post-infarction Ventricular Septal Defect

Rupture of the interventricular septum is the second most common site of cardiac rupture. It causes a ventricular septal defect (VSD). The infarct is always transmural and can be anterior or posterior. The rupture usually occurs between 2 and 4 days after the infarct. Anterior VSD is caused by occlusion of the left anterior descending artery and is located in the distal one-half of the septum. Posterior VSD results from occlusion of the dominant right coronary artery and the rupture is usually located in the proximal one-half of the posterior part of the septum. Posterior VSD is often associated with extensive right ventricular infarction when the right coronary artery is dominant.

Most patients who develop post-infarction VSD go into heart failure and/or cardiogenic shock. For this reason, the best approach is urgent surgery. Patients in cardiogenic shock require stabilization with intra-aortic balloon pump, vasodilators, inotropes and assisted ventilation if necessary. Coronary angiography should be performed immediately after hemodynamic stabilization and surgery soon after. Hemodynamically stable patients should have surgery on an urgent basis because they can deteriorate anytime; once multi-organ failure ensues, mortality rises dramatically.

Surgery consists of myocardial revascularization and repair of the VSD. The original techniques of ruptured septum repair consisted of infarctectomy and reconstruction of the septum with Dacron patches as illustrated in Fig. 45.1.

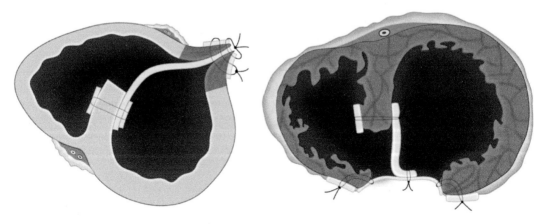

Fig. 45.1 Original techniques of postinfarction VSD repair consisted of infarctectomy and reconstruction of the ventricular wall with Dacron patches

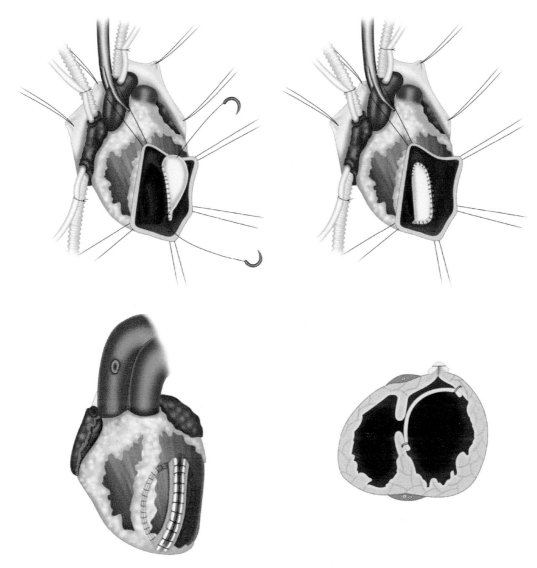

Fig. 45.2 Infarct exclusion technique to repair anterior: an incision is made through the infarcted wall and a patch of pericardium is sutured to exclude the infarcted area

The operative technique of infarct exclusion (Figs. 45.2 and 45.3) was introduced in the mid-1980s, and in our hands, made a major difference in survival, particularly in patients with posterior VSD who historically had a higher operative mortality than anterior VSD.

A report from The Society of Thoracic Surgeons Database on all patients with post-infarction VSD from 1999 to 2010 disclosed 2876 patients operated on at 666 centers in the United States with an average of 0.09–3.7 patients per year, per unit. Thus, very few surgeons operate on more than one patient per year, with the majority operating on one patient with post-infarction VSD every 4 years. For this reason it is difficult to develop expertise in managing and operating on these patients. The operative mortality in that cohort was 54.1% (1077 of 1990) if the repair was performed within 7 days of the MI and 18.4% (158 of 856) if the repair was performed

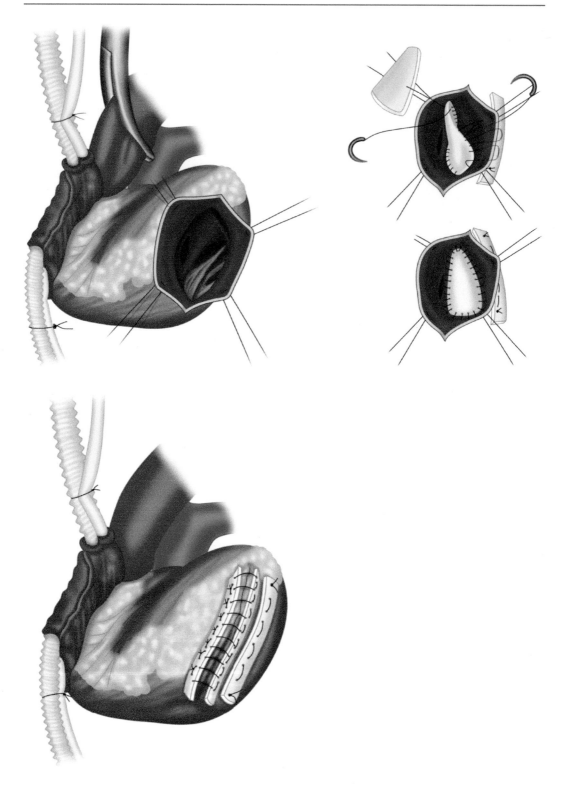

Fig. 45.3 Infarct exclusion technique of posterior VSD

more than 7 days from the MI. In our experience, the operative mortality was dependent on the patient's clinical presentation before surgery. Thus, repair of post-infarction VSD in hemodynamically stable patients was associated with an operative mortality of 10–20%; it was as high as 40–50% in patients in cardiogenic shock. Operative survivors had good long-term survival, particularly if ventricular function was not severely impaired and complete revascularization was performed at the time of the septal repair.

Transcatheter closure of postinfarction VSD using various types of devices has been successful in a small number of patients but it certainly is a promising technique.

Further Reading

1. Radford MJ, et al. Ventricular septal rupture: a review of clinical and physiologic features and an analysis of survival. Circulation. 1981;64:545–53.
2. David TE, Dale L, Sun Z. Postinfarction ventricular septal rupture: repair by endocardial patch with infarction exclusion. J Thorac Cardiovasc Surg. 1995;110:1315–22.
3. Arnaoutakis GE, et al. Surgical repair of ventricular septal defect after myocardial infarction: outcomes from The Society of Thoracic Surgeons National Database. Ann Thorac Surg. 2012;94:436–44.
4. Heiberg J, et al. Long-term outcome after transcatheter closure of postinfarction ventricular septal rupture. J Interv Cardiol. 2014;27:509–15.

Surgery for End-Stage Heart Disease and Heart Transplantation

46

Vivek Rao

Main Messages

1. Cardiac transplantation remains the gold-standard for the treatment of end-stage heart failure in eligible patients.
2. In surgical candidates, surgical revascularization and an appropriately performed left ventricular reconstruction procedure can provide survival benefit.
3. Perioperative management including myocardial protection, judicious fluid management, and attention to renal function is imperative in these high risk patients.

Congestive heart failure remains the only cardiovascular diagnosis increasing in prevalence in the developed world. The gold standard for the treatment of end-stage heart disease not amenable to any other form of conventional therapy is cardiac transplantation [1]. Unfortunately, limited organ availability precludes heart transplantation for many patients who would otherwise benefit from this therapy. Therefore, several centers have re-evaluated the role of high-risk surgical "alternatives" to transplantation. Although few of these procedures

V. Rao (✉)
Peter Munk Cardiac Centre, Toronto General Hospital, Toronto, ON, Canada
e-mail: vivek.rao@uhn.ca

have been evaluated formally for long term durability, the potential to delay the need for transplantation for even a few years is appealing. For centers with the resources to provide mechanical circulatory support (see Chap. 48), high-risk interventions can be performed in patients with ventricular assist device (VAD) backup [2].

Most patients in this population suffer from ischemic cardiomyopathy and may potentially benefit from one or more of the following "conventional" procedures: coronary artery bypass grafting (CABG), mitral valve repair/replacement, and left ventricular reconstruction.

Diagnosis

The role of ischemia in patients with end-stage cardiomyopathy remains controversial [3]. In the absence of any other known causes for heart failure (i.e. acute myocarditis, flail mitral valve), coronary angiography is recommended to rule out underlying coronary artery disease (CAD). Often, CAD is diffuse and wide-spread and not amenable to conventional revascularization. However, even in the presence of graftable CAD, the decision to operate on a patient with severe left ventricular dysfunction can be difficult. The STICH (Surgical Therapy for Ischemic Congestive Heart failure) trial was a large, multicenter, international trial designed to specifically address the benefits of revascularization +/− left ventricular reconstruction in patients with ischemic cardiomyopathy [4, 5]. The primary results of the trial were reported in 2009 and 2011 for the Hypothesis 2 and 1 arms respectively. A follow-up study (STICHES or STICH–extended study) was recently published in 2016 and extended the observations in the Hypothesis 1 arm [6].

Hypothesis 1 tested the efficacy of surgical revascularization over medical therapy, while Hypothesis 2 evaluated the added benefits of surgical ventricular reconstruction. The initial Hypothesis 1 results published in 2011 were confounded by the large number of patients who crossed over from medical therapy to surgery within the first year after randomization. As a result, the intention to treat analysis was negative; however, the as-treated analysis demonstrated a benefit to surgery. Interestingly, the results from the follow-up STICHES study demonstrated a significant benefit to surgery even with an intention to treat analysis. Compared to optimal medical therapy, surgical intervention reduced overall mortality, cardiovascular mortality and rehospitalizations due to heart failure (Fig. 46.1). Perhaps most striking are the various sub-studies that demonstrate the benefit of surgical intervention regardless of symptom state, underlying LV function, the presence of viability, or induced ischemia [7, 8].

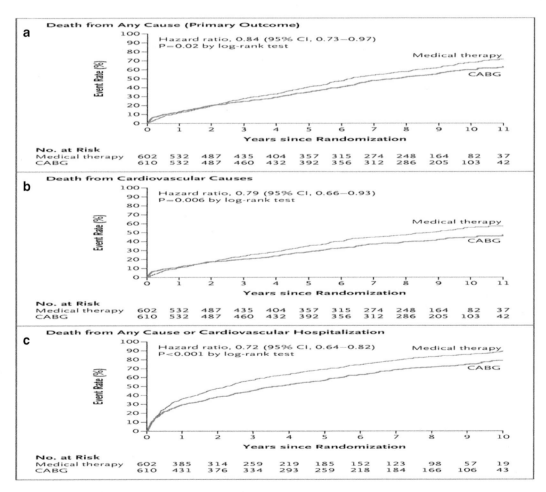

Fig. 46.1 Surgical revascularization versus optimal medical therapy in the STICHES (Surgical Treatment of Ischemic Congestive Heart Failure—Extended Study) trial. Surgery resulted in significant reductions in mortality and cardiovascular readmissions (reprinted with permission from Velasquez E, et al. N Engl J Med)

When CAD is amenable to surgical revascularization, most centers advocate risk stratification with viability testing. The most reliable tests for viability are Positron Emission Tomography (PET), employing radioactive carbohydrates (FDG), or Magnetic Resonance Imaging (MRI) with gadolinium infusion. Delayed enhancement with gadolinium implies fixed, non-viable tissue. In addition to the viability assessments, MRI provides intricate details about cardiac structure and function, and can differentiate between ischemic dyskinetic segments of viable myocardium and true aneurysmal formation. While the presence of viability or induced ischemia reduces the risk of surgery (and conversely increases the benefit), STICHES demonstrated that surgery provides benefit even in their absence. However, these tests are important when deciding to intervene on marginal candidates. For example, an otherwise healthy patient with good graftable targets but no viability should still be offered surgery. In contrast, a patient with multiple comorbidities and no viability or inducible ischemia should likely be managed medically. However, surgery should be considered if this same high risk patient has evidence of viability and/or inducible ischemia.

Transthoracic echocardiography provides invaluable information with respect to global and regional ventricular function, valvular morphology and function, and transverse/descending aortic atheroma. TEE should be a routine intraoperative adjunct for all surgical procedures in patients with end-stage heart failure.

For transplant eligibility, several screening tests are performed to identify significant comorbidities which may preclude successful transplantation [1]. Table 46.1 lists the most commonly performed screening evaluations.

Although each transplant program may have their own criteria for transplant eligibility, there are a few standard contraindications: (1) Fixed pulmonary hypertension, defined arbitrarily as >4 Woods units, a mean transpulmonary gradient (mean pulmonary arterial pressure – pulmonary capillary wedge pressure) >14 mmHg, or a systolic pulmonary to systemic artery pressure ratio >0.5; (2) recent (<5 years) malignancy; (3) active

Table 46.1 Commonly performed screening investigations to assess candidacy for heart transplantation

Routine	Additional
Consultations	
Cardiology	Dental Surgery
Cardiovascular Surgery	Chaplaincy
Psychiatry	Respirology
Social Work	Transplant Immunology
Transplant Coordinator	Transplant ID
Anesthesia	Hepatology
	Neurology
	Hematology/Oncology
	Gastroenterology
Investigations	
Right and Left Heart Catheterization	Liver Biopsy
Transthoracic Echocardiogram	Nerve Conduction Study
Electrocardiogram	GI Endoscopy
Pulmonary function tests	Bone marrow examination
Arterial blood gases	Chest CT
Chest X-ray	Abdominal US or CT
Cardiopulmonary Exercise Testing	
Laboratory tests	
ABO blood type and screen	Protein electrophoresis
CBC, ESR, smear, reticulate	Stool for parasites, C&S, blood
PT, PTT, INR, bleeding time	
Electrolytes, Creatinine	
Urinalysis, 24 h Creatinine Clearance	
Thyroid function tests	
Liver function tests	
Blood glucose (fasting, 2 h PC)	
Cholesterol, triglycerides	
Antibody screen (HBV, HCV, HIV)	
HLA typing	
Anti-HLA antibodies (PRA panel)	
Antibody titres (CMV, EBV, HSV, Toxo)	

systemic infection; (4) major systemic illness (i.e. diabetes, amyloidosis, hemochromatosis); and (5) other end-organ failure. Relative contraindications include peripheral vascular disease, age > 65, emotional instability, and demonstrated lack of compliance to medical regimens. It is important to realize that most patients would still benefit from cardiac transplantation, but that the chronic shortage of suitable donor organs forces transplant programs to rationalize care to those patients most likely to derive long-term benefit. Potential candidates are assessed by a multidisciplinary committee to allow for the equitable distribution of these scarce resources.

Surgical Techniques

CABG

STICHES has now proven the benefit of revascularization in patients with isolated heart failure symptoms without angina [6]. Often, the left anterior descending artery (LAD) is completely occluded, and even if graftable, supplies infarcted territory. Therefore, the author prefers to employ the LITA graft to an important lateral wall target. Similarly, the right coronary artery (RCA) is often found to be diffusely diseased or chronically occluded with no discernible targets. In these instances, an acute marginal branch can often be found which supplies important perfusion to the right ventricular free wall and interventricular septum.

Meticulous delivery of cardioplegia is extremely important in these cases as patients have little reserve for inadequate myocardial protection. Retrograde cardioplegia may be beneficial, especially in cases where the LAD is chronically occluded. The use of special induction or reperfusion strategies, such as terminal hot shots or amino-acid enriched reperfusates, may also be of benefit (see Chap. 34).

Mitral Valve Repair

Patients with congestive heart failure often have evidence of significant mitral insufficiency. The mitral valve leaflets are normal, or at most mildly thickened in the majority of patients. The mechanism leading to mitral insufficiency is usually annular dilatation and/or chordal tethering.

Bolling and colleagues have reported encouraging results with mitral valve repair in patients with poor ejection fraction due to a variety of etiologies [9]. However, the durability of these procedures remains uncertain as the 2 year freedom from recurrent MR is only 70%. Two recent NIH-sponsored trials evaluated the role of mitral valve surgery in moderate and severe ischemic regurgitation [10, 11]. The moderate MR study demonstrated no additional benefit to mitral repair in addition to surgical revascularization, although there was less residual MR in the repair group [10]. The severe MR trial compared repair to replacement and found no significant differences in the primary outcome of LV size; however, recurrent MR was much more likely in the repair arm [11]. Therefore, these results suggest that mitral repair be considered in patients with moderate functional MR, but that formal mitral valve replacement with preservation of the subvalvular apparatus is preferred for more severe regurgitation.

In patients with coexisting renal insufficiency (a common comorbidity in this patient population) the benefits of mitral valve repair must be weighed against the risk of a prolonged and complex operation. Certainly, if there is evidence of myxomatous disease in one or both leaflets suggesting the need for a complex repair, one may elect to proceed with formal mitral valve replacement with preservation of all subvalvular structures.

Left Ventricular Reconstruction

The role of LV reconstruction for patients with true or false aneurysms of the left ventricle is clearly established. However, for patients with akinetic areas comprising a mixture of muscle and scar tissue, the role of left ventricular repair is less defined. The second major hypothesis of the STICH trial was to determine the role of LV reconstruction for patients with ischemic cardiomyopathy [4]. The initial report by Jones et al suggested that there was absolutely no benefit to the addition of LV reconstruction in patients undergoing surgical revascularization for ischemic cardiomyopathy. This report generated a large amount of controversy due to the inconsistencies in patient recruitment (not all patients had an adequate assessment of anterior wall viability) and the performance of the reconstruction (LV volume reduction was a fraction of that observed in the RESTORE registry) [12].

The DOR procedure was initially described in 1989 [13]. Most surgeons now employ a modification of the originally described technique in which the LV defect is plicated with a purse-string suture prior to patch closure. Mickleborough and colleagues have also reported promising clinical results using a modified linear closure [14]. Figures 46.2 and 46.3 illustrate the DOR repair and the Mickleborough closure.

A subsequent sub-study of STICH by Michler and colleagues demonstrated that an adequately performed LV reconstruction led to survival benefit in the STICH population [15]. Those patients who displayed a postoperative LVESVI of less than 70 ml/m^2 had a lower 4 year mortality compared to those patients who received CABG alone (Fig. 46.4). Thus, as in almost all aspects of cardiac surgery, a procedure is only beneficial if it is done correctly and in the appropriate patients. Based upon this data, we continue to offer LV reconstruction to those patients with a dilated LV and a large area of non-viable anterior wall. We strive to reduce the predicted postoperative LVESVI to less than 70 ml/m^2.

Transplantation

Experimental organ transplantation began in the early 1900s with the work of Dr. Charles Guthrie and Dr. Alexis Carrel on extrathoracic heterotopic canine transplant. Until the development of cardiopulmonary bypass in 1958, the technique for orthotopic cardiac transplantation could not be perfected. Critical research by Shumway's group at Stanford paved the way for the first human transplant performed by Barnard in 1967.

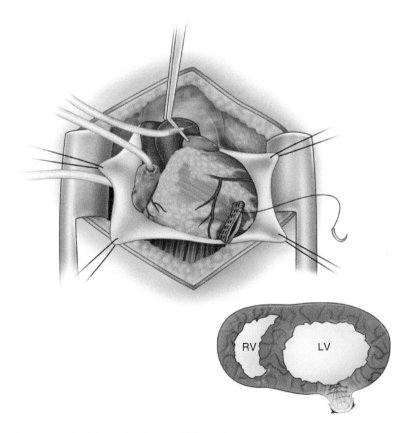

Fig. 46.2 Modified linear (Mickleborough) closure of left ventricular aneurysms

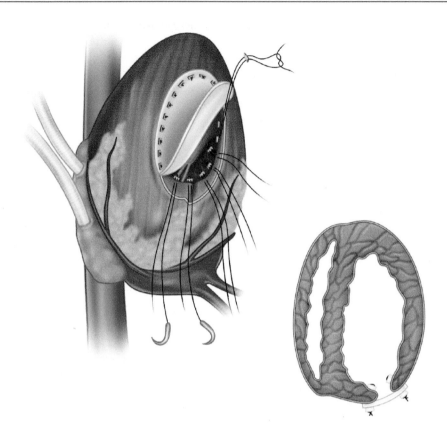

Fig. 46.3 Modified DOR repair of left ventricular aneurysms

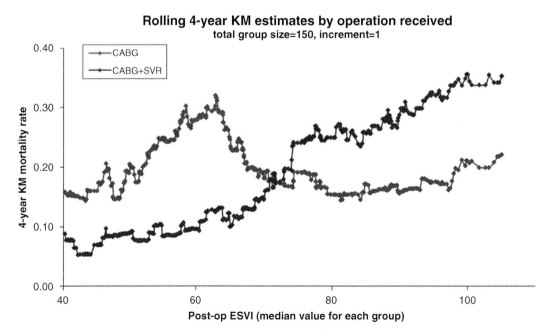

Fig. 46.4 The importance of a complete LV reconstruction. Patients who achieved a postoperative left ventricular end-systolic volume index (LVESVI) of less than 70 ml/m² displayed significantly lower 4 year mortality (reprinted with permission from Michler RE, et al. J Thorac Cardiovasc Surg)

After an initial flurry of activity, the procedure became virtually abandoned due to recalcitrant rejection and infection. The introduction of cyclosporine in the 1970s revolutionized all solid organ transplants and ushered in the second era of heart transplantation.

More recently, the field has been energized by the introduction of heart transplantation from donors who have suffered circulatory arrest, in contrast to the more traditional donors who have had neurologic determination of death. At present, donation after circulatory determination of death requires ex-vivo cardiac perfusion to assess and evaluate the grafts function prior to implant [16].

The initial technique described by Shumway consisted of a biatrial anastomosis employing a cuff of recipient left and right atria. Advances in suture technology and surgical technique has led to the adoption of the cava-cava technique and in some centers, complete orthotopic transplantation with cuffs of left and right pulmonary veins sewn to the donor left atrium (Fig. 46.5).

Perioperative Considerations

Regardless of the surgical intervention involved, patients with end-stage heart disease require careful attention to perioperative fluid and blood product administration. In patients presenting in florid heart failure and gross volume overload, consideration should be made to delay operative intervention until renal, pulmonary and cardiac function is optimized. When emergency surgery is required, it is often useful to incorporate a hemodialysis or ultrafiltration circuit in the cardiopulmonary bypass circuit to achieve significant hemoconcentration and avoid the detrimental effects of perioperative anemia. For potential transplant candidates, consideration must be made of the immunologic costs of blood product utilization. Platelet transfusions in particular can lead to HLA sensitization and greatly increase the risk of rejection episodes.

Although most patients present with evidence of left ventricular dysfunction, right ventricular failure is a devastating and highly fatal

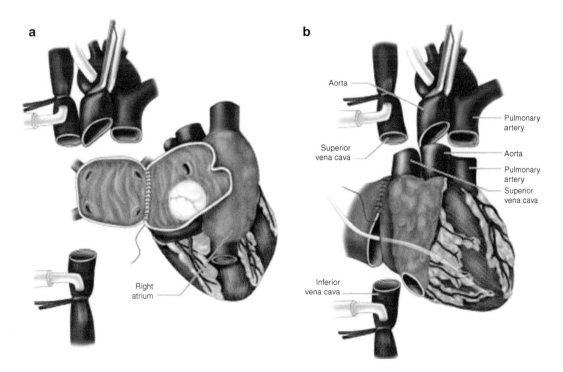

Fig. 46.5 Bicaval technique for orthotopic heart transplantation

complication. Meticulous detail to hemostasis will minimize blood product utilization. The cytokine release associated with transfusion has been directly correlated to right ventricular failure. Inadequate myocardial protection may also lead to significant right ventricular dysfunction (especially in situations where the RCA territory is incompletely revascularized). The author prefers a strategy of preventing RV failure as opposed to treating a hemodynamically labile patient. The prophylactic use of milrinone, a phosphodiesterase inhibitor, has proven to be a useful adjunct in these critically ill patients. A loading dose of 3–5 mg is delivered directly into the pump circuit at the onset of reperfusion. The hypotension associated with this loading dose is usually manageable with increased pump flow rates or intermittent vasoconstrictor support. If needed, a continuous infusion can be initiated during the attempt to wean from cardiopulmonary bypass.

As mentioned previously, renal insufficiency is a common comorbid condition in this patient population. To date, there have been no successful renal protective strategies validated in prospective, randomized clinical trials. Nevertheless, many institutions tend to administer low dose dopamine (2–4 µg/kg/min) throughout cardiopulmonary bypass and in the early postoperative period. Other strategies currently under investigation include N-acetylcysteine and vasopressin infusions, pulsatile cardiopulmonary bypass flows, and the BNP analogue nesiritide.

References

1. Mehra MR, Canter CE, Hannan MM, et al. The 2016 International Society for Heart Lung Transplantation listing criteria for Heart Transplantation: a 10 year update. J Heart Lung Transplant. 2016;35:1–23.
2. Kawajiri H, Manlhiot C, Ross H, et al. High risk cardiac surgery as an alternative to transplant or mechanical support in patients with end-stage heart failure. J Thorac Cardiovasc Surg. 2017;154:517–25.
3. Doenst T, Velazquez EJ, Beyersdorf F, et al. The STICH Investigators. To STICH or not TO STICH—We know the answer, but do we understand the question? J Thorac Cardiovasc Surg 2005; 129: 246-249
4. Jones RH, Velazquez EJ, Michler RE, et al. The STICH Investigators. Coronary bypass surgery with or without surgical ventricular reconstruction. N Engl J Med. 2009;360:1705–1171
5. Velazquez EJ, Lee KL, Deja M, et al. Coronary-artery bypass surgery in patients with left ventricular dysfunction. N Engl J Med. 2011;364:1607–16.
6. Velazquez EJ, Lee KL, Jones RH, et al. Coronary-artery bypass surgery in patients with ischemic cardiomyopathy. N Engl J Med. 2016;374:1511–20.
7. Bonow RO, Maurer JG, Lee KL, et al. Myocardial viability and survival in ischemic left ventricular dysfunction. N Engl J Med. 2011;364:1617–25.
8. Panza JA, Holly TA, Asch FM, et al. Inducible myocardial ischemia and outcomes in patients with coronary artery disease and left ventricular dysfunction. J Am Coll Cardiol. 2013;61:1860–70.
9. Romano MA, Bolling SF. An update on mitral repair in dilated cardiomyopathy. J Card Surg. 2004;19:396–400.
10. Michler RE, Smith PK, Parides MK, et al. Two year outcomes of surgical treatment of moderate ischemic mitral regurgitation. N Engl J Med. 2016;374:1932–41.
11. Goldstein D, Moskowitz AJ, Gelijns AC, et al. Two year outcomes of surgical treatment of severe ischemic mitral regurgitation. N Engl J Med. 2016;374:344–35.
12. Athanasuleas CL, Buckberg GD, Stanley AW, et al. Surgical ventricular restoration: The Restore Group Experience. Heart Fail Rev. 2004;9:287–97.
13. Dor V, Saab M, Coste P, Kornaszewska M, Montiglio F. Left ventricular aneurysm: a new surgical approach. Thorac Cardiovasc Surg. 1989;37:11–9.
14. Mickleborough LL, Merchant N, Ivanov J, Rao V, Carson S. Left ventricular reconstruction: early and late results. J Thorac Cardiovasc Surg. 2004;128:27–37.
15. Michler RE, Rouleau JL, Al-Khalidi HR, et al. Insights from the STICH trial: change in ventricular size after coronary artery bypass grafting with or without surgical ventricular reconstruction. J Thorac Cardiovasc Surg. 2013;146:1139–45.
16. Dhital KK, Iyer A, Connellan M, et al. Adult heart transplantation with distant procurement and ex-vivo preservation of donor hearts after circulatory death: a case series. Lancet. 2015;385:2585–91.

Lung and Heart-Lung Transplantation: Surgical Technique and Postoperative Considerations

47

Andrea Mariscal, Marcelo Cypel,
and Shaf Keshavjee

Main Messages
1. Outcomes following transplantation are impacted by donor characteristics.
2. Donor management standardization has had positive impact on organ utilization rates.
3. Clinical, psychological, and social features are all considered when patients are put on a lung transplant waitlist.
4. Postoperative care of a lung or heart-lung transplant patient should be managed by an interdisciplinary team including transplant surgeons, transplant pulmonologists, intensivists, infectious disease specialists, transplant coordinators, nurses, pharmacologists, physical therapists, nutritionists, pain management specialists, and social workers.

A. Mariscal · M. Cypel · S. Keshavjee (✉)
Toronto Lung Transplant Program,
Toronto General Hospital,
University Health Network,
University of Toronto, Toronto, ON, Canada
e-mail: shaf.keshavjee@uhn.ca

Donor

Donor Selection Criteria

It is well known that the donor characteristics can have an impact on short and long-term outcomes after transplantation. The criteria for ideal lung donors are described in Table 47.1. These criteria were established in the early days of lung transplantation. These include among others: donor age under 55, smoking history of less than 20 pack-years, clear chest x-ray, arterial partial pressure of oxygen (PaO_2/FiO_2) ratio greater than 300 mmHg, no history of chest trauma or cardiopulmonary surgery and absence of microorganisms in sputum gram stain [1]. Since then, most of the large transplant centers have adapted to include extended criteria donors to be able to enlarge the donor pool. There is a lack of prospective controlled studies that establish the exact risk and limits of using more extended-criteria donor lungs, but most centers now support their use based on studies showing similar outcomes [2, 3]. It is always important to balance the risk of death on waiting list when choosing to use extended criteria donors [4–6].

Donor Management

Lungs are especially vulnerable organs in terms of donor management. Only 15–25% of poten-

© Springer Nature Switzerland AG 2021
D. C. H. Cheng et al. (eds.), *Evidence-Based Practice in Perioperative Cardiac Anesthesia and Surgery*, https://doi.org/10.1007/978-3-030-47887-2_47

tially recoverable lungs are transplanted [7]. Brain death donors, which are the majority of the donors that are currently being used for lung transplantation, are at high risk of developing pulmonary injury [8]. The process of brain death induces a systemic inflammatory response by liberating pro-inflammatory factors. There is also a release of catecholamine as an attempt to increase cerebral perfusion, which translates into systemic hypertension and high left side heart pressure which can exacerbate the neurogenic pulmonary edema [9, 10]. Ventilator induced injury, injury related to gastric aspiration, and ventilator associated pneumonia are other common occurrences that can further affect the lung quality and compromise the potential donor lung [8].

The standardization of donor management has been shown to have positive results in terms of organ utilization rates [11, 12]. Goals in donor management during the pre-recovery phase have been established and they are mostly related to maintaining donor hemodynamic stability in order to be able to preserve as many organs as possible for transplantation. These goals include: mean airway pressure, oxygenation, pH, electrolytes, urine output, with single vasopressor and central venous pressure [11].

For thoracic organs, minimization of vasopressor use and avoiding high partial pressures of oxygen have been shown to have an important effect on utilization rates according to a study published by Franklin et al in 2010 [11].

In 2013 Munshi et al. reviewed donor management in the ICU and preservation in lung transplant and they summarized the following recommendations to maximize the donor pool : ventilation with tidal volume (V_T) of 6–8 ml/kg; fraction of inspired oxygen (FiO_2) 50%; positive end expiratory pressure (PEEP) of 5–10 cm H_2O; central venous pressure of 6–8 mmHg; vasopressin as initial vasopressor (with norepinephrine, epinephrine or phenylephrine as second line treatment in case of hemodynamic instability); and methylprednisolone and other hormone therapy replacement [8]. The technique of lung preservation followed by the Toronto Lung Transplant Program is summarized in Table 47.1.

Table 47.1 Technique of lung preservation followed by the Toronto Lung Transplant Program

Technique of lung preservation	
Donor lung protection	
Methylprednisolone	2 g IV to donor
Perfadex® (LPD, Low Potassium Dextran) solution	50 ml/kg, 4 °C pulmonary artery flush
PGE₁	500 mg direct injection into pulmonary artery
PGE₁	500 mg in flush solution
Lungs are stored at 4 °C in the inflated state ($FiO_2 > 0.5$) for transport	
Intraoperative lung protection	
Keep lung cool using a cooling jacket during implantation	
Clear blood and secretions and *gently* reinflate (25 cm H_2O) prior to reperfusion	
Gradually release pulmonary artery clamp over 10 min (modified reperfusion technique)	
Wash out flush solution and de-air through atrial anastomosis	

Donor Surgery

Before starting the donor procedure, a bronchoscopy should be performed to clear secretions and look for signs of infection, aspiration or lesions that can compromise the lung. After the bronchoscopy and during the donor surgery, the donor should be ventilated using FiO_2 50%, PEEP of 5 cm H_2O and V_T of 8 ml/kg. A median sternotomy incision is performed, pleural spaces are examined, and a complete recruitment is performed by gently massaging the lungs while the anesthesiologist inflates them to a sustained pressure of up to 30 cm H_2O. Deflation capacity is evaluated by recruiting the lungs with 20–30 cmH_2O for 30 s followed by disconnecting the endotracheal tube to room air. After this assessment, the retrieval surgeon updates the findings along with the estimated cross-clamp time to the recipient surgeon.

The pericardium is opened, the superior vena cava is dissected and encircled using a 0-silk tie, and the ascending aorta is separated from the pulmonary artery (PA). To secure the PA flush cannula, a purse string suture of 4-0 polypropylene suture is placed in the PA (halfway between the

PA valve and the bifurcation). Approximately 5 min before cannulation, heparin (300 IU/kg) is given to the donor. At that time, the cold low potassium dextran solution (LPD) (Perfadex®) containing PGE_1 (500 mcg) should be prepared and hung 30 cm above the level of the heart. Three to 5 min after the heparin is given, the PA cannula is inserted into the PA making sure the tip of the cannula is located proximal to the PA bifurcation; the PA cannula is then connected to the perfusion line. A bolus of prostaglandin E_1 (500 mcg in 10 ml normal saline) is injected directly into the main PA. After the PGE_1 administration, the blood pressure should drop; the aorta is then cross-clamped, the superior vena cava is ligated, and the inferior vena cava is transected above the diaphragm. The tip of the left atrial appendage is transected to vent the left atrium. The preservation flush is initiated. The LPD solution is drained into the pleural space providing topical cooling to the lungs. After four liters of anterograde flushing, the flush solution usually appears clear and both lungs look blanched.

After completing the pulmonary flush, the heart is excised first. The PA is transected at the point of the PA cannulation site. The aorta, IVC and SVC are transected. The pulmonary veins are exposed by lifting the heart, and the left atrium incision is initiated midway between the right inferior pulmonary vein and the coronary sinus. The incision is then extended under direct vision maintaining the pulmonary veins in sight at all times, making sure an appropriate atrial cuff is left on the left atrium of the heart as well as on the pulmonary vein cuff on the lung side. After the heart is removed from the surgical field, a one liter retrograde flush of the lung with LPD is performed using an 18-20 French inflated Foley catheter to deliver 250 ml into each of the pulmonary veins.

After the retrograde flush, the inferior pulmonary ligaments are divided, the esophagus is localized, and the dissection continues following the anterior wall of the esophagus all the way to the aorta on the left side and the azygos vein on the right side; both are transected. The trachea is encircled after mobilizing all mediastinal tissue.

The trachea is stapled twice with a TA-30 stapler after a recruitment with an FiO_2 of 50% and a sustained airway pressure of approximately 15–20 cmH_2O. At the time of stapling, the lungs should be about 75% inflated. The trachea is transected between the two stapler lines to avoid field contamination. The lungs are placed in a triple bag with three liters of 4 °C Perfadex®. This bag is then placed on ice in a cooler for transportation.

Special Considerations for Donation After Cardiac Death (DCD) Lung Retrieval

While the withdrawal of life support is performed (usually in the ICU) the donor retrieval team waits in the operating room. The donor usually receives heparin (500–1000 U/kg) 5–10 min before withdrawal, a nasogastric tube should be inserted, and the donor head of the bed should be elevated to avoid aspiration after the donor extubation. The donor is transferred to the OR after declaration of death. As soon as the donor arrives in the operating room, they are re-intubated and standard donor ventilation (V_T of 8–10 ml/kg, FiO_2 of 50% PEEP of 5 cm H_2O) is initiated. A rapid bronchoscopy is performed to clear secretions and evaluate for signs of aspiration. A median sternotomy incision is performed, the pericardium is opened, the PA is cannulated and the lungs are recruited. PGE_1 (500 mcg) is injected into the PA and 3–5 cardiac manual compressions are performed. The pulmonary flush is started and performed the same way as in brain death donors. After the lungs are outside the body the surgeon examines them carefully.

Recipient Back Table: Donor Lung Dissection

Lungs are placed in a basin, and two towels wet with Perfadex® are used to wrap the lungs to keep them cool, while exposing the hilum and middle mediastinal structures. The lungs are separated by dividing the midline between the pulmonary veins and the mediastinal tissue. The airway is divided without dissecting the peribronchial tissue. A GIA 60 stapler is placed across the left bronchus at the carina. The hilar structures are prepared, dissecting the PA until the first branch and trimming it. Finally, at the time of implantation, the bronchus is opened at the stapler line and trimmed to one ring proximal to the lobar bifurcation. Dissection of the peri-bronchial tissue should be avoided, and a flap of peribronchial tissue should be preserved to buttress the anastomosis.

Recipient

Selection of Lung Transplant Candidates

The decision to put a patient on a lung transplant waitlist is complex and involves recipient characteristics including clinical, psychological and social features; as well as considerations regarding the program itself and geographic elements. In 2015 the International Society of Heart and Lung Transplantation published a consensus document for the selection of lung transplant candidates [13]. The general criteria that an adult candidate should have in order to be placed on a wait list include: >50% risk of death from lung disease within 2 years without a lung transplant; >80% of probability of surviving at least 90 days after a lung transplant; and > 60% probability of 5-year survival post-transplant taking into consideration the overall medical condition.

Absolute contraindications for a lung transplant include: history of recent malignancy (less than 2 years for a low risk of recurrence malignancy or less than 5 years for other types of cancer); untreatable dysfunction of another major organ (unless a combined transplant is the option); uncorrected atherosclerotic heart disease with ischemia or dysfunction (including coronary artery disease that cannot be revascularized); acute myocardial instability (sepsis, myocardial infarction); bleeding diathesis; chronic infection with high virulence or resistant microbes poorly controlled (or active *Mycobacterium Tuberculosis*); severe chest wall or spinal deformity that causes severe restriction; obesity (body mass index >35 kg/m^2); history of non-adherence to medical treatment;

psychiatric or psychological issues that are associated with inability to cooperate; no reliable social structure; functional status severely limited; poor rehabilitation potential; and substance abuse (alcohol, tobacco and other drugs). Relative contraindications include age >75; obesity or malnutrition; severe osteoporosis; history of extensive chest surgery; and patients with highly resistant infections including *Burkholderia cenocepacia*, HIV, Hepatitis B and C (depending on the center's experience), among others.

Recipient Surgery

A radial arterial line and an intravenous line are placed before intubation with a double lumen endotracheal tube. A bronchoscopy is performed to confirm the endotracheal tube position, examine airway anatomy, and obtain baseline microbiological cultures. A central line and a Swan Ganz pulmonary artery (PA) catheter are placed in the neck.

In bilateral lung transplants, the side that receives the least blood flow (determined by a preoperative quantitative pulmonary ventilation and perfusion scan) should be the first to be transplanted, although there are other donor and recipient characteristics that can influence that decision. The chest, abdomen and bilateral groins should be prepped in the sterile field to allow access to the femoral vessels if the patient needs to go on extracorporeal support. For a bilateral lung transplant the patient is positioned supine with arms abducted.

A single lung transplant is performed through a standard posterolateral thoracotomy or through an anterior thoracotomy (this approach has the advantage of having faster access to central cannulation in case of urgent need). Bilateral lung transplant is usually performed through a transverse fourth intercostal space thoracosternotomy (clamshell) but it may also be performed using separate bilateral anterior thoracotomies without dividing the sternum. The mammary vessels are ligated and transected. If the sternum is divided it should be divided transversely with the saw held obliquely to improve stability after the closure with sternal wires.

All adhesions, if present, should be mobilized. A pneumonectomy is performed. During the dissection, extra care should be taken to avoid injuring the phrenic and laryngeal nerve. The PA is dissected first followed by the superior pulmonary vein. The ligament is divided up to the inferior pulmonary vein. The pericardium can be opened if central cannulation is needed. The PA is encircled making sure the Swan-Ganz catheter is not in that side. The PA is manually occluded for a few minutes to test hemodynamic stability. The pulmonary veins are isolated and the first branch of the PA is encircled and tied with 2-0 silk ties and divided. The PA and pulmonary veins are stapled and divided as distally as possible. The bronchus is dissected and transected. The edge is freshed with a scalpel trimming it short and close to the carina. Two 3-0 PDS sutures are placed at the corners between the membranous and the cartilaginous part of the bronchus. The bronchus should be cut short (two rings from the carina). Bleeding from the bronchial vessels is controlled making sure the future blood supply is not compromised. All secretions from inside the bronchus are suctioned.

The bronchial anastomosis is performed first. The donor bronchus is trimmed one ring from the lobar division without trimming the peribronchial tissue. A cooling jacket is placed inside the recipient chest to keep the lung cool during the surgery. It is important to avoid handling the airways as much as possible. The donor bronchial membrano cartilaginous junction is attached to the recipient using the previously placed holding sutures. The membranous part of the bronchus is sutured using a running 4-0 polypropylene suture, and the cartilaginous airway is anastomosed with interrupted 4-0 Prolene sutures placed 2–3 mm apart. A bronchoscopy is performed immediately after finishing the airway anastomosis to inspect its integrity and to suction any blood and secretions.

To perform the PA anastomosis, a vascular clamp is first positioned proximally on the PA, and the staple line is removed. A 5-0 polypropylene suture is placed in each edge of the PA as stay sutures; the position of the first branch should be used to orient the position of the PA to avoid torsion. The anastomosis is performed using the running 5-0 polypropylene suture interrupted in two places in a continuous manner. Before tying the sutures on the front wall, in order to be able to de-air the PA, an angiocatheter is inserted into the PA lumen and 10–15 ml of saline is instilled.

In order to perform the atrial anastomosis, the venous stumps are grasped with Judd-Allice clamps and a left atrial clamp is positioned proximally on the left atrium. The venous staple lines are removed and the orifices are joined to form a single atrial orifice. Two 4-0 polypropylene sutures are placed, one at each corner. The anastomosis is performed using a horizontal everting mattress to perform endothelial to endothelial apposition [14]. The suture is left untied at the anterior midpoint of the anastomosis until reperfusion for de-airing purposes.

The cooling jacket is then removed and the graft is ventilated using a sustained airway pressure of 20 cm H_2O until reperfusion, and then pressure control ventilation mode limiting the peak airway pressure to 15–20 mmHg, $FiO_2 < 50\%$, and PEEP of 5 cm H_2O. After complete expansion of the lung is reached, the PA clamp is partially open to slowly reperfuse the lung guaranteeing protective low pressure to the lung for the first 10 min during reperfusion. The atrial anastomosis suture is tied after de-airing. After completely opening the PA clamp, the patient is ventilated under pressure control mode or with tidal volumes of 5–7 ml/kg and PEEP of 5 cm H_2O.

The patient is allowed to stabilize for 10–15 min before the second lung is implanted in the same manner. Two chest tubes are positioned in each pleural space. Two straight tubes are placed toward the apex in the chest, and the curve chest tubes are placed along the diaphragm on each side.

Hemostasis should be carefully checked before the chest closure. The clamshell incision is closed using four figure of eight intercostal sutures on each side that are tied prior to closing the sternal wires. The sternum is approximated using three sternal wires.

Use of Cardiopulmonary Bypass or Extracorporeal Lung Support (ECLS or ECMO)

Extracorporeal membrane oxygenation (ECMO) is increasingly being used as a bridge to transplant by many lung transplant programs [15, 16]. Less than 40% of patients need cardiopulmonary support during lung transplantation. It is usually limited to patients who are unable to tolerate unilateral ventilation or patients suffering from pulmonary hypertension. There are currently lung transplant centers that use cardiorespiratory support routinely for all lung transplant procedures with reported good outcomes [17]. The routine use of cardiopulmonary devices is justified by the potential beneficial effect of a more controlled reperfusion, ensuring low PA pressures over longer periods of time [18, 19].

Traditionally, cardiopulmonary bypass (CPB) was the cardiorespiratory support device used intraoperatively for lung transplantation; however, extracorporeal lung support (ECLS or ECMO) is currently being used as a standard support technique in more and more centers, providing advantages such as less anticoagulation needed and less systemic inflammatory response, as recently reported by the Toronto Lung Transplant Group [20]. CPB is still required for patients who also need cardiac repair requiring heart arrest or in emergency situations with massive bleeding.

Heart-Lung Transplant Procedure

The heart-lung transplant procedure is performed through a clamshell incision. The clamshell incision gives better exposure to the entire thorax, including the posterior mediastinum and pleural spaces. This exposure has decreased the incidence of postoperative hemorrhage.

For heart-lung transplantation, the patient is cannulated for CPB in the standard fashion (ascendant aorta near the base of the innominate artery and bicaval venous cannulation). CPB is established and the heart is excised. The aorta is cross-clamped and transected just above the level of the valve. The pericardium is opened laterally anterior to and parallel with both phrenic nerves. The posterior wall of the left atrium is divided in the midline between the left and right pulmonary veins. The pulmonary vein and the rest of the left atrial dissection is surgically completed extra-pericardially, posterior to the phrenic nerve pedicles. The PA is divided at the bifurcation and a button of tissue is left on the ductus arteriosus to preserve the recurrent nerve. The pulmonary arteries are dissected laterally. The superior and inferior vena cava are transected well onto the atrium leaving a generous cuff for bicaval anastomoses. Both main bronchi are stapled and divided. The carina and stapled main bronchi are left in situ at this point. Once the heart and both lungs are excised, meticulous hemostasis is achieved while the surgeon has complete exposure of the posterior mediastinal bed.

Once the field is ready for implantation of the heart lung block, the carina is dissected with minimal mobilization of the distal trachea to preserve its blood supply. The trachea is trimmed one ring above the carina. The donor heart-lung block is positioned in the chest. The right lung is placed through the right pericardial window that was created behind the right phrenic nerve and similarly the left lung is slipped into the left chest through the pericardial window on the left side. The tracheal anastomosis is then performed using a running 4-0 PDS suture on the membranous wall and interrupted 3-0 prolene sutures on the cartilaginous wall, in an end-to-end fashion. The pre-tracheal donor and recipient tissues are approximated on the anterolateral aspect of the anastomosis to buttress it. Ventilation is then initiated using a protective mode (low volume—5 ml/kg at a rate of six breaths per min with a FiO_2 of 0.5)

The aorta is anastomosed using a running 4-0 polypropylene suture. Bicaval anastomoses are the preferred anastomosis for the venous side. The heart is aggressively de-aired and the aortic cross-clamp is released. The patient is weaned off CPB. Careful hemostasis is confirmed prior to closure.

Postoperative Care

The postoperative care of the lung (LTx) or heart-lung (HLTx) transplant patient can be challenging, and it should be performed by a multidisciplinary team that includes transplant surgeons, intensivists, transplant pulmonologists, and infectious disease specialists. Transplant coordinators, nurses, pharmacologists, pain management specialists, physical therapists, nutritionists, and social workers are also important members of the team.

Early Postoperative Care

Early postoperative care begins after the transplant while the patient is still in the operating room. During this period, the main areas of focus are hemodynamic management, ventilatory support, immunosuppression, and prevention of infection. After the operation is completed, the double lumen endotracheal tube is exchanged for a single lumen tube and a bronchoscopy is performed in order to assess the airway anastomosis and to clear the airway of blood and secretions.

After the surgical procedure, meticulous attention must be paid to the hemodynamic optimization of the patient. Cardiac output, filling pressures and systemic vascular resistance (SVR) should be measured. Lung transplant patients often present with a low systemic vascular resistance state that can be a manifestation of systemic inflammatory response syndrome related to reperfusion injury. These patients respond better to a vasopressor (norepinephrine) to restore vascular tone than to volume. The aim is to achieve a euvolemic state.

The central venous pressure (CVP) and capillary wedge pressure (PCWP) are kept as low as possible to maintain a mean blood pressure >65 mmHg with adequate urine output. Often the low SVR state persists for 12–24 h, and a continuous infusion of norepinephrine ± dopamine is required. Patients with elevated pulmonary artery pressures preoperatively tend to be more hemodynamically labile and more difficult to manage

Ventilatory Support and Weaning

The type of transplant (single or bilateral) and the underlying lung disease should be taken into consideration before choosing a ventilation and weaning strategy after transplant. The ultimate goal is to avoid respiratory acidosis and maintain satisfactory oxygenation. Optimal protective ventilation has been shown to reduce the incidence of primary graft dysfunction and infections after transplantation. A baseline arterial blood gas is obtained on a FiO_2 of 1.0, positive end-expiratory pressure (PEEP) of 5 cm H_2O on arrival in the ICU.

A lung protective ventilation strategy using low tidal volumes (VT <6 ml/kg based on donor predicted body weight) and moderate levels of positive end-expiratory pressure (PEEP < 10 cm H_2O) has been generally adopted—based on the experience with this strategy in patients suffering from acute respiratory distress syndrome. The respiratory rate should be regulated to maintain appropriate minute ventilation. Some level of hypercapnia is acceptable for patients with history of preoperative chronic hypercapnia (cystic fibrosis, emphysema). In the case of a single lung transplant, the strategy changes depending on the underlying disease. PEEP is usually kept very low (less than 5 cm H_2O) or avoided. This is even more important in patients with emphysema or other obstructive lung diseases, to avoid air trapping in the native lung.

The ventilator weaning strategy is different for patients suffering from pulmonary hypertension. These patients often need to be kept sedated for 24–48 h to avoid episodes of pulmonary hypertension and hemodynamic instability as these patients often exhibit.

The use of short-acting agents for sedation is recommended in order to be able to extubate the patient as soon as possible. Most patients can be weaned and extubated within the first 6–12 hours after lung transplantation. This prevents nosocomial infections and allows the patient to start rehabilitation. All patients should start with early chest physiotherapy and incentive spirometry as well as early ambulation.

Hemodynamic Management

Persistent postoperative hypotension is commonly seen. The target of fluid management is to maintain a euvolemic state, maintaining adequate intravascular volume. Pulmonary capillary wedge pressure should be maintained as low as possible (5–15 mmHg), and urinary output should be carefully monitored. For fluid replacement, colloids are usually a better option: 5% or 25% Albumin as needed; plasma or red blood cells (the fluids of choice) as needed for volume replacement; and coagulaopathy correction or hemoglobin correction. Blood products are generally administered in order to maintain a hemoglobin of 90–100 mg/L. Inhaled nitride oxide (iNO) is frequently used to help with oxygenation, and in patients with primary or secondary pulmonary hypertension.

Systemic hypotension can be caused by systemic vasodilation produced by cytokine release or medications. In this case short acting alpha-agonists are the preferred treatment. Other causes of systemic hypotension are blood loss, severe myocardial injury, infection and pneumothorax.

Supraventricular arrhythmias (supraventricular tachycardia or atrial fibrillation) after lung transplantation are common. Beta blockers and calcium channel blockers are the medications of choice for these patients. Amiodarone is generally avoided because of the idiosyncratic secondary toxic effects that can affect the lung, but is sometimes used as a last resort in patients who do not respond to electrical cardioversion, beta blockers and calcium channel blockers. Anticoagulants may be necessary for patients with atrial fibrillation.

Management of Primary Graft Dysfunction

Primary graft dysfunction (PGD) is an acute lung injury syndrome that can develop in the early postoperative period, generally during the first 3 days after lung transplantation. One of the major contributors to PGD is ischemia reperfusion lung injury. The clinic manifestation of PGD is hypoxemia and pulmonary infiltrates on the chest x-ray. PGD is the predominant cause of death during the initial post-transplant period and it also pre-disposes the patient to chronic lung allograft dysfunction [21].

Protective lung ventilation has shown to reduce PGD. Inhaled nitric oxide has been used to treat severe forms of primary graft dysfunction. It has shown to improve oxygenation and reduce pulmonary hypertension. Extracorporeal membrane oxygenation (ECMO) is an option for patients with severe PGD who do not respond to less aggressive measures. It should be instated early if more conservative measures are failing, in order to support the patient until the acute lung dysfunction recovers.

Immunosuppression

The first immunosuppressant is administered intraoperatively (methylprednisolone 500 mg iv on induction of anesthesia). Postoperatively, immunosuppression includes three drugs: steroid (methylprednisolone 0.5 mg/kg/day for 3 days and then prednisone 0.5 mg/kg/day from day four to 14, then taper 5 mg/week to 20 mg/day); a calcineurin inhibitor (cyclosporine 5 mg/kg po twice daily, target level 250–350 until 6 months), or tacrolimus 0.03 mg/kg po twice daily (target level 10–20 ng/ml in the first 6 months and 10 ng/ml subsequently); and a cell proliferation inhibitor (azathioprine 1.5 mg/kg/day po, or mycophenolate mofetil 2–3 g po daily in divided doses). The preoperative, intraoperative and early postoperative immunosuppression protocol used by the Toronto Lung Transplant Program is shown in Table 47.2.

Anticoagulation

Lung transplant patients are at moderate risk of suffering postoperative venous thromboembolism (VTE). Thus, anticoagulation is desirable, as bronchial anastomotic healing depends on microcirculatory blood flow through pulmonary–bronchial collaterals and VTE/pulmonary embolism prophylaxis is also necessary. Venous thromboembolism prophylaxis can start immediately post-transplant unless bleeding is a concern.

Table 47.2 Preoperative, intraoperative and early postoperative immunosuppression protocol followed by the Toronto Lung Transplant Program

Preoperative	
Calcineurin inhibitor	
Cyclosporine	5 mg/kg PO on arrival
Tacrolimus	0.05 mg/kg PO on arrival
Intraoperative	
Glucocorticoid	
Methylprednisolone	500 mg IV on induction
Early postoperative	
Glucocorticoid	
Methylprednisolone	0.5 mg/kg/day for 3 days
Prednisone	0.5 mg/kg/day from day 4, tapering 5 mg/every week until 0.25 mg/kg/day
Calcineurin inhibitor	
Cyclosporine	5 mg/kg bid PO adjusted to target level
Tacrolimus	0.1 mg/kg PO bid, follow by target levels
Nucleotide blocking agent	
Azathioprine	1.5–2.0 mg/kg/day NG/PO
Mycophenolate mofetil	1–1.5 g bid in IV
Monoclonal antibody	
Basiliximab (Simulec)	Usually not for induction but may be used if delayed on cyclosporine or tacrolimus is desirable.

PO, by mouth; IV, intravenous; bid, twice a day; NG, nasogastric

Most of the patients receive low dose subcutaneous unfractionated heparin.

Infection Prophylaxis

Infection is one of the major causes of morbidity and mortality after lung transplantation. Infection prophylaxis against bacteria, virus and fungus starts perioperatively and is empirically administered for the first 72 h. The antibiotics are then discontinued or adjusted according to any positive donor or recipient cultures available. An example of an antibiotic scheme used by the Toronto Lung Transplant Program is shown in Tables 47.3 and 47.4. If there was a concern of a possible infectious infiltrate in the donor lung or positive cultures are obtained, then antibiotic treatment is continued for 14 days. Patients with

Table 47.3 Infection treatment and prophylaxis for non-cystic fibrotic patients after lung transplantation followed by the Toronto Lung Transplant Program

Infection treatment and postoperative prophylaxis
Piperacillin – Tazobactam 3.375 g IV q6h for 3 days
If clinical concern: switch to culture directed antibiotic.
If no clinical concern: step - down to one of the following:
Ceftriaxone 1 g IV q24h
Amoxicillin – Clavulanate 875 mg PO q12h
Moxifloxacin 400 mg PO/IV q24h (if penicillin/ cephalosporin allergy)
If cultured organism not sensitive to any step - down antibiotics:
Piperacillin/tazobactam
If penicillin allergy:
Ciprofloxacin 400 mg IV q12h
Vancomycin 1 g IV q12

PO, by mouth; IV, intravenous; bid, twice a day; q6, every 6 h; q12, every 12 h; q24, every 24 h

Table 47.4 Infection treatment and prophylaxis for cystic fibrotic patients after lung transplantation followed by the Toronto Lung Transplant Program

Burkholderia cepacia Negative	
Ceftazidime	2 g IV q8h × 14 days
Meropenem	2 g IV q8h × 14 days
Tobramycin	160 mg bid Inhaled, or
Colistin	75 mg bid Inhaled for 3 months
+ Salbutamol	1–2 puffs Inhaled prior to above Tobramycin treatment (use whichever inhaled drug patient was receiving pre-transplant)

Burkholderia cepacia Positive	
Meropenem	2 g IV q8h × 21 days
Ceftazidime	2 g IV q8h × 21 days
Tobramycin	160 mg Inhaled bid
Azithromycin	500 mg IV daily × 21 days
Once discharged:	
Tobramycin inhaled 160 mg bid or Colistin inhaled 75 mg bid for 3 months	

IV, intravenous; Inh, inhaled; bid, twice a day; q6, every 6 h; q12, every 12 h; q24, every 24 h

cystic fibrosis or bronchiectasis are usually colonized with more resistant microorganisms and usually receive antibiotics according to previous sensitivities.

Lung and heart-lung transplantation are lifesaving procedures for patients with end stage pulmonary or combined pulmonary and cardiac failure. Optimal results depend on careful donor and recipient selection and careful attention to the many details of these complex procedures in very sick patients.

References

1. Orens JB, Boehler A, de Perrot M, Estenne M, Glanville AR, Keshavjee S, et al. A review of lung transplant donor acceptability criteria. J Heart Lung Transplant. 2003;22(11):1183–200.
2. Aigner C, Winkler G, Jaksch P, Seebacher G, Lang G, Taghavi S, et al. Extended donor criteria for lung transplantation—a clinical reality. Eur J Cardiothorac Surg. 2005;27(5):757–61.
3. Sommer W, Kuhn C, Tudorache I, Avsar M, Gottlieb J, Boethig D, et al. Extended criteria donor lungs and clinical outcome: results of an alternative allocation algorithm. J Heart Lung Transplant. 2013;32(11):1065–72.
4. Pierre AF, Keshavjee S. Lung transplantation: donor and recipient critical care aspects. Curr Opin Crit Care. 2005;11(4):339–44.
5. Botha P. Extended donor criteria in lung transplantation. Curr Opin Organ Transplant. 2009;14(2):206–10.
6. Van Raemdonck D, Neyrinck A, Verleden GM, Dupont L, Coosemans W, Decaluwe H, et al. Lung donor selection and management. Proc Am Thorac Soc. 2009;6(1):28–38.
7. Tuttle-Newhall JE, Krishnan SM, Levy MF, McBride V, Orlowski JP, Sung RS. Organ donation and utilization in the United States: 1998-2007. Am J Transplant. 2009;9(4 Pt 2):879–93.
8. Munshi L, Keshavjee S, Cypel M. Donor management and lung preservation for lung transplantation. Lancet Respir Med. 2013;1(4):318–28.
9. Yeung JC, Keshavjee S. Overview of clinical lung transplantation. Cold Spring Harb Perspect Med. 2014;4(1):a015628.
10. Lopau K, Mark J, Schramm L, Heidbreder E, Wanner C. Hormonal changes in brain death and immune activation in the donor. Transpl Int. 2000;13(Suppl 1):S282–5.
11. Franklin GA, Santos AP, Smith JW, Galbraith S, Harbrecht BG, Garrison RN. Optimization of donor management goals yields increased organ use. Am Surg. 2010;76(6):587–94.
12. Patel MS, De La Cruz S, Sally MB, Groat T, Malinoski DJ. Active donor management during the hospital phase of care is associated with more organs transplanted per donor. J Am Coll Surg. 2017;225(4):525–31.
13. Weill D, Benden C, Corris PA, Dark JH, Davis RD, Keshavjee S, et al. A consensus document for the selection of lung transplant candidates: 2014—an update from the Pulmonary Transplantation Council of the International Society for Heart and Lung Transplantation. J Heart Lung Transplant. 2015;34(1):1–15.
14. de Perrot M, Keshavjee S. Everting mattress running suture: an improved technique of atrial anastomosis in human lung transplantation. Ann Thorac Surg. 2002;73(5):1663–4.
15. Shafii AE, Mason DP, Brown CR, Vakil N, Johnston DR, McCurry KR, et al. Growing experience with extracorporeal membrane oxygenation as a bridge to lung transplantation. ASAIO J. 2012;58(5):526–9.
16. Mason DP, Boffa DJ, Murthy SC, Gildea TR, Budev MM, Mehta AC, et al. Extended use of extracorporeal membrane oxygenation after lung transplantation. J Thorac Cardiovasc Surg. 2006;132(4):954–60.
17. Marczin N, Royston D, Yacoub M. Pro: lung transplantation should be routinely performed with cardiopulmonary bypass. J Cardiothorac Vasc Anesth. 2000;14(6):739–45.
18. McRae K. Con: lung transplantation should not be routinely performed with cardiopulmonary bypass. J Cardiothorac Vasc Anesth. 2000;14(6):746–50.
19. Zangrillo A, Garozzo FA, Biondi-Zoccai G, Pappalardo F, Monaco F, Crivellari M, et al. Miniaturized cardiopulmonary bypass improves short-term outcome in cardiac surgery: a meta-analysis of randomized controlled studies. J Thorac Cardiovasc Surg. 2010;139(5):1162–9.
20. Machuca TN, Collaud S, Mercier O, Cheung M, Cunningham V, Kim SJ, et al. Outcomes of intraoperative extracorporeal membrane oxygenation versus cardiopulmonary bypass for lung transplantation. J Thorac Cardiovasc Surg. 2015;149(4):1152–7.
21. Porteous MK, Diamond JM, Christie JD. Primary graft dysfunction: lessons learned about the first 72 h after lung transplantation. Curr Opin Organ Transplant. 2015;20(5):506–14.

Ventricular Assist Devices

48

Vivek Rao

Main Messages

1. Patient selection and preoperative optimization are key. In acutely ill patients (INTERMACS category 1–2), consider short-term support or ECMO as a bridge to an implantable device.
2. In relatively stable patients (INTERMACS 3 and 4), consider optimization of volume status prior to VAD implant as this will reduce the risk of postoperative RV failure.
3. Even with an excellent hemodynamic response to VAD therapy, wean from inotropic support slowly to avoid a precipitous decline in RV function.
4. Institute early postoperative anticoagulation and blood pressure management to avoid severe adverse events such as pump thrombosis and stroke.

Congestive heart failure remains the only cardiovascular diagnosis increasing in prevalence in the developed world. The gold standard for the treatment of end-stage heart disease not amenable to any other form of conventional therapy is cardiac transplantation. Unfortunately, limited organ availability precludes heart transplantation for many patients who would otherwise benefit from this therapy. Ventricular assist devices (VADs) were introduced to provide mechanical circulatory support to critically ill patients until a suitable donor organ could be found. Several short term (days to weeks) and long term (months to years) devices are now in use with acceptable, albeit not ideal, clinical outcomes [1].

The successful use of mechanical circulatory support as a "bridge" to transplantation has led to permanent or "destination" therapy, whereby VAD implant represents the definitive treatment for non-transplant eligible patients with refractory heart failure. The clinically significant benefits were documented in REMATCH (Randomized Evaluation of Mechanical Assistance for the Treatment of Congestive Heart Failure) [2]. However, the overall poor survival at 2 years with the initial large pulsatile device did not lead to a significant adoption of this technology. Not until the current generation continuous-flow pumps were introduced and approved for use in non-transplant candidates did the use of VAD therapy dramatically rise (Fig. 48.1) [3].

While certain centres have reported impressive recovery of native myocardial function while on VAD support (enabling device explant), this remains a rare occurrence in the general experience [4]. Ongoing research is attempting to augment the native myocardial response to LVAD

V. Rao (✉)
Peter Munk Cardiac Centre, PMB 4-457,
Toronto General Hospital, Toronto, ON, Canada
e-mail: vivek.rao@uhn.ca

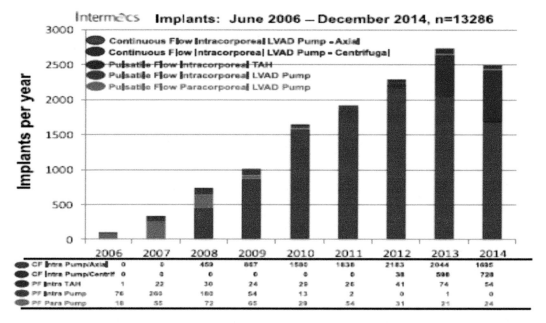

Fig. 48.1 Annual volume of mechanical circulatory support device implants. From the 7th INTERMACS report (reprinted with permission from Kirklin et al. J Heart Lung Transplant, 2015)

unloading using therapies such as allogeneic stem cell transplant; however, the results are still pending [5].

Regardless of the type of VAD system employed, there are several pre-, peri- and post-operative considerations when managing a critically ill patient dependent upon mechanical circulatory support. Careful patient selection remains the predominant key to clinical success.

Indications for Mechanical Circulatory Support

Mechanical circulatory support is now considered the standard of care for certain patients with acute or chronic heart failure. Device selection is dependent upon several factors including presenting illness, likelihood of short term recovery, neurologic status and body size. The overriding indication in all patients, however, remains inadequate cardiac function to preserve end-organ perfusion. Classical hemodynamic criteria include: pulmonary capillary wedge pressure >20 mmHg, systolic blood pressure <80 mmHg and a cardiac index <2.1 L/min/m^2, despite

optimal fluid and inotropic management. In patients with chronic heart failure awaiting heart transplantation, other factors may also favor earlier consideration of VAD insertion in an otherwise stable patient. These include blood type 0 and weight > 100 kg (suggesting prolonged wait for donor organ), oliguria or azotemia, inotrope dependency, refractory pulmonary hypertension or onset of malignant arrhythmias. Table 48.1 lists the currently available and most commonly employed ventricular assist devices.

Key considerations for device selection in potential surgical candidates include eligibility for transplantation (see Chap. 48), likelihood for recovery and potential need for biventricular support. ECMO (extracorporeal membrane oxygenation) has been deliberately excluded from this list as any patient who requires pulmonary support in addition to circulatory assistance should likely receive ECMO until lung function improves to the point that isolated cardiac support is feasible. In addition, with improved ECMO technology that permits less intensive anticoagulation, many centres have adopted ECMO as the first line of therapy in INTERMACS (Interagency Registry for Mechanically Assisted

Table 48.1 Commonly available ventricular assist devices

Name	Type	Mechanism	Duration	Percutaneous	Position
TandemHeart	BiVAD	Centrifugal	Days	Yes	Paracorporeal
Impella	BiVAD	Axial	Days	Yes	Paracorporeal
Centrimag	BiVAD	Centrifugal	Weeks	No	Paracorporeal
HeartMate 2	LVAD	Axial	Years	No	Implantable
Syncardia	TAH	Pulsatile	Months	No	Implantable
HeartWare	LVAD	Centrifugal	Years	No	Implantable
Jarvik 2000	LVAD	Axial Flow	Years	No	Implantable
HeartMate III	LVAD	Centrifugal	Years	No	Implantable

Table 48.2 INTERMACS (Interagency Registry for Mechanically Assisted Circulatory Support) Scale for Classifying Patients with Advanced Heart Failure [6]

Profiles	Definition	Description
INTERMACS 1	"Crash and burn"	• Hemodynamic instability in spite of increasing doses of catecholamines and/or mechanical circulatory support • Critical hypoperfusion of target organs (severe cardiogenic shock)
INTERMACS 2	"Sliding on inotropes"	• Intravenous inotropic support with acceptable blood pressure • Rapid deterioration of kidney function, nutritional state, or signs of congestion
INTERMACS 3	"Dependent stability"	• Hemodynamic stability with low or intermediate doses of inotropics, worsening of symptoms, or progressive kidney failure
INTERMACS 4	"Frequent flyer"	• Temporary cessation of inotropic treatment is possible, but the patient suffers from frequent symptom recurrences and typically with fluid overload
INTERMACS 5	"Housebound"	• Complete cessation of physical activity, stable at rest, but frequently with moderate water retention and some level of kidney dysfunction
INTERMACS 6	"Walking wounded"	• Minor limitation on physical activity and absence of congestion while at rest • Easily fatigued by light activity
INTERMACS 7	"Placeholder"	• Patient in NYHA functional class II or III • No current or recent unstable water balance

Circulatory Support, Table 48.2) class 1 patients [6]. These patients are critically ill and hemodynamically unstable requiring high dose inotropic support. Often these patients are at imminent risk of circulatory collapse or have been recently resuscitated and remain labile. Percutaneous ECMO provides the fastest method of stabilizing hemodynamics and is likely the most cost-effective manner in which to assess neurologic status and end-organ injury [7].

Preoperative Considerations

As mentioned previously, patient selection is paramount to clinical success following VAD insertion. Many authors have derived risk factor screening scores using multivariable logistic regression analyses to assist in patient selection. The most recent HeartMate 2 risk factor score by Cowger et al incorporates the newer generation continuous flow LVADs in contrast to many of the older scores that evaluated the first generation pulsatile pumps [8]. Note that even "low risk" patients face an operative mortality considerably higher than that of most conventional cardiac surgical procedures, reflecting the burden of their critical illness. In addition to these comorbidities, careful anesthetic and surgical evaluation of the potential VAD candidate should include the following:

1. Assessment of coagulation profile, including sickle cell status in appropriate patients. Blood bank should be notified and blood products

reserved (usually 4 units PRBC, 4 units FFP and 10 units platelets for *uncomplicated* VAD cases).

2. Determination of any co-existing infection which may lead to device endocarditis. If an infection is identified and appropriately treated, VAD insertion can usually proceed safely. However, in septic patients with no clear source of infection, VAD insertion is associated with high mortality.

3. Transesophageal echocardiography to rule out intracardiac shunts. Even minor atrial septal defects should be closed at the time of LVAD insertion as they can lead to significant right to left shunts and hypoxia postoperatively. The incomplete ventricular unloading with the current generation continuous-flow VADs may permit small ASDs to be managed conservatively. However, in the event of postoperative RV failure, a persistent septal defect may prove problematic to manage and thus if identified perioperatively most surgeons advocate closure.

4. Transesophageal echocardiography to evaluate cardiac valves. Significant aortic insufficiency MUST be addressed at the time of LVAD insertion as it can lead to a blind loop phenomenon with poor "real" cardiac output. Aortic stenosis is usually irrelevant unless recovery is anticipated, in which case bioprosthetic replacement is preferred as mechanical valves are prone to thrombose, even with therapeutic anticoagulation (due to lack of normal transvalvular flows). The treatment of mitral insufficiency remains controversial as most devices that completely unload the left ventricle eliminate residual mitral insufficiency. However, for axial flow devices and in situations where recovery is anticipated, several authors recommend repair or replacement of the mitral valve. Due to the normal transmitral flow, mechanical valves can be employed with appropriate postoperative anticoagulation. Mitral stenosis can lead to poor VAD filling and should be addressed with mitral valve replacement. Secondary tricuspid insufficiency is common in patients with biventricular failure and may complicate management in patients with iso-lated left-sided support. However, in most cases as the pulmonary vascular resistance decreases with mechanical support, the tricuspid regurgitation abates [9–11].

5. Surgically amenable coronary artery disease is common in patients with ischemic cardiomyopathy. In patients receiving isolated left ventricular support, care must be taken to optimize right ventricular performance. Thus, any RCA lesions should be revascularized at the time of LVAD insertion, or conversion to biventricular support may be necessary. A chronically occluded RCA has usually been well collateralized and thus may not require attention at the time of VAD implant.

6. Ventricular arrhythmias are common and are usually eliminated by cardiac decompression following institution of mechanical support. However, in patients with isolated left sided support, a failing right ventricle can produce hemodynamically significant arrhythmias. Although arrhythmias (both atrial and ventricular) are usually well tolerated, they often lead to decreased LVAD flows and a loss of normal physiologic responses to increased workload. Persistent atrial fibrillation may also lead to thrombus formation and should therefore be treated with early pharmacologic or electrical cardioversion.

Perioperative Considerations

Antibiotic prophylaxis is usually dependent on institutional colonization but commonly includes protection against gram-positive organisms. Most devices can be inserted via a standard median sternotomy, but some authors have reported lateral thoracotomy approaches to VAD insertion in patients with multiple previous sternotomies [12]. In critically ill patients, cardiopulmonary bypass (CPB) is initiated early to stabilize hemodynamics, but in more stable patients VAD insertion can often be performed without the need for CPB. Once on CPB, inotropic support is usually halved (not discontinued) and vasopressin infusions started (2–6 units/h depending upon the degree of vasoplegia).

While most of the long term devices are designed for LV apical cannulation, the short term devices can be configured to provide inflow via the right (for RVAD) or left atrium. However, even with short term devices (such as the CentriMag), ventricular cannulation is preferred to improve decompression (and likelihood of recovery), optimize flow, and prevent potential thrombus formation across the atrioventricular valves. The PREVENT investigators have developed a strategy for perioperative management that has proven to reduce severe adverse events such as pump thrombus and stroke [13]. While the PREVENT study evaluated the HeartMate 2 device, certain principles apply across all devices, such as early anticoagulation including bridging with heparin, avoiding low pump speeds, and strict blood pressure control. More specific to the HeartMate 2 is the orientation of the pump housing and inflow cannula (Fig. 48.2)

Intraoperative transesophageal echocardiography is also useful to reassess valvular function, rule out right-left intracardiac shunts, and aid in de-airing following device implantation. Weaning from CPB is a coordinated effort involving perfusion, anesthesia, surgery and the VAD controller. Devices should never be activated if CPB flows are greater than 2 L/min for risk of air entrainment and subsequent cerebral embolus. Heparin anticoagulation is fully reversed with protamine (even in devices that subsequently require anticoagulation). Blood product administration is common at this point due to inherent coagulation abnormalities present in heart failure patients.

Mean arterial pressure can be labile and volume responsive. We aim to titrate MAP between 65 and 75 mmHg. Higher pressures may lead to intracerebral bleeding while lower pressure can adversely affect RV function [14, 15]. It is important to note the differential response to afterload across the various implantable devices. In general, the HVAD is the most sensitive to afterload followed by the HeartMate 3, with the least sensitive device being the axial flow HeartMate 2. In the case of HVAD, we commonly see a 10 mmHg rise in MAP correspond to 0.5 L/min drop in flow.

Postoperative Considerations

In the early postoperative period, normal hemodynamic monitoring is employed in addition to continuous evaluation of VAD function. Coagulopathy is common, but persistent chest tube drainage should prompt early surgical exploration. The aortic anastomosis is the most common site of postoperative bleeding. When VAD output is below desired limits (2 L/min/m²), the differential diagnosis includes hypovolemia, tamponade and RV failure (in cases of isolated LVAD support). If volume status is adequate (CVP > 15 mmHg) and tamponade had been ruled out (by TEE or re-exploration), then RV failure is the likely cause of poor LVAD output. Milrinone, dobutamine and nitric oxide are all useful pharmacologic adjuncts to the management of postoperative RV failure. In approximately 15% of cases, temporary right sided VAD support may be required [16]. Usually, RV function recovers with LVAD support due to improvements in pulmonary vascular resistance. Thus, in most cases temporary RVAD support can be withdrawn after 3–5 days.

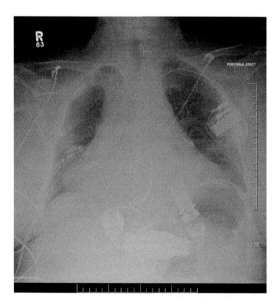

Fig. 48.2 Chest X-ray depicting ideal placement of a HeartMate 2 (Abbott Medical Inc) left ventricular assist device. Note the horizontal orientation of the pump housing and the angulation of the inflow cannula into the apex of the left ventricle oriented parallel to the interventricular septum

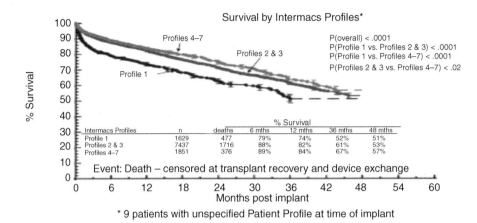

Intermacs Continuous Flow LVAD/BiVAD Implants: 2013 – 2016, n = 10,726

Fig. 48.3 Survival stratified by INTERMACS class. From the 7th INTERMACS report (reprinted with permission from Kirklin et al. J Heart Lung Transplant, 2015)

Clinical Outcomes

The overall operative mortality associated with VAD insertion has fallen significantly with the current generation devices, and is approximately 5–10% (Fig. 48.3) [17]. Most programs now routinely discharge their LVAD patients and maintain outpatient therapy while awaiting heart transplantation. A very small number of these patients suffer from fatal or transplant-precluding complications (stroke) prior to transplant. Due to the improved physiology secondary to VAD support, outcomes following transplant are better in this population compared to patients undergoing transplant without VAD support [18].

Late complications while on VAD support are often device specific but include driveline infections, pocket infections, thromboembolic events and HLA sensitization. The latter complication can significantly increase the risk of acute rejection following cardiac transplantation.

To facilitate potential myocardial recovery, most programs now reinstitute anti-failure therapy (beta blockade, ACE inhibition, etc.). The Harefield group has also reported promising results with clenbuterol, a beta-agonist that promotes myocyte hypertrophy [19]. Unfortunately, predicting which patients will recover native car-

diac function (and maintain it for a prolonged duration) remains a mystery and thus many patients eventually proceed to transplantation.

Mechanical circulatory support has now become established as a standard of care for the treatment of acute and chronic heart failure. The next-generation of devices are smaller, less morbid and are designed to have greater durability than the presently available VADs. As the technology continues to improve, it is likely that mechanical circulatory support will 1 day provide a real alternative to conventional transplantation.

References

1. Raju S, MacIver J, Foroutan F, Alba C, Billia F, Rao V. Long term use of left ventricular assist devices: a report on clinical outcomes. Can J Surg. 2017;60:236–2462.
2. Rose EA, Gelijns AG, Moskowitz AJ, et al. Randomized evaluation of mechanical assistance for the treatment of congestive heart failure (REMATCH) study group. Long term mechanical left ventricular assistance for end-stage heart failure. N Engl J Med. 2001;345:1435–43.
3. Slaughter MS, Rogers JG, Milano CA, et al. Advanced heart failure treated with continuous flow left ventricular assist device. N Engl J Med. 2009;361:2241–51.

4. Hon JK, Yacoub MH. Bridge to recovery with the use of left ventricular assist device and clenbuterol. Ann Thorac Surg. 2003;75:S36–41.

5. Ascheim DD, Gelijns AC, Goldstein D, et al. Mesenchymal precursor cells as adjunctive therapy in recipients of contemporary left ventricular assist devices. Circulation. 2014;129:2287–96.

6. Alba AC, Rao V, Ivanov J, Ross HJ, Delgado DH. Usefulness of the INTERMACS scale to predict outcomes post-mechanical assist device placement. J Heart Lung Transplant. 2009;28:827–33.

7. Singal RJ, Singal D, Bednarczyk J, et al. Current and future status of extracorporeal cardiopulmonary resuscitation for in-hospital cardiac arrest. Can J Cardiol. 2017;33:51–60.

8. Cowger J, Sundareswaran K, Rogers JG, et al. Predicting survival in patients receiving continuous flow left ventricular assist devices: the HeartMate 2 risk score. J Am Coll Cardiol. 2013;61:313–21.

9. Cowger J, Rao V, Massey T, et al. Comprehensive review and suggested strategies for the detection and management of aortic insufficiency in patients with a continuous flow left ventricular assist device. J Heart Lung Transplant. 2015;34:149–57.

10. Goldraich L, Kawajiri H, Foroutan F, et al. Tricuspid valve annular dilatation as a predictor of right ventricular failure after implantation of a left ventricular assist device. J Card Surg. 2016;31:110–6.

11. Goodwin M, Nemeh HW, Borgi J, Paone G, Morgan J. Resolution of mitral regurgitation with left ventricular assist device support. Ann Thor Surg. 2017;104:811–8.

12. Cheung A, Bashir J, Kaan A, Kealy J, Moss R, Shayan H. Minimally invasive off-pump explant of a continuous flow left ventricular assist device. J Heart Lung Transplant. 2010;29:808–10.

13. Maltais S, Kilic A, Nathan S, et al. PREVENtion of HeartMate II pump thrombosis through clinical management: the PREVENT multi-center study. J Heart Lung Transplant. 2017;36:1–12.

14. Lampert BC, Eckert C, Weaver S, et al. Blood pressure control in continuous flow left ventricular assist devices: efficacy and impact on adverse events. Ann Thorac Surg. 2014;97:139–46.

15. Nassif ME, Tibrewala A, Raymer DS, et al. Systolic blood pressure on discharge after left ventricular assist device insertion is associated with subsequent stroke. J Heart Lung Transplant. 2015;34:503–8.

16. Kormos RL, Teuteberg JJ, Pagani FD, et al. Right ventricular failure in patients with the Heartmate 2 continuous flow left ventricular assist device: incidence, risk factors and effect on outcomes. J Thorac Cardiovasc Surg. 2010;139:1316–24.

17. Kirklin JM, Naftel DC, Pagani FD, et al. Seventh INTERMACS annual report: 15000 patients and counting. J Heart Lung Transplant. 2015;34:1495–504.

18. Alba AC, McDonald M, Rao V, Ross HJ, Delgado DH. The effect of left ventricular assist devices on long-term post-transplant outcomes: a systematic review of observational studies. Eur J Heart Fail. 2011;13:785–95.

19. Birks EJ, Tansley PD, Hardy J, et al. Left ventricular assist device and drug therapy for the reversal of heart failure. N Engl J Med. 2006;355:1873–84.

Left Ventricular Aneurysm

49

Tirone David

Main Messages
1. The incidence of LVA is declining because of thrombolysis and urgent revascularization after myocardial infarction.
2. More common and difficult to manage is ischemic cardiomyopathy with akinetic walls and dilated ventricle.
3. A faster heart rate is often required after LVA repair or left ventricular restoration in the early postoperative period.
4. Operative mortality depends on patient characteristics and comorbidities, though it has fallen dramatically over the past 5 decades to less than 10%.

The treatment of ischemic heart disease continues to be a challenge, with an ever-increasing number of patients presenting with congestive heart failure. In patients with coronary artery disease and a previous myocardium infarct, the necrotic muscle is replaced by fibrous tissue, and if the necrosis is large enough, an area of akinesis or dyskinesis develops. To compensate for the loss of contractile myocardium, the ventricle dilates and undergoes adverse remodeling. Depending on the extent of scarring and other factors, the infarcted myocardium may undergo significant thinning and form a ventricular aneurysm (LVA). In anterior myocardial infarction, the anterior, septal and inferoseptal areas of the ventricle dilate with an increase in both longitudinal and short axis, which may cause distortion of the anterior papillary muscle with consequent mitral regurgitation (MR). In inferior wall infarction, the short axis is increased more than the longitudinal axis, which accounts for more frequent associated MR.

LVA were commonly seen in the early days of cardiac surgery, but the incidence is declining since the introduction of thrombolysis and early revascularization after myocardial infarction. Ischemic cardiomyopathy with akinetic walls and dilated ventricle is more common now and is difficult to manage.

Diagnosis

Akinetic and dyskinetic segments of the left ventricle can be identified by contrast ventriculography or echocardiography; however, magnetic resonance imaging (MRI) is probably the best method to determine segments that are scarred and thinned, and to determine if surgical

T. David (✉)
The University Health Network,
Toronto, ON, Canada
e-mail: Tirone.David@uhn.ca

© Springer Nature Switzerland AG 2021
D. C. H. Cheng et al. (eds.), *Evidence-Based Practice in Perioperative Cardiac Anesthesia and Surgery*, https://doi.org/10.1007/978-3-030-47887-2_49

resection is advisable. These patients also need coronary angiography and echocardiography to assess MR.

Indications for Surgery

Surgery is indicated to control symptoms of congestive heart failure, ventricular dysrhythmias, ongoing ischemia, MR, or thromboembolism due to ventricular thrombus on an akinetic segment.

Left Ventricular Aneurysmectomy and Ventricular Restoration

Resection of large dyskinetic segments of the left ventricle, particularly anterior aneurysms, has been performed since the early days of cardiac surgery. By 1985 surgeons began to understand the importance of reconstructing the left ventricle to restore its normal size and shape by suturing a Dacron patch of appropriate size and shape along the area of scarred and normal myocardium. This technique improved the outcomes of the operation. In addition, it opened the door to expand this approach to patients with large akinetic segments without obvious aneurysm— the so-called surgical ventricular restoration—to reduce ventricular volume and restore the ventricular elliptical shape. This technique has not been standardized, and surgeons use a variety of approaches to restore the shape of the left ventricular cavity. All of these techniques involve an incision into the diseased anterior wall, an exclusion of the entire diseased segment, and a reduction in ventricular cavity size. In the majority of patients, reconstruction is done on the anterior portion of the left ventricle. However, reconstruction has also been performed on the posterior wall after circumflex or dominant right coronary artery occlusion. Most of these patients undergo concomitant coronary artery bypass, and a number also need mitral valve repair or replacement.

Postoperative Care

In the early postoperative period, patients undergoing repair of LVA or left ventricular restoration often require a faster heart rate, preferably by means of atrial pacing and increased filling pressures to maintain adequate blood pressure and cardiac output. Inotropes are often needed and sometimes an intra-aortic balloon pump is useful during the first couple of days. As the heart adapts to the repair, diuresis can be started to remove excessive fluid, particularly if the patient was in heart failure prior to surgery. The aim is to get the patient as dry as possible without compromising renal function. Ventricular dysrhythmias should be treated with amiodarone and sometimes a beta blocker. If the renal function is normal, an angiotensin converting enzyme inhibitor is started. It may also be advisable to anticoagulate these patients with warfarin sodium during the first 3 to 6 months to reduce the risk of thromboembolism. Upon discharge, these patients should be followed by an expert in heart failure and adjust their management of sodium and fluid restriction and medications.

Clinical Outcomes

Operative mortality has fallen significantly during the past 5 decades, and is certainly lower than 10%; however, it varies widely depending on the patient population and comorbidities. Predictors of operative death include advanced age, female gender, advanced functional class, emergent operations, incomplete revascularization, left ventricular ejection fraction <30%, concomitant mitral valve replacement, pulmonary hypertension and impaired renal function. Late survival is largely dependent on the residual ventricular function and extensiveness of coronary artery disease. Early series showed a survival of approximately 35% at 10 years [1, 2].

The prospective, randomized STITCH trial of 1000 patients with left ventricular ejection fraction ≤35% and suitable anatomy for ventricular restoration showed no survival benefit over myocardial revascularization alone. Several individual series showed that ventricular restoration in properly selected patients improves symptoms and long-term survival [3].

References

1. Jatene AD. Left ventricular aneurysmectomy: resection or reconstruction. J Thorac Cardiovasc Surg. 1985;89:321–31.
2. DiDonato M, et al. Akinetic versus dyskinetic postinfarction scar: relation to surgical outcome in patients undergoing endoventricular circular patch plasty repair. J Am Coll Cardiol. 1997;29:1569–75.
3. Jones RH, et al. Coronary bypass surgery with and without surgical restoration. N Engl J Med. 2009;360:1705–17.

Part V

Cardiac Surgical Recovery Unit and Postoperative Complications

Fast Track and Ultra-Fast Track Cardiac Surgery Recovery Care

50

Janet Martin, Daniel Bainbridge, and Davy C. H. Cheng

Main Messages

1. Fast-track cardiac anesthesia is the standard of cardiac surgery recovery care. In order to successfully achieve reduced time to extubation and ICU length of stay, without adverse patient outcomes, fast-track care requires a coordinated, multi-component approach across the full spectrum of perioperative care pathways.

2. This has prompted a shift from recovering patients in the traditional intensive care unit manner, with ventilation weaning protocols and intensive observation, to management more in keeping with the recovery room practice of early extubation and rapid discharge.

3. The goal of a postcardiac surgery recovery model is a postoperative unit that allows variable levels of monitoring and care based on patient needs, particularly with the current era of minimally invasive cardiac surgery procedures and cardiology interventional procedures.

J. Martin (✉)
Department of Anesthesia & Perioperative Medicine, Schulich School of Medicine & Dentistry, Western University, London, ON, Canada

Department of Epidemiology & Biostatistics, Schulich School of Medicine & Dentistry, Western University, London, ON, Canada

Centre for Medical Evidence, Decision Integrity & Clinical Impact (MEDICI), Schulich School of Medicine & Dentistry, Western University, London, ON, Canada

WHO Collaborating Centre for Global Surgery, Anesthesia & Perioperative Care, Schulich School of Medicine & Dentistry, Western University, London, ON, Canada
e-mail: jmarti83@uwo.ca

D. Bainbridge
Department of Anesthesia and Perioperative Medicine, Schulich School of Medicine and Dentistry, Western University, London, ON, Canada

London Health Sciences Centre, University Hospital, London, ON, Canada

D. C. H. Cheng
Department of Anesthesia & Perioperative Medicine, Schulich School of Medicine & Dentistry, Western University, London, ON, Canada

Centre for Medical Evidence, Decision Integrity & Clinical Impact (MEDICI), Schulich School of Medicine & Dentistry, Western University, London, ON, Canada

WHO Collaborating Centre for Global Surgery, Anesthesia & Perioperative Care, Schulich School of Medicine & Dentistry, Western University, London, ON, Canada

© Springer Nature Switzerland AG 2021
D. C. H. Cheng et al. (eds.), *Evidence-Based Practice in Perioperative Cardiac Anesthesia and Surgery*, https://doi.org/10.1007/978-3-030-47887-2_50

4. An enhanced recovery cardiac surgery pathway is discussed.
5. Example order sets for postoperative care are provided in Appendix D (Fast-Track Post Cardiovascular Surgery Post-Op Multi-Phase Order) and Appendix B (Cardiovascular Surgery Post-Op) of this textbook.

Recovery Models for Post-operative Care

With the growing practice of fast-track cardiac anesthesia (FTCA), routine cardiac surgical patients can be extubated within 1–6 h, and off-pump coronary artery bypass (OPCAB) and TAVI patients can be extubated in the operating room, or shortly less than 4 h after the procedure. Some centres have adopted an ultra-fast track approach to extubation (less than 1 h). The latter approach has not yet been proven to further improve cost savings and patient safety. Ultra-fast track extubation is discussed further in Chaps. 5, 7, 27, 35 of this textbook. To maximize the potential benefits of fast-track care, alternative recovery models are necessary (Fig. 50.1). In the parallel model, patients are admitted directly to a cardiac recovery area (CRA) where they are monitored, with 1:1 nursing care, until tracheal extubation. Following this, the level of care is reduced to reflect the patients requirements: nursing ratios are reduced to 1:2 or 1:3 for extubated patients. Any patients requiring overnight ventilation are transferred to the ICU for continuation of care. The predominant drawback with the parallel model is the separation of the CRA and the ICU, which leads to two separate nursing units, and the requirement to transfer patients between physically separate areas. The integrated model overcomes these limitations by admitting all patients to the same physical area. The goal is a postoperative unit allowing variable levels of monitoring and care based on the needs of the patient [1–3]. The ultra-fast track model bypasses critical care, and the

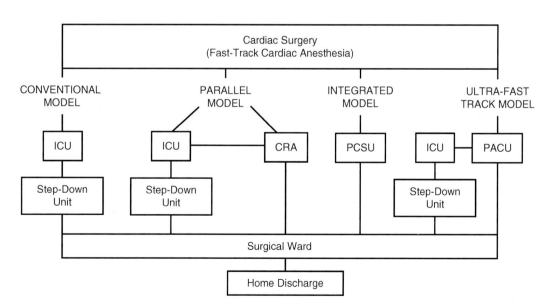

Fig. 50.1 Post-cardiac surgical recovery models. *ICU* intensive care unit, *CRA* cardiac recovery area; *PCSU* post-cardiac surgical unit, *PACU* post-anesthetic care unit. Modified with permission from Bainbridge D, Cheng D. Current evidence on fast track cardiac recovery Management. Eur Heart J Suppl. 2017;19(Suppl A), A3–A7

patient moves directly into the post-anesthetic care unit. The patient is then transferred to the surgical ward if they meet discharge criteria, or transferred to the ICU if they fail. This pathway becomes feasible as more and more cardiac patients receive sedation or ultra-fast track surgery to be extubated in the operating room or shortly in the PACU . The major limitation to this model is ensuring adequate nursing capacity and skills for this patient population. Variations on the ultra-fast track recovery model include the use of the ICU coronary care unit instead of the PACU, with the intent to discharge the patient to the ward 2–3 h after surgery. Ultra-fast track recovery models are frequently used for transfemoral transcatheter aortic valve implantation cases where sedation anesthesia is used [4]. Fast track (FT) recovery management is a multidisciplinary process using multimodal management techniques to improve the efficiency and safety of postoperative patient management, while using available resources appropriately.

Postoperative Care for FTCA Patients

Enhanced Recovery After Cardiac Surgery

The Society for Enhanced Recovery After Cardiac Surgery's (ERAS® Cardiac) mission is to optimize the perioperative care of cardiac surgical patients [5]. ERAS protocols are designed to achieve early recovery in patients and the evidence-based consensus statements for perioperative cardiac surgical care can be considered for institutional ERAS pathways in patients undergoing heart surgery (Table 50.1) [6]. In general, this perioperative pathway is reasonable to apply in cardiac surgery patients.

Postoperative Transfer of Care

Upon arrival in the CRA initial management of cardiac patients consists of ensuring stable patient vitals and an efficient transfer of care from OR staff to CRA staff. The anesthesiologist should relay patient history, conduct of anesthesia, blood product use, ease of bypass wean, inotropes, urine output, TEE findings and any associated complications. In addition, the most recent potassium, hemoglobin, glucose, $PaCO_2$, pH, and bicarbonate. Initial routine lab work should include electrolytes, complete blood count, arterial blood gas, coagulation profile (INR, aPTT), creatinine, urea, and glucose. An ECG and CXR should also be ordered. The patients Hb should be assessed as anemia occurs in the face of dilution and ongoing blood loss. Blood transfusions should be individualized to each patient but certainly should be initiated if the Hb falls below 70 mg/dl. Potassium is usually low following bypass especially if diuretics are given intraoperatively. Hypokalemia contributes to increased automaticity and may lead to ventricular ectopies, ventricular tachycardia, or ventricular fibrillation. Treatment consists of potassium infusions (20 meq of potassium in 50 ml run over 1 h) until the potassium exceeds 3.5 meq/ml. Increasing the potassium to 5.0 meq/ml may reduce the frequency of ventricular ectopy if problematic. Chest tube drainage should be checked every 15 min on arrival to aid detection of coagulopathic states. Initial treatment consists of 50–100 mg of iv protamine over 2-4 h to ensure complete heparin reversal, especially if heparinized pump blood has been given post protamine reversal in OR. The patient's temperature should be recorded on arrival and active measures instituted to warm the hypothermic patient. This improves coagulation, decreases oxygen consumption incurred by shivering and aids in early extubation.

Pain control following bypass surgery has become a renewed concern as patients are given fewer narcotics and heavy sedation is weaned earlier in the postoperative period. Intravenous morphine is still the mainstay of treatment for post bypass patients. The most common method is patient demanded, nurse delivered iv morphine. In patients at low risk for renal or bleeding complications low dosage NSAIDs assist in pain control and reduce morphine use.

Table 50.1 The Society for Enhanced Recovery After Cardiac Surgery's (ERAS® Cardiac) perioperative recommendations

Class of Recommendation (Strength)[a]	Level of Evidence (Quality)[b]	Recommendations
PREOPERATIVE		
Class I	C-LD	Preoperative screening for smoking and hazardous alcohol consumption is recommended. Consumption should be stopped 4 weeks before elective surgery.
Class IIa	B-NR	Prehabilitation is beneficial for patients undergoing elective cardiac surgery with multiple comorbidities or significant deconditioning.
	C-LD	Preoperative assessment of hemoglobin A1c and albumin is reasonable to be performed.
	C-LD	Correction of nutritional deficiency, when feasible, can be beneficial.
	C-LD	Patient engagement through online or application -based systems to promote education, compliance, and patient reported outcomes can be useful.
Class IIb	C-LD	A clear liquid diet may be considered to be continued up until 4 hours before general anesthesia.
	C-LD	Carbohydrate loading may be considered before surgery.
INTRAOPERATIVE		
Class I	A	Tranexamic acid or epsilon aminocaproic acid should be administered for on-pump cardiac surgical procedures to reduce blood loss.
	B-R	A care bundle of best practices should be performed to reduce surgical site infection.
Class IIa	B-R	Rigid sternal fixation can be useful to reduce mediastinal wound complications.
Class III (harm)	B-R	Hyperthermia (>37.9) while rewarming on CPB and in the early postoperative period is potentially harmful and should be avoided.
POSTOPERATIVE		
Class I	B-R	Perioperative glycemic control is recommended.
	B-R	Goal-directed therapy should be performed to reduce postoperative complications.
	B-NR	A multimodal, opioid -sparing, pain management plan is recommended postoperatively.

Table 50.1 (continued)

	B-NR	A multimodal, opioid -sparing, pain management plan is recommended postoperatively.
	B-NR	Postoperative systematic delirium screening is recommended at least once per nursing shift.
	B-NR	Maintenance of chest tube patency without breaking the sterile field is recommended to prevent retained blood complications.
	B-NR	Persistent hypothermia (T<35oC) after CPB should be avoided in the early postoperative period. Additionally, hyperthermia (T>38oC) should be avoided in the early postoperative period.
Class IIa	B-R	Biomarkers can be beneficial in identifying patients at risk for acute kidney injury.
	B-NR	Insulin infusion is reasonable to be performed to treat hyperglycemia in all patients in the perioperative period.
	B-NR	Early extubation strategies after surgery are reasonable to be employed.
	C-LD	Chemical thromboprophylaxis can be beneficial following cardiac surgery.
Class III (no benefit)	A	Routine stripping of chest tubes is not recommended.

Reproduced with permission from: Engelman DT, et al. Guidelines for Perioperative Care in Cardiac Surgery: Enhanced Recovery After Surgery Society Recommendations. JAMA Surg. 2019 May 4. doi: 10.1001/jamasurg.2019.1153. Copyright© 2019 American Medical Association. All rights reserved

[a]Class of Recommendation: I (strong): benefit many times greater than risk; IIa (moderate): benefit much greater than risk; IIb (weak): benefit greater than risk; III: no benefit (moderate): benefit equal to risk; III: harm (strong): risk greater than benefit

[b]A: High-quality evidence from multiple RCTs, meta-analysis of high-quality RCTs, one or more RCTs corroborated by registry studies; B-R: Moderate-quality evidence from multiple RCTs, meta-analysis of moderate-quality RCTs; B-NR: Moderate-quality evidence from one or more well-designed, well-executed nonrandomized studies or observational studies; C-LD: Randomized or nonrandomized observational or registry studies with limitations of design or execution

Rick Factors for Delayed Extubation, Prolonged ICU LOS and Mortality

The main benefit associated with fast-track cardiac anaesthesia is a clinically important reduction in time to extubation and ICU length of stay, without an increased risk of mortality or major complications after surgery [7]. Several studies have examined perioperative risk factors predictive of delayed extubation, prolonged ICU stay due to medical complications (greater than 48 h) and mortality in FTCA patients. Preoperative risk factors for delayed extubation include advanced age, and female sex. Postoperative risk factors include intra-aortic balloon pump use (IAPB), inotrope infusions, postoperative bleeding, and atrial arrhythmia. Preoperative risk factors for prolonged ICU LOS included both advanced age and female sex, as well as a recent history of myocardial infarction (MI). Preoperative risk factors for mortality include female sex, emergency surgery, and poor left ventricular function [8].

Management of Postoperative Complications

Management of postoperative complications are detailed in Chaps. 52–63 of this text. Complications are frequent post cardiac surgery. Many are transient, such as atrial fibrillation, but some (stroke, renal failure) are long-lasting catastrophic events that seriously affect the functional status of a patient. The incidence and predisposing risk factors are well studied for many of these complications. Many of these complications have specific management issues, which may improve recovery after surgery (Table 50.2) [9].

As postoperative bleeding is one of the major risk factors in delayed extubation and increased morbidity and mortality, a comprehensive approach in perioperative blood management in cardiac surgery is essential. Table 50.3 outlines a summary of recommendations in drugs, technologies and techniques for minimally invasive and conventional cardiac surgery [10].

Summary

Management of cardiac surgical patients is constantly evolving with new minimally invasive cardiac procedures and interventional procedures, as well as robotic and hybrid surgical approaches. Fast-track management depends on the careful selection of patients preoperatively based on surgical procedure, and patient comorbidities and risk factors. FT management continues through the intraoperative period with the intent for early extubation until proven otherwise by intraoperative and postoperative risk factors. A dedicated postoperative cardiac surgical and anesthesia critical care team is best to recognize and manage potential complications [11]. Finally, a designated cardiac surgery recovery unit with well-established best practice postoperative protocols will ensure the optimal postoperative care and recovery of these patients.

Table 50.2 Management of complications after cardiac surgery

Complications	Management
Bleeding/Chest re-exploration	Volume resuscitation Protamine infusion Tranexamic acid Correct coagulopathy: Platelet, FFP, Cryoppt Correct pH, electrolytes Normothermia Surgical exploration
Atrial Fibrillation	Rate control: calcium channel blockers, β-blockers, digoxin Rhythm control: amiodarone, sotalol, procainamide Thromboembolic prophylaxis: for atrial fibrillation > 48 hours
Left Ventricular Failure/Right Heart Failure	Increase preload, crystalloid volume Increase myocardial contractility: Inotropes (epinephrine, milrinone, norepinephrine) Reduce afterload (drugs, inhaled PGE, nitric oxide) Methylene blue in refractory vasoplegic shock Mechanical support: intra-aortic balloon pump; ECMO
Sternal Wound Infection/Debridement	Surgical debridement of all nonviable tissue and removal of all foreign material Wound lavage with antibiotics Deep wound cultures obtained (if feasible) Initial antibiotic therapy targeted at the most frequently isolated organisms (*Staphylococcus aureus* and coagulase negative Staphylococci)
Renal Failure/Dialysis	Remove the causative agent (nonsteroidal anti-inflammatory drugs, antibiotics) Hemodynamic support if necessary Hydration Supportive care
Delirium	Usually self-limited Requires close observation May require sedatives (midazolam, lorazepam)
Stroke	Supportive treatment Avoid potential aggravating factors (hyperglycemia, hyperthermia, and severe anemia)

Table 50.3 Summary of recommendations in perioperative blood management

Class of Recommendation (Strength)	Level of Evidence (Quality)	Recommendations
Lysine Analogs in Cardiac Surgery		
Class I	A	The lysine analogs Ɛ-aminocaproic acid (Amicar) and tranexamic acid (TA) reduce exposure to allogeneic blood in patients undergoing CPB cardiac surgery. These agents are recommended routinely as part of a blood conservation strategy in patients undergoing cardiac surgery.
Class IIb	C	It is important not to exceed maximum recommended TA dosages (50-100 mg/kg) because of potential neurotoxicity, particularly in elderly and open-heart procedures.
Class III	A	Aprotinin is not recommended in adult cardiac surgery until further studies on its safety profile.
Tranexamic Acid (TA) for OPCAB		
Class I	A	TA is recommended as part of a blood conservation strategy in patients undergoing OPCAB surgery.
Class IIb	C	TA dosing in OPCAB surgery needs further study particularly with regard to possible neurotoxicity such as seizures.
Desmopressin		
Class I	A	Use caution with DDAVP infusion rate to avoid significant hypotension.
Class IIa	A	DDAVP may be considered for prophylaxis in CABG surgery, in particular, for patients on ASA within 7 days or prolonged CPB more than 140 minutes.
Topical Hemostatics		
Class IIa	A	Routine use of topical antifibrinolytics in cardiac surgery is not recommended.
Class IIb	C	Topical fibrin sealant may be considered in clinical situations where conventional approaches of surgical and medical improvement of hemostasis are not effective, that is, with bleeding problems more local than generalized.
FVIIa		
Class IIa	A	Prophylactic use of FVIIa cannot be recommended because of a significant increase in the risk of thromboembolic events and stroke.

(continued)

Table 50.3 (continued)

Erythropoietin (EPO) + Iron		
Class IIa	A	It is reasonable to administer EPO preoperatively (2Y4 weeks) to increase red blood cell mass in patients who are anemic or refuse blood products (Jehovah's Witness) or as a blood management strategy.
Antiplatelet Agents Before Cardiac Surgery		
Class I	A	In stable elective CABG with no DES, clopidogrel should be discontinued 5 days preoperatively.
Class IIa	B	ASA may be continued until surgery.
	B	Direct-acting P2Y12 receptor antagonist may be a better alternative than clopidogrel in ACS patients undergoing CABG surgery.
Class IIb	C	In stable elective CABG with DES less than 1 year old, consider continuing clopidogrel or heparin as a bridge to surgery.
Antiplatelet Agents After Cardiac Surgery		
Class IIb	B	In stable CABG surgery (non -ACS patients), the routine use of postoperative clopidogrel with ASA is not warranted.
Acute Normovolemic Hemodilution (ANH)		
Class IIa	A	ANH can be considered in selected patients (adequate preoperative hemoglobin level) to reduce post -CPB bleeding.
Class IIb	B	Routine use of ANH in unselected patients cannot be recommended.
Retrograde Autologous Priming (RAP)		
Class I	A	RAP can be recommended as a blood conservation modality to reduce allogeneic blood transfusion in cardiac surgery.
Cell Salvage (CS)		
Class I	A	Routine use of CS is recommended in operations where an increased blood loss is expected.
Class IIa	A	CS should be used throughout the entire operation and not merely as a replacement for cardiopulmonary bypass cardiotomy suction.
Biocompatible Coated Cardiopulmonary Bypass (CBP) Circuit		
Class IIb	A	The routine use of biocompatible coated CPB circuitry may be considered as part of a multimodal blood conservation program. However, the heterogeneity of surface -modified products, anticoagulation management, and CPB technique does not significantly impact surgical blood loss and transfusion needs.

Table 50.3   (continued)

Miniaturized Cardiopulmonary Bypass		
Class IIa	A	MECC can be considered as a blood conservation technique to reduce allogeneic blood exposure; *however, issues related to heparinization management and biocoat remain to be clarified.*
Ultrafiltration		
Class IIb	A	The use of ultrafiltration may be considered for blood conservation; however, impact on clinically relevant outcomes remains unproven and issues related to different technologies and timing of ultrafiltration remain to be clarified.
Platelet Plasmapheresis		
Class IIa	A	It is reasonable to consider platelet plasmapheresis for blood management in cardiac surgery.
Point-of-Care (POC) Technology		
Class IIb	A	The evidence is too premature to recommend POC technology for routine use because its use has not been shown to impact clinical outcome.
Minimally Invasive Techniques		
Class IIa	A	Whereas minimally invasive cardiac procedures are not primarily selected for blood management, the reduced allogeneic blood exposure should be considered in the balance of benefits and risks when selecting the appropriate surgery for the patients.

ACS, acute coronary syndrome; ASA, acetylsalicylic acid; CABG, coronary artery bypass grafting; DES, drug-eluting stent; FVIIa, factor VIIa; MECC, miniaturized extracorporeal circuit; OPCAB, off-pump coronary artery bypass; see Table 50.1 for definitions of Class of Recommendation and Level of Evidence

Reproduced from: Menkis A, Martin J, Cheng D, et al. Drug, Devices, Technologies, and Techniques for Blood Management in Minimally Invasive and Conventional Cardiothoracic Surgery. A Consensus Statement from the International Society for Minimally Invasive Cardiothoracic Surgery (ISMICS) 2011. Innovations: Technology and Techniques in Cardiothoracic and Vascular Surgery 2012; 7(4):1–14

References

1. Cheng DC, Byrick RJ, Knobel E. Structural models for intermediate care areas. Crit Care Med. 1999;27:2266–71.
2. Brown MM. Implementation strategy: one-stop recovery for cardiac surgical patients. AACN Clin Issues. 2000;11:412–23.
3. Zakhary W, Turton E, Ender J. Post-operative patient care and hospital implications of fast track. Eur Heart J Suppl. 2017;19(Suppl A):A18–22.
4. Bainbridge D, Cheng D. Current evidence on fast track cardiac recovery management. Eur Heart J Suppl. 2017;19(Suppl A):A3–7.
5. Engelman DT, Boyle EM, Williams JB, et al. Enhanced Recovery After Surgery (ERAS): An Expert Consensus Statement in Cardiac Surgery. In: Abstract presented at the Enhanced Recovery After Surgery (ERAS®) session held on Saturday, April 28th, 2018, during the American Association for Thoracic Surgery (AATS), San Diego, CA.
6. The Society for Enhanced Recovery After Cardiac Surgery [website]. Available from https://www.eras-cardiac.org/
7. Wong WT, Lai VKW, Chee YE, Lee A. Fast-track cardiac care for adult cardiac surgical patients. Cochrane Database Syst Rev. 2016; (9):CD003587. https://doi.org/10.1002/14651858.CD003587.

8. Wong DT, Cheng DC, Kustra R. Risk factors of delayed extubation, prolonged length of stay in the intensive care unit, and mortality in patients undergoing coronary artery bypass graft with fast-track cardiac anesthesia: a new cardiac risk score. Anesthesiology. 1999;91:936–44.

9. Bainbridge D, Cheng D. Fast track management and outcomes. In: Kaplan JA, Reich DL, editors. Cardiac anesthesia: for cardiac and noncardiac surgery. 7th ed. Philadelphia, PA: Saunders; 2016.

10. Menkis A, Martin J, Cheng D, et al. Drug, devices, technologies, and techniques for blood management in minimally invasive and conventional cardiothoracic surgery. A consensus statement from the International Society for Minimally Invasive Cardiothoracic Surgery (ISMICS) 2011. Innovations. 2012;7(4):1–14.

11. Cheng DC. Fast track cardiac surgery pathways: early extubation, process of care, and cost containment. Anesthesiology. 1998;88:1429–33 (editorial).

Atrial and Ventricular Arrhythmia Management

51

Yatin Mehta and Dheeraj Arora

Main Messages

1. Atrial arrhythmias are quite common in the perioperative period, and can vary from sinus arrhythmia to supraventricular tachycardia. They can be benign, but may also cause hemodynamic instability.
2. Arrhythmias during the perioperative period are major causes of morbidity and mortality in cardiac and non-cardiac surgery.
3. Optimal monitoring and vigilance during the perioperative period is required for the detection of arrhythmia.
4. Most arrhythmias can be managed with correction of the reversible causes, such as electrolyte and acid base disturbances, mechanical causes, and hypothermia and ventilation problems.
5. Life threatening and malignant arrhythmia should be treated promptly with regard to the available protocols and guidelines.
6. A supraventricular tachycardia (SVT) is an umbrella term used to describe any tachycardia (heart rate >100 bpm) originating from bundle of His or above. Management varies from immediate cardioversion to pharmacological therapy depending upon patient's hemodynamic profile.
7. Atrial fibrillation (AF) is the most common arrhythmia after cardiac surgery—particularly after coronary artery surgery—with an incidence of 30%. Management includes cardioversion, pharmacotherapy and anticoagulation therapy.
8. Ventricular arrhythmias are more common during the perioperative period in patients with preexisting cardiac disease, and are usually considered life threatening. They originate from sites distal to the bundle of His and are characterized by wide QRS complexes greater than 110 ms. Common ventricular arrhythmias are premature ventricular contractions (PVC), ventricular tachycardia (VT) and ventricular fibrillation (VF).
9. Management of VT depend on the type; whether it is with palpable pulse or pulseless (cardiac arrest). For pulse-

Y. Mehta (✉) · D. Arora
Medanta Institute of Critical Care and Anesthesiology, Medanta The Medicity, Sector-38, Gurgaon, Haryana, India

© Springer Nature Switzerland AG 2021
D. C. H. Cheng et al. (eds.), *Evidence-Based Practice in Perioperative Cardiac Anesthesia and Surgery*, https://doi.org/10.1007/978-3-030-47887-2_51

less VT, the universal algorithm for cardiac arrest (i.e. advanced cardiac life support (ACLS)) should be followed.

10. AV conduction disorder is commonly seen after myocardial infarction, drug intake (digoxin, beta blockers, calcium channel blockers), inflammation or fibrosis of the conduction system, and post cardiac valvular surgery. They are usually benign, and if hemodynamically significant, may require pacemaker insertion.

Cardiac arrhythmias are the most frequent perioperative cardiovascular abnormalities in patients undergoing cardiac and non-cardiac surgery. They are one of the major causes of hemodynamic instability in the perioperative period, due to their alteration of the cardiac output (CO). The overall reported incidence is up to 70% in patients undergoing general anesthesia [1]. The incidence in cardiac and non-cardiac surgery is up to 60% and 90% respectively [2, 3]. Immediate diagnosis and intervention prevent any fatal complication in the perioperative period.

The normal ECG consists of P, QRS and T wave that correspond to mechanical events during the cardiac cycle. P wave is formed by atrial contraction due to firing of Sino-Atrial (SA) and electrical impulses, which are passed through internodal tracts to the atrioventricular (AV) node.

After this, atrial repolarization occurs (which is often obscured by the larger QRS complex due to ventricular depolarization). PR interval (0.16 s) denotes the interval between atrial and ventricular contraction. Ventricular depolarization is due to transmission of electrical impulses to conducting fibres in the bundle of His to the ventricular apices. The impulses are then carried in the Purkinje fibres to initiate ventricular contraction. The normal QRS duration is <0.12 s. Ventricular repolarization is represented by ST segment and T wave.

Perioperative Considerations

Perioperative arrhythmia particularly prevalent in high risk patients, such as elderly patients with comorbidities undergoing elective and emergency surgery, and can have significant long-term implications. Preoperative examination of the patient should focus on diagnosing the patient at risk, and identifying other factors such as coronary artery or valvular heart disease, electrolyte imbalance and hormonal or autonomic disturbances. Any arrhythmia (e.g. atrial fibrillation (AF)) in the postoperative period may cause a low CO state, leading to congestive heart failure, stroke or myocardial infarction and other end organ damage. Perioperative arrhythmia may be due to patient factors, or can be anesthesia or surgical procedure related.

Main pathogenesis of arrhythmia are [4]:

- **Pathological**—Injury or damage to the cardiac conduction systems.
- **Re-entry**—May precipitate a wide variety of supraventricular and ventricular arrhythmias.
- **Automaticity**—Abnormal atrial or ventricular depolarization during the periods of action can potentially lead to arrhythmias.
- **Ion channel mechanism**—As these channels are mainly responsible for depolarization, change in ion channels may lead to arrhythmias.
- **Ectopic or irritable foci**

Factors Predisposing Patients to Perioperative Arrhythmia [5]

- Underlying heart disease (ischemic or valvular heart disease, cardiomyopathy, heart failure).
- Electrolyte or acid-base disorder (hypokalemia, hyperkalemia, hypomagnesemia, hypercalcemia, acidosis).
- Endocrine disorders (thyrotoxicosis, pheochromocytoma).
- Intracranial bleed (subarachnoid hemorrhage).
- Drugs (digoxin, beta blockers, calcium channel blockers, theophylline, antidepressants).

Reversible Causes of Perioperative Arrhythmia [6]

- Hypoxaemia, Hypercarbia.
- Acidosis, electrolyte imbalances.
- Hypotension.
- Mechanical irritation—Pulmonary artery catheter, chest tube, handling of heart during cardiac surgery.
- Hypothermia.
- Adrenergic stimulation (light anesthesia), intraoperative traction, oculocardiac reflex, dental or carotid surgery.
- Proarrhythmic drugs—Volatile anesthetics, inotropic agents, etc.
- Myocardial ischemia.

Common Arrhythmias During the Perioperative Period-

Supraventricular arrhythmia Bradyarrhythmia; supraventricular tachycardia; atrial flutter; atrial fibrillation.

Ventricular arrhythmia Premature ventricular contraction (PVC); ventricular tachycardia (VT) nonsustained/ sustained; ventricular fibrillation (VF); Torsades de pointes.

Management of Perioperative Arrhythmia

Primary management of perioperative arrhythmia consists of treatment of reversible causes such as metabolic abnormalities, surgical causes, inadequate depth of anesthesia, etc. After addressing the cause, a 12 lead electrocardiograph (EKG) should be obtained. In the EKG, one should look for the following points [7]:

- What is the heart rate?
- Is the rhythm regular or irregular?
- Is there a P wave for each QRS?
- Is the QRS normal or abnormal?
- Is the rhythm dangerous or benign?
- Is treatment necessary? If so, with what?

After addressing above points, exact nature and severity of the arrhythmia is established and management should be focused accordingly.

Atrial Arrhythmia

Atrial arrhythmia is quite common in the perioperative period. It can be benign, but may also cause hemodynamic instability. It may vary from sinus arrhythmia to supraventricular tachycardia.

Sinus Arrhythmia

In sinus arrhythmia, there is a sinus rhythm but with variable R-R interval. It can be a normal finding, especially in young patients, and alters with respiration. It is usually of no concern perioperatively, and requires no treatment. It may be observed in lighter planes of anesthesia [8].

Sinus Tachycardia

Sinus tachycardia is the most common arrhythmia in the perioperative period. It is a sinus rhythm with normal P-QRS-T complexes and morphology, but with a rate of more than 100 bpm. It is further classified as-

- **Physiologic sinus tachycardia**: Appropriate increased sinus rate in response to exercise and other situations that increase the sympathetic tone.
- **Inappropriate sinus tachycardia**: Sinus heart rate >100 bpm at rest, with a mean 24-h heartrate >90 bpm not due to appropriate physiological responses or primary causes such as hyperthyroidism or anemia.

The cause may be multifactorial (increased sympathetic activity secondary to pain, anxiety, hypovolemia, fever, anemia, hypoxia, hypercarbia, low cardiac output states, sepsis and thyrotoxicosis). It may also be secondary to drugs such as inotropes, or other drugs such as atropine, ephedrine, aminophylline and salbutamol. Sustained tachycardia can lead to short diastolic time, which may result in myocardial ischemia, especially in a patient with compromised coronary reserve [7]. The treatment is usually to address the precipitating agent, and beta blockers should be reserved for patients with coronary artery disease. Metoprolol (2.5–5 mg IV repeated every two minutes if required, to a total of 15 mg) and esmolol 500 mcg/kg bolus then infusion 50–300 mcg/kg/min can be used [9].

Sinus Bradycardia

Sinus bradycardia is a sinus rhythm with normal P-QRS-T complexes and morphology with a heart rate of less than 60 bpm. It is usually benign and due to increased vagal tone, or secondary to medications such as narcotics with anesthetic agents, beta blockers, amiodarone, etc. It may be observed secondary to pain, nausea, vasovagal and carotid sinus syndromes, hypoxemia, hypothermia, hypothyroidism and raised intracranial pressure. Other cardiac causes are myocardial infarction and sick sinus syndrome [10]. It does not require any treatment if hypotension is not associated. If hypotension or low CO state is present, reversible causes should be treated first. Medical treatment includes atropine 0.5 mg IV boluses to a total of 3 mg or glycopyrrolate 0.1 mg IV bolus repeated every two to three min if required, and adrenaline or isoprenaline infusion. Resistant bradycardia may require temporary pacemaker (transvenous / transcutaneous) as a transit measure before permanent pacemaker insertion [10].

Premature Atrial Contractions

Premature atrial contractions (PACs) or atrial ectopics are due to an impulse originating from an ectopic focus in either atria. It manifests as an aberrant P wave which is sometimes hard to locate, being lost in the QRS or the preceding T wave. It is usually benign and hemodynamically insignificant, and sometimes may precede supraventricular arrhythmia. PAC do not require any treatment unless hemodynamically, significant which can be managed with beta blockers.

Supraventricular Tachycardia

A supraventricular tachycardia (SVT) is an umbrella term used to describe any tachycardia (heart rate >100 bpm) originating from bundle of His or above. It includes inappropriate sinus tachycardia, atrial tachycardia (focal or multifo-cal), junctional tachycardia, AV nodal reentrant tachycardia (AVNRT), or accessory pathway reentrant tachycardia. ECG features include abnormally shaped P waves, often outnumbering QRS complexes, while in multifocal atrial tachycardia there are three or more P wave morphologies with irregular QRS complexes. Junctional tachycardia has a rate of 150–200 bpm with P waves either buried or closely following the QRS complex.

SVT is relatively common in adult Americans, with 89,000 newly diagnosed cases each year, accounting for approximately 50,000 emergency department visits each year [11].

Management of SVT includes differentiation from potentially life threatening ventricular tachycardia. Narrow complex tachycardia should also be differentiated from other forms of atrial tachycardia (Fig. 51.1).

If the patient is hemodynamically unstable, immediate synchronized direct current (DC) cardioversion (Fig. 51.2) with 200 Joules (J) should be done (Class I) [9]. If the patient is hemodynamically stable, the initial management should include carotid sinus massage (Class I) that will cause increased vagal activity by activating baroreceptors leading to transient AV block, also helping to differentiate between SVT, atrial flutter, and atrial fibrillation (AF) [9]. Following this, pharmacological therapy [9] should be considered if the patient is not responding to the above methods.

- **Adenosine** (Class I)—A rapidly acting endogenous purine nucleoside with an ultra-short action. It can terminate the arrhythmia, and has a quick onset and an extremely short half-life (10 s). It should be avoided in asthmatics and Wolff Parkinson White (WPW) syndrome [9].
- **Non-dihydropyridine calcium channel blockers** (Class IIa)—Verapamil, diltiazem.
- **Beta-1 blockers** (Class IIA)—Metoprolol, esmolol (Fig. 51.2).
- **Amiodarone** (Class IIA)—Can also be used if the patient is not responding. Dose is 150 mg over 10 min followed by infusion 0.5–1 mg/min for next 24 h.

Fig. 51.1 Differential diagnosis for adult narrow QRS tachycardia. AV indicates atrioventricular; AVNRT, atrioventricular nodal reentrant tachycardia; AVRT, atrioventricular reentrant tachycardia; ECG, electrocardiogram; MAT, multifocal atrial tachycardia; and PJRT, permanent form of junctional reentrant

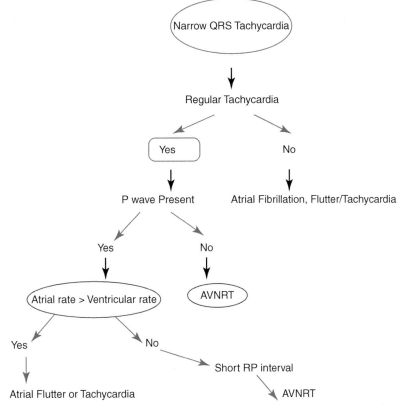

Fig. 51.2 Acute treatment of regular SVT of unknown mechanism

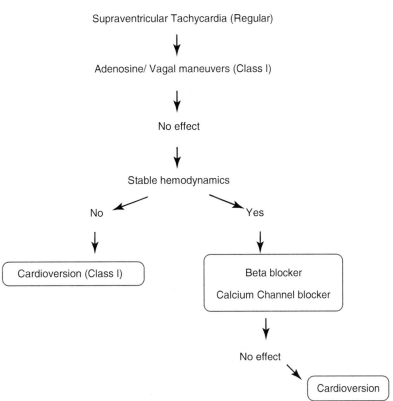

- **Ibutilide**—Contraindicated if QTc> 440 ms. Dose is 1 mg over 10 min and can be repeated after 10 min.
- **Digoxin**—Dose is 0.25–0.5 mg bolus and can be repeated 0.25 mg with maximum dose of 1 mg over 24 h. It should be avoided in renal dysfunction and AV blocks.
- **Ivabradine**—Dose is 5 mg orally twice daily dose. It should be avoided in heart failure, hepatic failure and hypotension

Atrial Flutter

Atrial flutter is due to electrical impulse re-entry into the atria. It is a regular atrial arrhythmia at a rapid rate that is usually associated with a conduction block. It is characterized by saw-tooth flutter waves preceding narrow QRS complexes and a regular rhythm. The flutter waves are best seen in inferior leads (II, III, aVF) or V1. Commonly, the atrial rate is 300 bpm with an AV conduction ratio of 2:1 giving a ventricular rate of 150 bpm. Both atrial flutter and atrial tachycardia can occur with any kind of AV block (e.g. 2:1, 3:1, etc.) and may predispose the patient to thromboembolism.

Management depends upon the hemodynamics of the patient (Fig. 51.3). Synchronized DC cardioversion (Class IB) should be done in hypotensive patients. In hemodynamically stable patients, the management involves ventricular rate control, conversion to sinus rhythm and long-term anticoagulation for prevention of embolic stroke. Ventricular rate control can be achieved by beta-1 blockers, non-dihydropyridine calcium channel blockers (Class IB), and digoxin. Amiodarone (Class IIA) may also be effective in patients with reduced LV function. Recently, oral dofetilide or intravenous ibutilide (Class IA) have been found to be useful for acute pharmacological cardioversion in patients with atrial flutter [9]. Intravenous ibutilide converts atrial flutter to sinus rhythm in approximately 60% of cases.

Atrial Fibrillation

Atrial fibrillation (AF) is an irregularly irregular rhythm that is often rapid. There is absence of P waves with irregularly irregular QRS complexes with a wandering baseline. It is an independent and uncoordinated atrial electrical activity, with a ventricular rate dependent on the intermittent AV node transmission. As atrial contraction contributes to 30–40% of normal ventricular filling, fast AF (>90 bpm) may lead to reduction in ventricular filling, cardiac output and hypotension. Moreover, reduction in diastolic time due to fast ventricular rate may lead to myocardial ischemia.

It is the most common arrhythmia after cardiac surgery, and in particular after coronary artery surgery the incidence is 30% [12]. It may

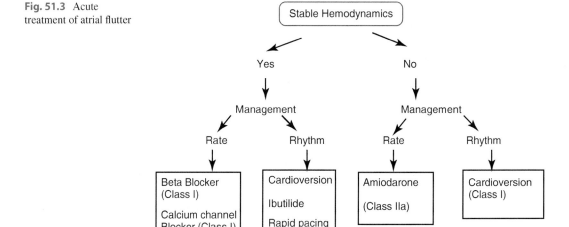

Fig. 51.3 Acute treatment of atrial flutter

be present in association with heart failure, ischemic heart disease, mitral valve disease, cardiomyopathy, electrolyte abnormalities, sepsis and congenital heart diseases such as atrial septal defect. AF is a risk factor for the development of left atrial thrombus leading to thromboembolic episodes.

Initial management of AF includes correction of the underlying cause. Synchronized DC cardioversion should be done in hemodynamically unstable patients with new-onset AF and can be repeated if it recurs. Elective cardioversion should be performed on hemodynamically stable patients. Management involves ventricular rate control, conversion to sinus rhythm and long-term anticoagulation for prevention of embolic stroke [13]. Ventricular rate control can be achieved by beta blockers, non-dihydropyridine calcium channel blockers, and digoxin. Amiodarone may also be used in patients with reduced left ventricular (LV) function. Other medications such as procainamide can be used with continuous QRS monitoring for evidence of QT prolongation, and ibutilide or flecainide are recommended in presence of an accessory pathway in hemodynamically stable patients. Sotalol and ibutilide should be used with caution as they can precipitate Torsades de pointes if the QTc exceeds 500 ms [14]. In AF more than 3 days old, along with rate control, anticoagulation prophylaxis should be started.

Ventricular Arrhythmia

Ventricular arrhythmias are more common during the perioperative period in patients with pre-existing cardiac disease, and are usually considered as life threatening. Ventricular arrhythmias originate from sites distal to the bundle of His and are characterized by wide QRS complexes greater than 110 ms.

Premature Ventricular Contractions

Premature ventricular contractions (PVCs) are ectopic beats originating from below the AV node, and impulses originating from an ectopic focus located in the ventricular myocardium; therefore, there is no P wave preceding the QRS complex. Moreover, ectopic impulse is not con-

ducted via the fast conducting normal pathway, producing a wide abnormal shaped QRS complex (>120 ms). It can be unifocal, multifocal, or alternate with sinus beats in every second (bigeminy) or third (trigeminy) beat [7]. Multifocal PVC may lead to generation of ventricular tachycardia (VT).

Primary management should focus on the reversible underlying problems such as hypoxemia, hypotension, hypoventilation, hypokalemia, hypothermia and avoiding mechanical stimulation [15]. Pharmacological therapy includes intravenous lidocaine with bolus of 1–1.5 mg/kg followed by infusion of 1–4 mg/min. Procainamide and bretylium have also been used as second line therapy. External pacing may be required if PVC occurs in association with sinus bradycardia.

Ventricular Tachycardia

VT is defined as three or more consecutive PVCs with the rate exceeding 100 beats/min [15]. Classical VT is characterized by wide-QRS complexes (>120 ms) with a regular rhythm. It may be associated with both adequate perfusion or shock state and may progress into VF ultimately leading to sudden cardiac death (SCD) [16]. Common causes of VT include acute myocardial infarction or ischemia, cardiomyopathy (dilated or hypertrophic), valvular heart diseases, mitral valve prolapse, myocarditis, or electrolyte imbalance.

A VT is called non-sustained (NSVT) if the duration is less than 30 s, and is called accelerated idioventricular rhythm for single morphology QRS complexes at a rate less than 120 beats/min. Both these forms of VT generally do not require any treatment. However, in hemodynamically significant NSVT, amiodarone (300 mg iv bolus) should be considered [16].

Recurrent sustained VT, especially when polymorphic, may be an indicator of incomplete reperfusion or recurrence of acute ischemia and it may disintegrate into VF. Typical ECG signs of VT are absence of typical RBBB or LBBB morphology, extreme axis deviation ("northwest axis"), broad QRS complexes (>160 ms), AV dissociation and capture or fusion beats (Fig. 51.4).

Management of VT depends on the type; whether it is with palpable pulse or pulseless (cardiac arrest). For pulseless VT, universal algorithm for cardiac arrest, i.e. advanced cardiac life support (ACLS), should be followed (Fig. 51.5).

Management of VT with pulse with unstable hemodynamics requires immediate DC cardioversion (Class Ic) [16]. Cardioversion is also indicated if the patient is not responding to anti-

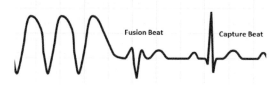

Fig. 51.4 Ventricular tachycardia with capture and fusion beats

arrhythmic drugs. Correction of underlying electrolyte abnormalities and ischemia should be done with a target serum potassium level of 4.5–5 mmol/L.

Pharmacological therapy is indicated for stable VT, depending on LV function of the patient. If LV function is good, then VT can be managed with amiodarone or lignocaine. Procainamide, propafenone, mexiletine and quinidine may be used with caution if the patient is not responding, as they may cause sinus node dysfunction. Sotalol may also be used for arefractory wide QRS tachycardia. However, in patients with LV dysfunction, only amiodarone or lignocaine is recommended [16].

Other nonpharmacological methods, such as overdrive pacing and catheter ablation therapy (Class Ib) [17], or implantable cardioverter-defibrillator insertion (Class Ic), should be considered for refractory cases [16]. Stellate

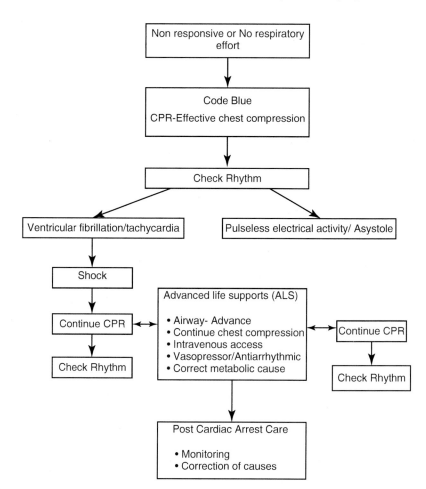

Fig. 51.5 Universal algorithm for cardiac arrest (advanced cardiac life support)

Ganglion block has also been successfully used in refractory cases.

Ventricular Fibrillation

VF is a life threatening arrhythmia characterized by abrupt onset of chaotic, irregular waveforms of different shape, duration and amplitude with no recognizable QRS T waves. There is no ventricular output during the arrhythmia, leading to a pulseless situation with loss of consciousness within seconds.

Management includes urgent initiation of universal algorithm for cardiac arrest (Fig. 51.5) [16]. Medication will only be effective after restoration of the sinus rhythm. Lidocaine, esmolol and amiodarone are primarily used as prophylactics for VF.

Torsades de pointes

Torsades de pointe ("twisting of points") is a type of polymorphic VT. EKG findings include constantly changing QRS morphology, alternating from positive to negative, and QRS amplitude varying, such that the complexes appear to twist around the baseline.

Treatment consists of correction of reversible causes, and the drug of choice is intravenous magnesium sulphate 1–2 g over one to two minutes. Isoprenaline and overdrive pacing can be used in recurrent Torsades de pointes [15].

AV Conduction Disorders

AV conduction disorder is commonly seen after myocardial infarction, drug intake (digoxin, beta blockers, calcium channel blockers), inflammation or fibrosis of the conduction system and post cardiac valvular surgery. AV conduction disorders observed during perioperative period are as follows:

1. **Prolonged PR-interval**—Characterized by a PR interval exceeding 200 ms and each P-wave followed by a QRS. It is benign and asymptomatic and does not require any treatment [18].
2. **Second-degree AV block**—In this type, some atrial impulses fail to be conducted to the ventricles. It is of two types: Mobitz type I and type II.

- **Mobitz type I** (Wenckebach Phenomenon)—Characterized by a progressive prolongation of PR-interval until a P-wave is not followed by a QRS, producing a pause on the EKG. As the PR-interval lengthens, the R-R interval shortens. It is generally benign and does not require any treatment.
- **Mobitz type II**—The PR-intervals remain constant and there is an abrupt failure of a P wave to get conducted, resulting in a P wave with no following QRS, resulting in P:QRS ratio >1. When the P:QRS ratio is 3:1 or more, it is referred to as high-grade second-degree AV block. It may be seen after anterior wall MI and post valvular surgery, and may progress to complete heart block. Pacemaker insertion may be required in high grade blocks [7, 18].

3. **Complete AV block**—The atria and ventricles function independently leading to AV dissociation, thus none of the P wave is conducted to the ventricles. EKG shows constant P-P and R-R intervals and the P waves bear no relationship to QRS complexes. Patient is symptomatic with a low CO state manifested as dyspnea on exertion or syncope. It is commonly observed after inferior wall MI, aortic valve surgery (particularly after calcific aortic stenosis) and congenital heart surgery. Permanent pacemaker insertion is required if the block is persistent [18].

Arrhythmia After Cardiac Surgery

Arrhythmia, especially atrial tachycardia, is frequent after cardiac surgery. The morbidity and mortality depends upon the duration, ventricular response rate, underlying cardiac function, and comorbidities of the patient [19]. Structural heart disease, age, LV function and inflammation are important risk factors for arrhythmia. Moreover, ischemic injury due to CPB and cross-clamp times, type of cardioplegia, and CABG surgical technique are also important determinants during cardiac surgery. Preservation of the anterior epicardial fat pad also tends to decrease atrial arrhythmia [19]. Surgical techniques that decrease inflammation, such as off-pump CABG and minimally invasive cardiac surgery, have less incidence of arrhythmia [20].

Complex congenital cardiac surgery also tends to have arrhythmia after surgical correction, sometimes warranting CPB circuit integrated with extracorporeal membrane oxygenation (ECMO) support [21]. ECMO along with cardiac surgical support decreases the incidence of arrhythmia from 36 to 16% [21].

Preoperative intra-aortic balloon pump (IABP) in patients with poor LV function and refractory angina of unstable hemodynamics have lower incidence of postoperative low CO and ventricular arrhythmia. IABP helps by improving the myocardial oxygen supply/demand ratio by increasing diastolic filling of coronary artery, hemodynamic stability during induction of anesthesia, and improving graft flow post CPB period [22]. Moreover, gentle manipulation of the heart, shorter aortic cross clamp time, maintaining electrolyte balance, and preventing hypoxia, hypercarbia, acidosis and hypothermia also prevent arrhythmia.

References

1. Forrest J, Rehder K, Cahalan M, Goldsmith C. Multicenter study of general anesthesia III. Predictors of severe perioperative adverse outcomes. Anesthesiology. 1992;76:3–15.
2. Katz RL, Bigger JT Jr. Cardiac arrhythmias during anaesthesia and operation. Anesthesiology. 1970;33:193–213.
3. Bertrand CA, Steiner NJ, Jameson AG, et al. Disturbances of cardiac rhythm during anesthesia and surgery. JAMA. 1971;216:1615–7.
4. Kumar P, Clark M. Clinical medicine. 3rd ed. Cardiac arrhythmias 1994. ELBS 554–5, 566–8.
5. Hollenberg SM, Dellinger RP. Noncardiac surgery: postoperative arrhythmias. Crit Care Med. 2000;28:N145–50.
6. Thompson A, Balser JR. Perioperative cardiac arrhythmias. Br J Anaesth. 2004;93:86–94.
7. Feeley TW. Management of perioperative arrhythmias. J Cardiothorac Vasc Anesth. 1997;11(2):10–5.
8. Pomfrett CJD, Barrie JR, Healy TJ. Respiratory sinus arrhythmia: an index of light anaesthesia. Br J Anaesth. 1993;71:212–7.
9. Page RL, Joglar JA, Al-Khatib SM, et al. 2015 ACC/AHA/HRS guideline for the management of adult patients with supraventricular tachycardia: a report of the American College of Cardiology/American Heart Association Task Force on Clinical Practice Guidelines and the Heart Rhythm Society [published online September 16, 2015]. J Am Coll Cardiol. 2016;67(13):e27–e115.
10. Gill HS, Gill JS. Causes, diagnosis and therapeutic strategy in bradyarrhythmias. In: Oxford textbook of critical care. Oxford: Oxford University Press; 2016. p. 730–6.
11. Al-Khatib SM, Page RL. Acute treatment of patients with supraventricular tachycardia. JAMA Cardiol. 2016;1(4):483–5. https://doi.org/10.1001/jamacardio.2016.1483.
12. Villareal RP, Hariharan R, Li BC, et al. Postoperative atrial fibrillation and mortality after coronary artery bypass surgery. J Am Coll Cardiol. 2004;43:472–8.
13. Frendl G, Sodickson AC, Chung MK, Waldo AL, Gersh BJ, Tisdale JE, et al. 2014 AATS guidelines for the prevention and management of perioperative atrial fibrillation and flutter for thoracic surgical procedures. J Thorac Cardiovasc Surg. 2014;148:e153–93.
14. Olshansky B, Rosenfeld LE, Warner AL, Solomon AJ, O'Neill G, Sharma A, et al. The atrial fibrillation follow-up investigation of rhythm management (AFFIRM) study; approaches to control rate in atrial fibrillation. J Am Coll Cardiol. 2004;43:1201–8.
15. Zipes DP, Camm J, Borggrefe M, Buxton AE, Chaitman B, Fromer M, et al. ACC/AHA/ESC 2006 guidelines for management of patients with ventricular arrhythmias and the prevention of sudden cardiac death. Circulation. 2006;114:e385–484.
16. Priori SG, Lundqvist CB, Mazzanti A, et al. 2015 guidelines for the management of patients with ventricular arrhythmias and the prevention of sudden cardiac death. Eur Heart J. 2015;36:2793–867. https://doi.org/10.1093/eurheartj/ehv316.
17. Carbucicchio C, Santamaria M, Trevisi N, Maccabelli G, Giraldi F, Fassini G, Riva S, Moltrasio M, Cireddu M, Veglia F, Della BP. Catheter ablation for the treatment of electrical storm in patients with implantable cardioverter-defibrillators: short- and long-term outcomes in a prospective single-center study. Circulation. 2008;117:462–9.
18. Knight J, Sarko J. Conduction disturbances and cardiac pacemakers. In: Textbook of critical care. Philadelphia, PA: Elsevier Saunders; 2011. p. 587–93.
19. Peretto G, Durante A, Limite LR, Cianflone D. Postoperative arrhythmias after cardiac surgery: incidence, risk factors, and therapeutic management. Cardiol Res Pract. 2014;2014:615987, 15 pages. https://doi.org/10.1155/2014/615987.
20. Tomic V, Russwurm S, Möller E, et al. Transcriptomic and proteomic patterns of systemic inflammation in on-pump and off-pump coronary artery bypass grafting. Circulation. 2005;112(19):2912–20.
21. Peer SM, Costello JP, Klein JC, Engle AM, et al. Twenty-four hour in-hospital congenital cardiac surgical coverage improves perioperative ECMO support outcomes. Ann Thorac Surg. 2014;98:2152–8.
22. Kang N, Edwards M, Larbalestier R. Preoperative intraaortic balloon pumps in high-risk patients undergoing open heart surgery. Ann Thorac Surg. 2001;72:54–7.

Cardiac Surgery Advanced Life Support (CS-ALS)

52

Osama Sefein, Jeff Granton, Dave Nagpal, Cheryl Kee, and Jian Ray Zhou

Main Messages
1. Most cardiac arrests after cardiac surgery are caused by reversible causes. Rapid recognition and treatment will save lives. The main pillars of management are early defibrillation, pacing, and resternotomy.
2. The time to chest reopening as outlined in the STS Consensus Statement is 5 min from starting external cardiac massage (ECM), if return of spontaneous circulation (ROSC) is not achieved. From a practical point of view, the resternotomy process must start immediately on cardiac arrest to achieve the 5 min target. Each institution's practice protocol may vary based on the comfort level and aggressiveness of surgical intervention in the ICU.
3. It is crucial to have a simple and clear protocol that is familiar to and practiced by the health care team to coordinate care and improve key treatment times. Implementing simulation-based training for the care team will increase knowledge and skills retention, and improve teamwork, communication, and care flow.

O. Sefein · J. R. Zhou
Department of Anesthesia and Perioperative Medicine, Western University, London, ON, Canada

J. Granton
Department of Anesthesia and Perioperative Medicine, Western University, London, ON, Canada

Critical Care Medicine, London Health Sciences Centre, London, ON, Canada

D. Nagpal (✉)
Division of Critical Care Medicine, London Health Sciences Centre, London, ON, Canada

Department of Surgery, Western University, London, ON, Canada
e-mail: dave.nagpal@lhsc.on.ca

C. Kee
Critical Care Medicine, London Health Sciences Centre, London, ON, Canada

Cardiac arrest after cardiac surgery is a unique situation. The standard Advanced Cardiac Life Support (ACLS) protocol [1] may not always apply and, in fact, can potentially cause harm to cardiac surgery patients. The European Resuscitation Council published a formal practice guideline for resuscitation post-cardiac surgery [2], yet many North American cardiac surgery centers do not have a dedicated cardiac arrest protocol for this special patient population. To address this apparent deficiency, the *Society of Thoracic Surgeons (STS) Expert Consensus for the Resuscitation of Patients Who Arrest After Cardiac Surgery* was published in 2017 [3], and

© Springer Nature Switzerland AG 2021
D. C. H. Cheng et al. (eds.), *Evidence-Based Practice in Perioperative Cardiac Anesthesia and Surgery*, https://doi.org/10.1007/978-3-030-47887-2_52

serves as an update to the 2015 European Resuscitation Council guidelines for the post-cardiac surgery population [2].

Evidence suggests that patients who experience cardiac arrest after cardiac surgery are sufficiently different from other patients to warrant their own treatment algorithm to optimize survival [3]. Based on data from European centers, the incidence of cardiac arrest after cardiac surgery is 0.7–2.9%, while in the United States the incidence varies between 0.7% and 8% [3]. Survival to discharge after in-hospital cardiac arrest is relatively high at 60–79% [4] among cardiac surgery patients, in contrast to 22.7% for all in-hospital cardiac arrests [5].

Why is the survival rate higher in the cardiac surgery population? First, a high proportion of cardiac arrests are caused by reversible etiologies: 25–50% are due to ventricular fibrillation (VF), pulseless ventricular tachycardia (VT), cardiac tamponade, or severe hypovolemia secondary to massive hemorrhage. Second, the majority of cardiac arrests occur in an intensive care unit, where vigilant monitoring and skilled help is readily available. Finally, protocol-based arrest management improves the speed of accurate diagnosis and guides appropriate treatment of the arrest situation. We believe that by establishing and following a dedicated post-cardiac surgery resuscitation guideline such as the Cardiac Surgery Advanced Life Support (CS-ALS), rates of patient survival to discharge will improve.

This chapter describes the important aspects of the CS-ALS, highlights the key roles in CS-ALS, and reviews the evidence for the protocol implemented in the Cardiac Surgery Intensive Care Unit at London Health Sciences Centre (LHSC).

Resuscitation Goals

The three key resuscitation goals in CS-ALS include:

1. Quick definitive therapy:
   (a) Defibrillation or pacing before external cardiac massage (ECM).
   (b) Re-sternotomy within 5–10 min. This is an important goal as CPR is ineffective in tamponade and severe hypovolemia. Moreover, internal cardiac massage (ICM) can be more effective than external cardiac compression.
2. Rapid diagnosis and treatment of reversible causes of cardiac arrest.
3. Early declaration of surgical emergency to ensure rapid surgical response. This would include early surgeon bedside presence and rapid operating room preparation for chest opening and re-exploration.

Six Key Roles

Leadership and organization are considered the most important keys to success in managing cardiac arrest. Proper training of the resuscitation team so all team members are familiar with their responsibilities and roles on the team is crucial.

There are six key roles in resuscitating the cardiac surgery patient. This list may be expanded to eight roles to include two additional members who perform resternotomy, if indicated. The key roles are described below:

1. Team Leader: the team leader is a medical expert who manages the cardiac arrest team and conducts the management of the arrest, ensuring the protocol is followed and every role is filled. In addition, the team leader ensures the team quickly prepares for resternotomy when indicated.
2. Defibrillation and Pacing: this team member is responsible for administering shocks or pacing as required. This is often the bedside nurse who is the first responder to the arrest. If emergency re-sternotomy is performed, this team member should ensure that internal defibrillator paddles are available and connected, and the appropriate energy level (10–20 J) is selected for internal defibrillation.
3. External Cardiac Massage: high quality compressions is defined by a compression rate of 100–120 per min at a depth of 2–2.5 in. The quality of compressions can be guided by tar-

geting a systolic blood pressure of greater than 60 mmHg on arterial pressure tracing. External cardiac massage should be delayed for up to 1 min to allow a trial of defibrillation or pacing, where appropriate. The member performing compressions should be switched out every cycle to prevent fatigue and diminishing compression quality.

4. Airway Management: the airway role is often filled by a respiratory therapist. Airway management includes delivery of 100% oxygen by bag valve mask or a definitive airway. This member must also exclude airway issues including pneumothorax, hemothorax, or endotracheal tube migration, dislocation, or blockage.

5. Coordinator: the coordinator is responsible for coordinating the activities peripheral to the bedside. The role is typically filled by the charge nurse or senior nursing unit leader. The coordinator ensures the resternotomy cart is at the bedside for potential resternotomy as soon as a cardiac arrest is called, directs available personnel, and calls for additional assistance including the cardiac surgeon, the operating room charge nurse, the anesthesiologist, and the perfusionists.

6. Resternotomy Team (roles 7 and 8): Once the cardiac arrest has been identified and resuscitation is underway, the resternotomy team (which includes a cardiac surgeon and surgical assistant) dons gowns and gloves, and prepares for resternotomy as soon as the arrest fails to respond to initial therapy.

CS-ALS Protocol

The CS-ALS protocol should be applied to all cardiac surgery patients who arrest within the first ten postoperative days. Beyond the tenth day, the arrest team leader must weigh the risks and benefits of resternotomy due to the postoperative intrathoracic adhesions [3]. The LHSC Cardiac Surgery Intensive Care Unit's CS-ALS protocol is presented in Fig. 52.1.

As with all cardiac arrest management, the crucial steps are recognizing the arrest, identifying the rhythm, calling for help, and early defibrillation.

External Cardiac Massage (ECM)

One of the major shifts in CS-ALS compared to ACLS is the delay to start external cardiac massage for up to 1 min in favour of definitive therapy (Table 52.1).

ECM is less preferred in the cardiac surgery population because of evidence of cardiovascular and thoracic injuries due to compressions on an unstable sternum. In a meta-analysis, up to 11% of patients have multiple CPR-associated injuries, and 3–7% have major injuries including sternal fracture (15%), rib fractures (32%), pericardial injury (8.9%), and cardiac chamber laceration or rupture (0.6%) [6].

When ECM is started, compressions should be performed per standard ACLS protocol at a rate of 100–120 per min and at a depth of 2–2.5 in., allowing for complete chest recoil, avoiding all interruption [1]. If arterial line monitoring is available during the arrest, effective ECM quality can be ensured by targeting a systolic blood pressure greater than 60 mmHg.

Defibrillation and Pacing Before Compressions

If the cause of arrest is VF or pulseless VT, the definitive therapy is defibrillation. Current guidelines recommend the delivery of three sequential shocks of 200 J biphasic. In a recent meta-analysis, the success rates of the first shock at achieving a perfusion rhythm was 78%, declining to 35% with the second shock, and 14% with the third shock. The fourth shock had minimal likelihood of success with a rate of less than 10% [7].

If the three stacked shocks fail to achieve return of spontaneous circulation (ROSC), ECM should be started as a bridge to early emergency resternotomy to facilitate internal cardiac massage and internal defibrillation by an experienced provider (Class I-B) [3]. A systematic review involving 22 studies published in 2008 by the European Association for Cardio-Thoracic Surgery showed no evidence of survival benefit from ECM prior to defibrillation for in-hospital cardiac arrest [8]. An in-hospital cardiac arrest

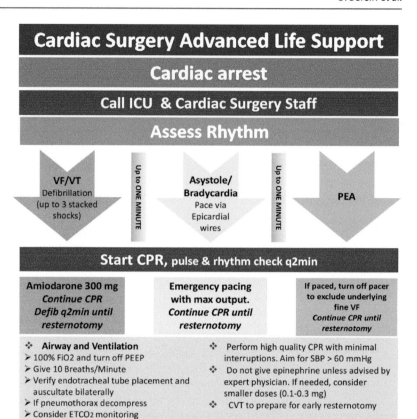

Fig. 52.1 London Health Sciences Centre Cardiac Surgery (LHSC) advanced life support protocol. *VF/VT* ventricular fibrillation/ventricular tachycardia, *PEA* pulseless electrical activity, *CPR* cardiopulmonary resuscitation, *Defib* defibrillate, *FiO2* fraction of inspired oxygen, *ETCO₂* end-tidal carbon dioxide; *SBP* systolic blood pressure, *CVT* cardiovascular and thoracic surgery, *ICU* intensive care unit, *IABP* Intra-aortic balloon pump, *VADs* ventricular assist devices, *RV* right ventricle, *OR* operating room

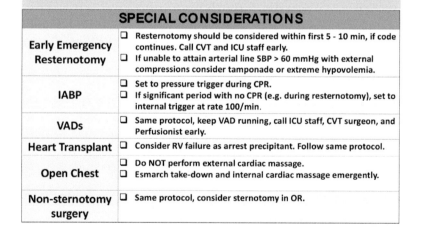

study of 6789 patients found early defibrillation within 1–2 min was an important predictor of survival [9].

If the cause of cardiac arrest is asystole or severe bradycardia, definitive therapy is electrical pacing with epicardial wires (Class IIa) [3]. Pacing should be performed in DDD mode at a rate of 80–100 beats per min with maximum output (Class I-C) [3]. Most pacemakers have an emergency function that defaults to this setting. In the absence of epicardial pacing wires, external pacing pads should be considered.

In the case of PEA arrest, any pacemaker activity must be turned off to rule out underlying VF (Class IIA-C) [3], and ECM should be started immediately if no definitive therapies are warranted.

Table 52.1 Comparison of ACLS and CS-ALS

ACLS Recommendations for arrest	CS-ALS Recommendations for post cardiac surgery arrest
Ventricular fibrillation or pulseless ventricular tachycardia	
Immediate external cardiac massage	Defibrillation first if available within 1 minute
External cardiac massage → single shock → external cardiac massage x 2 minutes before repeating shock	Three stacked shocks before external cardiac massage
Asystole or profound bradycardia	
External cardiac massage → vasopressor	DDD pacing at maximum outputs if available within 1 min → external cardiac massage
All pulseless cardiac arrest	
Epinephrine 1000 ug every 3-5 min	No epinephrine during arrest or reduce the dose to 100 ug for prearrest patients
Use specific roles under direction of team leader	Use 6 key roles during arrest management
	Rapid resternotomy if no response to initial therapy

ACLS Advanced cardiac life support, *CS-ALS* Cardiac surgery advanced life support

Airway Management

The main goals of airway management in cardiac arrest is the prevention of hypoxia which can be accomplished by delivering 100% oxygen by bag-valve mask ventilation or via a definitive airway; however, positive end-expiratory pressure (PEEP) should be avoided to improve passive venous return. End-tidal CO_2 monitoring should be used whenever possible. Equally important is the active exclusion and management of airway related causes of arrest including tension pneumothorax, massive hemothorax, or inadvertent extubation. Early intubation may be considered to secure the airway prior to resternotomy and assist with transfer back to the OR.

Medication Management

Another departure from standard ACLS protocols is in medication management, especially with atropine and epinephrine. Atropine has no role in CS-ALS for severe bradycardia and asystole due to a lack of evidence of benefit.

Epinephrine and vasopressin are potentially harmful post-cardiac surgery due to the high risk of fatal bleeding at suture lines from the hypertensive rebound after ROSC. Other possible harms from epinephrine boluses are aortic rupture, myocardial dysfunction, worsening arrhythmia, increased myocardial oxygen demand, and coronary graft disruption. Furthermore, there are currently no placebo-controlled trials showing improved rates of neurologically intact survival to hospital discharge from any vasopressor use during resuscitation [1, 10]. Therefore, these vasoactive medications should only be ordered by an expert physician who is experienced in managing post-cardiac surgery cardiac arrest.

Intravenous amiodarone bolus of 300 mg should be administered to patients after failing three sequential shocks. All intravenous infusions, especially sedatives and hypotensive agents, should be stopped during resuscitation to avoid their hypotensive and negative inotropic effect. All infusions should also be checked for any possible drug errors. Vasosupportive medications can be restarted once medication error is ruled out in the event the patient regains ROSC.

Emergency Bedside Resternotomy

Early emergency bedside resternotomy is considered one of the pillars to definitive resuscitation in CS-ALS, after failing pacing, defibrillation, compressions, and treating other reversible etiology. Resternotomy preparation should start immediately upon ECM to reduce the time of cardiac compressions and its associated trauma. The goal is to perform resternotomy within 5–10 min of initiating external compressions [3, 11] so that direct hemostatic control and release of cardiac tamponade can occur.

Resternotomy also allows for internal cardiac massage (ICM) and internal defibrillation. Internal massage has been shown to double the cardiac output compared to external compressions, leading to superior coronary and cerebral perfusion, increase the rate of ROSC, and improve the rate of survival compared with ECM [11, 12].

Every cardiac surgical ICU should have a dedicated and simplified resternotomy cart and kit. A simplified resternotomy kit allows for quicker workflow and less distractions. Each kit should be stocked with a sterile suction, scalpel, wire cutter, heavy needle holder, and a single-piece sternal retractor (Fig. 52.2).

A drape and skin prep tray also allows for quicker patient preparation (Fig. 52.3).

Additional surgical instruments including sutures, sponges, and needle drivers can be available in a separate complete kit. More detailed surgical repair should be performed in the operating room once the patient is successfully resuscitated. Additional antibiotic dosing and an aseptic washout may be considered in these patients.

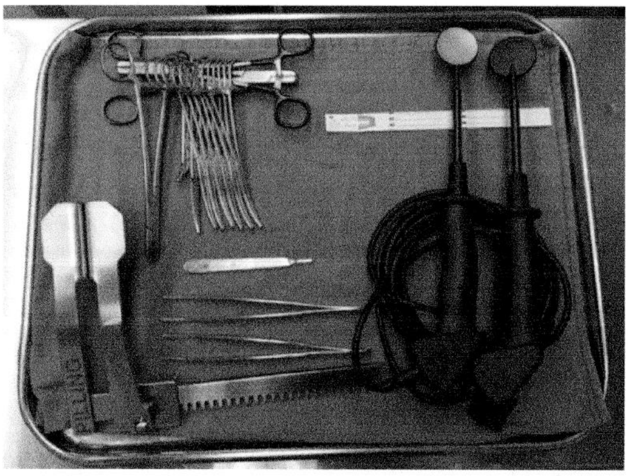

Fig. 52.2 Resternotomy tray with essential instruments and internal defibrillator paddles

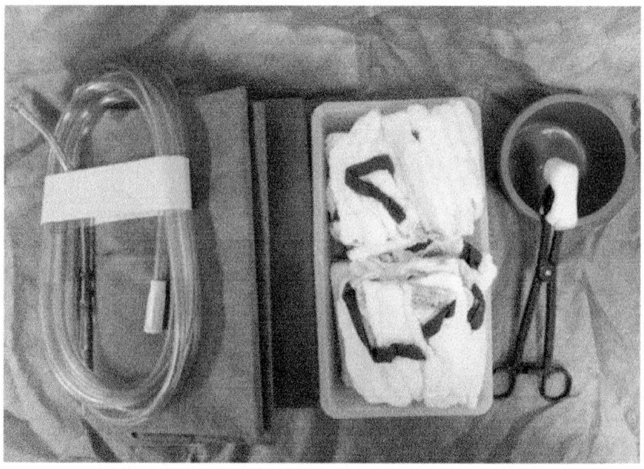

Fig. 52.3 Drape and skin prep tray

The best results from resternotomy occurs within the first ten postoperative days; beyond this, adhesions develop which make resternotomy more challenging and hazardous. After 10 days postoperatively, the decision to reopen should be made by a senior surgeon [3].

Extracorporeal Membrane Oxygenation (ECMO) Post Cardiac Arrest

ECMO should be considered for cardiac surgery patients who have reversible causes for cardiac arrest. A small study in 1994 showed 56% survival among patients with refractory VF despite open chest cardiopulmonary resuscitation who were then successfully rescued on ECMO in the ICU [13].

Special Considerations in CS-ALS

1. *Intra-Aortic Balloon Pump (IABP)*:

   The IABP should be set to "pressure trigger" so that the timing of inflation and deflation coincide with mechanical cardiac massage. When chest compressions are interrupted, such as during resternotomy, the IABP should be set on internal mode at 100 cycles/min until cardiac massage resumes [3].
2. *Ventricular Assist Devices (VADs)*:

   Patients with VADs experience cardiac arrest for similar reasons as non-VAD patients.

In addition, they may also suffer from mechanical VAD failure and right ventricular (RV) failure, in the case of left ventricular assist devices. The role of ECM is less clear as data is limited to sporadic case reports suggesting that chest compressions can damage the device and cardiac chambers. On the other hand, mechanical compressions may decompress a dilated failing RV, and more importantly, may provide life-sustaining circulation when the VAD has failed. Mabvuure and Rodrigues reported in their systematic review that there is not enough data to support harm or benefit from ECM in VAD patients, and that more research is needed [14]. Balancing the above potential risks and benefits, we recommend CPR in VAD patients.

A potential challenge faced in the management of patients with VADs is the identification of cardiac arrest and subsequently ROSC when invasive monitoring is not available due to the non-pulsatile flow characteristics of the device. There are several different ways to identify cardiac arrest in this patient population including signs of low cerebral perfusion such as loss of consciousness, low invasive arterial blood pressure measurements similar to the central venous pressure, loss of Doppler wave form over major arteries, inappropriate flow parameters on the device screen, loss of end tidal CO_2 waveform in mechanically ventilated patients, and echocardiographic evidence of device and ventricular failure.

VAD patients should be managed as outlined in the CS-ALS protocol. ECMO support should be considered in patients who arrest more than ten days postoperatively.

3. *Post-Transplant Patients*:

In cases of cardiac arrest after heart, heart-lung or double lung transplantation, the same recommendations should be followed including resternotomy. Fresh sternotomy after previous clamshell or bilateral thoracotomy incisions should be performed by an expert surgeon.

4. *Open Chest Patients*:

Patients who are managed by delayed chest closure also fall under the CS-ALS protocol.

When performing compressions, the force should be directed at the midpoint of the chest over sternal packing. Lower force is usually required to generate an adequate systolic blood pressure target on arterial line monitoring.

Access for internal cardiac massage is simpler in open chest patients as there are no wires to remove. Care must be taken during packing removal to prevent injury to adherent grafts or underlying right-sided cardiac structures. Occasionally, the pericardial packing can cause cardiac arrest by tamponade, which is resolved by packing removal.

5. *Non-sternotomy Patients*:

While non-sternotomy cardiac surgeries involving minimally invasive thoracotomies or mini-sternotomies are unique, the CS-ALS protocol may still apply because chest compressions can cause the same complications as in full sternotomy patients. If a fresh sternotomy is required, this should be performed by a trained surgeon.

References

1. Link MS, Berkow LC, Kudenchuk PJ, Halperin HR, Hess EP, Moitra VK, Neumar RW, O'Neil BJ, Paxton JH, Silvers SM, White RD, Yannopoulos D, Donnino MW. Adult advanced cardiovascular life support 2015 American Heart Association guidelines update for cardiopulmonary resuscitation and emergency cardiovascular care. Circulation. 2015;132: S444–64.
2. Soar J, Nolanb JP, Böttiger BW, Perkins GD, Lott C, Carli P, Pellis T, Sandroni C, Skrifvars MB, Smithl GB, Sunde K, Deakin CD. European resuscitation council guidelines for resuscitation 2015. Resuscitation. 2015;95(2015):100–47.
3. Dunning J, Levine A, Ley J, Strang T, Lizotte DE, Lamarche Y, Bartley T, Zellinger M, Katz N, Arora RC, Dembitsky W, Cheng AM, Lonchyna VA, Haft J, Deakin CD, Mitchell JD, Firestoneq S, Bakaeen FG. The society of thoracic surgeons expert consensus for the resuscitation of patients who arrest after cardiac surgery. Ann Thorac Surg. 2017;103:1005–20.
4. Gosev I, Nikolic I, Aranki S. Resuscitation practice in cardiac surgery. J Thoracic Cardiovasc Surg. 2014;148(4):1152–6.
5. Mancini ME, Diekema DS, Hoadley TA, Kadlec KD, Leveille MH, McGowan JE, Munkwitz MM, Panchal AR, Sayre MR, Sinz EH. Part 3: ethical issues: 2015

American Heart Association guidelines update for cardiopulmonary resuscitation and emergency cardiovascular care. Circulation. 2015;132:S383–96.

6. Miller AC, Rosati SF, Suffredini AF, Schrump DS. A systematic review and pooled analysis of CPR-associated cardiovascular and thoracic injuries. Resuscitation. 2014;85(6):724–31.

7. Richardson L, Dissanayake A, Dunning J. What cardioversion protocol for ventricular fibrillation should be followed for patients who arrest shortly post-cardiac surgery? Interact Cardiovasc Thorac Surg. 2007;6(2007):799–805.

8. Lockowandt U, Levine A, Strang T, Dunning J. If a patient arrests after cardiac surgery is it acceptable to delay cardiopulmonary resuscitation until you have attempted either defibrillation or pacing? Interact Cardiovasc Thorac Surg. 2008;7(2008):878–87.

9. Chan PS, Krumholz HM, Nichol G, Nallamothu BK. Delayed time to defibrillation after in-hospital cardiac arrest. N Engl J Med. 2008;358:9–17.

10. Tsagkatakia M, Levineb A, Strangc T, Dunning J. Should adrenaline be routinely used by the resuscitation team if a patient suffers a cardiac arrest shortly after cardiac surgery? Interact Cardiovasc Thorac Surg. 2008;7(2008):457–63.

11. Makay JH, Powell SJ, Osgathorp J, Rozario CJ. Six-year prospective audit for chest reopening after cardiac arrest. Eur J Cardiothorac Surg. 2002;22(2002):412–25.

12. Twomey D, Das M, Subramanian H, Dunning J. Is internal massage superior to external massage for patients suffering a cardiac arrest after cardiac surgery? Interact Cardiovasc Thorac Surg. 2008;7(2008):151–7.

13. Rousou JA, Engelman RM, Flack JE, Deaton DW, Owen SG. Emergency cardiopulmonary bypass in the cardiac surgical unit can be a lifesaving measure in postoperative cardiac arrest. Circulation. 1994;90(5 Pt 2):II280–4.

14. Mabvuure NT, Rodrigues JN. External cardiac compression during cardiopulmonary resuscitation of patients with left ventricular assist devices. Interact Cardiovasc Thorac Surg. 2014;19(2014):286–9.

Tamponade and Chest Re-opening

53

Amit Korach and Benjamin Drenger

Main Messages

1. The incidence of chest reopening due to postoperative mediastinal bleeding is in the range of 2–5% following cardiac surgery.
2. Cardiac tamponade is primarily a clinical diagnosis. Transesophageal Echocardiography (TEE) is highly sensitive and specific in the diagnosis of cardiac tamponade if readily available. Traditional diagnostic tools such as chest X-ray and transthoracic echocardiography are rarely helpful.
3. Significant mediastinal bleeding or tamponade are best treated by chest re-opening in the operating room.
4. In the setting of hemodynamic instability and cardiac tamponade or significant bleeding, bedside chest re-opening is indicated.
5. In case of dehiscence of the sternum, re-wiring is indicated.
6. Etomidate and ketamine are the preferred anesthetic agents for the management of tamponade or significant postoperative bleeding.

In the early postoperative period, chest reopening after cardiac surgery is indicated in various settings, including:

- Uncontrolled surgical site bleeding/ tamponade.
- Treatment of acute surgical problems such as coronary artery graft occlusion, replacement or repair of valve malfunction, or pseudoaneurysm of the aorta.
- Dehiscence of the sternum.
- Deep sternal wound infection.

In this chapter, we will focus on chest re-opening for bleeding/tamponade.

Patients undergoing cardiac surgery are at high risk for postoperative bleeding. Most patients are treated with medications that interfere with platelet adhesion/function or with the coagulation system, such as aspirin, P2Y12 receptor inhibitors, warfarin or heparin. In addition, factors associated with hemodilution, cardiopulmonary bypass

A. Korach (✉)
Department of Cardiothoracic Surgery, Hadassah-Hebrew University Medical Center, Jerusalem, Israel
e-mail: ramitk@hadassah.org.il

B. Drenger
Department of Anesthesiology and Critical Care Medicine, Hadassah-Hebrew University Medical Center, Jerusalem, Israel

© Springer Nature Switzerland AG 2021
D. C. H. Cheng et al. (eds.), *Evidence-Based Practice in Perioperative Cardiac Anesthesia and Surgery*, https://doi.org/10.1007/978-3-030-47887-2_53

(CPB), patient cooling and systemic full heparinization, increase bleeding tendency.

Changes in platelets, red blood cells and components of the inflammatory and the hemostatic system continue well into the postoperative period. Platelets are not only consumed; their activation results in degranulation, with release of adenosine diphosphate (ADP), together with other factors and receptors expression on their surface, leading to aggregation and permanent dysfunction. These changes occur in the immediate postoperative period when, initially, platelets rapidly adhere to exposed subendothelial areas in surgical sites or in coronary artery grafts, followed by gradual platelet recovery, and then rebound thrombocytosis by the seventh postoperative day.

Moreover, during cardiac surgery, the sternum is divided and the intra pericardial vessels are exposed, resulting in potential bleeding. Significant postoperative bleeding after cardiac surgery with or without re-exploration of the surgical site is associated with adverse patient outcome and greater hospital costs [1–3].

The incidence of significant postoperative bleeding necessitating chest reopening is in the range of 2–5%, and even higher in some reports. Risk factors vary; however, preoperative anticoagulation treatment, advanced age, high Euroscore, valve surgery and prolonged CPB time are the most common [4–6].

Preoperative Evaluation

In the process of evaluating potential candidates for cardiac surgery, a past medical history of bleeding tendency or known coagulation disorders should be elucidated. CBC and basic coagulation studies should be routinely performed. In recent years, more and more patients are receiving treatment with dual antiplatelet medications (usually aspirin in combination with P2Y12 receptor antagonists such as clopidogrel, prasugrel or ticagrelor). Others are receiving treatment with warfarin derivatives, low molecular weight heparin or novel oral anticoagulants. These anticoagulants vary in mechanism of action, half-life and the effect on the patient's

ability to form blood clots. Cessation of aspirin treatment before cardiac surgery is not associated with markedly reduced bleeding. Cessation of novel oral anticoagulants for 24–48 h before surgery is mandatory. Differing data exist regarding bleeding tendency in patients treated with P2Y12 receptor antagonists. Most studies demonstrated significant perioperative bleeding, re-exploration rate, and higher mortality in patients treated with clopidogrel or ticagrelor in addition to aspirin before cardiac surgery [7, 8]. Some studies demonstrated no significant difference [9]. Administration of preoperative aspirin does not increase the bleeding rate nor the risk of death following coronary artery bypass (CABG) surgery [10]. The 2014 ESC/ EACTS guidelines on myocardial revascularization recommend postponing non emergent CABG surgery for at least 5 days (plavix or ticagrelor) to 7 days (prasugrel) in patients receiving P2Y12 receptor antagonists [11].

Operative Care

In order to prevent surgical site bleeding, meticulous surgical technique and minimizing tissue dissection is essential. Intraoperative administration of tranexamic acid reduces postoperative bleeding and the need for chest re-opening [12]. Maintaining normothermia during CPB and complete reversal of heparin with protamine sulfate are essential. Administration of coagulation substances such as platelets, fresh frozen plasma, or cryoprecipitate is not routine. In some cases, where severe coagulation disorder are anticipated, such as operations using deep hypothermia and circulatory arrest or when there is a pre-existing coagulopathy, coagulation factors or platelet administration are indicated after heparin reversal. To avoid accumulation of blood in the pericardial sac, leading to cardiac tamponade, adequate drainage is mandatory. Our routine is placing one #36Fr chest tube and one more #28-36Fr tubes in the anterior and inferior mediastinum respectively.

The anesthesiologist may predict the risk for postoperative bleeding on arrival to the cardiac surgery intensive care unit, by performing thromboelastography with platelet mapping

(TEG-PM™, Haemonetics Corp., Braintree, MA) assay towards the end of the operation, after protamine has been administered and the ACT has returned to baseline values. Such an estimate of postoperative bleeding tendency provides information on whether to institute preventive measures [13].

The volume of bleeding through the chest tubes upon arrival in the cardiac surgery intensive care unit should be quantified. If substantial bleeding is observed, the differential diagnosis should include residual heparin rebound effect, coagulopathy related to consumption of coagulation factors, and fibrinolysis or platelets dysfunction due to the residual effects of APD therapy. Residual heparin effect can be confirmed with heparinase TEG, which may discern patients who may benefit from an additional dose of protamine. Prolonged R value in TEG indicates delay in clot formation and should be treated with fresh frozen plasma administration, while fibrinolysis may benefit from an additional dose of antifibrinolytic therapy, with aminocaproic acid or tranexamic acid. The maximum amplitude (MA) may be analyzed by TEG platelet mapping either with arachidonic acid (AA), to detect residual effect of aspirin on clot strength, or with adenosine diphosphate (ADP) for residual effect of clopidogrel. A depressed MA spun is best treated with platelet transfusion [14].

In case of significant postoperative bleeding in the presence of low platelet count (less than 50,000) or high elevated INR or PTT, platelets or fresh frozen plasma should be administered, respectively. Since hypothermia is associated with coagulopathy, maintaining normothermia is essential to prevent postoperative bleeding.

In some cases, bleeding persists despite adequate control of blood pressure, temperature and coagulation studies. In these cases, reopening of the chest is considered. Indications for reopening of the chest due to persistent post cardiac surgery bleeding varies between institutions and surgeons. Traditionally, chest reopening after cardiac surgery was indicated when chest tube drainage was greater than 500 ml during the first hour, 400 ml during each of the first 2 h, 300 ml during each of the first 3 h, 1000 ml during the first 4 h, 1200 ml during the first 5 h, or sudden onset massive bleeding [15]. Over the past two decades, the increased understanding that post cardiac surgery allogeneic blood transfusion is associated with greater postoperative morbidity and mortality was the impetus for surgeons lowering the threshold for chest re-opening [4, 16].

Tamponade

Cardiac tamponade is the physiological expression of rapid fluid or blood accumulation in the pericardial sac, resulting in the secondary appearance of dyspnea, tachycardia, muffled heart sounds, hypotension, and distended jugular neck veins. A common clinical sign is pulsus paradoxus, a change in intensity of peripheral pulse on palpation. The physiological explanation is the change in intra-pericardial pressure due to spontaneous inspiration, which causes an increase in the capacity of the pulmonary bed. The presence of excessive external compression by blood or fluid on the heart, on one hand, and the negative intra-pleural pressure during inspiration, cause an exaggerated venous return to the heart with septal bulging toward the left ventricle with reduced ejection fraction [17].

Non-specific diagnostic features of tamponade include enlarged silhouette of the heart on chest X-ray and reduced QRS amplitude on ECG. A more specific characteristic feature on the ECG tracing is electrical alternans, a cyclical alternation in QRS complex amplitude. Gradual accumulation of pericardial fluid will initially result in myocardial stiffness, followed by decreased volumes and even collapse of the right and later the left ventricle, with a decrease in cardiac output.

After cardiac surgery, the classic signs and symptoms of tamponade might be different from other chest cavity pathological conditions. Due to bleeding and "third spacing," intravascular volume, (i.e. preload), is reduced. Positive pressure ventilation decreases preload even more than under spontaneous respiratory conditions. Moreover, unlike other conditions where fluid (usually serous) is accumulated in a close pericardial sac with equal distribution of intra-pericardial pressure, this is not the case after cardiac surgery. In most cases, the pericardial space is left open at the end of surgery. Therefore, blood clots are not evenly distributed in the pericardial sac, resulting in elevated intrapericardial pressures in some locations and normal pressures in other areas. For example, accumulation of blood clots in the posterior pericardium might impair the filling of the left atrium or left ventricle with no significant physiological effect on right side pressures.

Tamponade is first and foremost a clinical diagnosis. Low blood pressure, elevated pulmonary artery or right atrial pressures always increase suspicion of tamponade. Signs of a low cardiac output state resulting in systemic hypoperfusion as evidenced by oliguria, metabolic acidosis, low mixed venous blood saturation and reduced skin temperature increase suspicion in the post cardiac surgery setting. The suspicion is obviously higher when large amounts of blood is drained through the mediastinal chest tubes. Sudden cessation of drainage from the mediastinal chest tubes is always a concern, since the chest tubes might be occluded by clots. Even moderate bleeding after cardiac surgery can result in tamponade.

Non-clinical diagnostic tools are rarely helpful in post-cardiac surgery tamponade. In some cases, wide mediastinal silhouette is present on chest X-ray. TTE is usually not helpful due to technical issues including lung hyperinflation, limited window for imaging and the presence of mediastinal chest tubes. Transesophageal echocardiography (TEE) is helpful since it is more sensitive and specific than TTE in diagnosing tamponade. It might reveal not only major accumulation of fluid or blood, but also smaller localized blood accumulation, which may lead to right ventricle wall collapse. However, since TEE is invasive and may not always immediately available in the cardiac surgery intensive care unit (CSICU), its application is limited when rapid diagnosis of post cardiac surgery tamponade is required. A large volume of pericardial fluid without clots or fibrous strands can result in the phenomenon of "swinging heart" which may be visible on the TEE examination. This manifests as a pendular swinging of the heart from side to side within the pericardium, which correlates with the alternation of QRS complex on ECG [18].

Treatment

Once the diagnosis of post cardiac surgery tamponade or persistent bleeding is made, the definitive treatment is chest re-opening for the purpose of exploration of the pericardial sac, removing blood clots, and controlling bleeding sites. The procedure should be performed in the ideal setting; the cardiac operating room. In case of severe hemodynamic compromise, bedside exploration in the cardiac surgery intensive care unit is performed.

When the patient is emergently transferred to the cardiac surgery operating room, he/she is placed on the operating room table in supine position, dressings are removed, and the chest is prepped in the standard fashion, as for the original surgery. To avoid potential contamination of the surgical field, we leave the chest tubes and pacing wires outside the field (Fig. 53.1).

The skin, subcutaneous sutures, and sternal wires are cut and removed. The goal is to release tamponade as quickly as possible and stop massive bleeding. We carefully spread the sternal edges, the sternal retractor is placed, and the mediastinum is explored. Blood clots are removed from the surgical field. In order to avoid damage to coronary artery grafts, special attention should be given when blood clots are removed, since the

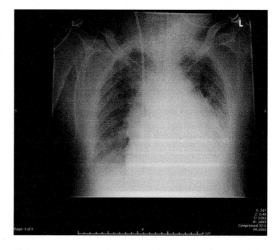

Fig. 53.1 Post cardiac surgery chest X-ray demonstrating wide mediastinum. Highly suggestive for tamponade

grafts are not always clearly visible. Rinsing the clots with warm 0.9% NaCl solution is helpful in this process. After freeing the pericardial space from blood and clots, we place pericardial stay sutures to enhance pericardial exploration. We meticulously look for the bleeding source in the entire surgical field including the large vessels, chambers of the heart suture lines, coronary artery grafts and anastomoses, mammary artery bed, small mediastinal vessels and the sternum. In 60–80% of the cases, "surgical bleeding" is found, advocating for early re-exploration [4, 19]. In other cases, coagulopathy with diffuse bleeding is diagnosed. In up to 25% of chest re-opening cases after cardiac surgery, no obvious bleeding source was identified [20]. Following adequate drainage of the surgical field and bleeding control, the chest tubes are rinsed to ensure patency and the chest is closed in the usual fashion. In rare cases of severe coagulopathy, the surgical field is packed and closure of the sternum is delayed.

In case of severe hemodynamic compromise due to uncontrolled bleeding or tamponade, transferring the patient to the operating room might not be safe. In such cases, chest re-opening should be performed in the cardiac surgery intensive care unit. The bedside procedure goal is to relieve the high intra-pericardial pressure and control major bleeding sites.

In rare cases, definitive bleeding control is not possible under intensive care unit conditions. In this situation, local bleeding control should be achieved and the patient transferred to the operating room for definitive care.

The intensive care unit setting for post cardiac surgery patients should have the capacity to perform bedside chest reopening. In addition to the regular intensive care unit equipment, conditions and materials for the procedure include, clean (sterile) environment, direct light, sterile sheets and gowns and a complete sterile set of operating room instruments.

The "number 1 rule" for the intensive care unit physician in such a situation is to "call for help!" Ideally, the appropriate staffing at the patient bedside includes: two surgeons, an anesthesiologist, two operating room nurses, and two intensive care unit nurses (one outside the room). In general, the technique for cardiac surgery intensive care chest re-opening is the same as if performed in the operating room.

Despite low blood pressure, general anesthesia is mandatory. To avoid further complications, strict sterile environment and standard surgical care should be the rule. Following chest re-opening and removal of blood clots to relieve tamponade, a major bleeding source is sought.

When the patient's hemodynamic status is stable and bleeding control is achieved, it is generally safe to place the sternal wires and close the chest in the ICU.

Chest Reopening for Dehiscence of the Sternum

In rare cases the healing of the sternum after cardiac surgery is insufficient. Potential causes are inappropriate approximation of the sternum, deviation from midline when opening the sternum, "fragile" sternum (elderly patients, long term steroid treatment), central obesity, and elevated intermittent intrathoracic pressure such as in deep cough and infection.

Non-union of the sternum might result in paradoxical movement of the chest wall and impaired breathing mechanism. The timing for diagnosis is from few days to weeks after surgery, although it is usually made during the first two postoperative weeks. Symptoms may vary. Some patients are asymptomatic, some experience mid chest pain, while others complain of shortness of breath. Physical examination revels separation of the sternal edges and an "unstable sternum", exaggerated by cough. Chest X-ray usually demonstrates malposition of the sternal wires (Fig. 53.2). In some cases, the sternal wires are interrupted. CT scan is more sensitive than chest X-ray in diagnosing dehiscence of the sternum.

The treatment of sternal dehiscence depends on the degree of instability and patient symptoms. If symptoms are mild and only minimal separation of sternum exists, adequate pain

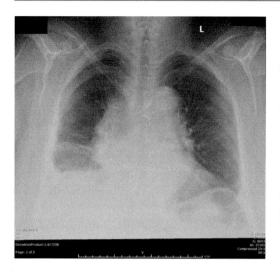

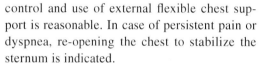

Fig. 53.2 Malposition of the sternal wires, a result of a broken sternum

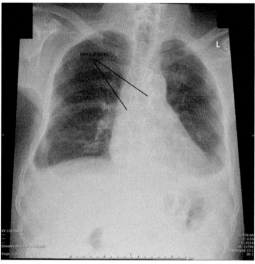

Fig. 53.3 Vertical wires placed along the lateral edge of the sternum

control and use of external flexible chest support is reasonable. In case of persistent pain or dyspnea, re-opening the chest to stabilize the sternum is indicated.

The procedure is performed under general anesthesia. The chest is prepped and draped for resternotomy. The sternal wires are removed and the sternum and the mediastinum are assessed. Even if pus is not present, we routinely culture the mediastinal fluid for potential bacterial contamination. In most cases, few unilateral or bilateral fractures of the sternum are present.

Our technique was first reported by Robicsek et al. in 1977 and has been widely used since [21]. In brief, it consists of supporting the lateral edges of the fractured side of the sternum with vertical running wires in a figure of eight configuration. This is followed by approximation of the edges of the sternum with horizontal wires passed lateral to the vertical ones. In this wire configuration, the horizontal tension on the sternum is transferred to the vertical sternal wires (Fig. 53.3). Failure of this method rarely occurs. In case of failure, use of other sternal fixation devices is considered. These methods include placement of metal plates and screws and are not widely used.

Chest Reopening for Sternal Wound Infection

Deep sternal wound infection following cardiac surgery is very well characterized [22]. Variability between institutions and geographical areas exists. The Society of Thoracic Surgeons Adult Cardiac Surgery Database reports an incidence of 1%. Many risk factors for deep sternal wound infection are reported such as chronic obstructive pulmonary disease, uncontrolled diabetes, use of bilateral internal mammary arteries, prolonged cardiopulmonary bypass time, obesity, congestive heart failure, and emergency surgery [23, 24].

In most cases of deep sternal wound infection, reopening of the chest is indicated. The purpose of the procedure is to remove foreign material (sternal wires) and debride necrotic and infected tissue. In some cases, chest reconstruction with a muscle or omental flap is indicated.

The procedure is performed under general anesthesia. The chest is prepped and draped in the usual sterile fashion. The chest is approached via the previous incision. The sternal wires are carefully removed. Due to the infected mediastinal process and potentially fragile cardiac tissue, extreme caution is taken when the sternal edges are separated. Necrotic and infected tissue is debrided. The sternum is debrided; the extent is dependent on the degree of involvement in the infectious process. A mediastinal drain is placed and the chest closed either primarily or with a muscle or omental flap.

Anesthetic Management of Cardiac Tamponade

The four pillars of the anesthetic management are:

1. Positive-pressure mechanical ventilation or high PEEP may compromise a patient's hemodynamic state by reducing cardiac filling and thus cardiac output. Therefore, either spontaneous breathing or mechanical ventilation with a high respiratory rate and low tidal volume, plus low peak inspiratory pressures is preferred.
2. Fluid and blood products management in tamponade is important in the hypotensive and hypovolemia state; in spite of the elevated filling pressures that represent external pressure on the heart, measured fluid challenge is necessary to maintain adequate stroke volume. However, in acute tamponade, caution should be taken since excessive fluid load may aggravate the bi-ventricular interdependence.
3. Inotropic support is an important resuscitative measure. The use of norepinephrine will maintain sympathetic tone, and will avoid bradycardia and anesthetic drugs-induced vasodilation.
4. The choice of anesthetic drugs should emphasize the use of drugs which rapidly induce deep anesthetic state, but with the least vasodilatory effects. Ketamine and etomidate are the drugs of choice; their administration should be incremental, in response to effect.

Ketamine is a phenylcyclidine derivative, and NMDA receptor antagonist, which induces a dissociative general anesthesia. It seems that its sympathomimetic effects, and its ability to increase noradrenaline release from nerve endings, contribute to the increase in blood pressure and heart rate. Those actions together with the minimal depression of ventilation are its main advantages. Its psychological side effects, such as hallucinations and delirium, require the co-administered of midazolam once the patient is hemodynamically stable.

Etomidate is a general anesthesia induction drug with remarkable hemodynamic stability. It does not inhibit sympathetic tone or myocardial contractility and as such, its effects on blood pressure and heart rate are minimal. Patients with cardiac tamponade, who are unstable hemodynamically, can safely be anesthetized by etomidate or ketamine.

In summary, chest re-opening after cardiac surgery is rarely indicated. It is performed in various settings such as bleeding/tamponade, dehiscence of the sternum, or deep sternal wound infection. In patients who receive dual antiplatelet therapy immediately prior to surgery, the anesthesiologist may perform thromboelastography testing with platelet mapping, to predict the risk for postoperative bleeding on arrival to the CSICU. Surgical site bleeding following cardiac surgery should be treated immediately, preferably in the operating theater, before fully realized tamponade with hemodynamic instability further deteriorate myocardial function. When clinical signs of tamponade are manifested, if possible, the CSICU physician or the anesthesiologist should avoid initiating positive pressure ventilation until the pericardial space has been drained. If general anesthesia is needed, spontaneous ventilation is ideal, and ketamine, with its respiratory sparing effect, is the drug of choice. To reduce the risk of hypotension, anesthetic induction should be postponed until the surgical team is ready to make their incision.

References

1. Ranucci M, Bozzetti G, Ditta A, Cotza M, Carboni G, Ballotta A. Surgical reexploration after cardiac operations: why a worse outcome? Ann Thorac Surg. 2008;86:1557–62.
2. Dacey LJ, Munoz JJ, Baribeau YR, Johnson ER, Lahey SJ, Leavitt BJ, et al. Reexploration for hemorrhage following coronary artery bypass grafting: incidence and risk factors. Northern New England Cardiovascular Disease Study Group. Arch Surg. 1998;133:442–7.
3. Alstrom U, Levine LA, Stahle E, Svedjeholm R, Friberg O. Cost analysis of re-exploration for bleeding after coronary artery bypass graft surgery. Br J Anaesth. 2012;108:216–22.
4. Vivacqua A, Koch CG, Yousuf AM, Nowicki ER, Houghtaling PL, Blackstone EH, Sabik JF 3rd. Morbidity of bleeding after cardiac surgery: is it blood transfusion, reoperation for bleeding, or both? Ann Thorac Surg. 2011;91:1780–90.
5. Dyke C, Aronson S, Dietrich W, Hofmann A, Karkouti K, Levi M, et al. Universal definition of perioperative bleeding in adult cardiac surgery. J Thorac Cardiovasc Surg. 2014;147:1458–63.
6. Unsworth-White MJ, Herriot A, Valencia O, Poloniecki J, Smith EE, Murday AJ, et al. Resternotomy for bleeding after cardiac operation: a marker for increased morbidity and mortality. Ann Thorac Surg. 1995;59:664–7.
7. Biancari F, Airaksinen KE, Lip GY. Benefits and risks of using clopidogrel before coronary artery bypass surgery: systematic review and meta-analysis of randomized trials and observational studies. J Thorac Cardiovasc Surg. 2012;143:665–75.
8. Schotola H, Bräuer A, Meyer K, Hinz J, Schöndube FA, Bauer M, et al. Perioperative outcomes of cardiac surgery patients with ongoing ticagrelor therapy: boon and bane of a new drug. Eur J Cardiothorac Surg. 2014;46:198–205.
9. Ebrahimi R, Dyke C, Mehran R, Manoukian SV, Feit F, Cox DA, et al. Outcomes following pre-operative clopidogrel administration in patients with acute coronary syndromes undergoing coronary artery bypass surgery: the ACUITY (acute catheterization and urgent intervention triage strategy) trial. J Am Coll Cardiol. 2009;53:1965–72.
10. Myles PS, Smith JA, Forbes A, Silbert B, Jayarajah M, Painter T, et al. Stopping vs. continuing aspirin before coronary artery surgery. New Engl J Med. 2016;374:728–37.
11. Authors/Task Force members, Windecker S, Kolh P, Alfonso F, Collet JP, Cremer J, Falk V, et al. ESC/EACTS Guidelines on myocardial revascularization. The Task Force on Myocardial Revascularization of the European Society of Cardiology (ESC) and the European Association for Cardio-Thoracic Surgery (EACTS). Eur Heart J. 2014;35:2541–619.
12. Myles PS, Smith JA, Forbes A, Silbert B, Jayarajah M, Painter T, et al. Tranexamic acid in patients undergoing coronary-artery surgery. New Engl J Med. 2017;376:136–48.
13. Chowdhury M, Shore-Lesserson L, Mais AM, Leyvi G. Thromboelastograph with platelet mapping (TM) predicts postoperative chest tube drainage in patients undergoing coronary artery bypass grafting. J Cardiothorac Vasc Anesth. 2014;28:217–23.
14. Preisman S, Kogan A, Itzkovsky K, Leikin G, Raanani E. Modified thromboelastography evaluation of platelet dysfunction in patients undergoing coronary artery surgery. Eur J Cardiothorac Surg. 2010;37:1367–74.
15. Kirklin JW, Barratt-Boyes BG. Cardiac surgery. New York: Wiley; 1986. p. 158–9.
16. Cheng DHC, David T. Perioperative care in cardiac anesthesia and surgery. Philadelphia: Lippincott Williams and Wilkins; 2006. p. 376–7.
17. Odor P, Bailey A. Cardiac tamponade: anaesthesia tutorial of the week 283, March 2013.
18. Akkerhuis JM, Hersbach FMRJ. Images in clinical medicine. Swinging heart. N Engl J Med. 2004;351:e1.
19. Karthik S, Grayson AD, McCarron EE, Pullan DM, Desmond MJ. Reexploration for bleeding after coronary artery bypass surgery: risk factors, outcomes, and the effect of time delay. Ann Thorac Surg. 2004;78:527–34.
20. Canadyova J, Zmeko D, Mokracek A. Re-exploration for bleeding or tamponade after cardiac operation. Interact Cardiovasc Thorac Surg. 2012;14:704–7.
21. Robicsek F, Daugherty HK, Cook JW. The prevention and treatment of sternum separation following open-heart surgery. J Thorac Cardiovasc Surg. 1977;73:267–8.
22. Garner JS, Jarvis WR, Emori TG, Horan TC, Hughes JM. CDC definitions for nosocomial infections. Am J Infect Control. 1988;16:128–40.
23. Lazar HL, Vander Salm T, Engelman R, Orgill D, Gordon S. Prevention and management of sternal wound infections. J Thorac Cardiovasc Surg. 2016;152:962–72.
24. Braxton JH, Marrin CA, McGrath PD, Ross CS, Morton JR, Norotsky M, et al. Mediastinitis and long-term survival after coronary artery bypass graft surgery. Ann Thorac Surg. 2000;70:2004–7.

Renal Failure and Dialysis

54

Anne D. Cherry, Benjamin Y. Andrew,
Jamie R. Privratsky, and Mark Stafford-Smith

Main Messages

1. Acute kidney injury (AKI) is common after cardiothoracic surgery and associated with significantly increased postoperative morbidity and mortality. Unfortunately, AKI is poorly predicted by current risk models.
2. AKI diagnosis in cardiothoracic surgery patients is based primarily on serum creatinine rise. Current consensus criteria can delay recognition of a renal insult up to 48 h. A search is underway to identify more useful early AKI biomarkers.
3. Dialysis and renal transplant are currently the only therapies that improve renal function. Therefore, a strategy of renal risk avoidance is most important to protect the kidneys as part of overall cardiothoracic surgical care.
4. A renal best practices approach has been shown to reduce AKI burden among patient cohorts, however individual patients will still sustain AKI.
5. Care of patients with confirmed AKI involves primarily supportive measures. In some circumstances early renal replacement therapy may improve patient outcomes.

Diagnosis and Classification

Consensus diagnostic criteria for cardiac surgery-associated acute kidney injury (CS-AKI) align with those used across other clinical settings. The three most commonly employed include: (1) RIFLE ("R"isk, "I"njury, "F"ailure, "L"oss, "E"nd-stage kidney disease); (2) AKIN ("A"cute "K"idney "I"njury "N"etwork); and (3) KDIGO ("K"idney "D"isease: "I"mproving "G"lobal "O"utcomes) criteria (Table 54.1) [1]. While each definition differs in the specifics for staging AKI, all use serum creatinine and/or urine output criteria. KDIGO is the most recent, and incorporates components of both RIFLE and AKIN, utilizing both *relative* and *absolute* serum creatinine changes as well as acute (48-h) and chronic (7 day) time windows (Table 54.1). Finally, the Society of Thoracic Surgeons definition of acute renal failure has been used to advanced understanding of renal dysfunction following cardiac surgery. This definition is clas-

A. D. Cherry · B. Y. Andrew · J. R. Privratsky
M. Stafford-Smith (✉)
Department of Anesthesiology, Duke University
School of Medicine, Durham, NC, USA
e-mail: mark.staffordsmit@duke.edu

© Springer Nature Switzerland AG 2021
D. C. H. Cheng et al. (eds.), *Evidence-Based Practice in Perioperative Cardiac Anesthesia and Surgery*, https://doi.org/10.1007/978-3-030-47887-2_54

Table 54.1 Consensus acute kidney injury definitions and classification systems [1]

	Serum creatinine	Urine output
RIFLE criteria		
Risk	Increase in SCr to ≥1.5 times baseline *or* decrease in GFR by >25% within 7 days	<0.5 mL/kg/h for >6 h
Injury	Increase in SCr to >2 times baseline *or* decrease in GFR by >50% within 7 days	<0.5 mL/kg/h for >12 h
Failure	Increase in SCr to >3 times baseline *or* decrease in GFR by >75% within 7 days, *or* increase in SCr to ≥4 mg/dL with an acute rise of 0.5 mg/dL	<0.3 mL/kg/h for >24 h *or* anuria for 12 h
Loss	Complete loss of kidney function requiring dialysis for >4 weeks	
ESRD	Complete loss of kidney function requiring dialysis for >3 months	
AKIN criteria		
Stage 1	Increase in SCr by ≥0.3 mg/dL *or* increase in SCr to ≥1.5 times baseline within 48 h	<0.5 mL/kg/h for ≥6 h
Stage 2	Increase in SCr to >2 times baseline within 48 h	<0.5 mL/kg/h for ≥12 h
Stage 3	Increase in SCr to >3 times baseline within 48 h *or* increase in SCr to ≥4 mg/dL with a rise of 0.5 mg/dL within 24 h *or* initiation of dialysis	<0.3 mL/kg/h for ≥24 h *or* anuria for ≥12 h
KDIGO criteria		
Stage 1	Increase in SCr by ≥0.3 mg/dL within 48 h *or* increase in SCr to ≥1.5 times baseline within 7 days	<0.5 mL/kg/h for ≥6 h
Stage 2	Increase in SCr to >2 times baseline within 7 days	<0.5 mL/kg/h for ≥12 h
Stage 3	Increase in SCr to >3 times baseline within 7 days *or* increase in SCr to ≥4 mg/dL *or* initiation of dialysis	<0.3 mL/kg/h for ≥24 h *or* anuria for ≥12 h

RIFLE "R"isk, "I"njury, "F"ailure, "L"oss, "E"nd-stage kidney disease, *AKIN* "A"cute "K"idney "I"njury "N"etwork, *KDIGO* "K"idney "D"isease; "I"mproving "G"lobal "O"utcomes, *GFR* glomerular filtration rate, *SCr* serum creatinine, *ESRD* end stage renal disease

sified by either an increase in serum creatinine three times greater than baseline *or* an increase in creatinine to ≥4 mg/dL *or* a new dialysis requirement. Differences in these AKI definitions must be considered when comparing incidence and severity of AKI across studies using different criteria.

For all major consensus AKI criteria, accumulation of serum creatinine reflects reductions in glomerular filtration rate, which serves as a surrogate marker for overall impaired renal function. However, the relationship between glomerular filtration rate and serum creatinine is non-linear in nature (Fig. 54.1). Serum creatinine accumulation following renal insult may require up to 48 h for clinical recognition of AKI. Furthermore, important renal insults may never achieve sufficient elevation to meet diagnostic thresholds: small changes in serum creatinine are significantly associated with mortality following cardiac surgery [3, 4].

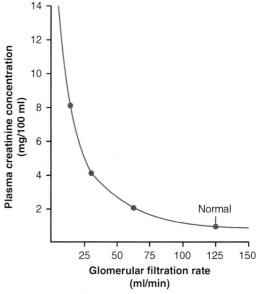

Fig. 54.1 Relationship between glomerular filtration rate and serum creatinine. With permission from [2]

Although oliguria criteria are included in all consensus definitions of AKI, there is limited and conflicting evidence on the additional diagnostic value of oliguria early after cardiac surgery, and perioperative AKI studies often limit diagnostic criteria to creatinine benchmarks only. Postoperative oliguria is common and may simply represent an appropriate homeostatic response to hypovolemia rather than a pathologic response to renal injury (i.e. acute renal "success") [5]. The addition of urine output to serum creatinine (AKIN) criteria does increase AKI incidence, but may or may not add prognostic value for long-term outcome [6, 7].

In summary, while defined originally in non-surgical populations, consensus diagnostic AKI criteria effectively capture important risk related to renal insult in the perioperative setting. However, these tools overlook smaller AKI in post-cardiac surgery patients that are still clinically important. Finally, the value of oliguria as an AKI diagnostic tool in the early postoperative period is an area of uncertainty.

Epidemiology

Worldwide, the incidence of CS-AKI is 22.3% [8]. Most CS-AKI is of low severity (i.e. stage 1; 13.6%) with a minority of cases reaching more severe stages [8]. AKI incidence varies by procedure, with aortic (29%) and valvular (27.5%) operations yielding higher rates than isolated coronary artery bypass graft (CABG; 19%) procedures [8].

Etiology and Pathophysiology

The development of CS-AKI is influenced by a number of different factors. Examining the pathophysiology in a stepwise manner begins with (1) an understanding of normal renal physiology, including the paradoxical vulnerability of the kidney to ischemic insult, followed by (2) the major mechanisms of renal injury. These mechanisms of injury will then be framed in the context of (3) major perioperative risk factors and (4) clinical and laboratory diagnostic biomarkers.

Renal Physiology and Vulnerability

Relative to other visceral organs, the kidney has reduced ischemic tolerance due to both its anatomical circulation and blood flow regulation. Countercurrent capillary circulation in the renal medulla allows for physiologic urine concentration, but also allows oxygen "escape" from entering to exiting capillaries. Furthermore, while the kidney receives 20% of cardiac output, the majority is shunted away from the vasa recta and renal medullary tissue. Collectively, these factors are responsible for the normal presence of renal medullary hypoxia, with a physiologic medullary resting oxygen tension of 10–20 mmHg [9]. Nonpulsatile flow during cardiopulmonary bypass may further exacerbate the imbalance between medullary and cortical perfusion [10].

The normal myogenic autoregulatory reflexes responsible for regulation of renal blood flow act through modulation of afferent arteriolar tone to divert systemic blood towards renal filtration at lower pressures, while protecting glomeruli from excessive flow at higher pressures. Notably, this system is primarily regulated by the need for glomerular filtration rather than, as for most homeostatic perfusion mechanisms, by oxygen demand. Renal oxygen supply-demand is also interesting, in that increased renal blood flow does increase overall oxygen delivery to the tissue, but also increases oxygen demand, through increased glomerular filtration and need for solute reuptake.

Mechanisms of Renal Injury

Ischemia-Reperfusion Injury
Ischemia-reperfusion (I/R) injury can occur at many stages during cardiac surgery. Examples include renal arterial hypoperfusion in the setting of systemic hypotension or cardiogenic shock, but also extended periods of low flow during cardiopulmonary bypass (CPB) despite acceptable mean blood pressures. There is also growing evidence that renal *venous* abnormalities such as congestion due to elevated central venous pressure may also contribute importantly to CS-AKI pathophysiology [11]. Finally, infarcts related to

renal artery dissection or embolic phenomena, such as from detached atheroma, thrombus, tumor, or infection, may contribute.

Nephrotoxic Agents

A number of nephrotoxic agents, both exogenous and endogenous, can contribute to the pathophysiology of CS-AKI. Endogenous toxin production is typically due to release of nephrotoxic free hemoglobin or myoglobin during surgical intervention. In the case of cardiac surgery, exposure of erythrocytes to the CPB circuit also induces damage to the cells, releasing free hemoglobin into the plasma. Free hemoglobin contributes to renal injury through (1) production of free radicals; (2) precipitation with Tamms-Horsfall proteins in the collecting system; and (3) induction of renal arteriole vasoconstriction through depletion of nitric oxide [5]. Furthermore, damage to erythrocytes increases circulating iron, which contributes to the production of reactive oxygen species. Indeed, cardiac surgery patients who develop AKI have significantly elevated levels of plasma free hemoglobin during and after separation from CPB [12]. Furthermore, postoperative elevation of serum myoglobin (a known AKI risk factor) is common in cardiac surgical patients, and may represent subclinical rhabdomyolysis [13].

Inflammation

Inflammatory AKI is a well described phenomenon that is relevant to CS-AKI [5, 14]. Studies in adult and pediatric populations have identified associations between both pre- and postoperative inflammatory markers and CS-AKI risk [15, 16]. It is worth noting in the context of cardiac surgery that inflammation is inherently interconnected with I/R, since I/R leads to downstream upregulation of pro-inflammatory mediators.

Risk Factors

Risk factors for CS-AKI are present in the preoperative, intraoperative, and postoperative periods (Table 54.2). Many are non-modifiable,

Table 54.2 Risk factors for post-cardiac surgery AKI [17–24]

| *Preoperative* |
| Age |
| Gender (female) |
| Elevated pulse pressure |
| Isolated systolic hypertension |
| Labile blood pressure |
| History of hypertension |
| History of diabetes mellitus |
| History of congestive heart failure |
| History of chronic obstructive lung disease |
| History of hyperlipidemia |
| History of chronic kidney disease |
| History of peripheral vascular disease |
| Anemia |
| History of myocardial infarction |
| History of smoking |
| Genetic predisposition |
| *Intraoperative* |
| Complex procedure (i.e. combined CABG + valve) |
| Emergent surgery |
| Extended duration of CPB |
| Extended duration of aortic cross-clamping |
| Multiple episodes of CPB |
| Intraoperative furosemide administration |
| Intraoperative inotrope administration |
| Intraoperative RBC transfusion |
| Extreme anemia during CPB |
| *Postoperative* |
| Postoperative inotrope administration |
| Postoperative diuretic administration |
| Postoperative vasoconstrictor administration |
| Postoperative RBC transfusion |
| Cardiogenic shock |

CABG coronary bypass graft surgery, *CPB* cardiopulmonary bypass, *RBC* red blood cell

but may improve risk prediction, and others are modifiable to mitigate risk. A number of pre- and intraoperative clinical risk score tools have been developed to allow for potential preemptive management in at-risk patients. In general, models that predict new renal replacement therapy (RRT) are more useful than those predicting AKI [17, 25], because pre-existing CKD combined with AKI particularly increases risk for RRT. Of RRT prediction tools, the Cleveland Clinic model [26] has shown superior discrimination [27].

Chronic Kidney Disease and Other at-Risk Populations

Chronic Kidney Disease

CKD is defined either as a reduced glomerular filtration rate (GFR) below 60 mL/min/1.73 m^2 *or* evidence of kidney damage that is present for >3 months [28]. CKD staging, using disease etiology and levels of both eGFR and albuminuria, allows for risk stratification and prognostication. Early mild renal insufficiency is commonly masked with a normal serum creatinine due to adaptive hyperfiltration. This may cause further glomerular damage and progression of renal failure. Complications of CKD include, among others: (1) volume overload; (2) hyperkalemia; (3) metabolic acidosis; (4) hypertension; (5) anemia; (6) dyslipidemia; and (7) bone mineral disorders. CKD patients are at increased risk for developing additional CS-AKI [2].

Aging

After age 50, overall kidney volume declines [29], with accelerated cortical volume loss (and also diminishing medullary volume in women). On a micro-anatomic level, the aging kidney shows signs of nephrosclerosis and a decline in the number of functional nephrons [30]. Glomerular filtration rate declines accordingly, by roughly 0.75 mL/min per year after age 30 [31]. These changes make aging kidneys vulnerable to injury and increase risk for CS-AKI [5].

Hypertension

Hypertension is implicated both as an etiologic contributor to renal dysfunction, and also as a pathologic sequela of CKD. Persistent hypertension causes several adaptive micro-anatomic changes within the kidney, including vessel wall thickening, sclerosis and damage to the glomerular filtration barrier [32]. Hypertension diagnosis has been implicated as a preoperative risk factor for CS-AKI in some analyses [17].

Diabetes

Diabetic kidney disease progresses through distinct pathophysiologic stages [33]. Initial glomerular hyperfiltration is followed by a period of normal filtration without albuminuria. Gradually microalbuminuria develops (with normal glomerular filtration), followed by macroalbuminuria and progressive glomerular filtration decline and CKD. Several analyses of cardiac surgical cohorts have identified preoperative diabetes as a significant risk factor for CS-AKI and RRT [17, 34].

Biomarkers

The creatinine-based diagnosis of AKI trails, rather than anticipates, AKI onset. Diagnosis can be delayed up to 48 h. As such, a number of earlier AKI biomarkers are currently being studied for better and earlier prediction of injury; however, none have been uniformly validated and widely adopted in the clinical setting. These newly developed AKI biomarkers are expressed during the continuum of renal injury. Some are relevant to the acute pre-injury kidney stress phase that typically precedes renal structural damage and subsequent overt GFR loss [35]. Thus, there are AKI biomarkers that detect: (1) kidney stress; (2) impaired function without structural damage; (3) structural damage with intact function; and (4) both structural damage with loss of function [36]. Each are discussed in the paragraphs below. Furthermore, how these biomarkers could be used to identify the phase of renal injury in hopes of guiding interventions to prevent further injury is outlined in Fig. 54.2.

Kidney Stress

The two primary kidney stress biomarkers are insulin-like growth factor-binding protein 7 (IGFBP7) and tissue inhibitor of metalloproteinases-2 (TIMP-2), both of which act to arrest the G$_1$ phase of the cell-cycle. Meta-analysis shows the product of the concentration of these two biomarkers in the urine (i.e. TIMP2 * IGFBP7) measured shortly after cardiac surgery to be predictive of subsequent AKI [37].

Fig. 54.2 Structure of the current biomarker paradigm. Combinations of damage and functional biomarkers allow for more specific identification of the pathophysiology underling renal dysfunction. Representative examples of each type of biomarker combination are shown in each quadrant. *With permission* from [36]

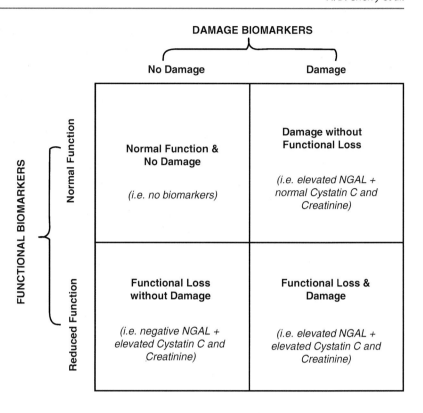

Kidney Damage

There are three major biomarkers indicative of renal damage: (1) neutrophil gelatinase-associated lipocalin (NGAL); (2) interleukin-18 (IL-18); and (3) kidney injury molecule-1 (KIM-1).

NGAL, a small protein with notable upregulation in instances of acute renal tubular injury, is measured as an AKI biomarker either after excretion into the urine, or release into the plasma. Meta-analysis has indicated modest discrimination of urinary NGAL for CS-AKI (composite AUC 0.72 [0.66–0.79]). Similar results were seen for circulating plasma NGAL (composite AUC 0.71 [0.64–0.77]) [38].

Expression and release of KIM-1 is induced within the proximal tubule after renal injury. Urine levels of KIM-1 perform similarly to NGAL in discrimination for CS-AKI (composite AUC 0.72 [0.59–0.84]).

Finally, in the context of renal insult, IL-18 is a pro-inflammatory cytokine involved in the evolution of tubular ischemia. As a biomarker for CS-AKI, urine levels of IL-18 parallel both KIM-1 and NGAL (composite AUC 0.66 [0.56–0.76]) perform similarly [38].

Kidney Function

Both serum creatinine and urine output, the consensus AKI diagnostic metrics, act as surrogates for renal filtration function. However, due to the non-linear relationship between glomerular filtration rate and serum creatinine (Fig. 54.1), early aberrations in GFR may not easily be detected through changes in serum creatinine level. Furthermore, as there is an approximately 48-h lag between renal functional decline and detectible accumulation of serum creatinine, the ability of creatinine as a biomarker to promptly inform preemptive changes in clinical management is limited. A clinically available alternate to serum creatinine is Cystatin C, a cysteine protease inhibitor protein produced by all nucleated cells. This biomarker is freely filtered by the glomerulus and subsequently completely reabsorbed in the renal tubules. Unfortunately, a recent large meta-analysis found that postoperative Cystatin C measured in the urine showed a lack of discrimination for AKIN CS-AKI (composite AUC 0.63 [0.37–0.89]) and only modest discrimination when measured in the plasma (composite AUC 0.69 [0.63–0.74]) [38].

Preoperative Period

While the majority of cardiac surgery-associated renal insults occur intraoperatively, preoperative planning affords opportunities to identify modifiable factors that may reduce renal insult. These include: (1) surgical planning; (2) identification and management of cardiorenal syndrome; and (3) minimizing exposure to nephrotoxic agents.

Procedure Selection and Surgical Planning

Postoperative AKI risk has been associated with many procedural characteristics including: (1) emergent operations; (2) redo operations; (3) valve replacement operations; (4) longer duration of CPB; and (5) operations utilizing circulatory arrest. Non-surgical alternatives may be preferable for patients with highest renal risk, and alternate surgical approaches may reduce CS-AKI risk for lower risk patients.

Minimally Invasive Procedures
Compared to their *traditional* counterparts, *minimally invasive* cardiac surgical approaches may limit renal insult through reduced invasiveness and attenuated physiologic stress. Main efforts in this regard are: (1) CPB avoidance; and (2) reduced tissue damage.

Avoidance of Cardiopulmonary Bypass
There was early speculation that avoidance of extracorporeal circulation through off-pump strategies would reduce AKI rates, but many randomized studies of on vs. off-pump CABG have failed to demonstrate major reductions in postoperative RRT rates [39]. However, other studies do report reduced overall AKI rates with off vs. on-pump CABG [40, 41]. Interpretation of these results is further complicated by those who question whether aortocoronary bypass graft surgery goals are equivalently achieved by off-pump approaches.

Retrospective comparisons of off and on-pump CABG approaches must account for the fact that patient characteristics may not be similar between groups; with a baseline tendency for off-pump CABG patients to be healthier with reduced renal risk. Stratification of patients according to renal risk is helpful in exploring the relationship between CS-AKI and CPB. In patients with preoperative CKD stage 4, off-pump CABG procedures are associated with reduced mortality and need for RRT [42], but in patients with established ESRD, there does not appear to be a short or long-term benefit [43]. Thus, in the majority of patients, CPB avoidance does not appear to confer important renoprotection; however, some evidence suggests that off-pump CABG may be associated with reduced risk for patients with stage 4 CKD, but not those with ESRD.

Reduction of Tissue Trauma
Through the use of smaller incisions (i.e. mini-thoracotomy or mini-sternotomy) and catheter-based technology during cardiac surgery, *minimally invasive* surgical approaches may diminish tissue trauma. The avoidance of tissue trauma theoretically limits the related inflammatory renal insult. In addition, *minimally invasive* procedures may have shorter recovery times, and less exposure to nephrotoxic insults.

Smaller Incisions: Mini-thoracotomy/Mini-sternotomy
In contrast to a traditional median sternotomy incision, mitral and aortic valve surgery can be performed via mini-thoracotomy or mini-sternotomy approaches. However, it is unclear whether these minimally invasive approaches result in less postoperative renal injury. Early retrospective analyses of mitral and aortic valve surgeries via mini-sternotomy suggested improvements in CS-AKI rates [44, 45]. However, subsequent retrospective studies have not confirmed reductions in either CS-AKI rate or new RRT requirement [46, 47]. As with off-pump CABG, minimally invasive valve procedures may benefit patients with pre-existing CKD [48].

Endovascular Approaches

Postoperative AKI in endovascular stenting for *abdominal* aortic aneurysm repair (EVAR) has been extensively studied, with somewhat conflicting results. Several large propensity-matched retrospective studies have shown a reduced burden of CS-AKI for endovascular vs. open repair [49, 50], but data suggest similar rates of postoperative RRT [51]. However, disentangling any potential renal benefit, potentially attributable to less invasive procedures, from their ability to expand the pool of eligible surgical candidates is problematic (e.g. comorbidities, high-risk vascular lesions, the potential for compromised renal blood flow). Thus, endovascular approaches for *aortic* aneurysm repair may reduce CS-AKI, but based on available evidence the decision to utilize endovascular versus open approaches to intervene on high-risk lesions should not be based on reducing renal risk.

Relative to abdominal EVAR, the relationship of endovascular *thoracic* aortic aneurysm repair (TEVAR) with renal outcomes is less extensively studied. The largest retrospective study to date found no difference in renal complication rate for endovascular versus open repair [52], but smaller studies demonstrated a reduction in renal injury with either endovascular repair [53] or a hybrid approach (aortic debranching and endovascular repair) [54]. However, in patients with aortic arch aneurysmal disease, studies have found no difference in AKI rate or requirement for new RRT [55, 56].

In patients requiring aortic valve replacement due to aortic stenosis, transcatheter replacement (TAVR) is rapidly becoming more common. Although TAVR was initially limited to high-risk patients, it is also now an acceptable alternative to SAVR for intermediate-risk patients [57]. Importantly, a large randomized trial of intermediate risk patients found that TAVR patients had significantly reduced AKI rates compared to surgical AVR (SAVR) [58]. Renal risk appears to be related to (1) procedural characteristics and (2) preoperative renal function. Regarding procedural characteristics, a meta-analysis reported that when compared to patients undergoing trans-femoral TAVR, those receiving trans-api-cal TAVR had an elevated risk of CS-AKI [59]. Trans-apical TAVR is typically reserved for patients with unfavorable anatomy (e.g. small femoral vessels or heavily calcified aorta); such patients are likely also at higher risk of renal injury, which may partially explain this finding. Regarding baseline renal function, one retrospective review observed that worse preoperative renal function prior to surgery was incrementally associated with elevated postoperative mortality in SAVR but *not* TAVR [60]. Thus, TAVR appears to be favorable relative to SAVR regarding renal risk, but particularly with a trans-femoral approach. Again, it appears that patients with baseline renal dysfunction may benefit the most from less invasive aortic valve replacement.

Cardiorenal Syndrome

The cardiovascular and renal systems interact in such a manner that dysfunction in one is often associated with derangements of the other. This phenomenon, known as cardiorenal syndrome (CRS), is divided into five distinct subtypes [61]: Types 1 and 2 are renal dysfunction due to cardiac dysfunction; Types 3 and 4 are cardiac dysfunction resulting from renal dysfunction; and Type 5 is combined cardiac and renal dysfunction due to systemic insult.

Types 1 and 2 CRS involve impairments of renal function resulting from acute or chronic heart failure, respectively. In these settings, the kidney acts as a "sentinel" organ, with its functional decline reflecting overall limited cardiac output, and with its consequent neuro-hormonal adaptation, reduced renal perfusion, and sometimes renal venous congestion related to right ventricular dysfunction; together contributing to impaired renal function [62]. Notably, renal dysfunction with CRS types 1 and 2 involves reduced GFR but otherwise *no* structural renal disease. In cardiac surgery populations, preoperative type 1 CRS is most commonly related an acute cardiac event (e.g. cardiogenic shock related to a myocardial infarction). In contrast, type 2 CRS is often a presenting feature of patients with chronic heart failure who are being considered for LVAD placement or heart transplant.

Types 3 and 4 CRS involve cardiac dysfunction resulting from acute or CKD, respectively. In type 3 CRS, AKI causes fluid overload, accumulation of toxic metabolites, and systemic inflammation, which together contribute to cardiac dysfunction [62]. In type 4 CRS, CKD results in accelerated hypertension and atherosclerosis, both of which lead to pathologic left ventricular hypertrophy and subsequent cardiac dysfunction. In cardiac surgery populations, type 3 CRS is often seen postoperatively due to post-cardiac surgery AKI or overt renal failure; whereas type 4 CRS is frequently encountered preoperatively, in the setting of ESRD or progressing CKD.

Finally, CRS type 5 is due to simultaneous dysfunction of both the heart and kidney due to a systemic insult (i.e. sepsis, diabetes mellitus, cirrhosis, lupus, vasculitis, etc.). Type 5 CRS can occur perioperatively in the setting of significant infection or multi-system organ failure. It can also occur as a consequence of cardiac arrest, where there has been a global ischemic insult.

Preoperative Optimization

Pharmacotherapy

Since the majority of studies examining the perioperative management of chronic pharmacotherapies and their effect on post-cardiac surgery renal outcomes are retrospective in nature, there is limited high quality evidence to guide clinical practice. Available studies have focused mostly on management of diuretics, renal-angiotensin system (RAS) blockers, statins, beta blockers, and the timing of surgery relative to intravenous contrast agent exposure.

With respect to preoperative diuretics, two retrospective analyses in cardiac surgical populations suggest increased risk with chronic loop diuretic therapy for both mortality and CS-AKI [63, 64]. With regard to perioperative management, consideration should be given to holding diuretics (e.g. for well-controlled hypertension). Of note, this adverse association does not include thiazide diuretics.

Although chronic RAS blocker therapy (i.e. angiotensin converting inhibitors and angiotensin receptor blockers) is common to treat hypertension or slow the progression of CKD, evidence to guide their use or discontinuation preoperatively in cardiac surgery patients is confusing: studies have shown both positive and negative effects. In patients taking preoperative RAS-blockers, one large meta-analysis (of mainly retrospective studies) found an increased risk for both CS-AKI and mortality [65]. In contrast, another meta-analysis (including both cardiac and general surgical patients) found no association. Finally, a meta-analysis of a single RCT and only propensity-matched retrospective studies found RAS-blockers to have a net-protective effect [66]. Thus, the relationship between preoperative RAS-blockers and CS-AKI is unclear based on available data. Further studies are necessary to define the role for these agents in the perioperative period.

Finally, the preoperative use of statins or beta blockers in the perioperative period surrounding cardiac surgery has been more intensely studied. A meta-analysis of nine RCTs examining the use of preoperative statins found no net-benefit with respect to either prevention of CS-AKI or RRT [67]. A large retrospective analysis found no association between preoperative beta-blocker therapy and CS-AKI [68]. Thus, these agents do not appear to have any relation to perioperative renal outcomes.

Intravenous Contrast Exposure

Contrast nephropathy is a well-recognized complication of intravenous dye administration that has long been thought to contribute to CS-AKI, particularly when emergent surgery immediately follows imaging procedures. In terms of guidelines, a large retrospective meta-analysis assessing surgical timing relative to contrast exposure reflects general dogma that 24 h delay (relative to longer delay) is sufficient to reduce renal risk [69]. Retrospective data suggests elevated CS-AKI rates up to 7 days following dye exposure [70].

However, with the advent of less toxic contrast agents and lower dosing strategies, it is important to readdress concerns over perioperative contrast dye exposure. Contrast exposure during diagnostic computed tomography (CT) scans emergency room patients is not associated with increased AKI [71, 72], but these results may not apply in cardiac surgery patients, who typically require higher contrast loads, followed by the added renal insult from emergent surgery [73]. Additionally, patients with diabetes and/or CKD are at higher risk for contrast nephropathy. Pretreatment with sodium bicarbonate or oral acetylcysteine prior to contrast exposure does not appear to be helpful [74].

Remote Ischemic Preconditioning

Remote ischemic pre-conditioning (RIPC) involves the intentional application of brief cycles of mild ischemia and reperfusion at one site to trigger protection (through yet to be fully defined mechanisms) against subsequent clinically significant I/R injury at another location. An example of strategic RIPC involves repeated blood pressure cuff inflations to interrupt blood supply to the arm to provide renal protection. The potential value of RIPC in preventing CS-AKI has been well-studied. A meta-analysis of 12 trials found no difference in AKI rates between patients randomized to RIPC or sham prior to cardiac surgery [75]. Post-hoc sub-group analyses did demonstrate lower AKI rates in three trials where propofol was *not* used, suggesting that this agent may attenuate or mask the effect of RIPC. Furthermore, in high-risk patients, RIPC was associated with reduced 3 months risk for major adverse kidney events (MAKE; a composite outcome including persistent renal dysfunction, new RRT, and mortality) [76]. RIPC appears safe in these high-risk patients, but there is insufficient evidence to support its routine use as a renoprotective strategy.

Intraoperative Period

A number of intraoperative interventions aimed at renoprotection have been studied in the context of CS-AKI, many of which have failed to show significant results.

Renal Response to Surgery and Anesthesia

Declining urine output is often utilized as an indirect marker of hypovolemia. However, during surgery and anesthesia, even normovolemic patients may have decreased urine output, often to rates that meet consensus AKI diagnostic thresholds. Such changes are related to the perioperative fluctuations in blood pressure, renal blood flow, glomerular filtration and tubular function. For example, upon induction of anesthesia, a modest drop in both blood pressure and cardiac output is associated with a similar decline in glomerular filtration and intraoperative urine output. Even when there is a hypertensive response to surgical stimulation, the resulting increase in glomerular filtration is often exceeded by the opposing effect of stress-related anti-diuretic hormone (ADH) release on urine production.

These concepts also apply to urine production during CPB, where urine output is highly predicted by mean arterial perfusion pressure but does *not* predict risk for CS-AKI. This finding is consistent across perioperative settings: studies both in cardiac and non-cardiac surgical populations have found that intraoperative oliguria is *not* predictive of postoperative renal dysfunction [6].

Renal Response to Cardiopulmonary Bypass

During CPB, intrarenal vasoconstriction and shunting reduces renal blood flow. Combined with hemodilution, this reduced flow decreases renal oxygen delivery by as much as 20%, which in turn obliges an increase in renal oxygen extraction. These findings are exacerbated during the period of weaning from CPB, as oxygen consumption again increases in the setting of hemodilution and reduced oxygen delivery [77] (Fig. 54.3).

Intraoperative Monitoring

Beyond standard cardiovascular monitoring, no additional monitors have been shown to reduce

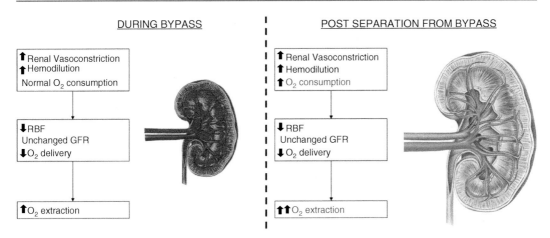

Fig. 54.3 Renal functional changes both during and following cardiopulmonary bypass in patients undergoing cardiac surgery (Cherry et al.)

CS-AKI. While several putative early AKI bio-markers have been identified, including both small molecules (e.g. Cystatin C, TIMP, KIM-1, etc.) and Doppler metrics of renal blood flow (e.g. renal resistive index [78]), none have yet been proven to reliably identify AKI in the operating room setting.

Anesthetic Agents and Other Perioperative Medications

The effects of anesthesia on blood pressure and cardiac output generally lead to reductions in glomerular filtration and urine output. While no anesthetic agents have true renoprotective properties, several anesthetic strategies are associated with a reduced risk of CS-AKI. Importantly, some medications that may be administered perioperatively have nephrotoxic characteristics.

Thoracic epidural analgesia, in combination with general anesthesia, is a strategy that may reduce risk for CS-AKI [79]. Retrospective studies of thoracotomy procedures have reported similar observations. Mechanistically, thoracic epidural anesthesia blocks the adrenergic stress-response to surgery, including alpha adrenergic receptors that modulate renal vasoconstriction and vasodilation.

Avoiding intraoperative use of pharmacologic agents with known nephrotoxic effects may also reduce the risk for CS-AKI. These include, but are not limited to: radiographic contrast dye; antibiotics (e.g. aminoglycosides, cephalosporins); loop diuretics (e.g. furosemide); anti-rejection transplant medications (e.g. calcineurin inhibitors); and non-steroidal anti-inflammatory drugs. While administration of these agents may be unavoidable, keeping to the lowest dose possible is an effective renoprotective strategy.

Potentially nephrotoxic agents such as aprotinin and colloid starch solutions are now rarely used in clinical practice following studies showing increased risk for renal insult [80]. Notably, while lysine analogs utilized for their antifibrinolytic effects (epsilon-aminocaproic acid, tranexamic acid) cause proteinuria, use of these agents is *not* associated with postoperative AKI [81].

Volatile anesthetic agents such as methoxyflurane and enflurane, now seldom available, are associated with polyuric renal insufficiency, attributed to the inorganic fluoride levels related to their metabolism [82]. Notably, sevoflurane metabolism also releases fluoride ions, and "compound A" which also is potentially nephrotoxic. However, in human studies, sevoflurane use has not been associated with postoperative AKI risk.

Intravenous Fluid Administration

Fluid Selection

While no strong evidence exists supporting any particular colloid or crystalloid solution as renoprotective during the perioperative period, the KDIGO guidelines suggest the use of isotonic crystalloid [83]. Chloride-rich crystalloid solutions (i.e. normal saline) increase the risk for hyperchloremic metabolic acidosis which, in turn, is associated with several renal responses (reduced renal blood flow and glomerular filtration, increased afferent arteriolar tone, modulation of renin secretion). Although poorly studied in cardiac surgery, in critically ill patients, a chloride-restrictive fluid policy (vs. chloride-liberal) was associated with reduced rate of AKI in one study [84], but a subsequent RCT (buffered crystalloid vs. normal saline) did not confirm this observation [85].

Fluid Management Strategy

Fluid management strategies in cardiac surgical patients to maintain euvolemia minimize renal risk through avoidance of complications related to hypovolemia (e.g. decreased renal perfusion) and hypervolemia (e.g. venous congestion). In the setting of AKI, venous hypertension is associated with increased mortality risk [86]. In a cardiac surgery cohort, elevated central venous pressure 6 h postoperatively predicted both risk for renal failure and mortality, even at central venous pressure values <10 mmHg [87].

Various protocolized fluid management strategies exist (e.g. "goal-directed", "restrictive"). Goal-directed therapy involves interventions guided by monitoring modalities (esophageal Doppler, transesophageal echocardiography, serial lactate levels) to optimize perfusion through management of preload (fluids), afterload (vasopressor administration) and contractility (inotrope administration). A meta-analysis of RCTs examining perioperative goal-directed therapy found that patients receiving goal-directed therapy had a reduced AKI rate. However, the overall difference in fluid administration was small (median difference of 555 mL), and the greatest reduction in AKI risk was noted

in studies when inotropes were used without strategic fluid administration [88]. These results suggest that cautious fluid resuscitation to maintain euvolemia perioperatively, complemented by administration of appropriate vasoactive agents (see next section) may be the best approach to maintaining perfusion.

Inotrope and Vasopressor Selection

While evidence comparing CS-AKI risk for each vasoactive agent is limited, numerous retrospective analyses suggest inotropic agent use in general is associated with increased risk for CS-AKI. Notably, retrospective studies cannot disentangle AKI risk related to inotropes from other perioperative considerations that often require inotrope therapy but also carry renal risk (e.g. sepsis). Nevertheless, inotropes are utilized effectively in the context of goal-directed therapy where, as previously discussed, they are associated with reduced renal risk. In a survey of 26 German Heart Centers, ICUs with the lowest CS-AKI rates patients preferred norepinephrine as a vasopressor (vs. epinephrine or dopamine) and avoided dopamine (vs. epinephrine) as an inotropic agent [89]. Notably, these findings align with other recent studies involving vasoactive agent selection: the SOAP II trial found norepinephrine superior to dopamine for patients with cardiogenic shock [90]; and, the rank order of preferred vasoactive agents in the Surviving Sepsis Campaign guidelines include norepinephrine as the first line vasopressor, followed by epinephrine and vasopressin, with only limited indications for dopamine and phenylephrine [91].

Anemia and Transfusion Management

Retrospective studies investigating anemia at various time-points throughout cardiac surgery (pre-, intra-, during CPB and postoperatively) have consistently identified very low hematocrit values as an AKI risk factor [18, 19, 92]. The largest body of evidence involves extreme hemodilution during CPB; some studies report an "inflection point" in escalating renal risk below a threshold hematocrit of approximately 21% [93]. This has been used by some to support a transfusion trigger at this level. Interestingly, the TRICS III trial found a transfusion trigger of 7.5 g/dl to be non-inferior relative to a higher threshold (9.5 g/dl) in cardiac surgery patients, with regards to renal failure and other major complications [94]. This is important, since transfusion itself is preferably avoided since it is independently associated with elevated AKI risk [95, 96]. Interestingly, neither the advanced age of transfused red blood cells, the use of cell saver technology to avoid transfusion, nor the co-occurrence extreme anemia with low blood pressure during CPB (pump flow maintained) appear to affect AKI risk [92, 97–100]. However, a meta-analysis of randomized trials of cardiac surgery studies suggests that leukocyte filtration of red blood cells prior to transfusion may considerably reduce (fivefold) AKI risk [101]. While there is general support for avoidance of extreme anemia and transfusion, and these two factors consistently predict CS-AKI risk, curiously no studies to date have examined the renoprotective value of pre-operative optimization strategies that correct anemia.

Glucose Management

Current perioperative insulin therapy recommendations advise administration to meet target glucose levels of 150–200 mg/dL. "Rigorous" glucose control protocols with intensive insulin therapy (e.g. serum target 80–100 mg/dL), used intra- and/or postoperatively, *have not* proven to be renoprotective compared to this more conventional approach to glucose control (i.e. target 150–200 mg/dl) [102–104]. Furthermore, such intense regimens are associated with an approximate fivefold increased risk of severe hypoglycemia (<40 mg/dL) [104], and were linked with increased risk of stroke and 30-day postoperative mortality in one randomized study [102].

Notably, *retrospective* cardiac surgery studies frequently report associations of intraoperative hyperglycemia with CS-AKI risk even after accounting for such conditions as diabetes, but such studies presumably do not account for other sources of AKI risk that may also be related to renal risk (e.g. metabolic syndrome).

Cardiopulmonary Bypass Management

Since during CPB there are changes in renal perfusion (i.e. increased medullary hypoxia) and the systemic inflammatory and stress hormone responses that may add to CS-AKI risk, questions over optimal perfusion strategies persist. Beyond the risks of anemia and transfusion (see above) various aspects of CPB management potentially related to CS-AKI are presented below: (1) blood pressure management; (2) pulsatile vs. non-pulsatile flow; and (3) temperature management.

Blood Pressure Management During CPB

Results from a randomized trial comparing renal risk for two mean CPB blood pressure targets (75–85 vs. 50–60 mmHg) found no difference in CS-AKI rates [105]. Notably, CPB flow was maintained at the same rate in both groups. Similarly, numerous large retrospective analyses failed to identify significant relationship between the cumulative degree and duration of hypotension (<50–55 mmHg) during CPB with flow maintained (with or without anemia) and CS-AKI risk [92, 106–108].

Temperature Management on CPB

Since *hypothermia* is a major component of organ protection during renal transplant surgery, it seems logical as a strategy to reduce CS-AKI. However, a randomized study of 298 CABG surgery patients comparing CPB target temperatures (28–30 °C vs. 35.5–36.5 °C) found no renoprotective effect [109]. In contrast, *hyperthermia* has been linked with increased CS-AKI risk in retrospective analyses, both during CPB (cumulative duration of arterial outlet temperature >37 °C vs. 36–37 °C) and postoperatively

[110, 111]. Collectively, these findings suggest that avoidance of over-aggressive CPB rewarming strategies may be advisable and that lowering CPB temperature targets does not importantly influence renal risk.

CPB Circuit Priming

Components of CPB priming fluid have been sparsely studied as related to risk for CS-AKI. In two small randomized trials there was no relationship between adding mannitol for patients with or without CKD and CS-AKI [112, 113].

Postoperative Period

Immediate Operative Versus Ongoing Versus New AKI

During the early postoperative period CS-AKI limited primarily to intraoperative insult typically manifests as a serum creatinine rise that peaks on the second or third day, and subsequently returns to preoperative values. Even small increases serum in creatinine that meet no consensus definition for AKI diagnosis are associated with poorer outcomes (i.e. are important) [3, 4]. Beyond intraoperative renal insult, numerous postoperative factors may additionally predispose patients to AKI. For example, surgical complications such as postoperative hemorrhage and low cardiac output syndrome may create ongoing renal insult. Other important non-surgical considerations may also add to AKI risk, most notably exposure to nephrotoxic agents and postoperative infection or sepsis.

Renoprotective Strategies

Beyond RRT for renal failure, there are no effective treatments for established CS-AKI and care is generally supportive in nature. Attention to nutrition is important, as patients with AKI *and* malnutrition are at increased risk for mortality [114]. Particularly in the setting of RRT, both caloric and protein requirements may be elevated [7]. Even if RRT is not required, KDIGO guidelines for patients with AKI include targeted caloric intake.

As highlighted, although a number have been investigated for established CS-AKI, and promising preclinical evidence suggests promise, there are to date no effective pharmacotherapies available for established CS-AKI. A meta-analysis of studies utilizing furosemide to treat established AKI found no reduction in hospital mortality or new RRT requirement [115]. The use of "renal-dose" intravenous dopamine infusion (1–3 µg/kg/min) has also been investigated, since this augments renal vasodilation, glomerular filtration, and natriuresis. However, several meta-analyses of randomized controlled trials in both cardiac and non-cardiac surgical populations have identified no advantage regarding mortality, renal function, or rate of AKI [116, 117]. Fenoldopam is a more selective dopamine-1 receptor agonist than dopamine that elicits similar renal effects while limiting concomitant adrenergic activation. In patients with established AKI, a multi-center RCT provides strong evidence against the use of fenoldopam, with increased risk of hypotension but a lack of any benefit (RRT requirement or mortality) [118]. While preliminary prophylactic studies suggested potential benefit to prevent post-cardiac surgery RRT, these analyses all had concerns raised [119]. Interestingly, the largest randomized trial of prophylactic fenoldopam (24-h postoperative infusion) for patients at high renal risk was associated with reduced risk for CS-AKI [120]. A recent multi-center RCT in patients with CS-AKI found that use of allogeneic human mesenchymal stem cells did not reduce time to recovery of renal function [121]. Taken together, despite the vast numbers of trials evaluating renoprotective agents, there are no specific CS-AKI therapeutics currently available.

In the context of no effective therapies, a bundle of treatments aimed at supportive care and avoidance of nephrotoxic agents, such as the "KDIGO bundle", holds the most promise for reducing CS-AKI [122]. Meersch and colleagues randomized cardiac surgical high renal risk patients to usual care or the KDIGO bundle and reported improvements in hemodynamics, glycemic control, and the frequency and severity of

CS-AKI with the KDIGO bundle [122]. Such coordinated care is intuitive, aimed at supportive interventions and avoidance of further renal insult appears to be the most effective renoprotective strategy currently available.

Renal Replacement Therapy

The severity of AKI following cardiac surgery sometimes requires the implementation of RRT. Assessment of a patient for RRT includes the following: (1) indications and timing; (2) modality; (3) dosing and desired end points; (4) anticoagulation regimens; and (5) RRT membrane characteristics. Considerations surrounding these issues are presented in Table 54.3.

Table 54.3 Renal replacement therapy

	Recommendations and evidence
Indications	Core indications: 1. Intractable fluid overload 2. Hyperkalemia (e.g., >6.5 mEq/L) 3. Clinical signs or symptoms of uremia 4. Metabolic acidosis (e.g., pH < 7.1)
Timing of initiation	In the presence of core indications: • Immediate initiation is recommended In the absence of core indications: • Existing evidence is unclear, although the trial most applicable to the cardiac surgical population (ELAIN) suggests a mortality and renal recovery benefit with early initiation [119]
Modality	While no strong evidence exists supporting one RRT modality over another (CRRT vs. IHT), CRRT may allow for increased hemodynamic stability
Dosing	Intermittent HD: 3.9 Kt/V per week, divided over sessions CRRT: effluent volumes of 20–25 mL/kg/h (no advantage of higher rates)
Anticoagulation	IHT: unfractionated heparin or LMWH (no difference in risk for bleeding or filter clotting) CRRT: citrate regional anticoagulation (reduced bleeding and filter clotting vs. systemic heparin)

Indications and Timing

There is general consensus regarding threshold clinical and laboratory findings that represent RRT indications for patients with CS-AKI. These include otherwise unmanageable fluid overload, hyperkalemia (e.g. >6.5 mEq/L), severe metabolic acidosis (e.g. pH < 7.1), and other clinical signs of uremia. Notably, the degree of fluid overload at RRT initiation in critically-ill patients is associated with subsequent mortality, suggesting that preemptive RRT may particularly benefit the fluid-overloaded patient [123]. In the absence of such emergent criteria, evidence for optimal timing of RRT initiation is less clear. RCTs comparing early vs. delayed RRT initiation in critically ill patients have generated conflicting results. The AKIKI trial found no mortality difference in early (KDIGO stage 3 diagnosis) vs. late (standard RRT criteria) initiation [124]; the ELAIN trial reported a lower 90-day mortality risk, increased renal recovery rate, shorter duration of RRT requirement, and decreased hospital length of stay when RRT was initiated earlier (KDIGO stage 2 vs. stage 3) [125]. Furthermore, the ELAIN trial found benefits with early RRT initiation out to 1 year (renal mortality, major adverse kidney events, and renal recovery) [126]. However, further trials are needed to confidently claim benefits from early RRT since a recent meta-analysis involving surgical (cardiac and non-cardiac) and non-surgical patients (10 RCTs, 1636 patients) found no association between early RRT and mortality (30-day, 60-day, 90-day, in-hospital) or dialysis at day 90 [127].

RRT Modality

Of the various strategies available, most commonly postoperative RRT is delivered through either continuous RRT (CRRT) or intermittent hemodialysis (IHD). Prolonged intermittent RRT and peritoneal dialysis are other options that are sometimes selected postoperatively. Among the three CRRT strategies, hemofiltration (convection), hemodialysis (diffusion) or hemodiafiltration (convection and diffusion), no modality has demonstrated superior outcomes. Some studies suggest improved renal recovery with CRRT vs. IHD but this was not evident in meta-analyses of

RCTs and prospective cohort studies [128]. Other potential benefits of CRRT compared to IHD include improved hemodynamic stability, better net fluid removal and improved clearance of inflammatory mediators. While the relationship of these factors with important outcomes is unclear, intuitively hemodynamic stability may be desirable for cardiac surgical patients. Nonetheless, most of the aforementioned evidence is not derived specifically from cardiac surgery studies.

In some hospitals, availability of CRRT may be limited due to technical and personnel issues since this requires intensive nurse monitoring and care. Prolonged intermittent RRT (PIRRT) involves extended periods of RRT, using IHD machines, resembling CRRT while minimizing staffing needs [129]. Meta-analyses of studies comparing mortality and renal recovery with PIRRT (vs. CRRT) have found neither to be superior [130].

RRT Dose and End Points

The KDIGO guidelines (2012) for CRRT suggest an effluent volume target of 20–25 mL/kg/h, while the IHD goal is 3.9 Kt/V per week, divided over intermittent sessions. Limited evidence exists to guide the frequency of administration of IHD as studies comparing intensive (i.e. daily) and less-intensive (i.e. every other day) IHD regimens show conflicting results [131, 132]. For CRRT, studies have found that higher delivery rates conferred no further mortality benefit or difference in rate of dialysis dependence [133].

Discontinuation of RRT is based on renal recovery reflected by resolution of oliguria, declining serum creatinine levels in the presence of a stable RRT schedule, or other evidence of improved creatinine clearance (e.g. elevated urine creatinine levels).

Anticoagulation for RRT

In general, anticoagulation is preferred for patients receiving RRT since extracorporeal filtration units can thrombose with either IHD or CRRT. However, specific to cardiac surgical patients, anticoagulation poses other significant risks (e.g. postoperative bleeding) [83]. CRRT implementation without anticoagulation has been described for patients with documented bleeding disorders. Notably, in the case of *consumptive* coagulopathy, laboratory measurements of anticoagulation may falsely suggest a reduced thrombosis risk. To prolong the functional life of dialysis filters (i.e. clot-free) without anticoagulation, flow rates should remain high.

The anticoagulation strategy selected to prolong the RRT circuit lifespan following cardiac surgery depends on the RRT modality selected and patient factors. For CRRT, since citrate regional anticoagulation effectively prolongs the circuit lifespan with fewer significant bleeding complications, this approach is preferred to systemic heparin administration when there is a high risk of hemorrhage [83, 134]. In contrast, for patients receiving IHD, the use of unfractionated heparin or low-molecular-weight heparin (LMWH) is generally recommended [83]. Unfractionated heparin and LMWH for intermittent RRT are equivalent in their bleeding risk and provide equally effective circuit thrombosis protection [135].

Notably, when dialysis patients receiving heparin experience premature filter clotting, the presence of heparin-induced thrombocytopenia (HIT) should always be suspected [136]. In this context, if HIT necessitates discontinuation of heparin anticoagulation, the high risk of thrombosis with HIT makes initiating an alternate strategy preferable to ceasing anticoagulation altogether. Administration of a direct thrombin inhibitor (e.g. argatroban) or factor Xa inhibitor (e.g. fondaparinux) is recommended [83].

Renal Recovery

The potential for renal recovery varies among patients and appears to be independent from vulnerability to, or degree of CS-AKI. While variably defined, better renal recovery following CS-AKI has been associated with reduced postoperative mortality [137, 138]. In this regard, early (within 7 days) and late (up to 90 days) renal recovery following AKI are differentiated from the development of so called "persistent acute kidney disease" and CKD [139]. Renal recovery generally reflects repopulation of proximal tubular epithelium primarily by uninjured endogenous tubular cells [140]. In some instances, damaged renal tubules undergo maladaptive repair including persistent inflammation, fibrosis, and reduction in vascular density which may lead to CKD [139]. Patient risk factors for poor renal recovery include: advanced age; pre-existing CKD; and comorbid conditions (hypertension, diabetes, cardiac disease) [139]. Although at an early stage, biomarkers that can predict renal recovery potential are currently being investigated.

References

1. Thomas ME, Blaine C, Dawnay A, Devonald MA, Ftouh S, Laing C, et al. The definition of acute kidney injury and its use in practice. Kidney Int. 2015;87(1):62–73.
2. Hall J. Guyton and hall textbook of medical physiology. 12th ed. Philadelphia: Saunders; 2011.
3. Kork F, Balzer F, Spies CD, Wernecke KD, Ginde AA, Jankowski J, et al. Minor postoperative increases of creatinine are associated with higher mortality and longer hospital length of stay in surgical patients. Anesthesiology. 2015;123(6):1301–11.
4. Lassnigg A, Schmidlin D, Mouhieddine M, Bachmann LM, Druml W, Bauer P, et al. Minimal changes of serum creatinine predict prognosis in patients after cardiothoracic surgery: a prospective cohort study. J Am Soc Nephrol. 2004;15(6):1597–605.
5. O'Neal JB, Shaw AD, Billings FT. Acute kidney injury following cardiac surgery: current understanding and future directions. Crit Care (Lond). 2016;20(1):187.
6. McIlroy DR, Argenziano M, Farkas D, Umann T, Sladen RN. Incorporating oliguria into the diagnostic criteria for acute kidney injury after on-pump cardiac surgery: impact on incidence and outcomes. J Cardiothorac Vasc Anesth. 2013;27(6):1145–52.
7. Petaja L, Vaara S, Liuhanen S, Suojaranta-Ylinen R, Mildh L, Nisula S, et al. Acute kidney injury after cardiac surgery by complete KDIGO criteria predicts increased mortality. J Cardiothorac Vasc Anesth. 2016;31(3):827–36.
8. Hu J, Chen R, Liu S, Yu X, Zou J, Ding X. Global incidence and outcomes of adult patients with acute kidney injury after cardiac surgery: a systematic review and meta-analysis. J Cardiothorac Vasc Anesth. 2016;30(1):82–9.
9. Karhausen J, Stafford-Smith M. The role of nonocclusive sources of acute gut injury in cardiac surgery. J Cardiothorac Vasc Anesth. 2014;28(2):379–91.
10. Stafford-Smith M, Grocott HP. Renal medullary hypoxia during experimental cardiopulmonary bypass: a pilot study. Perfusion. 2005;20(1):53–8.
11. Gambardella I, Gaudino M, Ronco C, Lau C, Ivascu N, Girardi LN. Congestive kidney failure in cardiac surgery: the relationship between central venous pressure and acute kidney injury. Interact Cardiovasc Thorac Surg. 2016;23(5):800–5.
12. Billings FT, Ball SK, Roberts LJ, Pretorius M. Postoperative acute kidney injury is associated with hemoglobinemia and an enhanced oxidative stress response. Free Radic Biol Med. 2011;50(11):1480–7.
13. Benedetto U, Angeloni E, Luciani R, Refice S, Stefanelli M, Comito C, et al. Acute kidney injury after coronary artery bypass grafting: does rhabdomyolysis play a role? J Thorac Cardiovasc Surg. 2010;140(2):464–70.
14. Mauricio Del Rio J, Nicoara A, Swaminathan M. Neuroendocrine stress response: implications for cardiac surgery-associated acute kidney injury. Rom J Anaesth Intensive Care. 2017;24(1):57–63.
15. Zhang WR, Garg AX, Coca SG, Devereaux PJ, Eikelboom J, Kavsak P, et al. Plasma IL-6 and IL-10 concentrations predict AKI and long-term mortality in adults after cardiac surgery. J Am Soc Nephrol. 2015;26(12):3123–32.
16. de Fontnouvelle CA, Greenberg JH, Thiessen-Philbrook HR, Zappitelli M, Roth J, Kerr KF, et al. Interleukin-8 and tumor necrosis factor predict acute kidney injury after pediatric cardiac surgery. Ann Thorac Surg. 2017;104(6):2072–9.
17. Kristovic D, Horvatic I, Husedzinovic I, Sutlic Z, Rudez I, Baric D, et al. Cardiac surgery-associated acute kidney injury: risk factors analysis and comparison of prediction models. Interact Cardiovasc Thorac Surg. 2015;21(3):366–73.
18. Oprea AD, Del Rio JM, Cooter M, Green CL, Karhausen JA, Nailer P, et al. Pre- and postoperative anemia, acute kidney injury, and mortality after coronary artery bypass grafting surgery: a retrospective observational study. Can J Anaesth. 2017;65(1):46–59.
19. Swaminathan M, Phillips-Bute BG, Conlon PJ, Smith PK, Newman MF, Stafford-Smith M. The association of lowest hematocrit during cardiopulmonary bypass with acute renal injury after coronary artery bypass surgery. Ann Thorac Surg. 2003;76(3):784–91; discussion 92.
20. Aronson S, Fontes ML, Miao Y, Mangano DT, Investigators of the Multicenter Study of Perioperative Ischemia Research G, Ischemia R, et al. Risk index for perioperative renal dysfunction/failure: critical dependence on pulse pressure hypertension. Circulation. 2007;115(6):733–42.
21. Aronson S, Boisvert D, Lapp W. Isolated systolic hypertension is associated with adverse outcomes from coronary artery bypass grafting surgery. Anesth Analg. 2002;94(5):1079–84.

22. Aronson S, Avery E, Dyke C, Varon J, Levy J. Blood pressure lability during cardiac surgery is associated with adverse outcomes. Am Soc Anesthesiol. 2008;FL2008.

23. Jiang W, Teng J, Xu J, Shen B, Wang Y, Fang Y, et al. Dynamic predictive scores for cardiac surgery-associated acute kidney injury. J Am Heart Assoc. 2016;5(8).

24. Stafford-Smith M, Li YJ, Mathew JP, Li YW, Ji Y, Phillips-Bute BG, et al. Genome-wide association study of acute kidney injury after coronary bypass graft surgery identifies susceptibility loci. Kidney Int. 2015;88(4):823–32.

25. Huen SC, Parikh CR. Predicting acute kidney injury after cardiac surgery: a systematic review. Ann Thorac Surg. 2012;93(1):337–47.

26. Thakar CV, Arrigain S, Worley S, Yared JP, Paganini EP. A clinical score to predict acute renal failure after cardiac surgery. J Am Soc Nephrol. 2005;16(1):162–8.

27. Englberger L, Suri RM, Li Z, Dearani JA, Park SJ, Sundt TM 3rd, et al. Validation of clinical scores predicting severe acute kidney injury after cardiac surgery. Am J Kidney Dis. 2010;56(4):623–31.

28. KDIGO. KDIGO 2012 Clinical practice guideline for the evaluation and management of chronic kidney disease. Kidney Int Suppl. 2013;3(1).

29. Wang X, Vrtiska TJ, Avula RT, Walters LR, Chakkera HA, Kremers WK, et al. Age, kidney function, and risk factors associate differently with cortical and medullary volumes of the kidney. Kidney Int. 2014;85(3):677–85.

30. Denic A, Glassock RJ, Rule AD. Structural and functional changes with the aging kidney. Adv Chronic Kidney Dis. 2016;23(1):19–28.

31. Lindeman RD, Tobin J, Shock NW. Longitudinal studies on the rate of decline in renal function with age. J Am Geriatr Soc. 1985;33(4):278–85.

32. Mennuni S, Rubattu S, Pierelli G, Tocci G, Fofi C, Volpe M. Hypertension and kidneys: unraveling complex molecular mechanisms underlying hypertensive renal damage. J Hum Hypertens. 2014;28(2):74–9.

33. Mora-Fernandez C, Dominguez-Pimentel V, de Fuentes MM, Gorriz JL, Martinez-Castelao A, Navarro-Gonzalez JF. Diabetic kidney disease: from physiology to therapeutics. J Physiol. 2014;592(18):3997–4012.

34. Parolari A, Pesce LL, Pacini D, Mazzanti V, Salis S, Sciacovelli C, et al. Risk factors for perioperative acute kidney injury after adult cardiac surgery: role of perioperative management. Ann Thorac Surg. 2012;93(2):584–91.

35. Fischer S, Salaunkey K. Cardiac surgery-associated acute kidney injury. Curr Anesthesiol Rep. 2017.

36. Murray PT, Mehta RL, Shaw A, Ronco C, Endre Z, Kellum JA, et al. Potential use of biomarkers in acute kidney injury: report and summary of recommendations from the 10th acute dialysis quality initiative consensus conference. Kidney Int. 2014;85(3):513–21.

37. Jia HM, Huang LF, Zheng Y, Li WX. Diagnostic value of urinary tissue inhibitor of metalloproteinase-2 and insulin-like growth factor binding protein 7 for acute kidney injury: a meta-analysis. Crit Care (Lond). 2017;21(1):77.

38. Ho J, Tangri N, Komenda P, Kaushal A, Sood M, Brar R, et al. Urinary, plasma, and serum biomarkers' utility for predicting acute kidney injury associated with cardiac surgery in adults: a meta-analysis. Am J Kidney Dis. 2015;66(6):993–1005.

39. Moller CH, Penninga L, Wetterslev J, Steinbruchel DA, Gluud C. Off-pump versus on-pump coronary artery bypass grafting for ischaemic heart disease. Cochrane Database Syst Rev. 2012;3:CD007224.

40. Cheungpasitporn W, Thongprayoon C, Kittanamongkolchai W, Srivali N, O'Corragain OA, Edmonds PJ, et al. Comparison of renal outcomes in off-pump versus on-pump coronary artery bypass grafting: a systematic review and meta-analysis of randomized controlled trials. Nephrology (Carlton, Vic). 2015;20:727–35.

41. Polomsky M, He X, O'Brien SM, Puskas JD. Outcomes of off-pump versus on-pump coronary artery bypass grafting: impact of preoperative risk. J Thorac Cardiovasc Surg. 2013;145(5):1193–8.

42. Chawla LS, Zhao Y, Lough FC, Schroeder E, Seneff MG, Brennan JM. Off-pump versus on-pump coronary artery bypass grafting outcomes stratified by preoperative renal function. J Am Soc Nephrol. 2012;23(8):1389–97.

43. Chen JJ, Lin LY, Yang YH, Hwang JJ, Chen PC, Lin JL, et al. On pump versus off pump coronary artery bypass grafting in patients with end-stage renal disease and coronary artery disease – a nation-wide, propensity score matched database analyses. Int J Cardiol. 2017;227:529–34.

44. McCreath BJ, Swaminathan M, Booth JV, Phillips-Bute B, Chew STH, Glower DD, et al. Mitral valve surgery and acute renal injury: port access versus median sternotomy. Ann Thorac Surg. 2003;75(3):812–9.

45. Antonic M, Gersak B. Renal function after port access and median sternotomy mitral valve surgery. Heart Surg Forum. 2007;10(5):E401–7.

46. Gilmanov D, Bevilacqua S, Murzi M, Cerillo AG, Gasbarri T, Kallushi E, et al. Minimally invasive and conventional aortic valve replacement: a propensity score analysis. Ann Thorac Surg. 2013;96(3):837–43.

47. Furukawa N, Kuss O, Aboud A, Schonbrodt M, Renner A, Hakim Meibodi K, et al. Ministernotomy versus conventional sternotomy for aortic valve replacement: matched propensity score analysis of 808 patients. Eur J Cardio-thorac Surg. 2014;46(2):221–6.. discussion 6-7

48. Valdez GD, Mihos CG, Santana O, Heimowitz TB, Goldszer R, Lamas GA, et al. Incidence of postoperative acute kidney injury in patients with chronic kidney disease undergoing minimally invasive valve surgery. J Thorac Cardiovasc Surg. 2013;146(6):1488–93.

49. Edwards ST, Schermerhorn ML, O'Malley AJ, Bensley RP, Hurks R, Cotterill P, et al. Comparative effectiveness of endovascular versus open repair of ruptured abdominal aortic aneurysm in the medicare population. J Vasc Surg. 2014;59(3):575–82.

50. Siracuse JJ, Gill HL, Graham AR, Schneider DB, Connolly PH, Sedrakyan A, et al. Comparative safety of endovascular and open surgical repair of abdominal aortic aneurysms in low-risk male patients. J Vasc Surg. 2014;60(5):1154–8.

51. Becquemin JP, Pillet JC, Lescalie F, Sapoval M, Goueffic Y, Lermusiaux P, et al. A randomized controlled trial of endovascular aneurysm repair versus open surgery for abdominal aortic aneurysms in low- to moderate-risk patients. J Vasc Surg. 2011;53(5):1167–73.. e1

52. Gopaldas RR, Huh J, Dao TK, LeMaire SA, Chu D, Bakaeen FG, et al. Superior nationwide outcomes of endovascular versus open repair for isolated descending thoracic aortic aneurysm in 11,669 patients. J Thorac Cardiovasc Surg. 2010;140(5):1001–10.

53. Lee HC, Joo HC, Lee SH, Lee S, Chang BC, Yoo KJ, et al. Endovascular repair versus open repair for isolated descending thoracic aortic aneurysm. Yonsei Med J. 2015;56(4):904–12.

54. Murphy EH, Beck AW, Clagett P, DiMaio JM, Jessen ME, Arko FR. Combined aortic debranching and thoracic endovascular aneurysm repair (TEVAR) effective but at a cost. Arch Surg. 2009;144(3):222–7.

55. Yoshitake A, Okamoto K, Yamazaki M, Kimura N, Hirano A, Iida Y, et al. Comparison of aortic arch repair using the endovascular technique, total arch replacement and staged surgery dagger. Eur J Cardio-thorac Surg. 2017;51(6):1142–8.

56. Kawatou M, Minakata K, Sakamoto K, Nakatsu T, Tazaki J, Higami H, et al. Comparison of endovascular repair with branched stent graft and open repair for aortic arch aneurysmdagger. Interact Cardiovasc Thorac Surg. 2017;25(2):246–53.

57. Reardon MJ, Van Mieghem NM, Popma JJ, Kleiman NS, Sondergaard L, Mumtaz M, et al. Surgical or transcatheter aortic-valve replacement in intermediate-risk patients. N Engl J Med. 2017;376(14):1321–31.

58. Leon MB, Smith CR, Mack MJ, Makkar RR, Svensson LG, Kodali SK, et al. Transcatheter or surgical aortic-valve replacement in intermediate-risk patients. N Engl J Med. 2016;374(17):1609–20.

59. Wang J, Yu W, Zhou Y, Yang Y, Li C, Liu N, et al. Independent risk factors contributing to acute kidney injury according to updated valve academic research consortium-2 criteria after transcatheter aortic valve implantation: a meta-analysis and meta-regression of 13 studies. J Cardiothorac Vasc Anesth. 2017;31(3):816–26.

60. Nguyen TC, Babaliaros VC, Razavi SA, Kilgo PD, Guyton RA, Devireddy CM, et al. Impact of varying degrees of renal dysfunction on transcatheter and surgical aortic valve replacement. J Thorac Cardiovasc Surg. 2013;146(6):1399–406.. discussion 13406-7

61. Umanath K, Emani S. Getting to the heart of the matter: review of treatment of cardiorenal syndrome. Adv Chronic Kidney Dis. 2017;24(4):261–6.

62. Shamseddin MK, Parfrey PS. Mechanisms of the cardiorenal syndromes. Nat Rev Nephrol. 2009;5(11):641–9.

63. Metz LI, LeBeau ME, Zlabek JA, Mathiason MA. Acute renal failure in patients undergoing cardiothoracic surgery in a community hospital. WMJ. 2009;108(2):109–14.

64. Renyolds A, White W, Stafford-Smith M, Grichnik K, Sickeler R, Gray M, et al. The relationship of loop diuretics with acute kidney injury and mortality after cardiac surgery. Anesth Analg. 2013;113(Suppl) (SCA3).

65. Yacoub R, Patel N, Lohr JW, Rajagopalan S, Nader N, Arora P. Acute kidney injury and death associated with renin angiotensin system blockade in cardiothoracic surgery: a meta-analysis of observational studies. Am J Kidney Dis. 2013;62(6):1077–86.

66. Cheungpasitporn W, Thongprayoon C, Srivali N, O'Corragain OA, Edmonds PJ, Ungprasert P, et al. Preoperative renin-angiotensin system inhibitors use linked to reduced acute kidney injury: a systematic review and meta-analysis. Nephrol Dial Transplant. 2015;30(6):978–88.

67. Xiong B, Nie D, Cao Y, Zou Y, Yao Y, Qian J, et al. Preoperative statin treatment for the prevention of acute kidney injury in patients undergoing cardiac surgery: a meta-analysis of randomised controlled trials. Heart Lung Circ. 2017;26(11):1200–7.

68. O'Neal JB, Billings FT, Liu X, Shotwell MS, Liang Y, Shah AS, et al. Effect of preoperative Beta-blocker use on outcomes following cardiac surgery. Am J Cardiol. 2017;120(8):1293–7.

69. Hu Y, Li Z, Chen J, Shen C, Song Y, Zhong Q. The effect of the time interval between coronary angiography and on-pump cardiac surgery on risk of postoperative acute kidney injury: a meta-analysis. J Cardiothorac Surg. 2013;8:178.

70. Kim K, Joung KW, Ji SM, Kim JY, Lee EH, Chung CH, et al. The effect of coronary angiography timing and use of cardiopulmonary bypass on acute kidney injury after coronary artery bypass graft surgery. J Thorac Cardiovasc Surg. 2016;152(1):254–61.. e3

71. Aycock RD, Westafer LM, Boxen JL, Majlesi N, Schoenfeld EM, Bannuru RR. Acute kidney injury after computed tomography: a meta-analysis. Ann Emerg Med. 2017.

72. Hinson JS, Ehmann MR, Fine DM, Fishman EK, Toerper MF, Rothman RE, et al. Risk of acute kidney injury after intravenous contrast media administration. Ann Emerg Med. 2017;69(5):577–86.e4.

73. Azzalini L, Candilio L, McCullough PA, Colombo A. Current risk of contrast-induced acute kidney injury after coronary angiography and intervention: a reappraisal of the literature. Can J Cardiol. 2017;33(10):1225–8.

74. Weisbord SD, Gallagher M, Jneid H, Garcia S, Cass A, Thwin SS, et al. Outcomes after angiography

with sodium bicarbonate and acetylcysteine. N Engl J Med. 2017;378(7):603–14.

75. Pierce B, Bole I, Patel V, Brown DL. Clinical outcomes of remote ischemic preconditioning prior to cardiac surgery: a meta-analysis of randomized controlled trials. J Am Heart Assoc. 2017;6(2):e004666.

76. Zarbock A, Kellum JA, Van Aken H, Schmidt C, Kullmar M, Rosenberger P, et al. Long-term effects of remote ischemic preconditioning on kidney function in high-risk cardiac surgery patients: follow-up results from the renal RIP trial. Anesthesiology. 2017;126(5):787–98.

77. Lannemyr L, Bragadottir G, Krumbholz V, Redfors B, Sellgren J, Ricksten SE. Effects of cardiopulmonary bypass on renal perfusion, filtration, and oxygenation in patients undergoing cardiac surgery. Anesthesiology. 2017;126(2):205–13.

78. Regolisti G, Maggiore U, Cademartiri C, Belli L, Gherli T, Cabassi A, et al. Renal resistive index by transesophageal and transparietal echo-Doppler imaging for the prediction of acute kidney injury in patients undergoing major heart surgery. J Nephrol. 2016;30:243–53.

79. Scott NB, Turfrey DJ, Ray DA, Nzewi O, Sutcliffe NP, Lal AB, et al. A prospective randomized study of the potential benefits of thoracic epidural anesthesia and analgesia in patients undergoing coronary artery bypass grafting. Anesth Analg. 2001;93(3):528–35.

80. Myburgh JA, Finfer S, Bellomo R, Billot L, Cass A, Gattas D, et al. Hydroxyethyl starch or saline for fluid resuscitation in intensive care. N Engl J Med. 2012;367(20):1901–11.

81. Stafford-Smith M. Antifibrinolytic use during cardiac and hepatic surgery makes tubular proteinuria-based early biomarkers poor tools to diagnose perioperative acute kidney injury. Am J Kidney Dis. 2011;57(6):960; author reply-1.

82. Mazze RI. Methoxyflurane revisited: tale of an anesthetic from cradle to grave. Anesthesiology. 2006;105(4):843–6.

83. KDIGO Clinical Practice Guideline for Acute Kidney Injury. Kidney International Supplements. 2012;2(1).

84. Yunos NM, Bellomo R, Hegarty C, Story D, Ho L, Bailey M. Association between a chloride-liberal vs chloride-restrictive intravenous fluid administration strategy and kidney injury in critically ill adults. JAMA. 2012;308(15):1566–72.

85. Young P, Bailey M, Beasley R, Henderson S, Mackle D, McArthur C, et al. Effect of a buffered crystalloid solution vs saline on acute kidney injury among patients in the intensive care unit: the SPLIT randomized clinical trial. JAMA. 2015;314(16):1701–10.

86. Zhang L, Chen Z, Diao Y, Yang Y, Fu P. Associations of fluid overload with mortality and kidney recovery in patients with acute kidney injury: a systematic review and meta-analysis. J Crit Care. 2015;30(4):860.e7–13.

87. Williams JB, Peterson ED, Wojdyla D, Harskamp R, Southerland KW, Ferguson TB, et al. Central venous pressure after coronary artery bypass surgery: does it predict postoperative mortality or renal failure? J Crit Care. 2014;29(6):1006–10.

88. Prowle JR, Chua HR, Bagshaw SM, Bellomo R. Clinical review: volume of fluid resuscitation and the incidence of acute kidney injury – a systematic review. Critical care (Lond). 2012;16(4):230.

89. Heringlake M, Knappe M, Vargas Hein O, Lufft H, Kindgen-Milles D, Bottiger BW, et al. Renal dysfunction according to the ADQI-RIFLE system and clinical practice patterns after cardiac surgery in Germany. Minerva Anestesiol. 2006;72(7–8):645–54.

90. De Backer D, Biston P, Devriendt J, Madl C, Chochrad D, Aldecoa C, et al. Comparison of dopamine and norepinephrine in the treatment of shock. N Engl J Med. 2010;362(9):779–89.

91. Dellinger RP, Levy MM, Rhodes A, Annane D, Gerlach H, Opal SM, et al. Surviving sepsis campaign: international guidelines for management of severe sepsis and septic shock: 2012. Crit Care Med. 2013;41(2):580–637.

92. Sickeler R, Phillips-Bute B, Kertai MD, Schroder J, Mathew JP, Swaminathan M, et al. The risk of acute kidney injury with co-occurrence of anemia and hypotension during cardiopulmonary bypass relative to anemia alone. Ann Thorac Surg. 2014;97(3):865–71.

93. Karkouti K, Beattie WS, Wijeysundera DN, Rao V, Chan C, Dattilo KM, et al. Hemodilution during cardiopulmonary bypass is an independent risk factor for acute renal failure in adult cardiac surgery. J Thorac Cardiovasc Surg. 2005;129(2):391–400.

94. Mazer CD, Whitlock RP, Fergusson DA, Hall J, Belley-Cote E, Connolly K, et al. Restrictive or Liberal red-cell transfusion for cardiac surgery. N Engl J Med. 2017;377(22):2133–44.

95. Karkouti K, Wijeysundera DN, Yau TM, Callum JL, Cheng DC, Crowther M, et al. Acute kidney injury after cardiac surgery: focus on modifiable risk factors. Circulation. 2009;119(4):495–502.

96. Haase M, Bellomo R, Story D, Letis A, Klemz K, Matalanis G, et al. Effect of mean arterial pressure, haemoglobin and blood transfusion during cardiopulmonary bypass on post-operative acute kidney injury. Nephrol Dial Transplant. 2012;27(1):153–60.

97. Lacroix J, Hebert PC, Fergusson DA, Tinmouth A, Cook DJ, Marshall JC, et al. Age of transfused blood in critically ill adults. N Engl J Med. 2015;372(15):1410–8.

98. Heddle NM, Cook RJ, Arnold DM, Liu Y, Barty R, Crowther MA, et al. Effect of short-term vs. long-term blood storage on mortality after transfusion. N Engl J Med. 2016;375(20):1937–45.

99. Cooper DJ, McQuilten ZK, Nichol A, Ady B, Aubron C, Bailey M, et al. Age of red cells for transfusion and outcomes in critically ill adults. N Engl J Med. 2017;377(19):1858–67.

100. Wang G, Bainbridge D, Martin J, Cheng D. The efficacy of an intraoperative cell saver during car-

diac surgery: a meta-analysis of randomized trials. Anesth Analg. 2009;109(2):320–30.

101. Scrascia G, Guida P, Rotunno C, de Luca Tupputi Schinosa L, Paparella D. Anti-inflammatory strategies to reduce acute kidney injury in cardiac surgery patients: a meta-analysis of randomized controlled trials. Artif Organs. 2014;38(2):101–12.

102. Gandhi GY, Nuttall GA, Abel MD, Mullany CJ, Schaff HV, O'Brien PC, et al. Intensive intraoperative insulin therapy versus conventional glucose management during cardiac surgery: a randomized trial. Ann Intern Med. 2007;146(4):233–43.

103. Wiener RS, Wiener DC, Larson RJ. Benefits and risks of tight glucose control in critically ill adults: a meta-analysis. JAMA. 2008;300(8):933–44.

104. Yamada T, Shojima N, Noma H, Yamauchi T, Kadowaki T. Glycemic control, mortality, and hypoglycemia in critically ill patients: a systematic review and network meta-analysis of randomized controlled trials. Intensive Care Med. 2017;43(1):1–15.

105. Azau A, Markowicz P, Corbeau JJ, Cottineau C, Moreau X, Baufreton C, et al. Increasing mean arterial pressure during cardiac surgery does not reduce the rate of postoperative acute kidney injury. Perfusion. 2014;29(6):496–504.

106. Abel RM, Buckley MJ, Austen WG, Barnett GO, Beck CH Jr, Fischer JE. Etiology, incidence, and prognosis of renal failure following cardiac operations. Results of a prospective analysis of 500 consecutive patients. J Thorac Cardiovasc Surg. 1976;71(3):323–33.

107. Urzua J, Troncoso S, Bugedo G, Canessa R, Munoz H, Lema G, et al. Renal function and cardiopulmonary bypass: effect of perfusion pressure. J Cardiothorac Vasc Anesth. 1992;6(3):299–303.

108. Smeltz AM, Cooter M, Rao S, Karhausen JA, Stafford-Smith M, Fontes ML, et al. Elevated pulse pressure, intraoperative hemodynamic perturbations, and acute kidney injury after coronary artery bypass grafting surgery. J Cardiothorac Vasc Anesth. 2017;32:1214–24.

109. Swaminathan M, East C, Phillips-Bute B, Newman MF, Reves JG, Smith PK, et al. Report of a substudy on warm versus cold cardiopulmonary bypass: changes in creatinine clearance. Ann Thorac Surg. 2001;72(5):1603–9.

110. Newland RF, Tully PJ, Baker RA. Hyperthermic perfusion during cardiopulmonary bypass and postoperative temperature are independent predictors of acute kidney injury following cardiac surgery. Perfusion. 2013;28(3):223–31.

111. Newland RF, Baker RA, Mazzone AL, Quinn SS, Chew DP, Perfusion Downunder C. Rewarming temperature during cardiopulmonary bypass and acute kidney injury: a multicenter analysis. Ann Thorac Surg. 2016;101(5):1655–62.

112. Yallop KG, Sheppard SV, Smith DC. The effect of mannitol on renal function following cardiopulmonary bypass in patients with normal preoperative creatinine. Anaesthesia. 2008;63(6):576–82.

113. Smith MN, Best D, Sheppard SV, Smith DC. The effect of mannitol on renal function after cardiopulmonary bypass in patients with established renal dysfunction. Anaesthesia. 2008;63(7):701–4.

114. Fiaccadori E, Lombardi M, Leonardi S, Rotelli CF, Tortorella G, Borghetti A. Prevalence and clinical outcome associated with preexisting malnutrition in acute renal failure: a prospective cohort study. J Am Soc Nephrol. 1999;10(3):581–93.

115. Ho KM, Sheridan DJ. Meta-analysis of frusemide to prevent or treat acute renal failure. BMJ. 2006;333(7565):420.

116. Kellum J, Decker J. Use of dopamine in acute renal failure: a meta-analysis. Crit Care Med. 2001;29(8):6.

117. Friedrich J, Adhikari N, Herridge M, Beyene J. Meta-analysis: low-dose dopamine increases urine output but does not prevent renal dysfunction or death. Ann Intern Med. 2005;142(7):15.

118. Bove T, Zangrillo A, Guarracino F, Alvaro G, Persi B, Maglioni E, et al. Effect of fenoldopam on use of renal replacement therapy among patients with acute kidney injury after cardiac surgery: a randomized clinical trial. JAMA. 2014;312(21):2244–53.

119. Landoni G, Biondi-Zoccai GG, Marino G, Bove T, Fochi O, Maj G, et al. Fenoldopam reduces the need for renal replacement therapy and in-hospital death in cardiovascular surgery: a meta-analysis. J Cardiothorac Vasc Anesth. 2008;22(1):27–33.

120. Cogliati AA, Vellutini R, Nardini A, Urovi S, Hamdan M, Landoni G, et al. Fenoldopam infusion for renal protection in high-risk cardiac surgery patients: a randomized clinical study. J Cardiothorac Vasc Anesth. 2007;21(6):847–50.

121. Swaminathan M, Stafford-Smith M, Chertow GM, Warnock DG, Paragamian V, Brenner RM, et al. Allogeneic mesenchymal stem cells for treatment of AKI after cardiac surgery. J Am Soc Nephrol. 2017;29(1):260–67.

122. Meersch M, Schmidt C, Hoffmeier A, Van Aken H, Wempe C, Gerss J, et al. Prevention of cardiac surgery-associated AKI by implementing the KDIGO guidelines in high risk patients identified by biomarkers: the PrevAKI randomized controlled trial. Intensive Care Med. 2017;43(11):1551–61.

123. Bouchard J, Soroko SB, Chertow GM, Himmelfarb J, Ikizler TA, Paganini EP, et al. Fluid accumulation, survival and recovery of kidney function in critically ill patients with acute kidney injury. Kidney Int. 2009;76(4):422–7.

124. Gaudry S, Hajage D, Schortgen F, Martin-Lefevre L, Pons B, Boulet E, et al. Initiation strategies for renal-replacement therapy in the intensive care unit. N Engl J Med. 2016;375(2):122–33.

125. Zarbock A, Kellum JA, Schmidt C, Van Aken H, Wempe C, Pavenstadt H, et al. Effect of early vs delayed initiation of renal replacement therapy on mortality in critically ill patients with acute kidney injury: the ELAIN randomized clinical trial. JAMA. 2016;315(20):2190–9.

126. Meersch M, Kullmar M, Schmidt C, Gerss J, Weinhage T, Margraf A, et al. Long-term clinical outcomes after early initiation of RRT in critically ill patients with AKI. J Am Soc Nephrol. 2017;29(3):1011–9.

127. Bhatt GC, Das RR. Early versus late initiation of renal replacement therapy in patients with acute kidney injury-a systematic review & meta-analysis of randomized controlled trials. BMC Nephrol. 2017;18(1):78.

128. Schneider AG, Bellomo R, Bagshaw SM, Glassford NJ, Lo S, Jun M, et al. Choice of renal replacement therapy modality and dialysis dependence after acute kidney injury: a systematic review and meta-analysis. Intensive Care Med. 2013;39(6):987–97.

129. Bellomo R, Baldwin I, Fealy N. Prolonged intermittent renal replacement therapy in the intensive care unit. Crit Care Resusc. 2002;4(4):281–90.

130. Zhang L, Yang J, Eastwood GM, Zhu G, Tanaka A, Bellomo R. Extended daily dialysis versus continuous renal replacement therapy for acute kidney injury: a meta-analysis. Am J Kidney Dis. 2015;66(2):322–30.

131. Schiffl H, Lang SM, Fischer R. Daily hemodialysis and the outcome of acute renal failure. N Engl J Med. 2002;346(5):305–10.

132. Network VNARFT, Palevsky PM, Zhang JH, O'Connor TZ, Chertow GM, Crowley ST, et al. Intensity of renal support in critically ill patients with acute kidney injury. N Engl J Med. 2008;359(1):7–20.

133. Combes A, Brechot N, Amour J, Cozic N, Lebreton G, Guidon C, et al. Early high-volume hemofiltration versus standard care for post-cardiac surgery shock. The HEROICS study. Am J Respir Crit Care Med. 2015;192(10):1179–90.

134. Liu C, Mao Z, Kang H, Hu J, Zhou F. Regional citrate versus heparin anticoagulation for continuous renal replacement therapy in critically ill patients: a meta-analysis with trial sequential analysis of randomized controlled trials. Crit Care (Lond). 2016;20(1):144.

135. Lim W, Cook DJ, Crowther MA. Safety and efficacy of low molecular weight heparins for hemodialysis in patients with end-stage renal failure: a meta-analysis of randomized trials. J Am Soc Nephrol. 2004;15(12):3192–206.

136. Lasocki S, Piednoir P, Ajzenberg N, Geffroy A, Benbara A, Montravers P. Anti-PF4/heparin antibodies associated with repeated hemofiltration-filter clotting: a retrospective study. Crit Care (Lond). 2008;12(3):R84.

137. Swaminathan M, Hudson CC, Phillips-Bute BG, Patel UD, Mathew JP, Newman MF, et al. Impact of early renal recovery on survival after cardiac surgery-associated acute kidney injury. Ann Thorac Surg. 2010;89(4):1098–104.

138. Thongprayoon C, Cheungpasitporn W, Srivali N, Kittanamongkolchai W, Sakhuja A, Greason KL, et al. The association between renal recovery after acute kidney injury and long-term mortality after transcatheter aortic valve replacement. PLoS One. 2017;12(8):e0183350.

139. Forni LG, Darmon M, Ostermann M, Oudemans-van Straaten HM, Pettila V, Prowle JR, et al. Renal recovery after acute kidney injury. Intensive Care Med. 2017;43(6):855–66.

140. Venkatachalam MA, Weinberg JM, Kriz W, Bidani AK. Failed tubule recovery, AKI-CKD transition, and kidney disease progression. J Am Soc Nephrol. 2015;26(8):1765–76.

141. Brown JR, Parikh CR, Ross CS, Kramer RS, Magnus PC, Chaisson K, et al. Impact of perioperative acute kidney injury as a severity index for thirty-day readmission after cardiac surgery. Ann Thorac Surg. 2014;97(1):111–7.

142. Pickering JW, James MT, Palmer SC. Acute kidney injury and prognosis after cardiopulmonary bypass: a meta-analysis of cohort studies. Am J Kidney Dis. 2015;65(2):283–93.

143. Xu JR, Zhu JM, Jiang J, Ding XQ, Fang Y, Shen B, et al. Risk factors for long-term mortality and progressive chronic kidney disease associated with acute kidney injury after cardiac surgery. Medicine. 2015;94(45):e2025.

144. Brochard L, Abroug F, Brenner M, Broccard AF, Danner RL, Ferrer M, et al. An official ATS/ERS/ESICM/SCCM/SRLF statement: prevention and management of acute renal failure in the ICU patient: an international consensus conference in intensive care medicine. Am J Respir Crit Care Med. 2010;181(10):1128–55.

Neurologic Complications After Cardiac Surgery: Stroke, Delirium, Postoperative Cognitive Dysfunction, and Peripheral Neuropathy

Janet Martin and Davy C. H. Cheng

Main Messages

1. Neurologic complications including stroke, delirium, and seizures are associated with a longer hospital stay, a higher risk of discharge to long-term care facilities, and a higher risk of mortality in the short-term and longer-term.
2. Prevention and management strategies are required to minimize the risk of long-term neurologic dysfunction related to stroke, cognitive dysfunction, delirium, and peripheral neuropathy.
3. Most strokes that occur in the setting of cardiac surgery occur within 24–48 h, and intraoperative versus postoperative strokes have differing likely aetiologies and prognoses.
4. Valvular repairs (especially mitral valve intervention) and combined CABG and valve procedures have higher risk of stroke than CABG alone.
5. Prior cerebrovascular disease and atherosclerotic disease affecting the aorta or coronary arteries are important risk factors for perioperative stroke.
6. Management of ischemic stroke for cardiac surgical patients is similar to that in other settings, except tissue plasminogen activators are contraindicated after cardiac surgery due to risk of serious bleeding.
7. Delirium is relatively common postoperative complication, with multiple possible aetiologies and risk factors. Postoperative delirium is a risk factor for long-term neurocognitive dysfunction, especially if delirium is persistent after surgery, it is likely multifactorial. A minority of patients will have persistent neurocognitive dysfunction. Evaluation in these patients focuses on excluding a cerebrovascular

J. Martin (✉)
Centre for Medical Evidence, Decision Integrity and Clinical Impact (MEDICI), Schulich School of Medicine & Dentistry, Western University, London, ON, Canada

Department of Anesthesia & Perioperative Medicine, Schulich School of Medicine and Dentistry, Western University, London, ON, Canada

Department of Epidemiology & Biostatistics, Schulich School of Medicine & Dentistry, Western University, London, ON, Canada
e-mail: jmarti83@uwo.ca

D. C. H. Cheng
Centre for Medical Evidence, Decision Integrity and Clinical Impact (MEDICI), Schulich School of Medicine & Dentistry, Western University, London, ON, Canada

Department of Anesthesia & Perioperative Medicine, Schulich School of Medicine and Dentistry, Western University, London, ON, Canada

event and reversible toxic and metabolic conditions.

8. Peripheral nerve complications of cardiac surgery are less common (brachial plexopathy related motor-sensory deficits in upper extremities; intercostal neuropathy with localized pain or sensory deficits) or rare (phrenic neuropathy with prolonged ventilator dependence), and usually transient.

Introduction

Neurologic complications including delirium, acute confusion, and stroke remain one of the most feared complications after cardiac surgery. Neurologic complications may be associated with longer hospital stay, higher risk of discharge to long-term care facilities, and higher risk of multiple morbidities and death during the index hospital stay and after discharge [1].

This chapter will discuss neurologic complications in the post-cardiac surgical population across the following categories: Stroke, Delirium and other Neuropsychiatric Encephalopathies, Peripheral Neuropathies.

Stroke

Incidence The incidence of clinically apparent stroke after cardiac surgery depends on patient characteristics and type of procedure. The incidence of stroke is most commonly reported to be between 1.5 and 2.5% for patients undergoing closed-chamber cardiac procedures, based largely on observational studies [2]. A 2019 meta-analysis of stroke after cardiac surgery in randomized trials and prospective observational studies reported an overall rate of 2.08% [3]. The heterogeneity of stroke rates post-CABG of 1–5% reported across other studies can be largely explained by differences in procedure type, and

patient baseline risk [3, 4]. Epidemiologic studies suggest that the age-adjusted risk of perioperative stroke has likely decreased over the past few decades [5].

Timing Most clinically-relevant strokes in cardiac surgery patients occur within the first 2 days postoperatively, and of these, 30–50% occur intraoperatively, and 50–70% occur postoperatively [3, 5, 6]. While neuroimaging studies suggest a high incidence of silent cerebral ischemia after cardiac surgery, the clinical relevance of these surrogate markers of neurologic injury remain unknown, and consequently prevention of clinically-relevant stroke and neurologic complications remains the focus [2, 7].

Risk Factors A number of patient-related and procedure-related risk factors for perioperative stroke have been associated with increased risk of stroke. These should be further considered from the perspective of whether they are modifiable or non-modifiable risks (Table 55.1).

A number of risk scores have been developed to facilitate individual risk estimation for serious neurologic complications and death [8, 9]. While

Table 55.1 Risk factors for stroke

Patient-related risk factors	Procedure-related risk factors
Advanced age	Open chamber procedures (valve surgery)
Aortic atheroma	
Severe carotid stenosis	Combined procedures
Prior stroke or TIA	Prolonged CPB
Perioperative atrial fibrillation	Aortic instrumentation
	Increased temperature
Recent myocardial infarction or unstable angina	Emergency surgery
	Hemodynamic instability during CPB
Hypertension	Procedure related hypotension
Left ventricular dysfunction	Procedure-related arrhythmias
Low cardiac output syndrome	
Peripheral artery disease	
Female sex	
Diabetes	
Renal failure	

CPB cardiopulmonary bypass, *TIA* transient ischemic attack

these risk models vary in predictive validity, at the very least, their use may facilitate shared decision-making and informed consent on whether to undertake cardiac surgery in patients with known risk factors for stroke.

Etiology for Early Versus Delayed Stroke

It is important to distinguish between early onset stroke (during surgery or within 24 h of surgery) versus delayed stroke (>24 h after surgery). Since different mechanisms are thought to predominate, different approaches to preventing and managing stroke are proposed for early versus delayed stroke.

Intraoperative Stroke

The most likely modifiable factors for intraoperative stroke include cerebral hypoperfusion and athero-embolization.

Cerebral perfusion: to avoid cerebral hypoperfusion, blood pressure and cardiac output should be appropriately managed.

- While mean arterial pressures (MAP) between 50 and 70 mmHg are commonly recommended targets during CPB; however, recent evidence from randomized trials and observational research suggests that a higher MAP (80–100 mmHg) may decrease neurologic and cardiac complications [10, 11]. Larger clinical trials are required to provide definitive conclusions regarding the best MAP targets, within patient subgroups, and across different types of cardiac surgery.
- Embolization: Three major types of emboli pose a risk during cardiac surgery: thrombo-emboli, atheroemboli, and air emboli. Atheromatous debris may embolize from diseased aorta during clamping and unclamping of the ascending aorta, construction of proximal anastomoses in the ascending aorta, during excision of calcified valves, or during turbulent high-velocity blood flow from the aortic cannula within a diseased aorta. Gaseous emboli enter the arterial circulation

via open cardiac chambers, vascular cannulation sites, or arterial anastomoses. While the clinical relevance of small gaseous emboli remains contested, the risk associated with larger emboli is clearly related to immediate risk of stroke [12].

Efforts to reduce intraoperative stroke include minimizing aortic manipulation, reduction or eliminating cardiopulmonary bypass, and preoperative CT scan of the ascending aorta, duplex scanning of carotid arteries and epi-aortic ultrasound to inform morphologic risk [6].

Postoperative Stroke

Stroke that develops after cardiac surgery, but within the first 24 h, is most likely related to cardiogenic embolism related to atrial arrhythmias or other underlying heart disease. Key approaches to preventing postoperative stroke may include pharmacologic and nonpharmacologic AF prophylaxis (beta-blockers, magnesium, amiodarone, atrial pacing, posterior pericardiotomy), anticoagulation for prevention and treatment of clot formation, and elimination of left atrial appendage (ongoing randomized trials).

Preoperative use of the CHA_2DS_2-VASC score, or other consideration of risk factors, has been proposed to stratify risk for postoperative stroke, and may support preoperative discussions for shared decision-making regarding benefit-risk trade-offs associated with undergoing surgery [8].

Evidence for treatment of stroke in the post-cardiac surgical patient remains scarce. The following list suggests common approaches to management of post-cardiac surgery stroke, based on indirect evidence from stroke management in non-surgical patients, combined with current experience in the cardiac surgical setting:

- Management of inciting factors, such as atrial fibrillation, hypoxemia, hypoperfusion, intramural thrombus is key.
- Hypoxia, hyperoxia, hypotension, hypertension, hypoglycemia, hyperglycemia, and fever should be avoided

- Antiplatelet therapy with aspirin, clopidogrel or ticagrelor have been shown to improve outcomes in acute stroke and may also improve clinical outcomes related to graft patency in post-CABG patients, but with a small increased risk of bleeding [13].
- Pharmacologic thrombolytics, such as TPA and rPA, are contraindicated in patients with stroke after cardiac surgery due to risk of serious bleeding.
- Other mechanical reperfusion techniques may be considered for stroke in post-cardiac stroke on a case-by-case basis depending on patient stability and availability within the effective window of time.
- Supplemental oxygen should be reserved only for patients with hypoxia. Target SaO_2 levels should be between 92 and 96% [14]. Higher levels of SaO_2 (>96%) may be harmful, and routine supplemental oxygen in the absence of hypoxia is discouraged [14].
- In general, in patients not eligible for thrombolysis, blood pressure lowering is not recommended for acute ischemic stroke management, unless the patient has SBP > 220 mmHg or DBP > 120 mmHg diastolic, or perhaps slightly lower if the patient is at very high risk for myocardial infarction, dissection, or heart failure. Hypotension should be avoided, and if it occurs, should be treated with judicious fluid management, supine position, and if necessary, apply judicious use of vasopressors such as low dose phenylephrine.
- Fever has also been associated with worse outcomes in the acute stroke setting; antipyretics are generally recommended to manage fever in patients after stroke if temperature is elevated.
- Statin therapy is recommended for secondary prevention of cardiac and cerebrovascular events in post-cardiac surgical patients, and is especially important for those with a stroke history [13].
- Hyperbaric oxygen remains an investigational treatment for air emboli.

Intracranial Hemorrhage

Primary intracranial hemorrhage (ICH) is rare after cardiac surgery and is most commonly associated with complications of ischemic stroke, or surgery in the presence of anticoagulants that were not discontinued with sufficient duration before surgery. Importantly, endocarditis may be a risk factor for ICH, and may warrant delayed surgery until antibiotic therapy has reduced the risk, if hemodynamics allow.

Mortality After Stroke

Perioperative stroke is associated with lower short-term and long-term survival rates post-cardiac surgery. Operative mortality in patients experiencing stroke during or after cardiac surgery is approximately 29% for early stroke, and 18% for delayed stroke, compared with 2.4% for patients without stroke, according to a pooled analysis of clinical trials and prospective studies of cardiac surgery [3]. At mean follow-up of 8.25 years, the incident rate for late mortality was about 12% for early and 9% for delayed stroke, compared with 3.4% in patients without stroke. This corresponds to three- to fourfold increased risk of death in patients experiencing perioperative stroke versus those without stroke [3]. Stroke also places patients at risk for functional deficits, dependence, and prolonged rehabilitation needs.

Delirium

Delirium is an acute brain dysfunction characterised by disturbances in attention, awareness and cognition not explained by a pre-existing neurocognitive disorder. Delirium may present clinically as hypoactive (decreased alertness, motor activity, anhedonia) or hyperactive (agitated, combative). Early onset of delirium during the immediate postanesthetic period is referred to as 'emergence delirium'. Postoperative delirium may occur anytime after emergence up to 5 days postoperatively [15].

Delirium after cardiac surgery has been reported in 3–50% of patients postoperatively (depending on definitions and diagnostic instruments used), and 25% at 6 months to 1 year postoperatively [16–18]. However, it is important to note that pre-surgical cognitive impairment is present in about 20% of patients presenting for cardiac surgery [16]. Risk factors may include frailty, advanced age, malnutrition, pre-existing dementia, pre-existing cerebrovascular disease, prior stroke, alcohol use disorders, and sensory impairment. The pathophysiology of delirium post-CABG remains poorly defined and is an area of active research.

Studies indicate that postoperative delirium, particularly in elderly patients, is associated with poor outcomes, including increased risk of long-term cognitive dysfunction and functional decline and increased risk of death compared to patients who do not experience postoperative delirium. Delirium that is persistent after cardiac surgery is associated with greater risk for longer-term neurocognitive dysfunction and mortality [15, 19, 20].

Detecting and managing delirium remains a challenge, since it may be difficult to differentiate delirium from neurologic dysfunction related other conditions including stroke, transient ischemic attack, renal dysfunction, hepatic failure, and (less commonly) thyroid abnormalities.

Early detection of postoperative delirium is essential to ensure removal of triggering factors, and to guide treatment. All patients should be screened for agitation during emergence, typically using the Richmond Agitation-Sedation Scale (RASS) (Table 55.2) [21].

Table 55.2 Richmond Agitation-Sedation Scale to assess sedation depths

Score	Term	Description
+4	Combative	Overtly combative or violent; immediate danger to staff
+3	Very agitative	Pulls on or removes tube(s) or catheter(s) or has aggressive behavior toward staff
+2	Agitated	Frequent nonpurposeful movement or patient–ventilator dyssynchrony
+1	Restless	Anxious or apprehensive but movements not aggressive or vigorous
0	Alert and calm	
-1	Drowsy	Not fully alert, but has sustained (more than 10 s) awakening, with eye contact, to voice
−2	Light sedation	Briefly (less than 10 s) awakens with eye contact to voice
−3	Moderate sedation	Any movement (but no eye contact) to voice
−4	Deep sedation	No response to voice, but any movement to physical stimulation
−5	Unarousable	No response to voice or physical stimulation

Procedure

1. Observe patient. Is patient alert and calm (score 0)?
   Does patient have behavior that is consistent with restlessness or agitation (score +1 to +4 using the criteria listed above, under description)?
2. If patient is not alert, in a loud speaking voice state patient's name and direct patient to open eyes and look at speaker. Repeat once if necessary. Can prompt patient to continue looking at speaker.
   Patient has eye opening and eye contact, which is sustained for more than 10 s (score -1).
   Patient has eye opening and eye contact, but this is not sustained for 10 s (score -2).
   Patient has any movement in response to voice, excluding eye contact (score -3).
3. If patient does not respond to voice, physically stimulate patient by shaking shoulder and then rubbing sternum if there is no response to shaking shoulder.
   Patient has any movement to physical stimulation (score -4).
   Patient has no response to voice or physical stimulation (score -5).

Cite
Sessler, C. N., Gosnell, M. S., Grap, M. J., Brophy, G. M., O'Neal, P. V., Keane, K. A., Tesoro, E. P., & Elswick, R. K. (2002). The Richmond Agitation-Sedation Scale: validity and reliability in adult intensive care unit patients. *American Journal of Respiratory and Critical Care Medicine*, 166(10), 1338–1344

For the postoperative recovery setting, a number of delirium assessment tools have been assessed and validated. The Confusion Assessment Methods for the ICU (CAM-ICU) tool is more appropriate for detecting delirium in intubated patients (Fig. 55.1), while other tools are more appropriate for detecting delirium in non-intubated patients, such as the 3-Minute Diagnostic Interview for Confusion Assessment Method [3D-CAM], Confusion Assessment Method [CAM], and the Nursing Delirium Screening Scale (Nu-DESC) [15]. Delirium assessment tools are available for download at icudelirium.org and for non-ICU delirium assessment tools, see hospitalelderlifeprogram.org/delirium-instruments.

Delirium may present as a fluctuating course, and tools may have varied sensitivity and specificity depending on the timing of use, training of administrators using the tool, and due to inherent components of the tool itself. Performance of the tools in terms of predictive value requires additional study before one tool can be definitively promoted over others [15, 18].

Prevention and Treatment of Postoperative Delirium

While the etiology of delirium remains unknown, a number of factors have been postulated, including microemboli which may travel to the brain after aortic manipulation. Gas emboli from open chamber cardiac valve procedures has also been postulated as an important mechanism. Many patients have detectable microemboli on diffusion-weighted MRI; however, the relationship between microemboli and delirium or postoperative cognitive dysfunction remains tenuous, and related interventions to reduce microemboli

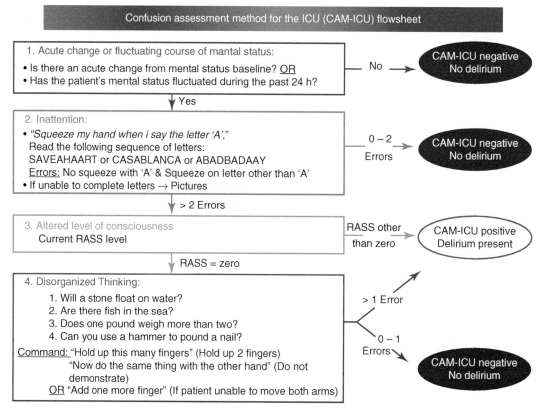

Fig. 55.1 Confusion assessment method for the ICU. Copyright 2002 © 2002, E. Wesley Ely, MD, MPH and Vanderbilt University, all rights reserved. Used with permission. Available at icudelirium.org

have not been definitively found to improve neurocognitive outcomes [18].

Dysregulation of oxygen delivery and utilization, and dysregulation of cerebral blood flow have also been an area of significant research. However, definitive conclusions about approaches to maintain target MAP or oxygen delivery remain in preliminary stages, again without definitive evidence to guide specific recommendations.

Research on whether off-pump instead of conventional on-pump bypass surgery reduces risk of delirium and postoperative cognitive dysfunction has been contradictory. While initial randomized trials suggested a protective effect of avoiding cardiopulmonary bypass, more recently, larger randomized trials and updated meta-analyses suggest that there may not be a relevant difference between off- and on-pump bypass surgery with respect to cognitive dysfunction [18].

Evidence generally supports temperature management (or, at least prevention of hyperthermia), and glucose homeostasis, preventing hypoxia and hyperoxia, and preventing hypertension or hypotension. Future evidence should focus on better defining specific optimal targets for temperature, glucose, cerebral oxygenation, and MAP [18].

Prevention of Delirium: Unmodifiable Versus Modifiable Risk Factors

A number of predisposing factors, many of which are non-modifiable, are associated with postoperative delirium, including increasing age, multiple comorbidities, alcohol abuse, drug abuse, frailty, pre-existing dementia or cognitive impairment, prior stroke, depression, renal dysfunction, diabetes, and heart disease [19].

Management of post-surgical delirium requires correcting any potentially reversible causes, identifying and managing triggers such as adequate pain control and patient orientation. The highest priority should be to prevent delirium through minimizing patient exposure to modifiable risk factors, including appropriate management of pain, blood pressure, glycemic control, sleep disruption, and environmental stress and stimulation perioperatively. In addition, since benzodiazepines and narcotics are associated with delirium, minimizing exposure to excessive doses while appropriately managing perioperative pain and anxiety remains a key part of delirium prevention. Table 55.3 outlines potentially modifiable perioperative risk factors for delirium in the cardiac surgical setting.

Table 55.3 Modifiable perioperative risk factors for postoperative delirium

Risk factor	Preoperative	Intraoperative	Postoperative
Alcohol abuse	✓		
Benzodiazepines	✓	✓	✓
Other high risk medications[a]	✓	✓	✓
Ketamine		✓	✓
Excessive opioids	✓	✓	✓
Hypoxemia (or hyperoxia)	✓	✓	✓
Arterial pressure management, MAP		✓	
Blood pressure control	✓	✓	✓
Cardiopulmonary bypass duration		✓	
Duration of procedure		✓	
Glycemic control	✓	✓	✓
Hemodilution		✓	
Sedation		✓	✓
Pain	✓	✓	✓
Sleep disruption	✓		✓
Sleep apnea	✓		✓
Temperature management		✓	✓
Infection	✓	✓	✓
Multi-component delirium management behavioural/environmental program[b]	✓	✓	✓

[a]See also Table 55.5
[b]See also Fig. 55.5

Prevention of Delirium: Processed EEG

A number of randomized trials have assessed whether anesthesia using processed EEG monitoring (i.e., BIS-guided monitoring) compared with usual care (monitoring anesthesia using clinical parameters and/or end-title anesthetic gas concentration-guided monitoring, ETAG) reduces total anesthetic exposure and postoperative delirium. Results of the randomized trials have been mixed, with some suggesting significant reduction and others showing no difference in postoperative delirium (Fig. 55.2) [23]. Reasons for the differences in outcomes may be related to differences in the comparison group (clinical vs. ETAG-guided anesthesia), differences in type of anesthesia and BIS targets, and differences in the way the BIS information was used. Furthermore, most of the studies were in the setting of non-cardiac surgery.

Given these challenges, the precise role of BIS for reducing risk of delirium remains unclear. On the other hand, BIS-guided anesthesia may reduce the risk of intraoperative awareness, and may be recommended for this purpose. Given the uncertainty in the evidence, and the heterogeneity in clinical trials in how BIS information was used, type of anesthesia provided, and what it was compared with, formal guideline statements for the use of BIS remain somewhat disparate [15, 19].

POQI 2020 guidelines for preventing postoperative delirium state: "There is insufficient evidence to recommend using processed EEG monitoring in older high-risk surgical patients undergoing general anesthesia to reduce the risk of postoperative delirium." [19] In their supporting meta-analysis of existing randomized trials of EEG monitoring versus usual care (Fig. 55.2), they found an overall incidence of delirium of 22.5%, and overall a reduction of incidence of delirium with EEG guided anesthesia versus usual care [RR 0.78, 95% CI 0.61–0.98; $I^2 = 70$], though the heterogeneity across trials was large (Fig. 55.2), and results were less definitive after excluding trials of sedation alone [RR 0.80, 95%CI 0.60–1.07; $I^2 = 78\%$] [19, 23].

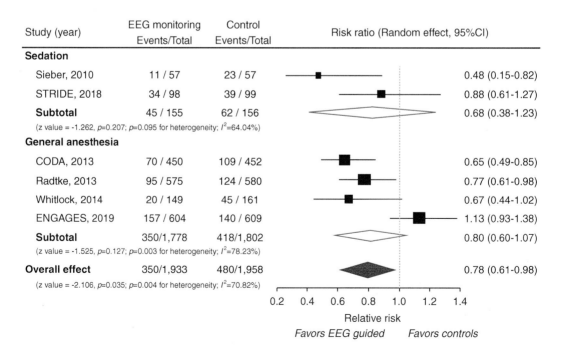

Fig. 55.2 Postoperative delirium for EEG-guided anesthesia versus usual care: meta-analysis of randomized trial (© Copyright permission from Perioperative Quality Initiative (POQI)) [23]

Prevention of Delirium: Dexmedetomidine and Other Anesthetics and Analgesic Regimens

In cardiac surgery settings, recent meta-analyses of randomized trials of perioperative use of dexmedetomidine for anesthesia and sedation have shown a significant reduction in the risk of postoperative delirium [OR 0.35, 95% CI 0.24–0.51], with similar reduction in cardiac surgery and non-cardiac surgery patients (Fig. 55.3) [24]. In these studies, dexmedetomidine was primarily used for postoperative recovery room and ICU sedation.

Studies of perioperative use of benzodiazepines have suggested increased risk of postoperative delirium [25]. Studies of other pharmacologic agents for the prevention of postoperative delirium have generally failed to show a significant reduction in the incidence of delirium, including studies of inhaled versus intravenous anesthesia (Table 55.4) [25, 26]. However, existing evidence remains under-powered, and suffers from lack of standardized definition of delirium [17, 25, 26].

Treatment of Delirium

Recent randomized trials and meta-analyses of pharmacologic agents (olanzapine, haloperidol, clonidine, dexmedetomidine, midazolam) have not shown clinically-relevant impact for the treatment of delirium in the postcardiac surgical population and in the general critical care setting [19, 27, 28].

Given the disappointing performance of drugs for the treatment of delirium, a number of non-pharmacologic interventions have been addressed in recent clinical trials, including sleep hygiene, ear plugs, music therapy, patient reorientation therapy, and multi-faceted programs with dedicated pathways, team-based approaches to promote co-management across the continuum of care, and devoted personnel to prevent, monitor, and manage delirium [15, 17, 19].

Pain management, sleep management, and control of excessive environmental stimuli are important modifiable risk factors for delirium, which are often forgotten in the busy recovery unit and ICU setting. Evidence to support specific approaches to non-pharmacologic interventions

is emerging, including sleep hygiene (dark room, regular sleep pattern to support circadian rhythm, ear plugs), music, patient orientation strategies, family/visitor education and support, and specific ventilation modes to improve sleep quality (Fig. 55.5). A number of ongoing studies will better inform which strategies work best for optimizing patient environment to reduce the risk of delirium [29–31].

Additionally, there are many drugs that predispose patients to delirium or cognitive dysfunction. These include benzodiazepines, antipsychotics, and centrally acting antihistamines, phenothiazines, antiemetics, and anticholinergics. Table 55.5 outlines some medications which have been associated with delirium or acute confusional states, especially in elderly patients.

Recent Guidelines and Recommendations

A number of anesthesia societies and working groups have published guidelines for the prevention and management of postoperative delirium [15, 19]. Most of these address mixed surgery settings, and are not specific to cardiac surgery. Readers are encouraged to use these guidelines with caution, given that the evidence for a number of the recommendations remains tenuous, and may change over time as evidence evolves. Of note, given the remaining debate (largely due to differences in interpretation of the existing evidence and its strengths and weaknesses), some of the statements contradict each other, especially with respect to the role of processed EEG to prevent delirium (not recommended for routine use to prevent delirium in ASA/POQI guidelines; but recommended for routine use by ESA Guidelines) [15, 19]. Another area of contradiction between guidelines relates to the role of antipsychotics for treatment of delirium postoperatively. Most guidelines do not recommend use of antipsychotics for treatment of postoperative delirium, due to lack of benefit shown in randomized trials, whereas ESA guidelines recommend antipsychotic use for treatment of delirium based on preliminary evi-

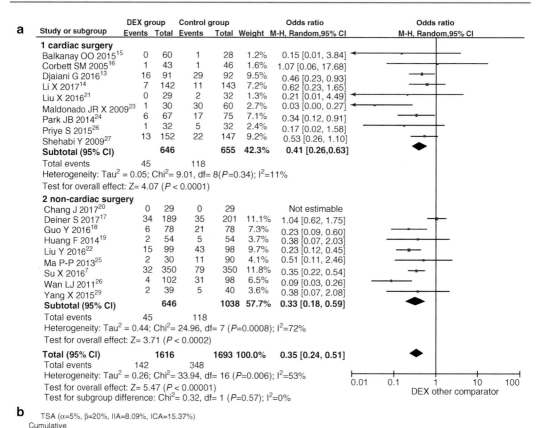

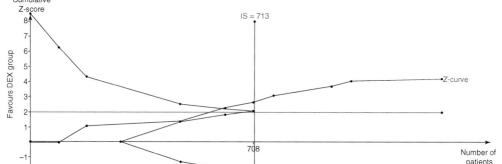

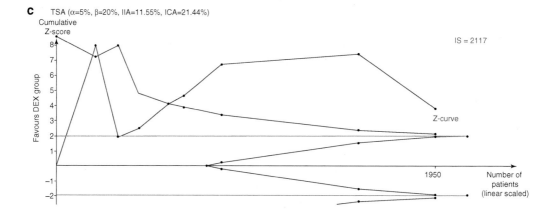

Table 55.4 Perioperative anesthetics for prevention of postoperative delirium on general anesthesia: results from a network meta-analysis

Treatments	OR	95% CI	I^2 statistic
Dexmedetomidine vs. Placebo	0.45	0.33–0.60	16%
Dexmedetomidine vs. Midazolam	0.11	0.04–0.28	27%
Dexmedetomidine vs. Propofol	0.23	0.07–0.73	45%
Propofol vs. Sevoflurane	0.54	0.15–1.99	73%
Propofol vs. Desoflurane	0.96	0.46–1.99	0%
Ketamine vs. Placebo	0.57	0.10–3.47	65%
Propofol vs.Midazolam	1	0.36–2.75	NE
Sevoflurane vs. Placebo	6.89	0.35–134.75	NE
Propofol vs. Placebo	NE	NE	NE
Sevoflurane vs. Desoflurane	NE	NE	NE

Test of consistency: $\text{Chi}^2(5) = 5.51$, $P = 0.357$
The direct evidence from pairwise meta-analysis (OR = odd ratio), 95% CI = (95% confidence interval) and information about heterogeneity (I^2 and heterogeneity variance τ^2). *NE* No estimate
Reprinted from the Journal of Clinical Anesthesia, 5;59, Cui Y, Li G, Cao R, Luan L, Kla KM, The effect of perioperative anesthetics for prevention of postoperative delirium on general anesthesia: A network meta-analysis, 89–98, Copyright 2019, with permission from Elsevier [25]

Table 55.5 Drugs that may predispose to delirium and acute confusional states [22]

Medication or class of medications	Examples	Rationale for avoiding
First-generation antihistamines	Diphenhydramine	Central anticholinergic effects
Phenothiazine-type antiemetics	Prochlorperazine, promethazine	Central anticholinergic effects
Antispasmodics/anticholinergics	Atropine, scopolamine	Central anticholinergic effects
Antipsychotics (first and second generation)	Haloperidol Droperidol	Risk of cognitive impairment, delirium, neuroleptic malignant syndrome, tardive dyskinesia
Benzodiazepines	Midazolam, diazepam	Risk of cognitive impairment, delirium
Corticosteroids	Hydrocortisone, methylprednisolone	Risk of cognitive impairment, delirium, psychosis
H2-receptor antagonists	Ranitidine Cimetidine	Risk of confusion, delirium
Metoclopramide		Extrapyramidal effects
Meperidine		Neurotoxic effects
Skeletal muscle relaxants	Cyclobenzaprine	Anticholinergic effects

dence. These contradictions highlight the challenges in distilling a heterogenous evidence base into definitive statements to guide practice, and which need to be revisited as evidence evolves.

The Perioperative Quality Initiative (POQI) 6 Workgroup recently released updated guidelines for postoperative delirium prevention. They recommend a comprehensive strategy that addresses preoperative, intraoperative and postoperative considerations (Fig. 55.4), using a multicomponent approach (Fig. 55.5). Their recommendations are summarized in Table 55.6.

Fig. 55.3 Postoperative delirium incidence for dexmedetomidine versus control. (**a**) Forest plot of postoperative delirium in randomized trials of dexmedetomidine versus control, subgrouped by cardiac surgery and non-cardiac surgery. (**b, c**) outline trial sequential analyses to demonstrate sufficiency of information size for cardiac surgery studies and non-cardiac-surgery studies. Creative commons open archive https://bjanaesthesia.org/article/S0007-0912(18)30447-1/fulltext

Fig. 55.4 A systematic
approach to prevent
delirium across the
continuum of pre, intra,
and postoperative care
[19]. (© Copyright
permission from
Perioperative Quality
Initiative (POQI))

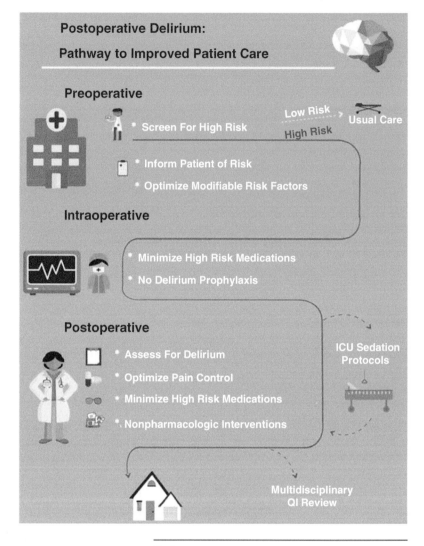

Fig. 55.4 A systematic approach to prevent delirium across the continuum of pre, intra, and postoperative care [19]. (© Copyright permission from Perioperative Quality Initiative (POQI))

Frailty and Delirium

Studies suggest that cardiac surgical patients who meet the definition of frailty before surgery are more likely to experience delirium after surgery. The precise role of routine screening for preoperative frailty and associated risk of dementia is an area of ongoing investigation for cardiac surgical patients, and future evidence should inform which frailty screening approaches and interventions in the preoperative setting are effective for mitigating risk of postoperative delirium [32]. Patients with frailty should be warned of their added risk for postoperative delirium.

Seizures

The reported incidence of seizures after cardiac surgery ranges from 0.01 to 3.5%, with diverse aetiologies including metabolic disturbance (hypoglycemia, hyponatremia), stroke, intracranial hemorrhage, drug toxicity (lidocaine, procainamide), and use of higher doses of the tranexamic acid [33].

Seizures may present as generalized tonic-clonic, focal seizures, or mixed. Seizures after cardiac surgery are associated with a twofold increase in length of stay and a 2.5-fold increase in risk of death, and potentially increased risk of delirium and longer-term risk of reduced quality

Fig. 55.5 Multicomponent interventions to decrease postoperative delirium [19]. (© Copyright permission from Perioperative Quality Initiative (POQI))

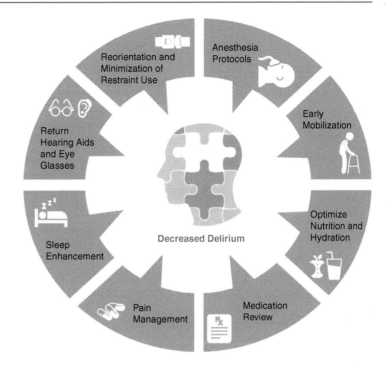

Table 55.6 Consensus statements and recommendations from POQI. (Reprinted with permission from: Hughes CG, Boncyk CS, Culley DJ, Fleisher LA, Leung JM, McDonagh DL, Gan TJ, McEvoy MD, Miller TE; Perioperative Quality Initiative (POQI) 6 Workgroup. American Society for Enhanced Recovery and Perioperative Quality Initiative Joint Consensus Statement on Postoperative Delirium Prevention. Anesth Analg. 2020 Jan 31) [19]

Statement	Strength[a]	LOE[b]
We recommend hospitals and health systems develop processes to reduce the incidence and consequences of postoperative delirium through an iterative multidisciplinary quality improvement process	Strong	D
We recommend that health care providers identify surgical patients at high risk for postoperative delirium	Strong	C
We recommend that surgical patients identified as high risk for postoperative delirium be informed of their risk	Weak	D
We recommend hospital and health systems develop a process to assess for postoperative delirium in older high-risk patients	Strong	C
We recommend the use of multicomponent nonpharmacologic interventions for the prevention of postoperative delirium in older high-risk patients	Strong	B
We recommend minimization of medications known to be associated with an increased risk of postoperative delirium in older high-risk surgical patients	Strong	C
There is insufficient evidence to recommend using processed EEG monitoring in older high-risk surgical patients undergoing general anesthesia to reduce the risk of postoperative delirium[c]	N/A	N/A
There is insufficient evidence to recommend specific anesthetic agents or doses to reduce the risk of postoperative delirium	N/A	N/A
There is insufficient evidence to recommend regional/neuraxial blockade as the primary anesthetic technique to reduce the risk of postoperative delirium	N/A	N/A
We recommend optimization of postoperative pain control to reduce the risk of postoperative delirium	Weak	C
There is insufficient evidence to recommend administration of prophylactic medications to reduce the risk of postoperative delirium	N/A	N/A
We recommend using ICU protocols that include sedation with dexmedetomidine to reduce the risk of postoperative delirium in patients requiring postoperative mechanical ventilation	Strong	B

EEG electroencephalogram, *GRADE* grading of recommendations assessment, development and evaluation, *ICU* intensive care unit, *LOE* level of evidence
[a]Strength of recommendation per GRADE process
[b]Level of evidence per GRADE process
[c]Additional evidence published after consensus conference which led to a change in recommendation statement

of life. Seizures are not always be easily recognized, and may be confused with shivering or non-seizure myoclonic movements. EEG should be considered for patients who remain unresponsive 24 h after surgery to detect non-convulsive seizure activity.

Avoidance of metabolic derangements and drug toxicity (i.e., lidocaine, procainamide) are key to reducing seizure risk. Importantly, tranexamic acid is often unrecognized as an avoidable risk factor for seizure, particularly for doses exceeding 80 mg/kg. The incidence of seizures associated with tranexamic acid use ranges from 0.5 to 7.3%, with higher risk associated with higher doses, older age, high disease severity score, renal dysfunction, and prior neurologic dysfunction. Most cases occur in open-chamber procedures (i.e., aortic valve repair/replacement). Seizures associated with tranexamic acid usually develop at 5–8 h after surgery, during weaning from sedation. Anesthetics including isoflurane and propofol, and sedation agents including benzodiazepines, are protective against seizures. Consequently, if seizures develop after tranexamic acid, they are most likely to occur around 5–8 h after surgery, when anesthetic effects have worn off, and during weaning from sedation. Importantly, neuromuscular blocking agents may mask the presence of seizures.

When considering the use of tranexamic acid to reduce bleeding risk, the expected magnitude of benefit in reduction of postoperative bleeding with tranexamic acid at moderate doses should be weighed against the corresponding risk of postoperative seizures [34].

Postoperative Cognitive Dysfunction (POCD)

Short term and long-term post-operative cognitive dysfunction (POCD) remains a concern after cardiac surgery. POCD typically includes disturbances in memory, attention, or executive function, varying in severity from subtle to clinically overt. Reports of POCD suggest an incidence ranging from 3 to 79% in the early weeks after CABG, and decreasing over the first year. This heterogeneity is likely related to issues of timing and method of measurement, as well as differences in patient baseline risk and procedural risk. Risk factors for POCD include hypertension, advanced age, previous stroke, carotid disease, pulmonary disease. For the majority of patients, early neurocognitive deficits typically resolve within 3–12 months after surgery; though longer-term deficits may persist, especially for more severe POCD [35]. POCD is associated with increased length of stay and increased in-hospital mortality risk.

Modifiable risk factors include intraoperative hypotension, intraoperative hypertension, prolonged hypoxemia, and postoperative hyperthermia. Avoiding these may mitigate the risk of POCD. Earlier reports suggesting that off-pump bypass surgery reduces the risk of on-pump bypass surgery have not been borne out in subsequent larger trials, and both on- and off-pump surgery are considered similar risk for POCD.

POCD that is reported after cardiac surgery may not be entirely attributable to nor unique to cardiac surgery. Risk of POCD should be interpreted in light of other studies comparing POCD post-cardiac surgery compared with other non-surgical adults with similar comorbid conditions. A study comparing neurocognitive function at 3–12 months in post-CABG patients versus those with coronary disease but no surgery, and versus those with no coronary disease, indicated that cognitive test performance of CABG patients did not differ from non-surgical patients with heart disease [35]. However, there is evidence to suggest the incidence of neurocognitive dysfunction after cardiac surgery is greater than after other types of surgery such as peripheral vascular surgery, suggesting that factors unique to cardiac surgery may be partly to blame [36–38]. Microemboli generated during heart and aorta manipulation (cannulation, suctioning) and inflammatory factors released during cardiac surgery have been proposed as potential risks for neurocognitive damage. Nevertheless, these remain controversial since studies have shown inconsistent correlation between microemboli detected on magnetic resonance imaging or biochemical analysis of inflammatory mediator concentrations intra- and postoperatively [18].

Late POCD

Whether CABG patients are at higher risk for long-term cognitive decline remains controversial. While a number of earlier non-comparative studies of CABG patients have suggested increasing incidence of cognitive decline with time, the more relevant question is whether these patients show accelerated decline relative to an age-matched and comorbidity-matched population. In more recent longitudinal studies comparing post-CABG patients with a control group of patients with coronary disease who did not undergo surgery, the rates of cognitive decline are similar, suggesting that late cognitive decline is not attributable to surgery, but rather to other factors such as underlying cerebrovascular disease or vascular dementia, or even heart disease itself (low cardiac output, heart failure) [39].

Peripheral Neuropathy

Peripheral neuropathy, presenting as numbness, pain, weakness, reduced reflexes, and/or reduced coordination in an upper extremity, has been reported in 2–15% of patients undergoing cardiac surgery. Neuropathy-associated pain indicates peripheral injury. Hemi-neuropathy, hemiparesis, and cranial nerve involvement indicates central injury (Table 55.7) [40, 41].

Typically, peripheral neuropathies improve or resolve within 1-month post-cardiac surgery. Consequently, conservative therapy for peripheral neuropathy including physical therapy for the purpose of continued use of the affected muscles to improve strength and flexibility while the neuropraxia resolves during the first weeks and months post-surgery. Less commonly, a pro-

Table 55.7 Neuropathy post-cardiac surgery [40, 41]

Symptom	Presumed etiology
Upper extremity (relatively common)	
Sensory disturbances in the fourth and fifth fingers	• Lower (medial) brachial plexus injury • Ulnar nerve injury at the elbow
Weakness in extensor indicis, abductor pollicis brevis	• Plexopathy involving lower cervical nerve roots (without ulnar nerve involvement)
Evaluation in these patients focuses on excluding a cerebrovascular event and reversible toxic and metabolic conditions	• Potentially related to brachial plexus traction, brachial plexus compression between the clavicle and rib during sternal retraction, or nerve injury during internal mammary artery dissection
Intercostal nerve (relatively common)	
Sternum or left anterolateral chest wall numbness, dysesthesia, burning	• Intercostal nerve injury may occur during ITA harvesting, usually resolving within 4 months. *Persistent in some patients at 1–2 years post-surgery*
Lower extremity (uncommon)	
Weakness or numbness in the leg, impaired gait	• Femoral nerve damage, potentially due to IABP insertion, local trauma, pseudoaneurysm, vascular occlusion or emboli
Diaphragm (rare)	
Diaphragm dysfunction (uncommon, especially given advances in surgical technique, reductions in use of iced slush for cooling)	• Phrenic nerve injury, potentially due to heart cooling methods (iced slush) or other direct injury. *May lead to prolonged dependence on ventilation* • Unilateral phrenic nerve injury typically occurs on same side as IMA graft *Bilateral phrenic nerve injury may require prolonged ventilatory support* **Note: Diaphragm dysfunction is not always due to phrenic nerve injury**
Dyskinesia (uncommon)	
Dyskinetic movement disorder (post-pump chorea)	• Uncertain regarding incidence; rare cases have been reported in children with congenital heart disease after cardiac surgery, and in a series of adults undergoing pulmonary endarterectomy with CABG. Symptoms occurred 1–3 days postoperatively and generally resolved within weeks to months

longed recovery period may be required if there is axonal involvement. Intercostal nerve injury may Clinically-apparent phrenic nerve injury may require 1–2 years for recovery. Typically, if neuropathic symptoms are not improving within 3–4 weeks post-surgery, nerve conduction studies and electromyography should be considered to guide further management.

Summary

Neurologic complications of cardiac surgery remain a common problem after cardiac surgery, and require prevention and management strategies to minimize the risk of long-term neurologic dysfunction related to stroke, cognitive dysfunction, delirium, and peripheral neuropathy.

- Most strokes that occur in the setting of cardiac surgery occur within 24–48 h.
- Intraoperative versus postoperative strokes have differing likely aetiologies and prognoses.
- Valvular repairs (especially mitral valve intervention) and combined CABG and valve procedures have higher risk of stroke than CABG alone.
- Mechanisms of intraoperative and postoperative ischemic stroke include cerebral hypoperfusion, artery-to-artery embolism, and cardiogenic embolism.
- Prior cerebrovascular disease and atherosclerotic disease affecting the aorta or coronary arteries are important risk factors for perioperative stroke.
- Management of ischemic stroke for cardiac surgical patients is similar to that in other settings, except tissue plasminogen activators are contraindicated after cardiac surgery due to risk of serious bleeding.
- Delirium is a relatively common postoperative complication, with multiple possible aetiologies and risk factors. Postoperative delirium is a risk factor for long-term neurocognitive dysfunction, especially if delirium is persistent after surgery, and it is likely multifactorial. A minority of patients will have persistent neurocognitive dysfunction. Evaluation in these patients focuses on excluding a cerebrovascular event and reversible toxic and metabolic conditions.
- Peripheral nerve complications of cardiac surgery are less common (brachial plexopathy related motor-sensory deficits in upper extremities; intercostal neuropathy with localized pain or sensory deficits) or rare (phrenic neuropathy with prolonged ventilator dependence), and usually transient.

References

1. Selnes OA, Gottesman RF, Grega MA, et al. Cognitive and neurologic outcomes after coronary-artery bypass surgery. N Engl J Med. 2012;366:250–7.
2. Messe SR, Acker MA, Se K, et al. Stroke after aortic valve surgery: results from a prospective cohort. Circulation. 2014;129:2253–61.
3. Gaudino M, Rahouma M, Di Muro M, Yanagawa B, Abouarab A, Demetres M, et al. Early versus delayed stroke after cardiac surgery: a systematic review and meta-analysis. J Am Heart Assoc. 2019;8:e012447.
4. McDonagh DL, Berger M, Mathew JP, Graffagnino C, Milano CA, Newman MF. Neurological complications of cardiac surgery. Lancet Neurol. 2014;13:490–502.
5. Tarakji KG, Sabik JF, Bhudia SK, Batizy LH, Blackstone EH. Temporal onset, risk factors, and outcomes associated with stroke after coronary artery bypass grafting. JAMA. 2011;305(4):381–90.
6. Hogue CW Jr, Murphy SF, Schechtman KB, Dávila-Román VG. Risk factors for early or delayed stroke after cardiac surgery. Circulation. 1999;100(6):642–7.
7. Patel N, Minhas JS, Chung EM. Risk factors associated with cognitive decline after cardiac surgery: a systematic review. Cardiovasc Psychiatry Neurol. 2015;12:370612. https://doi.org/10.1155/2015/370612.
8. Hu WS, Lin CL. Postoperative ischemic stroke and death prediction with CHA(2)DS(2)-VASc score in patients having coronary artery bypass grafting surgery: a nationwide cohort study. Int J Cardiol. 2017;241:120–3.
9. McKhann GM, Grega MA, Borowicz LM Jr, et al. Stroke and encephalopathy after cardiac surgery: an update. Stroke. 2006;37:562–71.
10. Sun LY, Chung AM, Farkouh ME, et al. Defining an intraoperative hypotension threshold in association with stroke in cardiac surgery. Anesthesiology. 2018;129:440–7.
11. Gold JP, Charlson ME, Williams-Russo P, Szatrowski TP, Peterson JC, Pirraglia PA, Hartman GS, Yao FS, Hollenberg JP, Barbut D, Hayes JG, Thomas SJ, Purcell MH, Mattis S, Gorkin L, Post M, Krieger KH, Isom OW. Improvement of outcomes after coronary artery bypass: a randomized trial comparing intra-

operative high versus low mean arterial pressure. J Thorac Cardiovasc Surg. 1995;110:1302–11. discussion 1311-4

12. Abu-Omar Y, Balacumaraswami L, Pigott DW, Matthews PM, Taggart DP. Solid and gaseous cerebral microembolization during off-pump, on-pump, and open cardiac surgery procedures. J Thorac Cardiovasc Surg. 2004;127(6):1759–65.

13. Hillis LD, Smith PK, Anderson JL, Bittl JA, Bridges CR, Byrne JG, Cigarroa JE, DiSesa VJ, Hiratzka LF, Hutter AM, Jessen ME, Keeley EC, Lahey SJ, Lange RA, London MJ, Mack MJ, Patel MR, Puskas JD, Sabik JF, Selnes O, Shahian DM, Trost JC, Winniford MD. ACCF/AHA guideline for coronary artery bypass graft surgery: a report of the American College of Cardiology Foundation/American Heart Association Task Force on Practice Guidelines. Developed in collaboration with the American Association for Thoracic Surgery, Society of Cardiovascular anesthesiologists, and Society of Thoracic Surgeons. J Am Coll Cardiol. 2011;58(24):e123–210.

14. Siemieniuk RAC, Chu DK, Kim LH, Güell-Rous MR, Alhazzani W, Soccal PM, Karanicolas PJ, Farhoumand PD, Siemieniuk JLK, Satia I, Irusen EM, Refaat MM, Mikita JS, Smith M, Cohen DN, Vandvik PO, Agoritsas T, Lytvyn L, Guyatt GH. Oxygen therapy for acutely ill medical patients: a clinical practice guideline. BMJ. 2018;363:k4169. https://doi.org/10.1136/bmj.k4169.

15. Aldecoa C, Bettelli G, Bilotta F, Sanders RD, Audisio R, Borozdina A, Cherubini A, Jones C, Kehlet H, MacLullich A, Radtke F, Riese F, Slooter AJ, Veyckemans F, Kramer S, Neuner B, Weiss B, Spies CD. European Society of Anaesthesiology evidence-based and consensus-based guideline on postoperative delirium. Eur J Anaesthesiol. 2017;34(4):192–214. https://doi.org/10.1097/EJA.0000000000000594.

16. Greaves D, Psaltis PJ, Ross TJ, Davis D, Smith AE, Boord MS, Keage HAD. Cognitive outcomes following coronary artery bypass grafting: a systematic review and meta-analysis of 91,829 patients. Int J Cardiol. 2019;289:43–9.

17. Vlisides P, Avidan M. Recent advances in preventing and managing postoperative delirium. F1000 Res. 2019;8(F1000 Facult Rev):607. Last updated May 2019.

18. Berger M, Terrando N, Smith SK, Browndyke JN, Newman MF, Mathew JP. Neurocognitive function after cardiac surgery: from phenotypes to mechanisms. Anesthesiology. 2018;129:829–51.

19. Hughes CG, Boncyk CS, Culley DJ, Fleisher LA, Leung JM, McDonagh DL, Gan TJ, McEvoy MD, Miller TE, for the Perioperative Quality Initiative (POQI) 6 Workgroup. American Society for enhanced recovery and perioperative quality initiative joint consensus statement on postoperative delirium prevention. Anesth Analog. 2020.

20. Saczynski JS, Marcantonio ER, Quach L, Fong TG, Gross A, Inouye SK, Jones RN. Cognitive trajectories after postoperative delirium. N Engl J Med. 2012;367(1):30–9. https://doi.org/10.1056/NEJMoa1112923.

21. Sessler CN, Gosnell MS, Grap MJ, Brophy GM, O'Neal PV, Keane KA, Tesoro EP, Elswick RK. The Richmond agitation–sedation scale. Am J Respir Crit Care Med. 2002;166(10):1338–44. https://doi.org/10.1164/rccm.2107138.

22. American Geriatrics Society. Beers criteria update expert panel. American Geriatrics Society 2015 updated beers criteria for potentially inappropriate medication use. J Am Geriatr Soc. 2015;63(11):2227–46.

23. Chan MRV, Hedrick TL, Egan TD, Garcia PS, Koch S, Purdon P, Ramsay MA, Miller TE, McEvoy MD, Gan TJ, on behalf of the Perioperative Quality Initiative POQI) 6 Workgroup. American Society for enhanced recovery and perioperative quality initiative joint consensus statement on the role of neuromonitoring in perioperative outcomes: electroencephalography. Anesth Analg. 2019. https://doi.org/10.1213/ANE.0000000000004502

24. Duan X, Coburn M, Rossant R, Sanders RD, Waesberghe JV, Kowark A. Efficacy of perioperative dexmedetomidine on postoperative delirium: systematic review and meta-analysis with trial sequential analysis of randomized controlled trials. Br J Anaesth. 2018;121:384–97.

25. Cui Y, et al. The effect of perioperative anesthetics for prevention of postoperative delirium on general anesthesia a network meta-analysis. J Clin Anesth. 2019;59:89–98.

26. Miller D, et al. Intravenous versus inhalational maintenance of anaesthesia for postoperative cognitive outcomes in elderly people undergoing noncardiac surgery. Cochrane Database Syst Rev. 2019;8:CD012317.

27. Burry L, Hutton B, Williamson DR, Mehta S, Adhikari NK, Cheng W, Ely EW, Egerod I, Fergusson DA, Rose L. Pharmacological interventions for the treatment of delirium in critically ill adults. Cochrane Database Syst Rev. 2019;9:CD011749.

28. Leigh V, Stern C, Elliott R, Tufanaru C. Effectiveness and harms of pharmacological interventions for the treatment of delirium in adults in intensive care units after cardiac surgery: a systematic review. JBI Database System Rev Implement Rep. 2019. https://doi.org/10.11124/JBISRIR-D-18-00010.

29. Lu Y, Li YW, Want L, Lydic R, Baghdoyan HA, Shi XY, Zhang H. Promoting sleep and circadian health may prevent postoperative delirium: a systematic review and meta-analysis of randomized clinical trials. Sleep Med Rev. 2019;48:101207.

30. Lewis SR, et al. Melatonin for the promotion of sleep in adults in the intensive care unit. Cochrane Database Syst Rev. 2019;5:CD012455.

31. Hu RF, et al. Non-pharmacologic interventions for sleep promotion in the intensive care unit. Cochrane Database Syst Rev. 2015;10:CD008808.

32. Kim DH, Kim CA, Placide S, Lipsitz LA, Marcantonio ER. Preoperative frailty assessment and outcomes at

6 months or later in older adults undergoing cardiac surgical procedures: a systematic review. Ann Intern Med. 2016;65:650–60.

33. Pataraia E, Jung R, Aull-Watschinger S, Skhirtladze-Dworschak K, Dworschak M. J Cardiothorac Vasc Anesth. 2018;32:2323–9.

34. Lecker I, Wang DS, Whissell PD, Avramescu S, Mazer CD, Orser BA. Tranexamic acid-associated seizures: causes and treatment. Ann Neurol. 2016;79(1):18–26.

35. McKhann GM, Grega MA, Borowicz LM Jr, Bailey MM, Barry SJ, Zeger SL, Baumgartner WA, Selnes OA. Is there cognitive decline 1 year after CABG? Comparison with surgical and nonsurgical controls. Neurology. 2005;65(7):991–9.

36. Clark RE, Brillman J, Davis DA, Lovell MR, Price TR, Magovern GJ. Microemboli during coronary artery bypass grafting. Genesis and effect on outcome. J Thorac Cardiovasc Surg. 1995;109(2):249.

37. Hogan AM, Shipolini A, Brown MM, Hurley R, Cormack F. Fixing hearts and protecting minds: a review of the multiple, interacting factors influencing cognitive function after coronary artery bypass graft surgery. Circulation. 2013;128(2):162–71.

38. Shaw PJ, Bates D, Cartlidge NE, French JM, Heaviside D, Julian DG, Shaw DA. Neurologic and neuropsychological morbidity following major surgery: comparison of coronary artery bypass and peripheral vascular surgery. Stroke. 1987;18(4):700–7.

39. Eggermont LH, de Boer K, Muller M, et al. Cardiac disease and cognitive impairment: a systematic review. Heart. 2012;98:1334–40.

40. UptoDate. Neurologic complications of cardiac surgery. Available at www.uptodate.com.

41. Welch MB, Brummett CM, Welch TD, et al. Perioperative peripheral nerve injuries: a retrospective study of 380,680 cases during a 10-year period at a single institution. Anesthesiology. 2009;111:490–7.

Difficult Weaning from Mechanical Ventilation and Tracheotomy Care

56

Martin Lenihan and George Djaiani

Main Messages

1. Prolonged mechanical ventilation occurs in up to 22% of cardiac surgical patients.
2. Weaning can be classified into three groups based on difficulty and duration: simple weaning, difficult weaning, and prolonged weaning.
3. Discontinuation of mechanical ventilation is largely based on clinical assessment.
4. Confounders in failure to wean patients include ventilator associated pneumonia; cardiac failure; delirium, ICU acquired weakness; nutritional status; acute respiratory distress syndrome; and transfusion-related lung injury.

M. Lenihan
Toronto General Hospital, University Health Network, University of Toronto, Toronto, ON, Canada

G. Djaiani (✉)
Department of Anesthesia and Pain Management, Toronto General Hospital, University Health Network, University of Toronto, Toronto, ON, Canada
e-mail: George.Djaiani@uhn.ca

Fast track cardiac anesthesia pathways are governing the current anesthesia/surgery field [1]. Pulmonary dysfunction is one of the leading causes of postoperative morbidity in the cardiac surgical population [2]. Postoperative pulmonary complications occur in 10–25% of patients, including 2.5% with severe pulmonary dysfunction, as well as acute respiratory distress syndrome (ARDS) [3], and tracheostomy care in 1.36% of patients [4]. Prolonged mechanical ventilation continues to be a significant part of overall postoperative morbidity with a reported incidence of up to 22% of patients [5]. The Society of Thoracic Surgeons promotes the extubation within 6 h of cardiac surgery as a quality of care benchmark [6].

Different thresholds have been chosen to delineate prolonged mechanical ventilation. Sharma et al. [5] suggested a 48-h time interval, given that the risk profile of cardiac surgical patients has changed over the past decades, with a higher proportion of elderly patients having multiple comorbidities and more complex cardiac surgical procedures. The prevalence of prolonged mechanical ventilation was 6.2% in the derivation, and 7.3% in the external validation cohorts, respectively [5]. Major predictors and risk factors for prolonged mechanical ventilation include:

- Previous cardiac surgery
- Cardiogenic shock
- Prolonged cardiopulmonary bypass time
- Chronic renal failure
- Peripheral vascular disease
- Atherosclerosis
- Diabetes mellitus
- Hypertension
- Presence of an intra-aortic balloon pump

Anesthesia, sternotomy, surgical manipulations, and use of cardiopulmonary bypass (CPB) create transient deleterious effects on pulmonary function. These are related to diminished functional residual capacity causing arterial hypoxemia due to ventilation/perfusion mismatch; reduced lung compliance increasing work of breathing and oxygen consumption; transient 50–75% reduction in vital capacity; as well as development of atelectasis and increased intravascular lung water. Changes in spirometric measurements and respiratory muscle strength may last up to 8 weeks after cardiac surgery.

Unplanned Re-intubation

In a recent study of approximately 18,500 cardiac surgeries, Beverly et al. [7] reported that the rate of unplanned postoperative re-intubations after cardiac surgery was 4% during the entire admission, with almost one-half of re-intubations occurring on day 5 or beyond postoperatively. The risk of re-intubation and failure to wean from mechanical ventilation is associated with increased age, frailty, chronic kidney disease, pre-existing pulmonary dysfunction, infections, previous cardiac surgery, and congestive heart failure.

Weaning from Mechanical Ventilation

Weaning is the gradual liberation from mechanical ventilation to spontaneous breathing allowing the patient to breathe without mechanical support [8]. According to its difficulty and duration,

weaning can be classified into three groups: simple weaning (successful extubation on the first attempt), difficult weaning (failure on the first attempt and requiring up to three Spontaneous Breathing Trials (SBT), or as long as 7 days from the first SBT) and prolonged weaning (failure on at least three attempts or >7 days from the first SBT) [8].

Clinical assessment is the basis in the decision to wean off ventilation [9]. Commonly, factors in the decision making include the verification of patients' hemodynamic stability, mental and cognitive status, ability to cough, resolution of the primary cause, nutritional status and specific parameters of lung mechanics [10]. To objectively assist the decision-making process in weaning off ventilation, several weaning predictors have been used [11]. Previous studies suggested that weaning protocols should be implemented in order to provide daily assessments of weaning-ready patients [12].

The rapid shallow breathing index and SBT are the most commonly used indices to assess readiness for extubation, however not all SBTs are performed with the same ventilator settings. There is a spectrum of positive end-expiratory pressure (PEEP) and pressure support levels used while performing SBTs; from T-piece trials (performed without PEEP or supplemental ventilator support) to "minimal ventilator settings" (often with a PEEP of 5 cm H_2O and pressure support ≤ 8 cm H_2O) [13].

In 2014, a Cochrane review examined the success of minimal support SBT versus T-piece trials in unselected patients undergoing mechanical ventilation [12]. The authors deemed that the quality of evidence was low due to "limitations in the design of the studies and imprecision in the effect estimates," and concluded that there was no difference with two approaches in success of weaning, need for re-intubation, or intensive care unit (ICU) mortality. Another Cochrane review noted that automated systems reduced prolonged mechanical ventilation and requirements for tracheostomy [14]. However, they are not in routine use in the vast majority of institutions.

The American Thoracic Society and the American College of Chest Physicians collaboratively developed evidence-based recommendations that addressed common clinical questions in the general ICU cohort of patients, which can be extrapolated to cardiac ICU. The goal of the guidelines is to assist clinicians in safely and effectively weaning patients from mechanical ventilation and to improve outcomes in critically ill patients. However, guidelines cannot take into account every possible individual clinical circumstance [15]. The following are a summary of recommendations:

Strength of Recommendation: conditional = 1; strong = 2

Certainty/Quality of Evidence: moderate = 3; low = 4; very low = 5

- For acutely hospitalized patients ventilated more than 24 h, we suggest that the initial spontaneous breathing trial (SBT) be conducted with inspiratory pressure augmentation (5–8 cm H_2O) rather than without (T-piece or CPAP) = 1.3
- For acutely hospitalized patients ventilated for more than 24 h, we suggest protocols attempting to minimize sedation = 1.4
- For patients at high risk for extubation failure who have been receiving mechanical ventilation for more than 24 h and who have passed am SBT, we recommend extubation to preventive non-invasive ventilation (NIV) = 2.3
- For acutely hospitalized patients who have been mechanically ventilated for >24 h, we suggest protocolized rehabilitation directed toward early mobilization = 1.4
- We suggest managing acutely hospitalized patients who have been mechanically ventilated for >24 h with a ventilator liberation protocol = 1.4
- We suggest performing a cuff leak test (CLT) in mechanically ventilated adults who meet extubation criteria and are deemed at high risk for postextubation stridor (PES) = 1.5
- For adults who have failed a CLT but are otherwise ready for extubation, we suggest administering systemic steroids at least 4 h before extubation; a repeated CLT is not required = 1.3

Patients with impaired cardiac function may require higher thresholds for extubation. It is common to perform SBTs in patients with marginal cardiac function without any supplemental support to assess the patient's ability to tolerate fully unsupported breathing. T-piece trials in this patient population may reveal acute pulmonary edema, arrhythmias, or hemodynamic instability that were not evident during minimal support trials due to the favourable effects of PEEP and/or pressure support on preload, afterload, and work of breathing [13]. T-piece trials in patients with impaired cardiac function may unmask the need for further optimization of preload and afterload, both before and after extubation, in order to prevent re-intubation events [13]. Some patients remain difficult-to-wean even though their acute illness and factors contributing to failure to wean have been resolved. In such patients, a tracheostomy is frequently indicated.

Potential Confounders in Failure to Wean Patients from Mechanical Ventilation

Ventilator Associated Pneumonia

The clinical criteria for ventilator associated pneumonia (VAP) are commonly based on the guidelines from the Centers for Disease Control and Prevention [16]. It is defined as the presence of new and/or progressive pulmonary infiltrates on a chest radiograph, plus two or more of the following: fever or hypothermia, leukocytosis, purulent tracheobronchial secretions, or a reduction in PaO_2/FiO_2 (partial pressure of arterial oxygen/fraction of inspired oxygen) of 15% or more in the previous 48 h [17]. A recent meta-analysis identified that the prevalence of VAP was 6.4% of all patients, and 35.2% of patients who were on mechanical ventilation for more than 48 h [18]. Risk factors such as New York Heart Association cardiac function class IV, pulmonary hypertension, chronic obstructive pulmonary disease, peripheral vascular disease, renal disease, emergency surgery, intra-aortic balloon counter pulsation, CPB time, aortic cross-clamp time, mechanical ventilation time, re-intervention, and re-intubation were closely related to the incidence of VAP [18]. The management of VAP is detailed in the 2016 Clinical Practice Guidelines by the Infectious Diseases Society of America and the American Thoracic Society [16].

Cardiac Failure

Heart failure and fluid balance are important predictors of failure to wean from mechanical ventilation, and should be optimized prior to planned extubation [13]. Cabello et al. [19] identified that heart failure was a cause of 42% of failures of SBTs in a large cohort of medical ICU patients. Currently, routine bedside assessments of focal lung-ultrasound and left ventricular diastolic function are used to determine readiness for weaning from mechanical ventilation. The focal lung-ultrasound can identify the presence of B-lines (a measure of degree of interstitial edema, and extra-vascular lung water), that have high negative predictive value (86%) for predicting extubation failure [20]. A higher E/e' ratio (measurement of diastolic dysfunction) may also signify a weaning failure [21], although a high heterogeneity of diastolic dysfunction criteria and different clinical scenarios may limit definitive conclusions linking diastolic dysfunction with weaning failure. Elective initiation of non-invasive ventilation immediately following extubation has been shown to reduce the incidence of respiratory failure in patients at risk, including those with underlying cardiac failure [22].

Delirium

Delirium is an acute change in cognitive functioning, characterized by inattention and associated with alterations in awareness and fluctuation in arousal, disorganized thinking, or altered level of consciousness that preferentially affects older adult patients. In the acutely ill cardiac patient, the incidence of delirium has been reported as high as 73%, depending on the type and sensitivity of delirium assessment [23]. When compared

with propofol, dexmedetomidine sedation reduced incidence, delayed onset, and shortened duration of postoperative delirium in elderly patients after cardiac surgery with an absolute risk reduction of 14%, and a number needed to treat of 7.1 [24]. Reduced incidence of postoperative delirium and shorter length of mechanical ventilation after cardiac surgery was confirmed in a recent meta-analysis of randomized controlled trials [25].

Most current studies favour the use of dexmedetomidine for patients with fast-track protocols, especially during the early postoperative period. Dexmedetomidine modulates undesirable increased sympathetic activity, and as a sedative agent, it does not affect the time to extubation because of its minimal effects on respiratory drive [26]. Furthermore, daily sedation interruptions in critically ill adult patients requiring ventilatory support may result in reduced duration of mechanical ventilation [27].

ICU Acquired Weakness

Weakness, critical illness neuropathy and/or myopathy, and muscle atrophy are common in critically ill patients. ICU-acquired weakness is associated with longer durations of mechanical ventilation and hospitalization, along with greater functional impairment for survivors [28]. Current guidelines recommend that a clinical diagnosis of ICU-acquired weakness is made by bedside evaluation of the muscle strength with the use of the Medical Research Council sum score [29]. This score appoints a value between 0 (no contraction at all) and 5 (normal muscle strength) for each of 12 muscle groups, including shoulder abduction, elbow flexion, wrist extension, hip flexion, knee extension, and dorsiflexion of the ankle, all scored bilaterally. The sum score ranges between 0 and 60, and the diagnosis is confirmed with a total score less than 48 [29]. Furthermore, diaphragmatic atrophy can become apparent in as little as 48 h after commencing mechanical ventilation as the work of breathing is totally assumed by a ventilator [30]. Limited data exists to support the benefit from specific inspiratory muscle training leading to reduced mechanical ventilation time and improved weaning rate [31].

Nutritional Status

Respiratory muscles, like skeletal muscles, are negatively affected by starvation and the catabolic state that contributes to malnutrition. Malnutrition can result in increased fatigability, decreased inspiratory and expiratory muscle strength, decreased endurance, and depletion of diaphragmatic muscle mass. A decrease in respiratory function results in an increase in respiratory muscle work, with increased energy demands, which further exacerbate the malnourished state [32]. Institution of nutritional support early, using appropriate calorie mix of fat and carbohydrates to maintain a respiratory quotient less than 1.0, is adopted in many centers worldwide.

Acute Respiratory Distress Syndrome

ARDS is a life-threatening form of respiratory failure characterized by inflammatory pulmonary edema resulting in severe hypoxemia. The severity of ARDS is classified according to the degree of hypoxemia as mild, moderate, or severe [33]. The incidence of ARDS varies from 0.17 to 2.5% and mortality from 15 to 91.6% after cardiac surgery [34]. Independent predictors of ARDS include sepsis, high-risk cardiac surgery, high-risk aortic vascular surgery, emergency surgery, cirrhosis, admission location other than home, increased respiratory rate ($\geq$30 breaths/min), FiO_2 greater than 35%, and SpO_2 less than 95% [35]. Recent meta-analyses have shown that preemptive application of protective ventilation strategies in both high-risk ICU and surgery patient populations can reduce the incidence of ARDS [36, 37]. With the understanding that mechanical ventilation itself can cause and potentiate lung injury, research has focused on ventilatory strategies and adjunctive measures aimed at mitigating ventilator-induced lung injury (Table 56.1) [33].

Table 56.1 An Official American Thoracic Society/European Society of Intensive Care Medicine/Society of Critical Care Medicine Clinical Practice Guideline: Mechanical Ventilation in Adult Patients with Acute Respiratory Distress Syndrome

The recommendations for the following interventions for the treatment of ARDS are strong:
- Mechanical ventilation using lower tidal volumes (4–8 ml/kg predicted body weight) and lower inspiratory pressures (plateau pressure, 30 cm H_2O) (moderate confidence in effect estimates)
- Prone positioning for more than 12 h/day in severe ARDS (moderate confidence in effect estimates)

The recommendation against the following intervention for the treatment of ARDS is strong:
- Routine use of high-frequency oscillatory ventilation in patients with moderate or severe ARDS (high confidence in effect estimates)

The recommendation for the following interventions for the treatment of ARDS is conditional:

Higher positive end-expiratory pressure in patients with moderate or severe ARDS (moderate confidence in effect estimates)

Additional evidence is necessary to make a definitive recommendation for/against the use of extracorporeal membrane oxygenation in patients with severe ARDS

Recruitment maneuvers in patients with moderate or severe ARDS (low confidence in effect estimates)

Transfusion-Related Acute Lung Injury

Transfusion-related acute lung injury (TRALI) is the leading cause of transfusion-related mortality. TRALI is defined as the occurrence of hypoxia and bilateral pulmonary infiltrates within 6 h of a transfusion, usually presenting with tachypnea, cyanosis, dyspnea and fever [38]. Its prevalence among cardiac surgical patients has been estimated at 2.4% with mortality ranging from 5% to 25% [38], contributing significantly to overall adverse outcomes [39].

Tracheostomy

Potential advantages of tracheostomy over orotracheal intubation include greater patient comfort, reduced requirement or discontinuation of sedatives, improved patient communication, decreased risk of confusion, and improved mobility and hemodynamic stability with possibly fewer ventilator associated complications. Complications related to tracheostomy include bleeding, hypoxia, oesophageal injury, tracheal stenosis, tracheal granulomas and death.

In the TracMan study (multicentre trial from over 70 ICUs), a cohort of general ICU patients were randomized to early (within 4 days) or late (after 10 days) tracheostomy when predicted ventilation time was longer than 7 days [40]. There was no difference in early and late mortality between the two groups. Additionally, only 45% of patients assigned to the late tracheostomy group received it, as the rest of patients were successfully weaned from mechanical ventilation [40]. In cardiac surgical patients, Puentes et al. [4] demonstrated that early tracheostomy (<7 days) was not associated with increased risk of sternal wound infection or dehiscence after cardiac surgery. This study was supported by a recent systematic review and meta-analysis confirming that there was no difference in the incidence of superficial or deep sternal wound infections with respect to early or late tracheostomy, however, a difference was noted when comparing percutaneous with open tracheostomy, with a threefold increase in the open group (3% vs. 9%) [41]. A recent Cochrane review also identified that compared to open tracheostomy, percutaneous tracheostomy reduced the rate of wound infection/stomatitis, and the rate of unfavourable scarring [42]. Even though there is no clear evidence to support a policy of early tracheostomy in cardiac surgical patients, the percutaneous tracheostomy is associated with preferable outcomes.

Postoperative pulmonary complications continue to occur in a significant proportion of cardiac surgical patients leading to prolonged mechanical ventilation and longer ICU stay. Patients with impaired cardiac function may require a higher threshold for extubation.

Various recommendations and clinical guidelines exist, however, the decision of attempting discontinuation of mechanical ventilation is often based on the clinical assessment with repeated attempts of trials and errors. Current research aims to focus on preventative factors aiming to decrease the incidence of postoperative pulmonary complications. Future areas of interest include the potential use of lung protective ventilation during CPB with a focus on preventive measures to decrease postoperative pulmonary complications.

References

1. Cheng DC. Fast track cardiac surgery pathways: early extubation, process of care, and cost containment. Anesthesiology. 1998;88(6):1429–33.
2. Nearman H, Klick JC, Eisenberg P, Pesa N. Perioperative complications of cardiac surgery and postoperative care. Crit Care Clin. 2014;30(3):527–55.
3. Ubben JFH, Lance MD, Buhre WF, Schreiber JU. Clinical strategies to prevent pulmonary complications in cardiac surgery: an overview. J Cardiothorac Vasc Anesth. 2015;29(2):481–90.
4. Puentes W, Jerath A, Djaiani G, Cabrerizo Sanchez R, Wasowicz M. Early versus late tracheostomy in cardiovascular intensive care patients. Anaesthesiol Intensive Ther. 2016;48(2):89–94.
5. Sharma V, Rao V, Manlhiot C, Boruvka A, Fremes S, Wasowicz M. A derived and validated score to predict prolonged mechanical ventilation in patients undergoing cardiac surgery. J Thorac Cardiovasc Surg. 2017;153(1):108–15.
6. Goeddel LA, Hollander KN, Evans AS. Early extubation after cardiac surgery: a better predictor of outcome than metric of quality? J Cardiothorac Vasc Anesth. 2018;pii:S1053–0770(17)31025-X. https://doi.org/10.1053/j.jvca2017.12.037.
7. Beverly A, Brovman EY, Malapero RJ, Lekowski RW, Urman RD. Unplanned reintubation following cardiac surgery: incidence, timing, risk factors, and outcomes. J Cardiothorac Vasc Anesth. 2016;30(6):1523–9.
8. Boles JM, Bion J, Connors A, et al. Weaning from mechanical ventilation. Eur Respir J. 2007;29(5):1033–56.
9. McConville JF, Kress JP. Weaning patients from the ventilator. N Engl J Med. 2012;367(23):2233–9.
10. Penuelas O, Thille AW, Esteban A. Discontinuation of ventilatory support: new solutions to old dilemmas. Curr Opin Crit Care. 2015;21(1):74–81.
11. Magalhaes PAF, Camillo CA, Langer D, Andrade LB, Duarte M, Gosselink R. Weaning failure and respiratory muscle function: what has been done and what can be improved? Respir Med. 2018;134:54–61.
12. Ladeira MT, Vital FM, Andriolo RB, Andriolo BN, Atallah AN, Peccin MS. Pressure support versus T-tube for weaning from mechanical ventilation in adults. Cochrane Database Syst Rev. 2014(5):Cd006056.
13. Kuhn BT, Bradley LA, Dempsey TM, Puro AC, Adams JY. Management of mechanical ventilation in decompensated heart failure. J Cardiovasc Dev Dis. 2016;3(4). pii: E33. https://doi.org/10.3390/jcdd3040033.

14. Rose L, Schultz MJ, Cardwell CR, Jouvet P, McAuley DF, Blackwood B. Automated versus non-automated weaning for reducing the duration of mechanical ventilation for critically ill adults and children. Cochrane Database Syst Rev. 2014(6):Cd009235.

15. Schmidt GA, Girard TD, Kress JP, et al. Liberation from mechanical ventilation in critically ill adults: executive summary of an official American College of Chest Physicians/American Thoracic Society clinical practice guideline. Chest. 2017;151(1):160–5.

16. Kalil AC, Metersky ML, Klompas M, et al. Management of adults with hospital-acquired and ventilator-associated pneumonia: 2016 clinical practice guidelines by the Infectious Diseases Society of America and the American Thoracic Society. Clin Infect Dis. 2016;63(5):e61–e111.

17. Garner JS, Jarvis WR, Emori TG, Horan TC, Hughes JM. CDC definitions for nosocomial infections, 1988. Am J Infect Control. 1988;16(3):128–40.

18. He S, Chen B, Li W, et al. Ventilator-associated pneumonia after cardiac surgery: a meta-analysis and systematic review. J Thorac Cardiovasc Surg. 2014;148(6):3148–55.

19. Cabello B, Thille AW, Roche-Campo F, Brochard L, Gomez FJ, Mancebo J. Physiological comparison of three spontaneous breathing trials in difficult-to-wean patients. Intensive Care Med. 2010;36(7):1171–9.

20. Soummer A, Perbet S, Brisson H, et al. Ultrasound assessment of lung aeration loss during a successful weaning trial predicts postextubation distress. Crit Care Med. 2012;40(7):2064–72.

21. de Meirelles Almeida CA, Nedel WL, Morais VD, Boniatti MM, de Almeida-Filho OC. Diastolic dysfunction as a predictor of weaning failure: a systematic review and meta-analysis. J Crit Care. 2016;34:135–41.

22. Corredor C, Jaggar SI. Ventilator management in the cardiac intensive care unit. Cardiol Clin. 2013;31(4):619–36.

23. Arora RC, Djaiani G, Rudolph JL. Detection, prevention, and management of delirium in the critically ill cardiac patient and patients who undergo cardiac procedures. Can J Cardiol. 2017;33(1):80–7.

24. Djaiani G, Silverton N, Fedorko L, et al. Dexmedetomidine versus propofol sedation reduces delirium after cardiac surgery: a randomized controlled trial. Anesthesiology. 2016;124(2):362–8.

25. Liu X, Xie G, Zhang K, et al. Dexmedetomidine vs propofol sedation reduces delirium in patients after cardiac surgery: a meta-analysis with trial sequential analysis of randomized controlled trials. J Crit Care. 2017;38:190–6.

26. Liu H, Ji F, Peng K, Applegate RL 2nd, Fleming N. Sedation after cardiac surgery: is one drug better than another? Anesth Analg. 2017;124(4):1061–70.

27. Burry L, Rose L, McCullagh IJ, Fergusson DA, Ferguson ND, Mehta S. Daily sedation interruption versus no daily sedation interruption for critically ill adult patients requiring invasive mechanical ventilation. Cochrane Database Syst Rev. 2014(7):Cd009176.

28. Jolley SE, Bunnell AE, Hough CL. ICU-acquired weakness. Chest. 2016;150(5):1129–40.

29. Kress JP, Hall JB. ICU-acquired weakness and recovery from critical illness. N Engl J Med. 2014;370(17):1626–35.

30. Grosu HB, Lee YI, Lee J, Eden E, Eikermann M, Rose KM. Diaphragm muscle thinning in patients who are mechanically ventilated. Chest. 2012;142(6):1455–60.

31. Daniel Martin A, Smith BK, Gabrielli A. Mechanical ventilation, diaphragm weakness and weaning: a rehabilitation perspective. Respir Physiol Neurobiol. 2013;189(2):377–83.

32. Doley J, Mallampalli A, Sandberg M. Nutrition management for the patient requiring prolonged mechanical ventilation. Nutr Clin Pract. 2011;26(3):232–41.

33. Fan E, Del Sorbo L, Goligher EC, et al. An official American Thoracic Society/European Society of Intensive Care Medicine/Society of Critical Care Medicine Clinical Practice Guideline: mechanical ventilation in adult patients with acute respiratory distress syndrome. Am J Respir Crit Care Med. 2017;195(9):1253–63.

34. Kogan A, Preisman S, Levin S, Raanani E, Sternik L. Adult respiratory distress syndrome following cardiac surgery. J Card Surg. 2014;29(1):41–6.

35. Kor DJ, Lingineni RK, Gajic O, et al. Predicting risk of postoperative lung injury in high-risk surgical patients: a multicenter cohort study. Anesthesiology. 2014;120(5):1168–81.

36. Gu WJ, Wang F, Liu JC. Effect of lung-protective ventilation with lower tidal volumes on clinical outcomes among patients undergoing surgery: a meta-analysis of randomized controlled trials. Can Med Assoc J. 2015;187(3):E101–9.

37. Serpa Neto A, Simonis FD, Barbas CS, et al. Association between tidal volume size, duration of ventilation, and sedation needs in patients without acute respiratory distress syndrome: an individual patient data meta-analysis. Intensive Care Med. 2014;40(7):950–7.

38. Rong LQ, Di Franco A, Gaudino M. Acute respiratory distress syndrome after cardiac surgery. J Thorac Dis. 2016;8(10):E1177–e1186.

39. Vlaar AP, Hofstra JJ, Determann RM, et al. The incidence, risk factors, and outcome of transfusion-related acute lung injury in a cohort of cardiac surgery patients: a prospective nested case-control study. Blood. 2011;117(16):4218–25.

40. Young D, Harrison DA, Cuthbertson BH, Rowan K, TracMan Collaborators. Effect of early vs late tracheostomy placement on survival in patients receiving mechanical ventilation: the TracMan randomized trial. J Am Med Assoc. 2013;309(20):2121–9.

41. Toeg H, French D, Gilbert S, Rubens F. Incidence of sternal wound infection after tracheostomy in patients undergoing cardiac surgery: a systematic review and meta-analysis. J Thorac Cardiovasc Surg. 2017;153(6):1394–400;e1397.

42. Brass P, Hellmich M, Ladra A, Ladra J, Wrzosek A. Percutaneous techniques versus surgical techniques for tracheostomy. Cochrane Database Syst Rev. 2016;7:Cd008045.

Infection, Sternal Debridement and Muscle Flap

57

Amine Mazine, Stefan O. P. Hofer, and Terrence M. Yau

Main Messages
1. Deep sternal wound infection is a rare but serious complication of cardiac operations performed through a median sternotomy.
2. *Staphylococcus aureus* and *coagulase negative Staphylococci* are the pathogens most commonly encountered in deep sternal wound infections.
3. The diagnosis of deep sternal wound infection is essentially clinical, but computed tomography can help determine the precise location and extent of the infectious process.
4. Prophylactic use of sternal reinforcement techniques may decrease the risk of sternal dehiscence and deep sternal wound infection in high-risk patients.
5. When deep sternal wound infection does occur, intravenous antibiotics and surgical debridement are the mainstay of therapy.
6. Sternal re-closure can be performed immediately after debridement, or following an interval of open chest management. Sternal closure is achieved either primarily or with the use of soft-tissue flaps. Vacuum-assisted closure therapy may improve outcomes.

A. Mazine
Division of Cardiac Surgery, Department of Surgery, University of Toronto, Toronto, ON, Canada
e-mail: amine.mazine@mail.utoronto.ca

S. O. P. Hofer
Department of Surgery, Division of Plastic and Reconstructive Surgery, University of Toronto, Toronto, ON, Canada

University Health Network, Toronto, ON, Canada
e-mail: stefan.hofer@uhn.ca

T. M. Yau (✉)
Division of Cardiac Surgery, Department of Surgery, University of Toronto, Toronto, ON, Canada

Peter Munk Cardiac Centre, Division of Cardiovascular Surgery, Toronto General Hospital, University Health Network, Toronto, ON, Canada
e-mail: terry.yau@uhn.ca

Since its introduction by Milton in 1897 [1], the median sternotomy has been the most commonly used approach for cardiac surgery. While fairly uncommon, infectious complications of this type of incision pose a significant challenge for cardiac surgeons, and remain associated with significant morbidity and mortality in the current era. This chapter focuses on the surgical management of deep sternal wound infections (DSWI).

Definition and Classification

Sternal wound dehiscence—i.e. sternal wound breakdown *without* clinical or microbiological evidence of infection—must be distinguished from sternal wound infection, in which there is clinical or microbiological evidence of infection of the presternal tissue, with or without sternal osteomyelitis and with or without mediastinal sepsis [2]. Sternal wound infections are further divided into superficial sternal wound infections (SSWI)—wound infection that is confined to the subcutaneous tissue—and DSWI—wound infection associated with sternal osteomyelitis, with or without infection of the retrosternal space. It is this latter entity that forms the focus of the present chapter.

The American Centers for Disease Control and Prevention (CDC) define DSWI in adults as any infection meeting *at least one* of the following criteria [3]:

1. Identification of an organism from mediastinal tissue or fluid by a culture or non-culture based microbiologic testing method.
2. Evidence of mediastinitis seen during surgery or histopathologic examination.
3. Presence of at least one of the following symptoms: fever (>38.0 °C), chest pain, or sternal instability, *in combination* with either
   (a) purulent drainage from mediastinal area
   (b) mediastinal widening on imaging test

Incidence and Risk Factors

The incidence of DSWI ranges from 0.75 to 1.44% in large observational studies [4, 5]. There is a large body of evidence documenting risk factors associated with DSWI [4, 6]. These can be broadly classified into preoperative, intraoperative and postoperative variables (Table 57.1).

The etiology of DSWI is multifactorial, and any factor contributing to impaired wound healing, poor bone healing, or increased risk of surgical site infection may be relevant. The risk is compounded when multiple risk factors are present concomitantly.

Table 57.1 Risk factors for deep sternal wound infection following cardiac surgery

Preoperative	Obesity, diabetes mellitus, COPD, CHF, renal failure, peripheral vascular disease, tobacco use, poor dental hygiene, older age, immunosuppression, malnutrition, osteopenia
Intraoperative	Untimely administration of antibiotic prophylaxis, intraoperative hyperglycemia, BIMA harvest, redo surgery, urgent surgery, excessive use of bone wax and electrocautery, prolonged duration of surgery
Postoperative	Re-exploration for bleeding, prolonged intensive care unit stay, prolonged duration of mechanical ventilation, transfusion, chest compressions

BIMA bilateral internal mammary artery, *CHF* congestive heart failure, *COPD* chronic obstructive pulmonary disease

While there is a clear association between sternal dehiscence and DSWI, it is unclear whether the sternal dehiscence predisposes to DSWI, or whether DSWI precipitates sternal dehiscence. Regardless, sternal wound healing is impaired if the edges of the sternum are not aligned appropriately. Several technical aspects contribute to poor sternal union, including an asymmetric sternotomy, bone ischemia due to excessive use of electrocautery, and failure to achieve proper alignment in patients with chest wall deformities [e.g. pectus excavatum, barrel chest in chronic obstructive pulmonary disease (COPD)]. Obese patients and women with macromastia are also at increased risk for sternal dehiscence and DSWI, due to the excessive tension being applied on the sternal closure by the chest wall, which can lead to sternal wire fracture or cutting through the sternum.

The impact of bilateral internal mammary artery (BIMA) harvest on the risk of DSWI has been widely studied, and remains controversial with various observational studies reporting diverging conclusions. This controversy is compounded by the potential interaction between BIMA harvest and other risk factors such as obesity, diabetes and technique of internal mammary artery harvest (i.e. skeletonized versus pedicled). In the Arterial Revascularization Trial (ART), which randomized 3102 patients to undergo coronary artery bypass grafting (CABG) using either BIMA or single internal mammary artery (SIMA), the risk of sternal wound infection was increased in the BIMA group, as was the rate of sternal reconstruction [7]. Similarly, in a meta-analysis of 32 observational studies which included 172,880 patients, of which 19,994 underwent BIMA harvest, the risk of sternal wound infection was significantly higher in the BIMA harvest group, as compared to the SIMA group [8]. This excessive risk was compounded by the presence of diabetes and old age, and mitigated by the use of a skeletonized harvest technique, such that the risk of sternal wound infection was not significantly different between patients who underwent skeletonized BIMA harvest and those who underwent SIMA harvest.

Microbiology and Pathogenesis

Staphylococcus aureus and *coagulase negative Staphylococci* are the organisms most commonly found in DSWI, representing approximately two thirds of all cases [9]. *Staphylococcus aureus* is often found in cases of perioperative contamination of the mediastinal space. It typically produces an aggressive systemic infection and is associated with more pronounced signs and symptoms of bacteremia [9]. In contrast, *coagulase negative Staphylococci* are most often found in the setting of DSWI associated with typical risk factors for sternal dehiscence, such as obesity and COPD. Infection with these organisms, which colonize the wound from the normal skin flora, is characterized by a slow and late onset, resulting in sternal wound dehiscence, but typically exhibiting a less pronounced systemic response.

Other less commonly encountered organisms in DSWI include Gram negative bacteria and fungi. These infections are usually associated with a prolonged intensive care unit (ICU) stay, and concomitant nosocomial infections (e.g. pneumonia, urinary tract infection, abdominal sepsis).

Diagnosis

The diagnosis of DSWI is essentially clinical. Typical manifestations include sternal tenderness and/or instability (often presenting with a characteristic "sternal click"), erythema, wound dehiscence, or purulent discharge, usually in the presence of leukocytosis and systemic symptoms such as fever, chills and signs of sepsis. Identification of staphylococcal bacteremia on blood cultures—in association with the aforementioned clinical findings—is virtually pathognomonic. Any fluid discharged from the wound should also be cultured. The diagnosis may be more challenging in patients who present with postoperative systemic symptoms in the absence of signs of sternal wound infection or dehiscence. In these patients, systemic manifestations typically precede sternal symptoms by a few days.

While the diagnosis of DSWI is primarily clinical, imaging can help determine the precise location and extent of the infectious process. Computed tomography is the imaging modality of choice, and is associated with excellent sensitivity and specificity, especially after the second postoperative week [10]. Computed tomography may also be useful in guiding needle aspiration and culture, although percutaneous interventions are usually eschewed in favor of early surgical intervention, permitting definitive diagnosis and therapy. Chest radiography is of limited utility, but may alert the clinician to early, indirect signs of DSWI such as sternal wire fracture. Patients with DSWI following valvular surgery may undergo transthoracic or transesophageal echocardiography to rule out concomitant endocarditis.

Prevention

A number of preoperative and perioperative measures can decrease the incidence of sternal wound dehiscence and infection. These include:

1. Encourage smoking cessation at least 6 weeks prior to surgery, if possible.

2. Encourage weight loss in obese patients prior to surgery, if possible.

3. Optimize nutritional status to promote wound healing.

4. Nasal colonization with *Staphylococcus aureus* has a prevalence of 10–15% in the normal population, and increases the risk of sternal wound infections [11]. Nasopharyngeal decontamination with intranasal application of mupirocin [12] or chlorhexidine gluconate [13] decreases the incidence of DSWI, and should be performed routinely.

5. Routine antibiotic prophylaxis should be administered within 30–60 min prior to skin incision. The antibiotics of choice are intravenous cefazolin (1 g if patient <80 kg, 2 g if patient >80 kg) or cefuroxime (1.5 g); intravenous vancomycin is preferred in patients with allergies to penicillin and/or cephalosporins, and in those who are at high risk for *methicillin-resistant Staphylococcus aureus.*

6. Topical antibiotic-eluting sponges may further decrease the risk of DSWI. In a meta-analysis of 14 studies which included a total of 22,135 patients—including 4672 patients from four randomized controlled trials (RCT)—retrosternal application of implantable gentamicin-collagen sponges prior to sternotomy closure was associated with a significant decrease in risk of both SSWI and DSWI. These findings were consistent between RCTs and observational studies [14].

7. Optimal perioperative glycemic control is of the utmost importance, both in patients with pre-existing diabetes and—to a lesser degree—in non-diabetic patients. Compared to intermittent subcutaneous insulin administration, use of a continuous insulin infusion to maintain blood glucose levels between 150 and 200 mg/dL (8.3–11.1 mmol/L) has been shown to decrease the incidence of DSWI in diabetic patients undergoing cardiac surgery [15].

8. In addition to the execution of a precise midline sternotomy, certain authors have advocated the parsimonious use of electrocautery and bone wax, but evidence regarding the efficacy of these measures is lacking.

9. Avoidance of BIMA harvest in high-risk patients, particularly diabetics with other risk factors for sternal wound dehiscence (e.g. obesity, COPD). Alternatively, skeletonized internal mammary artery harvest may mitigate the risk of DSWI in these patients.

10. Use of a sufficient number of sternal wires when closing the sternum [16].

11. Prophylactic use of sternal reinforcement techniques may decrease the risk of sternal dehiscence and DSWI in high-risk patients [17]. These techniques include alternative wiring methods [e.g. mattressed wires, figure-of-eight wiring or the Robicsek weaving technique (Fig. 57.1)] and rigid sternal fixation with sternal plates (Fig. 57.2). In a recently published multicenter randomized trial, sternotomy closure with rigid plate fixation resulted in significantly better sternal healing and fewer sternal complications at 6 months after surgery, compared with wire

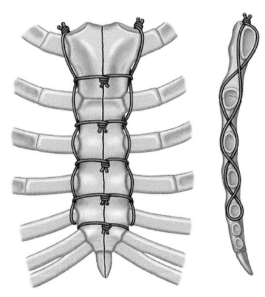

Fig. 57.1 Robicsek sternal closure technique. Reproduced with permission from Orgill DP. Surgical management of sternal wound complications. In: UpToDate, Butler CE (ed.). UpToDate, Waltham, MA (accessed September 2017). Copyright © 2017 UpToDate, Inc. For more information visit www.uptodate.com

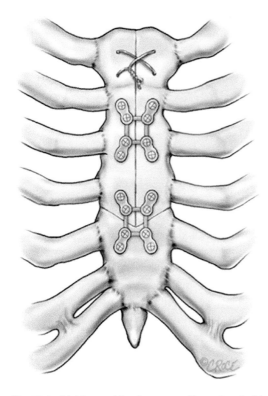

Fig. 57.2 Rigid sternal fixation system. Reproduced with permission from Russo MJ, et al. The Arrowhead Ministernotomy with Rigid Sternal Plate Fixation: A Minimally Invasive Approach for Surgery of the Ascending Aorta and Aortic Root. Minim Invasive Surg 2014;681371

cerclage [18]. While rigid plate fixation was associated with a trend toward greater index hospitalization costs, total costs at 6 months were equivalent between the groups, suggesting that this approach may be cost-effective.

12. External systems used to decrease the tension on the sternum, such as sternal vests and corsets, can be useful adjunctive measures, especially in high-risk patients [19].

Surgical Management

Superficial sternal wound infections without sternal involvement are treated with local wound care or operative debridement and re-approximation of the skin. Sternal dehiscence without evidence of infection can usually be treated with rewiring or plating. This section focuses on the management of DSWI.

As a general principle, the majority of patients suspected of having DSWI on the basis of clinical, microbiological and/or imaging findings should be taken to the operating room urgently for debridement and started on broad-spectrum antibiotics until results of wound culture and sensitivity are obtained.

Various therapeutic options are available for the management of DSWI—i.e. rewiring, sternal plate fixation, soft tissue flaps, negative pressure wound therapy—and treatment should be individualized. In an effort to provide evidence-based guidance regarding the use of these various treatment options, van Wingerden and colleagues developed the Assiduous Mediastinal Sternal Debridement & Aimed Management (AMSTERDAM) classification, a simple classification system based on two variables, namely sternal stability and sternal viability and stock [20].

Debridement, Irrigation and Wound Culture

Surgical debridement is the mainstay of therapy for sternal wound infections, and is indicated in the presence of necrotic tissue or purulent drainage. Thorough debridement of all nonviable tissue is essential, and all foreign material (e.g. sternal wires in the contaminated area) should be removed. The goal is preparation of the wound for reconstruction, and debridement should be carried out until well-vascularized, healthy looking bone edges are visualized. Total sternectomy is seldom necessary. Many centers advocate the use of wound lavage with antibiotics, although no RCT evaluating their effectiveness in sternal debridement has been published. Debridement of an infected sternal wound should be performed in the controlled environment of an operating room, and, whenever possible, with the collaboration of a plastic surgeon.

Deep wound cultures should be obtained whenever feasible. Initial antibiotic therapy is empirically targeted at the most frequently isolated organisms (i.e. *Staphylococcus aureus* and *coagulase negative Staphylococci*), and subsequent treatment is refined based on results of wound cultures and sensitivity testing.

Immediate Versus Delayed Closure

Following debridement, the sternum can be closed immediately, or after a period of open wound management. The decision is based on operative findings and patient characteristics. For example, immediate closure is more readily performed in a thin patient with intact sternal edges than in an obese patient with multiple sternal fractures. Regardless of timing—i.e. immediate versus delayed—sternal closure is achieved either primarily (with cerclage or rigid fixation) or with the use of soft-tissue flaps.

Primary Closure

Simple re-wiring with a mattressed, figure of eight, or cerclage wire technique is usually sufficient in the setting of malunion of the bone edges with an intact sternum. In the presence of multiple wire fractures—or in cases where sternal wires have cut through the sternum because of poor bone quality—the Robicsek technique or plate fixation can provide additional stability. Titanium plates can also be used prophylactically in high-risk patients [21].

Soft Tissue Flaps

The use of soft tissue flaps for sternal closure is reserved for patients with significant tissue deficits after debridement. Flap closure can be used for immediate or delayed closure, and is usually accomplished without bone re-approximation, as the resulting scar tissue typically leads to a stable anterior chest. Several options are available for sternal flap closure, including the use of the pectoralis major, rectus abdominis, and latissimus dorsi muscles, or an omental flap.

Pectoralis Major Flaps

Use of the pectoralis major muscle has become the most commonly used option for flap closure of anterior chest wall defects. Flaps derived from the pectoralis major rely on an understanding of this muscle's primary and secondary blood supplies, namely the thoracoacromial artery and perforators from the internal mammary artery, respectively.

Complete transposition of a large pectoralis major flap can be achieved by folding the muscle over itself, a maneuver that requires transection of the thoracoacromial artery and is therefore contra-indicated in patients who have had harvest of the ipsilateral internal mammary artery. Alternatively, advancement flaps can be created by elevating the entire pectoralis major muscle off the chest wall and, if required, detaching part or all of the muscle from its humeral and sternal attachments—while preserving the primary blood supply from the thoracoacromial artery. In most cases, both pectoral muscles are mobilized using this latter technique and the resulting bilateral flaps are used to cover the mediastinal defect. On one or both sides, the skin can be elevated over the first 6–8 cm off the pectoralis major muscle so that the free edge of the pectoralis major muscle can be used to fill the central sternal defect with well vascularized muscular tissue while the skin edges can be closed over the muscle. Further mobilization of the pectoral flap can be achieved by skeletonizing its vascular pedicle towards the origin of the thoracoacromial artery to create an extended island flap. With these techniques, additional muscle flaps are rarely required to provide coverage of the entire wound.

Omental Flaps

Omental flaps have a rich blood supply, attractive immunologic properties and the ability to adapt well to irregular defects. The omentum is pulled through an opening in the central diaphragm and affords good protection, whether used as a primary flap or as an adjunct to a muscular flap for additional coverage. Omental harvesting may be more complicated in obese patients or in those with previous abdominal surgery. In addition, there have been reports of donor-site complications such as abdominal wall herniation, diaphragmatic herniation, hematoma and/or seroma. Laparoscopic harvesting of the omentum is increasingly being used and may limit incisional complications.

Other Muscle Flaps

Other muscles that have been successfully used as muscular or myocutaneous flaps to cover sternal defects include the latissimus dorsi and rectus abdominis. Whereas the pectoralis major is thought to be the best muscle flap to cover defects in the superior third of the sternum, the rectus abdominis may confer superior coverage of the inferior third of the sternum if full muscular coverage is required, since the pectoralis major muscle usually does not reach the lowest portion of the sternal defect [22]. The rectus abdominis muscle is a rather thin muscle once transposed to the sternal defect and is best harvested as a vertical rectus abdominis musculocutaneous flap. Complications common to all flap closure techniques include hematoma, flap dehiscence, flap necrosis and recurrent infection.

Management of the Open Sternum

For patients who are not candidates for immediate closure due to ongoing infection requiring repeat debridement, the open sternum can be managed with conventional dressing changes—with or without closed antibiotic irrigation—or with vacuum-assisted closure (VAC) therapy.

Sternal Dressings

Open sternal wounds are dressed with moist saline soaked gauze placed over a barrier dressing (e.g. paraffin gauze) to protect the right ventricle. The entire wound is then covered with an elastic dressing (e.g. polyethylene plastic dressing). Soft suction drains may be placed in the wound, taking care to position them in a way that minimizes contact with the heart. Dressings should be changed in the operating room every 1–3 days for non-infected wounds, and more frequently—up to several times a day—if there is evidence of ongoing infection. In this latter situa-

tion, where frequent dressing changes are needed, they are usually carried out at the bedside for practical reasons. There is no proven efficacy for closed irrigation with antibiotics or disinfectant solutions in the setting of DSWI, and closed continuous wound irrigation should be avoided in patients with internal mammary artery grafts.

Vacuum-Assisted Closure Therapy

The concept of VAC therapy was introduced in 1997 by Morykwas and colleagues [23], and consists in a wound dressing system that continuously or intermittently applies subatmospheric local negative pressure through an open-pore polyurethane foam, covered with an adhesive drape. Vacuum-assisted closure therapy provides limited sternal stabilization, removes excess fluid, increases blood flow to the wound, and favors cellular organization and granulation tissue formation, thus facilitating wound healing. It can be used as a single-line modality followed by primary closure, or as a temporary measure aimed at preparing the wound for secondary flap closure. While no RCT has compared VAC therapy with conventional care in DSWI, VAC has been shown to decrease hospital length of stay and improve survival in a number of observational studies [24]. The most frequent complication associated with VAC therapy remains bleeding [25], and there have been rare reports of death by cardiac rupture [26]. Both of these risks can be mitigated by the application of a barrier paraffin dressing to cover the exposed right ventricle.

The optimal frequency of dressing changes and total duration of VAC therapy has not been established. The VAC sponge is typically changed every 2–3 days. Most clinicians discontinue the dressing once the wound is clean and has begun to granulate. The optimal timing of VAC cessation may be guided by C-reactive protein levels [27].

Conclusion

Deep sternal wound infections represent an infrequent but serious complication of cardiac surgery performed through a median sternotomy. Despite advances in surgical management, DSWI remains associated with significant morbidity and mortality in the current era. Strict adherence to established preventive measures is of paramount importance. When DSWI does occur, sternal debridement is the mainstay of therapy. Depending on the clinical situation, sternal closure is performed either immediately after debridement or following an interval of open wound management. Sternal closure is achieved either primarily (with sternal wires in a variety of configurations, or rigid fixation with plates and screws) or with soft tissue flaps. Vacuum-assisted closure therapy may improve outcomes.

References

1. Milton H. Mediastinal surgery. Lancet. 1897;1:872–5.
2. El Oakley RM, Wright JE. Postoperative mediastinitis: classification and management. Ann Thorac Surg. 1996;61(3):1030–6.
3. Centers for Disease Control and Prevention. Surveillance definitions for specific types of infections. Available at https://www.cdc.gov/nhsn/pdfs/pscmanual/17pscnosinfdef_current.pdf. Accessed 23 Sept 2017.
4. Borger MA, Rao V, Weisel RD, Ivanov J, Cohen G, Scully HE, et al. Deep sternal wound infection: risk factors and outcomes. Ann Thorac Surg. 1998;65(4):1050–6.
5. Gummert JF, Barten MJ, Hans C, Kluge M, Doll N, Walther T, et al. Mediastinitis and cardiac surgery—an updated risk factor analysis in 10,373 consecutive adult patients. Thorac Cardiovasc Surg. 2002;50(2):87–91.
6. Parisian Mediastinitis Study G. Risk factors for deep sternal wound infection after sternotomy: a prospective, multicenter study. J Thorac Cardiovasc Surg. 1996;111(6):1200–7.
7. Taggart DP, Altman DG, Gray AM, Lees B, Gerry S, Benedetto U, et al. Randomized trial of bilateral versus single internal-thoracic-artery grafts. N Engl J Med. 2016;375(26):2540–9.
8. Dai C, Lu Z, Zhu H, Xue S, Lian F. Bilateral internal mammary artery grafting and risk of sternal wound infection: evidence from observational studies. Ann Thorac Surg. 2013;95(6):1938–45.
9. Gardlund B, Bitkover CY, Vaage J. Postoperative mediastinitis in cardiac surgery - microbiology and pathogenesis. Eur J Cardiothorac Surg. 2002;21(5):825–30.
10. Jolles H, Henry DA, Roberson JP, Cole TJ, Spratt JA. Mediastinitis following median sternotomy: CT findings. Radiology. 1996;201(2):463–6.
11. Fynn-Thompson F, Vander Salm TJ. Methods for reduction of sternal wound infection. Semin Thorac Cardiovasc Surg. 2004;16(1):77–80.
12. Bode LG, Kluytmans JA, Wertheim HF, Bogaers D, Vandenbroucke-Grauls CM, Roosendaal R, et al. Preventing surgical-site infections in nasal carriers of Staphylococcus aureus. N Engl J Med. 2010;362(1):9–17.
13. Segers P, Speekenbrink RG, Ubbink DT, van Ogtrop ML, de Mol BA. Prevention of nosocomial infection in cardiac surgery by decontamination of the nasopharynx and oropharynx with chlorhexidine gluconate: a randomized controlled trial. JAMA. 2006;296(20):2460–6.
14. Kowalewski M, Pawliszak W, Zaborowska K, Navarese EP, Szwed KA, Kowalkowska ME, et al. Gentamicin-collagen sponge reduces the risk of sternal wound infections after heart surgery: meta-analysis. J Thorac Cardiovasc Surg. 2015;149(6):1631–40e1–6.
15. Furnary AP, Zerr KJ, Grunkemeier GL, Starr A. Continuous intravenous insulin infusion reduces the incidence of deep sternal wound infection in diabetic patients after cardiac surgical procedures. Ann Thorac Surg 1999;67(2):352–360; Discussion 60-2.
16. Kamiya H, Al-maisary SS, Akhyari P, Ruhparwar A, Kallenbach K, Lichtenberg A, et al. The number of wires for sternal closure has a significant influence on sternal complications in high-risk patients. Interact Cardiovasc Thorac Surg. 2012;15(4):665–70.
17. Bottio T, Rizzoli G, Vida V, Casarotto D, Gerosa G. Double crisscross sternal wiring and chest wound infections: a prospective randomized study. J Thorac Cardiovasc Surg. 2003;126(5):1352–6.
18. Allen KB, Thourani VH, Naka Y, Grubb KJ, Grehan J, Patel N, et al. Randomized, multicenter trial comparing sternotomy closure with rigid plate fixation to wire cerclage. J Thorac Cardiovasc Surg. 2017;153(4):888–96.e1.
19. Gorlitzer M, Wagner F, Pfeiffer S, Folkmann S, Meinhart J, Fischlein T, et al. Prevention of sternal wound complications after sternotomy: results of a large prospective randomized multicentre trial. Interact Cardiovasc Thorac Surg. 2013;17(3):515–22.
20. van Wingerden JJ, Ubbink DT, van der Horst CM, de Mol BA. Poststernotomy mediastinitis: a classification to initiate and evaluate reconstructive management based on evidence from a structured review. J Cardiothorac Surg. 2014;9:179.
21. Levin LS, Miller AS, Gajjar AH, Bremer KD, Spann J, Milano CA, et al. An innovative approach for sternal closure. Ann Thorac Surg. 2010;89(6):1995–9.
22. Davison SP, Clemens MW, Armstrong D, Newton ED, Swartz W. Sternotomy wounds: rectus flap versus modified pectoral reconstruction. Plast Reconstr Surg. 2007;120(4):929–34.
23. Morykwas MJ, Argenta LC, Shelton-Brown EI, McGuirt W. Vacuum-assisted closure: a new method for wound control and treatment: animal studies and basic foundation. Ann Plast Surg. 1997;38(6):553–62.

24. Petzina R, Hoffmann J, Navasardyan A, Malmsjo M, Stamm C, Unbehaun A, et al. Negative pressure wound therapy for post-sternotomy mediastinitis reduces mortality rate and sternal re-infection rate compared to conventional treatment. Eur J Cardiothorac Surg. 2010;38(1):110–3.

25. Petzina R, Malmsjo M, Stamm C, Hetzer R. Major complications during negative pressure wound therapy in poststernotomy mediastinitis after cardiac surgery. J Thorac Cardiovasc Surg. 2010;140(5):1133–6.

26. Abu-Omar Y, Naik MJ, Catarino PA, Ratnatunga C. Right ventricular rupture during use of high-pressure suction drainage in the management of poststernotomy mediastinitis. Ann Thorac Surg. 2003;76(3):974; Author reply 974–5.

27. Gustafsson R, Johnsson P, Algotsson L, Blomquist S, Ingemansson R. Vacuum-assisted closure therapy guided by C-reactive protein level in patients with deep sternal wound infection. J Thorac Cardiovasc Surg. 2002;123(5):895–900.

Palliative Care Post Cardiac Surgery

58

Valerie Schulz and Teneille Gofton

Main Messages

1. Incorporating palliative care principles in the perioperative and postoperative cardiac surgery period is recommended.
2. There are validated triggers for referral to specialist palliative care services for patients being cared for in medical and surgical critical care.
3. Adjunctive palliative care may help alleviate and manage symptoms such as dyspnea, delirium, pain, and provide support for challenging communication and decision-making in the cardiac surgery critical care unit.
4. Future research is needed to; advance palliative care knowledge, skills and roles within the cardiac surgery care team, and to align health system change with patient goals.

V. Schulz (✉)
Department of Anesthesia and Perioperative Medicine, Western University, London, ON, Canada
e-mail: Valerie.Schulz@lhsc.on.ca

T. Gofton
Department of Clinical Neurological Sciences, Western University, London, ON, Canada

Background

Advances in managing patients with heart diseases are expanding rapidly as evidenced throughout this book. While cardiac interventions may provide life extension, cardiac disease remains a leading cause of death [1]. The World Health Organization and American Heart Association, amongst others, report there is a growing need for palliative care services for patients with chronic diseases such as cardiovascular diseases [2, 3]. In addition, the aging population and those living with chronic illnesses increase the demand for cardiac procedures. Some patients require cardiac procedures to live longer, and if surgery is ineffective, may accept death over prolonged recovery periods that results in a move from independent to dependent living. Cardiac surgery recovery units (CSRU) exist to closely monitor patients post cardiac surgery to improve mortality risks, rather than to accept death as a normal acceptable outcome after a trial of cardiac therapy. The gap between the dying patient's wishes and expectations verses the health system's measured demands of survival is not reconciled. This chapter will review the components of a palliative care service and expose the discordance between a cure culture and a palliative culture. In doing so, we hope to encourage future research regarding the practical implementation of current guidelines

[2, 4] as cardiac surgery research, and policy and health services development evolves.

A palliative approach to care addresses the whole person and their preferences and expectations. Palliative care is a relationship-focused service that aims to identify patients with palliative needs, address their symptoms, provide communication and shared decision-making support by engaging patients, their substitute decision-makers (SDM) and health care teams, and supporting last days and hours care [5].

Case Vignette

A 73-year-old woman, who was living at home independently, with a history of mechanical aortic valve and double coronary bypass surgery 15 years ago, type 2 diabetes, hypertension and chronic kidney insufficiency, presented with severe mitral valve regurgitation requiring mitral valve replacement. In the postoperative period, the patient required renal replacement therapy due to acute kidney injury. After 2 days of anticoagulation for the mechanical valve, she was found to have right-sided hemiparesis and no verbal output. Neuroimaging demonstrated a large left hemispheric intracranial haemorrhage (ICH). The ICH led to a reduced level of consciousness, aphasia and dysphagia with associated aspiration, respiratory failure and a prolonged period of mechanical ventilation. During the period of mechanical ventilation, the patient suffered from critical illness neuromyopathy, delirium and fluctuating level of consciousness.

The patient's daughter was her substitute decision maker (SDM), and she found it difficult to watch her Mother struggle. She needed an update from the team, and began to wonder whether or not her Mother would be able to live independently once she recovered, as this was important to her Mother.

The Palliative Care Approach

Team-based palliative care aims to bring together primary care, cardiac care and palliative care to build a comprehensive care system for patients who require care within community, medical clinics and hospital systems [1]. These collaborative teams aim to align cardiac care in-context with the patient experiences and expectations. Evidence suggests that delaying the introduction of palliative care expertise for patients in need is associated with: poor symptom control and poor quality of life for a longer period of time; misconceptions regarding prognosis; treatments and care choices not in keeping with goals of care; and lack of preparation for end of life [6, 7]. Earlier palliative care discussions have not been shown to result in increased anxiety or depression related to discussions, and indeed patients having earlier palliative care discussions are more likely to forego ventilation or cardiopulmonary resuscitation and may have improved family bereavement [8].

Identifying Patients with Palliative Needs

There are different approaches for identifying people who would benefit from a palliative approach to care within a cardiac surgery ICU. Patients may be identified at the discretion of the primary care team or a more objective screening approach may be taken. Consensus statements and a growing evidence base in medical surgical intensive care units support the use of specific trigger criteria for referral to palliative services [9–11]. Triggers validated in medical/surgical intensive care units and also likely to be seen in a cardiac surgery ICU include the following criteria: (1) being admitted from skilled nursing facility, long term acute care, long term care with a ventilator, or home care with private duty nursing with activities of daily living dependencies; (2) end stage dementia, amyotrophic lateral sclerosis, Parkinson's disease and multiple sclerosis; (3) advanced or metastatic cancer; (4) admitted to ICU post-cardiac or respiratory arrest with neurological compromise post-arrest; (5) admitted to ICU with hospital length of stay greater than 5 days, or ICU readmission with same diagnosis within 30 days; and (6) team-perceived palliative care need based on poor prognosis and complex care (medical or social complexities) [9]. Additional triggers used in hospitalized patients, regardless of location, include: (1) difficult to control physical or psychological symptoms; (2) disagreement or uncertainty around the plan of care; (3) awaiting or ineligible for solid organ transplantation; (4) consideration for placement of a life supportive therapy or device such as transcutaneous feeding tube; (5) tracheostomy; (6) renal replacement therapy; (7) and left ventricular assist device or automated implantable cardioverter defibrillator [11]. Alternatively, the surprise question ("Would I be surprised if this patient died in the next year?") is also an evidence-based screening tool [12]. A patient with a complex postoperative course, multi-organ involvement and an uncertain prognosis is an ideal candidate for palliative care collaboration. Research supporting integration of a palliative approach to care specifically in the setting of cardiac surgery is limited, but will help guide future recommendations.

Frail patients are independently associated with postoperative complications and length of stay [13]. Frailty as a syndrome is being explored for patients in the perioperative period in order to create an approach to assessments, decision-making and management. Frailty includes unintended weight loss, exhaustion, weakness, slow walking speeds, physical decline, and accrued deficits in activities of daily living, dementia, depression, and physical comorbidities [13].

Frail patients undergoing either transcatheter aortic valve replacement (TAVR) or surgical aortic valve replacement (SAVR) experienced increased mortality and disability at 1 year. The Frailty-AVR Study aimed to determine the frailty tool that could identify which geriatric patients had increased risk of all-cause mortality or disability at 1 year. They noted the Essential Frailty Tool (EFT) used in older adults undergoing AVR could discriminate frail patients more predictably than other frailty tools. EFT reflects lower limb strength, cognition, anemia, and serum albumin. Of interest the authors comment on other predictive conditions that include; atrial fibrillation, oxygen dependent lung disease and kidney impairment, and especially dialysis dependence [14].

Common Symptoms

Pain

Evidence suggests that pain in the postoperative period after cardiac surgery is prevalent and frequently undertreated, especially in women [15]. Sources of pain include sequelae of the surgery itself in addition to procedural based pain in the CSRU. The assessment of pain in the postoperative period is, however, challenging because patients are often unable to communicate either adequately or at all during this time. Therefore, behavioral scales, such as the Behavioral Pain Scale (BPS) and the Critical Care Pain Observation Tool (CPOT) could improve pain assessments [16, 17]. Behaviour based scales are helpful, provided the observer is open to interpretation. For example, agitation can be caused not only by untreated pain, but also dyspnea, delirium, anxiety and so on. Pre-emptive analgesia is suggested for chest tube insertion or removal, or other procedures that may be associated with pain. Current guidelines [15, 18] suggest using non-opioid co-analgesics whenever possible, and if necessary, using intravenous opioid analgesics for non-neuropathic pain. For neuropathic pain, current guidelines suggest a trial of gabapentin or carbamazepine, and opioids may be needed to supplement the former. Interventions including the preoperative administration of pregabalin have been shown to reduce both acute and chronic postoperative pain associated with cardiac surgery [19].

Delirium

The incidence of delirium in the surgical ICU is frequently under-estimated. Prospective observational data from Canada demonstrates an incidence of 39%, specifically in a CSRU [20]. Bedside screening tools, such as the Intensive Care Delirium Screening Checklist (ICDSC) or the Confusion Assessment Method for the Intensive Care Unit (CAM-ICU) improve the ability to assess for and detect postoperative delirium, thereby facilitating management and resolution. The risk of delirium is increased by increasing age, a low preoperative serum albumin, a history of atrial fibrillation, perioperative stroke, ascending aortic replacement surgery, longer duration of procedure, and increased post-operative C-reactive protein concentration [20]. Prevention, identification and management of postoperative delirium are important because postoperative delirium in cardiac surgery patients is associated with worse cognitive outcomes 1 month following surgery [21]. There may however be some improvement in this dysfunction by 1 year. Delirium will also interfere with the acute rehabilitation process, as will depression and anxiety. Depression and anxiety should be approached by pharmacological and non-pharmacological means in order to optimize rehabilitation as well as the patient experience.

Sleep

Alterations in sleep patterns are frequently seen after cardiac surgery. Patients perceive the increased fragmentation of sleep and more frequent awakenings as poor sleep quality. Poor sleep quality may lead to decreased participation in rehabilitation therapies and increased delirium or irritability [22]. The cause of sleep disturbances in this setting are multifactorial and may include poorly managed pain or nausea and environmental factors, among others. There is little evidence to guide the selection of pharmacological sleep aids. Non-pharmacological therapies with some supportive evidence include the use of earplugs, sleeping masks, muscle relaxation, posture and relaxation training, white noise and music to reduce environmental interruptions, and educational strategies for patients [22].

Dyspnea

There is no evidence base specific to the management of dyspnea in the post cardiac surgery recovery unit. However, evidence based interventions aimed at relieving dyspnea in other areas of palliative medicine exist. Optimisation of ventilation strategies, management of pulmonary edema and cardiac function, as well as more conservative treatment such as blow by air or increased air circulation using a fan in the environment (if permitted) may all be effective in reducing dyspnea. Opioids such as hydromorphone or morphine used with appropriate dosing are also beneficial [23]. The mechanisms by which opioids relieve dyspnea are thought to include decreased oxygen requirements at rest, alterations in ventilator responses to carbon dioxide and hypoxia, and possible vasodilation of pulmonary vasculature, among other likely mechanisms [23].

Communication and Decision-Making

A systematic approach to communication and decision-making helps navigate meaningful patient-centered care for the dying patient [24]. These conversations are central components of palliative collaborative care with the primary team. Communication strategies are jurisdiction specific and may involve large teams, including, for example: the admitting cardiac surgical teams, social workers, ethicists, patients and families, and palliative care teams. Where appropriate, these conversations include concepts such as: breaking bad news, family meetings, advance care plans, advance directives, identifying substitute decision-making(SDM)/power of attorney for personal care, wishes and preferences, best interests, goals of care conversations, decision-making and so on. For example, frail, aging patients considering cardiac surgical care and/or their SDM(s) may benefit from support with these conversations and decision-making.

It is necessary to note that laws, ethics, language, clinical policy and practice vary amongst jurisdictions, adding complexity to research. Therefore, learn and use the rules and regulations applicable in your practice location. Jurisdictional variations may lead to confusion in practice.

Advance Care Planning and Goals of Care Discussions

The components of communication in palliative care vary dependent on practice location. Those applicable in the writers' jurisdiction are outlined in Wahl J. et al. 2016 [25]. Advance Care Plans (ACP) occur in advance of the patient disease and are not an informed consent for treatment. ACP's can only be determined by the capable patient, and is used to inform future decision-making by that patient's SDM(s) if the patient becomes unable to make his or her own decisions. Goals of Care (GOC) conversations occur in context of known disease to discuss care plans for the current situation. GOC conversations occur with the capable patient, or if the patient is not capable, these conversations occur with their SDM(s). ACP is a process that involves pre-planning. The GOC process involves the patient, and if appropriate, the SDM who considers the patient's wishes, values and beliefs relating to future treatments and care [25]. Although informed consent discussions are important and essential from providers of cardiac procedures, they are outside the scope of this chapter. However, informed consent and pre-planning, for example ACP and GOC, are inter-dependent and as health systems evolve, these could be considered simultaneously [25, 26].

Serious Illness Conversations

A systematic approach to conversations is a method to bring patients, families and providers together to participate in discussions regarding important concepts, such as prognostication and health care options guided by patient preferences for information and values. Online resources, such as the serious illness conversations framework, are being explored in multiple settings including chronic critical illness [27]. Guideline approaches to conversations have limitations with issues such as; prognostic uncertainty, shifting patient health state, and adjustments in care goals.

Do Not Resuscitate (DNR) Orders

When a patient has a DNR order in place prior to surgery, the American College of Surgeons and both the Canadian and American Societies of Anesthesiology advise that the involved physi-

cians conduct a required reconsideration of the DNR order prior to the surgery. This process includes reviewing the DNR with the patient/SDM; determining if the DNR applies in that specific situation; and, when appropriate, adjusting the DNR order according to informed, competent decision-making with individualized care plans [28]. The American Society of Anesthesiologists outlines three resuscitation alternatives: (1) full attempt at resuscitation; (2) limited attempt at resuscitation in relation to specific procedures; and (3) limited attempt at resuscitation in relation to the patient's goals and values [28]. The impact of patient resuscitation/DNR decision-making is not known.

Non-operative catheter-based cardiac interventions such as TAVR or VAD can serve as an example of the unresolved clash of cardiac surgery's goals to rescue patients verses palliative/ethical patient-centered care goals to limit resuscitation. These procedures are provided for patients considered too ill for cardiac surgery yet, if complications occur, a treatment option includes emergency cardiac surgery. Decision-making and planning regarding management of life-threatening complications or failure of the procedure is problematic [26]. Based on the principle of self-determination, Nurok suggests ideally that a collaborative team of providers align with patients and their designated SDM's to create an approach to care based on patient wishes, which could include limitations in resuscitation [26]. Limitations in resuscitation based on patient choices creates clinical, ethical and health system contradictions which have not yet been reconciled [26, 28].

Discussions regarding intraoperative resuscitation status are not straightforward. Important recent evidence demonstrates cardiac arrests in the operating room have better outcomes than cardiac arrests outside the operating room [29]. Intraoperative cardiac arrests are witnessed events with a known patient with an available provider [29]. This information will need to be considered in discussions regarding intraoperative resuscitation.

Role of Palliative Care on the Cardiac Care Team

The question of whether or not palliative care has a role in the care of patients receiving cardiac surgery has been answered by health policy. Guidelines call for the integration of palliative care services for some cardiac patient populations as an expectation. For example, ventricular assist device (VAD) guidelines outline in the facility criteria that the health care team *must* include: a cardiovascular surgeon, advanced heart failure cardiologist, program coordinator, social worker and *palliative care specialist* [4]. This guideline moves the discussion from whether or not palliative care has a place within cardiac surgery teams to how cardiac VAD providers can expand their teams to include and provide palliative care services. In addition, a decisive policy statement from the American Heart Association/American Stroke Association was published in 2016, titled: *Palliative Care and Cardiovascular Disease and Stroke* [2]. This policy statement identifies the rationale and outlines recommendations for the expansion of palliative care expertise and accepted integration into cardiac care, from the patient perspective to the system perspective. These policy statements underscore a pivotal shift in care, from the novel introduction of palliative care's distinct role in cardiac surgery recovery units, [30] to the expectation of an integrated system change within both palliative care and cardiac care to meet health care delivery demands.

Barriers

Although it seems intuitive that palliative services be readily available for patients within a cardiac surgery program, there are barriers to program implementation, such as underdeveloped awareness of what palliative care for non-cancer diseases is, and its value to patients, families, communities and health systems [3]. Policy-makers, health care providers and the public cultural and social practices are influenced by beliefs about death and dying [3].

Health care guidelines expecting palliative care to integrate with cardiac care have been developed despite paucity of specialized knowledgeable palliative care providers [31], and under the current mortality statistics reporting framework. Although mortality statistics account for risk factors, the data seems to ignore palliative patient wishes and patient health care choices [32]. Clinical and system discrepancies such as these need to be reconciled for cardiac surgery and palliative guideline integration to smoothly occur within patient care.

Case Conclusion

Throughout our patient's hospital stay, her condition slowly improved: renal function recovered such that intermittent hemodialysis could be stopped, there was near complete recovery of the left sided hemiparesis, communication gradually improved and the delirium cleared. At the time of hospital discharge, the patient required inpatient rehabilitation to address limitations in mobility secondary to the ICH, critical illness neuromyopathy, overall deconditioning and some residual communication impairments also associated with the ICH. After a lengthy admission for inpatient rehabilitation, the patient was able to return home but could no longer live independently because she required some assistance for activities of daily living and mild cognitive impairments remained. They are hoping she will continue to improve over the next year.

The integration of palliative care services within cardiac care teams is evolving. This integration aims to support patients with symptom concerns and complex decision-making needs. Guidelines supporting integration of palliative care and cardiac surgical care encourage opportunities for advances in patient care, and health system changes in both programs. Future research addressing discrepancies amongst, for example, patient values and preferences, cardiac surgical care and palliative care program integration efforts, and health system data management strategies will be pivotal for palliative care and cardiac surgical care integration. As advances in cardiac surgery bring desirable life extension, the precipice of inescapable human mortality looms over these advances; therefore, it behooves us blend these realities to create acceptable, realistic patient-centered cardiac surgical care.

Acknowledgements The academic support by the Department of Anesthesia and Perioperative Medicine, and Clinical Neurological Sciences, Western University.

References

1. Fendler TJ, Swetz KM, Allen LA. Team-based palliative and end-of-life care for heart failure. Heart Fail Clin. 2015;11(3):479–98.
2. Braun LT, Grady KL, Kutner JS, Adler E, Berlinger N, Boss R, et al. Palliative care and cardiovascular disease and stroke: a policy statement from the American Heart Association/American Stroke Association. Circulation. 2016;134(11):e198–225.
3. Palliative care: World Health Organization; 2017. Available from http://www.who.int/mediacentre/factsheets/fs402/en/
4. Ventricular Assist Devices (NCD 20.9.1). United Healthcare; 2016 October 12.
5. Goodlin SJ, Rich MW. End-of-life care in cardiovascular disease. London: Springer; 2015.
6. Smith TJ, Dow LA, Virago E, Khatcheressian J, Lyckholm LJ, Matsuyama R. Giving honest information to patients with advanced cancer maintains hope. Oncology (Williston Park, NY). 2010;24(6):521–5.
7. Heyland DK, Allan DE, Rocker G, Dodek P, Pichora D, Gafni A. Discussing prognosis with patients and their families near the end of life: impact on satisfaction with end-of-life care. Open Med. 2009;3(2):e101–10.
8. Wright AA, Zhang B, Ray A, Mack JW, Trice E, Balboni T, et al. Associations between end-of-life discussions, patient mental health, medical care near death, and caregiver bereavement adjustment. JAMA. 2008;300(14):1665–73.
9. Zalenski R, Courage C, Edelen A, Waselewsky D, Krayem H, Latozas J, et al. Evaluation of screening criteria for palliative care consultation in the MICU: a multihospital analysis. BMJ Support Palliat Care. 2014;4(3):254–62.
10. Mosenthal AC, Weissman DE, Curtis JR, Hays RM, Lustbader DR, Mulkerin C, et al. Integrating palliative care in the surgical and trauma intensive care unit: a report from the Improving Palliative Care in the Intensive Care Unit (IPAL-ICU) Project Advisory Board and the Center to Advance Palliative Care. Crit Care Med. 2012;40(4):1199–206.
11. Weissman DE, Meier DE. Identifying patients in need of a palliative care assessment in the hospital setting: a consensus report from the Center to Advance Palliative Care. J Palliat Med. 2011;14(1):17–23.
12. You JJ, Fowler RA, Heyland DK. Just ask: discussing goals of care with patients in hospital with serious illness. CMAJ. 2014;186(6):425–32.
13. Griffiths R, Mehta M. Frailty and anaesthesia: what we need to know. Contin Educ Anaesth Crit Care Pain. 2014;14(6):268–72.
14. Afilalo J, Lauck S, Kim DH, Lefevre T, Piazza N, Lachapelle K, et al. Frailty in older adults undergoing aortic valve replacement: the FRAILTY-AVR study. J Am Coll Cardiol. 2017;70(6):689–700.
15. Barr J, Fraser GL, Puntillo K, Ely EW, Gelinas C, Dasta JF, et al. Clinical practice guidelines for the management of pain, agitation, and delirium in adult patients in the intensive care unit. Crit Care Med. 2013;41(1):263–306.
16. Gelinas C, Johnston C. Pain assessment in the critically ill ventilated adult: validation of the Critical-Care Pain Observation Tool and physiologic indicators. Clin J Pain. 2007;23(6):497–505.
17. Young J, Siffleet J, Nikoletti S, Shaw T. Use of a behavioural pain scale to assess pain in ventilated, unconscious and/or sedated patients. Intensive Crit Care Nurs. 2006;22(1):32–9.
18. Busse JW, Craigie S, Juurlink DN, Buckley DN, Wang L, Couban RJ, et al. Guideline for opioid therapy and chronic noncancer pain. CMAJ. 2017;189(18):E659–66.
19. Bouzia A, Tassoudis V, Karanikolas M, Vretzakis G, Petsiti A, Tsilimingas N, et al. Pregabalin effect on acute and chronic pain after cardiac surgery. Anesthesiol Res Pract. 2017;2017:2753962.
20. Cereghetti C, Siegemund M, Schaedelin S, Fassl J, Seeberger MD, Eckstein FS, et al. Independent predictors of the duration and overall burden of postoperative delirium after cardiac surgery in adults: an observational cohort study. J Cardiothorac Vasc Anesth. 2017;31:1966–73.
21. Sauer AC, Veldhuijzen DS, Ottens TH, Slooter AJC, Kalkman CJ, van Dijk D. Association between delirium and cognitive change after cardiac surgery. Br J Anaesth. 2017;119(2):308–15.
22. Machado FS, Souza R, Poveda VB, Costa ALS. Non-pharmacological interventions to promote the sleep of patients after cardiac surgery: a systematic review. Rev Lat Am Enfermagem. 2017;25:e2926.
23. Kamal AH, Maguire JM, Wheeler JL, Currow DC, Abernethy AP. Dyspnea review for the palliative care professional: treatment goals and therapeutic options. J Palliat Med. 2012;15(1):106–14.
24. Ko DN, Blinderman CD. Withholding and withdrawing life-sustaining treatment (including artificial nutrition and hydration). In: Cherny N, Fallon M, Kaasa S, Portenoy RK, Currow DC, editors. Oxford textbook of palliative medicine. Oxford: Oxford University Press; 2015. p. 323–44.
25. Wahl JA, Dykeman MJ, Walton T. Health care consent, advance care planning, and goals of care practice tools: the challenge to get it right. Improving the last stages of life. Ontario: Commissioned by the Law Commission of Ontario; 2016.

26. Nurok M, Makkar R, Gewertz B. The ethics of interventional procedures for patients too ill for surgery. JAMA. 2017;317(4):359–60.

27. Serious illness care: Ariadne Labs. Available from https://www.ariadnelabs.org/areas-of-work/serious-illness-care/

28. Sumrall WD, Mahanna E, Sabharwal V, Marshall T. Do not resuscitate, anesthesia, and perioperative care: a not so clear order. Ochsner J. 2016;16(2):176–9.

29. Moitra VK, Einav S, Thies KC, Nunnally ME, Gabrielli A, Maccioli GA, et al. Cardiac arrest in the operating room: resuscitation and management for the anesthesiologist: part 1. Anesth Analg. 2017;126(3):876–88.

30. Schulz V, Novick RJ. The distinct role of palliative care in the surgical intensive care unit. Semin Cardiothorac Vasc Anesth. 2013;17(4):240–8.

31. Kirkpatrick JN, Hauptman PJ, Swetz KM, Blume ED, Gauvreau K, Maurer M, et al. Palliative care for patients with end-stage cardiovascular disease and devices: a report from the Palliative Care Working Group of the Geriatrics Section of the American College of Cardiology. JAMA Intern Med. 2016;176(7):1017–9.

32. Percutaneous coronary interventions (PCI) in New York State 2012–2014. New York: New York State Department of Health; 2017.

Routine Surgical Ward Care and Discharge Planning

Anthony Ralph-Edwards

Main Messages

1. Stable post-cardiac surgery patients who do not require ventilation are transferred to the surgical ward from the ICU within 24 h.
2. Standard considerations for management of patients on the surgical ward include wound care, nausea and vomiting, pain control, constipation, anticoagulation, atrial fibrillation prophylaxis and treatment, left ventricular dysfunction, coronary endarterectomy, and diabetes.
3. Discharge planning should occur before admission, and additional support for those who need it should also be arranged preoperatively.

General Care

Cardiac surgery patients who are hemodynamically stable and who do not need assisted ventilation are transferred out of the intensive care unit (ICU) to the surgical ward within 24 h. Prior to discharge, PA catheters, central venous lines and arterial lines are removed. Upon discharge from the ICU, a detailed summary of the operative and postoperative course in the ICU are provided, along with standardized ICU discharge orders to facilitate hospital ward care.

On the ward, vital signs are recorded every 4 h for the first 24 h and every 8 h thereafter, along with daily body weight. Urine output is monitored with a Foley catheter until its removal, typically on the second postoperative day (POD). All patients should be placed on a fluid restriction of 1500 mL/day following cardiac surgery, as many will have a positive fluid balance upon discharge from the ICU. Patients may have been fluid resuscitated immediately postoperatively and with increased production of antidiuretic hormone in the early postoperative period, patients are predisposed to fluid retention.

Typically, pleural, pericardial, and mediastinal chest drains are removed in the ICU after 24 h unless there is drainage in excess of 200 mL in 12 h. Blake drains are typically removed once the INR is >2.0. Prior to removal of chest tubes, an absence of air leak should be confirmed. Excess drainage or air requires further observation and/or intervention. Chest x-rays should be done within 3 h of chest drain removal. On the ward, telemetry is continued for an additional 24–48 h and can be discontinued after POD four, if there is an absence of cardiac dysrhythmia. External pacing wires are usually removed on the third or fourth POD, if the cardiac rhythm is stable. In

A. Ralph-Edwards (✉)
The University Health Network, Toronto, ON, Canada
e-mail: anthony.ralph-edwards@uhn.ca

patients being anticoagulated, wires should be removed when the international normalized ratio (INR) is <2.0. If patients are receiving intravenous heparin, the heparin should be discontinued for 2 h before the removal of the pacer wires and should be resumed 2 h following removal of the wires. Prophylactic enoxaparin or subcutaneous heparin should be held the morning prior to removal of pacing wires. Following pacer wire removal, patients should remain in bed for 30 min to 1 h and monitored for signs of active bleeding. Pacer wires should not be cut flush with the skin, but rather removed completely to minimize risk of late infection.

Early ambulation and respiratory exercises are critical to decreasing hospital stay following cardiac surgery. To minimize atelectasis, patients are instructed on respiratory exercises and incentive spirometry. Physiotherapy, occupational therapy and ward nursing staff will work with patients to ensure early mobilization and identify patients who would benefit from cardiac rehabilitation, either as an outpatient or inpatient.

Prior to discharge, hospital staff will provide classes for patients and families to outline instructions about the activities of daily living, exercise, diet, and follow-up care. In addition, a comprehensive booklet dealing with concerns during convalescence should be provided. The pharmacist provides a pre-discharge class for those patients going home with a warfarin prescription.

Routine Tests on the Ward

Standard postoperative orders include daily complete blood count, electrolyte concentration, and creatinine level during the first 3 days. The liver function test is evaluated in all patients starting statins or in those patients requiring anticoagulation if the evaluation was abnormal preoperatively or in the ICU. Once warfarin is started, the INR is checked daily. Electrocardiograms are taken daily during the first 3 days and on the day before discharge. Chest x-rays are done before and following the removal of chest tubes, as well as before discharge. Echocardiograms should be performed on all patients who have undergone valve surgery prior to discharge. All other tests are ordered as clinically indicated.

Wound Care

Surgical wounds are covered with sterile dressing until POD two. All wounds should be inspected daily. With increased use of endoscopic vein harvesting, leg wound infection rates are typically less than 5%. Early mobilization and Jackson Platt drains help minimize hematoma formation. Patients with a sternal click on palpation have a higher risk of dehiscence and/or infection. If a sternal click develops, patients are provided with a chest binder to give added stability when coughing and moving. In cases of instability, rewiring of the sternum should be undertaken.

Nausea and Vomiting

Following cardiac anesthesia, nausea and vomiting are common. While the etiology is multifactorial, minimizing or discontinuing contributory medications and administering antiemetics such as ondansetron can minimize postoperative nausea and vomiting. Ileus is common in patients receiving narcotics and abdominal distention can be decompressed with a nasogastric tube and limiting oral intake. Further imaging and laboratory tests should be considered with severe or persistent symptoms to rule out bowel ischemia, cholecystitis, liver failure or pancreatitis.

Pain Control

Management of pain is an important aspect of postoperative care. Hydromorphone 0.5–4 mg intravenously (IV) q 2–4 h is administered on the first and second POD. For younger patients, personal controlled analgesia (PCA) should be used and the patient followed by the Acute Pain Service. This will assist in early mobilization and minimize respiratory complications. High dose acetaminophen is used in all patients without liver dysfunction and all pain medications are switched to oral route once the patient is tolerating oral intake. Use of nonsteroidal anti-inflammatory drugs (NSAIDs) are effective for pain and can be used in patients who do not tolerate narcotics; however, they are contraindicated in patients with elevated creatinine levels, diabetics, or peptic ulcer disease. It is important to note literature suggests that selective COX-II inhibitor is contraindicated in cardiac surgical patients. For patients with a history of chronic opioid use, the acute pain service should be consulted preoperatively and patient-specific protocols should be instituted.

Constipation

Constipation is common in all patients because of narcotic administration. A bowel protocol should be in place and should include a daily laxative and enemas, as needed. We routinely use Colace, 100 mg PO b.i.d., and lactulose, 15–30 mL PO q.i.d.

Anticoagulation

Patients who undergo cardiac surgery may develop a hypercoagulable state postoperatively placing them at risk for thrombotic events. Postoperatively, prophylactic subcutaneous unfractionated heparin or low-molecular-weight heparin should be administered routinely. When the patient is ambulating adequately, prophylactic treatment is discontinued.

All patients with mechanical valves require permanent oral anticoagulation with warfarin sodium to maintain an INR of 2–3 for aortic prostheses and 2.5–3.5 for mitral valve prostheses. In some institutions, aspirin 81 mg daily is added to warfarin sodium. Patients with mechanical valves should be started on intravenous heparin or low-molecular-weight heparin following removal of chest drains and typically receive their first dose of warfarin sulfate on the second POD. Therapeutic partial thromboplastin time should be maintained until an INR of 2.0 is reached.

Patients who have had mitral valve replacement with a bioprosthesis or mitral valve repair should be anticoagulated for 3 months if they are in sinus rhythm or permanently if they are in chronic atrial fibrillation (AF). The INR should be maintained between 2 and 3. Patients who had aortic valve replacement with bioprostheses or biologic valves receive aspirin 81 mg, but do not need to be anticoagulated with warfarin sodium if they are in sinus rhythm. Some centers routinely use oral anticoagulation for bioprosthetic aortic valves during the first 3 months based on recent literature. Novel anticoagulation agents are avoided due to risk of thromboembolic and bleeding event rates.

All patients with chronic AF or with AF for >48 h of intermittent AF require oral anticoagulation with warfarin sodium. The target INR is 2.0–2.5. The patients should receive concurrent unfractionated or low-molecular-weight heparin until the INR is 2.0. If there is no valve prosthesis, patients can switch to a novel anticoagulation agent after 1–3 months.

Platelet count should be monitored in patients on heparin because of the risk of heparin-induced thrombocytopenia (HIT). If the platelet count drops >50% or below 100,000, a 4 T score should be calculated to assess the likelihood of HIT. Hematology should be consulted, heparin held, and a HIT assay should be ordered. If the patient with HIT requires ongoing anticoagulation, an alternative such as a direct thrombin inhibitor can be used.

Atrial Fibrillation Prophylaxis and Treatment

AF is a common complication following open-heart surgery, occurring in 10–40% of patients and can be associated with increased rates of death, complications and recurrent hospitalizations. Preoperative clinical predictors are age, sex, past history of AF, paroxysmal or new onset of AF, left ventricular dysfunction, congestive heart failure, withdrawal of β-blockers, and preoperative interatrial conduction delay. Operative predictors include the number of coronary artery bypass grafts, as well as concomitant heart valve surgery. Efforts to prevent AF postoperatively have included perioperative administration of β-blockers or amiodarone and use of Blake drains in the postoperative period. Some individuals use high dose Ascorbic acid. β-blockers are introduced by the second postoperative day and uptitrated once the patient is on the ward. In hemodynamically stable patients who develop new onset AF postoperatively, there is no evidence that rhythm control is superior to rate control with respect to short term outcomes. In patients with normal left ventricular function, use of β-blockers and/or amiodarone is preferred. If there are contraindications for β-blockers or amiodarone, a calcium channel blocker is used together with digoxin for rate control.

If the patient is hemodynamically compromised, patients are loaded with intravenous amiodarone and then switched to daily oral amiodarone. If necessary, electrical cardioversion is performed; unless the patient is medically pretreated, cardioversion is efficacious only for a limited period of time.

Resumption of sinus rhythm can often be achieved within 48 h. If sinus rhythm is not restored within 48 h, anticoagulation is mandatory. Patients who have mitral valve surgery and develop postoperative AF will remain on anticoagulants; thus these patients can be managed with rate controlled with less emphasis on sinus conversion due to the presence of anticoagulants for stroke prophylaxis. One strategy to decrease length of stay is to start warfarin on all patients who develop atrial fibrillation and reassess the need after 48–72 h.

Left Ventricular Dysfunction

For patients with considerable left ventricular dysfunction, angiotensin converting enzyme (ACE) inhibition should be reinstituted before intravascular euvolemia is achieved. A low dose can be introduced postoperatively and up-titration

is done by the outpatient cardiologist. Renal function must be carefully monitored because of the concomitant use of diuretics. For significant left ventricular dysfunction, the heart failure service should be consulted for medical optimization and follow up.

Coronary Endarterectomy

Approximately 30% of coronary arteries that underwent endarterectomy occlude within 1 year. Antiplatelet agents are important to enhance early- and late-patency rates. Aspirin is given immediately postoperatively if there are no signs of excessive bleeding and daily clopidogrel is initiated on the first postoperative day. The combination of aspirin and clopidogrel may be more efficacious than the combination of aspirin and dipyridamole.

Diabetes

Optimization of blood sugar starts preoperatively and blood sugar levels are maintained postoperatively using intravenous insulin. Once oral intake is tolerated, introduction of home glycemic control regimes can occur. The Endocrine Service should see all patients preoperatively and will follow all patients with type-1 or type-2 diabetes until discharge. Recent studies support moderate glycemic control as optimal for cardiac surgery patients, thus balancing the adverse effects of hyperglycemia and the hypoglycemia events.

Prophylaxis for Dressler Syndrome

All patients younger than 50 years who have undergone heart valve or aortic surgery should be placed on high-dose enteric-coated aspirin with gastric protection to prevent Dressler syndrome or post-pericardiotomy syndrome. The presence of a rub and ECG changes supportive of pericarditis should be assessed daily in all patients.

Discharge Planning

Discharge planning begins before admission. Elderly patients often require additional support in the community, which should be arranged preoperatively. Most patients can be safely discharged on the fifth or sixth POD. Criteria for discharge are:

- Afebrile for 24 h
- No signs of infection
- Weight at or below preoperative level
- No drainage from wounds
- Absence of heart failure
- Blood pressure and rhythm control
- Therapeutic anticoagulation plan
- Oxygen saturation satisfactory on room air
- Independent ambulation

Discharge medications for coronary artery bypass patients should include antiplatelet agents and statins. A hospital pharmacist, a knowledgeable nurse, or a physician should review all medications with the patient and family. Side effects and drug interactions should be outlined. A discharge letter describing the patient's surgery, hospital course, discharge medications, and follow-up care should be given to all patients, with copies sent to the family physician and the referring cardiologist. A schedule of appointments with the family physician, cardiologist, and surgeon should also be given. This provides seamless transition from in-hospital to community care.

A team based approach is required to optimize medical care for patients undergoing cardiac surgery and to minimize hospital length of stay. Early identification and treatment of common problems can minimize complications following cardiac surgery. Ensuring a continuity of care upon discharge from the cardiac surgery ward is critical to achieving excellent long-term patient outcomes.

Further Reading

1. Postoperative care. In Kouthoukos NT, Blackstone EH, Hanley FL, Kirklin JK. editors. Kirklin/Barratt-Boyes cardiac surgery, 4rd ed. Elesevier Health Sciences; 2013.
2. Martin DO, Saliba W, McCarthy PM, Gillinov M, Belden W, Nassir F, Marrouche NI, Natale A. Approaches to restoring and maintaining sinus normal rhythm. Cleve Clin J Med. 2003;70(3):S12–30.

Ward Complications and Management

60

Dave Nagpal and Sanjay Asopa

Main Messages
1. While individualized assessment is essential in perioperative care, checklists and protocols have improved efficiency and quality of care for routine surgical patients.
2. Surgical ward complications and management can pertain to wound healing; pulmonary concerns (atelectasis, pleural effusion, pneumonia, and pneumothorax); cardiovascular concerns (tachyarrhythmia, bradyarrhythmia, pericardial effusion and tamponade, and low cardiac output); as well as hematological, gastrointestinal, renal, and neurologic concerns (stroke, neuropsychiatric abnormalities, and peripheral neuropathy).

D. Nagpal (✉)
Division of Critical Care Medicine,
London Health Sciences Centre,
London, ON, Canada

Department of Surgery, Western University,
London, ON, Canada
e-mail: dave.nagpal@lhsc.on.ca

S. Asopa
Division of Cardiac Surgery, London Health Sciences
Centre, London, ON, Canada
e-mail: Sanjay.Asopa@lhsc.on.ca

Iterative improvements in pre-, peri-, and postoperative cardiac surgical care have allowed for excellent outcomes and an improved patient experience despite increasingly older and sicker patients being submitted for cardiac surgery. These improvements are due in large part to the combined efforts of surgical, medical, and allied health specialties' painstaking attention to detail along the entire continuity of care.

Recent emphasis on checklists and protocol-driven care has fostered efficiency and improved quality of care for the routine patient, however, individualized assessment and optimization remains essential for even the most routine "straight-forward" cases. Non-routine or complicated cases require particularly meticulous vigilance, with continuation of care strategies from the cardiac surgical intensive care unit, to ward convalescence, to acute hospital discharge. Reducing postoperative complications and improving patient satisfaction is paramount for ensuring not only the best care for patients currently undergoing cardiac surgery, but also for future cardiac surgical patients, and even for the specialty itself.

Pulmonary

Most routine early postoperative therapy focuses on prevention of pulmonary issues. Vital signs are routinely monitored, and supplemental oxy-

© Springer Nature Switzerland AG 2021
D. C. H. Cheng et al. (eds.), *Evidence-Based Practice in Perioperative Cardiac Anesthesia and Surgery*, https://doi.org/10.1007/978-3-030-47887-2_60

gen administered for oxygen saturations lower than 88–92%. Deep breathing and coughing, while splinting the sternotomy or thoracotomy incision with a pillow or folded flannel for comfort, is encouraged. The most common pulmonary complications encountered post cardiac surgeries are atelectasis, pleural effusion, pneumonia, and pneumothorax.

Atelectasis

Atelectasis is very common following cardiac surgery, seen in up to 80% of these patients [1]. Besides the usual postoperative atelectasis seen in most major surgical patients who require general anesthesia (which is due to prolonged supine operative positioning and postoperative pain, splinting, and slow mobility) cardiac surgical patients have specific reasons for the higher incidence of atelectasis. During CPB, the lungs are generally not ventilated, causing atelectasis, particularly when the pleurae are breached. The left lung may be more commonly involved during LITA harvest if the pleural space is opened and the lung packed down with sponges; this technique is discouraged in our institution. Postoperatively, pain from the surgical incision and chest tubes can contribute to splinting and poor cough efforts, further predisposing to atelectasis.

Significant atelectasis leads to poor gas exchange and reduced lung compliance that can cause or exacerbate respiratory failure. Management is therefore directed towards reexpansion of the atelectatic lung in the operating room and postoperatively. Although it is common practice to perform a recruitment maneuver on resumption of ventilation in the operating room, and again on arrival in the cardiac surgical recovery unit, it remains to be demonstrated that this is beneficial; harm has been demonstrated in the general intensive care population [2]. Following extubation, lung reexpansion is achieved by adequate analgesia, deep breathing and coughing exercises, and ambulation. Occasionally in refractory symptomatic atelectasis, incentive spirometry can be

helpful, and even non-invasive ventilation with non-invasive continuous positive pressure ventilation (CPAP) or bi-level positive airway pressure (BiPAP) may be necessary.

Pleural Effusion

Pleural effusion is very common after cardiac surgery. One series reported a 10% incidence of large effusions (occupying more than 1/4th of the hemithorax) [3]. They may be more common on the left side after a LITA harvest when the pleural space is breached. Predisposing factors include fluid shifts, hypoalbuminemia, inflammation, pneumonia or atelectasis. The majority of these patients are asymptomatic, but those with significant effusion volume may have exertional dyspnea, or may be difficult to wean off oxygen. Large or symptomatic effusions are treated with thoracentesis or a tube thoracostomy. Small or asymptomatic effusions are generally treated with diuretic therapy. If Dressler's Syndrome is suspected, colchicine is prescribed for 3 months; some institutions routinely utilize colchicine in all patients [4].

Pneumonia

Pneumonia post cardiac surgery is seen in 1–5% of patients. The cumulative incidence of pneumonia was reported at 2.4% in a recent series, of which one third occurred after discharge [5]. Identified risk factors were older age, lower hemoglobin level, chronic obstructive pulmonary disease (COPD), steroid use, operative time, and left ventricular assist device/heart transplant, prolonged mechanical ventilation, NG tube, and each unit of blood transfused. As would be expected, postoperative pneumonia was associated with a marked increase in mortality and length of hospital stay. Usual antimicrobial therapies for hospital-acquired pneumonia are utilized as per local hospital antibiograms, with infectious diseases service consultation as needed.

Pneumothorax

Postoperative pneumothorax is seen in 1.4% of patients post cardiac surgery [1]. Postoperative pneumothorax could be due to inadvertent injury to the lung during surgery or central venous catheter placement, air entrainment during chest tube removal, and/or barotrauma during ventilation (particularly in bullous emphysematous disease, or those with a need for high airway pressures to achieve ventilatory targets). Management is planned based on the cause, size, and clinical symptoms of the pneumothorax. We drain any pneumothorax which is enlarging, associated with subcutaneous emphysema, or greater than 25% of the lung field. Generally, we use 14-french pigtail catheters, but occasionally a traditional tube thoracostomy is required.

Cardiovascular

Common cardiovascular complications are arrhythmic; however, any myocardial, valvular, conduction, or pericardial pathology is possible following cardiac surgery. Tachyarrhythmia, bradyarrhythmia, pericardial effusion/tamponade, and low cardiac output state are the most common cardiovascular complications seen on the ward.

Tachyarrhythmia

Premature atrial or ventricular ectopic beats are very common post cardiac surgery; these are usually innocent, and nothing more than routine care is required. The most common arrhythmia seen after cardiac surgery is atrial fibrillation (AF), with an incidence of 30–40%. All postoperative patients are monitored with continuous telemetry for at least 48–72 h, and a 12 lead ECG is performed if there is a change in the rhythm. Targeting serum potassium above 4 mmol/L and magnesium above 1 mmol/L is purported to prevent arrhythmia, however evidence for this is weak [6].

Prophylactic beta blockers are started as soon as possible to prevent AF, and are first line therapy for postoperative AF. Although there is no benefit of amiodarone in most postoperative AF [7], an intravenous bolus of 150 mg is given for unstable AF, with a 5-day oral or intravenous load, followed occasionally by a daily maintenance dose for 1–2 months. Anticoagulation should be considered in patients with AF for more than 48 h.

Sustained ventricular arrhythmias are uncommon but can be due to electrolyte imbalance, ischemia, and/or electrophysiologic pathology (e.g. R on T phenomenon). Initial management follows advanced cardiovascular life support (ACLS) for any unstable arrhythmia. Thereafter, one must ensure no ongoing myocardial ischemia, correct serum electrolytes and metabolic concerns, review external pacing, and initiate amiodarone therapy when appropriate.

Bradyarrhythmia

Conduction abnormalities requiring pacing are dependent on the type of cardiac surgery, with an overall incidence of permanent pacing around 1.5%. Left bundle branch block (LBBB) and aortic valve replacement (AVR) on multivariate analysis are independent predictors of need for permanent pacing [8]. In patients undergoing AVR, permanent atrioventricular conduction disturbances are seen in 3–8% of cases [9]. We routinely use temporary epicardial wires for all cardiac surgical patients, which are generally removed after 4–5 days, or the day before discharge.

Pericardial Effusion and Tamponade

Pericardial effusion post cardiac surgery is very common, occurring in up to 80% of patients [10]. The incidence of persistent pericardial effusion at 30 days is around 8% [11]. Although the vast majority of these effusions are clinically inconsequential, the addition of an anticoagulant may increase the risk of tamponade [11]. In patients with significant pericardial effusion and hemodynamic instability, pericardiocentesis should be performed. Particularly with concomitant pleural effusions, Dressler's syndrome is suspected, and colchicine is prescribed.

Low Cardiac Output

Poor organ perfusion on the ward is generally assessed via clinical and biochemical parameters, since most patients will not have invasive monitoring data available. The components of low cardiac output etiology are assessed, including ineffective heart rate or rhythm and/or inadequate stroke volume. Inadequate stroke volume could be due to inadequate preload (intravascular volume depletion most common, but vasodilatory and obstructive shock states must be excluded); poor contractility (myocardial dysfunction); or increased afterload (hypertension or, less commonly, native or prosthetic aortic valvular dysfunction, systolic anterior motion of the mitral valve, or left ventricular outflow tract obstruction). Echocardiographic assessment aids in decision making.

Management targets the underlying cause. Inadequate preload (due to loss of vasomotor tone, increased capillary leak, blood loss and increased urine output) is corrected with volume replacement. After load reduction (hypertension) is managed with antihypertensive medications. Very rarely do patients with poor myocardial contractility need IV inotropic support in the ward environment. Heart failure medication titration with diuretic therapy, ACEI, aldosterone antagonists and beta blockers is usually helpful in those with cardiomyopathy when conservatively titrated. Echocardiographic assessment directs treatment of valvular and prosthetic valvular pathologies.

Hematological

All patients not on therapeutic anticoagulation for other reasons receive routine deep vein thrombosis (DVT) prophylaxis unless contraindicated, as DVT has been reported in up to 20% of patents going to cardiac rehabilitation programs [12]. The risk of pulmonary embolism was found to be 0.5–3.5% post cardiac surgery [13]. Risk factors for development of DVT include delayed mobilization, obesity, older age, history of DVT, and prothrombotic conditions.

Heparin induced Thrombocytopenia and Thrombosis (HITT) is uncommon, and diagnosis is difficult in patients immediately post cardiac surgery due to non-immune mediated, transient, asymptomatic thrombocytopenia. A secondary fall in the platelet count of $\geq$50% that begins between the fifth and tenth postoperative day is predictive of HITT [14]. Warkentin's 4 T score is used to risk stratify for HITT, but diagnosis and confirmation is by ELISA/SRA laboratory investigation. Thrombosis occurs in up to 50% of individuals with HITT, with venous more common than arterial thrombi. In a large series of hospitalized patients with HITT, bleeding was seen in approximately 6% [15]. Bleeding is rare unless the platelet count drops below 10,000/mL. Hematology is generally consulted in the management of these patients to provide post-discharge follow-up and guidance for duration of anticoagulation.

Gastrointestinal

Previously documented at 2–3%, a more recent large population-based study reported the incidence of GI complications following cardiac surgery to be higher (4.1%) [16]. GI complications post coronary artery bypass graft (CABG) increases inpatient mortality and the hospital length of stay.

Mesenteric ischemia after cardiac surgery is infrequent but can be catastrophic. Even with early recognition and treatment the outcomes are poor. The risk factors include duration on cardiopulmonary bypass (hypoperfusion), vasopressor agents (mesenteric bed vasoconstriction), intra-aortic balloon pump (IABP), and other sources of arterial atherosclerotic embolism, atrial fibrillation, and peripheral vascular disease (PVD). Even with early recognition and intervention nearly one in two patients die. Hyperamylasemia is seen in up to 65% of patients; however overt pancreatitis of unknown etiology (which is associated with an exceedingly high mortality risk) is seen in 0.4–3% of patients [17].

Patients receive proton pump inhibitors (PPI) or H2 blockers for 4–6 weeks post-surgery for gastric mucosal protection. Erosive upper GI bleeding tends to occur around postoperative day 10. Prolonged mechanical ventilation and raised INR are independent risk factors, whereas PPI use trends towards protection against GI bleed [18].

Renal

Acute kidney injury (AKI) is a common and important complication of cardiac surgery that is potentially associated with increased short-term and long-term mortality and morbidity. The incidence varies from 5 to 42%, and in severe cases of AKI there is three to eightfold higher perioperative mortality, prolonged length of stay in the ICU and hospital, and increased health care cost [19]. The risk of death associated with AKI remains high for 10 years after cardiac surgery regardless of other factors, even for those with complete renal recovery [20].

To date, there is no consensus on the definition of cardiac surgery associated AKI. Most researchers use the Acute Kidney Injury Network (AKIN) and/or the Risk, Injury, Failure, Loss, End Stage Kidney Disease (RIFLE) criteria to define AKI. The Kidney Disease: Improving Global Outcomes (KDIGO) criteria for AKI staging, which combines the RIFLE and AKIN criteria, has shown to be more sensitive in detecting AKI and predicting in-hospital mortality [21]. Novel serum and urinary biomarkers have demonstrated not only to predict subclinical AKI but also have a prognostic value [22]. However, the validity and application of these biomarkers to the cardiac surgical population at large remain untested.

The pathophysiology of cardiac surgery associated AKI is complex, and likely related to the multiple factors of renal ischemia (reperfusion injury, inflammation, oxidative stress, hemolysis, and nephrotoxins) that all contribute to AKI. Risk factors for AKI can be classified as patient related (age, preexisting renal disease, LV dysfunction, diabetes mellitus (DM), COPD, female gender, emergency surgery and IABP) and procedure related (use of CPB, combined procedures, X-clamp time, hemodilution, hemolysis, and pulsatile versus non-pulsatile flow) [21]. In the recent STS updates on outcomes and quality, the incidence of renal failure was reported to be 2.1% for patients undergoing CABG and 8.2% for patients with combined MVR and CABG [23].

Renal replacement therapy (RRT) is necessary in up to 5% of patients with AKI, and is associated with poor short and long term prognosis. Uncertainty persists regarding the optimal timing for initiation of RRT [21]; the KDGIO guidelines suggest initiation of RRT for life threatening changes in fluid status, electrolytes levels, and acid base balance. Generally, optimizing perfusion pressure, volume status, glycemic control, and avoiding nephrotoxic medications are the mainstay for management of AKI in postoperative patients [24].

Neurologic

Common neurological complications on the cardiac surgical ward can be divided into stroke, neuropsychiatric abnormalities, and peripheral neuropathy (see also Chap. 55).

Stroke

Perioperative stroke is a potentially devastating catastrophic complication of cardiac surgery. Compared to CABG, open-heart surgery such as valvular procedures carry a higher risk of stroke and transient/reversible ischemic neurological dysfunction, potentially due to particulate and air embolization. Risk factors associated with intraoperative stroke include PVD, redo cardiac surgery, deep hypothermic circulatory arrest (DHCA), older age, and prolonged CPB time. Factors associated with postoperative stroke include DM, female sex, and postoperative atrial fibrillation (POAF), suggesting that intra- and postoperative stroke could be due to different pathophysiological mechanisms [25].

Neuropsychiatric Abnormalities

The neuropsychiatric abnormalities encompass neurocognitive dysfunction, seizures, and delirium. They represent a spectrum of neurological dysfunction with varied presentation. Disturbances in memory, attention and other cognitive function can be seen in up to 70% of patients [25, 26]. Undiagnosed mild cognitive deficits, advanced age, hypertension, carotid disease, and previous stroke are risk factors for neurocognitive impairment, with intraoperative hypotension and cerebral micro emboli potentially contributing. Delirium is commonly seen in patients post cardiac surgery, the cause of which is thought to be multifactorial; but extracorporeal circulation, anesthetic medications, the ICU environment, and renal and hepatic dysfunction are known to contribute [25].

Peripheral Neuropathy

Peripheral nerve injury following cardiac surgery occurs in up to 15% of patients, and commonly includes phrenic nerves, brachial plexus, ulnar nerves, and saphenous nerves. Potential mechanisms include operating room positioning and padding, traction and compression during sternal retraction and IMA harvesting, and direct injury from local dissection of conduit or axillary artery exposure. Symptoms of paresthesia usually resolve in 3–6 weeks, suggesting neuropraxic injury due to myelin disruption, and these are therefore generally managed conservatively. In the uncommon event of axonal disruption or severe injury, symptoms persist, prompting further evaluation with electromyographic nerve conduction studies to confirm diagnosis and delineate site and extent of injury [27].

Given the lack of effective strategies to treat the above neurologic complications, management remains largely supportive, with physical and occupational therapy to attenuate the injury and/or improve functional status. Besides the most debilitating strokes, the majority of patients with perioperative stroke can fortunately recover adequate function to achieve a good quality of life. Delirium can be addressed with pharmacologic and non-pharmacologic strategies. Most neurological dysfunction is transient, with return of baseline neurocognitive and peripheral nerve function within months to 1 year.

Wound Healing

Sternal wounds are dressed and left covered for the first 48–72 h, unless dressings are soaked through. The donor vein harvest leg and radial artery arm are covered by compression dressings that are removed after the first 24 h post-surgery. Drains inserted in the leg or forearm are removed when drainage allows.

Sternal wound infections can be divided into superficial (SSWI) and deep sternal wound infections (DSWI). SSWI, which occurs in up to 8% of patients undergoing cardiac surgery, involves the skin, subcutaneous tissues and/or pectoral fascia; there is no bony involvement [28]. DSWI, which occurs in up to 2% of these patients, involves bone and the mediastinum. The Centres for Disease Control and Prevention defines DSWI as the presence of: (a) an organism isolated from culture of mediastinal tissue or fluid; (b) evidence of mediastinitis seen during operation; or (c) presence of chest pain, sternal instability, or fever (>38 °C), and purulent drainage from the mediastinum, or isolation of an organism present in a blood culture or a culture of the mediastinal area [29].

Although the incidence of SSWI is declining, it is associated with increased morbidity, mortality, length of hospital stay, and reduced long term survival, portending a significant economic burden. Similarly, the reported rate of DSWI from the 2013 STS database was 1%, but the associated mortality can be as high as 35% from some series [30, 31]. Most common microorganisms causing cardiac surgical wound infections are *staphylococcus epidermidis* (approximately 75% of cultured strains are methicillin resistant), and *staphylococcus aureus* [32].

Management of SSWI generally begins with antimicrobial therapy and enhanced wound care. Empiric gram positive coverage is appropriate for sternal wound infections, however, broad spectrum antibiotics with gram negative coverage may be preferred in massively obese patients with breast or abdominal pannus at the sternal incision site, or for infections of groin incisions. The wound is opened for appropriate dressing if an infected collection is identified or suspected. Negative pressure wound therapy (NPWT) may expedite wound healing when the wound is greater than 2 cm deep or if multiple wound-healing risk factors exist [33].

Patients complaining of undue sternal pain, discharging wounds with or without sternal insta-bility, and signs of systemic inflammation should alert one of a possible deep sternal wound prob-lem. In patients with suspicion of DSWI, a CT scan is performed to evaluate the mediastinum. In cases of sternal instability after 3–5 days of NPWT and antibiotics, one may consider sternal rewiring after drainage of any mediastinal collec-tion, debridement, and irrigation.

Prevention of wound infections is obviously favorable from all perspectives. Adherence to basic hand hygiene routines is imperative. Washing hands before and after patient assess-ment and care has helped reduce the rates of wound infection [34], and the use of gowning and gloving for patients with contact precau-tions reduces spread of drug-resistant organ-isms. Optimizing preoperative nutritional status, glycemic control, and achieving smoking cessa-tion reduces the risk of wound infection in patients undergoing cardiac surgical procedure.

Future Directions

Postoperative complications are unavoidable; even in perfectly optimized systems, the complexity and interplay of individual patient factors, human healthcare factors, systemic/institutional healthcare factors, and limitations of science and medicine will for the foreseeable future leave cardiac surgical patients at some degree of procedural risk. We nonetheless continue to strive for continuous quality improvement, with the ultimate laudable goal of 0% morbidity/mortality and 100% patient satisfaction.

Important areas for future investigation to optimize surgical outcomes include preoperative nutrition and physical conditioning; more accurate risk prediction scores to distinguish operative candidates from non-candidates including measures of frailty; continued refinement of operative and procedural techniques; advancement of specific cardiac surgical intensive care research to better guide acute care; improvement of protocol-directed care including early-warning systems for postoperative ward patients; and enhancing compliance with guideline-based pharmacologic treatment in the postoperative patient. With these and other directions of continuous quality improvement, our patients stand to receive the most effective, most durable, and most satisfying treatment available for their cardiovascular pathology.

References

1. Wynne R, Botti M. Postoperative pulmonary dysfunc-tion in adults after cardiac surgery with cardiopulmo-nary bypass: clinical significance and implications for practice. Am J Crit Care. 2004;13:384–93.
2. Gattinoni L, et al. Lung recruitment in patients with the acute respiratory distress syndrome. N Engl J Med. 2006;354:1775–86.
3. Light RW, et al. Prevalence and clinical course of pleural effusions at 30 days after coronary artery and cardiac surgery. Am J Respir Crit Care Med. 2002;166:1567–71.
4. Imazio M, et al. Colchicine for prevention of postperi-cardiotomy syndrome and postoperative atrial fibrilla-tion: the COPPS-2 randomized clinical trial. JAMA. 2014;312:1016–23.
5. Ailawadi G, et al. Pneumonia after cardiac surgery: experience of the National Institutes of Health/ Canadian Institutes of Health Research Cardiothoracic Surgical Trials Network. J Thorac Cardiovasc Surg. 2017;153:1384–91.
6. Kaplan M, Kut MS, Icer UA, Demirtas MM. Intravenous magnesium sulfate prophylaxis for atrial fibrillation after coronary artery bypass surgery. J Thorac Cardiovasc Surg. 2003;125:344–52.

7. Echahidi N, Pibarot P, O'Hara G, Mathieu P. Mechanisms, prevention, and treatment of atrial fibrillation after cardiac surgery. J Am Coll Cardiol. 2008;51:793–801.

8. Merin O, et al. Permanent pacemaker implantation following cardiac surgery: indications and long-term follow-up. Pacing Clin Electrophysiol. 2009;32:7–12.

9. Hassina B, et al. Pacemaker dependency after isolated aortic valve replacement: do conductance disorders recover over time? Interact Cardiovasc Thorac Surg. 2013;16:476–81.

10. Weitzman LB, Tinker WP, Kronzon I, Cohen ML, Glassman E, Spencer FC. The incidence and natural history of pericardial effusion after cardiac surgery—an echocardiographic study. Circulation. 1984;69:506–11.

11. Meurin P, et al. Evolution of the postoperative pericardial effusion after day 15: the problem of the late tamponade. Chest. 2004;125:2182–7.

12. Goldhaber SZ, Hirsch DR, MacDougall RC, Polak JF, Creager MA, Cohn LH. Prevention of venous thrombosis after coronary artery bypass surgery (a randomized trial comparing two mechanical prophylaxis strategies). Am J Cardiol. 1995;76:993–6.

13. Shammas NW. Pulmonary embolus after coronary artery bypass surgery: a review of the literature. Clin Cardiol. 2000;23:637–44.

14. Lillo-Le Louët A, et al. Diagnostic score for heparin-induced thrombocytopenia after cardiopulmonary bypass. J Thromb Haemost. 2004;2:1882–8.

15. Goel R, Ness PM, Takemoto CM, Krishnamurti L, King KE, Tobian AA. Platelet transfusions in platelet consumptive disorders are associated with arterial thrombosis and in-hospital mortality. Blood. 2015;125:1470–6.

16. Rodriguez F, Nguyen TC, Galanko JA, Morton J. Gastrointestinal complications after coronary artery bypass grafting: a national study of morbidity and mortality predictors. J Am Coll Surg. 2007;205:741–7.

17. Cardiac surgery in the adult, 5th ed. Lawrence and Cohn; 2016 Nov 11 .

18. Bhat M, et al. Prediction and prevention of upper gastrointestinal bleeding after cardiac surgery: a case control study. Can J Gastroenterol. 2012;26:340–4.

19. Ortega-Loubon C, Fernandez-Molina M, Carrascal-Hinojal Y, Fulquet-Carreras E. Cardiac surgery-associated acute kidney injury. Ann Card Anaesth. 2016;19:687–98.

20. Hobson CE, et al. Acute kidney injury is associated with increased long-term mortality after cardiothoracic surgery. Circulation. 2009;119:2444–53.

21. Wang Y, Bellomo R. Cardiac surgery-associated acute kidney injury: risk factors, pathophysiology and treatment. Nat Rev Nephrol. 2017;3:697–711.

22. Coca SG, et al. Urinary biomarkers of AKI and mortality 3 years after cardiac surgery. J Am Soc Nephrol. 2014;25:1063–71.

23. D'Agostino RS, et al. The society of thoracic surgeons adult cardiac surgery database: 2017 update on outcomes and quality. Ann Thorac Surg. 2017;103:18–24.

24. Elahi M, Asopa S, Pflueger A, Hakim N, Matata B. Acute kidney injury following cardiac surgery: impact of early versus late haemofiltration on morbidity and mortality. Eur J Cardiothorac Surg. 2009;35:854–63.

25. McDonagh DL, Berger M, Mathew JP, Graffagnino C, Milano CA, Newman MF. Neurological complications of cardiac surgery. Lancet Neurol. 2014;13:490–502.

26. Newman MF, et al. Longitudinal assessment of neurocognitive function after coronary-artery bypass surgery. N Engl J Med. 2001;344:395–402.

27. Welch MB, et al. Perioperative peripheral nerve injuries: a retrospective study of 380,680 cases during a 10-year period at a single institution. Anesthesiology. 2009;111:490–7.

28. Ridderstolpe L, Gill H, Granfeldt H, Ahlfeldt H, Rutberg H. Superficial and deep sternal wound complications: incidence, risk factors, and mortality. Eur J Cardiothorac Surg. 2001;20:1168–75.

29. https://www.cdc.gov/nhsn/pdfs/pscmanual/17pscnosinfdef_current.pdf. Accessed 20 Aug 2017.

30. Hillis LD, et al. ACCF/AHA guideline for coronary artery bypass graft surgery. A report of the American College of Cardiology Foundation/American Heart Association Task Force on Practice Guidelines. Developed in collaboration with the American Association for Thoracic Surgery, Society of Cardiovascular Anesthesiologists, and Society of Thoracic Surgeons. J Am Coll Cardiol. 2011;58:e123–210.

31. Lazar HL, Salm TV, Engelman R, Orgill D, Gordon S. Prevention and management of sternal wound infections. J Thorac Cardiovasc Surg. 2016;152:962–72.

32. Sjögren J, Malmsjö M, Gustafsson R, Ingemansson R. Poststernotomy mediastinitis: a review of conventional surgical treatments, vacuum-assisted closure therapy and presentation of the Lund University Hospital mediastinitis algorithm. Eur J Cardiothorac Surg. 2006;30:898–905.

33. Baillot R, et al. Impact of deep sternal wound infection management with vacuum-assisted closure therapy followed by sternal osteosynthesis: a 15-year review of 23,499 sternotomies. Eur J Cardiothorac Surg. 2010;37:880–7.

34. Boyce JM, Pittet D. Guideline for hand hygiene in health-care settings: recommendations of the Healthcare Infection Control Practices Advisory Committee and the HICPAC/SHEA/APIC/IDSA Hand Hygiene Task Force. MMWR. 2002;51(RR16):1–44.

Pain Management After Cardiac Surgery

61

Kevin Armstrong and Qutaiba A. Tawfic

Main Messages
1. Despite advances in the understanding and treatment of pain, postsurgical pain management continues to be a major challenge.
2. The use of high doses of intravenous opioids reduces the likelihood of achieving fast track cardiac surgery recovery.
3. The identification of patients with chronic pain, and the pre-operative initiation of treatment can improve postoperative pain management.

Postsurgical pain management continues to be a major medical challenge despite the advances in understanding pain, and the pharmacological agents available in this field. Pain management is a critical matter in postoperative care. The adverse events that result from the under treatment of pain includes tachycardia, increased oxygen consumption, psychological consequences, impairment of function, thromboembolic events, pulmonary complications, prolonged hospital stay, and an increased risk of persistent postsurgical pain [1].

Traditionally, anesthesia for cardiac surgery has utilized high doses of intravenous opioids. A similar approach exists for post cardiac surgery pain management; that is, in recovery units, intravenous or intramuscular opioids are a predominant strategy. However, the liberal use of opioids may contribute to prolonged mechanical ventilation postoperatively. With the introduction of fast-track cardiac surgery, the use of balanced anesthesia, lower doses or short acting opioid analgesics, and multimodal analgesia in the postoperative period are more common [2]. Multimodal analgesia as part of fast-track regimens includes regional anesthesia, non-opioid systemic analgesics, and opioid analgesia [3].

Incidence and Intensity of Acute Pain After Cardiac Surgery

Post cardiac surgery pain may be very intense, especially during the first 2 postoperative days. A mean pain score of four on the numerical rating score (NRS) of 0–10 is to be expected. Pain that occurs following cardiac surgery has multiple generators. Risk factors for poorly controlled acute pain are not clearly defined, however, longer duration of surgery (>2 h), pre-existing anxi-

K. Armstrong · Q. A. Tawfic (✉)
Department of Anesthesia and Perioperative Medicine, London Health Sciences Centre, Schulich School of Medicine and Dentistry, Western University, London, ON, Canada
e-mail: Kevin.Armstrong@sjhc.london.on.ca; Qutaiba.Tawfic@lhsc.on.ca

© Springer Nature Switzerland AG 2021
D. C. H. Cheng et al. (eds.), *Evidence-Based Practice in Perioperative Cardiac Anesthesia and Surgery*, https://doi.org/10.1007/978-3-030-47887-2_61

ety, and young age (<60 year), can result in higher pain scores [3]. The location/type of surgery may also play a role [3].

Incidence and Risk Factors of Chronic Post-cardiac Surgery Pain

Multiple etiological factors and mechanisms are likely involved in the development of chronic post-surgical pain. The incidence of chronic post-cardiac surgery pain varies widely (21–55%). Chronic post-surgical pain (CPSP) is likely to originate from surgically induced damage of the peripheral nerves, as well as an active inflammatory response that results from tissue injury [3, 4]. The immune response involving the affected nerves can continue for months after acute inflammation has resolved, and this may contribute to the development of CPSP. During cardiac surgery, injury to the intercostal nerves may result in chronic pain. This damage can be a consequence of the incision, drainage tubes and sternal wires [4, 5].

There are many risk factors for CPSP and these include perioperative depression, anxiety, catastrophizing and other psychological vulnerability, female gender, heritable susceptibility, more extensive or prolonged surgery, poorly controlled acute postoperative pain, higher postoperative opioid requirement, neuropathic pain, pre-existing chronic pain, and surgical approach [4, 6]. The awareness and early recognition of high postoperative pain scores and CPSP is crucial if we are to have a positive impact for those susceptible to a poor pain outcome. In the complex perioperative environment in which cardiac surgery takes place, it is helpful to have a simple and validated scoring system to identify these patients [4].

Evaluation of Post-cardiac Surgery Pain

The American Society of Anesthesiologists (ASA) has published guidelines for acute postoperative pain management (2012). According to these guidelines, the process of postoperative pain management should begin at the time of preoperative evaluation by an anesthesiologist. This includes the identification of risk factors for difficult to control acute postoperative pain and the development of CPSP. These factors are described above [4, 6]. During the postoperative phase, pain evaluation requires the use of systematic assessment with valid and reliable scales. In addition to pain scores (such as NRS), the evaluation should include pain-associated symptoms, vital signs, and side effects related to pain medications [3].

Physiology of Pain Perception

A basic one-dimensional model can be used to demonstrate the perception of pain. In this model, the pain nociceptive process is defined as detection, transduction, conduction and transmission of noxious stimuli from the nociceptors to higher centres, where pain is ultimately perceived. However, the perceived intensity of pain by any given patient may be very different despite a seemingly similar stimulus. This difference can be explained by the two-dimensional model where inhibitory pathways act as a modulator to reduce pain transmission. These inhibitory neuronal pathways originate in the brainstem, descend through the spinal cord, and end in the substantia gelatinosa. Serotonergic and noradrenergic systems are the predominant neurological inputs involved in the inhibitory pathway. Psychological status is one of the factors that can augment or weaken the outflow from the descending inhibitory pathways. Pain perception is also affected by neuroplasticity which results from peripheral and/or central sensitization of the neurons, which can lead to hyperalgesia. The issues of neuroplasticity and sensitization are complex and involve multiple pathways; however, there are two concepts which are recognized as important and sites for intervention. The first is that inflammatory mediators released at the site of injury result in peripheral sensitization. The second involves activation of centrally located N-methyl-d-aspartate (NMDA) receptors, which causes an increased influx of calcium ions in spinal and supra-spinal neuronal cells. Peripheral and central sensitization play an important role in the conversion of acute pain to chronic pain [1, 7].

Pain Treatment Modalities After Cardiac Surgery

For many years, opioids via the parenteral route have been a mainstay for treating acute pain following cardiac surgery. However, postoperative pain management now is widely dependent on the concept of a multimodal analgesia regimen. This concept was introduced to improve the pain experience of patients, and reduce the incidence of side effects resulting from opioids. While opioids continue to be central to postoperative pain management, different analgesic medications and techniques can be used for management of acute postoperative pain after cardiac surgery [1, 3, 4]. ASA practice guidelines recommend the use of regional anesthesia, and around the-clock foundational analgesia (acetaminophen and NSAIDs) whenever possible. Also, optimizing the dose of analgesics to achieve maximum efficacy and reduce side-effects is recommended [1, 4, 6].

Foundational Analgesia

Unless contraindicated, ASA practice guidelines recommend that foundational analgesia (acetaminophen and NSAIDs) is to be used around the clock, "first on last off," for acute postoperative pain [6]. The use of foundational analgesia improves pain control, reduces opioid consumption, and decreases the incidence of opioid-induced adverse events. The combined use of acetaminophen and NSAIDs provides better analgesia in comparison to either drug alone [1, 8]. The analgesic effect of acetaminophen is mainly central with almost no peripheral analgesic, and no anti-inflammatory activity.

Acetaminophen is considered a safe and well tolerated analgesic medication. The main concern with acetaminophen is the risk of hepatotoxicity at higher doses. Dose adjustment may be recommended in patients of advanced age, hepatic impairment, end stage renal disease, malnutrition and high alcohol consumption. The analgesic efficacy of acetaminophen has been studied (1000 mg dose) and the number needed to treat (NNT) was found to be 3.8 for a 50% reduction of mild to moderate postoperative pain over 4–6 h in comparison to placebo [8].

Pettersson et al. [9], compared intravenous and oral acetaminophen in 77 postoperative coronary artery bypass graft (CABG) patients in an ICU setting. There was a lower postoperative opioid requirement in the IV group (17.4 ± 7.9 mg vs. with 22.1 ± 8.6 mg) (p = 0.016). The clinical significance of the opioid-sparing effect was not clear, because there was no difference in pain scores, or in the incidence of postoperative nausea and vomiting [9].

Fayaz et al. [10], studied the impact of combining non-specific NSAIDs and acetaminophen on 60 CABG patients over 24 h in the ICU postoperatively. Three groups received either combined acetaminophen and diclofenac, diclofenac alone, or placebo. Combined acetaminophen and diclofenac reduced opioid consumption by 45% when compared to diclofenac alone, and by 67% in comparison to placebo. Active treatment groups showed lower pain scores than placebo group at 12 and 24 postoperative hours, less postoperative nausea and vomiting, a shorter time to extubation, and better oxygenation following extubation [10].

Traditionally, there has been some avoidance of NSAIDs in pain management after cardiac surgery. The concerns have been an increased bleeding tendency, and the risk of renal injury after cardiopulmonary bypass. A number of investigators employing systematic reviews have considered the question of complications secondary to NSAIDs following cardiac surgery. Bainbridge et al. [11] reported reduced pain at 24 h with no significant increase in the risk of mortality, myocardial infarction, renal injury, or gastrointestinal hemorrhage in 1065 patients. McDaid et al. [12] reported decreased opioid consumption and decreased opioid related side effects. In 2017,

DeSouza [13] used pooled data from 5887 patients to show that perioperative use of NSAIDs did not increase the risk of death, myocardial infarction, stroke, renal impairment, mediastinitis, or bleeding.

COX2 inhibitors are not recommended for routine analgesia in the cardiac patient based on the work of Nussmeier et al. published in 2005. Using an RCT design, the risk of developing an adverse event was higher with COX2 inhibitors in comparison to placebo (7.4 vs. 4.0%). The risk of cardiovascular events with the COX2 inhibitors group (myocardial infarction, cardiac arrest, stroke, and pulmonary embolism) was four times higher than in the placebo group (2.0 vs. 0.5%) [14].

Opioids

In cardiac surgery, opioids have been administered postoperatively via oral and parenteral routes [intermittent IM/IV injections and patient-controlled analgesia (PCA)]. Both synthetic and semisynthetic opioids have been used for postoperative acute pain management (morphine, hydromorphone, oxycodone, fentanyl and tramadol). Ruetzler et al. showed that oral opioids can be as effective as IV opioids (same pain scores) with less total opioid consumption [15].

Bainbridge et al., included ten randomized trials (666 patients) in a meta-analysis to compare nurse-controlled-analgesia (NCA) and PCA after cardiac surgery. PCA significantly reduced pain scores at 48 h, but not at 24 h post-surgery. However, total opioid consumption was significantly higher with PCA at both 24 and 48 h [16].

Opioids cause several clinically significant adverse effects for the cardiac surgery patient when used for postoperative pain management. These effects include sedation, sluggish bowel movements, nausea and vomiting, pruritus, respiratory depression, and opioid-induced hyperalgesia. Higher doses of opioids are more likely to produce these adverse effects. Of particular interest is the effect on the respiratory system and consequently the time to extubation. It is these

outcomes which highlight the importance of using adjuvant analgesics (multimodal analgesia) to reduce opioid usage.

Gabapentinoids

Gabapentinoids (gabapentin and pregabalin) are anticonvulsants that are commonly used as adjuvant analgesics to treat both acute postoperative pain and chronic pain. These medications can improve postoperative analgesia, reduce opioid usage and reduce opioid-related side effects when used in conjunction with opioids [1]. Ucak et al., studied 40 CABG patients for acute and chronic postoperative pain. The intervention group in this RCT received 1200 mg/d of oral gabapentin before surgery and for 2 days afterwards. Gabapentin significantly reduced the intensity of pain in the first 72 h after surgery and reduced tramadol consumption in the first 24 h after extubation with no difference in the incidence of adverse events. There was no significant difference in chronic pain after 3 months [17]. In another study, Menda et al. studied the effect of single dose gabapentin 2 h before surgery. In this RCT, data from 60 CABG patients was analyzed. There was a 57% reduction in total morphine consumption at 48 h after surgery (6.7 mg vs. 15.5 mg in placebo group), lower pain scores at rest and during cough, and less nausea in the gabapentin group. However, there was over-sedation and the duration of mechanical ventilation was longer by 60 min in comparison to the placebo group [18].

Pesonen et al. studied 70 elderly patients (≥75 year) undergoing CABG or valve surgery. Participants received either placebo or 150 mg of pregabalin preoperatively and 75 mg twice daily for 5 postoperative days. The pregabalin group had an almost 50% reduction in opioid consumption during the 5 postoperative days. There was a lower incidence of pain during movement in the pregabalin group at 3 months postoperatively, but no difference in pain at rest. Time to extubation was 138 min longer in the gabapentinoid group. There was no difference in sedation scores and incidence of nausea and vomiting between the groups [19]. Gabapentinoids may positively contribute to the management of both acute and persistent pain. However, in the doses studied, there is evidence that the goals of fast track cardiac surgery may be hampered by it use.

Regional Anesthesia

As a strategy for acute pain management following cardiac surgery, regional anesthesia/analgesia has a number of attributes that contribute to the multimodal aspect of pain management. Over the years, a number of approaches have been proposed, adopted and subsequently fallen out of favour [20]. The complexities of modern preoperative cardiac surgical care are perhaps one causative factor which limits wide spread incorporation of these techniques. These include patient, provider, and system factors.

In its simplest form, regional analgesia involves the inhibition/modulation of neural transmission from the site(s) of injury to and within the central nervous system. This will address one aspect of acute pain management and possibly the development of CPSP. The primary agents are local anesthetics and are well known to clinicians. Traditionally, regional anesthesia is provided as one time injections or continuous catheter based techniques. Adjuvants are, at times, added to local anesthetics to augment/improve the effect. When successful, regional techniques are effective, have low negative impact and will potentially improve desirable outcomes with lower pain scores and opioid consumption [21]. When utilized as part of multimodal analgesia, evidence exists for better pain scores, earlier extubation and reduced opioid consumption. There is limited evidence that regional anesthesia reduces the length of stay. In the complex patient, this modality is definitely worth considering. However, in many settings, there are logistical issues regarding the provision and maintenance of this form of analgesia.

Epidural Analgesia

Thoracic epidural analgesia (TEA) is a well-known regional technique. The use of TEA has many positive attributes [22], however there are many challenges for its use in the general cardiac surgery population [20]. Of particular concern is the risk of an epidural hematoma, which is increased by the concurrent use of heparin, and full anticoagulation during on-pump procedures. Although the incidence of epidural hematoma is very rare, this concern has limited the widespread use of TEA in cardiac surgery. Svircevic et al. performed a meta-analysis of 28 studies, involving 2700 cardiac surgery patients. This study showed that the use of TEA reduces the risk of postoperative supraventricular arrhythmias and respiratory complications [23]. A more recent meta-analysis by Zhang et al. in 2015 included 25 RCTs (3062 patients). There was no significant difference in the risk of death, myocardial infarction, and stroke when TEA was utilized. However, an epidural technique reduced the risk of outcomes such as supraventricular arrhythmias, longer time to tracheal extubation and duration of time in the hospital or intensive care unit [24]. Despite these outcomes, the lack of reduction in death or myocardial infarction renders the routine use of TEA in cardiac surgery difficult to justify when balanced with the potential risks of epidural hematoma and paralysis, in the context of full heparinization.

Intrathecal Morphine

Meylan et al. published a meta-analysis concluding that intrathecal morphine without local anesthesia reduced postoperative pain intensity at rest and movement for 24 h and reduced opioid consumption for 48 h after cardio-thoracic surgery. The risk of pruritus and respiratory depression increased with intrathecal morphine [25]. This technique may have some utility in pain management for those undergoing cardiac surgery, since the technique is familiar to most anesthesiologists, and there is evidence for effectiveness.

Paravertebral Analgesia

The thoracic paravertebral block (TPVB) can be delivered as a single- or multiple-site injection, as well as a continuous catheter technique. It can be performed on one side or bilaterally. Continuous catheter techniques allow for delivery of regional analgesia for 2–3 postoperative days. It can be used for port based surgeries as well as thoracotomy and sternotomy. The interest in TPVB has increased because of the relatively lower risk of epidural hematoma compared with an epidural technique, in the setting of anticoagulation. The evidence shows that effective TPVB can reduce intraoperative opioid use and facilitate early extubation in the operating room in patients undergoing minimally-invasive cardiac surgery [26].

Peripheral Nerve Blocks

Other forms of peripheral regional anesthesia are potentially useful in cardiac surgery. However, thus far there has been limited research performed in this area. Those blocks which have been studied include intrapleural blocks, which have been demonstrated to reduce drainage site pain [27]. Similarly, continuous intercostal nerve blocks (ICB), and parasternal blocks can reduce opioid consumption and improve pain scores

[28]. The serratus anterior block has been used in the setting of thoracotomy and there is evidence to suggest that the results of this block are as effective as the TEA [29].

Postoperative Pain Management in Patients with Chronic Pain and Opioid-Tolerance

Patients with a history of chronic pain, opioid tolerance and addiction are more likely to have a difficult postoperative experience and thus require special care to increase the likelihood of good postoperative pain control and a smooth postoperative recovery. The use of preoperative anti-pro-nociceptive medications (such as gabapentinoids, ketamine and i.v. lidocaine) is advised in these cases. Also, the inclusion of regional anesthesia may add positively to the management of challenging patients. These patients are at a higher risk to develop CPSP and all the required measures should be taken to reduce the risk of this problem (Table 61.1) [4].

There are a number of factors at play when making informed decisions about post cardiac surgery pain management. These include surgical technique, patient populations, expectations of health care systems, and goals for length of stay. The processes involved in perioperative care are challenging, many, and varied. In this highly resourced and multidisciplinary setting, coordination of care is a significant challenge. As surgical techniques evolve, the analgesic requirements also change. Therefore, a tailored, multimodal

Table 61.1 Recommendations for pain management in patients with opioid-tolerance [4]

Preoperative preparation	• Identify high-risk patients • Review preoperative treatment of pre-existent pain • Arrange educational material/session for the patients and their family
Intraoperative action	• Regional anesthesia should be considered if possible • Use adjuvant analgesics to reduce opioid requirement and hyperalgesia
Postoperative interventions	• Continue multimodal analgesia (regional analgesia, around the clock acetaminophen and NSAIDs, gabapentinoids and opioids through PCA • Neuropathic pain medications for neuropathic pain
Post-discharge follow-up	• Flag high-risk patients for CPSP • Communicate with surgeon and family physician regarding discharge medication • Use neuropathic pain medications in case of persistent neuropathic pain • If possible, to arrange an extended follow-up and pain care after surgery

approach to analgesia will be useful to the patient and the teams who provide care. In today's environment, incorporating a multimodal approach into care pathways is recommended. When the health care teams understand the analgesic plan and limitations to these plans, there is an opportunity for improved care. Expansion to the surgeon's office, clinics, and preoperative clinics will allow for the development, communication, and implementation of appropriate plans.

References

1. Tawfic QA, Faris AS. Acute pain service: past, present and future. Pain Manag. 2015;5(1):47–58.
2. Myles PS, Daly DJ, Djaiani G, Lee A, Cheng DC. A systematic review of the safety and effectiveness of fast-track cardiac anesthesia. Anesthesiology. 2003;99(4):982–7.
3. Cogan J. Pain management after cardiac surgery. Semin Cardiothorac Vasc Anesth. 2010;14(3):201–4.
4. Tawfic Q, Kumar K, Pirani Z, Armstrong K. Prevention of chronic post-surgical pain: the importance of early identification of risk factors. J Anesth. 2017;31(3):424–31.
5. Mailis A, Umana M, Feindel CM. Anterior intercostal nerve damage after coronary artery bypass graft surgery with use of internal thoracic artery graft. Ann Thorac Surg. 2000;69:1455–8.
6. American Society of Anesthesiologists Task Force on Acute. Pain Management. Practice guidelines for acute pain management in the perioperative setting: an updated report by the American Society of Anesthesiologists Task Force on Acute Pain Management. Anesthesiology. 2012;116:248–73.
7. Heinricher MM, Tavares I, Leith JL, Lumb BM. Descending control of nociception: specificity, recruitment and plasticity. Brain Res Rev. 2009;60(1):214–25.
8. Oscier CD, Milner QJ. Peri-operative use of paracetamol. Anaesthesia. 2009;64:65–72.
9. Pettersson PH, Jakobsson J, Owall A. Intravenous acetaminophen reduced the use of opioids compared with oral administration after coronary artery bypass grafting. J Cardiothorac Vasc Anesth. 2005;19:306–9.
10. Fayaz MK, Abel RJ, Pugh SC, Hall JE, Djaiani G, Mecklenburgh JS. Opioid-sparing effects of diclofenac and paracetamol lead to improved outcomes after cardiac surgery. J Cardiothorac Vasc Anesth. 2004;18:742–7.
11. Bainbridge D, Cheng DC, Martin JE, Novick R, Evidence-Based Perioperative Clinical Outcomes Research (EPiCOR) Group. NSAID-analgesia, pain control and morbidity in cardiothoracic surgery. Can J Anaesth. 2006;53(1):46–59.
12. McDaid C, Maund E, Rice S, Wright K, Jenkins B, Woolacott N. Paracetamol and selective and non-selective non-steroidal anti-inflammatory drugs (NSAIDs) for the reduction of morphine-related side effects after major surgery: a systematic review. Health Technol Assess. 2010;14(17):1–153.
13. de Souza BF, Mehta RH, Lopes RD, Harskamp RE, Lucas BD Jr, Schulte PJ, Tardif JC, Alexander JH. Nonsteroidal anti-inflammatory drugs and clinical outcomes in patients undergoing coronary artery bypass surgery. Am J Med. 2017;130(4):462–8.
14. Nussmeier NA, Whelton AA, Brown MT, Langford RM, Hoeft A, Parlow JL, Boyce SW, Verburg KM. Complications of the COX-2 inhibitors parecoxib and valdecoxib after cardiac surgery. N Engl J Med. 2005;352:1081–91.
15. Ruetzler K, Blome CJ, Nabecker S, Makarova N, Fischer H, Rinoesl H, Goliasch G, Sessler DI, Koinig H. A randomised trial of oral versus intravenous opioids for treatment of pain after cardiac surgery. J Anesth. 2014;28(4):580–6.
16. Bainbridge D, Martin JE, Cheng DC. Patient-controlled versus nurse-controlled analgesia after cardiac surgery—a meta-analysis. Can J Anaesth. 2006;53:492–9.
17. Ucak A, Onan B, Sen H, Selcuk I, Turan A, Yilmaz AT. The effects of gabapentin on acute and chronic postoperative pain after coronary artery bypass graft surgery. J Cardiothorac Vasc Anesth. 2011;25(5):824–9.
18. Menda F, Köner O, Sayın M, Ergenoğlu M, Küçükaksu S, Aykaç B. Effects of single-dose gabapentin on postoperative pain and morphine consumption after cardiac surgery. J Cardiothorac Vasc Anesth. 2010;24(5):808–13.
19. Pesonen A, Suojaranta-Ylinen R, Hammarén E, Kontinen VK, Raivio P, Tarkkila P, Rosenberg PH. Pregabalin has an opioid-sparing effect in elderly patients after cardiac surgery: a randomized placebo-controlled trial. Br J Anaesth. 2011;106(6):873–81.
20. Ziyaeifard M. A review of current analgesic techniques in cardiac surgery. Is epidural worth it? J Cardiovasc Thorac Res. 2014;6(3):133–40.
21. Neuburger PJ. A prospective randomized study of paravertebral blockade in patients undergoing robotic mitral valve repair. J Cardiothorac Vasc Anesth. 2015;29(4):930–6.
22. Rodrigues ES. Robotic mitral valve repair: a review of anesthetic management of the first 200 patients. J Cardiothorac Vasc Anesth. 2015;29(4):930–6.
23. Svircevic V, van Dijk D, Nierich AP, Passier MP, Kalkman CJ, van der Heijden GJ, Bax L. Meta-analysis of thoracic epidural anesthesia versus general anesthesia for cardiac surgery. Anesthesiology. 2011;114:271–82.
24. Zhang S, Wu X, Guo H, Ma L. Thoracic epidural anesthesia improves outcomes in patients undergoing cardiac surgery: meta-analysis of randomized controlled trials. Eur J Med Res. 2015 Mar 15;20:25. https://doi.org/10.1186/s40001-015-0091-y.

25. Meylan N, Elia N, Lysakowski C, Tramer MR. Benefit and risk of intrathecal morphine without local anaesthetic in patients undergoing major surgery: meta-analysis of randomized trials. Br J Anaesth. 2009;102:156–67.

26. Neuburger PJ, Chacon MM, Luria BJ, Manrique-Espinel AM, Ngai JY, Grossi EA, Loulmet DF. Does paravertebral blockade facilitate immediate extubation after totally endoscopic robotic mitral valve repair surgery? Innovations (Phila). 2015;10(2):96–100.

27. Mashaqi B. Local anesthetics delivered through pleural drainages improve pain and lung function after cardiac surgery. Thorac Cardiovasc Surg. 2015;66(2):198–202.

28. Dowling R. Improved pain control after cardiac surgery: results of a randomized, double-blind, clinical trial. J Thorac Cardiovasc Surg. 2003;126(5):1271–8.

29. Khalil A. Ultrasound-guided serratus anterior plane block versus thoracic epidural analgesia for thoracotomy pain. J Cardiothorac Vasc Anesth. 2017;31(1):152–8.

Post Cardiac Surgery Rehabilitation

62

Neville Suskin, Charles Faubert, and Robert McKelvie

Main Messages

1. Cardiac rehabilitation consists of multidisciplinary patient care, with the goal to improve cardiovascular health by addressing a wide variety of issues pertaining to diet, exercise, psychological well-being and secondary prevention. In patients with coronary artery disease, it aims to stabilize and possibly decrease disease progression.

2. The first phase of cardiac rehabilitation begins immediately after cardiac surgery in the hospital setting, with staged physical activity resumption and patient information and support. After a post-discharge convalescence period, inpatient or outpatient programs follow. The typical duration for outpatient programs is 3–6 months. A lifelong process of lifestyle change begins when these supervised programs end.

3. Cardiac rehabilitation is shown to be of great benefit in regard to cardiovascular and quality-of-life outcomes in a wide variety of cardiac disease populations, and must be routinely prescribed to almost all postoperative cardiac surgery patients.

4. Despite solid evidence and widespread guideline recommendations, cardiac rehabilitation programs remain underutilized. All professionals involved in the care of patients with heart disease share the responsibility to enroll patients in these programs.

5. Older and/or vulnerable patients awaiting elective cardiac surgery may be considered for pre-habilitation (preoperative cardiac rehabilitation). Preoperative reconditioning aims to reduce postoperative complications and hospital length-of-stays, and to improve the patient's transition from the hospital to the community after their surgery.

N. Suskin (✉)
Cardiac Rehabilitation and Secondary Prevention Program, Division of Cardiology, Schulich School of Medicine and Dentistry, Western University, London, ON, Canada

St. Joseph's Health Care London, London, ON, Canada
e-mail: neville.suskin@lhsc.on.ca

C. Faubert
Hôpital Maisonneuve-Rosemont, Montreal, QC, Canada

R. McKelvie
St. Joseph's Health Care London, London, ON, Canada

Heart Failure, Cardiac Rehabilitation and Secondary Prevention Program, Division of Cardiology, Schulich School of Medicine and Dentistry, Western University, London, ON, Canada

© Springer Nature Switzerland AG 2021
D. C. H. Cheng et al. (eds.), *Evidence-Based Practice in Perioperative Cardiac Anesthesia and Surgery*, https://doi.org/10.1007/978-3-030-47887-2_62

Recent decades have seen a significant decline in cardiovascular disease (CVD) due to improved interventional therapy, pharmacological treatment and risk factor management. A number of interventions to prevent CVD have been shown to be cost-effective [1]. As stated by the European Association of Cardiovascular Prevention and Rehabilitation, "Cardiac patients after an acute event, intervention or diagnosis with a chronic heart condition deserve special attention to restore their quality of life, to maintain or improve functional capacity. They require counseling to prevent event recurrence, by adhesion to a medication plan and adoption of a healthy lifestyle" [2].

Cardiac rehabilitation (CR) is defined as "a multi-factorial and comprehensive intervention in secondary prevention, designed to limit the physiological and psychological effects of CVD, manage symptoms, and reduce the risk of future CV events" [3]. Around the central goals of improving outcomes and quality of life, exercise training, psychological issues, nutritional optimization and risk-factor control are addressed with patients. The typical CR team is multidisciplinary, working closely with a CR physician to optimize the individual patient's risk factors.

CR is of particular importance to cardiac surgery patients, both to implement effective secondary prevention measures early in the postoperative course and to help patients regain their pre-morbid functional level.

Objectives of Cardiac Rehabilitation Programs

In general, CR programs aim to improve patient fitness, to promote autonomy and the ability to resume normal activities after a cardiac event or intervention. In some studies, CR has been associated with reduced mortality [4].

Indications for Cardiac Rehabilitation Programs

The following post cardiac surgery diagnoses are accepted indications for CR [4]:

- Coronary artery bypass surgery
- Cardiac valve surgery
- Cardiac transplantation
- Ventricular assist device implantation

The Phases of Cardiac Rehabilitation and the Role of Professionals Working in Immediate Peri- and Postoperative Care

Cardiac surgery postoperative care has changed dramatically over the past decades. Where patients used to have a relatively prolonged postoperative hospital length-of-stay (LOS), the duration of stay has been significantly lowered by technical progress and administrative desire to cut costs. For coronary artery bypass graft (CABG) patients, the average LOS decreased from 11 to 8 days across the US from 1988 to 2005 [5]. With these changes, parts of the rehabilitation process that were formerly done in the hospital are now performed on an outpatient basis.

Traditionally, CR programs have been divided in the following four phases. We present them to help readers understand usual program structure, however it should be noted that some guidelines (Canadian, for example) use other terminology [4].

Phase 1: Immediate Inpatient Postoperative Period

Since the 1960s it has been known that bed rest significantly decreases exercise capacity. Early mobilization is now considered key to minimizing postoperative deconditioning [6]. The first phase of CR begins in the very early postoperative period. It aims to avoid inactivity and to maintain or improve pulmonary capacity and muscular strength [7].

As a result of sternotomy, most post cardiac surgery patients exhibit a restrictive disturbance with lowered pulmonary volumes, which can impact ventilation and oxygenation. Respiratory physiotherapy is in widespread use, although evidence for its use remains equivocal [7].

Healthcare professionals working with postoperative cardiac surgery patients should promote early ambulation and enrolment in CR programs, and reinforce the importance of healthy lifestyle habits in their discussions with patients.

Phase 2: Early Outpatient Phase

Immediately after their discharge from the hospital, patients are encouraged to start with short bouts of activity, initially around 10 min of continuous activity a few times a day. They then progress slowly to 30–40 min of continuous activity, three to five times a week. The easiest and most commonly prescribed exercise modality is walking. Post-sternotomy patients should exclude upper limb exercises, including resistance training, until the sternum is stable—approximately 2 months after the surgery [4].

This phase lasts for the few weeks between discharge and the beginning of the supervised CR program. Patients should begin activity gradually, as stated above. Ideally, delays between surgery and program intake should be short, as longer wait times are correlated with diminished positive outcomes. For post-CABG patients, preferable wait times have been established at 30 days from surgery [8].

Phase 3: Supervised Cardiac Rehabilitation Programs

Phase 3 consists of the supervised CR program. A full description of the usual components of these programs is found further in this chapter. While many models exist, typical outpatient programs last from 3 to 6 months [4].

Phase 4: Lifelong Changes

When patients complete the supervised CR program the expectation is they will continue the lifestyle changes. The time spent in the supervised CR program should promote the

necessary lifestyle changes required by the patient. There should be discussion with the patient about how they can best maintain an active and healthy lifestyle, including smoking cessation, adequate diet and sufficient exercise.

Components of Cardiac Rehabilitation Programs (Fig. 62.1)

Initial Patient Assessment

Typically, outpatient CR programs begin in the weeks following hospital discharge. Involving patients in a timely fashion following hospital discharge is important because there is some evidence that delayed entry into CR can negatively impact patient outcomes. For example, an observational study of 1241 patients referred for CR demonstrated lesser benefits regarding weight management and exercise capacity for patients whose intake to programs was over 30 days after hospital discharge when compared to patients with earlier intakes [9].

At the CR program intake visit, patients meet with a physician who reviews their medical history and performs a physical examination. An ECG is performed, and most programs have patients undergo symptom-limited exercise stress testing, either on a treadmill or cycle ergometer, with the addition of expired gas analysis (CPET) in some centres [10, 11]. Data from this test helps set the exercise prescription for exercise training and may help to detect safety issues.

Risk factors are assessed, including lipids, blood pressure, diabetes mellitus, and if required, smoking cessation. Medications are reviewed and optimized if patients are not at evidence-based targets.

Programs can be either home-based or centre-based. Home-based programs provide additional flexibility to patients and can be as effective as centre-based programs [12]. This can be particularly useful in certain categories of patients, for instance those with scheduling conflicts due to work obligations or those who have issues attending the CR Centre, because of distance.

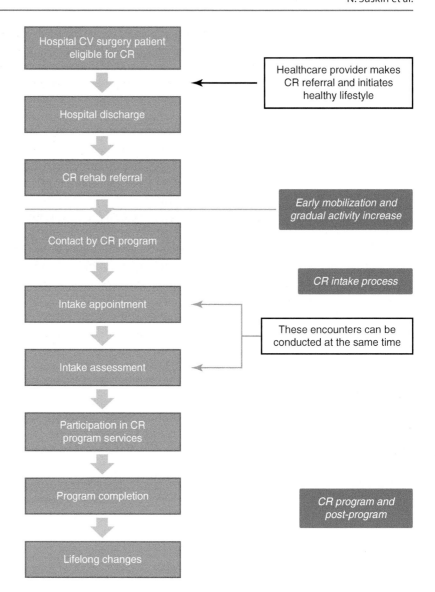

Fig. 62.1 Cardiac rehabilitation patient flow for CV surgery patients

Exercise Training and Physical Activity Counseling

Upon entering Cardiac Rehab programs, patients are stratified for exercise safety in categories outlined in the AHA Exercise Standards Guidelines [13]:

- Class A patients are apparently healthy and free of cardiac disease. Postoperative cardiovascular patients rarely fit into this category.
- Class B patients have presence of known, stable CVD with low risk for complications with vigor-

ous exercise, but slightly greater than for apparently healthy individuals. A typical example would be a post-CABG patient with complete revascularization and normal heart function.

- Class C patients are those at moderate to high risk for cardiac complications during exercise or those unable to self-regulate activity or to understand recommended activity level. This category could include, for instance, a heart failure patient with NYHA Class II or III symptoms, or patients with incomplete revascularization and inducible ischemia at low workloads.

- Class D patients have unstable disease with activity restriction. These patients typically do not undergo CR programs as exercise is contraindicated for them, and goal of care should be to restore them to Class C or better.

The majority of patients entering CR Programs will be categorized as either Class B or C [14]. Upon intake, they undergo exercise counseling that emphasizes the beneficial long-term effects of exercise for risk-factor control and its many positive effects. Moderate-intensity aerobic exercise for 30–60 min per session is usually suggested, preferably daily or at least 3–4 days a week. During the initial phases of the program, exercise supervision can be recommended, which may include ECG, blood pressure and/or heart rate monitoring. Class B patients can be monitored and supervised until they understand their desirable activity levels— usually 6–12 sessions. Home-based exercise programs can also be appropriate for patients from this category, in which case supervision only occurs during initial patient encounters. Although no strong evidence for this practice exists, and many CR models do not use ECG monitoring with exercise after the intake exercise stress test [4], American Heart Association Guidelines suggest that Class C patients can be supervised with ECG monitoring until they understand what level of activity is safe, and until the medical team determines that the activity level is effective and well-tolerated, usually for at least 12 sessions [14].

An exercise mode is determined with consideration to patient preference, and may include, for example, walking, jogging, cycling, and rowing. It is important to select a mode of physical activity that is enjoyable for patients to maximize the chances of them keeping up with physical activity once programs end. Programs traditionally focused on moderate intensity continuous training. Interest in high-intensity interval training (HIIT) as an alternative in patients with CVD has emerged in recent years. HIIT alternates short periods of intense aerobic exercise with recovery periods, and appears to be safe and at least as effective as moderate intensity training, although more research is still needed [15].

Resistance training can be included in CR programs, as increased strength has additional benefits to purely aerobic training. Post-sternotomy patients often have chest wall symptoms that require individualized strength training strategies, once the 2-month period required for sternal stabilization has passed.

Nutritional and Weight Counseling

Most CR programs should include nutritional assessment and education with a nutritionist/dietitian. An initial appointment will include analysis of dietary patterns, caloric intake, lipid and other macronutrient intake. Dietary goals will be reviewed with patients. Weight is assessed, and overweight status is determined either by BMI (>25) or waist circumference (>94 cm in men or >80 cm in women). Obesity is defined as BMI > 30 or waist circumference > 102 cm in men and >88 cm in women. Weight reduction is recommended to obese and overweight patients, with a usual target of 5–10% total weight loss [2].

Healthy food choices are reviewed with patients, including what to avoid and healthy alternatives—for instance, replacing saturated fats with mono- and polyunsaturated fats from vegetable and marine sources.

Adherence to the Mediterranean Diet can also be promoted by CR programs. This diet has attracted much attention in recent years, starting from the observation that European countries located around the Mediterranean Sea have lower CVD incidence and prevalence than North American and Northern European countries. It is characterized by a high intake of olive oil, fruit, nuts, vegetables, and cereals; a moderate intake of fish and poultry; a low intake of dairy products, red meat, processed meats, and sweets; and wine in moderation, consumed with meals [16]. Some evidence exists supporting the Mediterranean diet for the primary [16] and secondary [17] prevention of CVD.

Risk Factor Management: Smoking Cessation, Blood Pressure Control, Diabetes Control, Lipids Optimization

As part of CR programs, all smokers are counseled to stop smoking with interventions that can include education, referral to smoking cessation programs and pharmacotherapy.

Lipid levels are measured, and treatment optimized to specific targets that have demonstrated benefits in patients with CVD. Blood pressure is assessed, with hypertension managed as required through lifestyle modification and pharmacotherapy when needed.

Patients with diabetes mellitus require special attention regarding nutrition counseling and exercise prescription. Their dietary counseling is different than for general cardiovascular patients, and special attention is given to the carbohydrate content of foods and to hypoglycemia if patients are on at-risk medication. Exercise prescription must also consider the risk of hypoglycemia with exercise, and assess hypoglycemia awareness in patients and the possible need for additional snacks before or after exercise.

Psychosocial Support

Anxiety and depression are frequent and under-recognized complications of CVD. They occur in up to 20% of patients after a myocardial infarction [18], and between 30 and 40% of post-CABG patients [19]. Consequently, it is important that patients who undertake CR programs should be screened with standardized tools for psychological distress, including depression. Individual or group education sessions on adjustment to heart disease, stress management, and health-related lifestyle changes may be offered. Psychologists can provide invaluable help to patients with difficulty adjusting to their new health status [2].

The Prehabilitation Model

Elective cardiovascular surgery can be scheduled weeks or months in advance, whether the planned surgery is for CABG for stable CAD or an aortic valve replacement surgery for slowly progressive severe aortic stenosis. Patients who are waiting for their surgery often reduce their physical activity because of symptoms, but also because of anxiety and fear [20].

The prehabilitation model—"prehab"—aims to optimize patient function while awaiting an upcoming intervention. The goals include optimizing nutrition, implementing appropriate exercise training, and exploring psychological issues. Few stuides exist regarding the clinical impact of prehab in cardiovascular surgery patients. In one study, 249 patients awaiting elective CABG were randomized to either an 8-week preoperative cardiac prehab program or to usual care [21]. Prehab included two exercise sessions per week and education classes on risk factor modification. Participants in the intervention group experienced shorter intensive care unit (ICU) and hospital LOS and an improved quality of life. It is however notable that participants in that study were younger and do not represent the typical frail patients whom we might typically consider for prehab.

As of this writing, prehab programs are not widespread, and the limited evidence that is available does not clearly indicate which patients may benefit the most from this intervention. Randomized controlled trials in cardiovascular surgical populations are currently underway and may clarify the role of prehab in this population in the near future [22].

Specific Cardiovascular Surgical Populations

CABG

The value of CR is very well established in patients who are recuperating from a CABG. Following surgery it is important to involve the patient in CR to manage the risk factors that were initially responsible for the CAD that required surgery. CR programs help to manage these risk factors, including exercise training to improve exercise capacity and thus limit the progression of atherosclerosis.

A 2016 updated Cochrane systematic review and meta-analysis that included 63 studies with

14,486 participants who underwent either percutaneous coronary intervention (PCI) or CABG found a reduction in cardiovascular mortality (relative risk: 0.74; 95% confidence interval: 0.64–0.86) and the risk of hospital admissions (relative risk: 0.82; 95% confidence interval: 0.70–0.96) with exercise-based CR, though no reduction in all-cause mortality, myocardial infarction, and revascularization was found [23]. In a number of the randomized studies included in the Cochrane meta-analysis (14/20), higher levels of health-related quality of life were demonstrated after exercise-based CR compares with control subjects. At least one observational study specific to post-CABG patients has suggested a reduction in long-term mortality (reported as 12.7% absolute risk reduction at 10 years in one study [24]).

Base on this evidence, current guidelines from the American College of Cardiology Foundation/ American Heart Association give a grade IA recommendation for CR for all patients who undergo CABG [25]. This recommendation is mirrored by the current guidelines on myocardial revascularization (that include PCI or CABG) from the European Society of Cardiology/European Association for Cardio Thoracic Surgery [26], who gave a Class IIA recommendation for CR after CABG and a class IA recommendation for advice on lifestyle changes, including smoking cessation, regular physical activity, and a healthy diet.

Valve Replacement

As most valvular disease is now degenerative in nature [27], patients who undergo valve replacement therapy tend to be of advanced age, and tend to have much comorbidity—cardiovascular and otherwise. Many of them are classified NYHA III or IV preoperatively [28]. Without CR, the average NYHA improvement at 6 months postoperatively is one class [29]. Prototypical valvular surgery patients often exhibit deep preoperative deconditioning, and would logically benefit greatly from an exercise program that aims to improve function.

However, evidence remains scarce in this population. A 2016 Cochrane review found only two studies eligible for review, with 148 total participants, and concluded that CR may improve exercise capacity in this population, but lacked evidence to draw a conclusion regarding other outcomes including mortality and cardiovascular events [30].

Current European guidelines for heart valve surgery recommend exercise training as part of postoperative rehabilitation, especially if the postoperative course is complicated by heart failure [31]. No mention of CR is made in the ACC/ AHA guidelines [32, 33]. As no international guidelines or consensus statements concerning the recommendation of CR to this specific population exist, it remains based mainly on expert opinion. A more recent cost-effectiveness study suggested that CR programs are likely to be cost-effective for society, suggesting that benefits are worthy of the extra costs of providing CR [34].

Program structure for valve surgery patients usually mirrors that of post-CABG patients, as they experience similar postoperative challenges, like pleural effusions, neurological or respiratory complications, and surgical site-related issues [4].

Heart Transplant

Heart transplant patients usually have a rapid rise in their exercise capacity in the months following the transplant, but remain with lower exercise capacity and worse long-term outcomes than normal adults. Most studies on this population show maximal VO_2 levels of only 50–70% of expected levels in the months and years after surgery [35]. A combination of preop and postop conditions contribute to limited exercise capacity—transplant patients typically have marked preoperative deconditioning due to severe heart failure, and chronotropic incompetence secondary to cardiac denervation (higher resting heart rate and lower heart rate response to exercise). They are also treated with medications that can alter cardiovascular and muscular physiology, including high-dose corticosteroids that may induce myopathy.

A 2017 Cochrane Database review found moderate-quality evidence from nine trials showing that exercise-based CR increased exercise capacity compared with a no-exercise control, although there was no impact on health-related quality of life (HRQoL) in the short term [36]. Overall, clinicians should understand that replacing a malfunctioning heart will not reverse a patient's exercise limitations by itself, as peripheral factors that were a consequence of long-standing heart disease need to be addressed, and CR programs may do so.

Timeliness of enrolment into CR appears to be important, as was shown in a trial that demonstrated improved cardiopulmonary exercise measures with enrolment 2 weeks after surgery compared to an unstructured therapy at home [37].

Patients should be referred to CR for prehabilitation prior to their transplant to familiarize themselves with the different exercise modes and to facilitate early post-transplant rehabilitation [38]. This program typically includes aerobic and resistance training, which are safe when supervised in this population.

Availability and Underutilization of Cardiac Rehabilitation Programs

Despite the strength of the aforementioned evidence, CR remains underutilized and is unequally available in different countries. A 2014 review found CR services in fewer than 40% of all countries, including only 68% of the countries defined as high income by the World Bank [7]. Even in resource-rich countries, CR is underutilized despite supporting evidence. Although reports vary in their estimates, a 2011 Presidential Advisory from the American Heart Association mentions utilization rates of only 14–35% in survivors of a myocardial infarction and less than 31% in post-CABG surgical patients [39].

All healthcare professionals who work in the care of CV surgical patients have a duty to promote a healthy lifestyle and management of risk factors. Referrals to CR programs should be routine in this population.

References

1. Ades PA, Pashkow FJ, Nestor JR. Cost-effectiveness of cardiac rehabilitation after myocardial infarction. J Cardiopulm Rehabil. 1997;17(4):222–31.
2. Piepoli MF, Corrà U, et al. Secondary prevention through cardiac rehabilitation: from knowledge to implementation. A position paper from the Cardiac Rehabilitation Section of the European Association of Cardiovascular Prevention and Rehabilitation. Eur J Cardiovasc Prev Rehabil. 2010;17(1):1–17. https://doi.org/10.1097/HJR.0b013e3283313592.
3. Piepoli MF, Corrà U, Dendale P, et al. Challenges in secondary prevention after acute myocardial infarction: a call for action. Eur J Prev Cardiol. 2016;23:1994–2006.
4. Stone JA, Arthur HM, Suskin N, editors. Canadian guidelines for cardiac rehabilitation and cardiovascular disease prevention: translating knowledge into action. 3rd ed. Winnipeg, MB: Canadian Association of Cardiac Rehabilitation; 2009. isbn:978-0-9685851-3-9.
5. Swaminathan M, Phillips-Bute BG, Patel UD, et al. Increasing healthcare resource utilization after coronary artery bypass graft surgery in the United States. Circ Cardiovasc Qual Outcomes. 2009;2(4):305–12.
6. Saltin B, Blomqvist G, Mitchell JH, Johnson RL, Wildenthal K, Chapman CB. Response to exercise after bed rest and after training. Circulation. 1968;38:VII1–78.
7. Turk-Adawi K, Sarrafzadegan N, Grace SL. Global availability of cardiac rehabilitation. Nat Rev Cardiol. 2014;11:586–96.
8. Grace SL, Poirier P, Norris CM, Oakes GH, Somanader DS, Suskin N, Canadian Association of Cardiac Rehabilitation. Pan-Canadian development of cardiac rehabilitation and secondary prevention quality indicators. Can J Cardiol. 2014;30(8):945–8. https://doi.org/10.1016/j.cjca.2014.04.003.
9. Johnson DA, Sacrinty MT, Gomadam PS, et al. Effect of early enrollment on outcomes in cardiac rehabilitation. Am J Cardiol. 2014;114(12):1908–11.
10. Piepoli MF, Corrà U, Benzer W, et al. Secondary prevention through cardiac rehabilitation: from knowledge to implementation. A position paper from the Cardiac Rehabilitation Section of the European Association of Cardiovascular Prevention and Rehabilitation. Eur J Cardiovasc Prev Rehabil. 2010;7(1):1–17. https://doi.org/10.1097/HJR.0b013e3283313592.
11. Balady GJ, Williams MA, Ades PA, et al. Core components of cardiac rehabilitation/secondary prevention programs: 2007 update. A scientific statement from the American Heart Association Exercise, Cardiac Rehabilitation, and Prevention Committee, the Council on Clinical Cardiology; the Councils on Cardiovascular Nursing, Epidemiology and Prevention, and Nutrition, Physical Activity, and Metabolism; and the American Association

of Cardiovascular and Pulmonary Rehabilitation. Circulation. 2007;115:2675–82.

12. Anderson L, Sharp GA, Norton RJ, et al. Home-based versus centre-based cardiac rehabilitation. Cochrane Database Syst Rev. 2017;6:CD007130. https://doi.org/10.1002/14651858.CD007130.pub4.

13. Fletcher G, Ades P, Kligfield P, et al. Exercise standards for testing and training: a scientific statement from the American heart association. Circulation. 2013;128(8):873–934. https://doi.org/10.1161/CIR.0b013e31829b5b44.

14. Fletcher GF, Balady GJ, Amsterdam EA, et al. Exercise standards for testing and training: a statement for healthcare professionals from the American Heart Association. Circulation. 2001;104:1694–740.

15. Elliott AD, Rajopadhyaya K, Bentley DJ, et al. Interval training versus continuous exercise in patients with coronary artery disease: a meta-analysis. Heart Lung Circ. 2015;24:149–57.

16. Estruch R, Ros E, Salas-Salvadó J, et al. Primary prevention of cardiovascular disease with a Mediterranean diet. NEJM. 2013;369(7):676–7. https://doi.org/10.1056/NEJMc1306659.

17. Sikic J, Stipcevic M, Vrazic H, et al. Nutrition in primary and secondary prevention of cardiovascular risk in the continental and Mediterranean regions of Croatia. BMC Cardiovasc Disord. 2017;17(1):247. https://doi.org/10.1186/s12872-017-0678-z.

18. Milani RV, Lavie CJ, Cassidy MM. Effects of cardiac rehabilitation and exercise training programs on depression in patients after major coronary events. Am Heart J. 1996;132(4):726–32.

19. Tully PJ, Baker RA. Depression, anxiety, and cardiac morbidity outcomes after coronary artery bypass surgery: a contemporary and practical review. J Geriatr Cardiol. 2012 Jun;9(2):197–208.

20. Sawatzky J-AV, Stammers AN, Kehler DS, et al. Prehabilitation program for elective coronary artery bypass graft surgery patients: a pilot randomized controlled study. Clin Rehabil. 2014;28(7):648–57. https://doi.org/10.1177/0269215513516475.

21. Arthur HM, Daniels C, McKelvie R, Hirsh J, Rush B. Effect of a preoperative intervention on preoperative and postoperative outcomes in low-risk patients awaiting elective. Ann Intern Med. 2000;133(4):253–62. https://doi.org/10.7326/0003-4819-133-4-200008150-00007.

22. Stammers AN, Kehler DS, Afilalo J, et al. Protocol for the PREHAB study—pre-operative rehabilitation for reduction of hospitalization after coronary bypass and valvular surgery: a randomised controlled trial. BMJ Open. 2015;5:e007250. https://doi.org/10.1136/bmjopen-2014-007250.

23. Anderson L, Oldridge N, Thompson DR, et al. Exercise-based cardiac rehabilitation for coronary heart disease: Cochrane systematic review and meta-analysis. J Am Coll Cardiol. 2016;67(1):1–12.

24. Goel K, Pack QR, Lahr B, et al. Cardiac rehabilitation is associated with reduced long-term mortality in patients undergoing combined heart valve and CABG surgery. Eur J Prev Cardiol. 2015;22:159–68.

25. Hillis LD, Smith PK, Anderson JL, et al. 2011 ACCF/AHA guideline for coronary artery bypass graft surgery: a report of the American College of Cardiology Foundation/American Heart Association Task Force on Practice Guidelines. Circulation. 2011;124:e652–735.

26. Windecker S, Kolh P, Alfonso F, et al. 2014 ESC/EACTS guidelines on myocardial revascularization: the task force on myocardial revascularization of the European Society of Cardiology (ESC) and the European Association for Cardio-Thoracic Surgery (EACTS) developed with the special contribution of the European Association of Percutaneous Cardiovascular Interventions (EAPCI). Eur Heart J. 2014;35:2541–619.

27. Nkomo VT, Gardin JM, Skelton TN, et al. Burden of valvular heart diseases: a population-based study. Lancet. 2006;368(9540):1005–11.

28. Khan JH, McElhinney DB, Hall TS, et al. Cardiac valve surgery in octagenarians improving quality of life and functional status. Arch Surg. 1998;133:887–93.

29. Carstens V, Behrenbeck DW, Hilger HH. Exercise capacity before and after cardiac valve surgery. Cardiology. 1983;70:41–9.

30. Sibilitz KL, Berg SK, Tang LH, et al. Exercise-based cardiac rehabilitation for adults after heart valve surgery. Cochrane Database Syst Rev. 2016;3:CD010876. https://doi.org/10.1002/14651858.CD010876.pub2.

31. Butchart EG, Gohlke-Bärwolf C, Antunes MJ, et al. Recommendations for the management of patients after heart valve surgery. Eur Heart J. 2005;26:2463–71.

32. Nishimura RA, Otto CM, Bonow RO, et al. 2014 AHA/ACC guideline for the management of patients with valvular heart disease: executive summary: a report of the American College of Cardiology/American Heart Association Task Force On Practice Guidelines. Circulation. 2014;129:2440–92. https://doi.org/10.1161/CIR.0000000000000029.

33. Nishimura RA, Otto CM, et al. 2017 AHA/ACC focused update of the 2014 AHA/ACC guideline for the management of patients with valvular heart disease: a report of the American College of Cardiology/American Heart Association Task Force on Clinical Practice Guidelines. Circulation. 2017 Jun 20;135(25):e1159–95. https://doi.org/10.1161/CIR.0000000000000503.

34. Hansen TB, Zwisler AD, Berg SK, et al. Cost-utility analysis of cardiac rehabilitation after conventional heart valve surgery versus usual care. Eur J Prev Cardiol. 2017 May;24(7):698–707. https://doi.org/10.1177/2047487317689908.

35. Ades PA, Savage PD, Brawner CA, et al. Aerobic capacity in patients entering cardiac rehabilitation. Circulation. 2006;113(23):2706–12.

36. Nytrøen K, Gullestad L. Exercise after heart transplantation: an overview. World J Transplant. 2013 Dec 24;3(4):78–90. https://doi.org/10.5500/wjt.v3.i4.78.

37. Anderson L, Nguyen TT, et al. Exercise-based cardiac rehabilitation in heart transplant recipients. Cochrane Database Syst Rev. 2017;4:CD012264. https://doi.org/10.1002/14651858.CD012264. pub2.

38. Piña IL, Apstein CS, Balady GJ, et al. Exercise and heart failure: a statement from the American Heart Association Committee on exercise, rehabilitation, and prevention. Circulation. 2003;107(8):1210.

39. Balady G, Ades P, Bittner V, et al. Referral, enrollment, and delivery of cardiac rehabilitation/secondary prevention programs at clinical centers and beyond. A presidential advisory from the American Heart Association. Circulation. 2011;124(25):2951–60.

Appendices: Example Order Sets and Embedded Modules

© Springer Nature Switzerland AG 2021
D. C. H. Cheng et al. (eds.), *Evidence-Based Practice in Perioperative Cardiac Anesthesia and Surgery*, https://doi.org/10.1007/978-3-030-47887-2

Appendix A Cardiovascular Surgery Pre-Op

DO NOT THIN FROM HEALTH RECORD

Provider (SIGNATURE)	Date	Time
Provider (PRINT)		
Processor	Date	Time
Nurse	Date	Time

CARDIO SURG - Cardiovascular Surgery, Pre-Op

Inc	Req	ORDER	SPECIAL INSTRUCTIONS
Diet			
X		Surgery Clear Fluids	
		Up until 3 hours prior to surgery, max 500 mL. May take medications with sips.	
Activity			
		Activity as Tolerated	
Vital Signs			
		Vital Signs	
		per protocol (Def)	
		daily	
		q1 hour.	
		q12 hours.	
		q2 hours.	
		q3 hours.	
		q30 days	
		q30 minutes	
		q4 hours.	
		q6 hours.	
		q8 hours.	
		weekly	
Patient Care			
		Communication Order	
		If radial artery surgery, place all identification arm bands, allergy bands, and IVs in DOMINANT non surgical ARM	
		Communication Order	
		initiate coronary artery bypass graft pathway	
		Discontinue Telemetry	
		prior to transfering to the operating room	
		Peripheral IV Insertion	

Inc	Req	ORDER	SPECIAL INSTRUCTIONS
		Saline Lock Insertion	
X		Weight	
		ONCE, morning of surgery	
Continuous Infusions			
		lactated ringers	
		IV continuous, 75 mL/hr (Def)	
		IV continuous, 50 mL/hr	
		IV continuous, 100 mL/hr	
		IV continuous, 125 mL/hr	
		sodium chloride 0.9%	
		IV continuous, 75 mL/hr (Def)	
		IV continuous, 50 mL/hr	
		IV continuous, 100 mL/hr	
		IV continuous, 125 mL/hr	
Medications			
		Venous Thromboembolism Prophylaxis module to be implem when this powerplan is being used for the initial admission orderset. (Note)	
		COMMON - Venous Thromboembolism (VTE) Prophylaxis ((LHSC-UH, VC, PW, STEGH, TDMH)	
		Consider holding: calcium channel blocker, ACE inhibitor, beta blocker, ARB, oral hypoglycemics, insulin, non acetylsalicylic acid anti-platelets, anticoagulants, non acetylsalicylic acid anti-coagulants (Note)	
X		chlorhexidine 4% topical soap	
		1 application, soap, TOPICAL, BID (Def)	
		Comments - If BMI less than 30 use 2 skin preps, starting with the first one the night before surgery and one the morning of surgery. If BMI equal to or greater than 30 use 5 skin preps starting 2 days prior to surgery in am and pm including morning of surgery. Discontinue chlorhexidine after last skin prep.	
		5 application, soap, TOPICAL, as directed	
		Comments - If BMI less than or equal to 30 use 2 skin preps, 1 the night before surgery, one the morning of surgery. If BMI greater than 30 use 5 skin preps starting 2 days prior to surgery in am and pm including morning of surgery.	
Antimicrobials			
		ceFAZolin	
		2 g, injection, IV, on CALL, for: 1 dose	
		Comments - Dose #1 send to OR with patient, to be given prior to procedure	
		ceFAZolin	
		2 g, injection, IV, on CALL, for: 1 dose	
		Comments - Dose #2 send to OR with patient, to be given 3 hours into procedure	

		vancomycin	
		1 g, injection, IV, on CALL, infuse over 60 min, for: 1 dose	
		Comments - START DRUG WHEN PATIENT CALLE	
		PICS PREVENA STUDY protocol (Nov 25, 2019 - Sept 30, (Note)	
		ceFAZolin	
		2 g, injection, IV, on CALL, for: 1 dose, PICS PREVENA STUDY (Def)	
		Comments - Dose #1 send to OR with patient, to be given prior to procedure. For weight less than 120 kg.	
		3 g, injection, IV, on CALL, for: 1 dose, PICS PREVENA STUDY	
		Comments - Dose #1 send to OR with patient, to be given prior to procedure. For weight greater than or equal to 120 kg.	
		ceFAZolin	
		2 g, injection, IV, on CALL, for: 1 dose, PICS PREVENA STUDY (Def)	
		Comments - Dose #2 send to OR with patient, to be given 4 hours into procedure. For weight less than 120 kg.	
		3 g, injection, IV, on CALL, for: 1 dose, PICS PREVENA STUDY	
		Comments - Dose #2 send to OR with patient, to be given 4 hours into procedure. For weight greater than or equal to 120 kg.	
		vancomycin	
		1 g, injection, IV, on CALL, infuse over 60 min, for: 1 dose, PICS PREVENA STUDY (Def)	
		Comments - START DRUG WHEN PATIENT CALLE OR. For weight less than 85 kg	
		1.5 g, injection, IV, on CALL, infuse over 90 min, for: 1 dose, PICS PREVENA STUDY	
		Comments - START DRUG WHEN PATIENT CALLE OR. For weight greater than or equal to 85 kg	
Laboratory			
X		Complete Blood Count (CBC)	
		Now, T;N, Blood	
X		Electrolytes,Serum,Plasma (LYTE)	
		Now, T;N, Blood	
X		Creatinine (CRE)	
		Now, T;N, Blood	
X		Urea (U)	
		Now, T;N, Blood	
X		Glucose,Random (GLUR)	
		Now, T;N, Blood	
X		LIPIDS (Chol, Trig, HDL, LDL)	
		Now, T;N, Blood	
X		Glycated Hemoglobin (GLYHB)	

		Now, T;N, Blood	
X		Alanine Aminotransferase (ALT)	
		Now, T;N, Blood	
X		Aspartate Aminotransferase (AST)	
		Now, T;N, Blood	
X		Bilirubin, Total (BILT)	
		Now, T;N, Blood	
X		Alkaline Phosphatase (ALP)	
		Now, T;N, Blood	
X		INRPTT	
		Now, T;N, Blood	
X		Group and Screen	
		Now, T;N, Blood	
Diagnostic Imaging			
X		Chest PA/Lat	
		pre-op cardiac surgery	
X		ECG 12 Lead	
		T;N	
		US Carotid Doppler Bilat	
		to rule out stenosis	
		Echo Routine	
		RESP - Inpatient Pulmonary Function (PF) (Module)	
Consults			
		Consult to Physician	
		Service: Anesthesia	

Last Modified: 2020/01/03

A.1 Inpatient Pulmonary Function

DO NOT THIN FROM HEALTH RECORD

Provider (SIGNATURE)	Date	Time
Provider (PRINT)		
Processor	Date	Time
Nurse	Date	Time

RESP - Inpatient Pulmonary Function (PF) (Module)

Inc	Req	ORDER	SPECIAL INSTRUCTIONS
		Other Diagnostic Testing/Treatment	
		Full Pulmonary Function Tests	
		Respirology consult REQUIRED for Full PFTs	
		Consult to Physician	
		Service: Respirology	
		Full Pulmonary Function Tests (Spirometry, Lung Volumes, DLCO, Blood Gas)	
		Full Pulmonary Function Test Without Blood Gas (Spirometr Lung Volumes, DLCO)	
		Individual Pulmonary Function Tests	
		DO NOT ORDER individual: Spirometry, Lung Volumes or Bl Gas if Full PFT was ordered above	
		Spirometry	
		Pre and Post Bronchodilator	
		Seated and Supine (FVC)	
		MIPS and MEPS	
		Lung Volumes	
		Lung Volumes by Body Plethysmography	
		Estimate of Shunt Fraction	
		Flow Volume Loop (calc. for upper airway obstruction)	
		Blood Gas	
		Home O2 Assessment	

Last Modified: 2015/09/15

Appendix B Cardiovascular Surgery Post-Op

DO NOT THIN FROM HEALTH RECORD

Provider (SIGNATURE)	Date	Time	
Provider (PRINT)			
Processor	Date	Time	
Nurse	Date	Time	

CARDIO SURG - Cardiovascular Surgery, Post-Op, Critical Care

Inc	Req	ORDER	SPECIAL INSTRUCTIONS
Resuscitation Status			
		Please ensure the resuscitation documentation is completed/reviewed	
Alerts			
		Airborne Precautions	
		Contact Precautions	
		Droplet Precautions	
		Droplet/Contact Precautions	
Diet			
X		NPO	
Activity			
X		Activity as Tolerated	
		Up in chair for meals Post-Op day 1	
X		Dangle Legs at Bedside	
		prior to chest tube removal	
Vital Signs			
X		Vital Signs	
		per protocol (Def)	
		daily.	
		q1 hour.	
		q12 hours.	
		q2 hours.	
		q3 hours.	
		q30 days	
		q30 minutes	
		q4 hours.	
		q6 hours.	
		q8 hours.	
		weekly	
X		Temperature	

Inc	Req	ORDER	SPECIAL INSTRUCTIONS
		q4 hours.	
X		Continuous Oxygen Saturation	
X		Cardiac Monitoring	
		Assessment ICU	
X		Central Venous Pressure Monitoring	
		q1 hour.	
X		Systolic Blood Pressure Target	
Patient Care			
X		NO BP or Blood work	
		or IV start in radial graft arm until POD #7	
X		Oxygen Therapy	
X		Oxygen Titration	
		Target: SpO2 greater than or equal to 92% (Def)	
		Target: SpO2 88-92% for CO2 Retention	
X		POC Specimen LABEL - Blood Gas	
		Blood Gas - Arterial	
X		Urinary Catheter to Urometer	
X		Intake and Output	
		q1 hour.	
X		Notify Provider	
		if urine output less than 20 mL for 2 consecutive hours, call CSRU team.	
		Cardiac Output	
		q4 hours., and PRN	
X		Chest Tube Care/Monitor	
		Water-Seal Suction -20 cm, Notify provider if total drainage greater than 150 mL/hour x 2 hours	
X		Arterial Line Care and Monitoring	
X		Central Line Care	
		Discontinue Arterial Line	
		discontinue femoral line at 4 hours post-op if stable and INR/PTT are within normal range	
X		Convert IV to Saline Lock	
		when drinking well	
		Drain/Tube Care	
		Other:, endoscopic drain, remove morning of POD#1	
		Drain/Tube Care	
		for endoscopic sites	
X		Do Not Remove Dressing - Reinforce Only	
		x 48 hours for surgical site dressings	
X		Wound Care	

		When chest dressing removed, cleanse with normal saline & apply dry gauze dressing lightly and secured as long as patient is monitored	
		Tensor Bandages	
		Remove and re-wrap tensor bandages each shift. Discontinue tensor wrap (arm or leg) post op day #2.	
X		Communication Order	
		pacer wires secured and visible if present	
		Pacemaker Settings Temporary Transvenous/Epicardial	
		Epicardial, VVI, Ventricular (mV) 2, Atrial (mA) 0, Atrial (mV) 0	
		CARDIO - Intra-Aortic Balloon Pump (IABP) (Module)	
		CARDIO SURG - RVAD/LVAD/Centrimag/HeartMate II/Hear Post-Op, Critical Care (Module)	
		CARDIO SURG - Lumbar Drain with Elephant/Frozen Eleph Trunk Procedure (Module)	
		CARDIO SURG - Extracorporeal Membrane Oxygenation, E (Module)	
X		sodium chloride 0.9% arterial line flush	
		500 mL, intra-ARTERIAL, to keep line open, Total volume (mL): 500	
X		dextrose 5%-sodium chloride 0.9%	
		1,000 mL, IV continuous, 80 mL/hr	
		lactated ringers	
		IV continuous, 100 mL/hr	
		Comments - for one hour. Reduce to TKVO ONLY if patient on inotropes or vasopressors.	
Medications			
X		COMMON - Venous Thromboembolism (VTE) Prophylaxis ((LHSC-UH, VC, PW, STEGH, TDMH)	
X		CRIT CARE - Electrolyte Replacement (Module)	
X		CRIT CARE - Insulin Infusion (Module)	
X		CARDIO SURG - Ventilation and Rapid Wean (Module)	
		CRIT CARE - Sedation (Module)	
		COMMON - Warfarin (Coumadin) Daily Dosing (Module)	
X		sodium chloride 0.9% flush	
		3 mL, syringe, IV direct, as directed, PRN Other: See Comments	
		Comments - peripheral device maintenance	
X		sodium chloride 0.9% flush	
		10 mL, injection, IV direct, as directed, PRN Other: See Comments	
		Comments - central device maintenance	
Analgesics			
X		acetaminophen	
		650 mg, tab, ORAL, q6 hours, for: 3 day, Start: T;N	
		Comments - max 4 g acetaminophen in 24 hr from all sources	
X		acetaminophen	

		650 mg, tab, ORAL, q6 hours, PRN for pain, Start: T+3;0600	
		Comments - max 4 g acetaminophen in 24 hr from all sources	
		HYDROmorphone injection	
		0.4 mg, injection, IV direct, q30 minutes PRN for pain	
		Comments - until extubated, give 0.4 mg for severe pain, give 0.2 mg for moderate pain	
		HYDROmorphone	
		0.5 mg, tab, ORAL, q3 hours PRN for pain, for: 5 day	
		1 mg, tab, ORAL, q3 hours PRN for pain, for: 5 day	
		2 mg, tab, ORAL, q3 hours PRN for pain, for: 5 day	
Antiplatelets			
		acetylsalicylic acid	
		81 mg, EC tab, ORAL, ONCE, Start: T;N+360	
		Comments - Give 6-24 hours post op when patient is extubated.	
X		acetylsalicylic acid	
		81 mg, EC tab, ORAL, daily, Start: T+1;0800	
		Comments - If platelet count less than 100,000 or blood loss greater than 100 mL in any hour, verify with MD before administering acetylsalicylic acid.	
		acetylsalicylic acid	
		150 mg, supp, RECTAL, ONCE	
		Comments - 6 hours post op. If platelet count less than 100,000 or blood loss greater than 100 mL in any hour, verify with MD before administering acetylsalicylic acid.	
		clopidogrel	
		75 mg, tab, ORAL, daily, Start: T+4;0800	
		ticagrelor	
		90 mg, tab, ORAL, BID, Start: T+4;0800	
Antimicrobials			
		ceFAZolin	
		1 g, injection, IV, q8 hours, for: 48 hr	
		Comments - For aortic or valve surgery give for a total of 48 hours. For all other cardiac surgery give one dose of antibiotics post chest tube removal (to a maximum of 48 hours)	
		vancomycin	
		1 g, injection, IV, q12 hours, infuse over 60 min, order duration: 48 hr	
		Comments - For aortic or valve surgery give for a total of 48 hours. For all other cardiac surgery give one dose of antibiotics post chest tube removal (to a maximum of 48 hours)	
Antiemetics/GI Prophylaxis			
X		ondansetron injection	
		4 mg, injection, IV direct, q8 hours, PRN for nausea or vomiting (Def)	

		4 mg, injection, IV, q8 hours, PRN for nausea or vomiting	
X		pantoprazole injection	
		40 mg, injection, IV, daily, infuse over 30 min, Start: T+1;0800	
		Comments - if no enteral route available	
X		lansoprazole	
		30 mg, DR cap, ORAL, daily, Start: T+1;0800	
		Comments - if enteral route available	
Bowel Routine			
X		senna	
		8.6 mg, tab, ORAL, bedtime, for: 2 dose, Start: T+2;2200	
X		senna	
		8.6 mg, tab, ORAL, bedtime, PRN for constipation, Start: T+4;2200	
X		bisacodyl	
		10 mg, supp, RECTAL, ONCE, Start: T+3;0800	
		Comments - if no bowel movement since surgery	
X		bisacodyl	
		10 mg, supp, RECTAL, daily, PRN for constipation, Start: T+2;0800	
Critical Care Medications			
		nitroglycerin 50 mg in 250 mL dextrose 5% premix	
		dextrose 5% premix diluent (titrate)	
		Titration Range: 0-150 mcg/min, Routine, titrate	
		nitroglycerin -additive	
		50, mg, Every Bag	
		EPINEPHrine 1 mg in 50 mL dextrose 5% premix	
		dextrose 5% premix diluent (titrate)	
		Titration Range: 0 - 5 mcg/min, Routine, titrate, Contact Physician when high dose required	
		EPINEPHrine - additive	
		1, mg	
		milrinone 40 mg in 40 mL diluent premix	
		premix diluent	
		IV continuous	
		Comments - Usual range 0-0.25 mcg/kg/min	
		milrinone - additive	
		40 mg, mcg/kg/min	
		norepinephrine 4 mg in 50 mL dextrose 5% premix	
		dextrose 5% premix diluent (titrate)	
		Titration Range: 0-7 mcg/min	
		norepinephrine - additive	
		4, mg	
		vasopressin 50 units in 50 mL dextrose 5%	

		dextrose 5% in water (titrate)	
		Titration Range: 0-2.4 unit/hr, IV continuous	
		vasopressin - additive	
		50 units, Every Bag	
Laboratory			
X		Complete Blood Count (CBC)	
		STAT, T;N, Blood	
X		Electrolytes,Serum,Plasma (LYTE)	
		STAT, T;N, Blood	
X		INRPTT	
		STAT, T;N, Blood	
X		Creatinine (CRE)	
		STAT, T;N, Blood	
X		Urea (U)	
		STAT, T;N, Blood	
X		Magnesium,Serum,Plasma (MG)	
		STAT, T;N, Blood	
X		Phosphate (PHO)	
		STAT, T;N, Blood	
X		Complete Blood Count (CBC)	
		Routine, T;N+240, Blood	
X		INRPTT	
		Routine, T;N+240, Blood	
X		Electrolytes,Serum,Plasma (LYTE)	
		Routine, T;N+240, Blood	
X		Urea (U)	
		Routine, T;N+240, Blood	
X		Creatinine (CRE)	
		Routine, T;N+240, Blood	
X		Glucose,Random (GLUR)	
		Routine, T;N+240, Blood	
X		Magnesium,Serum,Plasma (MG)	
		Routine, T;N+240, Blood	
X		Phosphate (PHO)	
		Routine, T;N+240, Blood	
X		CBC Nurse order when	
		chest tube drainage greater than 150 mL/hour x 2 hours	
X		INRPTT Nurse Order When	
		chest tube drainage greater than 150 mL/hour x 2 hours	
Post-Op Day #1			
X		Complete Blood Count (CBC)	
		AM Routine, T+1;0300, Blood, Frequency: ONCE	
X		Electrolytes,Serum,Plasma (LYTE)	
		AM Routine, T+1;0300, Blood, Frequency: ONCE	

X		Magnesium,Serum,Plasma (MG)	
		AM Routine, T+1;0300, Blood, Frequency: ONCE	
X		Urea (U)	
		AM Routine, T+1;0300, Blood, Frequency: ONCE	
X		Glucose,Random (GLUR)	
		AM Routine, T+1;0300, Blood, Frequency: ONCE	
X		Phosphate (PHO)	
		AM Routine, T+1;0300, Blood, Frequency: ONCE	
X		Creatinine (CRE)	
		AM Routine, T+1;0300, Blood, Frequency: ONCE	
X		INRPTT	
		AM Routine, T+1;0300, Blood	
Diagnostic Imaging			
X		Xray Nurse order when	
		order chest xray post chest tube removal	
X		Xray Nurse order when	
		post-op day #1 if chest tubes are not being removed	
Other Diagnostic Testing/Treatment			
X		ECG Nurse order when	
		if change in cardiac rhythm	
X		ECG 12 Lead in 1 Day	
		Reason: Other, post op cardiac surgery	
X		ECG 12 Lead in 3 Days	
		Reason: Other, post op cardiac surgery	
Allied Health			
		Dietitian Referral	
X		Physiotherapy Referral	

Last Modified: 2018/02/22

B.1 Ventilation and Rapid Wean

DO NOT THIN FROM HEALTH RECORD

Provider (SIGNATURE)	Date	Time
Provider (PRINT)		
Processor	Date	Time
Nurse	Date	Time

CARDIO SURG - Ventilation and Rapid Wean (Module)

Inc	Req	ORDER	SPECIAL INSTRUCTIONS
Patient Care			
X		VAP Reduction Protocol	
		(VTE Module/head of bed 30 degrees/Sedation Module/chlorhexidine mouthwash)	
		VAMAAS	
X		Ventilation Routine	
		pH: 7.30 - 7.4, SpO2: Greater than 92%, Vt 6-8 mL/kg Predicted Body WT	
		Ventilation Prescribed Parameters	
		Ventilation Acute Respiratory Distress Syndrome ARDS	
X		Communication Order	
		Discontinue mechanical ventilation when patient extubated	
		Consider Lung Recruitment Maneuver for hypoxemia with lu atelectasis or Adult Respiratory Distress Syndrome (ARDS)	
		Lung Recruitment Maneuver	
		Prone Position	
X		POC Blood Gases	
Medications			
X		chlorhexidine 0.12% mouthwash	
		15 mL, mouthwash, ORAL, BID	
		ipratropium CFC free 20 mcg/inh inhalation aerosol	
		12 puff, inhaler, INHALE, q1 hour, PRN, for intubated patients	
		salbutamol 100 mcg/inh inhalation aerosol	
		12 puff, inhaler, INHALE, q1 hour, PRN, for intubated patients	
		Consider neuromuscular blockade for all patient with ARDS who have a PaO2/FiO2 ratio less than 150	

Inc	Req	ORDER	SPECIAL INSTRUCTIONS
Laboratory			
X		Conditional If/Then	
		If ventilatory changes, Then order Blood gases as indicated	
X		Blood Gas (BG)	
		Routine, T;N, ART or CAP	
Microbiology			
		Sputum C&S (RESP)	
		Tracheal Aspirate, Frequency: post procedure	
Diagnostic Imaging			
		Conditional If/Then	
		If patient intubated or acute change in ventilation or oxygenation status, Then order chest x-ray daily	
X		Chest AP Portable	
		Routine, Check endotracheal tube placement, Contact CSRU 17440	

Last Modified: 2015/01/26

B.2 Venous Thromboembolism (VTE) Prophylaxis

DO NOT THIN FROM HEALTH RECORD

Provider (SIGNATURE)	Date	Time
Provider (PRINT)		
Processor	Date	Time
Nurse	Date	Time
Height	Weight	Time

COMMON - Venous Thromboembolism (VTE) Prophylaxis (Module)			

Inc	Req	ORDER	SPECIAL INSTRUCTIONS
Patient Care			
		** To complete the VTE assessment you MUST complete on the following orders**	
		VTE Prophylaxis Not Required	
		Hospital stay is less than 72 hours	
		Patient already on anti-coagulants	
		Patient ambulating well	
		Other	
		VTE Prophylaxis is Contraindicated	
		Active Bleeding	
		Acquired Bleeding Disorder	
		Coagulopathy	
		Procedure expected in next 12 hours	
		Recent cranial, spinal, or eye surgery	
		Subarachnoid/Intracerebral Hemorrhage	
		Thrombocytopenia	
		Untreated Inherited Bleeding Disorder	
		Other	
		VTE Prophylaxis Moderate/High Risk	
		Active cancer or cancer treatment	
		Acute medical illness	
		Autoimmune disorders	
		Heart failure	
		Hypercoagulable state	
		Immobility	
		Increasing Age	
		Major Surgical Procedure	
		Major trauma or spinal cord injury	

Inc	Req	ORDER	SPECIAL INSTRUCTIONS
		Orthopaedic surgery	
		Pregnancy/ less than 6 weeks postpartum	
		Previous VTE/Family history of VTE	
		Stroke	
		Other	
		VTE Prophylaxis and Bleeding Moderate/High Risk	
		Active Bleeding	
		Acquired Bleeding Disorder	
		Coagulopathy	
		Procedure expected in next 12 hours	
		Recent cranial, spinal, or eye surgery	
		Subarachnoid/Intracerebral Hemorrhage	
		Thrombocytopenia	
		Untreated Inherited Bleeding Disorder	
		Other	
		Mechanical Prophylaxis	
		NOTE: ONLY select mechanical prophlyaxis if clinically indicated. ONLY consider discontinuing IPC and/or antiembolic stockings after first dose of dalteparin or heparin.	
		Graduate compression stockings have shown to be ineffectiv to prevent venous thromboembolism among stroke patients, and they might be associated with a higher risk of deep vein thrombosis	
		Further evidence to antiembolic stocking risk	
		Further evidence to antiembolic stocking risk	
		Intermittent Pneumatic Compression (IPC) Device	
		Sequential Compression Device	
		Discontinue Sequential Compression Device	
		Only discontinue SCD after the first dose of dalteparin or heparin	
		Discontinue Intermittent Pneumatic Compression (IPC) Devi	
		Only discontinue IPC and/or antiembolic stockings after the first dose of dalteparin or heparin	
		Medications	
		These products can induce thrombocytopenia therefore consider ordering CBC	
		dalteparin	
		5,000 units, syringe, SUBCUTANEOUS, daily (Def)	
		5,000 units, syringe, SUBCUTANEOUS, daily, Requested Start Date/Time T+1;0800	
		dalteparin	
		2,500 units, syringe, SUBCUTANEOUS, daily (Def)	
		2,500 units, syringe, SUBCUTANEOUS, daily, Requested Start Date/Time T+1;0800	

		dalteparin	
		7,500 units, syringe, SUBCUTANEOUS, daily (Def)	
		7,500 units, syringe, SUBCUTANEOUS, daily, Requested Start Date/Time T+1;0800	
		heparin	
		5,000 units, injection, SUBCUTANEOUS, q8 hours (Def)	
		5,000 units, injection, SUBCUTANEOUS, q8 hours, Start: T+1;0800	
		Parkwood choose the ""syringe"" sentence below. (Note)	
		heparin	
		5,000 units, syringe, SUBCUTANEOUS, q8 hours (Def)	
		5,000 units, syringe, SUBCUTANEOUS, q8 hours, Requested Start Date/Time T+1;0800	
		For Ischemic Stroke Only:	
		enoxaparin	
		40 mg, syringe, SUBCUTANEOUS, daily	
Laboratory			
		Complete Blood Count (CBC)	
		Routine, T;N, Blood	
		Complete Blood Count (CBC)	
		Routine, T;N, Blood	
		Complete Blood Count and Differential (CBCD)	
		Routine, T;N, Blood	
		Complete Blood Count (CBC)	
		AM Routine, T+1;0300, Blood, Frequency: q48 hours for 14 day	
		Complete Blood Count (CBC)	
		AM Routine, T+1;0300, Blood, Frequency: q48 hours for 14 day	
		Complete Blood Count and Differential (CBCD)	
		AM Routine, T+1;0300, Blood, Frequency: q48 hours for 14 day	

Last Modified: 2016/08/04

B.3 Electrolyte Replacement

DO NOT THIN FROM HEALTH RECORD

Provider (SIGNATURE)	Date	Time
Provider (PRINT)		
Processor	Date	Time
Nurse	Date	Time

CRIT CARE - Electrolyte Replacement (Module)

Inc	Req	ORDER	SPECIAL INSTRUCTIONS
Alerts			
X		Communication Order	
		Electrolyte replacement orders should not be used for patients with: renal failure, creatinine greater than 200 umol/L or severe Oligura, unless pt is on CRRT or specifically ordered.	
X		Notify Provider	
		if potassium is less than or equal to 2.9 mmol/L	
X		Notify Provider	
		if contraindications exist and electrolyte orders cannot be carried out.	
Patient Care			
X		Conditional If/Then	
		If electroyle replacement administered, Then send electroyle serum/POC blood gas plus 2 hours post replacement	
Medications			
Phosphate Replacement:			
X		potassium phosphate	
		30 mmol, injection, IV, as directed, PRN Other: See Comments, infuse over 2 hr	
		Comments - Serum phosphate less than 0.8 mmol/L and Potassium less than or equal to 3.5 mmol/L with Central Venous access. Phosphate 30 mmol as potassium salt in 100 mL of IV solution over 2 hours. Provides 44 mmol of potassium. Continue replacement therapy until goal met.	
X		potassium phosphate	
		30 mmol, injection, IV, as directed, PRN Other: See Comments, infuse over 4 hr	
		Comments - Serum phosphate less than 0.8 mmol/L and Potassium less than or equal to 3.5 mmol/L with peripheral venous access.Phosphate 30 mmol as potassium salt in 500 mL of IV solution over 4 hours. Provides 44 mmol of potassium. Continue replacement therapy until goal met.	
X		sodium phosphate	
		30 mmol, injection, IV, as directed, PRN Other: See Comments, infuse over 2 hr	

		Comments - Serum phosphate less than 0.8 mmol/L and Potassium greater that 3.5 mmol/L. Phosphate 30 mmol as sodium salt in 100 mL of IV solution over 2 hours via peripheral or central venous catheter. Provides 40 mmol of sodium. Continue replacement therapy until goal met.	
X		sodium acid phosphate	
		1,000 mg, EFF tab, NG TUBE, as directed, PRN Other: See Comments	
		Comments - Serum phosphate less than 0.8 mmol/L and potassium greater that 3.5 mmol/L and patient tolerating enteral feeds. Continue replacement therapy until goal met.	
Potassium Replacement			
X		potassium chloride injection	
		40 mmol, injection, IV, as directed, PRN for Other: See Comments, infuse over 1 hr	
		Comments - Potassium less than or equal to 3.2 mmol/L with central venous access. Potassium Chloride 40 mmol in 100 mL IV solution over 1 hour. Continue replacement therapy until goal met.	
X		potassium chloride injection	
		10 mmol, injection, IV, as directed, PRN for Other: See Comments, infuse over 60 min	
		Comments - Potassium less than or equal to 3.2 mmol/L with peripheral venous access. Potassium Chloride 10 mmol in 100 mL IV solution over 1 hour x 4 doses. Continue replacement therapy until goal met.	
X		potassium chloride 20 mmol/15 mL oral liquid	
		40 mmol, liquid, NG TUBE, as directed, PRN Other: See Comments	
		Comments - Potassium less than or equal to 3.2 mmol/L and patient tolerating enteral oral feeds. Continue replacement therapy until goal met.	
X		potassium chloride injection	
		20 mmol, injection, IV, as directed, PRN for Other: See Comments, infuse over 60 min, for: 2 dose	
		Comments - Potassium greater than 3.2 and less than or equal to 3.5 mmol/L with central venous access. Potassium Chloride 20 mmol in 100 mL IV solution over 1 hour. Continue replacement therapy until goal met.	
X		potassium chloride injection	
		10 mmol, injection, IV, as directed, PRN for Other: See Comments, infuse over 60 min	
		Comments - Potassium greater than 3.2 and less than or equal to 3.5 mmol/L with peripheral venous access. Potassium Chloride 10 mmol in 100 mL IV solution over 1 hour x2 doses. Continue replacement therapy until goal met.	
X		potassium chloride 20 mmol/15 mL oral liquid	
		20 mmol, liquid, NG TUBE, as directed, PRN Other: See Comments	

		Comments - Potassium greater than 3.2 and less than 3.5 mmol/L and patient tolerating enteral feeds. Continue replacement therapy until goal met.	
Magnesium Replacement			
X		magnesium sulfate	
		2,000 mg, injection, IV, as directed, PRN Other: See Comments	
		Comments - Magnesium less than 0.7 mmol/L. Magnesium sulfate 2 grams in 100 mL IV solution over 1 hour via central or peripheral venous access. Continue replacement therapy until goal met.	
Calcium Replacement			
X		calcium chloride	
		1 g, injection, IV, as directed, PRN for Other: See Comments	
		Comments - systemic ionized calcium less than 0.95 mmol/L. Calcium chloride 1 gram in 100 mL IV solution over 1 hour via central or peripheral venous access. Continue replacement therapy until goal met.	

Last Modified: 2017/05/26

B.4 Insulin Infusion

DO NOT THIN FROM HEALTH RECORD

Provider (SIGNATURE)	Date	Time
Provider (PRINT)		
Processor	Date	Time
Nurse	Date	Time

CRIT CARE - Insulin Infusion (Module)

Inc	Req	ORDER	SPECIAL INSTRUCTIONS
Admission			
		This protocol is NOT to be used for patients with diabetic ketoacidosis (during the first 48 hours post admission) or fulminant hepatic failure.	
Patient Care			
X		Communication Order	
		Initiate insulin infusion protocol if two consecutive blood glucose results are greater than 7.5 mmol/L	
X		Blood Glucose Target	
		4.5 - 6.5 mmol/L	
X		Communication Order	
		Ensure maintenance IV contains dextrose while on insulin infusion if patient not on enteral or parenteral nutrition	
Medications			
X		insulin regular infusion 1 unit/mL in 100 mL sodium chloride 0.9%	
		100 mL, IV continuous, titrate	
		Comments - refer to protocol	
		Ensure maintenance IV contains dextrose while on insulin infusion if patient not on enteral or parenteral nutrition (Note)	
X		dextrose 5%-sodium chloride 0.9%	
		1,000 mL, IV continuous, 75 mL/hr (Def)	
		Comments - until enterally fed and then reassess solution	
		1,000 mL, IV continuous, 100 mL/hr	
		Comments - until enterally fed and then reassess solution	
		1,000 mL, IV continuous, 125 mL/hr	

Inc	Req	ORDER	SPECIAL INSTRUCTIONS
		Comments - until enterally fed and then reassess solution	
X		dextrose 50% in water injection	
		12.5 g, syringe, IV direct, as directed, PRN for blood glucose	
		Comments - = 25 mL. For blood glucose less than 2.5 (Refer to protocol)	
X		dextrose 50% in water injection	
		5 g, syringe, IV direct, as directed, PRN for blood glucose	
		Comments - = 10 mL. For blood glucose 2.5-3 (Refer to protocol)	

Last Modified: 2017/05/26

B.5 CRIT CARE Sedation

DO NOT THIN FROM HEALTH RECORD

Provider (SIGNATURE)	Date	Time
Provider (PRINT)		
Processor	Date	Time
Nurse	Date	Time

CRIT CARE - Sedation (Module)		

Inc	Req	ORDER	SPECIAL INSTRUCTIONS
		Admission	
		This order set is for patients who do NOT require a deep level of sedation	
		Medications	
		propofol	
		20 mg, injection, IV direct, q2 minutes, PRN Other: See Comments	
		Comments - until target VAMAAS achieved.	
		propofol 2000 mg in 100 mL diluent	
		premix diluent infusion	
		Titration Range: 0-5 mg/kg/hr	
		Comments - NOTE DOUBLE STRENGTH OF PROP not exceed 5 mg/kg/hour. Change tubing every 12 hours. Wea as per protocol.	
		propofol - additive	
		2,000 mg, Every Bag	
		Comments - NOTE DOUBLE STRENGTH OF PROP	
		Consider Midazolam if propofol intolerance.	
		midazolam	
		2 mg, injection, IV direct, q5 minutes, PRN Other: See Comments	
		Comments - until target VAMAAS achieved.	
		midazolam 100 mg in 50 mL sodium chloride 0.9% premix	
		sodium chloride 0.9% premix diluent (infusion)	
		Titration Range: 0-10 mg/hr	
		Comments - Wean as per protocol	
		midazolam - additive	
		100 mg, Every Bag	
		Laboratory	
		Triglycerides,Serum (TRIG)	
		AM Routine, T+1;0300, Blood, Frequency: daily Mon,Wed,Fri a.m.	

Last Modified: 2020/06/15

B.6 Warfarin (Coumadin) Daily Dosing

DO NOT THIN FROM HEALTH RECORD

Provider (SIGNATURE)	Date	Time
Provider (PRINT)		
Processor	Date	Time
Nurse	Date	Time

COMMON - Warfarin (Coumadin) Daily Dosing (Module)

Inc	Req	ORDER	SPECIAL INSTRUCTIONS
Alerts			
		Prior to selecting an initial dose for Physician Daily Dosing, this Powerplan must be initiated. Subsequent daily warfarin doses can be entered as a single order.	
Medications			
		Please select ONE of the following for the initial dose:	
		warfarin	
		2.5 mg, tab, ORAL, daily, dose	
		warfarin	
		5 mg, tab, ORAL, daily, dose	
		warfarin	
		7.5 mg, tab, ORAL, daily, dose	
		warfarin	
		10 mg, tab, ORAL, daily, dose	
X		warfarin daily order	
		1 dose, -, ORAL, daily	
X		Do Not Administer IM Injections	

Last Modified: 2016/02/16

B.7 Intra-Aortic Balloon Pump (IABP)

DO NOT THIN FROM HEALTH RECORD

Provider (SIGNATURE)	Date	Time
Provider (PRINT)		
Processor	Date	Time
Nurse	Date	Time

CARDIO - Intra-Aortic Balloon Pump (IABP)	

Inc	Req	ORDER	SPECIAL INSTRUCTIONS
Alerts			
		Airborne Precautions	
		Contact Precautions	
		Droplet Precautions	
		Droplet/Contact Precautions	
Activity			
		Bedrest	
		Positioning: Elevate head of bed, less than or equal to 30 degrees	
		Bedrest	
		q2 hours., reposition patient	
Vital Signs			
		Vital Signs	
		q1 hour.	
		Neuro Vital Signs	
		q12 hours. (Def)	
		q1 hour., if level of consciousness altered	
		Arterial Line Care and Monitoring	
		arterial line tracing from console with balloon in 1:2 q shift	
		Peripheral Pulse Monitoring	
		q6 hours., radial pulse	
		Pedal Pulse Assessment	
		q1 hour on affected leg	
		Cardiac Monitoring	
		6 second rhythm strip printed q shift	
		Oxygen Saturation	
		Routine, continuous	
Patient Care			
		Oxygen Therapy	

Inc	Req	ORDER	SPECIAL INSTRUCTIONS
		Oxygen Titration	
		Target: SpO2 greater than or equal to 92% (Def)	
		Target: SpO2 88-92% for CO2 Retention	
		Intake and Output - Strict	
		q1 hour.	
		Urinary Catheter to Urometer	
		Notify Provider	
		if urine output less than 30 mL/hour x 2 hours	
		Wound Care	
		dressing change over IABP site as per central line protocol	
Medications			
		heparin 2 units/mL arterial line flush	
Laboratory			
		Complete Blood Count (CBC)	
		AM Routine, T+1;0300, Blood	
		Electrolytes,Serum,Plasma (LYTE)	
		AM Routine, T+1;0300, Blood	
		Urea (U)	
		AM Routine, T+1;0300, Blood	
		Creatinine (CRE)	
		AM Routine, T+1;0300, Blood	
		Group and Screen Nurse order when	
		prior to removal of IABP	
		INR Nurse order when	
		prior to removal of IABP	
Diagnostic Imaging			
		daily chest x-ray to assess position of IABP	
		Xray Nurse order when	
		order daily portable chest xray while balloon pump in SITU to assess position of IAB	
		Notify Provider	
		after daily chest x-ray complete	

Last Modified: 2015/01/26

Appendix C Transfer to Inpatient Unit

DO NOT THIN FROM HEALTH RECORD

Provider (SIGNATURE)	Date	Time	
Provider (PRINT)			
Processor	Date	Time	
Nurse	Date	Time	

CARDIO SURG - Transfer to Inpatient Unit

Inc	Req	ORDER	SPECIAL INSTRUCTIONS
		Resuscitation Status	
		Please ensure paper resuscitation form is completed/reviewed	
		Alerts	
		Precautions	
		Airborne Precautions	
		Contact Precautions	
		Droplet Precautions	
		Droplet/Contact Precautions	
		Diet	
X		Cardiac Diet LHSC	
		Activity	
X		Activity as Tolerated	
		Vital Signs	
X		Vital Signs	
		q4 hours., x 24 hours then QID (Def)	
		per protocol	
		daily	
		q1 hour.	
		q12 hours.	
		q2 hours.	
		q3 hours.	
		q30 days	
		q30 minutes	
		q6 hours.	
		q8 hours.	
		weekly	
X		Telemetry	
		Indication: Arrhythmia (known or suspected) for 5 day, then reassess	

Inc	Req	ORDER	SPECIAL INSTRUCTIONS
\multicolumn{4}{l}{Patient Care}
		Communication Order	
		Initiate Coronary Artery Bypass pathway	
		NO BP or Blood work	
		or IV start in radial graft arm until POD #7	
X		Oxygen Therapy	
X		Oxygen Titration	
		Target: SpO2 greater than or equal to 92% (Def)	
		Target: SpO2 88-92% for CO2 Retention	
X		Weight	
		daily 03:00	
X		Urinary Catheter to Urometer	
		q12 hour output x 48 hours then reasses	
X		Intake and Output	
		q12 hours.	
X		Discontinue Urinary Catheter	
		Discuss removal post op day #2 with team.	
X		Urinary Catheter Insertion	
		Reinsert catheter if has not voided 8-12 hours post removal and leave in if residual greater than 300 mL	
		Chest Tube Care/Monitor	
		Water-Seal Suction -20 cm, Call CVT if total drainage greater than 150 mL/hour x 2 hours	
		Discontinue Chest Tube	
X		Dressing Change	
		Remove chest tube pressure dressing in 48 hours post chest tube removal	
X		Dressing Change	
		Leave all initial dressings intact for 48 hours. Starting 48 hours post op cleanse sternal, radial, leg incision and pacer wires daily with sterile saline and cover with dry gauze until showering or continue to change sternal dressing if on telemetry.	
X		Convert IV to Saline Lock	
		When drinking well	
X		Communication Order	
		pacer wires secured and visible if present	
		POC Blood Glucose	
		Before Meals and at Bedtime for 24 hr	
		Pacemaker Settings Temporary Transvenous/Epicardial	
\multicolumn{4}{l}{Continuous Infusions}
X		dextrose 5%-sodium chloride 0.9%	
		1,000 mL, IV continuous, 80 mL/hr	

		Comments - Until drinking well	
Medications			
		COMMON - Warfarin (Coumadin) Daily Dosing (Module)	
X		sodium chloride 0.9% flush	
		3 mL, syringe, IV direct, as directed, PRN IV device maintenance	
		Comments - peripheral	
X		sodium chloride 0.9% flush	
		10 mL, IV direct, as directed, PRN IV device maintenance	
		Comments - central	
		amLODIPine	
		2.5 mg, tab, ORAL, bedtime	
X		ondansetron	
		4 mg, tab, ORAL, q8 hours, PRN for nausea or vomiting	
		lansoprazole	
		30 mg, DR cap, ORAL, daily	
		insulin aspart correctional dose HIGH	
		sliding scale, SUBCUTANEOUS, injection, before meals & bedtime (QID)	
		Comments - Blood Glucose Range (mmol/L) Less than/equal to 4 Implement Hypoglycemia management where applicable. Notify MRP within reasonable time frame for further orders or adjustment to existing orders 4.1-8 *0 units 8.1-10* *4 units 10.1 - 14* *6 units 14.1 - 17*	
		clopidogrel	
		75 mg, tab, ORAL, daily	
		Comments - POD 4	
		ticagrelor	
		90 mg, tab, ORAL, BID	
		Comments - POD 4	
Beta Blockers			
		metoprolol	
		12.5 mg, tab, ORAL, q12 hours (Def)	
		Comments - Hold if heart rate less than 60/min or SBP less than 100 mmHg	
		25 mg, tab, ORAL, q12 hours	
		Comments - Hold if heart rate less than 60/min or SBP less than 100 mmHg	
Laboratory			
X		Complete Blood Count (CBC)	
		AM Routine, T+2;0300, Blood	

X		Electrolytes,Serum,Plasma (LYTE)	
		AM Routine, T+2;0300, Blood	
X		Urea (U)	
		AM Routine, T+2;0300, Blood	
X		Creatinine (CRE)	
		AM Routine, T+2;0300, Blood	
		INR	
		AM Routine, T+1;0300, Blood, Frequency: daily.	
Diagnostic Imaging			
X		Xray Nurse order when	
		upon removal of chest tubes	
Allied Health			
		Dietitian Referral	
X		Physiotherapy Referral	

Last Modified: 2018/02/22

C.1 Subcutaneous Insulin Correctional Scale

DO NOT THIN FROM HEALTH RECORD

Provider (SIGNATURE)	Date	Time
Provider (PRINT)		
Processor	Date	Time
Nurse	Date	Time

ENDO - Subcutaneous Insulin Correctional Scale (Module)

Inc	Req	ORDER	SPECIAL INSTRUCTIONS
Alerts			
		Prolonged use of correctional scale insulin regimes as the sole form of insulin coverage is strongly discouraged if targets are not being met. Rapid transition to a regimen that includes basal insulin is usually appropriate. Correction scale insulin should never be used as the sole form of insulin therapy in type 1 diabetic patients.	
Patient Care			
		POC Blood Glucose	
		Other:, TID Before Meals (Def)	
		Before Meals and at Bedtime	
		q6h	
		Other:	
Medications			
		Discontinue all previous correctional insulin orders	
		Ensure all previous correctional scale insulins are discontinued	
		Correctional scale insulin should be the same type of short-acting insulin as the regularly scheduled insulin if applicable AND reassess glycemic control daily. If not achieving targets (blood sugars are greater than 10) scheduled insulin should likely be initiated.	
		LOW DOSE (sensitive) consider if total daily insulin dose less than 60 units/day or not on home insulin	
		insulin regular correctional dose LOW	
		insulin aspart correctional dose LOW	
		insulin lispro correctional dose LOW	
		MEDIUM DOSE (usual) consider if on 60 to 100 units/day	
		insulin regular correctional dose MEDIUM	

Inc	Req	ORDER	SPECIAL INSTRUCTIONS
		insulin aspart correctional dose MEDIUM	
		insulin lispro correctional dose MEDIUM	
		HIGH DOSE (resistant) consider if on more than 100 units/day	
		insulin regular correctional dose HIGH	
		insulin aspart correctional dose HIGH	
		insulin lispro correctional dose HIGH	
		CUSTOM DOSE	
		insulin regular correctional dose CUSTOM	
		insulin aspart correctional dose CUSTOM	
		insulin lispro correctional dose CUSTOM	

Last Modified: 2016/05/06

Appendix D Fast-Track Post Cardiovascular Surgery Post-Op Multi-Phase Order

DO NOT THIN FROM HEALTH RECORD

Provider (SIGNATURE)	Date	Time
Provider (PRINT)		
Processor	Date	Time
Nurse	Date	Time

CARDIO SURG - FAST TRACK Cardiovascular Surgery, Post-Op (Multi-Phase)			

Inc	Req	ORDER	SPECIAL INSTRUCTIONS
		Fast Track Post-Op Care	
		Resuscitation Status	
		Please ensure the resuscitation documentation is completed/reviewed	
		Diet	
X		NPO	
X		Advance Diet as Tolerated	
		to cardiac diet	
		to diabetic diet	
		Activity	
X		Dangle Legs at Bedside	
		4 hours post-op and prior to chest tube removal	
X		Activity as Tolerated	
		Up in chair for meals Post-Op day 1	
		Vital Signs	
X		Vital Signs	
		per protocol (Def)	
		daily	
		q1 hour.	
		q12 hours.	
		q2 hours.	
		q3 hours.	
		q30 days	
		q30 minutes	
		q4 hours.	
		q6 hours.	
		q8 hours.	
		weekly	
X		Cardiac Monitoring	
		Arrhythmia (known or suspected), lead 2 and V5	

Inc	Req	ORDER	SPECIAL INSTRUCTIONS
X		Central Venous Pressure Monitoring	
		on admission and q1 hour, discontinue prior to transfer to floor	
		Systolic Blood Pressure Target	
Patient Care			
X		Oxygen Therapy	
X		Oxygen Titration	
		Target: SpO2 greater than or equal to 92% (Def)	
		Target: SpO2 88-92% for CO2 Retention	
X		POC Blood Glucose	
		Before Meals and at Bedtime	
		Once	
X		POC Specimen LABEL - Blood Gas	
		Blood Gas - Arterial	
X		Urinary Catheter to Urometer	
X		Intake and Output	
		q1 hour.	
X		Notify Provider	
		if urine output less than 20 mL for 2 consecutive hours, call CVT or CSRU team	
X		Chest Tube Care/Monitor	
		Water-Seal Suction -20 cm, Notify provider if total drainage greater than 150 mL/hour x 2 hours	
X		Arterial Line Care and Monitoring	
X		Central Line Care	
X		Discontinue Arterial Line	
		discontinue prior to transfer to floor	
X		Convert IV to Saline Lock	
		when drinking well	
		Discontinue Chest Tube	
		remove chest tube POD #1 in morning	
Continuous Infusions			
X		dextrose 5%-sodium chloride 0.9%	
		IV continuous, 80 mL/hr	
X		sodium chloride 0.9% arterial line flush	
		intra-ARTERIAL, to keep line open, Total volume (mL): 500	
Medications			
X		COMMON - Venous Thromboembolism (VTE) Prophylaxis (LHSC-UH, VC, PW, STEGH, TDMH)	
		insulin aspart correctional dose HIGH	
		sliding scale, SUBCUTANEOUS, injection, with meals & bedtime (QID)	

		Comments - Blood Glucose Range (mmol/L) *Dose Less than/equal to 4* *Implement Hypoglycemia management where applicable. Notify* *MRP within reasonable time frame for further orders or* *adjustment to existing orders 4.1-8* *0 units 8.1-10* *4 units 10.1 - 14* *6 units 14.1 - 17*	
X		sodium chloride 0.9% flush	
		3 mL, syringe, IV direct, as directed, PRN IV device *maintenance*	
		Comments - Peripheral	
X		sodium chloride 0.9% flush	
		10 mL, injection, IV direct, as directed, PRN IV *device maintenance*	
		Comments - Central	
Antiplatelets			
X		acetylsalicylic acid	
		81 mg, EC tab, ORAL, ONCE, Start: T;N+360	
		Comments - give within the first 6 to 24 hours *post-op once patient extubated. If platelet count less* *than 50,000 or blood loss greater than 100 mL in any hour,* *verify with MD before administering acetylsalicylic acid.*	
X		acetylsalicylic acid	
		81 mg, EC tab, ORAL, daily, Start: T+1;0800	
		Comments - If platelet count less than 50,000 *or blood loss greater than 100 mL in any hour, verify with* *MD before administering acetylsalicylic acid.*	
		clopidogrel	
		75 mg, tab, ORAL, daily, Start: T+1;0800	
		Comments - If platelet count less than *100,000 or blood loss greater than 100 mL in any hour,* *verify with MD before administering.*	
Antimicrobials			
		ceFAZolin	
		1 g, injection, IV, q8 hours, for: 24 hr	
		vancomycin	
		1 g, injection, IV, q12 hours, infuse over 60 min, *for: 48 hr*	
		Comments - give one dose after removal of chest *tubes then discontinue*	
Antiemetics/GI Prophylaxis			
X		ondansetron	
		4 mg, tab, ORAL, q8 hours, PRN nausea or vomiting	
X		lansoprazole	
		30 mg, DR cap, ORAL, daily, Start: T+1;0800	
Beta Blockers			
		metoprolol	
		12.5 mg, tab, ORAL, q12 hours (Def)	

		Comments - Hold beta blocker if heart rate is less than 60/minute or SBP is less than 100 mmHg	
		25 mg, tab, ORAL, q12 hours	
		Comments - Hold beta blocker if heart rate is less than 60/minute or SBP is less than 100 mmHg	
		50 mg, tab, ORAL, q12 hours	
		Comments - Hold beta blocker if heart rate is less than 60/minute or SBP is less than 100 mmHg	
Bowel Routine			
X		senna	
		8.6 mg, tab, ORAL, bedtime, for: 2 dose, Start: T+2;2200	
X		senna	
		8.6 mg, tab, ORAL, bedtime, PRN constipation, Start: T+4;2200	
X		bisacodyl	
		10 mg, supp, RECTAL, ONCE, Start: T+3;0800	
		Comments - if no bowel movement since surgery	
X		bisacodyl	
		10 mg, supp, RECTAL, daily, PRN constipation, Start: T+2;0800	
		Fleet Enema	
		133 mL, enema, RECTAL, daily, PRN constipation	
		Comments - do not administer if serum creatinine is greater than 200 umol/L	
Laboratory			
X		Complete Blood Count (CBC)	
		Timed, T;N+30, Blood	
X		Magnesium,Serum,Plasma (MG)	
		Timed, T;N+30, Blood	
X		Phosphate (PHO)	
		Timed, T;N+30, Blood	
X		INRPTT	
		Timed, T;N+120, Blood	
X		Complete Blood Count (CBC)	
		Timed, T;N+240, Blood	
X		Electrolytes,Serum,Plasma (LYTE)	
		Timed, T;N+240, Blood	
X		Glucose,Random (GLUR)	
		Timed, T;N+240, Blood	
X		Urea (U)	
		Timed, T;N+240, Blood	
X		Creatinine (CRE)	
		Timed, T;N+240, Blood	
X		Magnesium,Serum,Plasma (MG)	
		Timed, T;N+240, Blood	
X		Phosphate (PHO)	
		Timed, T;N+240, Blood	

X		INRPTT Nurse Order When	
		chest tube drainage greater than 150 mL/hr x 2 hrs	
X		CBC Nurse order when	
		chest tube drainage greater than 150 mL/hr x 2 hrs	
Diagnostic Imaging			
X		Chest AP Portable	
		Post op Cardiac surgery	
X		Xray Nurse order when	
		post chest tube removal	
X		Xray Nurse order when	
		post op day #1 if chest tubes are not being removed	
Other Diagnostic Testing/Treatment			
X		ECG Nurse order when	
		if change in cardiac rhythm	
X		ECG 12 Lead	
		Reason: Arrhythmia Assessment	
X		ECG 12 Lead in 1 Day	
		Reason: Arrhythmia Assessment	
Consults			
		Acute Pain Service Consult	
		Anesthesiologist, Dr	
Allied Health			
		Dietitian Referral	
X		Physiotherapy Referral	
Discharge Planning			
X		Discharge Instructions	
		patient to be discharged from PACU or CSRU by the anesthesiologist, cardiac surgeon or CSRU intensivist	
Pain and Symptom Management			
X		COMMON - Acute Pain and Symptom Management Module	

Last Modified: 2018/09/17

D.1 Acute Pain and Symptom Management

DO NOT THIN FROM HEALTH RECORD

Provider (SIGNATURE)	Date	Time	
Provider (PRINT)			
Processor	Date	Time	
Nurse	Date	Time	

COMMON - Acute Pain and Symptom Management (Module)

Inc	Req	ORDER	SPECIAL INSTRUCTIONS
		Vital Signs	
		Vital Signs	
		per protocol (Def)	
		daily	
		q1 hour.	
		q12 hours.	
		q2 hours.	
		q3 hours.	
		q30 days	
		q30 minutes	
		q4 hours.	
		q6 hours.	
		q8 hours.	
		weekly	
		Patient Care	
		Communication Order	
		contact the surgical team for pain related issues once patient has been discharged from APS/Anesthesia	
		Medications	
		Analgesics	
		acetaminophen	
		650 mg, tab, ORAL, q6 hours (Def)	
		Comments - max 4 g acetaminophen in 24 hr from all sources	
		975 mg, tab, ORAL, q6 hours	
		Comments - max 4 g acetaminophen in 24 hr from all sources	
		640 mg, susp, NG TUBE, q6 hours	
		Comments - max 4 g acetaminophen in 24 hr from all sources	

Inc	Req	ORDER	SPECIAL INSTRUCTIONS
		960 mg, susp, NG TUBE, q6 hours	
		Comments - max 4 g acetaminophen in 24 hr from all sources	
		acetaminophen	
		650 mg, tab, ORAL, q6 hours, PRN pain (Def)	
		Comments - max 4 g acetaminophen in 24 hr from all sources	
		975 mg, tab, ORAL, q6 hours, PRN pain	
		Comments - max 4 g acetaminophen in 24 hr from all sources	
		640 mg, susp, NG TUBE, q6 hours, PRN pain	
		Comments - max 4 g acetaminophen in 24 hr from all sources	
		960 mg, susp, NG TUBE, q6 hours, PRN pain	
		Comments - max 4 g acetaminophen in 24 hr from all sources	
		ibuprofen	
		400 mg, tab, ORAL, q6 hours, PRN pain (Def)	
		Comments - Max dose: 3200 mg in 24 hours	
		200 mg, tab, ORAL, q6 hours, PRN pain	
		Comments - Max dose: 3200 mg in 24 hours	
		ketorolac	
		10 mg, tab, ORAL, q6 hours, for: 2 day	
		Comments - Do Not exceed 40 mg/day. Do Not give with other NSAIDs.	
		ketorolac	
		10 mg, tab, ORAL, q6 hours PRN pain, for: 2 day	
		Comments - Do Not exceed 40 mg/day. Do Not give with other NSAIDs.	
		ketorolac	
		30 mg, injection, IV, q6 hours, for: 2 day (Def)	
		Comments - Do Not exceed 120 mg/day. Do Not give with other NSAIDs.	
		15 mg, injection, IV, q6 hours, for: 2 day	
		Comments - Do Not exceed 120 mg/day. Do Not give with other NSAIDs.	
		ketorolac	
		30 mg, injection, IV, q6 hours PRN pain, for: 2 day (Def)	
		Comments - Do Not exceed 120 mg/day. Do Not give with other NSAIDs.	
		15 mg, injection, IV, q6 hours PRN pain, for: 2 day	
		Comments - Do Not exceed 120 mg/day. Do Not give with other NSAIDs.	
		naproxen	

		250 mg, tab, ORAL, q12 hours, for: 5 day (Def)	
		500 mg, tab, ORAL, q12 hours, for: 5 day	
		naproxen	
		250 mg, tab, ORAL, q12 hours, PRN pain, for: 5 day (Def)	
		500 mg, tab, ORAL, q12 hours, PRN pain, for: 5 day	
		gabapentin	
		100 mg, cap, ORAL, q8 hours, for: 5 day (Def)	
		100 mg, cap, ORAL, q12 hours, for: 5 day	
		200 mg, cap, ORAL, q8 hours, for: 5 day	
		200 mg, cap, ORAL, q12 hours, for: 5 day	
		300 mg, cap, ORAL, q8 hours, for: 5 day	
		300 mg, cap, ORAL, q12 hours, for: 5 day	

Analgesics: Opioids

		morphine	
		5 mg, tab, ORAL, q4 hours PRN pain, for: 7 day (Def)	
		10 mg, tab, ORAL, q4 hours PRN pain, for: 7 day	
		5 mg, syrup, ORAL, q4 hours PRN pain, for: 7 day	
		10 mg, syrup, ORAL, q4 hours PRN pain, for: 7 day	
		morphine injection	
		5 mg, injection, SUBCUTANEOUS, q3 hours PRN pain, for: 7 day (Def)	
		Comments - give 5 mg for severe pain, give 2.5 mg for moderate pain	
		7.5 mg, injection, SUBCUTANEOUS, q3 hours PRN pain, for: 7 day	
		Comments - give 7.5 mg for severe pain, give 5 mg for moderate pain	
		10 mg, injection, SUBCUTANEOUS, q3 hours PRN pain, for: 7 day	
		Comments - give 10 mg for severe pain, give 5 mg for moderate pain	
		morphine 12 hour (M-Eslon) extended release	
		15 mg, ER cap, ORAL, q12 hours, for: 7 day (Def)	
		30 mg, ER cap, ORAL, q12 hours, for: 7 day	
		HYDROmorphone	
		2 mg, tab, ORAL, q4 hours PRN pain, for: 7 day (Def)	
		4 mg, tab, ORAL, q4 hours PRN pain, for: 7 day	
		2 mg, liquid, ORAL, q4 hours PRN pain, for: 7 day	
		4 mg, liquid, ORAL, q4 hours PRN pain, for: 7 day	
		HYDROmorphone injection	
		1 mg, injection, SUBCUTANEOUS, q3 hours PRN pain, for: 7 day (Def)	
		Comments - give 1 mg for severe pain, give 0.5 mg for moderate pain	
		2 mg, injection, SUBCUTANEOUS, q3 hours PRN pain, for: 7 day	

		Comments - give 2 mg for severe pain, give 1 mg for moderate pain	
		traMADol	
		50 mg, tab, ORAL, q6 hours PRN pain, for: 7 day (Def)	
		Comments - Maximum 400 mg tramadol in 24 hr from all sources	
		50 mg, tab, ORAL, q12 hours PRN pain, for: 7 day	
		Comments - Maximum 400 mg tramadol in 24 hr from all sources	
		100 mg, tab, ORAL, q6 hours PRN pain, for: 7 day	
		Comments - Maximum 400 mg tramadol in 24 hr from all sources	
		100 mg, tab, ORAL, q12 hours pain, for: 7 day	
		Comments - Maximum 400 mg tramadol in 24 hr from all sources	
		oxyCODONE	
		5 mg, tab, ORAL, q4 hours PRN pain, for: 7 day (Def)	
		10 mg, tab, ORAL, q4 hours PRN pain, for: 7 day	

Analgesics: Combination Analgesics

		Communication Order	
		Patients may receive opioids without delay following intrathecal opioid administration	
		acetaminophen-caffeine-codeine 30 mg oral tablet	
		2 tab, tab, ORAL, q4 hours PRN pain, for: 7 day	
		Comments - give 2 tablets for severe pain, give 1 tablet for moderate pain -- Max 4 g acetaminophen in 24 hr from all sources	
		acetaminophen-oxycodone 325 mg-5 mg oral tablet	
		2 tab, tab, ORAL, q4 hours PRN pain, for: 7 day	
		Comments - give 2 tablets for severe pain, give 1 tablet for moderate pain.--max 4 g acetaminophen in 24 hr from all sources	
		acetaminophen-tramadol 325 mg-37.5 mg oral tablet	
		2 tab, tab, ORAL, q6 hours PRN pain, for: 7 day	
		Comments - Maximum dose: 8 tablets in 24 hr-- Max 4 g acetaminophen in 24 hr from all sources	

Antiemetics

		ondansetron	
		4 mg, tab, ORAL, q8 hours, PRN nausea or vomiting	
		Comments - Not to be given within 24 hours of granisetron.	
		ondansetron injection	
		4 mg, injection, IV, q8 hours, PRN nausea or vomiting	
		Comments - Not to be given within 24 hours of granisetron.	
		metoclopramide	
		10 mg, tab, ORAL, q6 hours, PRN nausea or vomiting	
		metoclopramide	
		10 mg, injection, IV, q6 hours, PRN nausea or vomiting	

		dimenhyDRINATE	
		25 mg, tab, ORAL, q4 hours, PRN nausea or vomiting (Def)	
		50 mg, tab, ORAL, q4 hours, PRN nausea or vomiting	
		dimenhyDRINATE injection	
		25 mg, injection, IV direct, q4 hours, PRN nausea or vomiting	
		dimenhyDRINATE injection	
		50 mg, injection, IV direct, q4 hours, PRN nausea or vomiting	
Antipruritic			
		hydrOXYzine	
		25 mg, cap, ORAL, q6 hours, PRN for itching (Def)	
		10 mg, cap, ORAL, q4 hours, PRN for itching	
		diphenhydrAMINE	
		50 mg, tab, ORAL, q4 hours, PRN itching (Def)	
		25 mg, tab, ORAL, q4 hours, PRN itching	
		naloxone	
		0.1 mg, injection, SUBCUTANEOUS, q1 hour, PRN itching	

Last Modified: 2019/08/19

Appendix E RVAD, LVAD, Centrimag, HeartMate II, HeartWare

DO NOT THIN FROM HEALTH RECORD

Provider (SIGNATURE)	Date	Time
Provider (PRINT)		
Processor	Date	Time
Nurse	Date	Time

CARDIO SURG - RVAD/LVAD/Centrimag/HeartMate II/HeartWare, Post-Op, Critical Care (Module)			

Inc	Req	ORDER	SPECIAL INSTRUCTIONS
Activity			
		Bedrest	
		Positioning: Elevate head of bed, to 30 Degrees	
X		Turn Patient	
		q2 hours., use rotation module in Total Care Sport or Total Care bed if hemodynamically unstable.	
X		Activity as Tolerated	
X		Dangle Legs at Bedside	
		prior to chest tube removal	
Vital Signs			
X		Vital Signs	
		per protocol (Def)	
		daily	
		q1 hour.	
		q12 hours.	
		q2 hours.	
		q3 hours.	
		q30 days	
		q30 minutes	
		q4 hours.	
		q6 hours.	
		q8 hours.	
		weekly	
X		Mean Arterial Blood Pressure Target	
		Comments - notify provider if MAP is greater than 85 mmHg after scheduled and prn antihypertensives administered	
Patient Care			
		Nitric Oxide	
		Communication Order	

Inc	Req	ORDER	SPECIAL INSTRUCTIONS
		Record hourly HeartWare and HeartMate device parameters on VAD flowsheet at bedside.	
		Communication Order	
		Record hourly Centrimag device parameters on VAD flowsheet at bedside.	
X		Intake and Output	
		q1 hour., 24 hour intake recorded and continue a CUMULATIVE fluid balance	
		Drain/Tube Care	
		Other:, HEARTMATE/HEARTWARE: Drive Line Care as central line protocol	
		Drain/Tube Care	
		Other:, CENTRIMAG: Cannula Care as per central line protocol	
		Communication Order	
		reposition flow probe (CENTRIMAG) sensor q shift	
		Communication Order	
		check if ICD was disabled during implantation, call ICD clinic to restart function	

Medications

Inc	Req	ORDER	SPECIAL INSTRUCTIONS
		Consider anticoagulation as per Centrimag/ HeartMate/HeartWare protocol (i.e. IV heparin, acetylsalicylic acid, warfarin, clopidogrel)	
		Review continuation of medications: Antiplatelet agents, anticoagulants, NSAIDs if ordering Heparin	
		Notify Provider	
		In the event of significant bleeding and stop heparin	
		dextrose 5% in water	
		1,000 mL, IV continuous, 75 mL/hr	
		heparin 20,000 units in 500 mL dextrose 5% premix	
		dextrose 5% premix diluent	
		500 mL, IV continuous	

| | | *Comments - Adjust heparin infusion as per following E.1 heparin nomogram* | |

PTT(sec)	Bolus	Hold	Rate Change	Recheck PTT
Less than 40	1000 units	0	+2 units/kg/hr	6 hours
40-49	0	0	+1.5 mL/hr	6 hours
50-64	0	0	No cha	6 hours

Inc	Req	ORDER	SPECIAL INSTRUCTIONS
		heparin - additive	
		20,000, units, Every Bag, unit/kg/hr	
		heparin bolus (40 units/mL)	
		1,000 units, injection, IV, as directed, PRN for Other: See Comments	
		Comments - for PTT less than 40 seconds. Administer from heparin infusion bag.	

Other Diagnostic Testing/Treatment			
		Echo Transoesophageal	
		Routine, T+1;N	
X		Echo Routine	
		T+5;N, Assess - Known Cardiac Condition, LVAD, assess cardiac function	

Last Modified: 2016/01/14

E.1 Heparin Nomogram—RVAD LVAD

PTT (sec)	Bolus	Hold	Rate Change	Recheck PTT
Less than 40	1,000 units	0	+2 units/kg/hr	6 hours
40-49	0	0	+1 unit/kg/hr	6 hours
50-64	0	0	No change	Next AM
65-74	0	0	-1 unit/kg/hr	6 hours
Greater than 75	0	60 min	-2 units/kg/hr	6 hours after restart

Appendix F Extracorporeal Membrane Oxygenation (ECMO)

DO NOT THIN FROM HEALTH RECORD

Provider (SIGNATURE)	Date	Time	
Provider (PRINT)			
Processor	Date	Time	
Nurse	Date	Time	

CARDIO SURG - Extracorporeal Membrane Oxygenation, ECMO (Module)

Inc	Req	ORDER	SPECIAL INSTRUCTIONS
Diet			
X		NPO	
		x 24 hours then reassess (for enteral feeding or TPN)	
Activity			
X		Activity as Tolerated	
		Bedrest	
		Positioning: Elevate head of bed, to 30 Degrees, as tolerated	
		Turn Patient	
		q2 hours., use rotation module in Total Care Sport or Total Care bed if hemodynamicaly unstable - while on ECMO	
Vital Signs			
		Mean Arterial Blood Pressure Target (mmHg)	
		Pulse Assessment	
		Colour-Sensation-Movement Checks	
		q1 hour., on affected limbs	
Patient Care			
X		ECMO Device Parameters	
		Frequency: q1 hours	
X		Conditional If/Then	
		If ECMO pump failure, Then clamp access and return cannulas, engage manual crank to ensure forward flow, then release clamps. Reassess patient for signs of adequate perfusion and notify perfusionist and MD.	
X		Drain/Tube Care	
		Other:, Cannula care as per VAD/ECMO dressing change procedure	
		Notify Provider	
		In the event of significant bleeding and stop heparin	
		Dressing Change	

Inc	Req	ORDER	SPECIAL INSTRUCTIONS
		reinforce tegaderm only for patients with an open chest	
		Communication Order	
		Chest X-ray to be done doing a straight lift for patients with an open chest	
X		Perfusion Support Scale	
		Perfusion Support: Class A-Perfusionist at bedside	
		Comments - Immediately post insertion, minimum 6 hours Severe hemodynamic instability requiring adjustments to ECMO flow Massive blood loss, possible cell saver, benefitting from rapid transfusion through ECMO circuit ECMO device alarm, circuit instability potentially requiring hardware change Other indications as agreed upon by the ECLS team	
		Perfusion Support: Class B-Perfusionist in hospital	
		Comments - No unplanned changes to ECMO circuit within last 6 hours as Class A Other indications as agreed upon by the ECLS team	
		Perfusion Support: Class C-Perfusionist on call	
		Comments - No unplanned changes to ECMO circuit within last 6 hours as Class B Other indications as agreed upon by the ECLS team	

Medications

Inc	Req	ORDER	SPECIAL INSTRUCTIONS
		heparin bolus (100 units/mL)	
		1,000 units, injection, IV, as directed, PRN	
		Comments - for pTT less than 40 seconds. Administer from heparin infusion bag	
		heparin 25,000 units in 250 mL dextrose 5% premix	
		dextrose 5% premix diluent	
		IV continuous	
		Comments - Adjust heparin infusion as per following F.1 heparin nomogram	

PTT(sec)	Bolus	Hold	Rate Change	Recheck PTT
Less than 40	1000 units	0	+2 units/kg/hr	6 hours
40-49	0	0	+1 units/kg/hr	6 hours

Inc	Req	ORDER	SPECIAL INSTRUCTIONS
		heparin - additive	
		25,000 units, 6 unit/kg/hr	

Other Diagnostic Testing/Treatment

Inc	Req	ORDER	SPECIAL INSTRUCTIONS
		Echo Transoesophageal	
		Routine, T+1;N, CSRU #17440, CSRU	
		Echo Routine	
		Routine, T+1;N, Assess - Known Cardiac Condition, ECMO, assess cardiac function, CSRU #17440, CSRU	

Last Modified: 2019/09/18

F.1 Heparin Nomogram—ECMO

PTT (sec)	Bolus	Hold	Rate Change	Recheck PTT
Less than 40	1,000 units	0	+2 units/kg/hr	6 hours
40-49	0	0	+1 unit/kg/hr	6 hours
50-64	0	0	No change	Next AM
65-74	0	0	-1 unit/kg/hr	6 hours
Greater than 75	0	60 min	-2 units/kg/hr	6 hours after restart

Appendix G Heart Transplant Post-Op Critical Care

DO NOT THIN FROM HEALTH RECORD

Provider (SIGNATURE)	Date	Time
Provider (PRINT)		
Processor	Date	Time
Nurse	Date	Time

CARDIO SURG - Heart Transplant Postop Critical Care (Module)

Inc	Req	ORDER	SPECIAL INSTRUCTIONS
		Vital Signs	
		Mean Arterial Blood Pressure Target	
		Respiratory Orders	
		Nitric Oxide	
		20 ppm	
		Medications	
		Antibiotics	
X		sulfamethoxazole-trimethoprim 800 mg-160 mg oral tablet	
		1 tab, tab, ORAL, daily Mon,Wed,Fri, Start: T+4;0800	
		Antiviral Agents	
X		ganciclovir	
		5 mg/kg, injection, IV, q12 hours, for: 30 day, Start: T+4;0800	
		Comments - re-assess dose for renal function, assess for oral suitability	
		Corticosteroids	
		Prednisone Taper must be ordered outside of the powerplan (Note)	
X		methylPREDNISolone sodium succinate	
		1 mg/kg, injection, IV, daily, for: 3 day	
		Comments - then assess for oral taper	
		Immunosuppression	
		Consider ordering Tacrolimus, Thymoglobulin, Basiliximab therapy	
X		mycophenolate mofetil	
		1,000 mg, injection, IV, q12 hours, infuse over 2 hr	
		Comments - change to 1000 mg ORAL BID when suitable for oral intake	
		tacrolimus	
		0.5 mg, cap, ORAL, q12 hours (Def)	

Inc	Req	ORDER	SPECIAL INSTRUCTIONS
		1 mg, cap, ORAL, q12 hours	
		Suggested dose of Thymoglobulin is 0.5 - 1.5 mg/kg (Note)	
		Thymoglobulin (rabbit)	
		0.5 mg/kg, injection, IV, ONCE, infuse over 6 hr	
		Comments - 0.22 micron in-line filter MUST be used to be run centrally ONLY	
		diphenhydrAMINE	
		50 mg, injection, IV, ONCE	
		Comments - To be given with thymoglobulin	
		acetaminophen	
		650 mg, tab, ORAL, ONCE, for: 1 dose	
		Comments - max 4 g acetaminophen in 24 hr from all sources. To be given with thymoglobulin	
Vasoactive Agents			
		Heart Rate Target (bpm)	
		isoproterenol 1 mg in 50 mL dextrose 5%	
		dextrose 5% in water (titrate)	
		Titration Range: 0-5 mcg/kg/min, IV continuous	
		isoproterenol - additive	
		1 mg	
Laboratory			
Liver Function/Enzymes			
X		Amylase,Total (AMY)	
		AM Routine, T+1;0300, Blood, Frequency: daily. 2 times	
X		Aspartate Aminotransferase (AST)	
		AM Routine, T+1;0300, Blood, Frequency: daily. 2 times	
X		Alkaline Phosphatase (ALP)	
		AM Routine, T+1;0300, Blood, Frequency: daily. 2 times	
X		Alanine Aminotransferase (ALT)	
		AM Routine, T+1;0300, Blood, Frequency: daily. 2 times	
X		Albumin,Serum,Plasma (ALB)	
		AM Routine, T+1;0300, Blood, Frequency: daily. 2 times	
X		Bilirubin,Total (BILT)	
		AM Routine, T+1;0300, Blood, Frequency: daily. 2 times	
X		Gamma Glutamyl Transferase (GGT)	
		AM Routine, T+1;0300, Blood, Frequency: daily. 2 times	

		Other	
X		Tacrolimus Level,Whole Blood (FK)	
		Routine, T;N, Blood, trough, Frequency: daily.	
		Comments - once tacrolimus started. Trough - half hour prior to dose	
X		Quantitative Epstein Barr Virus (QEBV)	
		Routine T;N, Frequency: weekly 4 week	
X		Quantitative Cytomegalovirus (QCMV)	
		Routine T;N, Frequency: weekly 4 week	
		HLA donor specific antibody (continue at month 1, month 3 and month 6)	
X		HLA Serum Archive (HLA Serum)	
		Routine, T;N, Blood	
X		HLA Luminex Ab workup (.LxAb wu)	
		Routine, T;N, Blood	
X		HLA DSA Workup (.DSA wu)	
		Routine, T;N, Blood	
		Diagnostic Imaging	
		Biopsy/Aspiration under Fluoro	
		Routine, Right heart catheterization	
		Consults	
X		Consult to Physician	
		Service: Infectious Disease-Day Team University, Reason: Transplant, Priority: ASAP (Provider must call)	

Last Modified: 2019/06/10

Appendix H Lumbar Drain with Elephant, Frozen Elephant Trunk Procedure

DO NOT THIN FROM HEALTH RECORD

Provider (SIGNATURE)	Date	Time
Provider (PRINT)		
Processor	Date	Time
Nurse	Date	Time

CARDIO SURG - Lumbar Drain with Elephant/Frozen Elephant Trunk Procedure (Module)

Inc	Req	ORDER	SPECIAL INSTRUCTIONS
Activity			
		Bedrest	
		Positioning: Elevate head of bed	
		Positioning: Do NOT elevate head of bed	
X		Turn Patient	
		q2 hours., use rotation module in Total care Sport or Total Care bed if hemodynamically unstable	
		Dangle Legs at Bedside	
		Clamp Lumbar drain while dangling patient	
		Activity as Tolerated	
		Clamp Lumbar drain with patient activity	
Vital Signs			
X		Spinal Cord Testing	
		q1 hour. 8 hr, then q2 hours for 8 hr, then q4 hours for a total of 48 hours, then daily (as long as there is no signs of spinal cord ischemia) - per Complex Aortic Reconstruction Surgery resource	
		Comments - document on spinal testing record	
X		Mean Arterial Blood Pressure Target	
		65 mmHg	
		Comments - if no bleeding MAP 70-80 mmHg overnight	
X		Blood Pressure	
		Record NIBP once in EACH arm on arrival. Manage Blood pressure using Right arm.	
Patient Care			
X		Notify Provider	
		if strength less than 4/5 in lower limbs	
X		Notify Provider	
		if lumbar drain disconnects	

Inc	Req	ORDER	SPECIAL INSTRUCTIONS
X		Notify Provider	
		if drainage from lumbar drain is more than 15 ml/hour or 0 mL/hour	
Drain Management			
X		Lumbar Drain Level	
		Set Drain To: +10 cm H20 (Def)	
		Set Drain To: +5 cm H20	
		Set Drain To: 0 cm H20	
		Lumbar Drain - Continuous Drainage	
		10 mL/hr (Def)	
		Comments - level transducer to the iliac crest. Notify physician if hourly maximum reached to decide whether or not to clamp lumbar drain for the remainder of the hour, then reopen drain for the next hour.	
		5 mL/hr	
		Comments - level transducer to the iliac crest. Notify physician if hourly maximum reached, to decide whether or not to clamp lumbar drain for the remainder of the hour, then reopen drain for the next hour.	
		15 mL/hr	
		Comments - level transducer to the iliac crest. Notify physician if hourly maximum reached, to decide whether or not to clamp lumbar drain for the remainder of the hour, then reopen drain for the next hour	
		Lumbar Drain - Clamped	

Last Modified: 2017/08/18

Appendix I Transapical Aortic Valve Implantation

DO NOT THIN FROM HEALTH RECORD

Provider (SIGNATURE)	Date	Time
Provider (PRINT)		
Processor	Date	Time
Nurse	Date	Time

CARDIO SURG - Transapical Aortic Valve Implantation (CSRU) Post-Op

Inc	Req	ORDER	SPECIAL INSTRUCTIONS
		Resuscitation Status	
		Please ensure the resuscitation documentation is completed/reviewed	
		Diet	
X		NPO	
X		Advance Diet as Tolerated	
		to cardiac diet	
		to diabetic diet	
		Activity	
X		Activity as Tolerated	
		4 hours post-op if patient stable	
		Comments	
X		Dangle Legs at Bedside	
		prior to chest tube removal	
		Vital Signs	
X		Vital Signs	
		per protocol (Def)	
		daily	
		q1 hour.	
		q12 hours.	
		q2 hours.	
		q3 hours.	
		q30 days	
		q30 minutes	
		q4 hours.	
		q6 hours.	
		q8 hours.	
		weekly	
X		Continuous Oxygen Saturation	
X		Cardiac Monitoring	

Inc	Req	ORDER	SPECIAL INSTRUCTIONS
		Arrhythmia (known or suspected), continuous ECG monitoring	
		Comments	
X		Systolic Blood Pressure Target (mmHg)	
X		Pedal Pulse Assessment	
		pedal pulse check q15 minutes x 4 ; then q30 minutes x 2	
Patient Care			
X		Oxygen Therapy	
X		Oxygen Titration	
		Target: SpO2 greater than or equal to 92% (Def)	
		Target: SpO2 88-92% for CO2 Retention	
X		POC Specimen LABEL - Blood Gas	
		Blood Gas - Arterial	
X		POC Blood Glucose	
		Before Meals and at Bedtime	
		q6h	
		Once	
X		Urinary Catheter to Urometer	
X		Intake and Output	
		q1 hour.	
		Comments	
X		Notify Provider	
		if urine output less than 20 mL for 2 consecutive hours, call CSRU team	
X		Chest Tube Care/Monitor	
		Water-Seal Suction -20 cm, Notify provider if total drainage greater than 150 mL/hour x 2 hours	
X		Arterial Line Care and Monitoring	
X		Central Line Care	
X		Convert IV to Saline Lock	
		when drinking well	
X		Groin Puncture Site Assessment	
		q15 minutes 4 times, then q30 minutes x 2	
X		Do Not Remove Dressing - Reinforce Only	
		groin puncture site and chest incision x 48 hours	
X		Dressing Change	
		Groin, when groin dressing removed, cleanse with normal saline and leave open to air	
X		Dressing Change	
		Chest, When chest dressing removed, cleanse with normal saline and apply dry gauze dressing lightly and secured as long as pt is monitored	
		Femoral Artery Cannulation Site Management	

		Pacemaker Settings Temporary Transvenous/Epicardial	
		Transvenous, VVI, Ventricular (mV) 2, Atrial (mA) 0, Atrial (mV) 0	
X		Weight	
		daily 03:00	
Continuous Infusions			
		Consider adequate hydration and avoidance of early diuretic administration for preservation of renal function.	
X		sodium chloride 0.9% arterial line flush	
		intra-ARTERIAL, to keep line open, Total volume (mL): 500	
X		dextrose 5%-sodium chloride 0.9% (D5/NS)	
		IV continuous, 80 mL/hr	
Medications			
		Prescriber should consider resuming pre-operative/home medications within the first 24 hours after operation. eg. anti-platelets, statins.	
X		COMMON - Venous Thromboembolism (VTE) Prophylaxis (LHSC-UH, VC, PW, STEGH, TDMH)	
X		CARDIO SURG - Ventilation and Rapid Wean (Module)	
		Consider immediate or early extubation	
		insulin aspart (NovoRapid) correctional dose HIGH	
		sliding scale, SUBCUTANEOUS, injection, with meals & bedtime (QID)	
		Comments - Blood Glucose Range (mmol/L) Dose Less than/equal to 4 Implement Hypoglycemia management where applicable. Not MRP within reasonable time frame for further orders or adjustment to existing orders 4.1-8 0 units 8.1-10 4 units 10.1 - 14 6 units 14.1 - 17	
X		sodium chloride 0.9% flush	
		10 mL, injection, IV direct, as directed, PRN IV device maintenance	
X		Communication Order	
		Avoid beta blockers and centrally-acting calcium channel blockers.	
Analgesics			
X		acetaminophen	
		650 mg, tab, ORAL, q6 hours, for: 3 day	
		Comments - max 4 g acetaminophen in 24 hr from all sources. Administer as soon as patient can swallow.	
X		acetaminophen	
		650 mg, tab, ORAL, q6 hours, PRN pain, Start: T+3;N	
		Comments - max 4 g acetaminophen in 24 hr from all sources.	
		HYDROmorphone injection	
		0.2 mg, injection, IV direct, q30 minutes PRN pain	
		Comments - until extubated.	

		HYDROmorphone	
		0.5 mg, tab, ORAL, q3 hours PRN pain, for: 48 hr	
		Comments - give 0.5 mg for severe pain, give 0.25 mg for moderate pain.	
		1 mg, tab, ORAL, q3 hours PRN pain, for: 48 hr	
		Comments - give 1 mg for severe pain, give 0.5 mg for moderate pain.	
		2 mg, tab, ORAL, q3 hours PRN pain, for: 48 hr	
		Comments - give 2 mg for severe pain, give 1 mg for moderate pain.	
Antiplatelets			
X		acetylsalicylic acid	
		81 mg, EC tab, ORAL, daily, Start: T+1;0800	
		Comments - Verify with MD if platelet count less than 50,000 or blood loss greater than 100 mL in any hour.	
Antimicrobials			
		In a patient where MRSA is not suspected, prescriber to consider a first or second generation cephalosporin.	
		Consider completion of surgical antibiotic prophylaxis within the first 24 hours post-op.	
		ceFAZolin	
		1 g, injection, IV, q8 hours, for: 24 hr	
		Comments	
		vancomycin	
		1 g, injection, IV, q12 hours, infuse over 60 min, for: 24 hr	
		Comments	
Antiemetics/GI Prophylaxis			
X		ondansetron	
		4 mg, tab, ORAL, q8 hours, PRN nausea or vomiting	
X		ondansetron injection	
		4 mg, injection, IV, q8 hours, PRN nausea or vomiting	
		Comments - while patient intubated	
X		lansoprazole	
		30 mg, DR cap, ORAL, daily, Start: T+1;0800	
Bowel Routine			
X		senna	
		8.6 mg, tab, ORAL, bedtime, for: 2 dose, Start: T+2;2200	
X		senna	
		8.6 mg, tab, ORAL, bedtime, PRN constipation, Start: T+4;2200	
X		bisacodyl	
		10 mg, supp, RECTAL, ONCE, Start: T+3;0800, if no bm since surgery	
		Comments - if no bowel movement since surgery	
X		bisacodyl	
		10 mg, supp, RECTAL, daily, PRN constipation, Start: T+2;0800	

		Vasodilators	
		nitroglycerin 50 mg in 250 mL dextrose 5% premix	
		dextrose 5% premix diluent (titrate)	
		Titration Range: 0-150 mcg/min, IV continuous	
		nitroglycerin -additive	
		50 mg	
		Laboratory	
X		Complete Blood Count (CBC)	
		STAT, T;N, Blood	
X		Electrolytes,Serum,Plasma (LYTE)	
		STAT, T;N, Blood	
X		INRPTT	
		STAT, T;N, Blood	
X		Magnesium,Serum,Plasma (MG)	
		STAT, T;N, Blood	
X		Phosphate (PHO)	
		STAT, T;N, Blood	
X		Complete Blood Count (CBC)	
		Routine, T;N+240, Blood	
X		Electrolytes,Serum,Plasma (LYTE)	
		Routine, T;N+240, Blood	
X		Urea (U)	
		Routine, T;N+240, Blood	
X		Creatinine (CRE)	
		Routine, T;N+240, Blood	
X		Glucose,Random (GLUR)	
		Routine, T;N+240, Blood	
X		Magnesium,Serum,Plasma (MG)	
		Routine, T;N+240, Blood	
X		Phosphate (PHO)	
		Routine, T;N+240, Blood	
		Post-Op Day #1	
X		Complete Blood Count (CBC)	
		AM Routine, T+1;0300, Blood	
X		Electrolytes,Serum,Plasma (LYTE)	
		AM Routine, T+1;0300, Blood	
X		Urea (U)	
		AM Routine, T+1;0300, Blood	
X		Creatinine (CRE)	
		AM Routine, T+1;0300, Blood	
		Diagnostic Imaging	
X		Chest AP Portable	
		post op TAVI, Contact CSRU 17440	
X		Xray Nurse order when	
		If Chest tube not removed Post-op day #1	
X		Xray Nurse order when	
		Post Chest tube removal	

		Other Diagnostic Testing/Treatment	
X		ECG Nurse order when	
		if change in cardiac rhythm	
X		Echo Routine	
		T+1;N, Aortic Regurgitation, post TAVI insertion, #13153, Cardiac surgery	
		Allied Health	
		Dietitian Referral	
X		Physiotherapy Referral	
		Routine	
		Comments	

Last Modified: 2019/05/16

I.1 Care of the Transapical TAVI Patient Post-Op

BACKGROUND
Patients are intubated in the OR for the procedure & some may be extubated prior to transfer to CSRU

PROCEDURE

Ensure that patient and <u>health care provider safety standards</u> are met during this procedure including:
• Risk assessment and appropriate PPE
• 4 Moments of Hand Hygiene
• Two patient identifications
• Safe patient handling practices
• Biomedical waste disposal policies

Admission from the OR	
Patient may be extubated on rebreather mask or may be intubated	• RT can place on nasal prongs if O2 saturation stable
Radial arterial line (AL) insitu	• Remove AL 3-4 hours after admission to CSRU or PACU
IV access	
Peripheral IV with D5/0.9 NaCl	• May be NS locked
Triple lumen catheter (R internal jugular)	• Placed in internal jugular vein above transvenous pacemaker insertion site
R internal jugular introducer (Introflux ™ 8.5 Fr)	• Capable of running a large volume bolus or blood products. May be used as a central line, rate of administration will vary if a different introducer is used • D5/0.9 NaCl TKVO (10-20 mls/hr) while in CSRU: Same day transfers: keep running while on transfer to inpatient ward • For POD1 CSRU: may lock central line May be central line locked while on inpatient ward (may be able to draw blood from this line if unable to obtain blood through peripheral access)

Cardiac pacing	
Temporary Transvenous Pacing 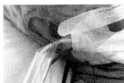 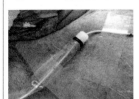 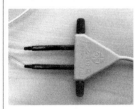 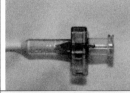	• Record catheter measurement at introducer connection so it be checked to make sure pacing catheter has not moved (ICU 12 hr. Nursing Assessment and Intervention flowsheet below the pacing information, check the PAC box and record the cm marking) • Check that tightener at introducer is secure • Check that tightener at end of sleeve cover is secure • Connections fully secured at black and red pins; red pins into connection cable (proximal lead to positive opening) • Attached to ventricular port on external pacemaker generator • Pacing threshold checked • Pacing rate set to backup rate of 40/bpm to transfer to inpatient ward (if same day transfer) If patient is paced: check to see if there is a hemodynamically stable underlying rhythm (to ensure patient safety for transfer to inpatient ward) • Remove 3 ml syringe from balloon port (tape to external pacing generator box); ensure balloon lock in open position (red marks in alignment)
TAVI orders	
Pacing	• If pacing, specific pacing orders should be completed (VVI, rate mA, sensitivity)
Vascular access: site care	• Both groins will have been accessed; procedure catheters will be through direct cut-down and supporting catheters will be through percutaneous arterial and venous sites • Vascular management will have specific strategies for R and L groin ordered (primary closure of artery or angioseal in percutaneous access, venous hemostasis managed with compression) • Nurse patient HOB < 30 degrees for 2 hrs. • Dressing check and pedal pulses q 15 mins X 4; q 30 min X 4; then q 1 hr x 3
Chest tube (transapical L minithoracotomy)	• Check chest tube connections, tighten & secure with tag tie • Check that suction is attached, indicator is visible, & dial is set at -20 cm
Transfer to inpatient ward	
Usual post-operative care	• Check to remove triple lumen catheter in AM POD 1 • Check to remove arterial line in AM POD 1 • Check to remove chest tube in AM POD 1
Transvenous temporary pacemaker	• If in situ, pacemaker may be off but attached if there is a stable heart rhythm • Introducer side arm may be central line locked
Medication reconciliation to be done prior to transfer CARDIO SURG-Transapical Aortic Valve Implantation (CSRU) Post-Op	• Do not discontinue the TAVI order set upon patient transfer (Echocardiogram & ECG)

Cheryl Kee NP, February 2018

Appendix J Transfemoral Aortic Valve Implantation

DO NOT THIN FROM HEALTH RECORD

Provider (SIGNATURE)	Date	Time
Provider (PRINT)		
Processor	Date	Time
Nurse	Date	Time
Height	Weight	Time

CARDIO SURG - Transfemoral Aortic Valve Implantation, Post-Op		

Inc	Req	ORDER	SPECIAL INSTRUCTIONS
		Resuscitation Status	
		Please ensure the resuscitation documentation is completed/reviewed	
		Diet	
X		NPO	
X		Advance Diet as Tolerated	
		to cardiac diet	
		to diabetic diet	
		Activity	
X		Dangle Legs at Bedside	
		4 hours post-op if patient stable	
X		Activity as Tolerated	
		4 hours post-op as tolerated	
		Vital Signs	
X		Vital Signs	
		per protocol (Def)	
		daily	
		q1 hour.	
		q12 hours.	
		q2 hours.	
		q3 hours.	
		q30 days	
		q30 minutes	
		q4 hours.	
		q6 hours.	
		q8 hours.	
		weekly	
X		Continuous Oxygen Saturation	

Inc	Req	ORDER	SPECIAL INSTRUCTIONS
		discontinue when pt transferred to the ward	
X		Cardiac Monitoring	
		Arrhythmia (known or suspected), continuous ECG monitoring	
X		Systolic Blood Pressure Target	
X		Pedal Pulse Assessment	
		pedal pulse check q15 minutes x 4 ; then q30 minutes x 2	
Patient Care			
X		Oxygen Therapy	
X		Oxygen Titration	
		Target: SpO2 greater than or equal to 92% (Def)	
		Target: SpO2 88-92% for CO2 Retention	
X		POC Specimen LABEL - Blood Gas	
		Blood Gas - Arterial	
X		POC Blood Glucose	
		Once	
		Before Meals and at Bedtime	
X		Urinary Catheter to Urometer	
X		Intake and Output	
		q1 hour.	
X		Notify Provider	
		if urine output less than 20 mL for 2 consecutive hours, call CSRU or CVT team	
X		Arterial Line Care and Monitoring	
X		Central Line Care	
X		Convert IV to Saline Lock	
		when drinking well	
X		Discontinue Arterial Line	
		within 2 hours post-op if stable	
X		Groin Puncture Site Assessment	
		q15 minutes x 4 ; then q30 minutes x 2	
X		Do Not Remove Dressing - Reinforce Only	
		groin puncture site; x48 hours	
X		Dressing Change	
		Groin, when groin dressing removed, cleanse with normal saline and leave open to air	
		Femoral Artery Cannulation Site Management	
		Pacemaker Settings Temporary Transvenous/Epicardial	
		Transvenous, VVI, Ventricular (mV) 2, Atrial (mA) 0, Atrial (mV) 0	
X		Weight	
		daily 03:00	

		Continuous Infusions	
X		sodium chloride 0.9% arterial line flush	
		intra-ARTERIAL, to keep line open, Total volume (mL): 500	
X		dextrose 5%-sodium chloride 0.9% (D5/NS)	
		IV continuous, 80 mL/hr	
		Medications	
		Prescriber should consider resuming pre-operative/home medications within the first 24 hours after operation. eg. anti-platelets, statins.	
X		COMMON - Venous Thromboembolism (VTE) Prophylaxis (LHSC-UH, VC, PW, STEGH, TDMH)	
		insulin aspart correctional dose HIGH	
		sliding scale, SUBCUTANEOUS, injection, with meals & bedtime (QID)	
X		sodium chloride 0.9% flush	
		10 mL, injection, IV direct, as directed, PRN IV device maintenance	
X		Communication Order	
		Avoid beta blockers and centrally-acting calcium channel blockers.	
		Analgesics	
X		acetaminophen	
		*650 mg, tab, ORAL, q6 hours, for: 3	3 day*	
X		acetaminophen	
		650 mg, tab, ORAL, q6 hours, PRN pain, Start: T+3;N	
		Antiplatelets	
X		acetylsalicylic acid	
		81 mg, EC tab, ORAL, daily, Start: T+1;0800	
		Antiemetics/GI Prophylaxis	
X		ondansetron	
		4 mg, tab, ORAL, q8 hours, PRN nausea or vomiting	
X		ondansetron injection	
		4 mg, injection, IV, q8 hours, PRN nausea or vomiting [Greater Than or Equal to 13 kg]	
X		lansoprazole	
		30 mg, DR cap, ORAL, daily, Start: T+1;0800	
		Bowel Routine	
X		senna	
		8.6 mg, tab, ORAL, bedtime, for: 2 dose, Start: T+2;2200	
X		senna	
		8.6 mg, tab, ORAL, bedtime, PRN constipation, Start: T+4;2200	
X		bisacodyl	
		10 mg, supp, RECTAL, ONCE, Start: T+3;0800	
X		bisacodyl	
		10 mg, supp, RECTAL, daily, PRN constipation, Start: T+2;0800	

Vasodilators			
		nitroglycerin 50 mg in 250 mL dextrose 5% premix	
		dextrose 5% premix diluent (titrate)	
		Titration Range: 0-150 mcg/min, IV continuous	
		nitroglycerin -additive	
		50 mg	
Laboratory			
X		Complete Blood Count (CBC)	
		STAT, T;N, Blood	
X		Electrolytes,Serum,Plasma (LYTE)	
		STAT, T;N, Blood	
X		INRPTT	
		STAT, T;N, Blood	
X		Magnesium,Serum,Plasma (MG)	
		STAT, T;N, Blood	
X		Phosphate (PHO)	
		STAT, T;N, Blood	
X		Urea (U)	
		STAT, T;N, Blood	
X		Creatinine (CRE)	
		STAT, T;N, Blood	
Post-Op Day #1			
X		Complete Blood Count (CBC)	
		AM Routine, T+1;0300, Blood	
X		Electrolytes,Serum,Plasma (LYTE)	
		AM Routine, T+1;0300, Blood	
X		Urea (U)	
		AM Routine, T+1;0300, Blood	
X		Creatinine (CRE)	
		AM Routine, T+1;0300, Blood	
Diagnostic Imaging			
		Chest AP Portable	
		Routine, post-op TAVI, Contact CSRU #17440	
Other Diagnostic Testing/Treatment			
X		ECG Nurse order when	
		if change in cardiac rhythm	
X		Echo Routine	
		T+3;N, Aortic Regurgitation, Post TAVI insertion, #13153, Cardiac Surgery	
Allied Health			
		Dietitian Referral	
X		Physiotherapy Referral	
		Routine	

Last Modified: 2019/02/25

J.1 Care of the Transfemoral TAVI Patient in Critical Care, PAC, and through inpatient ward or CCU

BACKGROUND

The Transfemoral Transcatheter Aortic Valve Implantation (TAVI) is a less invasive procedure for aortic valve replacement allowing for shorter post-operative recovery. Patients are intubated in the OR for the procedure and will be extubated prior to transfer from the OR.

PROCEDURE

Ensure that patient and health care provider safety standards are met during this procedure including:
- Risk assessment and appropriate PPE.
- 4 Moments of Hand Hygiene.
- Two patient identifications.
- Safe patient handling practices.
- Biomedical waste disposal policies.
- The 6th floor will send an inpatient bed to the Operating Room (OR) prior to the completion of the procedure. The patient will be transferred to the PACU or CSRU on this inpatient bed.

Admission from the OR:

- A nurse that has received TAVI education will be present.

- Link to 'Fast Track Cardiac: Transcatheter Aortic Valve Implantation (TAVI) Elective Protocol'

Admission from the OR	
Patient will be extubated on re-breather mask	• RT can place on nasal prongs if O2 saturation stable
Radial arterial line (AL) insitu	• Remove AL prior to transfer to CCU or inpatient ward
IV access	
Peripheral IV with D5/0.9 NaCl	• May be NS locked
Triple lumen catheter (R internal jugular)	• Placed in internal jugular vein above transvenous pacemaker insertion site
R internal jugular introducer (Introflux ™ 8.5 Fr)	• Capable of running a large volume bolus or blood products. May be used as a central line, rate of administration will vary if a different introducer is used • D5/0.9 NaCl TKVO (10-20 mls/hr) while in CSRU: Same day transfers: keep running while on transfer to inpatient ward • For POD1 CSRU: may central line lock May be central line locked while on inpatient ward (may be able to draw blood from this line if unable to obtain blood through peripheral access)

Cardiac pacing	
Temporary Transvenous Pacing 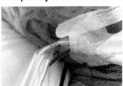 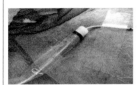 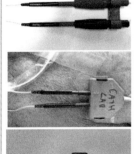	• Record catheter measurement at introducer connection so it can be checked to make sure pacing catheter has not moved (ICU 12 hr. Nursing Assessment and Intervention flowsheet below the pacing information, check the PAC box and record the cm marking or under significant findings on the Cardiac A&I flowsheet) • Check that tightener at introducer is secure • Check that tightener at end of sleeve cover is secure • Connections fully secured between black and red pins; red pins into connection cable (proximal lead to positive opening/red connector or + sign) • Attached to ventricular port on external pacemaker generator • Pacing rate set to backup rate of 40/bpm to transfer to inpatient ward • Remove 3 ml syringe from balloon port (tape to external pacing generator box); ensure balloon lock is in open position (red marks in alignment)

TAVI orders	
Pacing	• If pacing, specific pacing orders should be completed (VVI, rate mA, sensitivity)
Vascular access: site care	• Both groins or radial artery may have been accessed; procedure catheters will be through direct cut-down and supporting catheters will be through percutaneous arterial and venous sites • Vascular management will have specific strategies for R and L groin ordered (primary closure of artery or angioseal in percutaneous access, venous hemostasis managed with compression) or radial artery clamp • Nurse patient HOB < 30 degrees for 2 hrs • Dressing check and pedal pulses q 30 min X 4

Transfer to inpatient ward	
Usual post-operative care	• Recovered in PACU anticipated stay less than 2 hours; then transferred to inpatient ward or CCU as ordered • ***Ensure arterial line removed prior to transfer*** • Patient may be drinking clear fluids • Patient may dangle at bedside (3 to 4 hrs. postop) Continue dressing and pedal pulse assessments as per protocol • Telemetry
	• Discomfort may be managed with acetaminophen prn
Transvenous temporary pacemaker	• If in situ, pacemaker should be on at a minimum backup rate of 40/bpm for transfer to inpatient ward
Medication reconciliation to be done **prior to** transfer CARDIO SURG-Transfemoral Aortic Valve Implantation (CSRU) Post-Op	• Do not discontinue the TAVI order set upon patient transfer

Revised Cheryl Kee NP, Elizabeth McGowan, January 2019

Appendix K Mitraclip

DO NOT THIN FROM HEALTH RECORD

Provider (SIGNATURE)	Date	Time
Provider (PRINT)		
Processor	Date	Time
Nurse	Date	Time

CARDIO SURG - Mitraclip Post - Op

Inc	Req	ORDER	SPECIAL INSTRUCTIONS
Resuscitation Status			
		Please ensure paper resuscitation form is completed/reviewed	
Alerts			
		Airborne Precautions	
		Contact Precautions	
		Droplet Precautions	
		Droplet/Contact Precautions	
Diet			
X		Advance Diet as Tolerated	
		resume pre-procedure diet when ambulatory	
		Cardiac Diet LHSC	
		1500 ml Fluid Restriction	
Activity			
X		Bedrest with Bathroom Privileges	
		Positioning: Other:, May turn on side with Right leg straight. Limit physical activity during first day.	
X		Dangle Legs at Bedside	
		at 4 hours post-op if patient stable	
Vital Signs			
X		Vital Signs	
		per protocol (Def)	
		daily	
		q1 hour.	
		q12 hours.	
		q2 hours.	
		q3 hours.	
		q30 days	
		q30 minutes	
		q4 hours.	

Inc	Req	ORDER	SPECIAL INSTRUCTIONS
		q6 hours.	
		q8 hours.	
		weekly	
X		Pedal Pulse Assessment	
		q15 minutes x 4; q30 minutes x 4; then q1 hr x 2 hours	
X		Groin Puncture Site Assessment	
		q15 minutes x 4; q30 minutes x 4; then q1 hr x 2 hours	
Patient Care			
X		Cardiac Monitoring	
		Arrhythmia (known or suspected), On return to ward	
X		Oxygen Therapy	
X		Oxygen Titration	
		Target: SpO2 greater than or equal to 92% (Def)	
		Target: SpO2 88-92% for CO2 Retention	
X		Urinary Catheter Insertion	
		PRN	
X		Discontinue Urinary Catheter	
		when ambulatory	
X		Intake and Output	
		q12 hours.	
X		Notify Provider Vital Signs/Urine Output	
		Notify CCU or CSRU team, Urine Output less than 30 mL for 2 hours	
X		Arterial Line Care and Monitoring	
X		Discontinue Arterial Line	
		in AM if stable	
X		Convert IV to Saline Lock	
		when drinking well	
X		Discontinue Central Venous Line	
		Intrajugular line in AM if stable	
		Transfer out to floor	
		Patient to be discharged from CCU or CSRU by the anesthesiologist, cardiac surgeon or CSRU intensivist	
X		Discontinue Arterial Sheath	
		when ACT less than 169 seconds	
X		Return to Clinic	
		Return to Office/Clinic: 6 weeks, Reason: Post procedure Mitral Clip	
Continuous Infusions			
X		sodium chloride 0.9%	
		1,000 mL, IV continuous, 50 mL/hr	
		Comments - Convert to saline lock once diet resumed	

X		sodium chloride 0.9% arterial line flush	
		500 mL, intra-ARTERIAL, to keep line open, Total volume (mL): 500	

Medications			
X		COMMON - Venous Thromboembolism (VTE) Prophylaxis (LHSC-UH, VC, PW, STEGH, TDMH)	
		ENDO - Subcutaneous Insulin Correctional Scale (Module)	
X		sodium chloride 0.9% flush	
		3 mL, syringe, IV direct, as directed, PRN Other: See Comments	
		Comments - peripheral device maintenance	
X		sodium chloride 0.9% flush	
		10 mL, syringe, IV direct, as directed, PRN for Other: See Comments	
		Comments - central device maintenance	
X		acetylsalicylic acid	
		81 mg, EC tab, ORAL, daily	

Antimicrobials			
X		ceFAZolin	
		1 g, injection, IV, ONCE, Start: T;N+360	
		If allergic to cephalosporins or pencillins then choose Vancomycin (Note)	
		vancomycin	
		1 g, injection, IV, ONCE, infuse over 60 min, Start: T;N+360	

Bowel Routine			
X		bisacodyl	
		10 mg, supp, RECTAL, ONCE, Start: T+2;N	
		Comments - if no bowel movement since surgery	
X		lactulose	
		15 mL, syrup, ORAL, daily, for: 48 hr, Start: T+1;N	
X		bisacodyl	
		10 mg, supp, RECTAL, daily, PRN constipation, Requested Start Date/Time T+3;N	
X		lactulose	
		15 mL, syrup, ORAL, daily, PRN constipation, Requested Start Date/Time T+3;N (Def)	
		30 mL, syrup, ORAL, daily, PRN constipation, Requested Start Date/Time T+3;N	
		Fleet Enema	
		133 mL, enema, RECTAL, daily, PRN constipation	

Antiemetics/GI Prophylaxis			
X		ondansetron injection	
		4 mg, injection, IV direct, q8 hours, PRN nausea or vomiting	

		Laboratory	
X		Blood Gas Plus (BGP)	
		Routine, T;N	
X		Phosphate (PHO)	
		Routine, T;N, Blood	
X		Magnesium,Serum,Plasma (MG)	
		Routine, T;N, Blood	
X		Electrolytes,Serum,Plasma (LYTE)	
		Routine, T;N, Blood	
X		INRPTT	
		Routine, T;N, Blood	
X		Complete Blood Count (CBC)	
		AM Routine, T+1;0300, Blood	
X		Complete Blood Count (CBC)	
		Routine, T;N+240, Blood	
X		Electrolytes,Serum,Plasma (LYTE)	
		Routine, T;N+240, Blood	
X		Urea (U)	
		Routine, T;N+240, Blood	
X		Creatinine (CRE)	
		Routine, T;N+240, Blood	
X		Glucose,Random (GLUR)	
		Routine, T;N+240, Blood	
X		Magnesium,Serum,Plasma (MG)	
		Routine, T;N+240, Blood	
X		Phosphate (PHO)	
		Routine, T;N+240, Blood	
		Diagnostic Imaging	
X		Chest AP Portable	
		Routine, Post procedure Mitral Clip	
		Other Diagnostic Testing/Treatment	
X		ECG 12 Lead	
		Routine, Reason: Structural Heart Disease Assessment	
X		Echo Routine	
		Routine, Mitral clip, Post-op assessment	

Last Modified: 2016/03/07

Printed by Printforce, the Netherlands